Cajal's Degeneration and Regeneration
of the Nervous System

HISTORY OF NEUROSCIENCE

A series of books published by Oxford University Press
in cooperation with the Fidia Research Foundation

EDITORS

Pietro Corsi, D. Phil.
Edward G. Jones, M.D., D. Phil.
Gordon M. Shepherd, M.D., Ph.D.

1. Cajal on the Cerebral Cortex
   An Annotated Translation of the Complete Writings
   Javier DeFelipe and Edward G. Jones

2. Disturbances of Lower and Higher Visual Capacities
   Caused by Occipital Damage
   Walther Poppelreuter
   Translated by J. Zihl

3. Mind, Brain and Adaptation in the Nineteenth Century
   Cerebral Localization and its Biological Context from Gall to Ferrier
   Robert M. Young

4. The Enchanted Loom
   Chapters in the History of Neuroscience
   Edited by Pietro Corsi

5. Cajal's Degeneration and Regeneration of the Nervous System
   Translated by Raoul M. May
   Edited, with an Introduction and Additional Translations
   by Javier DeFelipe and Edward G. Jones

History of Neuroscience
No. 5

CAJAL'S
DEGENERATION AND REGENERATION OF THE NERVOUS SYSTEM

Translated by Raoul M. May
Edited, with an Introduction
and Additional Translations, by

JAVIER DeFELIPE
AND
EDWARD G. JONES

New York   Oxford
OXFORD UNIVERSITY PRESS
1991

Oxford University Press

Oxford New York Toronto
Delhi Bombay Calcutta Madras Karachi
Petaling Jaya Singapore Hong Kong Tokyo
Nairobi Dar es Salaam Cape Town
Melbourne Auckland

and associated companies in
Berlin Ibadan

Copyright © 1991 by Oxford University Press, Inc.

Published by Oxford University Press, Inc.,
200 Madison Avenue, New York, New York 10016

All rights reserved. No part of this publication may be reproduced,
stored in a retrieval system, or transmitted, in any form or by any means,
electronic, mechanical, photocopying, recording, or otherwise,
without the prior permission of Oxford University Press.

Library of Congress Cataloging-in-Publication Data
Ramón y Cajal, Santiago, 1852-1934.
[Estudios sobre la degeneración y regeneración
del sistema nervioso. English]
Cajal's degeneration and regeneration of the nervous system /
translated by Raoul M. May ; with an introduction and
additional translations by
Javier DeFelipe and Edward G. Jones.
p. cm. — (History of neuroscience ; no. 5)
Translation of : Estudios sobre la degeneración y regeneración
del sistema nervioso.
Includes bibliographical references and index.
ISBN 0-19-506516-6
1. Nervous system—Regeneration. 2. Ramón y Cajal, Santiago, 1852-1934.
Estudios sobre la degeneración y regeneración del sistema nervioso.
I. DeFelipe, Javier. II. Jones, Edward G., 1939- .
III. Title. IV. Title: Degeneration and regeneration of the nervous system.
V. Series.
[DNLM: 1. Nerve Degeneration. 2. Nerve Regeneration.
W1 HI85J no. 5 / WL 102 R175e]
QP363.5.R3513 1991 591.1'88—dc20
DNLM/DLC for Library of Congress 91-3890

2 4 6 8 9 7 5 3 1

Printed in the United States of America
on acid-free paper

For Alicia and Sue

"I succeeded in collecting some original observations that were not without value."

Santiago Ramón Cajal, 1917

Foreword

VIKTOR HAMBURGER

Of the two *magna opera* of Ramón y Cajal, the "Histology of the Nervous System" and "Degeneration and Regeneration of the Nervous System," only the latter has been translated into English, but, as the present editors point out, it was no longer widely available. J. DeFelipe and E. G. Jones have now reissued the translation of R. M. May that was first published in 1928. However, this new edition is much more than a reprint; the editors have enriched it substantially in several ways. They have written a detailed, informative introductory commentary to the text. They have added the translation of a lengthy chapter from Cajal's autobiography that deals with nerve degeneration and regeneration, and which gives a succinct overview of the author's observations and theoretical ideas concerning this topic. Furthermore, they have included the translation of parts of memorial lectures by one of Cajal's most prominent students, F. Tello, that deal with Cajal's work on nerve regeneration and provide valuable comments by an eyewitness and collaborator. And last, but not least, they have transformed Cajal's references, which were presented in footnotes and were not always complete, into an impeccable bibliography. Altogether, the editors have done the community of neuroscientists a great service by reviving this classic and giving it an attire that is worthy of the author.

The main body of the two volumes contains a wealth of observations covering all phases of the nerve regeneration process, as well as a comprehensive survey of the contributions of Cajal's contemporaries and of his students, to this topic. However, as the editors point out in their introductory commentary, Cajal's most original contribution is the theoretical interpretation of what he observed. For one, the new findings provided strong support for his axon outgrowth theory that at that time, in the early years of this century, faced renewed opposition. Early on, Cajal had realized that the axon outgrowth theory poses a fundamental problem: How do axons find their way to their targets? Or, in the case of nerve transection, how are the axons guided from the proximal to the distal stump? In his earlier work on the development of the retina he had formulated the theory that the target structures release chemical agents that attract the growth cones. At first he had referred to this theory as chemotaxis, but he later adopted the term *neurotropism*. In the case of peripheral nerve regeneration, the role of producing the attractants was assigned to the Schwann cells in the distal stump that are activated after nerve transection. Many observations and experimental results were cited by Cajal in support of his theory.

Neurotropism found wide acceptance in the early part of this century, but it gradually lost ground. This was due in part to the fact that critical experimental verification was not forthcoming; but, more importantly, a competing theory, the "contact guidance" theory of Weiss[1] gained more credibility. Early on, it had been established that axons require a solid substrate for their outgrowth. In the 1930s, in vitro experiments by Weiss had shown that when artificial "pathways" are created in the substrate, they are then pursued by growing axons. However, it was realized that purely mechanical guidance could not account for specificity of neuronal pathways and synaptic connections. In the 1940s, Sperry's chemoaffinity theory[2] was proposed to address this problem. It postulated specific chemical affinities between specific sets of neurons and their axons on the one side, and their pathways and synaptic connections with their targets on the other. Attraction at a distance seemed to have lost all credibility.

However, the last two decades have witnessed the revival of Cajal's original idea. A number of in vivo and in vitro experiments have provided clear evidence that axonal growth cones can be diverted from their path and guided to a source of chemical attractants. These experiments have reinstated neurotropism as an alternative to chemoaffinity—though the two theories are by no means mutually exclusive. If, indeed, modern developmental neurobiologists take neurotropism seriously again, then it will be worthwhile to record Cajal's detailed and prescient ideas about how neurotropism works. One finds many references relevant to this topic in the present work. His observations and experiments convinced him that neurotropism is a much more complex phenomenon than the phrase "attraction at a distance" suggests. He recognized two aspects that are conceptually separable though in fact often interwoven.

The first has to do with specificity; Cajal distinguishes between a nonspecific and a specific component in neurotropism. He states on p. 371:

> The orienting chemical stimuli are probably, so far as their selective power is concerned, both generic and specific. The attractive substance elaborated by the embryonic connective cells and by the cells of Schwann of the peripheral stump have a generic character, acting without distinction on all sprouts, while the attractive substances, given out by the spindles of Kühne, motor plates, cutaneous sensory

structures, etc. have a specific character, acting only on certain functional categories of regenerated axons.

The distinction between agents that are responsible for axon outgrowth, and highly specific agents responsible for synaptic connections is certainly valid, though the designation of the former as nonspecific may not be tenable. But it is truly remarkable that he anticipated the role of extraneous trophic agents in stimulating axon outgrowth, as well as the highly specific interaction between particular axon terminals and their synaptic sites, which later became a key element in the chemoaffinity theory.

The other aspect of neurotropism that Cajal subjected to a critical analysis is the distinction between the trophic function of the target-derived substances and their capacity to provide directional cues. The association of the two functions, epitomized in the term "trophic–tropic," is a recurrent theme in his writing. On p. 238 of the present work he speaks of:

> the great influence that the proximity of the peripheral stump has on the growth and orientation of the outgrowing newly formed fibers. We believe it likely that this action is exercised through ferments or stimulating substances formed by the rejuvenated cells of Scwann of the distal stump and poured out by the regions near the scar . . . These substances have not only an orienting function, but . . . they are also trophic in character, since the sprouts that have arrived at the peripheral stump are robust, show a great capacity for ramification and grow straight to their goal without vacillations, as though they were following an irresistible attraction.

The distinction between activating axonal outgrowth and giving it direction can be illustrated by a frequent observation he made: After nerve transection all axons of the proximal stump are activated to produce growth cones. Some go astray, that is, they fail to detect the directional cues, but most of them are guided to their targets.

As I have indicated, many of Cajal's original ideas have been confirmed by modern developmental neurobiology. The most outstanding instance is the experimental proof of the existence of neurotrophic agents, in the discovery of the Nerve Growth Factor (NGF) by R. Levi-Montalcini in the early 1950s. To mention only one of the crucial experiments[3]: When in tissue culture a source of NGF was placed in the proximity of a spinal or sympathetic ganglion, it stimulated a profuse outgrowth of fibers in all directions. This and many other experiments on embryos provided conclusive evidence for the reality of the "trophic" component of Cajal's neurotropic agents. Since then, NGF has become the prototype of neurotrophic factors in neurogenesis. However, Cajal's notion of a trophic agent was developed in the context of peripheral nerve regeneration: "The degenerated nerves of the peripheral stump give out into the scar some substance—an enzyme, nutritive substance, or other material, which stimulates the assimilation and growth of the sprouts in an opposite direction from the diffused current" (p. 308: see also previous quotation). It is therefore of great interest that in recent years a substantial increase of NGF was found in Schwann cells and other nonnervous cells in the distal stump, some time after nerve transection.[4] Furthermore, local application of NGF to the proximal cut surface reduced neuronal death in dorsal root ganglia.[5] There can be little doubt that NGF is an obligatory trophic agent for ganglia also in nerve regeneraton.

But the experiments mentioned so far gave no evidence of "attraction at a distance," a key element in Cajal's conception of neurotropism. However, two decades after the discovery of NGF, in the 1970s, it was found that NGF also has a neurotropic component. Tissue culture experiments provided convincing proof that axons of embryonic ganglionic neurons can be diverted from their path and attracted by a source of NGF.[6] Since then, similar trophic–tropic interactions have been discovered in other systems apart from NGF. Targets as unrelated as a brain center[7] and a nonnervous peripheral structure[8] can stimulate axon outgrowth in their appropriate source of innervation and attract the fibers at some distance. The future will show to what extent neurotropism, as defined by Cajal, contributes to pathfinding and synaptic connections.

Readers of the present work can detect other instances of Cajal's anticipation of themes that are being pursued by modern developmental neurobiologists. For instance, it did not escape his attention that regenerating fibers sometimes make inappropriate connections that are then corrected by withdrawal and resorption of the fiber and, in some instances, can lead to the death of the perikaryon.

> There is no doubt that at first many imperfect connections are formed and that many duplications and errors of distribution occur. But these incongruences are progressively corrected, up to a certain point, by two parallel methods of rectification. One of these occurs at the periphery and is the atrophy through disuse of superfluous and parasitic ramifications. . . . The other occurs in the ganglia and spinal centers; by this there would be a selection, due to the atrophy of certain collaterals, and the progressive disappearance of disconnected and useless neurons, of the sensory and motor fibers capable of being useful (p. 279).

We know now that indeed the withdrawal of fibers from incorrect connections can lead to neuronal death, but a much more frequent cause of neuronal death is the inadequate supply of trophic agents.

The seminal ideas of Ramón y Cajal relating to neurogenesis and nerve regeneration that were conceived around the turn of the century have served as guideposts to three generations of neuroscientists—an enduring testimony to his genius.

Notes

1. Weiss, P. 1934. *In vitro* experiments on the factors determining the course of the outgrowing nerve fiber. J. Exp. Zool. *68*:393–448.
2. Sperry, R. 1963. Chemoaffinity in the orderly growth of nerve fiber patterns and connections. Proc. Natl. Acad. Sci. *50*:703–10.
3. Levi-Montalcini, R., H. Meyer, and V. Hamburger. 1953. *In vitro* experiments on the effects of mouse sarcoma 180 and 37 on the spinal and sympathetic ganglia of the chick embryo. Cancer Res. *14*:49–57.
4. Heumann, R., S. Korsching, C. Bandtlow, and H. Thoenen. 1987. Changes of nerve growth factor synthesis in non-neuronal cells in response to sciatic nerve transection. J. Cell Biol. *104*:1623–31.
5. Fitzgerald, M., T. D. Wall, M. Goedert, and P. C. Emson. 1985. Nerve growth factor counteracts the neurophysiological and neurochemical effects of chronic sciatic nerve section. Brain Res. *332*:131–41.
6. Gundersen, R. W., and J. R. Barrett. 1979. Neuronal chemotaxis: chick dorsal-root axons turn toward high concentrations of nerve growth factor. Science *206*:1079–80.
7. Heffner, C. D., A. G. S. Lumsden, and D. D. M. O'Leary. 1990. Target control of collateral extension and directional axon growth in the mammalian brain. Science *247*:217–20.
8. Lumsden, A. G. S., and A. M. Davies. 1983. Earliest sensory nerve fibers are guided to peripheral targets by attractants other than growth factor. Nature *306*:786–88.

Preface

Santiago Ramón y Cajal's contributions to the study of degenerative and regenerative phenomena in the nervous system were largely made during two periods of sustained effort that, collectively, lasted little more than five years. Although begun earlier, the greater part of the work was carried out after the age of 55 years, subsequent to his winning the Nobel Prize in 1906, and when further honors were being showered on him. Neither the decline in energy level that accompanies middle age nor the distractions of high recognition were permitted to stand in the way of the new research program and the end result, summed up in the 1913–1914 Spanish and 1928 English editions of *Degeneration and Regeneration of the Nervous System*, is one of the most comprehensive studies of its kind ever made. Although Cajal initiated his research because he saw it as another avenue for providing objective proof of the validity of the neuron doctrine, his attention became more and more focused on phenomena that were indicative of abortive regeneration in the central nervous system and on experimental approaches that might give hints as to how this failure could be overcome. To some extent, he was overshadowed in this last by his favorite pupil, Francisco Tello; however, his contributions in the field loom almost as large as his enormous body of descriptive neurohistology in which not only the neuron doctrine, but also the doctrine of neurotropism and some of the fundamental rules of neurogenesis were founded.

Successive generations of neuroscientists have found inspiration in Cajal's book on degeneration and regeneration of the nervous system and for that majority who were unfamiliar with Spanish, Raoul M. May's 1928 English version has served as a standard reference work. Although the translation has been republished in facsimile form twice (in 1959 and 1968), there have been only limited printings and the book is not widely available. That rapidly growing population of developmental neurobiologists who represent one of the most exciting movements in modern neuroscience is thus denied access to a classic in the field. Accordingly, it was felt that a new edition would be valuable.

In producing this new edition, we have reproduced May's translation intact. Had we been making a new translation, we would probably replace a few out-of-date English expressions and older scientific words with modern equivalents, but the text does not suffer for a lack of modernization and the modern reader can be assured that it represents an accurate record of Cajal's ideas and data. Following the style of our *Cajal on the Cerebral Cortex*, we have added an editorial overview of this phase of Cajal's work, together with translations from the relevant passages of his autobiography (1917) and from his *¿Neuronismo o reticularismo?* (1933). Apart from providing English readers with the opportunity to learn what Cajal thought about this period in his research career and the significance of his observations, these translations fill in the large gaps in Craigie's (1937) English translation of the autobiography in which Craigie, in focusing on the personal side of Cajal's life, omitted virtually all details of what Cajal regarded as his major scientific contributions. We have also translated a lengthy excerpt from Tello's series of memorial lectures in honor of Cajal, made in 1935 shortly after the latter's death. In these, Tello gives a contemporary view of Cajal's work, although the reader will not fail to note his own claims to priority. In addition, following our earlier practice, we have verified the vast majority of Cajal's (and May's) references and they appear in complete form in the bibliography that concludes Part I of the book.

We are grateful to Jeffrey House of Oxford University Press, New York, for his support and to Sir Roger Elliott, secretary to the Delegates of the Press at Oxford, for his advice and help. We thank the president of the Consejo Superior de Investigaciones Científicas, Dr. Emilio Muñoz, Dr. Gustavo Villapalos, president of the Universidad Complutense of Madrid, the director of the Instituto Cajal, Dr. José Borrell, and Dr. F. Martínez-Tello for permission to translate and to republish certain material. We also thank members of the Cajal family who lent their support, Drs. M.-J. Besson, J. F. Horvat, and M. Sensenbrenner who helped with our enquiries regarding Raoul May, and Professor Viktor Hamburger for his interest and advice.

Finally, we are deeply indebted to Elizabeth Swanson and Philippa Jones for photographic and secretarial help.

Madrid   J.DeF.
Irvine, Calif.   E.G.J.
September 1990

Contents

PART I

CAJAL AND DEGENERATION AND REGENERATION OF THE NERVOUS SYSTEM

Section 1: Introduction, 3

1. Editors' commentary, 5

2. Material omitted from the original English edition, 19

Section 2: Cajal in his own Words—Translations from Biographical and Other Works, 25

3. From: *Recuerdos de mi vida*. Volume 2, Chapter 19 (1917), 27

4. From: *Recuerdos de mi vida*. Volume 2, Chapter 21 (1917), 45

5. From: *Recuerdos de mi vida*, Volume 2, Chapter 22 (1917) And: *Algunas observaciones contrarias a la hipótesis* syncytial *de la regeneración nerviosa y neurogénesis normal* (1920) and *Démonstration photographique de quelques phénomenes de la régénération des nerfs* (1926), 73

6. From: *¿Neuronismo o reticularismo?* (1933), 91

7. From: *Cajal y su labor histológica* by J. F. Tello (1935), 101

Section 3: Bibliography, 129

Subject Index to Part I, 155

Author Index to Part I, 159

PART II

DEGENERATION AND REGENERATION OF THE NERVOUS SYSTEM, VOLUMES I AND II

First Section: Traumatic Degeneration and Regeneration of the Nerves, 1

Second Section: Degeneration and Regeneration of the Nerve Centres, 397

PART I

CAJAL AND DEGENERATION AND REGENERATION OF THE NERVOUS SYSTEM

JAVIER DeFELIPE AND EDWARD G. JONES

SECTION ONE

INTRODUCTION

CHAPTER 1

Editors' Commentary

Santiago Ramón y Cajal's scientific career consisted of three major phases. In the first, before his somewhat fortuitous "discovery" of the Golgi technique in 1887 (see DeFelipe and Jones 1988), and during his period at the University of Valencia, he was occupied with studies of a rather general histological character carried out with conventional techniques. The second phase, largely contemporaneous with his stay in the University of Barcelona (1887–1892), was a period of intense activity in which the Golgi technique was used with great finesse to describe the cellular architecture and unravel the intrinsic circuitry of the cerebellum, cerebral cortex, hippocampal formation, diencephalon, retina, brainstem, and spinal cord (see references in Pérez de Tudela 1983). From these studies, indeed from the first two or three years of such studies, the foundations of the neuron doctrine (Waldeyer 1891; Cajal 1892c, 1894a,b) were firmly laid, and in 1906 Cajal was jointly awarded with Golgi, the ardent reticularist, the Nobel Prize for Physiology or Medicine. Cajal was to return intermittently to analytic studies in neurohistology throughout the remainder of his life, but even before the award of the Nobel Prize and some eight years after his move to the University of Madrid in 1892, his career was already entering its third major phase. In this phase he turned his attention mainly to the problem of degeneration and regeneration of the nervous system.

It is not without significance that this phase was also ushered in by the application of a new technique, that of reduced silver nitrate, which in this case he had perfected himself in 1903 (see DeFelipe and Jones 1988). As with the Golgi technique, it was the use of this new method, with its greater capacity to reveal detail, that permitted old questions to be answered and old and new controversies to be resolved.

Cajal makes it clear in his autobiography, the relevant parts of which we reproduce in Section 2, that he entered the field of neural regeneration with some reluctance and largely because he felt that the neuron doctrine was under attack. Within a year of his first paper on the subject (Cajal 1905a), however, he was embroiled in what he refers to as "the great controversy" (p.

324). In this he was to find arrayed against him, among others, his old archrival Hans Held (1907) and a vigorous debater in the person of Albrecht Bethe (1907a,b) (e.g., Cajal 1903a, 1908b). Much of the debate revolved around the nature of degeneration and regeneration in the peripheral nervous system, but Cajal, with his usual insight, saw that the issues raised had important implications for normal neural development and for any hopes of promoting regeneration in the central nervous system.

In turning his attention first to the regeneration of peripheral nerves, Cajal was thrown into a thirty year controversy that had raged between those whom he called monogenists and polygenists. The first of the theories, dating to Waller (1850) and Ranvier (1878) held that in the course of regeneration, the peripheral stump of a divided nerve was invaded by sprouts issuing from the cut fibers of the proximal stump which still retained continuity with their trophic centers, the cell somata. The implications of this for the neuron doctrine are obvious. The polygenists' view, dating to Vulpian (1866) and later championed by Bethe (1901a, 1903a), considered that new fibers were formed in the peripheral stump from the coalescence of linear chains of Schwann cells which later linked up with the fibers of the central stump. This is an application of an old developmental theory of Hensen (1864), later supported by Held (1909), that newly growing nerve fibers are formed in a similar manner. The implications of this for the neuron doctrine were also fraught with danger since it flew in the face of His's (1889, 1890) and Cajal's (1890a, 1892a) demonstration of the outgrowth of the axon from the embryonic nerve cell. On this, Cajal's whole theory of neurotropism, first enunciated in his 1892 study of the retina, was based.

The principal arguments adduced by Bethe and others were that growing axons could not be demonstrated crossing the scar joining the central and peripheral stump and especially that reinnervation of the peripheral stump and restoration of motor function could be demonstrated even when physical union of the two stumps was prevented (see chapters I and XVI of the present work). The first of these arguments can now be seen to have been based on the inability of techniques, prior to the introduction of reduced silver nitrate, to stain individual axons, and as a consequence of workers having to rely on the staining of the Schwann sheath or the myelin sheath. Obviously, both of these reappear only after the axons have crossed the gap and as innervation of the end organs is imminent. The second argument seemed particularly cogent to many contemporary scientists and, as Cajal points out both in his autobiography and in chapter I of the present work, even that strong supporter of the neuron doctrine, Van Gehuchten, was led to accept for a time the polygenist viewpoint because of it. Again from a modern perspective, we can see the results of Bethe's experiments as being a manifestation of the enormous capacity of regenerating nerve fibers to reach their targets by the most devious routes—a vindication, in fact, of Cajal's neurotropic theory; however, this was knowledge as yet unfamiliar to the scientists of the day.

Both of the points raised by Bethe against the monogenist viewpoint were easily demolished by Cajal's first application of the reduced silver nitrate method which enabled naked, growing axon sprouts to be revealed in continuity in thick sections. Here, he could see the growth cone, comparable to that of the embryonic axon which he had first identified in 1890, the initial growth of the sprouts devoid of Schwann cell covering, their passage around obstructions and across gaps, and their growth along the Schwann bands and tubes of the peripheral stump. With his first studies he was able to demolish the views of Bethe and within two years the monogenist viewpoint had won the day. Cajal's glee is apparent in the protracted metaphor with which in his autobiography he describes this victory in terms of a cavalry engagement culminating in Bethe's being unhorsed and quitting the field. The mode of innervation of the peripheral stump, as clearly seen in the reduced silver preparations, also furnished ammunition for dismissing what Cajal called the Hensen–Held theory of axon development and he was to use this repeatedly in his polemics with Held (Cajal 1907d, 1908a, 1933; and see the translation from ¿*Neuronismo o reticularismo?* in chapter 6).

It would be inappropriate to dismiss volume I of *Degeneration and Regeneration of the Nervous System* as being concerned only with the resolution of the problem of peripheral nerve regeneration and with the winning of a victory in support of the neuron doctrine. The volume contains much more of both a descriptive and theoretical character. Cajal's descriptions of the processes of nerve degeneration and regeneration are among the most comprehensive ever and cover nearly 300 pages of volume I. In these descriptions there is still much from which a modern neuroscientist can draw information and possibly the only point of discord is Cajal's unwillingness to accept that the myelin sheath is actually formed from the Schwann cells. In this he was obviously influenced by his knowledge that myelin is formed in the central nervous system in the absence of a supporting Schwann sheath. It would be wrong, however, to give Cajal sole credit for the elucidation of the phenomena that accompany nerve regeneration and repair, for he was competing with several very productive Italians and the Franco-Romanian group led by neurologist, Marinesco. One of the Italians, Perroncito, in fact made what was probably a more extensive study than Cajal of the early phenomena occurring in the central stump of a divided nerve. Cajal's quibblings over priority, on pp. 20 and 158 of Part II, seem to betray an awareness of the possibility of being "scooped"—something that was never far from Cajal's mind (DeFelipe and Jones 1988).

If volume I contains much of a descriptive nature that could arguably have been produced by any competent neurohistologist armed with the new method, its greatest impact derives from its development of the theory of neurotropism. This is always to the fore and it reveals Cajal at his best. In his studies of central neurogenesis, particularly in those on the retina in 1892, Cajal had formulated what he then called a theory of *chemotactism* in which he felt that the growth ("amoeboidism") and target finding by young axons had to be brought about by the presence of an "orienting" or "attracting" stimulus of a chemical nature. By 1905–1906 he had applied the theory to the whole field of neurogenesis, dropping the word *chemotaxis* in favor of Forssman's (1900) alternative, *neurotropism*. A further alternative, not adopted by Cajal, was Kappers' (1908b,c) *neurobiotaxis* which extended the principle to cell migration as well.

For Cajal, the principle of neurotropism was one of the fundamental laws of neurogenesis that had been established as the result of convergent work in the field of neural development and in that of pathological degeneration and regeneration. Throughout volume I he makes it clear that regeneration of severed axons has three elements: the capacity of cut axons to sprout; their capacity to grow propelled, as it were, from behind by the trophic influence of the parent soma (the *vis a tergo* of Held); and the influence of extrinsic factors, mechanical and chemical. In his studies of regeneration in peripheral nerves, which involved complete or partial transection, crushing, the placement of obstacles in the gap, cross reunion, inversions, and the introduction of neural and non-neural grafts, Cajal clearly identified the proliferating Schwann cells as the most likely source of neurotropic substances. He indicates that he had some concept of the necessity for receptors for these substances on the growth cones of the growing axons, a very modern point of view (p. 392). It is also clear that he realized the necessity for two kinds of tropic agent, a general type in the distal stump that promoted axon growth and specific types that assured innervation of the appropriate targets at the periphery. It is typical of his insight that he foresaw the possibility of reorganization of connections in the spinal cord as an adaptation to inappropriate reinnervation at the periphery, also a subject of modern appeal. His writing is full of characteristically vivid images. He speaks, for example, of axons "throwing themselves on the peripheral stump," of the "alluring or attracting substances," of axons "scenting the specific chemotactic fount," of the "nutritive and tutorial functions of the cells of Schwann," and there is another extended metaphor (p. 205) likening the reinnervation process to an obstacle race run in the dark.

The material for volume I is largely drawn from the series of papers on nerve regeneration published in the *Trabajos del Laboratorio de Investigaciones Biológicas de la Universidad de Madrid* between 1905 and 1908. By 1907, however, Cajal's student, Tello, had also become a major contributor to the field, particularly with his studies of degeneration and regeneration at the peripheral end organs, especially the motor end plates and muscle spindles (Tello 1907a,b). Cajal makes extensive use of Tello's data and after publication of Volume I of the Spanish version of the book in 1913, Tello was the principal experimentalist (Tello 1917; and see later). It is clear, however, from the additions made to chapter X of the English version (1928) that Cajal himself continued some experimental studies in the interim.

Volume II of *Degeneration and Regeneration of the Nervous System* clearly had its origins in a series of later studies carried out by Cajal on the central nervous system and published in the *Trabajos* mainly in 1906 and in 1910 and 1911. There are numerous additions from the studies of Tello and the work is fleshed out with a review of phenomena occurring in degenerating and transplanted peripheral ganglia to which Cajal added descriptions of original material.

The first part of volume II, on the sensory and sympathetic ganglia, is essentially a continuation of volume I and in it Cajal describes in detail the normal structure of ganglia, the effects of aging and of trauma, the capacity for regeneration, and experiments involving the transplantation of ganglia. Much of this is derived from papers by Cajal and his students and published between 1905 and 1910 (Cajal 1905b,c, 1906b,e, 1910b,c) plus his review paper of 1913 (Cajal 1913a; and see also Cajal 1913b), with substantial additions from the work of the Marinesco School and the Italians. In the course of this we learn that Cajal and Olóriz in 1897 were first to discover the satellite cells of the sensory ganglia (p. 399), that the term *neuroplasticity* was first introduced by Marinesco's student, Minea, in his 1909 thesis (p. 430), and Cajal seems to imply (p. 432) that *heterochrono-* and *homochronotransplantation* are his (Cajal's) words. Cajal concludes this part in a somewhat negative frame of mind about the possibilities for regeneration of transplanted ganglia, but perhaps the major element in this part is the introduction of the concept of a symbiotic relationship between neurons and satellite cells which is an extension of the neurotropic theory. The "neurobione" theory which is also developed further in the rest of volume II is perhaps less felicitous to modern ears. In this, Cajal postulates the presence of a fundamental unit of nerve cell cytoplasm on which the trophic influences of the Schwann cells may play and which forms the basis for neurofibrillar regeneration and reorganization. In reality, however, the theory is not too far removed from modern ideas of inductive phenomena and the regulation of gene expression for structural proteins.

Part II of volume II deals with the degeneration and regeneration of the spinal cord and its roots and of the optic nerve. In his autobiography (see Section 2 of this book), Cajal tells us that by late 1906, he was looking into the potential for regeneration in the central nervous system and much of the work covered in Part II derives mainly from his studies of 1906, 1910, and

1913 (Cajal 1906d, 1910b,d,e, 1911c, 1913b), with further additions from the Italian and Romanian investigators and from Tello (1907c, 1911a,b). This part of volume II finds Cajal in a more optimistic mood. He is clearly impressed by the frustrated regeneration of dorsal root fibers on reaching the spinal cord, by the influence of the ventral root environment over regenerating motor axons, and by the capacity for more extensive growth of regenerating central axons that come in contact with components of the dorsal or ventral roots. The frustrated and aborted regeneration in the spinal cord is, thus, seen by him as due to the lack of tropic substances and of the orienting environment normally provided in the regenerating peripheral nervous system by the Schwann cells. In the chapter on the optic nerve and retina, the primary sources are Tello (1907c, 1911b) and Leoz and Ortín (1913), but Cajal had made a number of additional relevant observations in his 1905–1906 papers and in the 1913 review. The main conclusion is that sprouting and attempted regeneration definitely occur in these structures, but that regeneration is frustrated and the sprouts reabsorbed. A note of hope is introduced, however, by the possibilities for stimulating optic nerve fiber regeneration by sciatic nerve grafts.

Part III of volume II, consisting of two chapters on the lesioned cerebellar cortex, is derived mainly from a paper by Cajal in 1911 (Cajal 1911a), although preliminary observations had been mentioned as early as 1907 (Cajal 1907c). From this work he derives the conviction that neurons of long axon, that is, the Purkinje cells, can survive as short axon neurons provided that their axon is cut beyond the first collateral. He feels that this collateral, in becoming hypertrophied and maintaining connections with other neurons of the same type, can not only preserve the damaged cell but may also help to compensate for the loss of efferent connectivity. It appears to us that the hypertrophy of the collateral and the localized axonal swellings at nodes of Ranvier reported by Cajal may be manifestations of redirected and obstructed axoplasmic flow. Of course, the concept of axoplasmic transport was unknown to Cajal. That Cajal may have had some inkling of this, however, is evident on page 668 where, in describing similar changes in the severed axons of cerebral cortical pyramidal cells, he likens the effects to those seen after placing a ligature on an artery.

Overall, Cajal was unimpressed by the limited capacity displayed by the cerebellar cortex for regeneration, seeing it as far less than in the spinal cord and even less than in the cerebral cortex, even in the neonatal animals that he preferentially used for his experimental studies. He states that the *"retraction ball*, which at first we believed might in time become transformed into a growth cone, represents an act of sedentary reaction, without any power of vanquishing the surrounding obstacles, or energy to form new paths. Something appears to be lacking . . . [something] . . . capable of rousing it from its apathy and quiescence" (pp. 614, 615). That something, that *ignotum quid* of Cajal is clearly the neurotropic influence.

The cerebellar chapters contain two other points of note. There are a number of interesting observations on the similarities between traumatic effects on cerebellar neurons and pathological states seen in cerebellar disease. These are mostly taken from the work of others, supplemented by his own observations on the human cerebellum and on the cerebellum of dogs infected with rabies. There are also observations on the reactions of basket axons and climbing fibers in which he emphasizes that the persistence of the latter in the presence of death of the underlying Purkinje cell is clearly a vindication of the neuron doctrine.

The final part of volume II occupies more than 100 pages and is devoted to the responses of the cerebral cortex to traumatic and infective insults. These chapters derive in large part from a series of papers published in 1910 and 1911 (Cajal 1910e, 1911b,c,d). In them, a modern reader will find much of interest. Cajal observes that the cerebral cortex is far more responsive in terms of its capacity for the display of regenerative phenomena than the cerebellar cortex but less reactive than the spinal cord. Despite this, and their failure to proceed to complete regeneration, the phenomena are similar to those seen in the peripheral nervous system. Moreover, he recognizes that many of the morphological changes occurring in axons due to traumatic lesions of the cerebrum are similar to these seen in degenerative diseases such as Alzheimer's disease and in inflammatory and compressive lesions in humans. The colonies of new fibers and terminal clubs found in senile plaques, for example, are seen by Cajal as regenerative effects similar to the ephemeral regenerative sprouting that he observed under experimental conditions.

One of the most interesting features of the cerebral cortex work is the lengthy account of Tello's (1911b) experiments on the transplantation of pieces of sciatic nerve into the cerebral cortex which are summarized by Cajal (pp. 728–744). In these experiments, provided the nerve grafts were taken from distal stumps in which Schwann cells were dividing, and the cerebral cortex was incised, a certain number of fibers of the white matter would invade the graft and some would apparently even acquire Schwann cell sheaths. This seems to peak with time and then degeneration ensues. To Cajal, any attempt to promote regeneration in the cerebral cortex and central nervous system generally will have to provide trophic substances capable of stimulating sprouting and the further growth of sprouts, as well as attracting and orienting (tropic) substances that would guide growing axons along appropriate pathways. He, therefore, saw Tello's experiments as pointing in the direction of the first set of substances, but recognized that discovery and utilization of the second set would be a far more difficult problem.

In summing up his work on regeneration in the spinal cord, cerebellum, and cerebral cortex, Cajal concludes that the regenerative phenomena observed are on the whole temporary reactions, "aborted restorative processes incapable of bringing about a complete and definitive repair of interrupted paths." This probably depends on the lack of neurotropic factors ("catalytic agents") and is, therefore, potentially a soluble problem. It cannot be denied that the central nervous system has the capacity to produce new axons although it is "impoverished" in comparison with the peripheral nervous system and the sprouts "lose their energy" once the process is initiated. Then, in a final typically insightful moment, he recognizes that the complexity of organization of the adult nervous system must also have demanded the presence of neurotropic agents in development (pp. 744–750).

The Spanish edition of *Degeneration and Regeneration of the Nervous System* appeared in two volumes in 1913 and 1914. The costs of publication were met by expatriate Spanish physicians then resident in Argentina who had undertaken to make a gesture in recognition of Cajal's winning the Nobel Prize (see chapter 2 of this book). Having been published by private subscription, the book had an understandably limited distribution. The files of Oxford University Press report that Cajal gave away virtually all copies. Plans to produce a larger printing were thwarted by the outbreak of World War I.

The present English translation, originally published by Oxford University Press, first appeared in 1928 and probably achieved a somewhat wider circulation than the original Spanish version. The translator, Raoul Michel May, was born of French parents in Sonora, Mexico, in 1900. He received his university education in the United States at Stanford, Johns Hopkins, and Harvard Universities, being awarded the Ph.D. from Harvard University in 1924. While working in the Zoological Laboratory at Harvard, he carried out two early studies of a non-neurological nature (May 1923–1924; Kropp and May 1924), the second of them at the suggestion of Samuel R. Detwiler, one of the founders of the American school of experimental embryology. Then, under the direct supervision of Detwiler, he turned to studies on nerve regeneration. One of these studies, on the role of innervation in the induction and maintenance of regenerating taste buds in the barbels of catfish (May 1925), contains a clear statement of the neurotropic hypothesis of Cajal. The second, dealing with the fate of optic nerve fibers subsequent to the transplantation of eye primordia in *Ambystoma* larvae (May and Detwiler 1926; May 1927a,b), is one of the first of its kind to address the issue of neurotropism in the guidance of nerve fibers to the brain.

May went to Paris in 1924 as Parker Fellow of Harvard University and worked in the Laboratoire d'Évolution des Êtres Organismes of the University of Paris. In 1925 he was appointed an American Field Service Fellow in the Laboratoire d'Anatomie Comparée at the Sorbonne. There he received his D.Sc. in 1928. At some time prior to this, according to Tello (1935), he spent an undetermined period in Cajal's laboratory. The files at Oxford University Press show that shortly after his arrival in Paris he approached the Press, indicating that he had "out of enthusiasm" made an English translation of Cajal's *Degeneración y Regeneración de los nervios* (1913), and *Degeneración y regeneración de los centros nerviosos* (1914) and, with Cajal's permission, was offering it to the Press for publication, Cajal having agreed to provide the blocks of the plates. May's translation was subjected to very substantial editorial revision by Sir Paul Harvey (1869–1948), a former diplomat and parliamentary secretary, who subsequently became compiler and editor of the *Oxford Companion to English Literature* (1932) and of the *Oxford Companion to Classical Literature* (1938). Harvey worked by comparing May's translation with a copy of the Spanish text provided by Sir Charles Sherrington, then Waynflete Professor of Physiology at Oxford. Additional improvements of a technical nature were made by H. M. Carleton, also a member of the University Laboratory of Physiology at Oxford and the author of a well-known textbook of histology. The two volumes were finally published in July 1928. Apparently they were never particularly popular and went out of print in 1944. Facsimile reprints were published in the United States in 1959 and 1968.

May remained at the University of Paris for the rest of his career, becoming director of the Laboratoire de Biologie Animale and later of the Laboratoire d'Anatomie Comparée at Orsay. He continued to work mainly on the nervous system, concerning himself with the chemical analysis of degenerating nerves and with the transplantation of neural and non-neural tissue (e.g., May 1957, 1960; May and Jeanmarie 1963). He achieved a reputation for his work in transplantation, during the course of which he coined the term "brephoplastic transplantation" to refer to the grafting of fetal tissue. Most of his work was published in French as short communications in the *Comptes Rendus de l'Academie des Sciences* of Paris. He died in 1968. We believe that the younger figure seated to the far left of Cajal in the photograph on page 265 of Albarracín's book *Santiago Ramón y Cajal o la Pasión de España* (1982), is May and that the photograph was taken at about the time of publication of the English translation of *Degeneration and Regeneration of the Nervous System*.

We have checked the translation, word for word, against the original Spanish and have found it to be generally literal, accurate, and highly readable. There are relatively few errors. Those few that we have detected are mainly in the methods chapter. The others could easily stem from typesetting or proofreading. A small number of short omissions or modifications of detail seem to have been mainly made in the interests of readability and do not materially affect the content. A number of words or expressions that May regularly uses have gone out of fashion in modern scientific English and we have suggested a list of alternatives, along with some corrections of obvious errors (Table 1). The only expression that perhaps requires special note is "innervation" which to May simply meant the invasion of a scar or peripheral stump of a severed nerve by regenerating axons. It does not imply reinnervation of a target organ and the restoration of functional continuity. Cajal's word for this was the more neutral "neurotization," which May probably avoided for its lack of euphony.

During preparation of the English edition, Cajal produced a number of notes to be appended to certain chapters in order to deal with developments that had occurred in the decade and a half that had ensued following

TABLE 1. Glossary of Unusual Terms

Agony, agonal: death struggle

Autochthonic neurons (page 407, line 5): intrinsic neurons

Bundles of Weismann: intrafusal muscle fibers

Catenary: chain- or ropelike

Commotion: concussion

Current: stream of fibers

Erethism: excessive stimulation

Functional expansion or prolongation: axon

Gibbous: humped or protuberant

Grumes: lumps or clots

Innervation, nervous reunion: invasion of the scar, peripheral stump of a cut nerve, or graft, not implying innervation of the target. Cajal uses "neurotization."

Lustrum: a period of five years

Neurocladism, neurocladic: the phenomenon of induction and branching of the processes of a nerve cell.

Neurone (page 598, last line): in this case means interneuron

Odogenesis: see neurocladism

Phlegmasia: inflammation

Phlogosis, phlogotic, phlogistic: inflammation, inflammatory

Pip (page 627, line 14): canine distemper

Ravelling, ravelled: fraying, frayed

Spindles of Kühne: muscle spindles

Spireme (page 623): tangled strands of chromosomal material. A term formerly applied to the first stage of mitosis when extended chromosome filaments have the appearance of a loose ball of yarn.

Spools: tangles

trophic and *[neuro] tropism:* Cajal uses these in the traditional senses of nourishing and orientation to a stimulus respectively. *Trophic* is applied in the sense of maintenance of axonal viability by the parent soma. *Neurotropism* is applied to include both induction of axon outgrowth and guidance towards a target, phenomena that many modern neuroscientists would tend to call "trophic."

Vegetation: sprouting. Usually in reference to the growth of dendrites.

CHAPTER 2

Material Omitted from the Original English Edition

Dedicatory*

Subscribed by the Commission of Spanish Physicians of Buenos Aires.

We, the physicians of Spanish origin, some graduated from the Universities of the mother country, others from the Faculty of Medicine of Buenos Aires, [and] scattered through the vast territory of the Republic of Argentina, have assembled with the laudable purpose of paying a modest tribute of admiration and respect to our compatriot, the scholar histologist Don Santiago Ramón y Cajal, [who has been] already honored by all that are most eminent and distinguished in the scientific world: individuals and corporations, Academies and Congresses, without respect to nationalities, races nor continents, reflecting the universality of the science and the [promptness and egalitarianism with which merit is recognized in modern times].

In deciding to do this, we have been influenced not so much by the [special nature] of scholarship as by the scholarship itself. If Dr. Cajal would have been eminent in other branches of human knowledge, we certainly would have admired him, but without feeling ourselves so deeply impressed; what is clear on reflection is that his talent stands out in sciences which did not seem to be of Spanish concern, judging by our neglect of them, and by the lack of affection and love with which we treat them, as if they could not derive from our essence and were beyond our intelligence and our means. Dr. Cajal, and this is the particular value that we refer to, so grateful in our hearts, counteracted at one stroke the prejudice, excessively accentuated among individuals at home and abroad, of our inability to cultivate the

---

*This dedication and the appended list of contributors in Table 2 did not appear in the 1928 English version.

experimental sciences, having effected with intelligence and admirable laboriousness, in a relatively short time, more discoveries than other investigators had made up till then and, what is even more valuable, he had given us the key with which henceforth we will be able to penetrate the mysterious caverns of cerebral structure, [which represents] the most noble and differentiated organ of the human being.

But, although we cannot follow this great work in all its details, it does not prevent us from glimpsing its immense significance. We, therefore, feel ourselves authorized to say that the studies made by Dr. Cajal on the cerebrum, cerebellum, and sensory organs, [but] especially those on the cerebrum, that great complex of confederate centers, interconnected by innumerable contacts that are opened for function or closed for rest, under the influence of stimuli originating in the environment or in our own organism, will give an exact basis to the growing science of psychic determinism and will explain affective, intellectual and volitional phenomena, with the same clarity with which nowadays Physics explains many phenomena of the cosmic world.

In our opinion, Cajal has not only the very great merit of having personally created a science but also of having disseminated it, circulating his discoveries among all the scholars of the world, putting in front of them, by means of clear and concise illustrations drawn by himself, those facts that deserved to be especially settled, and drawing their attention to new ones.

If [Cajal] had not proceeded in this manner, [that is to say] in revealing himself, would the foreign [scientists] have come to know him in time? Would the master have witnessed his apotheosis? Surely not; many years would have passed before his studies would have been appreciated as they deserved had they not been imposed by the vigor with which the author himself did it; had his work been recognized late, perhaps it would not reach the degree of perfection that we can nowadays appreciate, and who knows if Science would recognize so many eminent works of the scholar histologist, works that provoke the admiration of both natives and foreigners.

Illustrious master: You already know the feelings that have led us to carry out this collective demonstration, which we do not consider a reward, which would be without value, but as a proof of our admiration, of our empathy, and our affection for your person.

Accept it as such, and together with it our most fervent wishes that you can continue your immortal works for a long time; may you succeed in consolidating your brilliant school, which counts in its active list renowned personalities such as Pedro Ramón y Cajal, Claudio Sala, Blanes, Villa, Tello, C. Calleja, Achúcarro, G. Lafora, R. Illera, Sánchez, etc., all of whom it is also just to recall in this moment, so that you can be, finally, a witness to the resurgence of Spain, which is beginning to penetrate into all branches of human knowledge.

TABLE 2. List of the Physicians who contributed to the subscription in honor of Ramón y Cajal [See footnote p. 19]

Lista de los Sres. Médicos contribuyentes á la suscripción de homenaje á
RAMÓN Y CAJAL

NOMBRES	DOMICILIO	CANTIDAD $
Dr. Justo Carlé	Capital	50,00
» José González Pellicer	»	50,00
» Francisco Cobos	»	10,00
» Eladio Arrieta	»	50,00
» Anselmo O. de Retana	»	50,00
» Federico Iribarren	»	50,00
» Francisco Carisomo	»	50,00
» José M.ª Carrera	»	50,00
» Ignacio Imaz	»	50,00
» Avelino Gutiérrez	»	50,00
» Ramón Leiguarda	»	50,00
» José Torrontegui	»	50,00
» Esteban Molla Catalán	La Plata	50,00
» Mariano Centeno	Mercedes	50,00
» José J. Badia	Capital	50,00
» Egidio G. Ciano	Ayacucho	50,00
» Alfredo Lamas	Juárez	10,00
» Angel Gutiérrez	Capital	50,00
» José Pagés	»	50,00
» Crescencio Orcoyen	»	10,00
» Severiano P. Redondo	Paraná	50,00
» Alfredo Arines	Concordia	50,00
» Joaquín Aguirrezabala	Gualeguay	50,00
» José Dalmau	B. Blanca	50,00
» Regino Cavia	San Pedro	50,00
» Miguel Santamarina	Capital	50,00
» Camilo Clausolles	»	50,00
» Enrique Herráiz	25 de Mayo	50,00
» Javier Santero	Capital	10,00
» Antonio Mir	Magdalena	50,00
» Víctor Grau	T. Arroyos	10,00
» Ernesto Carbó	Capital	10,00
» N. Esquerdo	Tandil	10,00
» N. Alonso	Juárez	10,00
» José Fabres García	Bolívar	50,00
» L. Rivas Míguez	Capital	50,00
» J. B. Troncoso	»	50,00
» Arturo Galceran	»	50,00
» Andrés Bayón	»	10,00
» Emilio Cabello	»	50,00
» Anselmo Ruiz Gutiérrez	»	10,00
» Daniel Lizarralde	»	10,00
» Antonio Valdivieso	»	10,00
» Aniceto Poncela	»	10,00
» José Solá	»	40,00
» Ingnacio Blanes	»	40,00
» Carlos Magdalena	T. Lauquen	40,00
TOTAL $		1.800,00

And you, work of the scholar, on whom we have fixed our thoughts, looked after by him with special love, spread to all the winds the new ideas, and with them the glory of the master and of the mother country.

For the Commission,

Justo Carlé
President
Ignacio Imaz
Secretary

Author's Preface to the Spanish Edition*

The Nobel Prize with which the Carolinian Institute of Stockholm was pleased to recompense my modest scientific achievements was the signal, among physicians of Spanish race, for patriotic and enthusiastic testimonies of affection and consideration. But, among the homages received none did me more honor, because of its delicate and spiritual nature, than the tribute paid to the humble man of science by his medical compatriots of the Argentine Republic. They did not deem it sufficient to show their esteem by flattering me with an artistic diploma made the more valuable by their signatures, but, resolving that their noble sentiments should crystallize into something useful and permanent, they decided to print at their cost a book of ours, which was in need of publication.

Such was the origin of the present work. When I began it I believed that it would perhaps be useful to include in a general treatise the numerous memoirs that my pupils and myself (not forgetting the very valuable contributions made by illustrious foreign scholars) had devoted during the last few years to the difficult problem of the degeneration and regeneration of the nervous system. When I set to work, however, I saw that if the undertaking were to do justice to the magnitude and dignity of the homage, it could not consist merely of a compilation of published facts. In order, then, to honor as far as possible the objective initiative of my colleagues overseas, I set myself the task, by means of laboratory investigation of revising all the subjects previously studied, and also of making a special study of many doubtful or uncertain points. The present book constitutes, then, an extensive monograph, original in large part. It is obvious that by adopting this approach, the undertaking has required more time and effort

---

*This is a corrected version of May's slightly imperfect translation of the original preface.

than I had expected. The sickly state of my health has also contributed, with deplorable insistence, to the inevitable delay of publication.

It is a pleasure for me to record here my profound gratitude to my honorable and cultured friends of the Argentine Republic. I hope that the offering which I am sending them in return for their kindness will not be deemed too far below their own generosity. As a last resort, it consoles me to think that, among all the imperfections and deficiencies of [this] work, there will always be evident two excellent and laudable things: the noble and patriotic example of my countrymen from beyond the seas, and the good will and fraternal affection of the author.

Madrid, *July 10*, 1913

SECTION TWO

CAJAL IN HIS OWN WORDS—TRANSLATIONS FROM BIOGRAPHICAL AND OTHER WORKS

CHAPTER 3

From: *Recuerdos de mi vida,* Volume 2, Historia de mi labor científica, chapter 19, pages 453–475*

S. RAMÓN Y CAJAL
Madrid: N. Moya, 1917

[The chapter is entitled: Works of the triennium, 1905, 1906 and 1907. Investigations on the regeneration of nerves and central pathways. Controversy between the monogeneticists and polygeneticists. Neuronism rises triumphant over the charges brought against it by the devotees of the catenary theory. New studies on the origins of the nerve pathways in the embryo, that strengthened the neuron doctrine. Conclusive demonstrations that the neurofibrils of the nerve cell consist of relatively autonomous living entities.]

The years 1905 and 1906 are coincident will the zenith of my scientific career. During [those years] fortune smiled upon me to the extent that I reached the greatest heights to which a man of science can aspire; and in the said period, apart from communications of lesser importance, I carried out observations that were decisive for the consolidation of the neuron doctrine.

Let us start by referring briefly to the most fruitful of my Laboratory works during the cited biennium.

Yielding to [pressures] about which I will talk later, I first devoted my attention to elucidate the long disputed problem of the mode of regeneration of nerves and interrupted central nervous pathways; and afterwards (a task performed in the second half of 1906) to explore with the new technique [of

---

*Craigie's 1937 English translation is from the 1923 edition of the same work (Cajal 1923), but omits substantial portions of this.

reduced silver nitrate] the origins of the nerve fibers of the embryo, [which is] a subject intimately related to the foregoing.

Both studies were in response to certain prevailing attitudes. After a long period of quiet and almost undisputed sovereignty of the neuron doctrine, about which, as the reader will remember, I had had the good fortune to bring forward the main objective proofs, the old and almost forgotten error of *reticularism* and other similar speculative extravagances (*catenary theory*, etc.) were revived with incredible strength in certain schools. It could be said that certain minds, inclined towards mysticism, were disturbed by the simple and patent truths. Excessively haughty temperaments seem to be determined to overthrow fame, not [only] by the honorable and difficult way of discovering new facts but [also] by the much more comfortable and expedient way of denying or discounting, in the name of very risky prejudices, the most rigorously demonstrated facts. Such an anarchic and unfortunate passion, never entirely banished from the domain of biology, had, as I just said, reached its culminating point around 1900 to 1904. But then the fanatics of reticularism adopted a new tactic. Feeling, no doubt, but little confidence in achieving victory in the open field of adult neuronal morphology, they chose to impugne neuronism in the apparently more propitious fields of the *regeneration of nerves* and of *embryonic neurogenesis*.

Many were the bold adventurers eager for combat under the old flag originally unfurled in 1867 by Gerlach and Meynert. Discordant, and even antagonistic in many of their affirmations, they concurred only in a strange and unanimous feeling of aversion towards the doctrine of contact and of the independence of the nerve cells; a doctrine proved up to the hilt, as was known, lustrums ago, by His, Forel, us, Lenhossék, Retzius, Kölliker, Van Gehuchten, Lugaro, Waldeyer, Harrison, etc., in the field of normal histology and histogenesis; and by Waller, Münzer, Ranvier, Vanlair, Ziegler, Stroebe, Forssmann, Marinesco, Langley, Mott, Halliburton, Segale, Purpura, and many others in the sphere of degeneration and regeneration of the nerves. Except for the prestigious Professor Nissl and certain others, [it was mostly] enthusiastic youths who formed up in the ranks of reticularism, as much eager for reputation as they were naive observers. Let us remember, among them: Büngner, Joris, Huber, Sedgwig, Ballance, Wietting, Marchand, Galeotti and Levi, Monckeberg, Durante, O. Schültze, etc., some of whom worked prior to 1900.

[Albrecht] Bethe, professor in the University of Strasbourg, whose impressive studies on the neurofibrils of vertebrates had made him justly famous, turned out to be the leader and strategist of this gallant troop, by the dual rights of talent and gallantry of criticism. [Apart from the unquestionable authority of the cited scholar, his incomparable polemical skill, the ingeniousness of his technical resorts and even the brightness of his style, contributed powerfully to fascinate the University youth of Germany and of Italy. (In France and England, the reticular theory made few converts.) Although defending very different and personal [doctrines] of reticularism, also contributing their authority to this risky hypothesis, were H. Held of Leipzig; Professor Dogiel of Saint Petersburg, and the eminent Golgi of Pavia. With such advocates it was little wonder that it became fashionable to execrate and even smile at the neuron concept and at the theory of connection by contact, in spite of its being based, as we had stated, on the very accurate expression of innumerable concordant observations(1)].*

So fulminant and widespread did the contagion of reticularism become in 1903, thanks, above all, to the attractive hypotheses of A. Bethe, that the illustrious Waldeyer wavered in his neuronist faith; Professor Marinesco changed sides temporarily, and even the illustrious Van Gehuchten, [who was] one of the pillars of neuronism weakened (who would have thought it!); he, without renouncing the orthodox doctrine completely, made the following humiliating concession to the dissidents: "In the adult the nerve cell possesses a perfect individuality, [and is the] product of a single neuroblast; but in the pathological state, for example during the process of nervous regeneration, the new axons result from the fusion and differentiation of a chain of peripheral neuroblasts. . . ."

The foregoing will lead the reader to see the extent to which the danger grew. There were [even] some authors who considered the brilliant concept of His and Forel definitively buried. In short, the reticularist chimera became so pervasive and used in its inconsistent objections a language so arrogant and insolent, that the patience of the neuronists reached its limit. It was necessary to impose a corrective on the general aberration. Some scholars, being surprised at my silence and considering me perhaps to be the most obligated to come out in defense of the authority of the truth, wrote to me reproachfully: "What do you do?, how do you defend yourself?"

I have always felt an overwhelming repugnance towards idle polemics. With it one loses precious time which could be used profitably in collecting new facts. Who can ignore, anyway that the truth, however, defenseless, ends up by prevailing? But in the face of the crushing tide of error and in view of the repeated requests of my friends, I found myself compelled to halt in my path and descend to the arena, it being a great grief to me to have to spend two or three years in anatomicopathological researches, whose fruits could not do other than confirm the truth [already] demonstrated a long time ago by Waller, Ranvier, Vanlair, Stroebe, and many other scholars. At the end of the campaign, I had, however, the consolation of seeing that [I] had not entirely wasted my time. Besides strengthening several classical conclusions [that had been] somewhat uncertain because of methodological

---

*The text in brackets is not in the 1923 edition.

insufficiencies, I succeeded in collecting some original observations [that were] not without value.

It would be unjust to forget that I was not a solitary participant in this hard battle on behalf of the truth; several prestigious researchers also joined me; [they], like me, were exasperated by the boasting and rashness of the reticularists. Let us mention in first place Perroncito, the favorite pupil of Golgi, who also applied the new method [of reduced silver nitrate] to the subject; Lugaro, [neurologist and psychologist of great talent];* Medea, Marinesco and Minea, Tello, Nageotte, Krassin, etc. Needless to say the procedure of reduced silver nitrate contributed decisively to the triumph of the right cause; with regard to the debated subject, this possesses the inestimable advantage of staining completely and intensely the buds or sprouts of the mutilated axons (central stump), sprouts that it is feasible to follow comfortably in thick sections across the scar and through the peripheral stump up to the very [terminations].

Let us recall now some antecedents of the problem of regeneration of the nerves.

The pathologists and physiologists of the first half of the last century (Waller, Vulpian, Ranvier, Brown-Séquard, Münzer, etc.) made the following fact clear: when a nerve trunk is cut in a young mammal, the portion of this situated distal to the cut (the *peripheral stump*) rapidly degenerates and dies, the remains of the axon and myelin being progressively reabsorbed; while months later both the intermediate or internerve scar and the peripheral stump show numerous newly formed fibers that reestablish totally or partially the sensibility and motion of the paralyzed limb.

By virtue of what histological mechanism is the damaged peripheral stump restored and the nerve terminations in muscles and sensory surfaces regenerated?

All the proposed solutions centered on the following two: the *theory of continuity or monogenetic [theory]*, maintained by Waller, Münzer, Ziegler, Ranvier, Vanlair, Stroebe, Kölliker, Mott, Halliburton, Harrison, Lugaro, etc; and the *theory of discontinuity or polygenetic [theory]*, proclaimed by certain physiologists (Vulpian, Brown-Séquard, Bethe) and by a goodly number of pathological anatomists (Büngner, Wietting, Ballance, Stewart, Marchand, Medea, etc.).

The supporters of the first solution maintained that the newly formed fibers of the peripheral stump simply represent the prolongation, by means of progressive sprouting and growth, of the axons of the central stump, which would retain full vitality thanks to their continuity with the neuron of origin or *trophic center;* whereas the followers of polygenetism or the second theory, affirmed resolutely that the regenerated fibers result from

---

* Added in the 1923 edition.

the differentiation and successive tranformation of the ensheathing cells of the old nerve [fibers] (nucleus and protoplasm through division of the cells of Schwann). These cells, at the beginning, would be arranged in a solid protoplasmic chain or trunk, inside whose links axon segments would emerge progressively, by an act of differentiation, and would subsequently be fused into a continuous filament and, finally, joined together with the free ends of axons of the central stump.

[Needless to say, not only on account of my neuronist conviction but also from the point of view of irresistible tendencies, this explanation thoroughly revolted me. As a fervent believer in the unity of biological laws and persuaded that nature always proceeds in its operations with a spirit of strict economy, it did not enter my head that the organism, depending on its developmental state, uses two different and almost antagonistic mechanisms for the construction of the nerves. That is to say, if polygenetism were true for nervous regeneration, then during embryonic neurogenesis the axon represents the work of an individual neuroblast or young nerve cell but in pathological regeneration, the newly formed axon constitutes the product of innumerable cells of Schwann or *peripheral neuroblasts,* as some [authors] call them, except for the central axonic piece [which] is the product of an embryonic neuroblast. It is clear that this big contradiction did not occur to certain histologists; for them (Fragnito, Joris, Besta, Capobianco, Bethe, etc.), in both nerve regeneration and embryonic neurogenesis, the axon is produced by the fusion of innumerable originally independent cells (*catenary theory*). But such an assertion (acceptable to those histologists who had explored only the early phases of neurogenesis with simple methods that are useless for giving a clear and [dense] outline of axons in the process of formation) was unable to persuade those such as v. Lenhossék, Retzius, Edinger, Lugaro, Athias, and us, who had observed, thanks to the supreme revelations of the Golgi method, very clear and ineluctable images of the neuroblasts and of the axons during all their developmental moments; images peremptorily demonstrative, as we indicated in another chapter, of the *genetic unity* of the axons].*

Let us consider now some of the supposed evidence presented by Bethe and his principal corybants.

Bethe began his investigations by reproducing completely the experiments of Philippeaux and Vulpian, that is, by cutting out, in mammals a few days old, pieces of sciatic nerve and withdrawing and covering the stumps in such a way that any union was impossible and, therefore, any reestablishment of physiological continuity.

Working under the above-mentioned conditions, the said scholar de-

---

*The paragraph in brackets is not in the 1923 edition and neither it nor the succeeding five paragraphs appear in Craigie's translation.

clared that in a certain number of cases (not all, [which is] a very significant limitation), the macromicroscopic examination of the scar revealed an absolute interruption of the segments, at the same time that a more or less advanced regeneration of the peripheral [stump], [had occurred], as indicated by the fact of its physiological excitability. These observations, as well as the verification of all intermediate phases leading from Schwann cells to young nerve [fibers], phases already indicated by Büngner, led [Bethe] to suppose, like the latter [researcher], that the nerves radically and definitively separated from their trophic centers are capable of autoregeneration. Each axon, then, would represent the combined work of many cells of Schwann, in whose protoplasm, [once it had] reached maturity, the neurofibrils would be later differentiated, [which is a] positive sign of the appearance of nervous conductivity.

Bethe bases such radical polygenetism more on the results of physiological experiments than on precise histological observations. Thus, in [particular] cases of nerve section, when the autoregenerated peripheral stump is electrically excited, the animal, [although] insensitive to pain (an indication of lack of sensory communication), moves the muscles of the leg and foot; whereas, if the stimulated segment is the central no muscular contractions occur. The exceptions to this rule are interpreted by Bethe by supposing that, in spite of the precautions, fortuitous communications had been created between the two stumps.

More or less complete verifications of these conclusions were published not only by those affiliated with reticularism, but, as I said, even by such convinced neuronists as Marinesco and Van Gehuchten. [As can be seen, the epidemic was spreading and threatened to infect all minds.]*

In this [charged atmosphere] we undertook in 1905 our researches on the *regeneration of nerves* (2). They lasted for nearly two years, and were made in a great number of [different] animals (rabbit, cat, dog, etc.). The main conclusions of these studies are summarized in the following statements:†

1. When the sciatic nerve of a young mammal is cut and the animal is sacrificed several days after the operation, it is observed in preparations made with the [reduced silver nitrate method] that a great number of axons of the central stump are the seat of a very active phenomenon of sprouting. This sprouting is carried out in [one of] two manners; *a*, the new fiber or fibers possess the character of terminals, and sprout from the thickened stump of the old axon; *b*, the new fibers represent collateral branches originating at right angles or at an acute angle from the old axon. In both cases, the newly formed branches have an appearance similar to the fibers of Remak, that is to say, they lack a

---

* Added in the 1923 edition.
† These seven statements were not translated by Craigie.

myelin sheath, [and] invade the exudate interposed between the nerve stumps; they often branch [during] their course, and, finally, they end freely, preferentially as a *terminal club or bouton,* [which is] a kind of battering ram, [designed] to push the mesodermal cells [aside] and to forge a path through the future scar tissue (fig. 117, *C, b*) [*fig.1*].

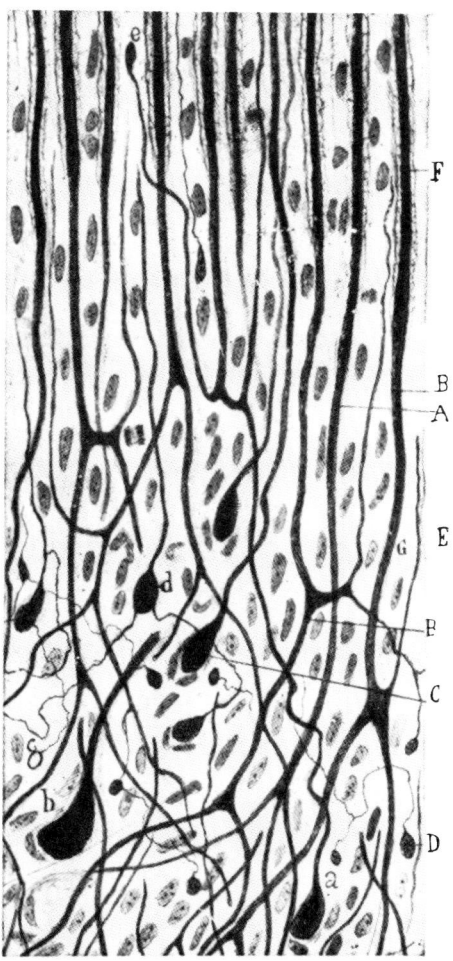

[*FIG. 1*] Fig. 117. Central stump and beginning of the intermediate scar of the sectioned sciatic nerve, examined three days after the operation. [Four days in *Degeneration and Regeneration of the Nervous System*—Eds.] Cat of a few days. *F*, fiber of the central stump; *a*, terminal branch arising from a pre-existent axon; [*C, b*, terminal boutons of the fibers that course through the scar; *d*, bouton from which new branches sprout.] [Phrase in brackets not found in the 1923 edition—Eds.]

The discovery of this terminal excrescence, confirmed later in the investigations of Perroncito, Marinesco, Nageotte, Sala, Tello, Dustin, Rossi, etc., has a certain importance for the resolution of the debated problem, since, thanks to the said terminal protoplasmic bouton, it is possible to determine exactly in sections not only the level which the regenerative process has reached, but also the origin and orientation of the newly formed axons. [This swelling is identical to our *growth cone* on the fibers of the embryo.]*

2. The newly formed nerve fibers, during their initial phases, and also their terminal boutons, lack nuclei or cells of Schwann; but from the third or fourth day on, the embryonic connective cells are attracted, and marginal nuclei appear around the naked axons. This formative precedence of the regenerated axons over the cells of Schwann, singularly imperils the catenary theory since it demonstrates that during the first phases of regeneration, the fibers completely lack the cellular chains (see figs. 117 and 118) [*figs. 1* and *2*].

3. Studying the course of the newly formed fibers during the six days following nerve interruption, it is easily recognized that the terminal clubs grow at random in the direction of least resistance: a great number of them retrograde, both inside the central stump in which they ascend greatly, and in the perineural territories; other groups of these [fibers], astray and errant, are obstructed in the face of the obstacles, trace complicated bends and are decidedly lost for the purposes of neurotization of the peripheral stump. Such stray axons, [which are] very abundant in cases of resection or of intentional separation of the nerve stumps, are characterized by a gigantic, encapsulated terminal club or sphere, [which is] frequently in the process of degeneration. These enormous terminal balls belong to fibers that are stopped in their growth (fig. 120, *c*) [*fig. 4*].

4. After ten or twelve days in adult animals, and after six or seven days in those a few weeks old, the young fibers [that are still on course] wander through the intercalated scar tissue, assail the sheaths of the peripheral stump, inside which they travel, moving aside in their passage the myelin debris not yet reabsorbed. At obstacles, the new fibers often divide, and the branches run flexuously, traveling indiscriminately through both the bands of Büngner and their interstices (fig. 119, *b, c*) [*fig. 3*].†

5. When, in repeating the experiment of Vulpian, Brown-Séquard, Bethe, etc., obstacles are interposed to prevent the immediate

---

* Added in the 1923 edition.
† In the 1923 edition, this figure was exchanged for another that we reproduce here as *fig. 3, bis.*

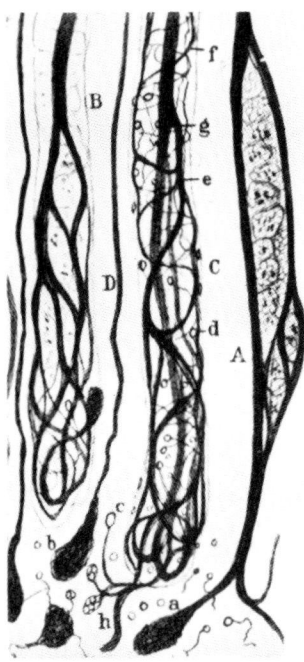

[*FIG. 2*] Fig. 118. Central stump of the sciatic nerve of a cat, in which the remains of the necrotic axon appear covered with branches generated by the living portion of the axon; these branches sometimes are unable to gain rapid access to the scar and generate complicated tangles (*B*, *C*). [The autopsy was made fifty-two hours after the operation.] [Phrase in brackets is not found in the 1923 edition—Eds.]

union of the stumps of a traumatically sectioned nerve, very advanced regeneration of the peripheral stump is frequently observed two or three months postoperatively. On examining this with the aid of our staining method, we observe in the interior of the peripheral nerve trunk, numerous young axons that always terminate at different levels, by means of a tiny growth bouton or by a fusiform thickening (fig. 119, *f*) [*fig. 3* and *fig. 3, bis, d*].

Exploration of the extensive and uneven scar that joins the separated nerve stumps does not reveal an absence of [single] nerve fibers, as the supporters of the catenary theory arbitrarily suggested, but a complicated nerve plexus, formed by small bundles of unmedullated fibers, and extending without interruption from the central to the peripheral stump.

6. The newly formed nerve fibers repeatedly divide in the scar and especially at the border of the peripheral stump, where frequently, each thick axon resolves itself into a *bouquet* of fine, small terminal

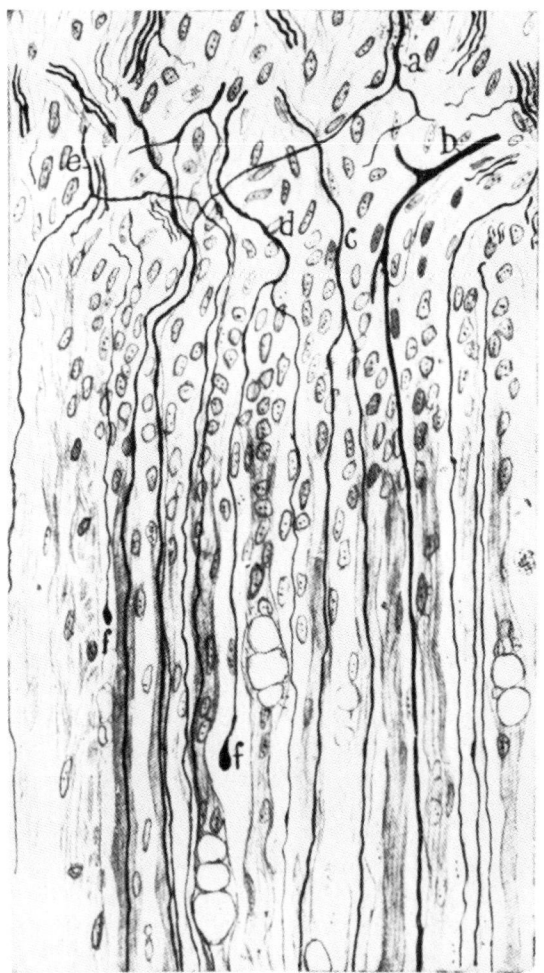

[*FIG. 3*] Fig. 119. Piece of scar and peripheral stump from a young cat [rabbit in *Degeneration and Regeneration of the Nervous System*—Eds.], whose sciatic nerve was sectioned seventy-two days before. Notice how the sprouts arriving at the said stump do not form chains, [but] penetrate either between or within the sheaths of the peripheral segment (old sheaths of Schwann), along which they grow rapidly (*f*). *A* [*upper*], scar; *B* [*lower*], peripheral stump. (The union of the stumps was impeded by mechanical obstacles.)

branches. The branches generated by each axon are not consigned to a single old [Schwann] tube, rather they are distributed in several of the empty sheaths; from which it results that, a group [of fibers] relatively deficient in afferent axons, can innervate a good deal of the

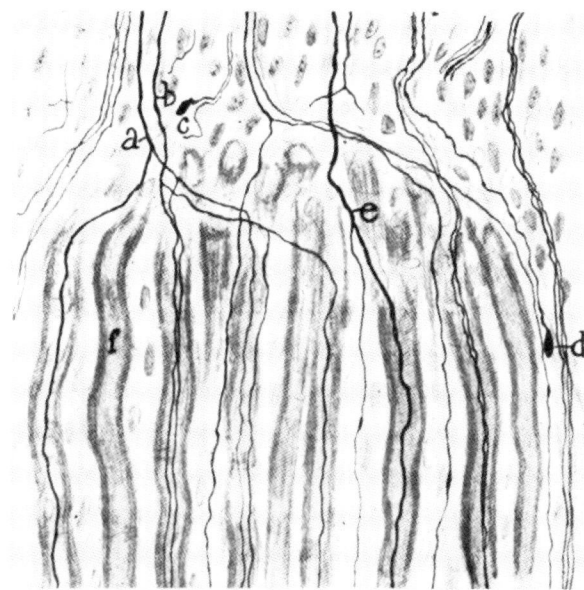

[*FIG. 3, bis*] Fig. 119. [The legend to this figure is the same as that to figure 3 except for A and B which were exchanged for: "*a, b*, newly formed fibers which travel through the scar; *e*, sprout bifurcating inside the peripheral stump; *d* and *c*, sprouts ending in small clubs."]

degenerated nerve (fig. 119, *b, d*) [*fig. 3* and *fig. 3 bis, b, e*]. Let us note that the above-mentioned branches, [which are] always oriented towards the periphery, as well as their free terminal clubs, are facts that are absolutely irreconcilable with the catenary theory.

7. The process of multiplication of the cells of Schwann of the peripheral stump is not for the purpose of producing chains of transformable elements leading to the autoregeneration of axons, as declared by Büngner and Bethe, but for the purpose of secreting stimulating substances, [which are] capable of attracting and guiding the young nerve fibers wandering through the scar towards the motor or sensory nerve terminations.

I have already said that a young Italian researcher, Aldo Perroncito (3), a disciple of the illustrious histologist of Pavia [Camillo Golgi], also used the reduced silver nitrate method (whose usefulness in anatomicopathological investigations was already reported by me in 1904), for the study of regeneration of nerves. The conclusions reached by this scholar coincided almost exactly with those of mine, except for his being able to detect the existence of divisions and of newly formed branches in the central stump at an earlier date than me, that is to say, from the second day following the section, and for having described perfectly the initial forms of the nerve bundles and tangles, indicated by several authors and described in detail by us (fig. 120 and 121, C) [*figs. 4* and *5*].

My above-mentioned work on the *Regeneration of Nerves* had as its essential aim [the purpose] of attaining objective proof that the new fibers appearing in the *peripheral stump* of a cut nerve unquestionably represent axon sprouts of the *central stump*. By contrast, we neglected somewhat the examination of the initial events of regeneration itself (behavior of the

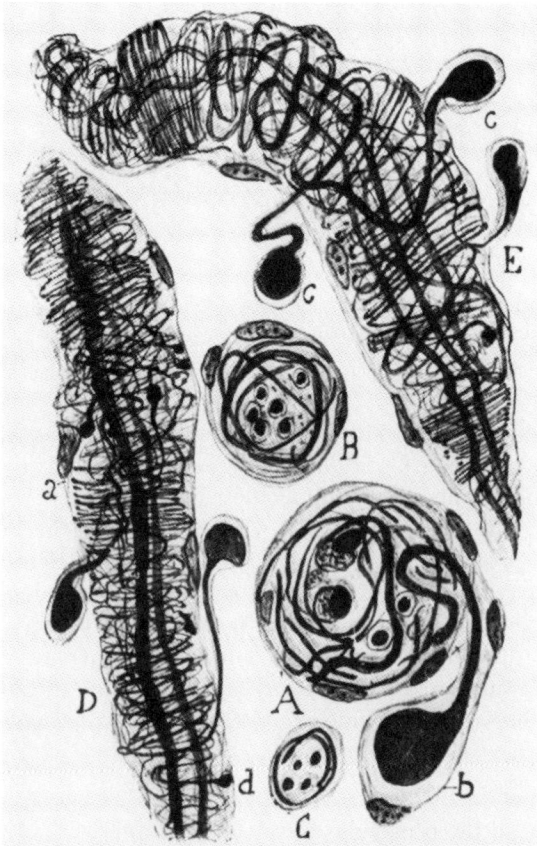

[*FIG. 4*] Fig. 120. Curious tangles of regenerated fibers created near the central stump or within it, on account of the obstacles that the sprouts encounter by ending in the scar. Many of these follow retrograde trajectories, tracing innumerable spirals. Some, finally, break the old membrane of Schwann, showing a thick terminal bouton [which] reveals the long [duration of the] obstruction (*c, d, b*).

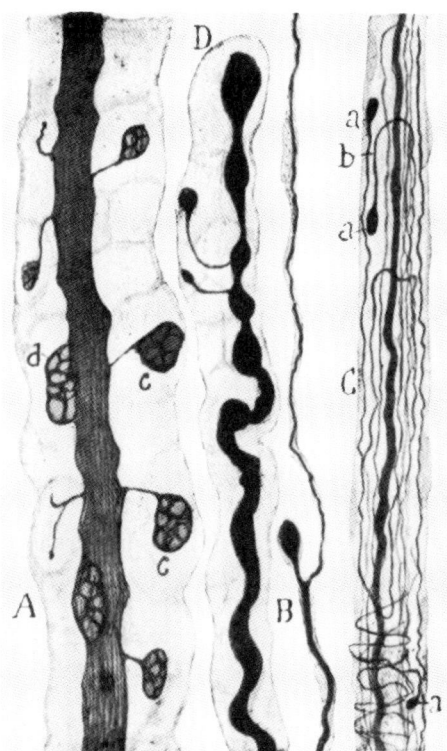

[*FIG. 5*] Fig. 121. Phenomena of aborted sprouting of the axons of the central stump. Cat [rabbit in *Degeneration and Regeneration of the Nervous System*—Eds.] of several weeks, seven [twenty-seven in *Degeneration and Regeneration of the Nervous System*—Eds.] days after the operation. *A*, tube with aborted buds; *B*, varicose axon with terminal ball; *C*, tube inside which the sprouts have produced bundles and complicated tangles.

axons of the central stump during the first two days), [which is] a subject well illustrated, as we said, by Perroncito. A certain communication published in 1907 (4) was directed at repairing this shortcoming. In it, in addition to confirming some interesting facts indicated by the young disciple of Golgi, we revealed:*

1. That the first sprouts of the central stump sprout preferentially at the level of the axonal thickenings adjacent to the *junctional disc*[†] (medullated axons).

---

*These four statements were not translated by Craigie.
[†] At the node of Ranvier.

2. That the axons of the peripheral stump do not die instantly when they are suddenly cut off from their trophic centers, rather, they pass, especially in the vicinity of the scar, through a certain agonal process, during which they attempt to form growth clubs, boutons, and ramifications, [which are] ephemeral and frustrated productions because they are not influenced by the lifegiving ferments emanating from the trophic center (the neuron with its nucleus).

3. That when the axon dies suddenly as in crushing or other traumatic injuries, the necrotic protoplasm, with a pale and granular appearance, is frequently invaded by isolated fibers of recent formation, which end by means of rings, handles, and other [structures] (see in fig. 123, *a, c, d*) [*fig. 7*], the curious intraaxonal sproutings of the neurofibrils engendered in the living portion of the axon). Such phenomena take place also in the peripheral stumps of the cut nerves (fig. 122, *a*) [*fig. 6*].

4. Finally, that these and other vegetative acts of isolated neurofibrils, as well as the above-mentioned phenomena of metamorphosis of the neurofibrillar skeleton of the neuronal soma (rabies, action of cold, etc), imply that the threads of the axon [that are] stainable with silver are composed of infinitesimal living entities, the *neurobiones;* [these are] capable of growing and multiplying with relative autonomy in the bosom of the neuroplasm, and capable of being arranged, depending on the circumstances, in intraaxonal colonies of variable architecture. The hypothesis of the *neurobiones,* which explained many structural changes in neurons, was received with interest by the authors.

Because of these works, a good number of authors returned to neuronism. Among the repentant we remember Dorhn, Levi, Marinesco, and Van Gehuchten. Then followed the confirmatory works of Guido Sala, Nageotte, Minea, Lugaro, Dustin, Sala and Cortese, Modena, and especially of Tello, to whom we owe a brilliant study on the *regeneration of the motor end plates* and sensory terminations (5). Nor should be forgotten those [authors] who, using other methods, supported monogenetism: Krassin, Mott and Halliburton, Stewart, Poscharisky, Edmont, Stuart, etc. Opinion reacted, finally, vigorously in favor of the classic doctrine of *continuous development or monogenesis.*

Even Albrecht Bethe, the champion battler of catenarism, who in his rejoinders was not exempt from vigor and acrimony, especially in a certain polemical work that appeared in 1907, showed himself to be quite conciliatory, since he did not deny outright the regenerative capacity of the fibers of the central stump nor the arrival of their sprouts at the frontier of the peripheral stump; he limited himself to defending the necessity for coopera-

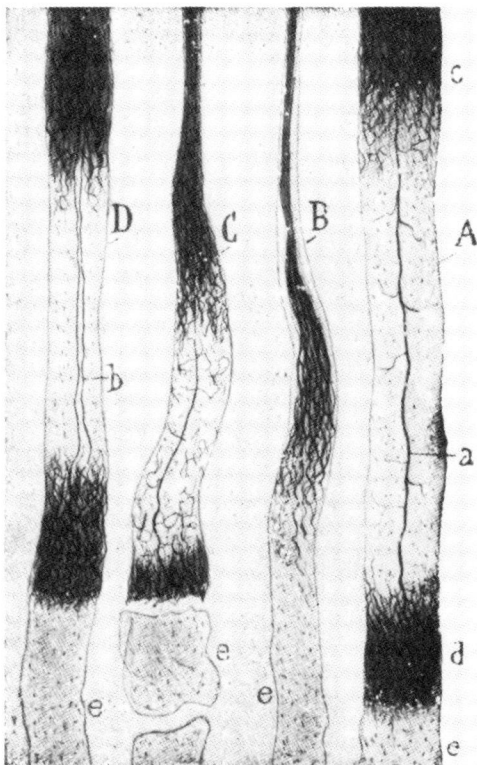

[*FIG. 6*] Fig. 122. Axons of the peripheral stump of a cut nerve. Note in the zone near the wound phenomena of survival and regeneration of the neurofibrils (*C, D*). (Cat, forty-eight hours [after] the operation.)

tion of the *cells of Schwann* of the latter segment in making nervous restoration effective. Sometime later, perhaps influenced by the irrefutable arguments provided by Perroncito, Lugaro, Marinesco, and us, the unhorsed physiologist of Strasbourg decided to abandon the field (6). *Victis honos!*

Let us add still that authorities as prestigious as Retzius, v. Lenhossék, Schiefferdecker, Edinger, Heidenhain, Verworn, Harrison, etc., who were witnesses at a distance, although with interested attention, of the incidents of the debate, adopted explicitly or implicitly in their writings the monogenetic doctrine or doctrine of continuity.

Needless to say the maltreated *neuron theory* passed the test strengthened and supreme. Far from finding, as its adversaries had anticipated, insuperable difficulties in the area of nerve regeneration, it found, to the contrary, new arguments in the light of which not a few enigmatic phenom-

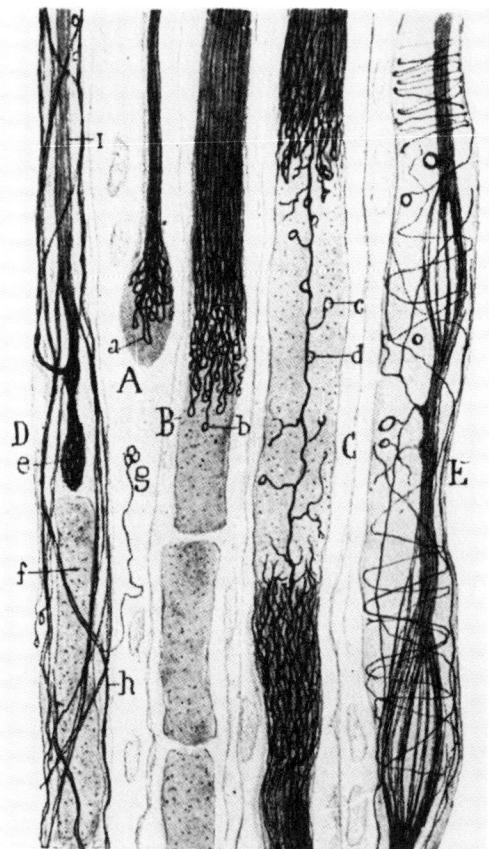

[*FIG. 7*] Fig. 123. Phenomena of intraaxonal sprouting of neurofibrils in axons mortified by compression with forceps (*a, b, d, c*). *D*, central portion of an axon from which emanate sprouts. (Fifty-two hours [after] the operation in a cat.)

ena of the structure and vegetative mechanisms of nerve protoplasm received unexpected elucidation.*

I yearned for testing the new formula [of reduced silver nitrate] in the analysis of the *degeneration and regeneration of the central pathways,* a subject about which an infinity of monographs had been published (Eichorst, Stroebe, Schiefferdecker, Kahler, Homén, Lowenthal, Ziegler, Coën, Barbacci, Lugaro, Nageotte, etc.).

Although with some differences of opinion, virtually all authors agreed

---

* At this point the text continues with Cajal's studies on neurogenesis, published in 1906. We continue the translation on page 473.

that regeneration of the *white matter* of the spinal cord, cerebrum, cerebellum, etc., is impossible, perhaps on account of the absence of the orienting elements or *cells of Schwann*. My observations, made on the *optic nerve and spinal cord*, confirmed at first the preceding conclusion; but demonstrated also that irregenerability is not an irrevocable and unavoidable law, but a secondary consequence of the unfavorable [nature of the] chemical millieu to the growth of sprouts. In the central stumps of the cut axons, *clubs and boutons of growth* are produced that penetrate into the scar; from these cones, prolixly subdivided secondary projections sometimes arise. However for unknown reasons, days after the lesion, the newly formed axonal sprouts wither without crossing the scar, and end up by being reabsorbed.

[The text continues with an account of a series of works published in 1907; one involves exploration of regeneration and degeneration in the fibers of the cerebrum and cerebellum (7) in which Cajal mentions "discovery of the so-called *ball of retraction* in the central stump of the axon and other curious phenomena"; finally, there is an account of two articles of a polemical character published in the *Anatomischer Anzeiger*. According to Cajal: "The former (8) constitutes an ardent and reasoned argument in favor of the neuron doctrine of His and Forel, being supported by an impressive array of concordant proofs deduced from the process of neurogenesis and from the mechanism of regeneration of the nerves." The second (9) is a response to perceived criticisms of Held regarding the development of neuroblasts and differentiation of neurofibrils.]

Cajal's Notes

1. Even in Spain this bitter fight between neuronists and antineuronists had repercussions. Two [friendly] provincial professors, no doubt, having heard of it from some French *Journal*, pealed the bells, declaring with ill concealed rejoicing that the neuron theory had gone down to history. And there was even another *dear* comrade who, protecting himself under the cloak of anonymity, took the liberty of addressing some coarsely insulting postcards to me. They thought innocently that with the fall of the neuron doctrine my modest scientific work would be definitively discredited. If the aforesaid professors would have taken the trouble to read me, they would have known that the neuron theory was created by His and Forel; from my harvest of facts I only contributed the demonstration of its authenticity. The impartial study of my books and numerous neurological monographs would also have shown them that if I were capable of feeling the fatuous pride of the inventor, I would proclaim not that I had forged such-and-such an hypothesis, but that I had discovered hundreds of facts [that had been] universally confirmed. And these facts, in spite of the fervent *patriotism* of my Spanish detractors, will last, so long as no

radical change occurs in the intimate organization of man and animals (and that will be rather difficult). [This footnote does not appear in the 1923 edition.]

2. An extensive account of our observations, illustrated with a profusion of figures, was published, under the title of Mecanismo de la degeneración y regeneración de los nervios, in *Trab Lab Invest Biol*, vol. 4, 1905. In the form of a summary these works appeared also in the *Boletín del Instituto de Alfonso XIII*, nos. 2 and 3, 1905. Finally, another complementary communication closes our investigation on the subject, namely: Les métamorphoses précoces des neurofibrilles dans la régénération et la dégénération des nerfs, *Trav Lab Rech Biol*, vol. 5, no. 2, 1907.

Let us also add that from the above mentioned studies, a German translation in the form of a book also emerged [Cajal, 1908 c] and, finally, our speech on being admitted to the Academy of Medicine of Madrid also dealt with the subject of the *Regeneration of the Nerves*. This speech, [which] was read on 30 June 1907 [Cajal 1907 e], was honored and lauded in a very beautiful speech of response by Don Federico Olóriz, the illustrious anatomist of San Carlos [Faculty of Medicine of Madrid].

3. A. Perroncito, Sulla questione della rigenerazione autogena della fibre nervose. Preliminary note. *Boll. Soc. Med-Chir*, Pavia, Seduta 19, Maggio, 1905 published in September of 1905. An extensive work with illustrations appeared in 1906, from which a translation was published in *Beitr Path Anat Allg Path*, vol. 62, 1907.

4. Cajal, Les métamorphoses précoces des neurofibrilles, etc., *Trav Lab Rech Biol* vol. 5, 1907.

5. F. Tello, Dégénération et régénération des plaques motrices après la section des nerfs, *Trav Lab Rech Biol, Univ Madrid*, vol. 5, 1907; F. Tello, La régénération dans les fuseaux de Kühne, *Trav Lab Rech Biol*, vol. 5, pt. 6, 1907.

6. He announced it to me several years later, not without a touch of melancholy, when he kindly acknowledged receipt of my two volume work, *Degeneración y regeneración del sistema nervioso*. [In the 1923 edition Cajal adds: "Recently, he affirms, with a nobility of character which does him honor, that in the majority of cases at least, the fibers of the peripheral stump come from the central [stump]" (see *Libro en honor de Santiago Ramón y Cajal*, 1923)].

7. Cajal, Note sur la dégénérescence traumatique des fibres nerveuses du cervelet et du cerveau. With 4 plates. *Trav Lab Rech Biol*, vol. 5, 1907.

8. Cajal, Die histogenetischen Beweisse der Neurontheorie von His und Forel. With 24 figures. *Anat Anz*, vol. 30, 1907.

9. Cajal, Nouvelles observationes sur l'évolution des neuroblastes avec quelques remarques sur l'hypòthese neurogénétique de Hensen-Held. With 16 plates. *Trav Lab Rech Biol*, vol. 5, 1907, and *Anat Anz*, vol. 37, 1908.

CHAPTER 4

From: *Recuerdos de mi vida*. Volume 2,
Historia de mi labor científica,
Chapter 21, pages 516–546

S. RAMÓN Y CAJAL
Madrid: N. Moya, 1917

[The chapter is entitled: *A brief account of the work carried out in the decade* (1907–1917). Studies on the comparative anatomy of the *cerebellum, medulla oblongata,* and origins of the *motor and sensory nerves* of fish, birds and mammals. Structure of the nucleus. Survival of neurons outside the organism. New investigations on *degeneration and regeneration* in the spinal cord, cerebrum and cerebellum. Experiments on the transplantation of nerves. Facts favorable to the neurotropic theory. Production of artificial nerves in transplanted ganglia.]

The investigations undertaken during the triennium 1910–1912 were quite diverse being dispersed over many and varied topics. We may cite: the *structure of the nucleus*, the *autolysis and survival of neurons*, the problem of *neurotropism*, the *transplantation of nerves and ganglia*, the technique of *staining the platelets of the blood*, methodological communications on the *demonstration of the endocellular apparatus of Golgi and of the neuroglia in the human, structure of the cerebellum*, etc. But the general subject to which I devoted years of persistent work and on which I collected data of greater value and superior theoretical importance, was that concerning the *degeneration and regeneration of the neurons and axons of the ganglia, cerebellum, cerebrum, and spinal cord*. As we will see later, the latter studies, which draw back a little the veil of the intimate physiology of the neurofibrillar reticulum, served to corroborate the old neurotropic hypothesis formulated by me in 1892 and received kindly by numerous authors.

At the foot of these pages we will give successively a list of the principal above-mentioned works. Here we shall expound, in chronological order, the most valuable objective conquests or theoretical deductions. [Here follows a description in outline of the various studies conducted by Cajal on the structure of the nucleus of nerve cells and on neuronal autolysis.]

4. The harvest of acquisitions in the field of the *degeneration and regeneration of the spinal cord* (1) was very copious and highly interesting. Some of the facts of which we are going to give a brief account represent, as we [have already] pointed out, arguments of inestimable value on behalf of the neurotropic doctrine. They prove that the creation of sprouts and their orientation through the different tissues, are conditioned by the liberation around the fibers and cells, of ferments which activate assimilation. These catalytic agents (*neurotropic substances*) are made by the embryonic *connective tissue;* but very especially by the *cells of Schwann* of the ordinary nerve [fibers] during the process of regeneration.

Under normal conditions, the above-mentioned attractants are lacking in the [central nervous system], so that regeneration of the fibers of the interrupted white matter is aborted. As soon as favorable experimental circumstances concur, however, the regenerative tendency, [which is] latent in the fibers of the [central nervous system] is aroused and develops extraordinary strength.

In the spinal cord such favorable conditions are often established, following the simultaneous section of the white matter and sensory and motor roots. The degeneration of the cells of Schwann initiates the liberation of neurotropic substances that diffuse into the territory of the spinal fasciculi and the axons, once sluggish and inert, actively grow; it is not rare to see them invading the interior of the roots and advancing through them over long distances. [This paradoxical invasion of the anterior roots by the fibers of the fasciculi when overexcited by trauma appears in figure 145 [*fig. 11*]. It is frequently observed that the fiber attracted by something that has diffused from the roots represents a newly formed collateral. By virtue of this unusual fact, the cord axons are provisionally transformed into motor axons.]* The same occurs in the cerebrum. If, as shown by Tello (2) in his brilliant experiments, a segment of a degenerated nerve is introduced into a cerebral wound, the axons belonging to the pyramids, [which are] the [fibers] most apathetic and resistant to any regenerative process, shake off their sluggishness, become turgid with activity and give off very long sprouts, which assail the nerve implant with the same

---

*Text in brackets was added to the 1923 edition of the *Recuerdos.*

aggressiveness and strength of growth that is characteristic of the sprouting of the interrupted sciatic nerve.

On a smaller scale, the connective tissue cells of scars also possess the capability of elaborating neurotropic materials during the initial phases (figs. 142 and 144, *B*) [*figs. 8* and *10*].

Such facts, which are of great biological importance, definitely refute the generally accepted dogma of the *essential irregenerability of the central pathways*.* Such a great productive incapacity constitutes a contingent and adventitious property, masked as we have said,

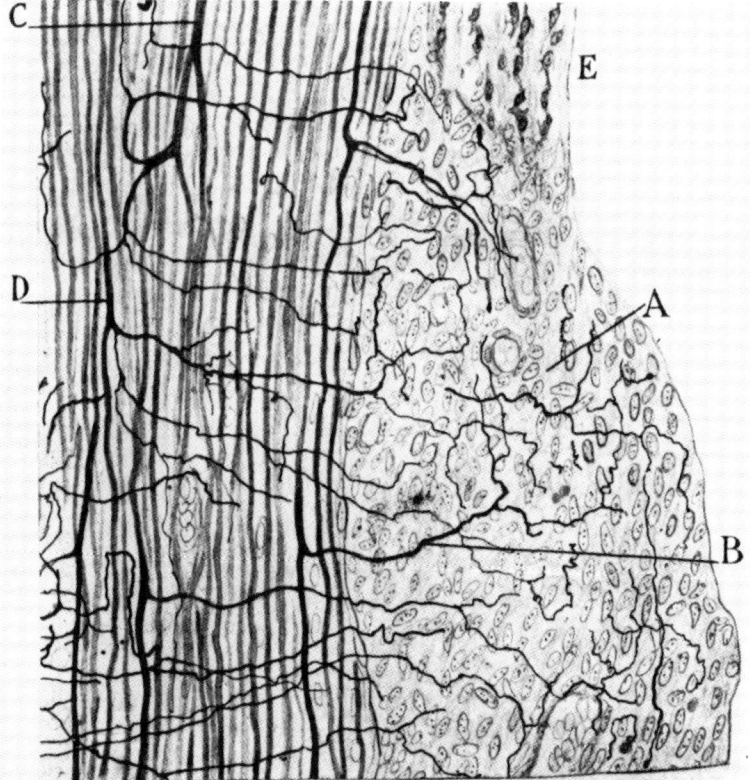

[*FIG. 8*] Fig. 142. Piece of the posterior column of the spinal cord of a young cat whose meninges suffered trauma followed by exuberant scar formation. *A*, embryonic scar; *B*, sprout that has penetrated it; *D*, longitudinal fibers of the white matter in the phase of productive irritation.

---

*The last sentence of this paragraph and the following text up to number 7 of the outline were omitted by Craigie in his English translation of the 1923 edition. Craigie reproduced no figures from this part of the *Recuerdos*.

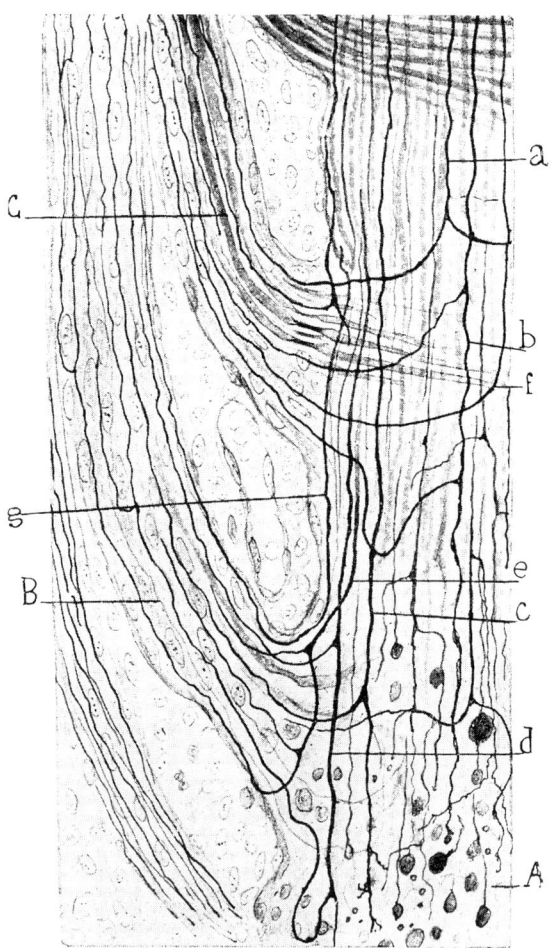

[*FIG. 9*] Fig. 143. Longitudinal section of the anterolateral [fasciculus of the] spinal cord of a cat of a few days, in which the lumbar cord was cut. *A*, border of the scar of the anterolateral cord; *B*, *C*, anterior roots, degenerated and invaded by newly formed cord branches; *a*, *b*, funicular fibers which gave off branches to the motor roots.

by the irremediable absence, inside the white and gray matter, of secretory sources of catalytic agents or orienting materials (3).

Among the proofs of such an important doctrine, the following, which are singularly expressive, have been extracted from my works on the *degeneration and regeneration of the spinal cord and nerve roots.*

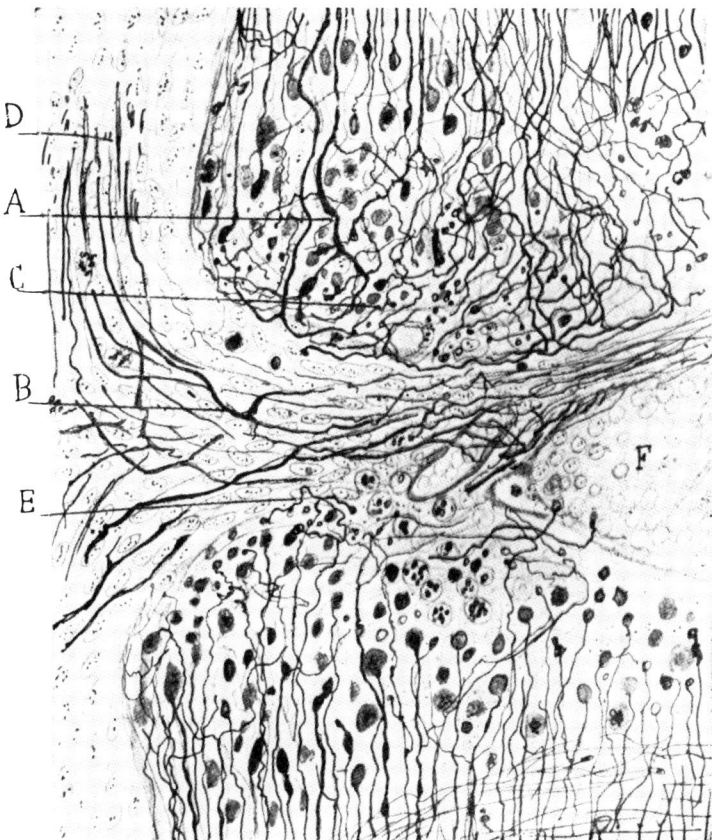

[*FIG. 10*] Fig. 144. Tranverse wound of the spinal cord. *A*, superior stump with sprouting fibers; *B*, scar invaded by sensory fibers of the posterior roots; *E*, central cyst of the wound.

a. When, in the course of manual labor, the *pia mater* is accidentally injured and a certain perispinal mass of scar tissue is created, on many occasions collateral sprouts are observed arising from [fibers] of the posterior cord, and even true terminal fibers, which emerge from the spinal territory and ramify prolixly in the bosom of the connective tissue. So, the latter is shown to be capable of arousing to some extent, the regenerative capacity of the axons and of attracting growth cones (fig. 142, *B*) [*fig. 8*].

b. When the Schwann cells of the nerve roots degenerate following a wound of the spinal cord and roots, or by propagation into the latter of traumatic spinal inflammation, the Schwann cells induce the

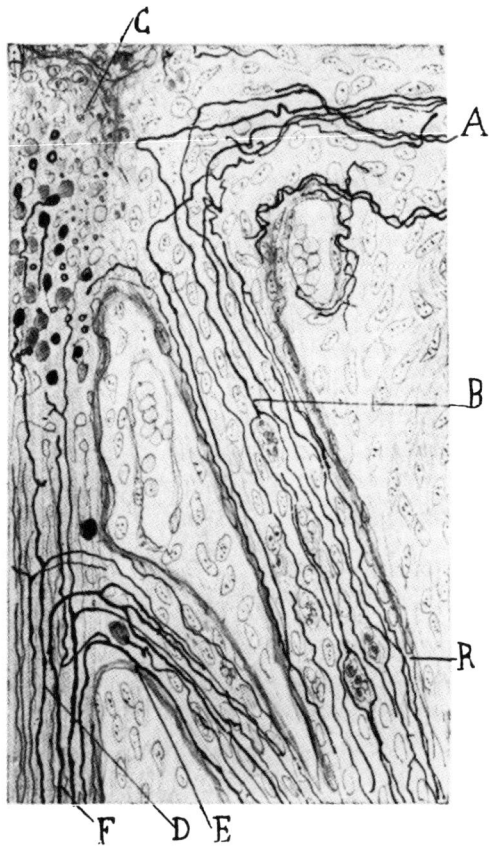

[FIG. 11] Fig. 145. Longitudinal section of the anterior roots of a cat in which a spinal wound was produced. A, sensory fibers of the scar invading a degenerated anterior root; B, invading fibers ramifying at the level of a fatty conglomeration; C, necrosed portion of the anterior cord in the neighborhood of the wound.

formation of sprouts in the white matter and exert a violent attraction on the sprouts towards the cells.

In figure 143, e, c [fig. 9], which reproduces a longitudinal section of the anterior cord, it can be seen how the funicular axons near the spinal wound, influenced by the inducements arriving from the degenerated anterior roots, emit branches that, after vigorous growth, penetrate into the roots, traveling [among] the cells of Schwann, or along their gaps, [the branches having been] converted into aberrant motor conductors (B, C).

Also instructive is the case reproduced in figure 145, A [fig. 11] in which one sees lost in the scar several recently formed axons (probably derived from the peripheral stump of a sectioned sensory root) inappropriately penetrating into a degenerated motor root (which is traveling in a centrifugal direction). [The new axons are] irreversibly attracted by the neurotropic substances elaborated by the cells of Schwann. The same occurs if the cut and degenerated roots are the posterior or sensory.

5. Not all of the deviated dorsal column fibers or sprouts arising from the lesioned motor and sensory roots (central stump, that is to say, the portion of the axon joined to the cell of origin) respond to neurotropic processes. Also having an influence on the dislocations of the sprouts are the absence of obstacles in a certain direction (the direction of least resistance) and a certain capacity for eruptive outgrowth gained by the newly formed fibers after they have been nourished for some time, or when they have been born in a field crammed with neurotropic substances.

a. For example, as we show in figure 146, *B, G* [*fig. 12*], exuberant sprouts, arising as collaterals of the lesioned motor roots, retrogradely invade the spinal cord to become aberrant funicular fibers. Their eventual collision with insurmountable obstacles sometimes bends the course of the sprouts during their intraspinal trajectory, leading to their division into ascending and descending branches (fig. 146, *A*) [*fig. 12*].

b. This kind of mechanical phenomenon explains, no doubt, the [example] shown in figure 147, *A, B* [*fig. 13*], which reproduces several degenerated sensory roots together with a completely necrosed segment of the posterior funiculus. Notice how the sprouts arising from the peripheral stump of the said roots (ganglionic side) penetrate into the spinal cord by virtue of their initial impulse (*vis a tergo*) and organize like a rudimentary posterior funiculus. The letters *K, H,* etc., indicate growth cones each advancing as a battering ram along the roots and through the interior of the posterior funiculus.

6. My studies on traumatized [central neural structures] (spinal cord, cerebrum, and cerebellum) revealed also the existence of notable *phenomena of compensation* or, if one prefers, of morphological adaptation of the neurons to the artificial physiological conditions promoted by the mutilation. When an axonal fragment is amputated from a nerve cell the [neuron] does not necessarily die, just as an individual deprived of a limb does not succumb; rather, it tries to get the best advantage from the new situation, eliminating the useless segment of the [fiber] (a kind of blind alley) and maintaining and reinforcing the collaterals, the last of which is converted into a terminal branch.

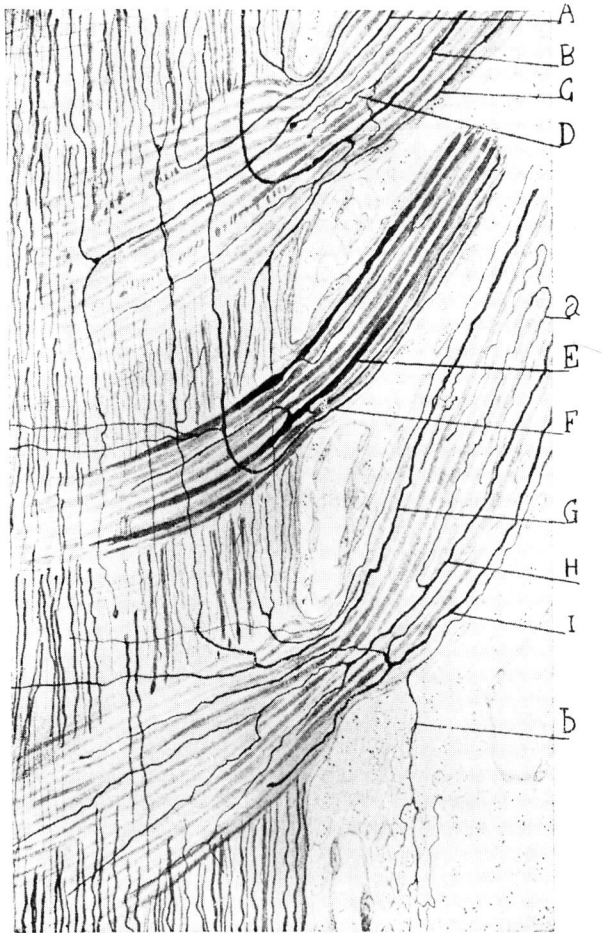

[*FIG. 12*] Fig. 146. Invasion of the spinal cord by retrograde motor collaterals originating from the extraspinal course of the anterior roots. Cat of a few days, sacrificed four days after section of the spinal cord. *A, B, C, D*, recurrent motor branches that invade the spinal cord; *E*, almost normal axon from which emanated two collaterals; *F*, branch that becomes longitudinal; *H, I*, invading branches several times divided.

Here are some instructive examples of such an interesting phenomenon, illustrated by semischematic drawings:

a. After the fibers of the spinal white matter are sectioned and in the absence of the *neurocladic* catalysts, the portion of the axon situated beyond the last collateral atrophies and reabsorbs, after

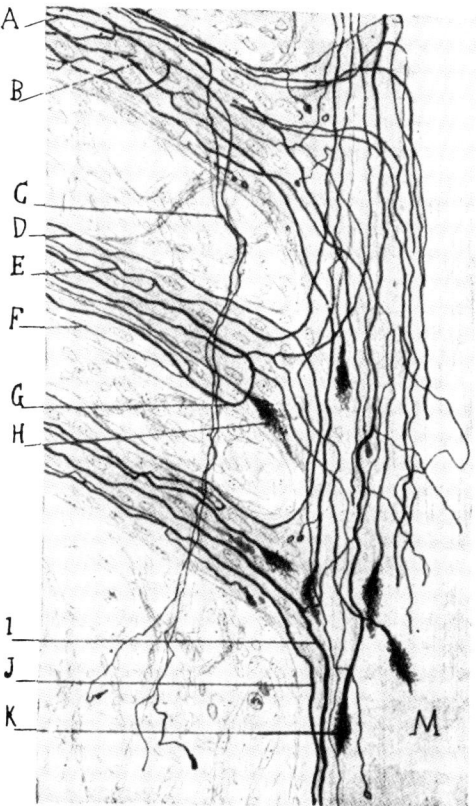

[FIG. 13] Fig. 147. Piece of the posterior cord and regenerated roots in a dog of a few days, the [lower part] of whose [cord] was lesioned in several parts. A, sensory roots; C, deviated sensory fibers; D, penetrating fiber which leaves the spinal cord; H, terminal club; E, fiber which gives off recurrent branches.

forming a retraction club (fig. 148, b, d) [*fig. 14*]. Note in figure 148, A [*fig. 14*] how said collateral hypertrophies becoming transformed into a terminal branch, perhaps because now it alone absorbs all the energy of the [impulse] previously dissipated by the expanded arborization.

b. Still more surprising cases of the cited morphological adaptation are found in the traumatized cerebellum and cerebrum, according to what we communicated in several extensive monographs (4). Because of this singular *modus vivendi*, it is possible to *transform experimentally a cell with long axon into a cell with short axon*. [Here is another fact which will seem paradoxical to [those researchers] who suppose that the architecture of the nervous centers

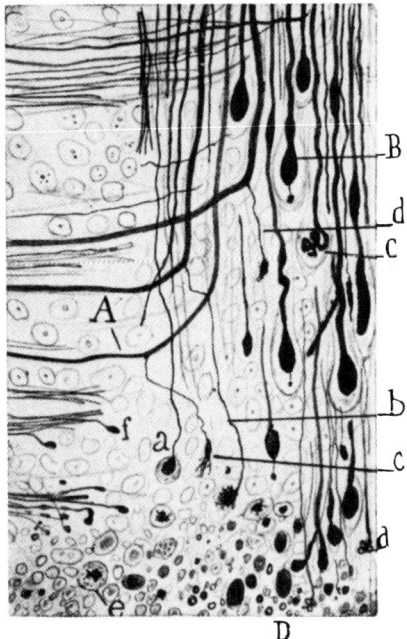

[*FIG. 14*] Fig. 148. Piece of the central stump of the spinal wound of a young cat, three days after the operation. A, thickened collaterals which will be transformed into terminals; a, b, c, longitudinal portions of the axons destined to disappear; B, retraction clubs.

is immutable and preestablished even in its smallest details.]* Let the following two examples suffice:

In figure 149, E, [D]† [*fig. 15*] from the cerebellum, we show how, thanks to the disappearance of the peripheral portion of the Purkinje cell axon, the nerve arborization is reduced to one or two notably hypertrophic initial collaterals. Henceforth, then, the cerebellar neuron cannot maintain [functional] commerce except with neighboring Purkinje cells with whose dendritic shafts the referred branches enter into contact (5).

Figure 150, A, D, C [*fig. 16*] shows the same metamorphic phenomenon in relation to the *cerebral pyramids*, whose axons were interrupted near the white matter. Notice how some [axon] collaterals close to the wound have been reabsorbed, no doubt attacked by traumatic degeneration; however, the undamaged [axon collaterals],

---

* Added to the 1923 edition.
† The original text incorrectly says G.

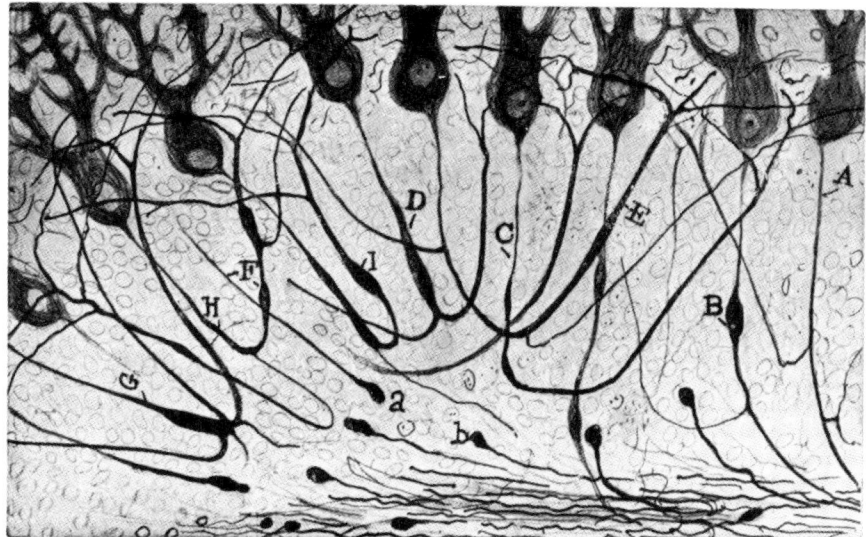

[*FIG. 15*] Fig. 149. Principal types of Purkinje axons of the cerebellum of a cat of twenty days, two days after trauma. This zone is found near the scar and the axons are drawn from two consecutive sections from the same region. *A*, normal axon; *B*, axon with varicosity; *C, D, E*, [*I*], axons of arciform type; [*a, b*] terminal club.

arising from the initial portion of the axon, have maintained their vitality, becoming notably hypertrophic and adapting an arciform configuration (*f*). The inititial phases of the adaptative process are shown in the cells *A* and *B*, where an axonal segment (*a, b*) in the process of atrophy still exists.

When the lesion affects the part of the axon from which the initial collaterals arise, these completely disappear and the axon exhibits a pointed stump (fig. 150, *e*) [*fig. 16*], which we named the *point of corrosion*. These neurons, severely mutilated, quickly degenerate and die.

The preceding facts reveal that the morphology of the nerve cell *does not obey an immanent and fatal tendency, maintained by heredity, as certain authors have defended, but it depends entirely on the physical and chemical circumstances present in the environment.**

7. From the point of view of *regeneration*, the cerebrum and cerebellum are incomparably less active than the ganglia and spinal

---

*Craigie's translation includes this paragraph but omits all the following pages up to the final three paragraphs of the chapter.

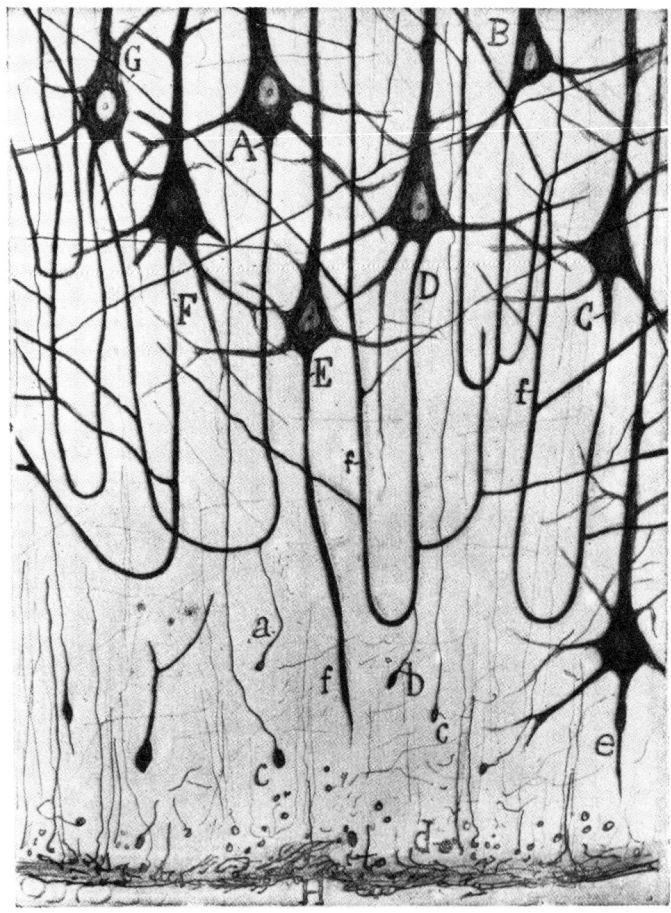

[FIG. 16] Fig. 150. Section of the motor cerebrum of a cat of twenty-five days, sacrificed twenty-four hours after the operation. A, D, medium pyramids with hypertrophic arciform collaterals and fine and atrophic axonal stumps (a, b); C, F, G, arciform pyramids whose peripheral axonal segment has disappeared; B, pyramid whose axon resolves itself into two recurrent arcs; H, wound.

cord. No histologist had been able to demonstrate with absolute certainty the reality of regenerative phenomena in the white matter of the former centers. For our part, by dint only of persistent explorations were we able, finally, to discover unquestionably active production of new fibers, although ephemeral and, therefore, frustrated. Such vicarious sprouting is exclusively observed in young animals (cat and dog of ten to twenty days) and at the levels of the varicosities along the trajectories and at the terminal clubs of the axons interrupted inside the white matter (central stumps). Two main varieties are presented:

a. From a thick, terminal (*retraction ball*) or en passant varicosity arise several fine and pale radiations that get lost in the neighboring territories where they ramify and end in a pale tip. Because it evokes the shape of the tortoise, I named such a singular disposition the *testudinoid apparatus* (fig. 151, E, F, H) [*fig. 17*].

b. At the frontiers of a necrosed axon segment, the surviving neurofibrils of the neighboring varicosity enter into active proliferation, generating certain tufts of small branches that invade the dead protoplasm (fig. 152, a) [*fig. 18*], where they end by means of boutons or rings. Because of its shape which somewhat recalls that of the *cuttlefish*, I baptized such an unusual disposition with the name of *cephalopodic apparatus*.

Figures 151 and 152 [*figs. 17* and *18*] excuse us from going into more details about these failed neoformations.

Fortuitous acts of incipient regeneration are very rare in the *cerebellum*. In spite of this, by dint of persistent experiments involving traumatic irritation of the Purkinje cells, and by choosing for this

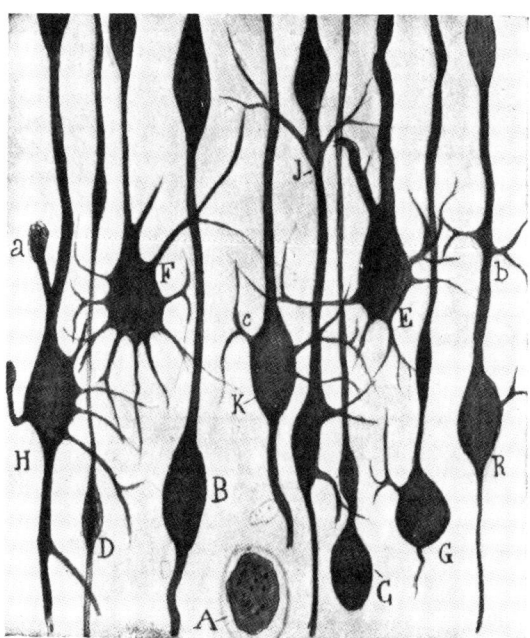

[*FIG. 17*] Fig. 151. Cerebrum of dog. Sprouts sprung from the varicosities of the central stump of the cerebral pyramids.

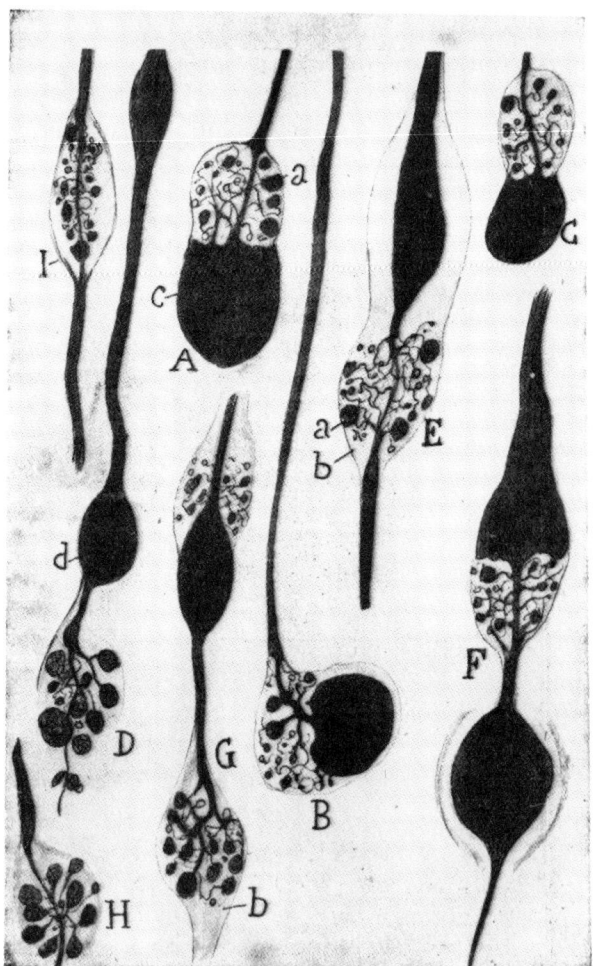

[*FIG. 18*] Fig. 152. Cerebrum of dog. Axons of the central stump with necrosed segments (*b*), into which penetrate *bouquets* of sprouting neurofibrils (*a*).

purpose mammals a few days old (cat and dog), I was able to perceive in these cells indubitable signs of sprouting. Let me indicate, among other dispositions of a failed neoformative nature, these two:

a. Transformation (with creation of abortive branches) of the [dendrites] of the Purkinje cells into an elegant *bouquet*, composed of fine pedicles crowned with reticulated boutons (fig. 153, *c*) [*fig. 19*]. In order to distinguish it from others, we call this singular modification *rosaliform metamorphosis*.

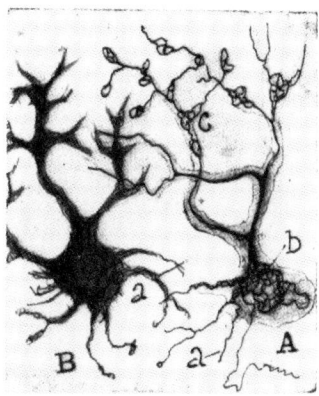

[*FIG. 19*] Fig. 153. Cerebellum of a cat of few days. Cells of Purkinje, excited by the trauma, from whose somata arise descending buds (*a*).

b. Emission, at the level of the soma, of thin, lateral or descending appendages ending at a short distance (fig. 153, *a*) [*fig. 19*] by means of a ring, clot, or varicosity. Certain [appendages] seem to contain a single neurofibril.

8. With regard to the *degenerative process of the fibers and cells of the cerebrum and cerebellum*, caused either by sectioning, or contusion, or by introduction of foreign bodies, the harvest of morphological dispositions collected was so copious and varied that it surpassed all my expectations. To relate all of them, even concisely, would require many pages. In order to avoid torturing the reader too much with interminable lists of descriptive paraphernalia, I will restrict myself to expounding certain outstanding data:

a. Corroborating and extending results, already indicated in 1907 (6), we demonstrated that every cerebral or cerebellar axon interrupted at a regular distance from the cell of origin, strongly reacts, forming at the level of its central segment or stump, a *terminal ball* or *club*, preceded by other spheres or varicosities extending like [the beads of] a rosary back to the last initial collateral (fig. 154) [*fig. 20*]. Almost all of these balls detach from the axon during the days following the lesion, successively becoming atrophied in the bosom of the gray matter, where they form agonal neurofibrillar colonies. One or two weeks after the lesion, only the more proximal varicosity of the undamaged portion of the axon remains, taking the form of a terminal club or bouton. This is the *retraction ball*, that clearly marks in a preparation from the cerebrum or cerebellum the direction in which the neuron of origin is to be found. The preceding mutations of the

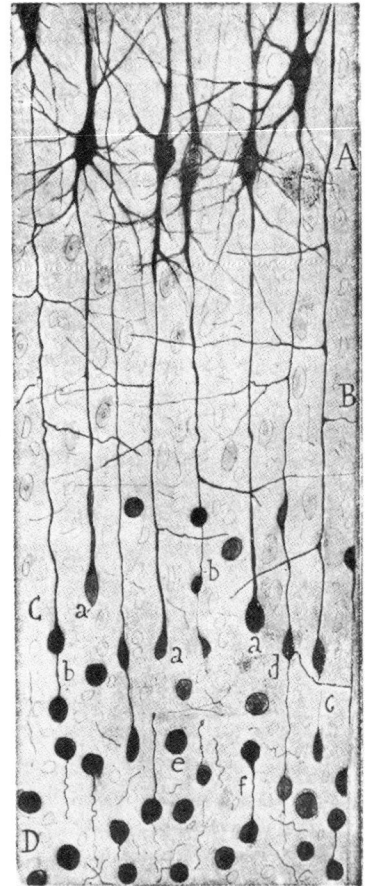

[FIG. 20] Fig. 154. Cerebral pyramids of a dog. Near the wound the interrupted axons (central stump) show rosaries of balls (B, C); D, free balls near the wound.

axon, together with the above-mentioned *autotomy* or act of elimination of the spheres, generically correspond to the process commonly designated by the authors *traumatic degeneration of the central stump* and [which] has been studied by means of inadequate techniques. In figure 156, B [*fig. 22*], we show several retraction clubs, belonging to Purkinje cells, eight days after the cut; and in figure 154 [*fig. 20*] we reproduce the process of beading and autotomy of the axons of the giant pyramids of the cerebrum.

b. The large balls detached by *autotomy* from robust axons, for a long time, maintain a central neurofibrillar [core] which in certain exceptional cases, demonstrated in figure 155, E, J, F [*fig. 21*], offer

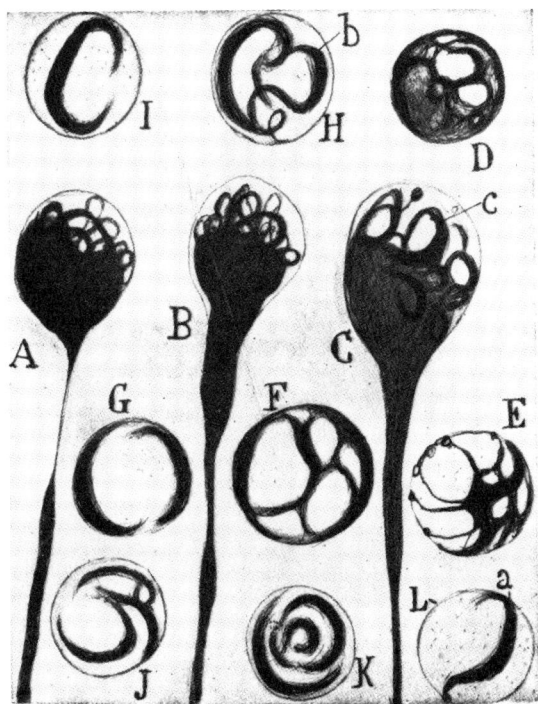

[*FIG. 21*] Fig. 155. Phenomena of neurofibrillar metamorphosis in the terminal clubs of cut cerebral axons (*A, B, C*) and in free balls (*G, F, E*). [The following is added to the 1923 edition: This demonstrates the temporary survival of the neurofibrils and of their constitutive granules.]

evident signs of survival and intraprotoplasmic sprouting. The cores are the *neurobiones,* that, before they die, make during their agony, frenzied efforts to reestablish the lost continuity with their sisters.

   c. My observations also revealed that the neurons which are exposed to compression, concussion, or trauma occurring in their vicinity, do not always suddenly succumb, victims of granular disintegration, but necrotize gradually, propagating the destructive process (7) from their superficial protoplasmic layers to the deeper ones. In figures 157, *A, E* and 158, *A, E* [*figs. 23* and *24*], we present patent examples of this gradual mortification of the cells of Purkinje of the cerebellum [and cerebral pyramids]. Notice in figure 160 *A, E* [*fig. 24*] from the contused cerebrum, a similar phenomenon of persistence of the perinuclear neurofibrils].* Observe how around the nucleus and

---

*Text in brackets was added to the 1923 edition. Note that fig. 160 of the 1923 edition corresponds to fig. 158 of the 1917 edition.

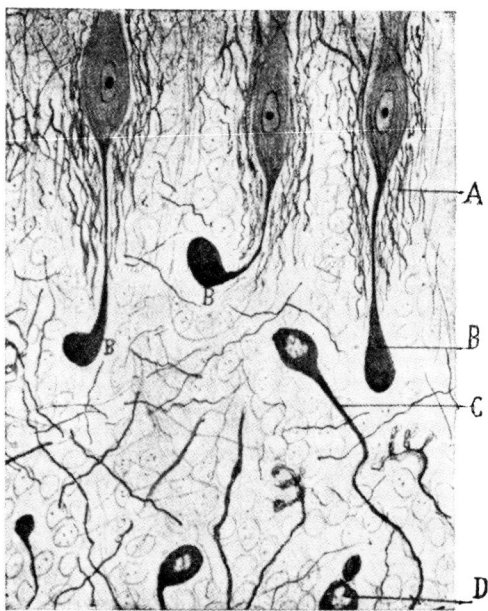

[*FIG. 22*] Fig. 156. Eight days after the lesion, the axons of the Purkinje cells (cerebellum of the adult rabbit) present *balls of retraction* (B). [This figure, unlike all the others used to illustrate the *Recuerdos,* is not in the present book.]

in the axis of the dendrites the protoplasmic framework tenaciously survives and, entering into formative excitation, its neurofibrils sometimes hypertrophy and acquire surprising and most varied configurations (fig. 157, *D, E*) [*fig. 23*].

d. Among the changed forms of the neurofibrillar framework lesioned by contusion and compression, there are often observed certain alterations, on the whole comparable to those characteristic of hibernating animals or of animals attacked by rabies (8). Many neurofibrils exhibit a *fusiform hypertrophy* while others completely disappear. The reader will find varied transitions between the mere hypertrophic process and the production of spindles in figure 158, *J, G* [*fig. 24*], which shows some cerebral pyramids taken from the vicinity of a wound complicated by the effects of severe contusion.

e. The above-mentioned works revealed likewise, a fact of certain heuristic interest (9), since it allows us to distinguish the dead axons from the *living*. I allude to the so-called *conserved fibers* (fig. 159, *d*) [*fig. 25*] [which are] segments of axons suddenly destroyed by the trauma, and apparently embalmed by the action of the exudate. They

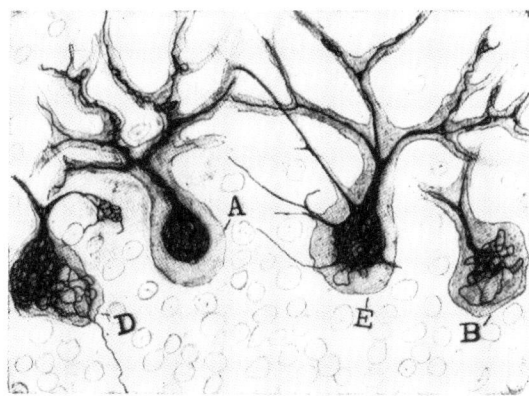

[*FIG. 23*] Fig. 157. Cells of Purkinje of the traumatized cerebellum. Notice at A, B, and E the presence of a damaged cortical zone with persistence of the perinuclear neurofibrils.

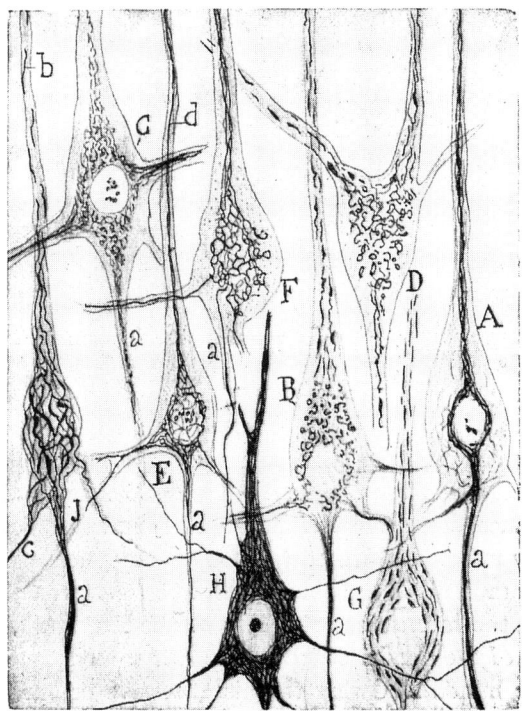

[*FIG. 24*] Fig. 158. Phenomena of neurofibrillar metamorphosis in the cerebral pyramids close to a contusion wound. A, persisting perinuclear neurofibrils; B, C, D, formation of handles and rings; J, neurofibrillar hypertrophy; G, fusiform state.

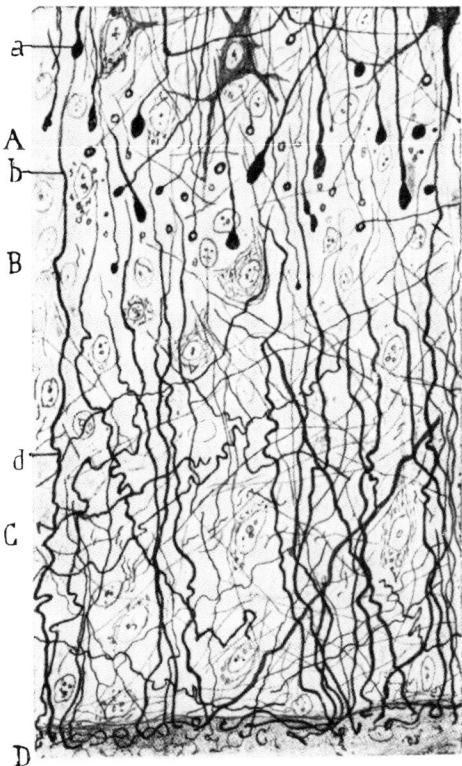

[*FIG. 25*] Fig. 159. Proximal border of a transverse wound of the cerebrum of a cat of one month, sacrificed twenty-one hours after the operation. *A*, living zone or zone of reaction; *B*, zone of corrosion; *C*, zone of preserved fibers; *D*, exudate of the wound; *a*, retraction club; *b*, tip of corrosion of a preserved fiber still joined to a healthy axon; *c*, floating tips of preserved fibers.

appear near the wounds, exhibiting all the attributes of normal axons, which they resemble because of their perfect stainability, cylindrical form, striated appearance, and lack of balls and varicosities. At first sight one mistakes them for living axons. They differ, however, in that they terminate at the border of the wound, and sometimes in the expanse of exudate by means of a hook (*c*) or in some spiral turns; they exhibit a more or less twisting trajectory, and finally, taper off towards the depth of the gray matter by means of a progressively pale *point of corrosion* (*b*).

In figure 159, *D* [*fig. 25*], we present the borders of a cerebral wound crossed by numerous *conserved fibers*. Notice how none of them shows a *retraction ball,* by contrast with the deeper situated living axons, all of which possess en passant varicosities and terminal clubs (*a*).

9. With regard to *pathological metamorphosis and the regenerative acts that occur in the sensory ganglia,* I published two works of investigation: one relating to *transplanted ganglia* (10) and another (in 1913) on the reactive phenomena that occur in [the ganglia] after the *avulsion* at a distance of the corresponding nerves [11].

Our studies on the fertile subject of *grafting of sensory ganglia,* confirmed, naturally, the very beautiful and important experiments of Nageotte concerning the metamorphosis of the [monopolar] neurons into multipolar neurons, the appearance of nervous nests, the cellular necrosis of the ganglionic center followed by the formation of *residual nodules,* etc., and added the following observations:

a. If instead of transplanting large ganglia [from young animals] under the skin of an adult animal, as Nageotte, Marinesco, Rossi, Dustin, etc., did (*homotransplantation*), very small ganglia (the terminal ones of the cauda equina) of newborn mammals are grafted under the skin of sibling animals (*homochronotransplantation*), the number of surviving nerve cells is much larger, even the inhabitants of the ganglionic center, surviving with their axons. Usually, in the experiments of Nageotte these processes appeared necrosed. Notice also, that the phenomena of creation and projection of new appendages acquire an unusual energy (fig. 159) [*fig. 25, bis*].*

b. As we note in figure 159, *A* [*fig. 25 bis*], the strength of growth and progression of the cited sprouts is such that they often penetrate the fibrous capsule of the grafted ganglion. Joined together in bundles, that are true small nerves, the sprouts cross the capsular barrier, lured without doubt by the neurotropic substances of the adjacent scarified tissue, and scatter in disorder in the connective tissue of the host, as though in search of their missing terminal territories (fig. 159, *D*) [*fig. 25, bis*].

c. In a similar manner are led the surviving axons of the ganglionic roots. Thanks to the smallness of the graft, almost all of them are kept alive and generate, mainly from the peripheral branch, aberrant small nerves that get lost in the neighboring territories of the host animal.

10. My experiments on *avulsion of the nerves* (11) external to and at a distance from the sensory ganglia, revealed a fact of some interest, namely: that it is possible to promote in the ganglionic neurons, by

---

*This is the second of two figures labeled 159 in the 1917 edition. The figure numbering is corrected in the 1923 edition.

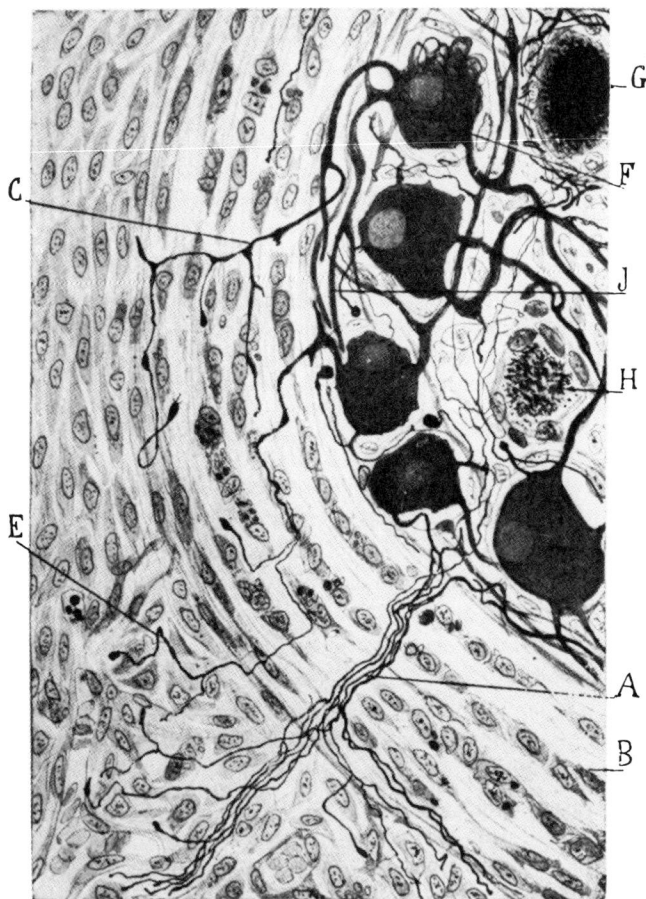

[*FIG. 25, bis*] Fig. 159. Piece of a transplanted small ganglion. *A*, nerve formation that crosses the ganglionic capsule (*B*) and invades the connective tissue of the host; *C*, *E*, newly formed branches that trace turns in the capsule; *G*, *H*, dead neurons; *F*, appendage directed to the interior of the ganglion.

simple concussion or mechancial vibration, all the curious phenomena of metamorphosis of the soma and production of sprouts observed by Nageotte in the grafted ganglia (creation of appendages, formation of pericellular *nests* and of tattered and lobulated cells, appearance of *residual nodules*, etc.).

When the avulsion affects the motor roots, at a distance from the spinal cord, there is promoted, among other effects already indicated by Sala and Cortese (who also worked with my technique), the formation of numerous sprouts, many of which, reversing direction in the interior of the root, penetrate the spinal cord, flooding the territory of the anterolateral cord with nerve branches.

Likewise, we revealed that wounds of the ganglia or the crushing of their roots give rise to active phenomena of sprouting in the sensory fibers and cells, with luxuriant formation of extraordinarily complicated nests.

11. Singularly expressive in favor of the *neurotropic theory*, were the results of my experiments on *transplantation and reimplantation of nerve trunks* (12) in the gap between the segments of the interrupted sciatic nerve. From these studies, at first confirmatory of those carried out by Lugaro, Marinesco, and Dustin, there follows an important conclusion: that the attractive tropic action of the cells of Schwann of the graft is closely bound up with the vitality of the same. Dead grafts (decomposed or altered by means of coagulant liquids, etc.) do not exert a neurotropic influence on the sprouts of the central stump of the cut sciatic nerve [see fig. 163 bis [*fig. 27*]];* thick and fresh grafts only attract the fibers towards their cortical or subneurilemmal layer, the territory where the cells of Schwann are maintained alive and active; finally, very thin and very fresh grafts, (reimplantation), whose [tissue] maintains entirely its physiological properties, are almost completely invaded by the sprouts circulating in the environment. In figure 160 [*fig. 26*], we reproduce the result of one of our experiments. Notice how the axons newly formed in the central stump of a sectioned nerve are concentrated at the proximal extremity of the graft (*e*), and traverse the full length of the graft to emerge, finally, on the opposite side and become insinuated into the peripheral stump of the sciatic [nerve] (*d*). Note, also the preference of the sprouts for the superficial layers of the grafted nerve, which are naturally the most vital and the most active, therefore, in the production of the attractive ferments. The axonal convergence, indicative of the exquisite sensitivity of the sprouts to the substances liberated by the graft, is a result singularly favorable for our neurotropic theory.†

12. In several studies on regeneration we had advanced the idea that the *giant balls,* observed at the free extremity of certain sprouts, were caused by the eventual obstruction or stoppage of the clubs; that the *withdrawals* were due to collision with insuperable obstacles and, finally, that the *divisions,* apart from the possible participation of multiple neurotropic sources, were also due to the butt of the [growth] cone against cells or cellular aggregates. Such interpretations seemed

---

*This figure appears only in the 1923 edition, but it is not mentioned in the text of either edition.

†"*The* neurotropic theory" in the 1923 edition.

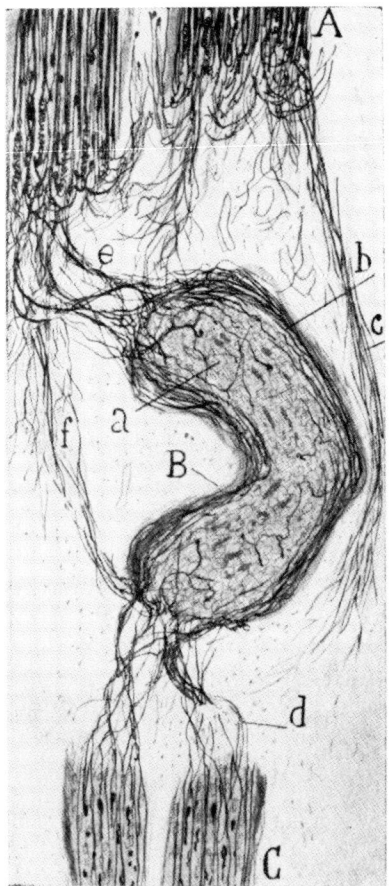

[*FIG. 26*] Fig. 160. Intercalation of a piece of nerve in a wound of the sciatic [nerve]. Note how the sprouts of the central stump are attracted to the two ends of the graft (*B*), inside which they run superficially. *A*, central stump; *C*, peripheral stump; *d*, fibers which, after going across the graft, penetrate the degenerated stump. [The following is added to the legend in the 1923 edition: *b*, obstructed ball from which arises an explorer projection (semischematic figure).]

probable but not indisputable: they were lacking decisive experimental evidence.

In order to bring this forward, in 1912 (13) we made some experiments directed at gradually narrowing the routes destined to receive the young axons to establish in them insurmountable obstacles. In this, we obtained complete satisfaction from the known procedure of *nerve ligatures*, combined with [nerve] section (fig. 161) [*fig. 28*].

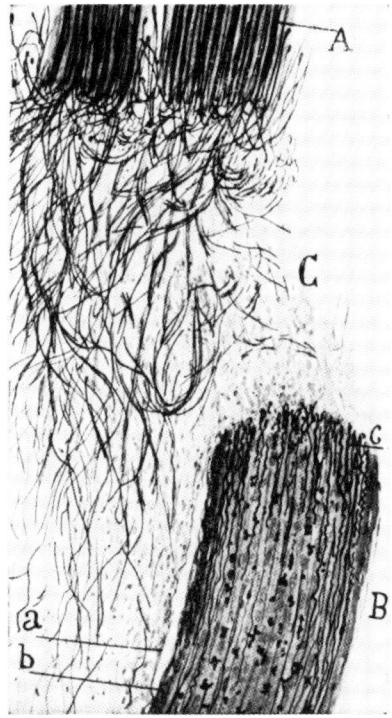

[*FIG. 27*] Fig. 163. Demonstration that a dead graft of a nerve (*B*) does not attract the sprouts (*C*) of the central stump, circulating in the scar.

From our work, considerably extended in the book on *degeneration and regeneration,* we extract two highly significant figures:

  a. Figure 161 [*fig. 28*] which reproduces schematically the effects of a moderately tight ligature, proves peremptorily *that any obstruction of the growth cone results in the modeling of a ball or club of variable thickness* (*b*). Sometimes, near the region of the ligature, that is to say in the maximum narrowness, the clubs give off thin explorer fibers [which are] in their turn promptly obstructed. In the same figure it can be seen that after colliding with the obstacle a few axons suddenly reverse direction, tracing handles whose convexity indicates the presence of the obstacle (*a*).

  b. Finally, figure 162 [*fig. 29*], shows a several times sectioned peripheral stump, [which] demonstrates that the divisions of the axons assailing old sheaths of Schwann (*B*) occur precisely at the level of the intermediate scars, that is to say in territories packed with connective [tissue] cells, which although irregularly distributed are

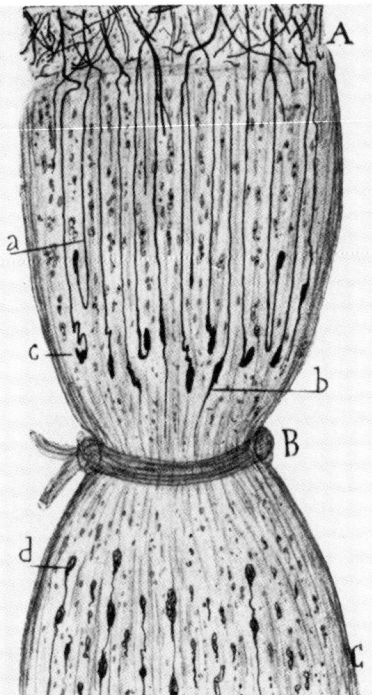

[*FIG. 28*] Fig. 161. Peripheral stump of a cut nerve. In the said stump and not far from the wound a tight ligature was made to obstruct the passage of the invading sprouts. *A*, internervous scar; *B*, ligature; *a*, *c*, insinuated sprouts in the degenerated peripheral stump; *C*, portion situated below the ligature, with agonal axons (*d*), in process of degeneration; *b*, obstructed ball from which arises an explorer projection (semischematic figure).

rich in neurotropic substances. The abundance of stimulating ferments to axonal growth and the presence of multiple obstacles constitute, then, the determinant conditions of the axonal ramifications.*

The majority of the preceding investigations on regeneration and degeneration were, as we have intimated, gathered together in an extensive work of two volumes, one of the most important and meticulous works that we have been able to undertake. We should be guilty of ingratitude if we did not remember that the printing of this work was sponsored by the generosity of the Spanish physicians of the Argentine Republic, who had the courtesy to

---

*The text of the 1917 edition ends at this point. The following paragraphs were added to the 1923 edition and were translated by Craigie.

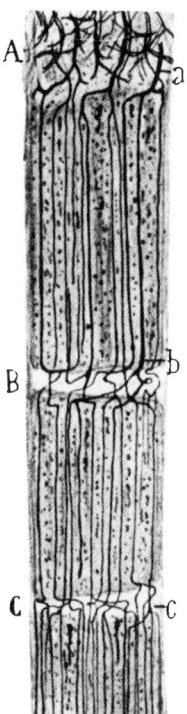

[*FIG. 29*] Fig. 162. Multisectioned sciatic nerve. *A*, principal scar, frontier of the living or central stump; *B, C*, nerve hemisections destined to create narrow scarred bands; *a, b, c*, ramifications of the sprouts at the level of the scars (semischematic figure).

write a forward. Because of the hyperbolic encomiums about my modest person, we do not reproduce it here.

Oh the noble, the nostalgic, the fervent emigrant compatriots, the flower of the race and mirror of silent perserverance and heroic industriousness!

In the middle of your tribulations, you dream of a great Spain, redeemed by culture and tolerance. I could almost say that you are the only great and good Spaniards that remain to us. Distance, the mitigator of feeling, has exalted in your spirit the sacred love of the mother country. Separated in space, but near to your heart, Spain appears in your retinae as a star of the first magnitude; not as she is, but as you desire her to be. Here is both a noble passion and a splendid program; because inasmuch as all wish it with sincere and deep emotion, Spain will return to occupy in the world the rank that she has lost.

Cajal's Notes

1. Cajal, Algunas observaciones favorables a la hipótesis neurotrópica. With 13 plates; Observaciones sobre la regeneración de la porción intramedular de las raíces sensitivas. With 5 plates; and Algunos hechos de regeneración parcial de la substancia gris de los centros nerviosos. With 11 plates. *Trab Lab Invest Biol,* vol. 8, 1910.

2. Tello, La influencia del neurotropismo en la regeneración de los centros nerviosos. With 8 plates. *Trab Lab Invest Biol,* vol. 9, 1911.

3. A methodical summary of the neurotropic theory, with exposition of all the arguments on which it rests, appeared on the occasion of the inauguration of the sessions of the *Sección de Ciencias Naturales,* in the meeting of the *Asociación para el Progreso de las Ciencias,* held in Zaragoza (1911). [What follows was added to the 1923 edition.] Nowadays the scholars tend to complicate the chemical action with electrical influences. In any case, and whichever is the chosen hypothesis, the fundamental postulate that the growth and orientation of the nerve sprouts is a function of the physiochemical conditions of the environment, will always remain unquestionable.

4. Cajal, Los fenómenos precoces de la degeneración neuronal en el cerebelo. With 18 plates; and Los fenómenos precoces de la degeneración traumática de los cilindros-ejes del cerebro. With 20 plates. *Trab Lab Invest Biol,* vol. 9, 1911.

5. The first author who in man found Purkinje cells reduced to their initial collaterals, was [U.] Rossi. His studies, verified with my technique, were applied to the cerebellum of a syphilitic alcoholic. Thanks to my investigations, it was shown clearly that the same dispositions can be experimentally produced in animals. The work of Rossi, published in *Trab Lab Invest Biol,* vol. 6, 1908, is entitled: *Per la rigeneration dei neuroni.* Similar facts were later confirmed in man by Marinesco and several other scholars.

6. Cajal, Note sur la dégénérescence traumatique des fibres nerveuses due cervelet et du cerveau. With 4 plates. *Trav Lab Invest Biol,* vol. 5, 1907; see also, Los fenómenos precoces de la degeneración neuronal en el cerebelo. With 8 plates. *Trab Lab Invest Biol,* vol. 9, 1911.

7. Cajal, Alteraciones de la substancia gris provocadas por conmoción y aplastamiento. With 6 plates. *Trab Lab Invest Biol,* vol. 9, 1911.

8. Ibid., vol. 3, 1904.

9. Cajal, Fibras nerviosas conservadas y fibras nerviosas degeneradas. With 9 plates. *Trab Lab Invest Biol,* vol. 9, 1911.

10. Cajal, Algunas observaciones favorables a la hipótesis neurotrópica. With 13 plates. *Trab Lab Invest Biol,* vol. 8, 1910.

11. Cajal, Fenómenos de excitación neurocládica en los ganglios y raíces nerviosas consecutivamente al arrancamiento del ciático. With 4 plates. *Trab Lab Invest Biol,* vol. 11, 1913.

12. Cajal, *Estudios sobre la degeneración y regeneración del sistema nervioso,* vol. 1, p. 537ff, 1913.

13. Cajal, Influencia de las condiciones mecánicas sobre la regeneración de los nervios. With 3 plates. *Trab Lab Invest Biol,* vol. 10, 1912.

CHAPTER 5

From: *Recuerdos de mi vida.* Volume 2,
Historia de mi labor científica,
Chapter 22, pages 564–567*

S. RAMÓN Y CAJAL
Madrid: N. Moya, 1917

and

Algunas observaciones contrarias
a la hipótesis *syncytial*
de la regeneración nerviosa y
neurogénesis normal,
Trab. Lab. Invest. Biol., Univ. Madrid
18 (1920):275–302

and

Démonstration photographique de quelques
phénomènes de la régénération des nerfs,
Trav. Lab. Rech. Biol., Univ. Madrid 24
(1926):191–213

S. RAMÓN Y CAJAL

---

*The greater part of this chapter was not translated by Craigie

Part I. The Publication of *Degeneration and Regeneration of the Nervous System*

[In chapter XXII of *Recuerdos de mi vida,* Cajal describes in his original book on *Degeneration and Regeneration of the Nervous System* in the following terms:] This voluminous work in two volumes and illustrated with 317 figures, [which were] copies of my preparations, constituted the main enterprise undertaken during the years 1912, 1913, and 1914. Such a considerable effort left me deeply tired since I not only had to compile synthetically all my investigations on the subject, but essentially make a new work. In the preface, I tried to justify my labor in the following terms: . . . [here Cajal reproduces the preface to the Spanish edition of *Degeneration and Regeneration of the Nervous System.* The text then continues as follows:]

The chapters [which are] the most enriched with new contributions are those that deal with the *phases of Wallerian degeneration in nerves and central pathways* (myelin and axon); the phenomena of *multiplication and transformation* of the cells of Schwann; the degenerative alterations of the *soldering discs, incisures of [Schmidt-] Lantermann and rings of Segall;* the fate of the non-neurotized *old sheaths of Schwann* of the peripheral stump; the *morphology and structure of the growth cone* within the *bands of Büngner* of the peripheral stump; the measurement of the *rate of growth* of the axon in the various terrains; the sequence of *atrophy of the axons of the central stump,* below the viable sprouts; the analysis of the exact site and form of *origin of the sprouts;* experiments in relation to *nerve and ganglionic grafts;* proof that *transplanted sympathetic ganglia* also show invading sprouts and residual nodules; the effects of the intercalation of obstacles in nerve wounds, with the aim of determining the changes of direction of the newly formed fibers; the phenomena of *proliferation of the neuroglia* in cerebral wounds; the *metamorphosis of the Golgi complex* in degenerative zones of spinal cord and cerebrum; and finally, the detailed exposition and discussion of a *hypothesis envisaged to explain the genesis and orientation* of nerve fibers in the embryo and of *aberrant sprouts* of normal and transplanted sensory ganglion cells.

The text is preceded by an enthusiastic and deeply felt dedication (probably written by that wise and admirable patriot, Dr. Avelino Gutiérrez, professor in the University of Buenos Aires), signed by forty-seven colleagues, spread throughout the whole territory of the Republic of Argentina. Needless to say each subscriber was opportunely delivered a copy [of the book] printed on special paper and affectionately dedicated.

What else might I do, to repay so noble and spiritual a gift, than to offer to my compatriots beyond the sea an original work, seriously thought out, and carefully illustrated and written!

[After the publication of the two volumes of the *Estudios Sobre la Degeneración y Regeneración del Sistema Nervioso* in 1913–1914, Cajal and his students continued to publish a number of works on degeneration and regeneration and many of these are referred to in notes added to the English version of the book. In the 1923 edition of *Recuerdos de Mi Vida,* Cajal singled out one of these works for further comment. The paper is entitled *Algunas observaciones contrarias a la hipótesis syncytial de la regeneración nerviosa y neurogénesis normal.* (Some observations against the syncytial hypothesis of nervous regeneration and normal neurogenesis) (Cajal 1920), and he describes it as follows:]

In this work is discussed the opinion recently defended by Nageotte, and in part, also by Marinesco, of the growth of the nerve sprouts through the neuroglial sheaths furnished by the cells of Schwann of the central and peripheral stumps, with the addition of a large volume of proof in favor of the free growth of the young axons. [At this point in the 1923 edition of the *Recuerdos,* Cajal inserts the following footnote:] Marinesco, in a recent monograph, has accepted our point of view expounded in the said article, and he has abandoned the *syncytial* hypothesis. (See Marinesco, "Le rôle des ferments oxidants pendant la croissance et la régénérescence des nerfs," *Rev Gen des Sciences,* XXXII year, Numbers 17–18, September, 1921.)

Among them I cite the invasion, by [axon] sprouts of the sectioned spinal cord, of the masses of adjacent scar tissue (in the spinal cord, cells of Schwann do not exist); the penetration into the spinal cord of newly formed fibers of the anterior and posterior roots (after previous section of these), without the escort of any covering or orientating element; the fact discovered by Tello and confirmed by Ortín and Arcaute of the dispersion and growth across the retina of sprouts originating in the wounded optic nerve fiber layer; the undoubted existence in the embryo (phase of the formation of the nerves) of independent axons circulating far away from any satellite cells; the experiments of the schools of Harrison and of Levi, Marinesco, etc., on the culture of nerves in plasma, where they grow naked or by passing close to threads of fibrin or an occasional mesodermal element, etc.

[Cajal's 1920 paper was translated almost completely as the additional note to chapter X of the English version of *Degeneration and Regeneration of the Nervous System* (pp. 249–264). Several paragraphs and three figures (figs. 7, 8, and 11) [*figs. 30, 31,* and *32*], however, were excluded. The most relevant omissions are as follows: In the introduction, just before note 1 on page 250 of the present work, the following paragraphs were omitted:]

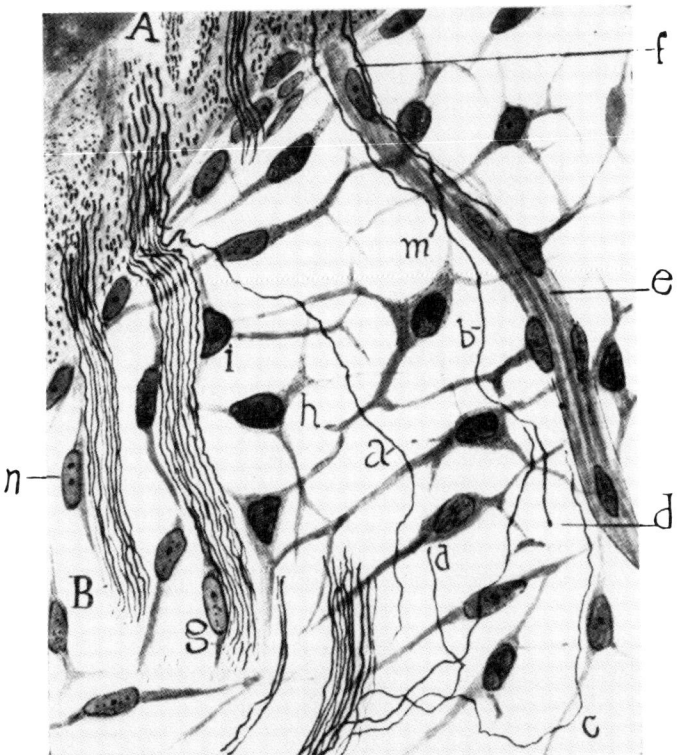

[*FIG. 30*] Fig. 7. Another section at a higher magnification of the same region and embryo reproduced in the previous figure [fig. 101*E*]. *A*, protuberance; *B*, bundles of the oculomotor [nerve]; *a, b, d,* isolated neurites; *e,* capillary; *m,* neurites that skirt [the small blood vessel]; *g, n,* early *lemnoblasts* surrounding the bundles; *h,* fibroblasts.

It is not our purpose to deal here with the whole complex problem of nervous regeneration; about it we have published numerous works. Besides, the matters subject to controversy will be discussed in the second edition of our book *Degeneration and Regeneration of the Nervous System* (1), the fruit of six years of persistent investigations, which, because it appeared in the Spanish language, and in part during the mournful period of the war, received little or no attention from the neurologists, [who were] distracted, naturally, by profound and distressing preoccupations.

For the present, we propose to deal only summarily and in the light of new observations with an aspect of the great problem of regeneration and neurogenesis; to examine whether, according to what Nageotte and Marinesco uphold formally, recently formed fibers are unable to travel in

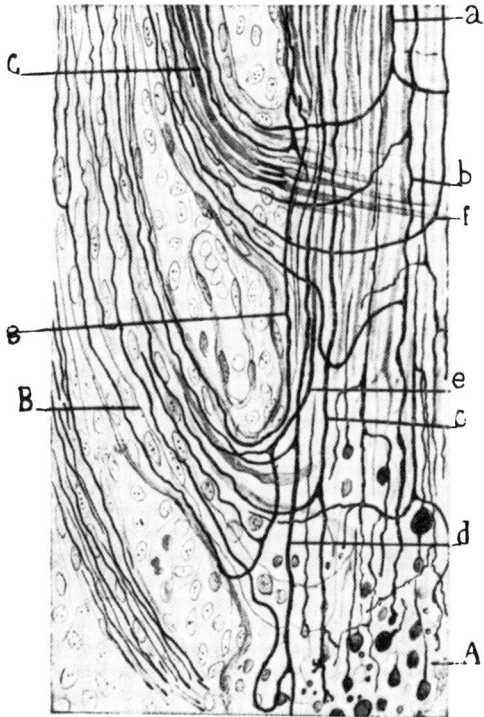

[*FIG. 31*] Fig. 8. Spinal cord of a young cat where, as a consequence of a cut, some bundles of the motor roots were lesioned. Notice how many fibers of the anterior fascicle are branched in front of the root bundles to which they send sprouts of great length. This fact, besides proving the neurotropic capacity of the degenerated anterior roots, demonstrates that the sprouts can travel freely in the spinal cord and without the cooperation of cells of Schwann.

isolation through the scar, requiring for their orientation a preestablished route of neuroglial conduits (proliferated *cells of Schwann* or *apotrophic* [cells] of Marinesco), or whether it is still permissible to accept, in disagreement with the opinion of the above scholars, that the sprouts run and are oriented, at least during their initial phase, with absolute independence of any ectodermal covering.

We will deal, thus, almost exclusively, with the *syncytial concept* expounded by Nageotte and Marinesco. The exceptional authority that these scholars possess, the brilliant neurological discoveries with which they are honored, and which we are the first to proclaim and admire, lend singular significance to their opinions, [and] justify our consideration.

Fortunately, our disagreements are with the interpretation of certain

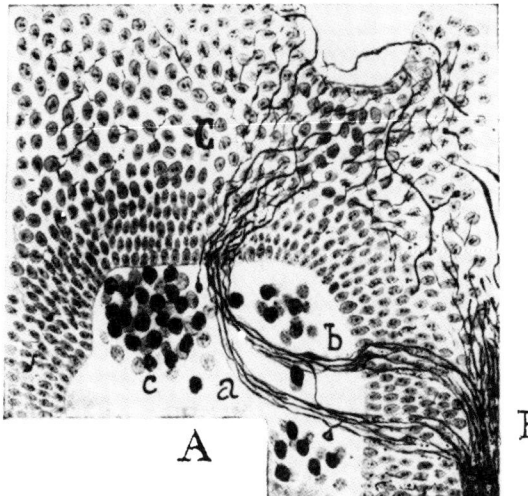

[*FIG. 32*] Fig. 11. Piece of a longitudinal section of a tadpole whose spinal cord was cut. *A*, very dilated ependymal cavity; *B*, fibers of the antero-lateral fascicle in the course of regeneration; *a, b*, newly formed bundles that cross the ependymal fluid without going astray; *C*, region of the spinal scar crossed by the sprouts. (The animal was sacrificed twelve days after the operation.)

secondary facts; nor are they absolutely irreconcilable provided that the theory of the *syncytium* can undergo some slight modification. We are glad to recognize that our agreement on the fundamental problems of the regenerative and neurogenic process is perfect or almost perfect.

With regard to the hypothesis of the *difference of electrical potential* as a primary condition for the emission and orientation of the nervous sprouts, formulated many years ago by Strasser in ontogenetic development and recently proposed by Ariëns Kappers, the distinguished neurologist of Amsterdam, to explain phylogenetic development (growth of the dendrites in direction of the sensitive or sensory afferent fibers), this will be examined carefully in other work.

But, before setting up some precise and unequivocal data, collected from both recent and older studies, against the theory of the neuroglial *syncytium*, let us state in some detail the view of the new supporters of the *syncytial* conception. . . . [The text then continues as in the note to chapter X of the present work.]

[Text referring to figure 7 [*fig. 30*] appeared just after the first paragraph of page 262:] The latter phenomenon is observed especially in figure 7 [*fig. 30*], drawn at a higher magnification than figure 6 [which corresponds to figure 101E of the present book, not shown here]. Notice how at the emergence from the protuberance (*A*), some fibers (*m*) flank the walls of an irregular blood vessel. Also in this figure, which corresponds to another section of the region of emergence of the oculomotor nerve, there are observed several isolated and completely naked nerve fibers (*a, b, c, d*), which although they run through plasmatic spaces do not lose their direction, since some of them are incorporated again into the most distal portion of the nerve bundles. Finally, here, as in the previous figures, the existence of marginal cells can be detected around the thick bundles (*g*), cells that do not differ at all, with the exception of their orientation, from the other embryonic connective tissue cells. Let us add also that around the protuberance there is a tight layer of flattened cells, [which are] probably the source of a future *pia mater*.

[Following the second paragraph on page 262, there appeared in the original article:] To illustrate here in detail the aforesaid cases, [which are] of great theoretical importance, would oblige us to lengthen this account indefinitely. I will limit myself to recommending to the supporters of the orientating *syncytium* and to the adversaries of neurotropism, the reading of the chapters of my referenced book on *Degeneration [and Regeneration]*, dealing with the axons of the posterior bundle which extend and prolixly ramify through the perispinal embryonic connective tissue (volume 2, figs. 217 and 221); the innervation of the anterior roots by means of axonal branches arising from the anterior column (fig. 8, *e, b*) [*fig. 31*]; the aforementioned experiments of Tello, who has provoked the growth of axons of the white matter of the cerebrum over great distances, by grafting pieces of peripheral nerve stump, or pieces of elder pith soaked in the sap extracted from a mature peripheral stump; the no less expressive observations of Tello (2), Arcaute and Leoz (3), recently confirmed by Urra in the birds, [which] demonstrate that under certain circumstances the axons of the retina, ordinarily unable to regenerate, grow enormously, cross all the layers of [the retina] and extend beyond the choroid; my observations about the production of artificial, naked sensory nerves in transplanted ganglia, nerves whose force of growth [is so great] that it enables them to pierce the strong ganglionic capsule and finally spread out through the scar (fig. 10, *A*) [fig. 169 of the present work, not shown here]; my findings of retrograde motor innervation of the spinal cord when the anterior roots are cut (fig. 9, *F, G*) [fig. 211 of the present work, not shown here], etc. (4). In all these cases, and many others that we do not cite in the interests of brevity, either the syncytial or apotrophic cells are completely lacking or they lie so far away from the place where the newly formed axons arise, that it is necessary to invoke an action at a distance, either from the embryonic connective tissue, or the *bands* of Büngner of a nerve [which are] more or less degenerated. These facts demonstrate, in addition, that the young axons in the process of turgidity and growth possess an enormous power of penetration, in the face of which obstacles sometimes yield that *a priori* appeared to us insurmountable.

[The text referring to figure 11 [*fig. 32*] appeared after the final sentence of point 8 on page 263:] Notice how near the scar (*C*) two bundles of newly formed fibers, originating in the anterolateral bundle (*B*), cross the wall of epithelial cells, cross the ventricular fluid, increasing in number through the exudate, penetrate again the spinal cord and disperse at the level of the scar (*C*) where ramifications and arrested balls are seen. In their passage through the ventricle, no cells accompany the axons (the swollen parts of these [axons] are thickenings of the trajectory due to arrests of growth); nevertheless, they are oriented as if they were attracted by some substance poured into the ventricle by the scar or by the interrupted region of the spinal cord. We possess numerous sections made by Sr. Lorente [de Nó], in which are observed similar phenomena of intraventricular straying and of more or less congruent rectification of the lost course.

[The 1920 paper ends with the following section, entitled "General Considerations and Conclusions":]

When investigators of great technical skill, helped by amply demonstrated scientific and neurological experience, support improbable interpretations, it is obvious that their judgment, so lucid and perspicacious on other occasions, has been interfered with by one of the following three motives: the use of inadequate methods; the deceptive appearance of fortuitous facts; or, finally, the fascination with some current hypothesis that distorts and deforms the objective truth.

In our modest opinion, these three perturbing influences have come together in the concept of the *syncytium*. The *seductive hypothesis* has been the *catenary theory* that, having been ejected from the redoubts of the front line, now takes refuge, shielded by the great authority of Held and other scholars, in the trenches of the *neuroglial chain* or *syncytial* cells of Schwann. It is appropriate to note, however, in relation to Nageotte, that it is mainly the risky lucubrations of Held, in his present attitude that have influenced the doctrine of the continuity of the Schwann cells of the normal [myelinated] fibers and of the enveloping cells of the fibers of Remak [unmyelinated axons].

It is not the occasion now to examine this point which figures in the program of my future investigations. I will note only that, until today, all of my efforts to demonstrate the cited continuity have failed, even [when] using very powerful selective procedures of impregnation. It will be prudent, therefore, to hold ourselves still bound to the old concept of Ranvier, until this question is definitely resolved.

The methodological insufficiency or inappropriateness rests on not having explored at this time, or having attached little importance to the precocious phenomena of regeneration of the central stump (noticed some time ago by Perroncito, us, and Marinesco). In effect, in favorable circumstances from the second day of the lesion, as we stated above, naked exploratory neurites (and even isolated bundles) crowned by clubs or fusiform swellings already penetrate the exudate, at an earlier period than the possible migration of the cells of Schwann. And if these early phases of the regeneration to which I allude have been explored—[although this cannot be assured] from the several communications of Nageotte—could not this scholar in his neurogenic investigations have fallen, as did Held, into the mistake of taking a simple phenomenon of stereotropism as evidence of an intraprotoplasmic or intrasyncytial position of the young neurites? It is obvious that such an illusion becomes impossible when [it is realized that] the enormous *syncytial* tubes or perifascicular sheaths are [only] constructed from the seventh day following the nerve section.

Another source of possible mistakes has been the excessive predilection shown by Nageotte for the [use] of transverse sections; [this is] a deceptive procedure used by us, not without great risks, in our former studies on regeneration, for, among other disadvantages, it possesses the very grave one of preventing us from discerning the origin of the nervous sprouts and the source of the perifascicular sheaths. Furthermore, given the almost inevitable refoldings of the nerve stumps and the unequal levels of section of each bundle (some well into the scar and others only a little), nothing is easier than taking for a precociously differentiated tubular syncytium, some advance bundle of the central stump, or a fascicle of the peripheral [stump]. With this we do not wish to deny that an expert and sagacious investigator like Nageotte had also resorted to the study of longitudinal sections as a control and to the several known techniques, in many of which he is an incomparable master.

Conclusions

1st. Both in ontogenetic development and in the [course of the] regenerative process in lesioned nerves and centers, the earliest sprouts or neurites penetrating the mesodermal tissues (*explorer axons* of Harrison) travel freely through the cellular interstices.

2nd. To each explorer fiber, several others with the same orientation are usually joined, by virtue of the *reciprocal stereotropism,* by means of which the neuritic bundles wandering through the scar are formed.

3rd. After some days (three or four in the chicken embryo, six or eight in the regenerative process), a nucleated membrane appears around the nerve fascicles. The origin of its constituent elements is still unknown in the embryo, in spite of the many investigations made in order to ellucidate it

(5). During the regenerative process it could very well originate from the same cells of Schwann proliferating from the stump, in accord with what Marinesco and Nageotte affirm and what we have expounded as a plausible hypothesis.

4th. This precocious sheath probably represents the rudiment of the *laminar membrane* of the nerves (the *sheath of Henle* of the isolated fibers). It corresponds no doubt to the tubular *syncytium* stained by iron haemotoxylin and demonstrable, with more or less clarity, by the neurofibrillar methods.

5th. Some time after the lesion (from six days upwards), or after the beginning of development (after the third or fourth day), the isolated axons also appear surrounded by a nucleated sheath, with the exception of the late growing fibers.

6th. The origin of the cells of Schwann or of the single sheaths of each fiber included in a bundle is a problem still not definitively resolved. The histogenetic mechanism recently described by Nageotte (regeneration of the nerves) may be accepted, nevertheless, as a probable hypothesis.

7th. The bundles possessing a nucleated sheath grow in thickness (regeneration), like the incipient nervous fascicles (ontogeny), by means of the arrival of numerous waves of late axons, which, by virtue of the reciprocal homotactism or stereotropism, make use of the early differentiated sheaths.

8th. We still think that the opinion of Nageotte, to the effect that during nervous regeneration with the immediate reunion of the stumps impeded, a *neuroglial nerve* always precedes a *neuritic* [nerve] is problematic. In our preparations in which the tubular bundles or *tracts* are shown clearly differentiated in the scar or near the distal stump, neurites are found within them [which are] more numerous the thicker the *syncytial* cord appears.

9th. The seductive theory of Nageotte, [which is] true in many cases, namely: that every adult nerve fiber in the [vicinity] of its terminal territory, lies separated from the mesoderm by a *syncytial* border of ectodermal origin, would only reach the level of a law if it should be proved that all the nervous arborizations (motor end plates, tendon organs of Golgi, [corpuscles] of Pacini, or Meissner, etc.) are surrounded by structures originating from the ectoderm. Our recent observations on the genesis of the sensory terminations (6) and the older ones of Tello, appear difficult to reconcile with this opinion.

10th. The results of the investigations of Nageotte and Marinesco are, in principle, as we indicated above, reconcilable with our idea of the normal and pathological neurogenetic mechanism, provided that it is accepted that the *syncytium* is formed, not before the explorer neurites but somewhat after, adapting to the nervous bundles, and conceding besides a somewhat greater participation of neurotropic influences in explaining the growth and common orientation of the sprouts and isolated bundles and their arrival in the peripheral stump. Needless to say that with it we do not pretend to prejudge the physicochemical nature of the neurotropism [which is] a question that will be definitively resolved only by future biochemical investigations. *Madrid, February 1921*

Part II. Cajal and Photography of the Nerves

[Cajal's last paper on the subject of degeneration and regeneration of the nerves appeared in the *Travaux du Laboratoire de Recherches Biologiques de l'Université de Madrid* in 1926 (Cajal 1926) under the title: "Démonstration photographique de quelques phénomènes de la régénération des nerfs." This paper is devoted to the illustration by photomicrographs of many of the phenomena of regeneration that he had elucidated and represented in drawings in his earlier publications. In this, we see another example of how Cajal, late in his career, turned to photography in order to provide further documentation and to offset real or imagined criticism made on technical grounds (see DeFelipe and Jones 1988). In the following paragraphs, we have translated the introduction and certain relevant sections of the 1926 paper.]

It is possible to reproduce accurately by means of photographs some acts of degeneration and regeneration of the nerves on the condition that the researcher renounces showing an ensemble image of the process [and limits himself] to reproducing certain axonal segments in the process of transformation, and above all, on the condition that the sections be thin and very flat. To this end, sections of 20 to 25 μm are excellent.

Unfortunately, while thin sections reveal certain details of the metamorphosis of axons, they are not suitable for perfectly demonstrative photomicrographs of the innervation of the peripheral segment, especially if we wish to detect, in a single section, the emergence of sprouts from the central stump, their course through the scar, and finally, their penetration into the peripheral segment.

All who have dealt with the process of regeneration know very well that the axons make considerable deviations and very complicated bends during their trajectory through the scar, and before arriving at their destination. Hence, if we wish to demonstrate the Wallerian doctrine or the [doctrine] of continuity, it is absolutely essential to make thick sections, provided, however, that they are well stained and transparent. They, thus, have to be 40 or even 45 μm thick, and it is also necessary to shorten, as much as possible, the distance between the two stumps by means of various operative devices. One such aid is *hemi-section* of the nerves. In this manner, we obtain a notable shortening of the scar and a reduction in the delays of growth and in the deviation of the sprouts. Another help is the insertion in the internerve cavities produced by retraction, of a living nerve segment freshly extracted from the same animal. Finally, another effective resort, [which is] well-known and frequently used by surgeons, consists of the suture of the distal and proximal segments. But this suture, [although] easy to carry out in mammals of some size, becomes very difficult and almost impracticable to carry out without causing grave nerve damage in the young rabbit or young cat, animals in which on account of the thinness of the nerves and the rapidity of the regenerative process, one finds the most appropriate conditions to reveal the invasion of the peripheral stump by the newly formed fibers (1).

For us, who would seek the demonstration of the essential facts of regeneration, that is to say, the origin and course of the sprouts invading the peripheral stump, almost all our good preparations (more than 500) made during the course of eight years of investigation, are much too thick and therefore inappropriate for photography. In examining these directly, they impose indisputably upon us the conviction of the *doctrine of continuity*, but few among them lend themselves to our obtaining persuasive photomicrographic proof. Even those [preparations] which seem to be the most favorable can only make clear some special points, as we shall see below.

Be that as it may and pointing out, not without surprise (2), that despite the tremendous labor of these last twenty years, there are still distinguished scholars who are, with greater or lesser reserve, partisans of autogeneous regeneration, we have decided to publish certain of our [photographic] evidence dealing largely with the mode of invasion of the scar and innervation of the peripheral stump (3).

We believe that these photographs, although not entirely decisive, offer a certain interest in relation to the question debated by the catenarists and the partisans of the Wallerian concept.

It is unnecessary to add that we do not consider these photographs technically perfect at all, not even passable. In spite of the long experience that we have in this sort of work (our first photomicrographs go back some fifty years, that is to say, to the almost legendary epoch of moist collodion), it has not been possible for us to contravene the inexorable laws of optics. It is well known that when a section is thick (40 μm or more) and contains [cells] disposed in several planes and oriented in diverse ways, little is achieved by trying to focus on one group of cells; the images of those that are situated above or below and not in focus project shadows that disturb the purity and sharpness of the image. The use of the diaphragm, absolutely essential in thick sections, and even more so when one makes use of the long focal length objective, often aggravates the damage and affects the plate by the annoying phenomenon of diffraction. When objectives of high numerical aperture (objective 1.30 of Zeiss with large diaphragm, etc.) are used, good overall photographs can never be obtained. We have therefore limited ourselves to the uncertain remedy of making a laborious choice of sections in which, a very rare thing, the newly formed nerve fibers are almost parallel, which allow one to pursue them, in spite of the complication of the plexus, over a sufficient length by means of long focal length objectives (0.65 and 0.30 of Zeiss).

But, leaving aside technical considerations which this is not the occasion to lay stress on, we have described some of the photographs obtained. Almost all of them, as the reader will see, are classified in two groups: namely, first, those that show the initial solitary advance of the sprouts through the scar, and second, those that reveal the innervation of the peripheral stump by means of fibers coming from the central stump (4).

[The text continues with descriptions of the nineteen figures that illustrate the paper. Unfortunately, the quality of these figures is not high and precludes satisfactory reproduction. Three of the most representative (figs. 8, 13, and 14) [*figs. 33, 34, and 35*] are however shown. The following paragraphs deal with these figures.]

. . . [page 199] On several occasions, the wandering of fibers in the scar has been described, those that grow in all directions, in particular when they collide with obstacles in their path, or when the distal stump is found very far away. Figure 8 [a] [*fig. 33*] gives us an example of these deviations; two details appear that are not without interest: one is the preferred trajectory in the scar of the fascicles in a direction transverse to the peripheral stump, as if they were searching for another fascicle of the same nerve, which was also cut at a rather long distance and could not be fitted into the same photograph (figure 8a) [*fig. 33*];* the other detail is the reluctance, often pointed out by ourselves, shown by the sprouts to traverse the massed pleiads of phagocytes that surround foreign bodies. This peculiarity can be well appreciated at [B], where an obliquely cut hair appears surrounded by serried connective [tissue] elements.

. . . [page 208] Figure 13 [*fig. 34*] deals with the reimplantation of a piece of sciatic nerve inserted between the two stumps of the same fascicle immediately after the cut. . . . The grafted segment comes from the sciatic nerve of the opposite leg of the same animal. The union was carried out rapidly, and the cat [which was the] subject of the experiment was sacrificed six days after the operation, showing, thanks to the exceptional narrowness of the scar, an excessively abundant neurotization of the distal stump. Therefore, nothing is easier, given such favorable conditions, than to observe the crossing, not only of free fibers but also of true fascicles, from the

---

*Not indicated in the figure.

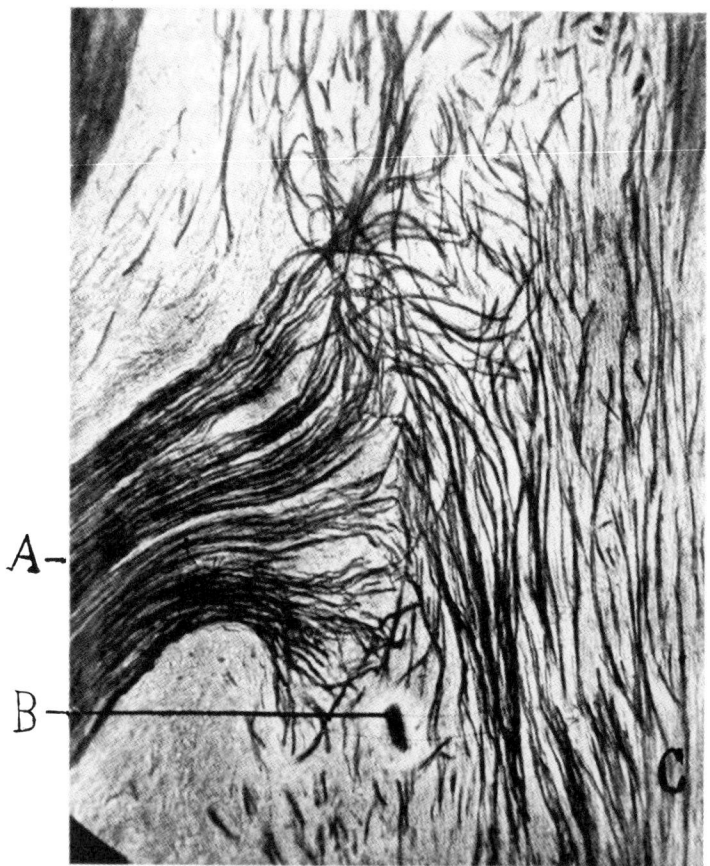

[*FIG. 33*] Fig. 8. *A*, central stump; *B*, hair; *C*, strayed fibers. (Rabbit sacrificed seven days after the operation.)

central segment to the peripheral (fig. 13, *a, b*) [*fig. 34*], inside which they had progressed almost a centimeter. The photograph does not show well the situation of the sprouts inside the distal stump; by contrast, direct observation showed that inside [the tubes formed by] the sheaths of Schwann, the majority of the fibers and especially the isolated fascicles, run between the *bands* of Büngner and that they are still without covering cells. It is unnecessary to multiply photographs of this kind, although we possess an abundant collection, corresponding to several varieties of section. All support conclusively the doctrine of continuity. But we will make an exception of the case illustrated in figure 14 [*fig. 35*]. It concerned a young cat whose sciatic nerve had been partially cut (with the aim of avoiding

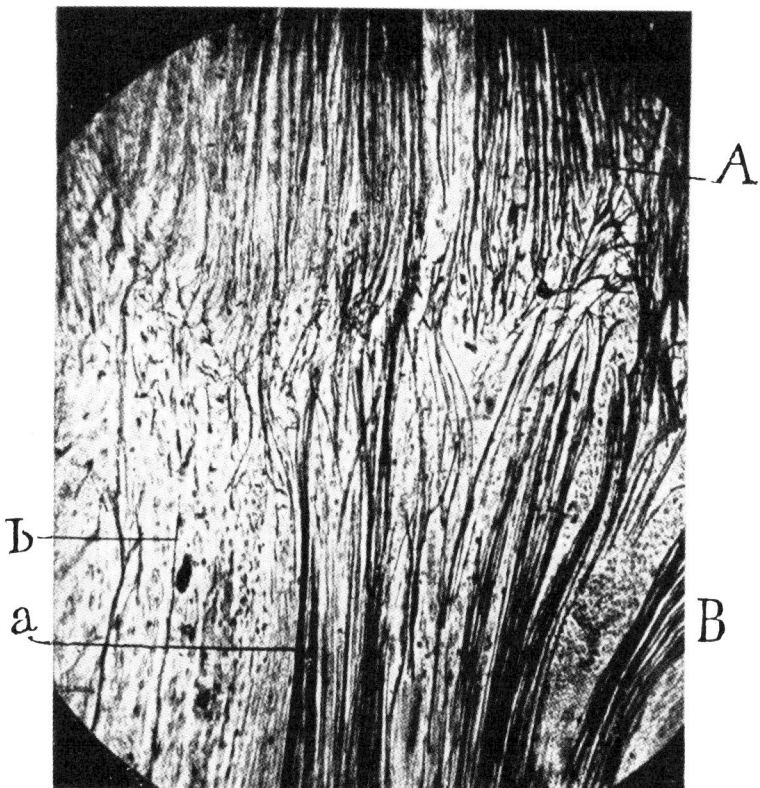

[*FIG. 34*] Fig. 13. *A*, central stump; *B*, neurotized graft; *a*, fascicle of newly formed fibers; *b*, an isolated fiber. (Cat sacrificed six days after the operation.)

excessive retraction) in three parts. The photomicrograph in question shows the neurotization of the first segment, which appears six days after the operation. The scar (*B*) was very narrow and in it is clearly seen the branching of many sprouts originating from the central stump (*A*) and penetrating, in most luxuriant contingents, the peripheral stump (*C*). . . .

[After the description of the nineteen figures the text continues on page 212 as follows:]

The above-mentioned facts prove sufficiently the implausibility of autogeneous regeneration inside the bands of Büngner. Later, if time and occasion permit, we will embark upon new experiments of nervous regeneration; but at that time, the goals will be exclusively photographic, that is to say, by making thin sections (from 15 to 30 μm) and by paying attention to the gold-toning. It is evident that the majority of such sections, given the nature of the question, will offer only a little of demonstrative value; but a

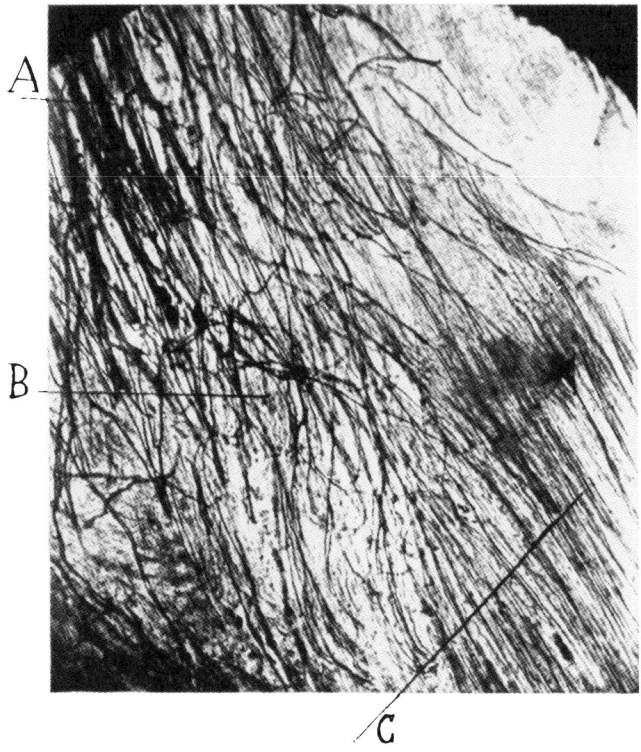

[*FIG. 35*] Fig. 14. *A*, central stump; *B*, scar; *C*, neurotized peripheral stump. (Photographic ocular Phoku of Zeiss.)

number of them will give an image that, if not perfect, will be at least sufficiently persuasive in relation to some of the much debated phenomena of the process of nervous regeneration.

In summary, and as a general conclusion of this short work, one might affirm:

First, that according to Waller, Ranvier, Vanlair, Perroncito, Lugaro, Harrison, Marinesco, Nageotte, Tello, Boeke, etc., the sprouts innervating the scar and peripheral stump originate from the axons of the central stump.

Second, that any precocious exploratory fiber, in the process of growth, runs freely. The individual or collective sheath develops later, six or seven days after the operation.

Third, that the free extremity of the sprouts in the phase of ameboidism, may adopt various forms, including those of the terminal veils, spreading over obstacles, both those that run inside the tubes of Schwann and those that are lost in the mesodermal tissues.

Fourth, that when the conditions are favorable, the innervation of the peripheral stump, also in the case of grafted nerve segments, is effected before the differentation of the bands of Büngner (five days after the operation).

Cajal's Notes to Part I

1. Cajal, *Estudios sobre la degeneración y regeneración del sistema nervioso*. With 317 plates. 2 vols., 1913 and 1914.
2. J. F. Tello, La régénération dans les voies optiques, *Trab Lab Invest Biol*, vol. 9, 1911.
3. Leoz [Ortín], and [L. R.] Arcaute, Procesos regenerativos del nervio óptico y retina con ocasión de injertos nerviosos, *Trab Lab Invest Biol*, vol. 11, fasc, 4, 1914.
4. Cajal, Algunas observaciones favorables a la hipótesis neurotrópica, *Trab Lab Invest Biol*, vol. 8, 1910.
5. Following the opinions of His, Kölliker, Graham Kerr, and other scholars, we proposed some time ago a mesodermal origin for the ontogeny of the cells of Schwann (Génesis de las fibras nerviosas en el embrión y observaciones contrarias a la teoría catenaria, *Trab Lab Invest Biol*, vol. 4, 1905–1906). It is true that the interesting experiments and observations of Harrison and v[on] Lenhossék later brought doubt to our mind. But at the present time, in the presence of much more demonstrative preparations than those obtained in the beginning, and with those obtained recently by Tello in the chicken embryo, we align ourselves unreservedly with the idea of a mesodermal origin of the *lemnoblasts* or *coleoblasts* (cells of Schwann), which could well arise, according to Tello's beliefs, from the cellular zone that surrounds the nerve centers during the earliest developmental phases. Once they become differentiated and infiltrate into the nerves, such cells would constitute perhaps a specific type [of cell] capable of proliferating indefinitely and of maintaining their newly acquired attributes.
6. Cajal, Acción neurotrópica de los epitelios. (Algunos detalles sobre el mecanismo genético de las ramificaciones nerviosas intraepiteliales, sensitivas y sensoriales), *Trab Lab Invest Biol,* vol. 17, 1919.

Cajal's Notes to Part II

1. Some scholars, who are of great authority and of recognized talent, seem to like to create grave experimental difficulties for the observation of the cardinal facts of regeneration, since they use large mammals (for example, the dog) or, for the same purpose, the regenerated nerve segments of man (wounds of war). Working under

such conditions, it is not only difficult, but *absolutely impossible* to arrive at a precise conception of the mechanism of innervation of the scar and of the distal stump.

2. Here we have left aside both any polemical intent, and the recent bibliography which can be found in the English edition, at present in press, of our work in two volumes: *Estudios sobre la degeneración y regeneración.* . . . (2 vols.,) Madrid, 1914. We are very sorry that we cannot offer this work, out of print already for eight years, to the scholars who, in these modern times, are engaged in the problem of degeneration.

3. See, for example, the very interesting recent works of Bethe and Spielmeyer.

4. Of course, all of these photomicrographs are without retouching.

CHAPTER 6

From: ¿*Neuronismo o reticularismo?* Las pruebas objectivas de la unidad anatómica de las células nerviosas

S. RAMÓN Y CAJAL
Archivos de Neurobiología 13
(1933): 217–291 and 579–646

[Published in 1954 as *Neuron Theory or Reticular Theory.
Objective Evidence of the Anatomical Unity of the Nerve Cells.*
Translated by M. Ubeda-Purkiss and C. A. Fox.
Madrid, Consejo Superior de Investigaciones Científicas]*

From chapter XII (pages 133–136)

B. The theory of autoregeneration and ensheathment in the restoration of sectioned nerves.

Today the arguments drawn from [experiments] of nerve regeneration have lost all their potential polemic value. This is not surprising. *Autoregeneration*, that is to say, the process of discontinuous generation of the axons from the cells of Schwann of the peripheral stump and without the collaboration of the trophic centers or neurons of origin, appeared at a time when there were no adequate methods for impregnating axons during the course of their continuous growth through the scar and distal segment of the sectioned nerve. But today, now that we possess formulas of great analytic efficiency, such a hypothesis is absolutely untenable (1) [*fig. 36*].† Further-

---

*We reproduce here, with the permission of the publisher and with a few corrections, the part of the translation that deals with the regeneration and degeneration of the nervous system (pages 133–143).

† This figure is not mentioned in the text.

more, it can be said that its few actual defenders reveal a state of mind favorable to compromise, as is shown by their many concessions to the doctrine of Waller, Ranvier, and Vanlair. We sincerely believe that, were it not for the deplorable ostentation that consequently ruins so many good intentions and sterilizes or paralyzes so many talents, acceptance of the monogenist theory would be absolute.

In summary, every sectioned nerve regenerates its axons by means of sprouts from the central stump which, as Tello proved, cross the scar and assail the peripheral stump to reach the external sensory and muscular terminations. Arriving at their destination, attracted no doubt by some substance (or physical influence as yet unknown) arising from the nuclei of the terminal apparatus, the destroyed motor arborization moulds itself anew (2).

Concerning the hypothesis of *ensheathment* of the newly formed axons through the scar, the old dispute between Bethe and his school and the new researchers is reduced to a question simply of timing. In the beginning the sprouts from the central stump emerge naked, and their ramifications

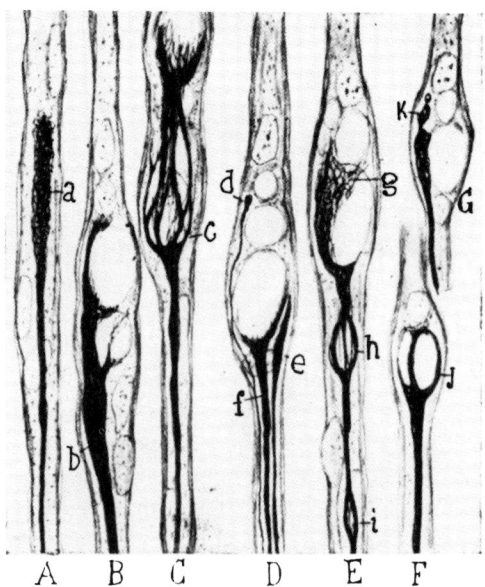

[*FIG. 36*] Fig. 67. Details of the course of the growth cones colliding with fat droplets of the [Schwann tubes] of the peripheral stump; *a, b, c, e,* growth cones. This refutes categorically the hypothesis of autoregeneration (or discontinuous regeneration). Young cat sacrificed five [days] after operation. The sprouts travel in the interior of the degenerated sheaths of Schwann.

course freely through the interstices of the connective [tissue] [*fig. 37*];*
but from the sixth or seventh day after the operation, satellite cells which
accompany them throughout their course and constitute a protective sheath,
arise. Although these adventitial cells are not guiding [cells] (the
Leitzellen of Held or the *apotrophiques* of Marinesco), their origin is a
problem that has still not been resolved. The majority of neurologists are
inclined to consider them as the progeny of Schwann's cells emigrating from
the central stump of the mutilated nerve (3).

For the justification of the neuron theory we should recall a fact proved
almost unanimously by all of the modern investigators: that anastomoses
between the sprouts growing out of the central stump have never been
found.

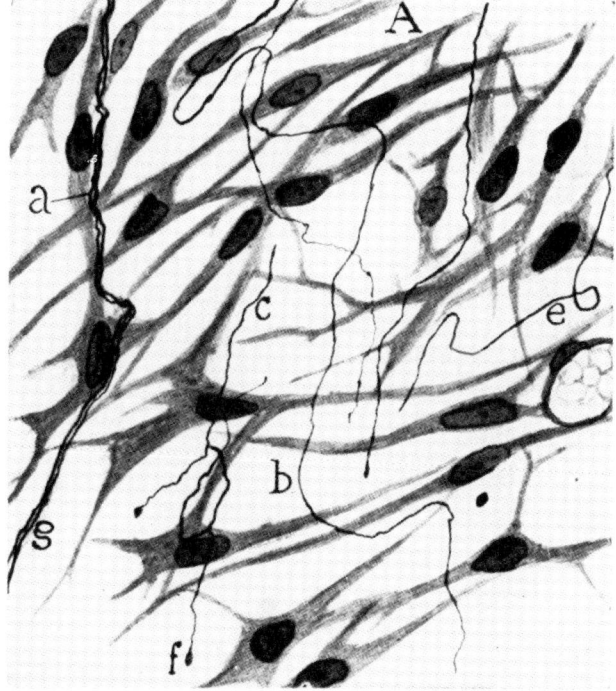

[*FIG. 37*] Fig. 68. Scar near the central stump of a cut nerve. The animal (cat) was sacrificed four days after section. *A*, fibroblasts; *a*, fine exploring sprouts which deviate around fibroblasts of the incipient scar; *b*, *c*, *e*, other sprouts which travel freely through the plasma exudate. Note the absence of a protective envelope in the fibers arising from the central stump.

---

*This figure is not mentioned in the text.

From chapter XII (page 137)

C. Regeneration in the [central nervous system]

Regeneration does not take place in the nervous centers. In favorable cases one may note phenomena of branching, degeneration and neuronal metamorphosis, but the reestablishment of the continuity of a sectioned neurite can never be observed. Curious and significant [in this regard] is the experiment carried out by Tello: When a piece of peripheral stump of a sectioned nerve (before the penetration of the sprouts) is introduced into a cerebral wound in the rabbit, a regenerative capacity appears in the apathetic neurites of the white matter. This demonstrates that the impotence of the central axons to restore the peripheral segment is neither fatal nor irremediable, but that is due, perhaps, to the absence of Schwann's cells in the process of rejuvenation (4).

Instead of this regenerative apathy, the central axons show numerous degenerating transformations, the principal one of which is the formation, close to or far away from the point of section, of a *ball* or *club of retraction* (Cajal) and the fragmentation [of the axons] in free balls ordinarily positioned close to the wound and distal to the initial [axon] collaterals. When the section is made in the region of the neurite from which the [latter] projections emanate, only a retraction club is produced which is almost inevitably followed by the death of the mutilated neuron (fig. 69, *D, G, F*) [*fig. 38*]. Some of these phenomena, [which are] easy to verify but neglected because they are troublesome to certain fashionable theories, have been confirmed by Miskolczy [1925] and other impartial authors.

From chapter XIII (pages 137–143)

II. Anatomicopathological facts favorable to the neuron theory. Persistence of the baskets and other pericellular terminations, etc.

The unity of the pathological reaction in neurons demands a clarifying restriction. Always when the disturbing causes (either traumatic or chemicobiological) affect the integrity of a single neuron, the reaction is perfectly autonomous. But as the morbid processes usually present a diffuse character and act upon large or small foci, it is difficult to verify the unity of the pathological reaction, that is to say, the degeneration of the neuron while

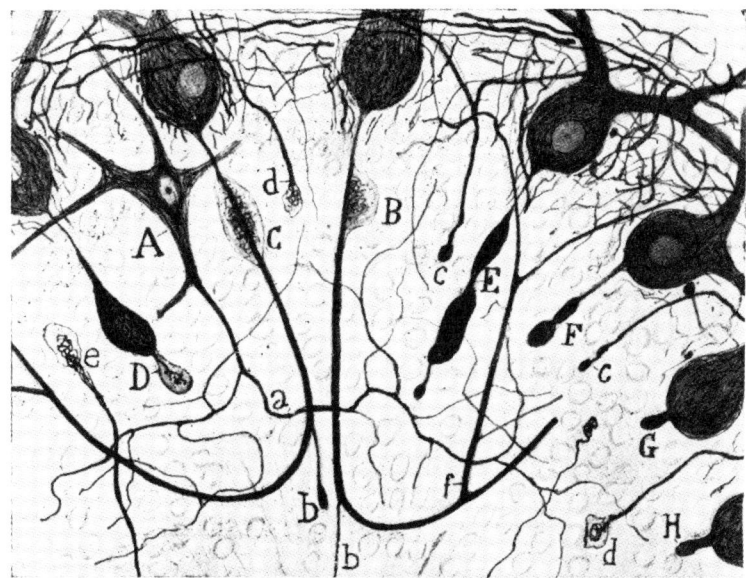

[*FIG. 38*] Fig. 69. Section of a cerebellar [folium]. Cat of twenty-five days, a day after section. *D, E, F*, varieties of double clubs; *G, H*, axon with retraction ball; *b*, continuation of the Purkinje axon terminating in a club; *c, d*, hypertrophied recurrent collaterals of Purkinje axons. In *F, G, H*, the baskets have disappeared.

leaving the integrity of the nervous arborizations [with which it enters into] contact. It is not surprising that neurons and the [neurologlial] and microglial cells with them are simultaneously affected either by microbial causes or by chemical conditions not always well understood.

There are examples, however, in which there appear here and there resistant groups of neurons or isolated neurons affected very little or not at all, despite the extent of the lesion (degenerative processes [caused] by circulatory disorders, absorption of toxins or poisons, microbial infections, senility).* Let us cite as examples *general paralysis,* Friedreich's *disease, senile dementia, rabies,* necrotic foci produced by *emboli* or *thromboses,* intoxication by alcohol (Rossi) or by lead salts (Villaverde), etc.

As an example of a convincing and well-known case let us mention the disappearance of the Purkinje cells [of the cerebellum] in *general paralysis* with maintenance of the *basket* and stellate cells of the molecular layer. This persistence, revealing the independence of the baskets and the cells they surround, can also be produced experimentally by sectioning the axons of the Purkinje cells at the level of the granular layer or even below as is shown

---

*The phrase in parenthesis is found only in the Spanish version.

in figure 70 [*fig. 39*] (5). This remarkable conservation of the baskets, despite the disappearance of the cells in connection with them has been described by Schob (6), and others, among them Río-Hortega (7), K. Schaffer, Kindberg, Cajal, Nageotte, Marinesco, Somoza, etc. The opposite phenomenon, that is, the destruction of the baskets (figs. 69 and 71) [*figs. 38 and 40*], has been observed by Bielschowsky (8) in *amaurotic idiocy*, the histological pathology of which has been masterfully studied by K. Schaffer (9), Bielschowsky, etc. Analogous cases of pathological dissociation between the Purkinje cells and the climbing fibers have been noted. Against the authors such as Wolff, Held, and others who claim anastomoses between

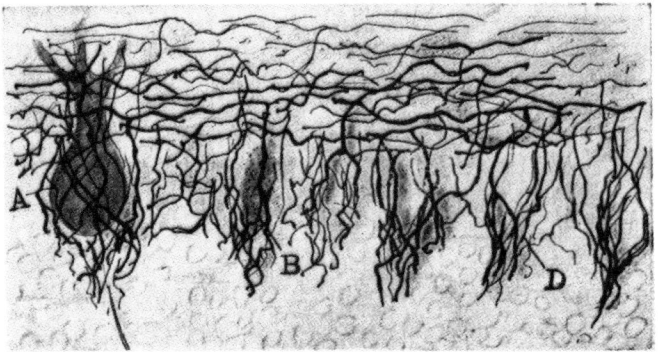

[**FIG. 39**] Fig. 70. Cat of twenty-five days, twenty-four hours after operation. *A*, nearly normal Purkinje cell; *B*, another in the process of atrophy and with a granular appearance; *D*, [axonal] baskets which surround the cavity where the destroyed bodies of Purkinje cells resided.

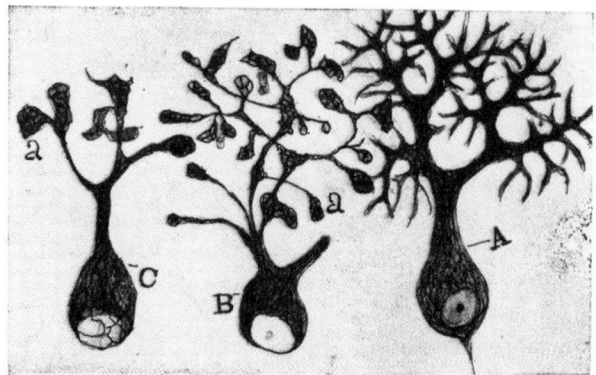

[**FIG. 40**] Fig. 71. Purkinje cells of a cat of twenty-five days, sacrificed two days after the traumatic lesion. *A*, normal cell; *B*, *C*, cells whose retracted dendrites terminate in reticulated clubs; *a*, terminal bulbs. The baskets have disappeared.

the dendrites of neighboring Purkinje cells (direct or indirect unions), is the process whereby degeneration and death of the axon (portion at a distance of the cell) of [the Purkinje] cells is followed by the conservation of the [dendritic arborization] and hypertrophy of the [axon] initial collaterals, a degenerative phenomenon that does not extend to the neighboring [cells] (Umberto Rossi [10] and many other authors). Even more expressive is a lesion of these [dendritic arborizations] which we observed in trauma of the cerebellar white matter (11). The dendritic arborization is transformed and shrunken, acquiring the form of a rose bush (rosaliform degeneration), but this curious retraction and metamorphosis does not spread to the adjoining cells (fig. 71) [*fig. 40*].

The fibers that make up a *basket* may also exhibit other important alterations that are significant for the thesis here defended. One of these is the hypertrophy and marked retraction of the terminal [axonal] branches observed in many pathological states, particularly in general paralysis and dementia praecox (Cajal). Another, also very expressive, consists of the total detachment of the nervous ramifications that withdraw themselves from the surrounded soma without leaving the slightest trace of communicating neurofibrillar bridges. Such an abnormality, quite frequent in the pathological histology of the cerebellum, was first observed in the rabid dog by G[arcía e] Izcara and us (1904). It is unnecessary to point out that both lesions represent strong arguments against the reticular hypothesis.

In very limited trauma of the cerebrum, cerebellum, etc. (punctures with a needle or very fine scalpel), it is common to find degenerated cells which stand out among the neighboring uninjured pyramids. Indeed, some of the pyramids, the axons of which were mutilated below the collaterals, show a curious reaction: the initial collaterals hypertrophy (this occurs also in the Purkinje cells of the cerebellum) and here is encountered the surprising case in which long axon cells are converted into short axon neurons (fig. 69, c, d) [*fig. 38*] (12).

Similar proofs of histopathologic discontinuity can easily be obtained in the spinal cord and even in the medulla oblongata, although here well-localized experimental lesions are more rare. Thus, recently, in our laboratory [De] Castro and De Juan destroyed a part of the *ventral nucleus* of the acoustic [nerve] in the rabbit. We studied the cells of the nucleus of the *trapezoid body* using the Bielschowsky method and noted two days after the operation that the *chalices* of Held became turgid, considerably hypertrophied, and exhibited a granular degeneration while the neurons the chalices surround did not suffer any apparent injury [and] conserved their neurofibrils, although these are not clearly visible.

By exhaustively consulting the bibliography one would find numerous examples similar to the ones mentioned.

Nevertheless, we cannot refrain from mentioning the experiments of

Lawrentjew (13) and [De] Castro (14), since they are modern and significant. The [latter] author has demonstrated that section of the afferent or preganglionic nerves of the sympathetic ganglia causes the disappearance of the pericellular and peridendritic arborizations after a rapid degenerative process (according to [De] Castro, from seven to twenty-four hours after section of the [pre]ganglionic fibers), while the cells of the sympathetic chain persist, appearing normal six or seven days after the operation. In the experiments of Lawrentjew, section of the vagus produces degeneration of the pericellular plexuses of the cardiac sympathetic neurons, [but the neurons] remain normal twenty-one days after the operation. Moreover, the nerve fibers arising from the autonomic cardiac ganglia, not being affected by the trauma, are preserved. Omitting here the debatable normality, as we said before, of certain atypical nervous nests (Nageotte and Cajal) of sensory and sympathetic cells, a problem [discussed] in modern times by P. Stöhr (15), let us recall the fact that fibers of spinal origin in contact with certain sympathetic neurons do not produce the least alteration in these cells, at least for some time, when they degenerate. This result confirms the physiological interpretations of Langley.

Obviously, such physiopathological persistence of the associated neurons is not endless. In reality, all the nervous elements in intimate connection suffer functionally, following lesion of the associated cells, and after months or years may undergo atrophy and degenerate because of disuse, provided that they do not have other connections capable of [maintaining] functional activity.

In any case, the fact that the elements which have lost their principal connections persist for a greater of lesser time constitutes a strong indication of the anatomical discontinuity of nerve cells.

We do not wish to cite here physiological results too well known and incompatible with the theories of the diffuse nets of Golgi, Apáthy, Bethe, and Held, particularly the latter scholar's new concept concerning the structure of the gray matter, etc. Let us limit ourselves to declaring that in accepting the more exaggerated syncytial hypotheses and extending them to the whole nervous system, all the local muscle reflexes, as well as the [specific] sensory impressions (chromatic, acoustic, tactile, spatial, etc.) and in fact everything that the physiologists, during fifty years of dogged and fruitful investigation, have taught us concerning localization in the nervous centers, are left without explanation. We would fall, therefore, into chaos or hopeless nihilism unless, to avoid complete disaster to our better founded concepts of connections, we were to invoke Dogiel's colonial hypothesis or something similar (anastomosis in pleiads or nervous regions). But these intracolonial anastomoses remain to be demonstrated and, even if we accepted them, they would clarify only in part the physiological and pathological processes.

Perhaps microdissection combined with tissue culture will in time have the last word. But up to the present it has not been possible, at least as far as we know, to apply it to the living nerve tissue of the [central nervous system]. The general impression of those who have worked with microdissection is, as Woollard (16) declares in commenting upon the results of Chambers' method (17), that the rarity of protoplasmic continuity ([as occurs in some] epithelia) suggests the idea that the bodies of animals, despite the almost metaphysical speculation of the partisans of the continuity theory, are actually composed of a cellular colony and that there is no necessity for changing any of our histophysiological ideas, as Held and Boeke [would have us do].

Cajal's Notes

1. Miskolczy notes rightly that the quarrel between the partisans of continuity and the autogeneticists arose from the difference in methods used. We are convinced that if Bethe (today virtually the only defender of discontinuous regeneration), before fixing his attitude on the question of regeneration had [been acquainted] with the silver procedures, [and] above all with the formulas of reduced silver nitrate which makes it possible to obtain transparent, thick sections, he would have defended the Wallerian thesis. Despite this, in his later works he gives proof of intellectual flexibility and scientific honesty by coming closer and closer to the theory of continuity. Nevertheless, he continues to defend as probable, in certain cases, the neoformation of nerve fibers, from the activities of the cells of Schwann of the peripheral stump. Spielmeyer also, for the same technical reasons, continues to maintain the autogenetic attitude. *See* Bethe, Zur theorie und Praxis der Verhheilung durchtrennten Nerven. Volume in honor of Doctor Cajal, 1922. Consult B. Spielmeyer: *Gesamte Neurol. Psychiatr.*, vol. 36, 1917. And his: *Histopathologie des Nervensystems*, Bd. I, 1922.

2. Tello, Dégénération et régénération des plaques motrices, etc., *Trav Lab Rech Biol*, vol. 5, 1907.

3. Those who desire orientation in the study of these questions should consult the papers of Bethe, Dustin, Lugaro, Perroncito, Marinesco, Spielmeyer, Tello, Rojas, Castro, Boeke, Miskolczy, etc., and particularly owr work: *Degeneración y Regeneración del Sistema Nervioso* (there is an English translation by Doctor May, Oxford: Oxford University Press, 1928).

4. Tello, La influencia del neurotropismo en la regeneración de los centros nerviosos. *Trab Lab Invest Biol* vol. 9, 1911.

5. Cajal, Les phénomènes precoces de la régénération neuronale dans le cervelet. *Trab Lab Invest Biol*, vol. 9, 1911.

6. Schob, *Arb Dtsch Forsch-Anstalt Psychiatr*, München, vol. 5, 1922.

7. Río-Hortega, *Trab Lab Invest Biol*, vol. 12, 1914.

8. Bielschowsky, Histopathologie der amäurotischen Idiotie, etc., *J Psychol Neurol*, vol. 26, 1921.

9. K. Schaffer, Tatsächliches und Hypothetisches aus der Histopathologie der infantil-amäurotischen Idiotie, [*Arch Psychiatr Nervenkr*, vol. 64], 1922.

10. U. Rossi, Per la rigenerazione dei neuroni. *Trab Lab Invest Biol*, vol. 6, 1908.

11. Cajal, Loc. cit *Trab Lab Invest Biol*, vol. 9, 1911.

12. Let us recall also the classical facts of Nissl's *chromatolysis* and the atrophy of the *motor nuclei* (Gudden's method) and finally, the late destruction of motor neurons in Van Gehuchten's method, all very individualized neuronal lesions, following section or excision of nerves.

13. Lawrentjew, Experimentelle-morphologische Studien über den feineren Bau des autonomen Nervensystems. *Mikros Anat. Forsch*, vol. 16, 1929.

14. De Castro, *Trav Lab Rech Biol*, vol. 26, 1930.

15. Ph. Stöhr, *Handbuch der mikroskopischen Anatomie des Menschen*, vol. 4, 1928. Heräusg. W. v. Mollendorf. *Note:* These bibliographical notes [13–15] are incomplete; to cite all of the authors who have stated these facts of anatomical dissociation would have required too much space.

16. Woollard, *Recent Advances in Anatomy*, 1927.

17. [R.] Chambers [and G. S. Renyi], The Structure of the Cells in Tissues as Revealed by Microdissection, [*Am*] *J. Anat.* vol. 35, 1925. It is known that this scholar, by means of an ingenious microdissection apparatus associated with the method of tissue culture, has been able to evaluate lesions following cellular laceration with extremely fine needles. The effects provoked by the trauma are transmitted from some cells to other cells when protoplasmic bridges exist between them, but they are not transmitted if the opposite is the case. For example, in the epithelium of the skin, lesions are propagated because of anastomoses; but the same is not true with epithelial or mesodermal cells [which lack] anastomoses.

CHAPTER 7

From: *Cajal y su labor histológica,* pages 155–184*

J. F. TELLO
Universidad Central, Madrid, 1935

Degeneration and Regeneration in the Nervous System.

The nervous system, when it reaches its maximum cellular differentiation, to a large extent loses its vegetative capacities, especially that of multiplication, having acquired, instead, an exquisite sensitivity to any pathogenic action [in response to which it is predisposed] to degenerate and die. However, from early times it has been known that although the cells are not capable of multiplication, [the] broken or altered axon can be repaired, reestablishing function when it is affected in the peripheral nervous system. Cajal dedicates more than twenty of the most important works of his third period to the study of degeneration and regeneration in the peripheral and central nervous system. [These have] an intimate relationship with neurogenesis and with the verification of facts and theories, that otherwise [would have] remained baseless.

The major portion of the results obtained in his works and in those of his pupils were gathered together in two volumes in his work *Estudios Sobre la Degeneración del Sistema Nervioso,* published in 1913 and 1914 by sub-

---

*This publication is a transcript of a series of memorial lectures given by Tello in the Faculty of Medicine of Madrid. Tello distinguishes three major periods during Cajal's scientific career: ". . . the first, from 1877 to 1887, included exploration of all the fields of Histology; the second, from 1887 to 1903, the most active and the most fertile in results, in which Cajal devoted himself to study of the nervous system with the Golgi method, and the third, from 1903 to his death, also very active and in which he preferentially utilized techniques that he himself created, above all that of reduced silver in its multiple forms." We have translated the pages that deal with the work on degeneration and regeneration of the nervous system carried out in the third phase.

scriptions raised among the Spanish physicians of the Argentine Republic, on the occasion of his having been awarded the Nobel Prize. In 1928, Dr. May, who had worked in his laboratory, published a second edition in English, considerably extended by Cajal by the inclusion of all the works appearing subsequent to the Spanish edition.

We will examine the results obtained first in the peripheral nervous system and then in the central.

Degeneration and Regeneration in the Nerves.

Since the time of Johannes Müller, it has been known to the field of physiology that nerves which have been separated from their centers lack excitability, but only in the works of Waller, in the middle of the last century, can the [relevant] histological data be found. [This was] still rudimentary because of the imperfection of [his] technique, but very accurate in its interpretation, [so that we may] repeat with Cajal, that in this matter, contrary to what is usual in science, error is modern and truth old. The nerves separated from their trophic centers degenerate, and the central stump, still in continuity with the trophic center, carries exclusively the burden of regeneration.

In keeping with the rate at which technique is improved, histological knowledge of the degeneration and regeneration of nerves was becoming increasingly more complete; a quite perfect description was already found in Ranvier (1871–1878) [and it was extended] by Vanlair, Stroebe, and other investigators. The myelin is condensed, the [nodes of Ranvier] and the Schmidt-Lantermann clefts becoming more perceptible, until [the myelin is] transformed into elongated oily droplets; the axon is fragmented, the pieces [of axon] that progressively disorganize being seen in the interior of the drops of lipid; the nuclei of the cells of Schwann multiply and the protoplasm of the cells increases, being insinuated between the pieces of myelin; finally, when the remains of myelin and axon have disappeared (the leukocytes having contributed to their disappearance), the peripheral fibers are reduced to protoplasmic cords. Degeneration of a more or less extensive piece of the central stump also occurs as a consequence of the traumatic inflammation, but above this zone, the fibers grow out in search of the peripheral stump, which sooner or later they penetrate, depending on the distance and the relationship between the two stumps; at the end of a variable time, fibers with all the normal characteristics are found.

Not long after the English physiologist [Waller], two eminent French physiologists, Philippeaux and Vulpian (1859), found electrical excitability to be reestablished and regeneration to have occurred in peripheral stumps that were kept separated from the central stump; and instead of considering the possibility that a communication existed between the two stumps that was impossible to demonstrate microscopically with the methods then known, they thought that the peripheral stump could have self-regenerated, naming the process autogenic regeneration. Although Vulpian (1874) later rather changed his opinion, the idea was supported by others, above all by Büngner (1891) and Bethe (1901). According to these authors, the protoplasmic cords resulting from the hypertrophy of the cells of Schwann, generally known by the name bands of Büngner, would produce the nerve fibers piecemeal and these would be joined to one another and to those that came from the central stump; but the fibers formed in the degenerated piece of the central stump would lack continuity with the old axons until their [eventual] fusion. The fundamental experiments on which this point of view was based involved the resection of large portions [of the nerve] and the use of devices that would prevent the arrival at the peripheral stump of fibers coming from the central stump, [followed by] checking the regeneration preferentially by means of physiological methods; the histological methods up till then used, except in a very few cases, were based mostly on the impregnation of normal or altered myelin; therefore, the [histological] pursuit of the fibers was very difficult during virtually the whole process of regeneration because of the lack of a myelin sheath.

But even with such limited resources, and on occasions resorting to very capricious procedures such as that of Golgi, as used by Purpura, investigators [like] Münzer, Langley and Anderson, and Lugaro, contradicted the polygenetic or catenary hypothesis.

With the introduction in 1903 of the neurofibrillar methods of Cajal and Bielschowsky, especially that of the former, the circumstances [surrounding] the problem rapidly changed, since because of the ease with which the axons could be block-stained and the capacity to use relatively thick sections, the pursuit of the new fibers turned out to be very easy. In 1905 the very important studies of Cajal and Perroncito on the regeneration of nerves appeared and in 1907 those of myself on the regeneration of the motor nerve terminations and of those in the spindles of Kühne,* completing the evolutionary cycle. Rapidly confirmed and completed by many others, the controversy between monogeneticists and polygeneticists has been declining, and at present the discrepancies rest less on the growth of the axon than on the roles played in the definitive regeneration by the several [other] elements of the nerve.

---

*The muscle spindles.

Degeneration.

From older times two forms of degeneration were known in the nerves: *trophic or Wallerian* [degeneration] due to the lack of influence of the cell of origin on the piece that is left isolated, and *traumatic* [degeneration] produced by the direct action of the trauma; as Cajal notes, the latter is found in both the central and peripheral stump, in the zone which has suffered directly the influence of the trauma.

Let us begin with the study of the *trophic form*. This degeneration necessarily falls on those constitutive elements of the nerves which [need] the central trophic action and cannot persist without it, that is to say, the axon and the myelin; but the cells of Schwann and the connective [tissue] elements, although they can live without this trophic action, do not remain indifferent; influenced by the changes in those factors, they in their turn become notably modified.

In the drawings that we are going to [show], taken from the works of Cajal, the phenomena that occur in a nerve in degeneration are admirably represented. The first perceptible alterations of the myelin were also the first to be recognized, since they can be shown by means of osmic acid and other lipid stains, as well as by staining with hematoxylin and aniline dyes. Twenty-four hours after the cut, the myelin begins to retract, the [nodes of Ranvier] and Schmidt-Lantermann clefts becoming more perceptible, and the remaining free spaces are occupied by the protoplasm of the cells of Schwann [which is] usually increased, particularly in the [perinuclear] region. In the following days, the retraction is accentuated, the spaces occupied by the protoplasm increasing in size, and the myelin fragments now appear as thick elliptic masses; these have been shown to contain a liquid, [which] according to Nageotte is exuded by the axon in degeneration, and they have been named *digestion chambers* because portions of the disintegrating axon are found in them; this is very clearly observed on the fourth day after the cut. At the same time that the retraction is accentuated, progressive fragmentation of the myelin takes place, [the myelin] appearing [as] numerous spherules of variable size, stained black by the osmic acid; during the second week, the oily detritus blackened by the osmic acid is most abundant, the myelin, disappearing little by little, by disintegration inside the protoplasm of the cells of Schwann or in that of leukocytes into which it has been [incorporated].

We have just seen that the spaces left by the myelin during its progressive degeneration, are going to be occupied by the increasingly abundant protoplasm of the cells of Schwann. The hypertrophy of these cells begins fourteen or sixteen hours after the nerve has been cut, first becoming perceptible around the nucleus, the [internodes] appearing covered by a continuous layer of protoplasm at twenty-four or thirty-six hours; after forty-eight hours the protoplasm reaches the axon. At four days the separations between the cells which formed each of the [nodes] have been erased, the fibers appearing as continuous protoplasmic cords, the enlarged portions of which contain as inclusions the digestive chambers and numerous oily drops. At this moment, the multiplication by mitosis of the nuclei of the cells of Schwann begins, although some have observed it earlier; the number of observable mitoses increases until the sixth or ninth day and decreases thereafter, [mitoses] being difficult to find in the third week. The nuclear multiplication is not followed by division of the protoplasm; a synctium is apparently created, with chains of nuclei [named] bands of Büngner being observed in it from the beginning of the second week [and], especially in the portions without nuclei, a longitudinal striation; [this] is reinforced, three or four weeks later, by another [which] is even more obvious [and] involves the sheath of Key and Retzius.* [The striations were the] sources of error to the polygeneticists.

At the beginning of the second week, leukocytes penetrate the bands; from the second day after the cut these cells have commenced being insinuated between the nerve fibers, phagocytosing and digesting the lipoid debris and taking on the classic appearance of the [compound] granular cells, so frequent in all destructive processes of the nervous system. For many [researchers] these cells would originate from the Schwann cells: Cajal, with Marinesco and Besta were convinced in their studies that they are true leukocytes, especially the polymorphonuclear cells. By the end of one month, it is difficult to find leukocytes in the interior of the bands.

If neurotization of the peripheral stump occurs, the phenomena that are shown by the above elements are mingled with those of regeneration; but if not, little by little the cells of Schwann become marginated in the tubes, as I described and as confirmed by Cajal; plasma spaces are formed and the tubes formed by the connective [tissue] sheaths persist for a greater or lesser time, all being later transformed into ordinary connective tissue.

Study of the phenomena that occur in the degeneration of the axon, could only be successfully carried out with the neurofibrillar methods, which have shown four phases in the destruction of the nerve fibers; moniliform state, granular disintegration of the neurofibrils, fragmentation, and reabsorption. The *moniliform state* appears very clearly; in the slide† it consists of a concentration of axonic material at certain points, which reveal themselves to be thickened and fusiform, with a notable thinning of the intermediate portions, the neuroplasm being impregnated more strongly than usual so that the fibers become more diffusely blackened. This alteration is very precocious, being sometimes visible at two or three

---

*The endoneurium.
†The reader should recall that Tello's account is the transcript of a lecture.

hours, although it usually begins at twelve hours. The granular disintegration of the neurofibrils was first seen by Monckeberg and Bethe and was confirmed by Cajal, Marinesco, us, Perroncito, etc., as a transformation of the neurofibrils into granules; in such a way the moniliform masses come to consist of agglomerations of granules appearing clearly after twenty-four hours or a little later. The rupture of the fibers at the level of the thinned parts constitutes the phase of fragmentation, in which the axons are retracted inside cavities with a helicoidal appearance. The speed at which the fragmentation occurs is very variable, as has been demonstrated by Cajal, Marinesco, and us, for weakly resistant fibers exist which at forty-eight hours are broken; others [more] resistant, by this time are found only in the granular phase and, finally, the unmedullated fibers stand out by their great resistance. The reabsorption of the axon fragments occurs generally with rather more speed in the fine fibers, masses which are stained black with silver eventually being found.

As I demonstrated in my work, degeneration appears almost simultaneously over the whole length of the peripheral stump, regardless of its length, something that is to be expected, because the cause of Wallerian degeneration is the lack of trophic stimulation from the nerve cell. The phases of degeneration are also similar in the motor and sensory terminations, as can be seen in the following slides.

In some cases we observe an interesting modification of the motor end plates, in which the [terminal] ramification seems to be concentrated; it is a terminal sphere, as if it were returning to the embryonic state, appearing like an agonal survival, similar to that discovered by Cajal in traumatic degeneration, as we will now see.

Traumatic degeneration is displayed in the zone of the nerve directly influenced by the action of the trauma, that is to say, supposing that the site of maximum effect corresponds to the point at which the separation of the two stumps occurred, in each of these there will exist a zone, more or less extensive, in which the traumatic action will operate; and it will decrease from the cut towards the periphery or towards the center, depending on whether the peripheral or central stump is affected. Naturally, in the corresponding zone of the peripheral stump there will be added both degenerative forms, trophic and traumatic, but in the central stump only the traumatic will exist, for which reason [Cajal] could study it in its greatest purity. [There], the principal difference between the two forms of nervous degeneration lies in the modifications of the axon; many fibers degenerate much faster [in traumatic] than in trophic [degeneration], no doubt because of the zone of infiltration corresponding to the inflammation (liquids, leukocytes, etc.); completely destroyed portions are found less than twenty-four hours after the trauma. In other [cases] the traumatic action is so intense that the portion directly influenced rapidly dies, undergoing a kind of coagulation that impedes the degenerative actions for a rather long time; under the microscope, these portions appear as if they were completely normal, except for a more intense staining, having been named by Cajal *conserved fibers;* above this part we can find in the same fibers another part showing rapid destruction and at a somewhat greater distance [the state] of *agonal reaction or the metamorphic segment.*

Except in the conserved fibers and in the portions of very rapid destruction, the axon survives for some time, during which, because of the influence of the trauma, there are produced modifications that resemble the regenerative processes with which we shall deal later; [the similarities] lie in the appearance of terminal clubs, in the fraying of the neurofibrillar stump, in the formation of two regenerative zones joined together by one or several very fine threads, which demonstrate, according to Cajal, a certain autonomy of the neurofibrils, [and] in the branching of fibrils inside the necrotic portions of the sheath. The rest of the fiber remains indifferent, until the phenomena of trophic degeneration arise, but frequently intermediate zones are found in which regenerative phenomena are observed that are less marked in the vicinity of the junctional discs.*

Regeneration.

In the central stump, the intermediate portion, between the traumatically degenerated and the indifferent portions, constitutes the zone of regeneration. As has been known since the time of Ranvier, the persisting part of the sectioned axon ends in a thickening, but the studies of Cajal have also shown (fig. 64) [*fig. 41*] that both the collaterals and all the [sprouted] fibers terminate in balls, spheres, or boutons of growth, identical to those discovered by Cajal in growing fibers during development; the works of the Master also demonstrated that in the vast majority of cases, the terminal ball of the primitive axons is rarely exploited in the regeneration, the regeneration usually occurring [through] the collateral or terminal sprouts, and almost always above the terminal ball.

The terminal thickening of the primitive fiber, during the first two hours, notably resembles the termination of the metamorphic zone of the peripheral stump, showing the appearance of a brush of neurofibrils; soon after, it forms a sort of concavity which embraces the degenerated part; from five hours on, it exhibits an olive-shaped disposition; but although this is the most frequent, the process does not occur with the same speed in all the fibers, [and it is possible] to find different phases in the same section. The zone of regenerative reaction is distinguished by its turgidity, by its more

---

* At the nodes of Ranvier. See page 42 of volume 1.

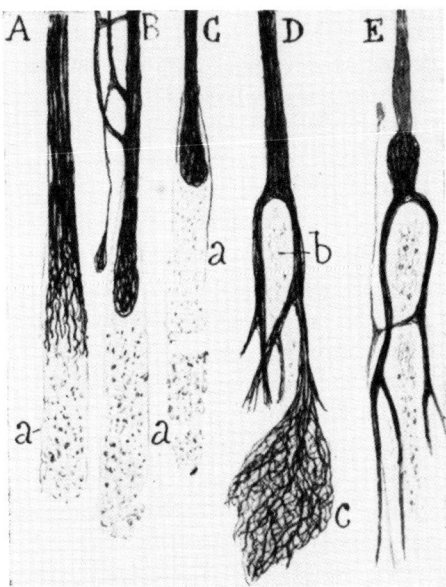

[*FIG. 41*] Fig. 64. Fibers of the central stump of the sciatic nerve of a cat fifty hours after section. Method of reduced silver nitrate (Cajal). *A*, axon with hypertrophied neurofibrils; *B*, *C*, axons whose ends, shaped like bulbs, are inserted into the disintegrated segment; *D*, *E*, axons from whose final bulbs new branches emerge.

intense impregnation with silver and by its capacity to produce sprouts.

The neoformation can be terminal or collateral. The former occurs sometimes as a direct growth of the fiber through its end, [such as] when one is dealing with unmedullated or finely medullated fibers (it being noted that the terminal club is prolongated directly or by means of branches arising from it, until it penetrates the coagulum that fills the cut, all the new fibers ending in clubs or rings). At other times there seems to be produced a fraying of the neurofibrils, [forming] tufts of neurofibrils that outline vacuolated portions and separate as they reach the end. On occasions, the terminal growth is indirect, since the terminal club degenerates, the persisting portion embracing it and forming a hairpin which grows at its ends, first inside the sheath of Schwann and later on the outside [and] branched.

The collateral neoformation appears in all cases in which the trauma has been intense and the necrotic portion relatively long; it looks as if the most proximal part of the metamorphic zone was partially lesioned and had lost the capacity to complete the regeneration that had started. The emissions of new fibers can take place at any site if the zone of emergence is close to the terminal club, but if it is distant they always arise at the level of a strangulation.* The study of this mode of neoformation which gives rise to very curious phenomena is the work of Perroncito and Cajal. The fibers growing inside the sheaths of Schwann describe numerous turns and engender the apparatuses of Perroncito, so named by Cajal and clearly [shown] in the slide. In many cases they are of notable complexity, presenting pathological forms of regeneration, which do not lead to any definitive result. Many of the new fibers of the regeneration, [however], are intratubal collaterals which invade the scar.

The new fibers, whether collaterals or terminals, begin to invade the *scar* from the third day (fig. 65, *D*) [*fig. 42*], this name being applied to the gap that remains between the two stumps, first [filled] by exudates and coagulated blood, and later mainly by connective tissue. Given the differential rate at which the sprouting occurs, the invasion is gradual, the faster sprouts penetrating first and the others later, [that is to say,] in the order in which they are produced, and they always end in clubs or rings. The fibers leave the nerve through the stump itself, or by going across the sheath, using little breaks in this, since in general, all forms of connective tissue sheath offer a great resistance to being pierced by the growing fibers, as we will see repeatedly; it is interesting that each of the interstices is used by a goodly number of fibers, as if the first fiber that arrived had attracted the later ones, a phenomenon [that is] frequent both in regeneration and in the genesis of the nervous system.

[During] most of the first week, the fibers which pass through the wound or the interval between the stumps are completely naked, which does not mean, as some [authors] would have deliberately attributed to Cajal and to those of us who have insisted on this phenomenon, that the fibers run through empty spaces, but rather that they are found frequently in exudates in which there are still no cells; or [even] if there are, they lack the path in which [fibers] have necessarily to travel; cells are seen frequently in the path of the fibers, but this does not happen in a constant manner and in the absence of parallelism between cells and fibers that would permit us to suppose such a relationship [to exist]. We have also found something similar in the formation of the nerves in the early stages of embryonic development; this is at present one of the most debated problems, [mainly] because [researchers] persist in not studying carefully the first phases of both processes; we will dwell later on this problem.

At the first moments [the axons] grow in the most varied directions, but later they are directed in increasingly straight lines towards the peripheral stump, forming bundles of fibers from which fibers that are directed to other bundles separate off to form kinds of chiasmata. The fibers of the bundles are either direct sprouts from the terminal buds or collaterals of the axons of the

---

* The node of Ranvier.

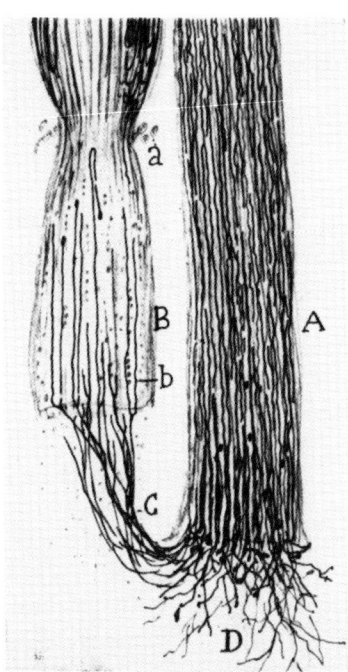

[*FIG. 42*] Fig. 65. Central stump of the sciatic nerve eight days after section and ligature of one of the halves at *a*. Method of reduced silver nitrate (Cajal). *A*, nonligated piece; *B*, degenerated piece in the ligated half; *D*, fibers dispersed in the scar; *C*, fasciculi that are directed to the degenerated piece.

central stump reunited by mutual attraction or by the common action of the orientational mechanisms, but a very great number result from the multiplication of the fibers in their course through the scar.

As Cajal has demonstrated, although all the newly formed fibers terminate in little clubs, not all can be considered growth clubs similar to those described by him and Lenhossék in embryos, since many, and particularly the largest and the ones most frequently observed by those who study these processes, are clubs stopped in their course [and] aborted or degenerated. For this reason, Perroncito, Da Fano, and Bethe do not concede to them a regenerative character, and Marinesco and Dustin consider them to be a manifestation of delayed growth; but numerous facts demonstrate the basis of the opinion of Cajal: particularly the termination in clubs of fibers which grow in tissue cultures [as shown] by Harrison and others, and the demonstration by myself that fibers which grow without obstacles in small nerves, inside or outside the old sheaths, and those that arrive at the old motor end plate to regenerate the motor endings, are found provided with small balls of growth.

Although the fibers need the influence of the [parent] cells to which they belong to grow and subsist, the nutritional influence of the tissue which supports them is indubitable; in this regard there are great differences among the different elements that can form the scar, the connective [tissue] being [evidently] the most favorable. In our experiments with grafts of nerves kept in the oven over a rather long time, or in Ringer's or Locke's solution, we observed that the connective [tissue] of the scar was not homogeneous, [since there] existed a peripheral zone of connective [tissue] apparently originating from the neurilemma or its vicinity, which did not show a [capacity] for the growth of nerve fibers, whereas, at the center, the connective [tissue] seemed to come from the interior of the nerve, and was an excellent medium for the nerve fibers.

According to Dustin the fibers could grow only along paths formed by the connective [tissue] cells (theory of *odogenesis*), but Cajal, us, and some others, although recognizing the influence of the cellular medium, could not accept such a definitive action, since in many cases, growth of the nerve fibers independent of the cells of the scar can easily be observed.

The interstices of small pieces of muscle included in the scar also offer a good field for the [survival] of nerve fibers, which wind repeatedly around the muscle fibers and branch many times; they also grow around fat fibers but find a great resistance, however, in blood clots and foreign bodies (silk, bone, etc.), although, from time to time, the fibers grow in the interstices, showing the influence of the *stereotropism* revealed by Harrison. In our experiments with grafts in the cerebral cortex, we saw the growth of fibers completely free of cells in the interstices of lycopodium.

As we have indicated, during the first week the fibers run through the scar, without a connective [tissue] or myelin sheath, but after this time one begins to find cells along the bundles of fibers, first in a discontinuous manner, later as a small membrane which covers the bundle, forming the sheath of Schwann corresponding to each of the fibers. These cells, according to some (Kölliker, Kölster, Stroebe, etc.) would be of a connective [tissue] nature, whereas for the majority of the polygeneticists they would come from the cells of Schwann of the nerve [and these] in turn would come from the ectoderm. Cajal, who in his first works was a supporter of the mesodermal theory, later, in view of the experiments of Harrison who had seen nerves grow uncovered by cells of Schwann in embryos in which the neural crest had been destroyed, is uncertain about it. I, as a consequence of my work in embryos, think that the cells of Schwann constitute a special lineage of cells. The continuous observation of mesodermal cells with [Golgi apparatus] impregnated with the reduced silver method of Cajal, has convinced me that not all the cells are of the same nature; in the mouse, those which appear more intensely impregnated and which have a somewhat different character, originate from the splachnopleure, accompany the nerves which grow in great quantities, [and] seem to form the chromaffin cells (as I expounded in the work for the public competition for the Chair of Histology) and the cells of the nerves; in the chicken, those that I saw around the fourth and fifth branchial arches, near the vagus, seem to produce the cells included in the carotid body, situated as a ganglion of the vagus in the upper part of the thorax, and the cells of the nerves. Hence, although we have not been able yet to establish the relationship in an indubitable way, it seems to us that those cells may also be cells of Schwann. The formation of the abdominal recticular cells of the mouse by the mesothelium is indubitable, but we have not been able to observe the origin from the epithelium of those of the branchial arches of the chicken, even in the first moments of their appearance.

The myelin appears much later. Cajal, who with his method observed it earlier than the other investigators, distinguishes it from the twenty-fifth day.

The arrival of the fibers at the *peripheral stump* will be more or less delayed depending on the distance that remains between the two stumps, the nature of the scar, the material included in it, the age of the animal, the [extent of the] necrotic portion, etc., but from ten to fifteen days (Cajal, Perroncito) fibers begin to enter the peripheral stump (fig. 66) [*fig. 3, bis* see Chapter 3].* The behavior of the fibers when they arrive differs, as Cajal has perfectly shown, depending on the state of the peripheral stump; it is possible to distinguish in this, neurotization which is late (from the twenty-fifth to thirtieth day) (fig. 67) [*fig. 43*] or early (from the tenth day), depending on a number of conditions that more or less delay the arrival of the fibers at the peripheral stump, which will be found [as a consequence] in different states of degeneration. If the [fibers] arrive late, then most of the remnants of the old fibers and of the myelin have disappeared, and abundant neurotropic substances exist, and, [if] the quantity of fibers that arrive is relatively scarce, these find a very easy path for their course; the fibers divide at the entrance to the peripheral stump, the branches entering different sheaths; [some sheaths contain] branches of several fibers and [some branches] run outside the sheaths. The course is rapid, and the fibers end in small spherical or olive-shaped clubs. If the arrival [of the fibers] is rapid, many appear at the same time, [and] many of these penetrate the sheaths or [run] among them without branching during their course,

---

*Tello's legend for this figure reads: Arrival of new fibers at the peripheral stump from the central. Method of reduced silver nitrate (Cajal). *f*, empty sheath; *a* and *b*, new fibers which are divided and enter the sheaths; *d*, growth club; *e*, fiber that is divided, one of the branches entering a sheath and the other running among [the sheaths].

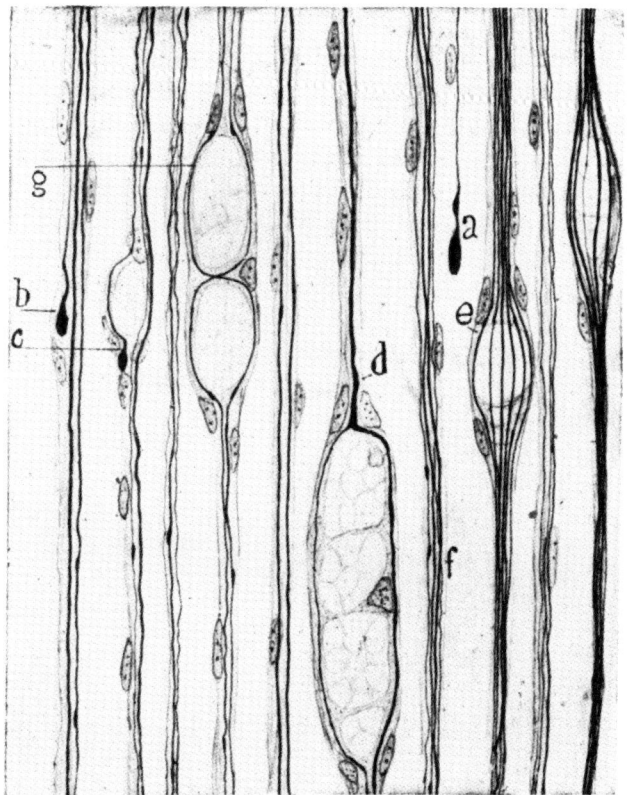

[*FIG. 43*] Fig. 67. New fibers in the peripheral stump twenty-seven days after the section. Method of silver nitrate (Cajal). *a*, intestinal club; *b*, straight club of a [fiber]; *c*, the same which has passed on oily droplet; *d*, axon which has divided on arriving at an oily droplet; *e*, bundle of fibers which outline an oily droplet; *f*, bundle of fibers; *g*, fibers that are passing between two droplets.

ending like debrided brushes or in sharp ends; along their route they frequently encounter myelin fragments which they outline. In spite of the obstacles, the growth of the fibers inside the sheaths is rapid, as though these stimulate [the fibers]. Another difference from late regeneration is the presence of old fibers still in the process of degeneration.

After a very variable length of time, depending mainly on the length of the peripheral stump, that is to say, the distance of the nerve termination from the point at which the nerve was cut, and many other circumstances (among which stand out any that might modify the emergence of the sprouts and the length and conditions of the scar), the fibers arrive at the [vicinity] of their termination (muscle, skin, etc). In my works on the regeneration of motor endings, I saw the fibers of the sciatic nerve, which had been sectioned halfway along the thigh of the rabbit, arrive at the triceps surae muscle, two and a half or three months after the section, and in animals a few days old from one and a half to two months; Boeke, who has confirmed to a large extent my observations, has found in the hypoglossal and the intercostal nerves shorter periods of one month and a half to two months; Cajal, who also confirmed my observations, saw them arrive, in animals a few days old, at forty days, and at twenty [days] in nerves of short length.

With the arrival of the nerves at their organs of distribution a rapid branching commences which can be by bifurcation or by the emission of collaterals; the new fibers that run through the empty nerves repair the old ramification to a state similar to the original, sending collaterals preferentially where formerly there were also collaterals and dividing into two fibers of similar [caliber], where there had been [such] divisions. After many repeated divisions, the fibers arrive at the final ramifications of the old nerve in which the fibers remain isolated, covered only by the sheaths of Henle and Schwann, which are the only [elements] persisting on their arrival, appearing like tubes filled with liquid or rather of a substance of lesser consistency than that forming the protoplasm of the cells of Schwann.

As soon as the fibers arrive at the termination of the sheaths, and in many cases before, they leave the sheaths and are directed to the protoplasmic-nuclear remains of the old end plates and to other nuclear agglomerations on the surfaces of the muscle fibers, in order to form the new terminations. This attraction of the nuclei and the end plates for the nerve fibers is indubitable, and I, myself, explain it in the context of the neurotropic doctrine, by the emission of substances that would act like an inducement, having influence, it is thought, not only on the arrival of the new fibers but [also] on the formation of the branches of the future arborizations; this modeling influence appears much clearer, as I have demonstrated, in the formation of the end plates during the embryonic period. In effect, the plate in its first moments shows only the fiber that has just penetrated ending in a small club, but later sprouts arise from this that finish up by forming a ramification like the original one. Frequently, a single free fiber can form several plates before it comes to an end, contrasting with what is observed in the distribution of a normal nerve and looking very much like the ramification of the fibers of embryos.

In the sensory terminations on the fascicles of Weissmann* of the muscles, I have found similar phenomena. Of course, the motor ending on those fibers regenerates exactly the same as the motor ending of the remaining fibers of the muscle; with regard to the true sensory termination it regenerates out of the [nerve] fibers that, once inside the old sheath of the

---

*The intrafusal fibers.

fascicle, abundantly ramify, forming bundles of fibers which outline the nuclear or central portions of the [intrafusal] fibers, showing thick intumescences.

Degeneration and Regeneration in the Nerve Centers.

The different histological constitution [of the gray and white matter] ensures that the degenerative and regenerative processes do not present the same characteristics in the white and gray matter, although in essence they are of the same character.

Degeneration in the White Matter

The most favorable place for the study of degeneration of the white matter is the spinal cord because of its simpler organization. If, for example, a cut is made in the white matter of the spinal cord, as we have seen in the nerves, two classes of alterations will be produced in the nerve fibers: one due to the direct action of the trauma, the traumatic degeneration described by Schiefferdecker, and the other due to the cutting off of the neurons which give origin to the fibers, the trophic degeneration of Waller or secondary degeneration.

The *traumatic degeneration*, like in the nerves, will be more or less extensive, depending on the nature and intensity of the trauma, the production of hemorrhages, etc., and it is observed to be similar at the two edges of the wound. Usually, it comprises an extent of one to two millimeters, and includes both a necrotic zone and a degenerative zone. In the necrotic zone, from the first hours fibers are found transformed into granular masses, which disappear very rapidly; if the action has been much more intense, we will also find preserved fibers, as in the similar cases of the nerves. In the degenerative zone we will see at intervals the swellings of the myelin sheath, which is transformed into ellipsoids and oily droplets, whereas the axon becomes rosary-like by the accumulation at certain places of argentophilic matter; the part of the axon (fig. 68, *D*) [*fig. 14* see chapter 4]* which is adjacent to the necrotic zone retracts, forming a club of retraction; this is

---

*Tello's legend for this figure reads: Central portion of the white matter of the spinal cord, three days after section. Method of silver nitrate (Cajal). *A*, thickened collaterals which are transformed into terminals; *a, b, c*, terminal portions of axons destined to disappear; *B*, club with an appendage; *C*, terminal glomerulus; *D*, border of the wound with detritus of axons and lipoids; *e*, free clubs which have become hyaline.

soon after separated from the rest of the fiber by a kind of autotomy, forming a new [club of retraction] which in turn undergoes autotomy, and so on until in this way both the unmedullated and fine medullated fibers in the whole degenerated zone are destroyed; [by contrast] in the thick medullated [fibers] the autotomy of the ball of retraction and of all the thickenings of the axon happen simultaneously. If we examine now the part of the degenerated segment adjacent to the normal zone, we find some phenomena that recall those affecting the metamorphic portion of the peripheral stump of a sectioned [peripheral] nerve, such as the appearance of certain thickenings with neurofibrillar cores and ramifications, and others with a hump shape, as if they had an inclination to emit branches. In the whole traumatically degenerated portion leukocytes are soon (after twenty-four hours) found that are loaded with myelin fragments, forming the [compound] granular cells, which have been known since older times [and] to whose formation the neuroglial cells will also later contribute.

Wallerian or secondary degeneration is difficult to distinguish in the early stages, since both ascending and descending fibers exist in the fasciculi of the spinal cord, [and] it is not easy to recognize which is really the peripheral stump, until total degeneration [allows one] to distinguish [between the central and peripheral]. Nevertheless, it has been possible to perform the study on the posterior columns and on others in which most fibers are ascending; in them it is seen that the degeneration occurs as in the nerves, with the formation of varicosities, followed by fragmentation and granular disintegration of the condensations. There are great differences in regard to the speed of the phenomenon among unmedullated, thin medullated, and thick medullated fibers; the latter degenerate much more rapidly than the others, appearing fragmented from the fourth to the eighth day, whereas the medium medullated [fibers] do so from the fourteenth to the eighteenth, and in the thin ones there is not the least sign of degeneration from the eighth to the tenth [days].

If the spinal cord is studied one or one and a half months after the cut, the [affected part] is found to be replaced by a scar, made up of neuroglia, some lipoidal fragments, a cyst, and a few [compound] granular cells; most of the latter have disappeared, as well as all the axonal fragments. The axons of the white matter close [to the cut] form arcs which penetrate into the gray matter, because of the degeneration of the whole portion of the fiber that was left without function, that is to say, up to the origin of the nearest persisting collateral.

With regard to the roots of the spinal cord, we will find in the extraspinal portions the same phenomena as in the nerves, whereas in the short intraspinal course [the phenomena] of traumatic inflammation will predominate.

Another portion of the nerve centers in which degenerative phenomena of the white matter are easily observable, because of the uniformity of its fibers, is the optic nerve. My work, confirmed by O. Rossi, Leoz [Ortín] and Arcaute, Cajal, and others, has demonstrated that on either side of a cut, the phenomena of traumatic degeneration are identical to those described in the spinal cord; also identical is the secondary degeneration of the peripheral stump, which in this case is the portion joined to the brain.

The cerebellum also is particularly useful for the study of degenerative phenomena, as Cajal repeatedly demonstrated in his works, because of the perfect organization of its fibers, and although it offers some slight peculiarities, what we have said about the spinal cord can be applied to it in broad outline, both for the traumatic degeneration and for the secondary degeneration of the distal stump.

In the degeneration of the white matter of the cerebrum some interesting details are found. Of course, as seen in the slide, in the region of traumatic degeneration the same zones exist as in the other centers, although the phenomenon of preserved fibers acquires more importance, [since] even complete dendrites and neurons are observed in this state. Also interesting is the great participation in the ball of retraction, as well as in the varicosities along the course [of the fiber], of the terminal glomerulus and of the spirals along the course.

Degeneration in the Gray Matter.

The cells of the portion of the gray matter of the nerve centers that suffers the direct action of the trauma undergo traumatic degeneration, which is revealed by several cellular alterations that vary with the severity of the action. In the most severely affected, necrosis is observed, with granular degeneration of the protoplasm and a failure to stain or little staining of the nuclei and Nissl granules; if the lesion is less severe and, consequently, the death of the cells slower, phenomena of reaction are found; these are represented by neurofibrillar hypertrophy, similar to that revealed in rabies by Cajal and García Izcara, [and by] neurofibrillar atrophy especially in the peripheral portion, the perinuclear meshwork persisting. With other methods, chromatolysis, margination of the nucleus, fragmentation of the Golgi complex, and vacuolation are observed.

From the point of view of the degeneration of the nerve cells, the spinal ganglia occupy a peculiar situation, since although they can be considered as centers, the presence of satellite cells and the intermingling of bundles of medullated fibers with cells of Schwann give them a special character. The neurons rapidly die on account of the intense action of the trauma [and] are soon transformed into masses of granular detritus that rapidly disappears, being replaced by groups of polyhedral cells and leukocytes which make up the residual nodules of Nageotte; the former stem from the satellite cells. In the most indirectly influenced [neurons], we found leech-shaped [neurons formed] because of the atrophy of the superficial neurofibrils, and other [forms] that arise on account of the progressive penetration of the neuron by the satellite cells, [for example], tearing, angular, retracted, and deformed [types], all of them described by Cajal. In the bundles of fibers we find degenerative phenomena exactly the same as those described in the peripheral nerves.

Regeneration in the White Matter.

The incapacity of the central nervous pathways to regenerate is a dogma accepted by science, although a good number of investigators have found indubitable phenomena of regeneration in lower vertebrates and even, to a lesser extent, in mammals. However, the study of all of these aborted phenomena of regeneration has only been capable of being carried out perfectly since we came to possess the neurofibrillar methods, for these have allowed us to see clearly the behavior of the nerve fibers; Nageotte and Marinesco indicated regenerative phenomena in the altered [dorsal] roots of tabetic [individuals], and Cajal inaugurated experimental investigations which were followed by many other [researchers].

In the stumps of the thin and medium fibers of the fasciculi of the spinal cord, near wounds, Cajal demonstrated indubitable phenomena of regeneration, above all in animals a few days old, this regenerative zone being characterized, as in the nerves, by the increase in thickness of the fibers, their greater stainability, and their striated appearance. In the eight-day-old dog, three or four days after section of the spinal cord, there is seen the production of branches that invade the borders of the wound, sometimes by terminal division at other times by the emission of terminal or collateral branches, as seen in the slides in which are gathered the main types. The process of new formation is stopped, or at least decreases, from the tenth to fourteenth day; the new fibers, having become atrophied, disappear by reabsorption.

If the portions of the fasciculi in which the above-mentioned regenerative phenomena occur are close to the roots of the spinal cord or if one is dealing with the intraspinal portions of the roots, the regenerative phenomena acquire even more intensity, as if the presence of the roots for some reason, can stimulate the growth of the fibers. The fibers of the sectioned motor roots, as Cajal has demonstrated, exhibit from the fourth day a prominent sprouting, forming branches, some of which, after following the path of the root, go through the [base] of the root and enter its extraspinal course; others do not succeed in crossing the [base] of the root and remain in the fasciculi. The branches entering the root continue the course [of the root], but emit numerous retrograde collaterals directed towards the spinal cord, which many succeed in penetrating, dividing, and giving branches; [some of these] follow the intraspinal path of the same root, [while] others become ascending or descending inside the fasciculi of the spinal cord. Of those stopped at the [base] of the root, many remain there, but others branch, giving off ascending or descending fibers.

The fibers of the [spinal cord] fasciculi also receive an intense stimulus to grow, probably because of the presence of the bands of Büngner of the root; the fiber is directed to the root from its termination or by one or two collateral branches, as seen in the slide.

In the dorsal root the regenerative phenomena are even more evident, as is to be expected, since the fibers that course through it are the axons of the [dorsal root] ganglion cells, and in their extraspinal portion they behave as [fibers] in the central stump of a nerve. The fibers are branched, heading for the spinal cord which many succeed in penetrating, becoming ascending or descending in the dorsal columns, and although in approximately *six percent* of the cases the fibers bifurcate when they penetrate, giving an ascending and a descending branch, this does not constitute a general rule, as [D']Abundo and Dustin claimed. Most of the fibers do not succeed in penetrating the spinal cord, remaining at the surface, where they begin to organize like a new dorsal column. Some fibers produce retrograde collaterals, and not a few fibers leave the root and penetrate the connective [tissue] of the scar, where they grow like the fibers of every nerve. Also, the fibers of the [dorsal columns] acquire, because of the influence of the roots, a great regenerative capacity, as seen in the slide, the extensive ramification being formed by a single fiber.

True regenerative phenomena in the optic nerve were revealed by me in 1907, as we indicated before, and were confirmed by O. Rossi, Leoz Ortín and Arcaute, and Cajal.* The central [diencephalic] stump, which in this case is the peripheral [stump] since it is the one that contains the pieces of fibers separated from their neurons of origin, shows in the metamorphic zone of fibers a frustrated regeneration, similar to that observed by Perroncito and Cajal in the peripheral stumps of nerves; fibers grow towards the scar, isolated or in bundles, these phenomena having a certain vitality because of the persistence of good perfusion due to the conservation of the central artery of the retina in [the retinal] stump. Although the vascular circumstances are the opposite in the peripheral stump, [which] is in this case the central [diencephalic stump] for the reason above indicated, the regenerative phenomena are still more intense than in the other [stump];

---

*The following, somewhat confused account of Tello is rendered far more clearly in Cajal's description of the same experiments on page 586 of the present work.

the turgidity of the zones of growth is greater, the fibers appearing thicker and the ramifications greater; very frequently a characteristic termination of the fibers is seen that we showed and which Cajal confirmed, namely the termination in fine balls and rings that gather together in groups, resembling racemes. In both stumps, all of these sprouts disappear by atrophy, no remains of them being found on the fortieth day.

O. Rossi, because he avoided section of the [central] artery of the retina, achieved even more significant regenerative phenomena in the retinal stump, and Weissfesler in the urodeles even observed the formation of a new [optic] chiasm.

In the cerebrum and cerebellum, the regenerative phenomena in the sectioned white matter are even more precarious since neither growth of fibers nor ramifications of any extent are found; the only manifestation that it is possible to show is the appearance of the testudinoid and cephalopodic formations, and the beginnings of an occasional collateral. The former consist of thick varicosities, from which arise diverging and short little branches, recalling the appearance of a tortoise with the feet extended; the latter are [made up of] small branches of the axon itself.

We have seen that the proximity of the [spinal] roots with their cells of Schwann notably stimulates the growth of the axons of the white matter in the cut spinal cord; in the other nervous centers, these circumstances are not immediately present, and it occurred to me to promote these conditions experimentally by putting peripheral nerves in front of the lesions of central nerve fasciculi. With this aim I addressed, in the first instance, the cerebral cortex.

Lugaro was the first to graft pieces of the sciatic nerve into the cerebral cortex of the dog one or two months old [but] without results. I used the rabbit as the experimental animal. In order to excite the potential tendency to growth, I introduced into wounds that I performed in the cerebral cortex, pieces of the peripheral stump of the sciatic nerve eight or fourteen days after it had been cut. [This was to ensure that] the fibers of the nerve would disappear (*empty graft*) [so as to avoid] error in the interpretation and to allow time for the formation of the bands of Büngner, which are the major source of neurotropic materials in the regeneration of the nerves. With such important modifications, we had the good fortune to see, when the graft was well incorporated, that the fibers of the white matter were penetrating the nerve and following long trajectories inside or among the bands of Büngner, depending on the degree of vitality that had been conserved in the graft. I also saw fibers penetrate pieces of elder pith impregnated with neurotropic substances.

Another very appropriate place for the study of regenerative phenomenon in the central pathways is the optic nerve, which, after all, is no more than a central nervous path; together with Dr. Leoz y Ortín, a skillful ophthalmologist and enthusiast for histological studies, I placed in the cut optic nerves of rabbits, pieces of empty sciatic nerves. Unfortunately, the movements of the eyeball, which we could not avoid, caused the graft to suffer alterations and deviations that prevented the connective [tissue] union of the optic nerve with the grafted piece of sciatic nerve; even under these unfavorable conditions, [however], we saw that the fibers of the optic nerve showed a greater regenerative tendency; in one case in which the nerves had remained close and joined by connective [tissue] and in which granular cells did not impede the penetration of the fibers, the latter had grown much more that in simple sections of the optic nerve and they were undoubtedly directed towards the graft. Three years later, Leoz together with Arcaute repeated the experiments and they were more successful in obtaining grafts with the optic nerve that remained joined from one end to the other, and they saw the penetration of the fibers of the optic nerve into the graft.

After this brief review of the regenerative phenomena in the nervous pathways of the white matter, and although the studies of Cajal and ourselves infer a certain optimism for the future, when it may be possible to find substances that by exciting the neurons would promote the regenerative tendency to a degree hitherto unknown, it is a fact that the regeneration in the white matter of the nervous centers is completely ineffectual.

Regeneration in the Gray Matter.

Let us see now what happens when wounds fall on the gray matter, [which is] of greatest interest from the point of view of the restoration of function and from that of the theory of free growth; [and let us see also] the phenomena of reaction of the distant neurons. Both classes of phenomena present a greater intensity in the ganglia as was to be expected because of their situation, half in the central and half in the peripheral [nervous system]. As seen in the slide, the phenomena consist of the emission of new processes called paraphytes by Nageotte [and] which arise from the soma or from the initial glomerulus, and more rarely in the emission of fibers that, divided or not, terminate in balls; at other times [there is] the formation of tangles around the nerve cells at the expense of the newly formed fibers that go backwards from the cut nerve fibers. The same phenomena, emission of paraphytes and branches and the formation of pericellular tangles and interstitial plexuses, are observed in ganglia in which the corresponding roots have been sectioned, without cutting the ganglia directly. But, where these manifestations of a regenerative nature reached greatest proportions, was in the experiments [involving] transplantation and *in vitro* culture of the ganglia, especially as made by Nageotte, Marinesco, and Cajal; in these, they excised spinal ganglia and put them underneath the skin or in the interior of parenchymatous organs, liver, etc. In the central zone of the ganglion [which was] the worst nourished, intense phenomena of neurophagia were produced, whereas at the periphery an intense sprouting was seen. In the cultures or, more correctly, in the ganglia kept in Ringer's or Locke's solution, the emission of thick branches from the soma and [axon] was also observed.

The phenomenon of neurocladism or emission of branches, so abundant in the ganglion cells, was not seen by Cajal in his repeated experiments on clean wounds of the spinal cord, in spite of the affirmation of O. Rossi; that is to say, in [experiments] that are not accompanied by bruising; only in an occasional case did he observe some fibers that had penetrated and seemed to ramify in the scar, but he showed himself to be doubtful in [this] interpretation, even reaching the point of suspecting that they might be preserved fibers. In spinal contusions, with or without a wound, it is easier to find [ventral horn] cells which appear to emit thickened branches and axons with apparent production of branches, and although Cajal thought, by comparison with what is normally found, that a true formation of branches was being dealt with, he could not exclude the possibility that they could indicate already existing collaterals.

In the retina, I demonstrated in 1907 indubitable regenerative phenomena; as a consequence of the section of the optic nerve, a retrograde degeneration of many fibers is produced that is observed in the layer of the optic nerve fibers at the thirteenth day, but with greater intensity at the fortieth day; [there is] thickening of the fibers and the production of branches that are disoriented in their trajectory and that terminate in little balls. In their disorientation, the new fibers go across the different layers of the retina, in a radial or oblique direction, becoming stopped at the level of the plexiform [layers] or in the pigment [layer]; sometimes they branch, from which we gave them the name of perforant fibers. Figures 3, 4, and 5 of that work* give a clear idea of this disorientation. These phenomena of induced [fiber branching] in the retina were confirmed in [1913] by Leoz and Arcaute who, thanks to the fortunate circumstance of having produced in occasional cases a traumatic inflammation of the sclera with a connective [tissue] scar, observed this sprouting and disorientation discovered by me, with a greater intensity; [this] is seen in figures 3 and 4 of their work which [show] many new fibers that reach the sclera or form plexuses in the original plexiform [layers], [that is to say], in the originally degenerated layers, giving rise, as Leoz and Arcaute say, to a kind of pseudo-retina. In

---

*Tello, J. F. (1907), La régénération dans les voies optiques. *Trav Lab Rech Biol*, Univ Madrid 5:237–248.

1923, our late lamented colleague Muñoz Urra also confirmed these discoveries of ours which, as we saw on other occasions, have great significance for the criticism of the theory of preestablished paths in the growth of nerve cells.

In the cerebellar and cerebral cortices not stimulated by neurotropic substances, the regenerative phenomena amount to little more than the survival and hypertrophy of the portion of axon from the first collateral existing above the section; this fact, already seen in the spinal cord, acquires in the cerebellum and cerebrum an interesting significance, since in the spinal cord the fiber of the white matter that [loses] a part of its course by degeneration, is still a link between different levels of the spinal cord, that is to say, it continues to belong to a cell with a long axon, although of shorter length; in the cerebellum and cerebrum, as the collaterals arise preferentially from the proximal part of the axon, the cells are transformed as Cajal demonstrated, into cells with short axons. This phenomenon is observed particularly in the cerebellum, where because of the thinness of the white matter it is difficult to lesion it without lesioning the adjacent gray [matter] and, epecially, the cells of Purkinje, [which are] so easy to see; in the slide (fig. 69) [*fig. 44*] are gathered different aspects of the modifications that those cells undergo as a consequence of the nearby trauma; the cells that, like the [one labeled] A,* have remained without collaterals, degenerate, showing curious transformations of their [dendritic] branches; in those that have conserved collaterals [A] the axon is notably hypertrophied in its [initial] portion and the cell persists indefinitely; it is as though the cell [thanks to these collaterals], had kept its function [although] no longer involved in the transmission of nervous commands to different centers but with [transmission] of the impressions of one cell of Purkinje to the neighboring [cells of Purkinje], as though it were a cell with a short axon.

An identical thing occurs in the cerebral cortex; the axons of the pyramids degenerate back to the first collateral, the pyramids being transformed, [and those which] become devoid of collaterals, as a consequence, are without possible function.

Neurotropism in Nerve Regeneration.

When we dealt with neurogenesis, we expounded the chemotactic hypothesis of Cajal to explain the orientation of the fibers during growth; experimental

---

*Not seen in the figure.

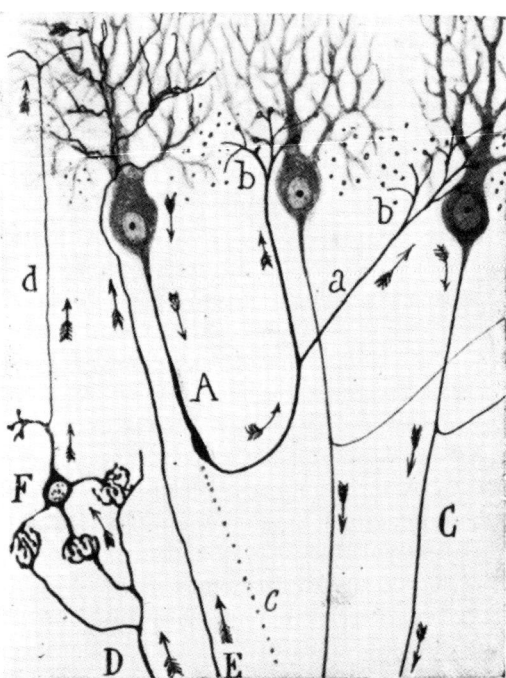

[*FIG. 44*] Fig. 69. Scheme that shows the path of the [impulses] in the cells of Purkinje which have been deprived of the peripheral portion of the axon (Cajal). *A*, arciform Purkinje cells; *D*, mossy fibers; *E*, climbing fiber; *F*, granule cell; *C*, normal axons of the cells of Purkinje; *c*, position that had been occupied by the disappeared axon.

confirmation came with the study of the regeneration of nerve fibers. Forssmann, in 1898, without having knowledge of the ideas of Cajal, maintained that fibers are directed towards the peripheral stump by a tropism of a chemical nature that he called *neurotropism*. Kappers (1920), who recognizes in Cajal "the merit of having stated the tropic character of that process and the tropic influence of the nerve element," explains these tropisms by the change of position of the nerve nuclei during phylogeny and calls the process *neurobiotaxis*.

Forssmann achieved the first experimental demonstration of neurotropism. In his first experiment, already mentioned, he sectioned the sciatic nerve of the guinea pig and introduced the central and peripheral stumps into opposite openings of a tube of straw, joined together by silk, observing after two months by means of the Weigert-Pal method, that the fibers of the central stump had reached the peripheral stump, neurotizing it through the thread; this was the normal simple case of regeneration of a sectioned nerve, apparently perfectly explicable by the tendency [of the fiber] to grow in a continuous manner from the cell of origin, the idea of Ranvier, Vanlair, Stroebe, etc., that was very popular at that time. In the second [experiment], he introduced the two ends of the sectioned sciatic nerve into the upper opening of the straw tube, the central directly and the peripheral by forcing it to make an arch; therefore, most of the length of the tube and especially the lower opening remained free. It seemed logical that, according to the above-mentioned ideas, the fibers of the central stump, which had a perfectly unobstructed growth path along the tube, would travel along it until they left it at the lower opening; yet nothing of this kind occurred; instead, after two months he found that the fibers of the central stump had turned back in search of the peripheral stump, describing a curve with a superior concavity, [and that] they had penetrated the peripheral stump, neurotizing it. This fundamental experiment, which demonstrated, in the most brilliant manner, the attraction that the peripheral stump exerts upon the fibers of the central stump was repeated in the most varied ways and in different [species], always with the same result by Forssmann, in trying to determine the influence of different factors on neurotropism, [such as] animal species, presence of threads, motor or sensory function of the stumps, etc.

The method of Weigert, used by Forssmann for the study of the fibers, did not permit him to see these until they had a myelin sheath, that is to say, when everything was already consolidated, and the several [developmental] phases are lacking [from his results] as a consequence.

Cajal, with his [reduced silver nitrate] method, made a very brilliant demonstration, studying the direction of the fibers from the first moments in the varied experiments gathered in his work on [degeneration and] regeneration [of the nervous system], from which we select the most obvious. The slide which is [now] projected (fig. 65) [*fig. 42*] represents an [experiment] in which the sciatic nerve was sectioned and then a ligature put on one of the bundles of the central stump; after eight days, the fibers of the central stump are directed to the degenerated point of the ligated bundle, penetrating into it and going through it up to the ligature where they draw back. This other slide differs from the previous one in that one of the bundles of the central stump was sectioned at two sites instead of being ligated; six days after the operation, the fibers from the two ends of the central stump get to the cut portions (which have the same significance as a peripheral stump), demonstrating the polar indifference of the new sprouts. In figure 70 [*fig. 45*], A corresponds to a complete section of the sciatic nerve in the lowest part of the thigh of a cat; a large piece of the central stump was extirpated and the rest was retracted up to the sciatic notch [by] pulling it out through the bundles of the gluteus [muscles] and [then] sutured underneath the skin; in spite of the great pains taken to prevent

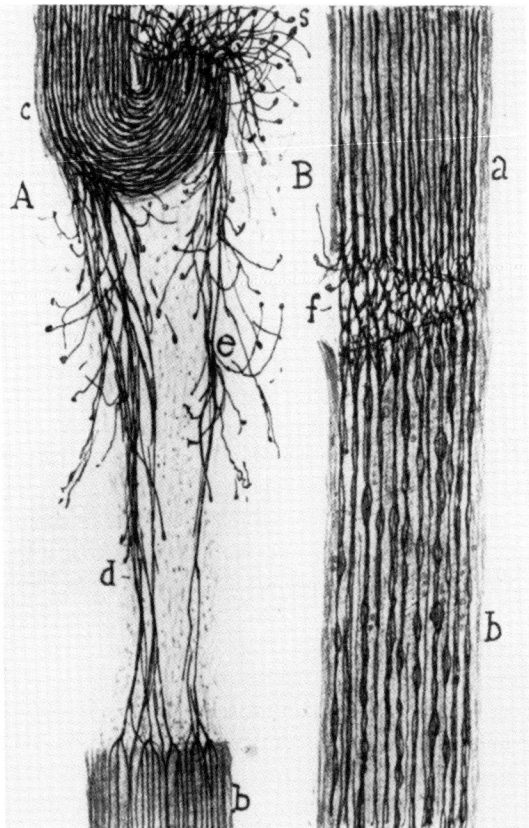

[*FIG. 45*] Fig. 70. Scheme that shows at *A* an extraordinarily difficult neurotization, and at *B* another very straightforward one; *a, c*, central stumps; *b*, peripheral stumps; *f*, scar.

regeneration, this occurred and there were fibers that neurotized the peripheral stump at the forty-eighth day. This experiment is very interesting because when it was made by the polygeneticists, since they could not follow the fibers well with the methods [that they] used and because they found new fibers in the peripheral stump, they deduced that an autogenic regeneration existed; repeated by Cajal with his methods, [it turns out] to be a clear demonstration of continuous growth.

Also, very demonstrative are the experiments in which another piece of nerve was grafted between the two stumps of the sectioned nerve; if the graft was alive, it attracted the fibers which went through it as if it were a peripheral stump (fig. 71) [*fig. 26* see Chapter 4];* if it was dead, it came to be indifferent to the sprouts (fig. 72) [*fig. 27* see Chapter 4].†

---

*Tello's legend for this figure reads: Graft of a nerve in a wound of the sciatic nerve of an adult rabbit, seventeen days after the operation. Method of reduced silver nitrate (Cajal). *A*, central stump; *B*, graft; *C*, peripheral stump; *a*, mortified central portion; *b*, living peripheral portion; *e* and *f*, streams of fibers towards the graft; *d*, fibers that have arrived at the peripheral stump after crossing the graft.

†Tello's legend for this figure reads: Graft of a nerve killed with chloroform, twelve days after the operation. Method of reduced silver nitrate (Cajal). *A*, central stump; *B*, dead graft; *C*, scar.

SECTION THREE

BIBLIOGRAPHY

[Cajal's and May's references appear in their original form as footnotes in the reproduction of the 1928 English version. Because these are incomplete by modern bibliographical standards, we reproduce them here in their complete form and after light editing and correction of any errors detected by us in checking those of the originals that we were able to verify. Those few that we were unable to verify are left in their original form and are so indicated. This list also contains any additional references made in Part I].

Achúcarro, N. (1909) Cellules allongées et Stäbchenzellen, cellules névrogliques et cellules granulo-adipeuses à la corne d'Ammon du lapin. *Trab Lab Invest Biol*, Univ. Madrid 7:201–215.

———. (1909–1910) Zur Kenntnis der pathologischen Histologie des Zentralnervensystems bei Tollwut. In: *Histologische und histopathologische Arbeiten über die Grosshirnrinde*. F. Nissl and A. Alzheimer (Eds.). Vol. 3. Jena: Fischer, pp. 43–199.

———. (1910a) Some pathological findings in the neuroglia and in the ganglion cells of the cortex in senile conditions. *Gov Hosp Insane Bull*, no. 2, Washington, D.C., pp. 81–90.

———. (1910b) Algunos datos relativos a la naturaleza de las células en bastoncito de la corteza cerebral humana obtenidos con el método de Cajal. *Trab Lab Invest Biol*, Univ Madrid 8:169–176.

———. (1913) Alteraciones del ganglio cervical superior en enfermedades cerebrales. *Bol Soc Españ Biol* 2:109–110.

———, and Gayarre, M. (1914) La corteza cerebral en la demencia paralítica con el nuevo método del oro y sublimado de Cajal. *Trab Lab Invest Biol*, Univ Madrid 12:1–38.

Agduhr, E. (1919–1920) Studien über die postembryonale Entwicklung der Neuronen, und die Verteilung der Neuriten in den Wurzeln der Spinalnerven. *J Psychol Neurol* 25:463–626.

Albarracín, A. (1982) *Santiago Ramón y Cajal o la Pasión de España*. Barcelona: Editorial Labor.

Alzheimer, A. (1907) Ueber eine eigenartige Erkrankung der Hirnrinde. *Zentralbl Nervenhlk Psych* 18:177–179.

———. (1909–1910) Beiträge zur Kenntnis der pathologischen Neuroglia und ihrer Beziehungen zu den Abbauvorgängen im Nervengewebe. In: *Histologische und histopathologische Arbeiten über die Grosshirnrinde*. F. Nissl and A. Alzheimer (Eds.). Vol. 3. Jena: Fischer, pp. 401–562.

Apáthy, I. (1907) Bemerkungen zu den Ergebnissen Ramón y Cajal's hinsichtlich der feineren Beschaffenheit des Nervensystems. *Anat Anz* 31:481–496.

Ballance, C. A., and Stewart, P. (1901) *The Healing of Nerves*. London: Macmillan.

Ballance, [C. A.], and Stewart, [P.] [1902] Le processus de réunion des nerfs. Travaux de neurologie chirurgicale, vol. 6, no. 3–4, December 1901. *Rev Neurol*, Paris, 10:860–861. [This is an abstract of a larger review of: Ballance, C. A., and Stewart, P. (1901) *The Healing of Nerves*. London: Macmillan.]

Banchi, A. (1906) Sullo sviluppo dei nervi periferici in maniera indipendente del sistema nervoso centrale. *Anat Anz* 28:169–176.

Berblinger, W. (1918) Über die Regeneration der Achsenzylinder in reserzierten Schufsnarben peripherer Nerven. *Beitr Path Anat Allg Path* 64:226–277.

Bethe, A. (1901a) Ueber die Regeneration peripherischen Nerven. *Arch Psychiatr Nervenkr* 34:1066–1073.

———. (1901b) Ueber die Regeneration peripherischen Nerven. 26. Wanderversammlung der südwestdeutschen Neurologen and Irrenärzte zu Baden-Baden am 8. und 9. Juni, 1901. [*See Neurol Centralbl* 20:720–725.]

———. (1903a) Zur Frage von der autogenen Nervenregeneration. *Neurol Centralbl* 22:60–62.

———. (1903b) *Allgemeine Anatomie und Physiologie des Nervensystems.* Leipzig: Thieme.

———. (1904) Die heutige Stand der Neurontheorie. *Dtsch Med Wochenschr* 30:1201–1204.

———. (1905) Ueber Nervenheilung und polare Wachstumserscheinungen aus Nerven. *Münchener Med. Wochenschr* 52:1228.

———. (1907a) Neue Versuche über die Regeneration der Nervenfasern. *Arch Physiol*, Bonn 116:385–478.

———. (1907b) Ein neuer Beweis für die leitende Funktion der Neurofibrillen. *Folia Neurobiol* 1:100–101.

———. (1908) Die Nervenregeneration und die Verheilung durchschnittener Nerven. *Folia Neurobiol* 1:63–76.

———. (1909) *Die Entwickelung der Nervengewebe bei den Wirbelthieren.* Leipzig: Barth.

———. (1922) Zur theorie und Praxis der Verheilung durchstrennter Nerven. In: *Libro en Honor de D.S. Ramón y Cajal.* Vol. 2. Madrid: Publicaciones de la Junta para el Homenaje a Cajal, pp. 31–35.

Bianchi, V. (1912) Alterazioni istologiche della corteccia cerebrale in seguito a focolai distruttivi ed a lesioni sperimentali. *Ann Neurol*, Napoli 30:61–91.

Bielschowsky, M. (1901) Zur Histologie der Compressionsveränderungen des Rückenmarks bei Wirbelgeschwulsten. *Neurol Centralbl* 20:300–305.

———. (1906) Ueber das Verhalten der Achsenzylinder in Geschwülsten des Nervensystems und in Kompressionsgebieten des Rückenmarks; ein Beitrag zur Kenntnis der Regeneration zentraler und peripherischer Nervenfasern. *J Psychol Neurol* 7:101–140.

———. (1908) Ueber den Bau der Spinalganglien unter normalen und pathologischen Verhältnissen. *J Psychol Neurol* 11:188–227.

———. (1909) Ueber Regenerationerscheinungen an zentralen Nervenfasern. *J Psychol Neurol* 14:131–149.

———. (1910) Allgemeine Histologie und Histopathologie des Nervensystems. In: *Handbuch der Pathologischen Anatomie des Nervensystems.* E. Flatau, L. Jacobsohn, and L. Minor (Eds.). Vol. 1. Berlin: Karger, pp. 3–90.

———. (1911) Zur Kenntnis der Alzheimerschen Krankheit präsenilen Demenz mit Herdsymptomen. *J Psychol Neurol* 18:273–292.

———. (1920–1921) Zur Histopathologie und Pathogenese der amäurotischen Idiotie mit besonderer Berücksichtigung der zerebellaren Veränderungen. *J Psychol Neurol* 26:123–199.

———, and Gallus, [?] (1913) Ueber tuberöse Sklerose. *J Psychol Neurol* 20:1–88.

———, and Unger, E. (1916–1918) Die Ueberbrückung grosser Nervenlücken. Beiträge zur Kenntnis der Degeneration und Regeneration peripherischen Nerven. *J Psychol Neurol* 22:267–318.

———, and Valentin, B. (1922–1923) Die histologischen Veränderungen in durchfrorenen Nervenstrecken. *J Psychol Neurol* 29:133–152.

Bikeles, G. (1904) Zur Frage der Regeneration im Rückenmark. *Neurol Centralbl* 23:559.
Biondi, G. (1910–1911) Sulla fina anatomia die ganglii annessi al simpatico craniano nell'uomo. *Riv Lab Anat Norm*, Rcalc Univ., Roma 16:135–148.
Boeke, J. (1913) Ueber die Regenerationserscheinungen bei der Verheilung von motorischen mit sensiblen Nervenfasern. *Anat Anz* 43:366–378.
———. (1921) Nervenregeneration und verwandte Innervationsprobleme. *Ergeb Physiol* 19:448–593.
Bok, S. T. (1915) Die Entwicklung der Hirnnerven und ihrer centralen Bahnen. Die stimulogene Fibrillation. *Folia Neurobiol* 9:475–565.
Bonfiglio, F. (1908) Di speciali reperti in un caso di probabile sifilide cerebrale. *Riv Sper Freniat*, Reggio–Emilia 34:196–199, 206.
Borst, M. (1904) Neue Experimente zur Frage nach der Regenerationsfähigkeit des Gehirns. *Beitr Path Anat Allg Path* 36:1–81.
Boveri, T. (1886) Beiträge zur Kenntnis der Nervenfasern. *Abhandl Baier Akad Wiss* 15:421–495.
Braus, H. (1905) Experimentelle Beiträge zur Frage nach der Entwicklung peripherer Nerven. *Anat Anz* 26:433–479.
Bravetta, E. (1909) Sopra alcune alterazione degli elementi nervosi nella demenza paralitica. *Boll Soc Med-Chir*, Pavia 23:445–451.
Bruch, C. (1855) Ueber die Regeneration durchschnittener Nerven. Vorläufige Mittheilung. *Z Wiss Zool* 6:135–138.
Büngner, O. von (1891) Ueber die Regeneration und Degenerationvorgänge an Nerven nach Verletzungen. *Beitr Path Anat Allg Path* 10:321–393.
Burrows, M. T. (1911) The growth of tissues of the chick embryo outside the animal body, with special reference to the nervous system. *J Exp Zool* 10:61–83.
Cajal, S. Ramón y. (1889) *Manual de Histología Normal y Técnica Micrográfica.* Valencia: Aguilar.
———. (1890a) A quelle époque apparaissent les expansions des cellules nerveuses de la moelle epiniere du poulet? *Anat Anz* 5:21–22, 609–613, 631–639.
———. (1890b) Sur l'origine et les ramifications des fibres nerveuses de la moelle embryonnaire. *Anat Anz* 5:85–95, 111–119.
———. (1892a) La rétine des vertébrés. *La Cellule* 9:121–246.
———. (1892b) Las defensas orgánicas en el epitelioma y carcinoma. *Bol Oficial Col Méd Madrid* 1:20–28.
———. (1892c) El nuevo concepto de la histología de los centros nerviosos. *Rev Ciencias Méd* 18:457–476.
———. (1894a) The Croonian lecture: La fine structure des centres nerveux. *Proc R Soc Lond [Biol]* 55:444–467.
———. (1894b) *Les Nouvelles Idées sur la Structure du Système Nerveux chez l'Homme et chez les Vertébrés.* French edition revised and enlarged by the author. Translated by L. Azoulay, preface by M. Duval. Paris: Reinwald.
———. (1896) Estudios histológicos sobre los tumores epiteliales. *Rev Trim Micrograf*, Madrid 1:83–112.

———. (1898) Estructura del kiasma óptico y teoría general de los entrecruzamientos de las vías nerviosas. *Rev Trim Micrográf,* Madrid 3:15–65.

———. (1899, 1904) *Textura del Sistema Nervioso del Hombre y de los Vertebrados.* 2 vols. in 3. Madrid: Moya.

———. (1903a) Consideraciones críticas sobre la teoría de Bethe, acerca de la estructura y conexiones de las células nerviosas. *Trab Lab Invest Biol,* Univ Madrid 2:101–128.

———. (1903b) Sobre un sencillo proceder de impregnacíon de las fibras interiores del protoplasma nervioso. *Arch Lat Med Biol,* Madrid 1:1–6.

———. (1904a) Algunos métodos de coloración de los cilindros-ejes, neurofibrillas y nidos nerviosos. *Trab Lab Invest Biol,* Univ Madrid 3:1–7.

———. (1904b) Notas preventivas sobre algunos métodos de coloración de los cilindros-ejes y ciertas variaciones normales y patológicas de los neurofibrillas. *Trab Lab Invest Biol,* Univ Madrid 3:1–5.

———. (1904c) Variaciones morfológicas normales y patológicas del retículo neurofibrilar. *Trab Lab Invest Biol,* Univ Madrid 3:9–15.

———. (1905a) Sobre la degeneración y regeneración de los nervios. Boletín del Instituto de Sueroterapia, Vacunación y Bacteriología de Alfonso XIII. 1:49–60, 113–119.

———. (1905b) Tipos celulares de los ganglios sensitivos del hombre y mamíferos. *Trab Lab Invest Biol,* Univ Madrid 4:1–35.

———. (1905c) Las células del gran simpático del hombre adulto. *Trab Lab Invest Biol,* Univ Madrid 4:79–104.

———. (1905d) *Manual de Anatomía Patológica General y Fundamentos de Bacteriología.* 4th ed. Madrid: Moya.

———. (1906a) Las metamorfosis de las neurofibrillas en la regeneración y degeneración de los nervios. *Rev Med Cir Fac Med Madrid* 1:43–54, 73–83, 107–115.

———. (1906 b) Mecanismo de la regeneración de los nervios. *Trab Lab Invest Biol,* Univ Madrid 4:119–210.

———. (1906c) Génesis de las fibras nerviosas del embrión y observaciones contrarias a la teoria catenaria. *Trab Lab Invest Biol,* Univ Madrid 4:227–294.

———. (1906d) Notas preventivas sobre la degeneración y regeneración de las vías nerviosas centrales. *Trab Lab Invest Biol,* Univ Madrid 4:295–301.

———. (1906e) Die Struktur der sensiblen Ganglien des Menschen und der Tiere. Anatomische Hefte. II Abtheilung. *Ergeb Anat Entw* 16:177–215.

———. (1906f) Genèse des fibres nerveuses de l'embryon et observations contraires à la théorie catenaire. *Trav Lab Rech Biol,* Univ Madrid 4:219–284.

———. (1907a) Die histogenetischen Beweise der Neuronentheorie von His und Forel. *Anat Anz* 30:113–144.

———. (1907b) Les métamorphoses précoces des neurofibrilles dans la régénération et la dégénération des nerfs. *Trav Lab Rech Biol,* Univ Madrid 5:47–104.

———. (1907c) Note sur la dégénérescence traumatique des fibres nerveuses du cervelet et du cerveau. *Trav Lab Rech Biol,* Univ Madrid 5:105–116.

———. (1907d) Nouvelles observations sur l'évolution des neuroblastes, avec quelques remarques sur l'hypòthese neurogénétique de Hensen-Held. *Trav Lab Rech biol*, Univ Madrid 5:169–215.

———. (1907e) *Regeneración de los Nervios*. Madrid: Real Acad. Med.

———. (1908a) Nouvelles observations sur l'évolution des neuroblastes, avec quelques remarques sur l'hypothèse neurogénetique de Hensen-Held. *Anat Anz* 32:1–25, 65–87.

———. (1908b) L'hypothèse de la continuité d'Apáthy. Résponse aux objections de cet auteur contre la doctrine neuronale. *Trav Lab Rech Biol*, Univ Madrid 6:21–90.

———. (1908c) *Studien über Nervenregeneration*. Translated by J. Bressler. Leipzig: Barth.

———. (1910a) Las fórmulas del proceder del nitrato de plata reducido y sus efectos sobre los factores integrantes de las neuronas. *Trab Lab Invest Biol*, Univ Madrid 8:1–26.

———. (1910b) Algunas observaciones favorables a la hipótesis neurotrópica. *Trab Lab Invest Biol*, Univ Madrid 8:63–136.

———. (1910c) Algunos experimentos de conservación y autolisis del tejido nervioso. Nota preventiva. *Trav Lab Invest Biol*, Univ Madrid 8:137–148.

———. (1910d) Observaciones sobre la regeneración de la porción intramedular de las raices sensitivas. *Trav Lab Invest Biol*, Univ Madrid 8:177–196.

———. (1910e) Algunos hechos de regeneración parcial de la substancia gris de los centros nerviosos. *Trab Lab Invest Biol*, Univ Madrid 8:197–236.

———. (1911a) Los fenómenos precoces de la degeneración neuronal en el cerebelo. *Trab Lab Invest Biol*, Univ Madrid 9:1–38.

———. (1911b) Los fenómenos precoces de la degeneración traumática de los cilindros-ejes del cerebro. *Trab Lab Invest Biol*, Univ Madrid 9:39–96.

———. (1911c) Fibras nerviosas conservadas y fibras nerviosas degeneradas. *Trab Lab Invest Biol*, Univ Madrid 9:181–216.

———. (1911d) Alteraciones de la substancia gris provocadas por conmoción y aplastamiento. *Trab Lab Invest Biol*, Univ. Madrid 9:217–254.

———. (1912a) Fórmula de fijación para la demostración fácil del aparato reticular de Golgi y apuntes sobre la disposición de dicho aparato en la retina, en las nervios y algunos estados patológicos. *Trab Lab Invest Biol*, Univ Madrid 10:209–220.

———. (1912b) El aparato endocelular de Golgi de la célula de Schwann y algunas observaciones sobre la estructura de los tubos nerviosos. *Trab Lab Invest Biol*, Univ Madrid 10:221–246.

———. (1912c) Sobre ciertos plexos pericelulares de la capa de los granos del cerebelo. *Trab Lab Invest Biol*, Univ Madrid 10:273–276.

———. (1912d) Influencia de las condiciones mecánicas sobre la regeneración de los nervios. *Trab Lab Invest Biol*, Univ Madrid 10:277–285.

———. (1913a) El neurotropismo y la transplantación de los nervios. *Trab Lab Invest Biol*, Univ Madrid 11:81–102.

———. (1913b) Fenómenos de excitación neurocládica en los ganglios y raíces nerviosas consecutivamente al arrancamiento del ciático. *Trab Lab Invest Biol*, Univ Madrid 11:103–117.

―――. (1913c) Sobre un nuevo proceder de impregnación de la neuroglia y sus resultados en los centros nerviosos del hombre y animales. *Trab Lab Invest Biol,* Univ Madrid 11:219–238.

―――. (1913d) Contribución al conocimiento de la neuroglia del cerebro humano. *Trab Lab Invest Biol,* Univ Madrid 11:255–315.

―――. (1913e) *Estudios sobre la Degeneración y Regeneración del Sistema Nervioso.* Vol. 1. *Degeneración y Regeneración de los Nerviosos.* Madrid: Moya.

―――. (1914) *Estudios sobre la Degeneración y Regeneración del Sistema Nervioso.* Vol. 2. *Degeneración y Regeneración de los Centros Nerviosos.* Madrid: Moya.

―――. (1917) *Recuerdos de mi Vida.* Vol. 2. *Historia de mi Labor Científica.* Madrid: Moya.

―――. (1919a) La desorientación inicial de las neuronas retinianas de axón corto. (Algunos hechos favorables a la concepción neurotrópica). *Trab Lab Invest Biol,* Univ Madrid 17:65–86.

―――. (1919b) Acción neurotrópica de los epitelios. (Algunos detalles sobre el mecanismo genético de las ramificaciones nerviosas intraepiteliales, sensitivas y sensoriales.) *Trab Lab Invest Biol,* Univ Madrid 17:181–228.

―――. (1920) Algunas observaciones contrarias a la hipótesis *syncytial* de la regeneración nerviosa y neurogénesis normal. *Trab Lab Invest Biol,* Univ Madrid 18:275–302.

―――. (1921) La innervación de las cicatrices. *El Siglo Médico* 68:1–2.

―――. (1923) *Recuerdos de mi Vida.* 3d ed. Madrid: Pueyo.

―――. (1926) Démonstration photographique de quelques phénomènes de la régénération des nerves. *Trav Lab Rech Biol,* Univ Madrid 24:191–213.

―――. (1928) *Degeneration and Regeneration of the Nervous System.* Translated by R. M. May. 2 vols. London: Oxford University Press.

―――. (1933) ¿Neuronismo o reticularismo? Las pruebas objetivas de la unidad anatómica de las células nerviosas. *Arch Neurobiol* 13:217–291, 579–646.

―――. (1937) *Recollections of My Life.* Translated by E. H. Craigie with the assistance of J. Cano. Philadelphia: American Philosophical Society. (Reprint. Cambridge, MA: MIT Press, n.d.)

―――. (1954) *Neuron Theory or Reticular Theory.* Translated by M. Ubeda Purkiss, and C. A. Fox. Madrid: Consejo Superior de Investigaciones Científicas.

―――. (1959) *Degeneration and Regeneration of the Nervous System.* Translated by R. M. May. 2 vols. New York: Hafner. (Reprint. 1968).

―――, and García, D. D. (1904) Las lesiones del retículo de las células nerviosas en la rabia. *Trab Lab Invest Biol,* Univ Madrid 3:213–266.

―――, and Illera, R. (1907) Quelques nouveaux détails sur la structure de l'écorce cérébelleuse. *Trav Lab Rech Biol,* Univ Madrid 5:1–12.

―――, and Olóriz, F. (1897) Los ganglios sensitivos craneales de los mamíferos. *Rev Trim Micrográf* 2:129–152.

Capparelli, A. (1904) La fina struttura delle fibre nervose. Atti dell' Academia Gioenia di scienze naturali di Catania. Serie 4, vol. 8 [not verified].

Catola, G., and Achúcarro, N. (1906) Ueber die Entstehung der Amyloidkorperchen im Zentralnervensystem. *Virchows Arch Pathol Anat* 184:454–469.

Catola, G. (1910) Alcuna nuove ricerche sulla struttura delle lacune di disintegrazione cerebrale. *Riv Patol Nerv Ment* 15:605–647.

Cattaneo, D. (1923) I fenomeni degenerativi e rigenerativi nelle vie visive in seguito a lesioni del nervo ottico. *Riv Patol Nerv Ment* 28:61–118.

Cattani, G. (1886) L'appareil de soutien de la myéline dans les fibres nerveuses périphériques. [Translated from *Atti R Accad Sci*, Torino. Vol. 21. 1886.] *Arch Ital Biol*, Turin 7:345–356.

Cerletti, U. (1905) Sopra alcuni rapporti tra le cellule a bastoncello (Stäbchenzellen) e gli elementi nervosi nella paralisi progressiva. *Riv Sper Freniat*, Reggio-Emilia 31:483–495.

Chambers, R., and Renyi, G. S. (1925–1926) The structure of the cells in tissues as revealed by microdissection. I. The physical relationships of the cells in epithelia. *Am J Anat* 35:385–402.

Child, C. M. (1921) *The Origin and Development of the Nervous System from a Physiological Viewpoint*. Chicago: University of Chicago Press.

Cipollone, L. T. (1897) Ricerche sull anatomia normale e patologica delle terminazioni nervesi nei muscoli striati. Supplemento agli Annali di Medicina navale. Rome: Berlero.

D'Abundo, G. (1907–1908) Dottrina metamerica e rigenerazione consecutiva allo strappo contemporaneo del prolungamento midollare di molteplici gangli intervertebrali nei primi tempi della vita extra-uterina. *Riv Ital Neuropatol Psch Elettroter* 1:353–368.

———. (1908–1909a) Di nuovo sul potere rigenerativo del prolungamento midollare dei gangli intervertebrali nei primi tempi della vita extra-uterina. *Riv Ital Neuropatol Psch Elettroter* 2:289–299.

———. (1908–1909b) Doctrine métamérique et régénération consécutive à l'arrachement simultané du prolongement médullaire de multiples ganglions intervertébraux dans les premiers temps de la vie extra-utérine. *Arch Ital Biol* 50:215–229.

———. (1911–1912) Ulteriori osservazioni sulla rigenerazione del tratto midollare dei gangli intervertebrali. *Riv Ital Neuropatol Psch Elettroter* 4:289–320.

Da Fano, C. (1907) A proposito delle nuove dottrine sulle modificazioni della struttura dei gangli spinali nella tabe. *Boll Soc Med-Chir*, Pavia 21:191–208.

Darkschewitsch, L. (1892) Ueber die Veränderungen in den centralen Abschnitt eines motorischen Nerven bei Verletzung des peripheren Abschnittes. *Neurol Centralbl* 11:658–668.

De Castro, F. (1920) Nota sobre algunas terminaciones aberrantes de fibras trepadoras estudiadas en el cerebelo del perro joven. *Trab Lab Invest Biol*, Univ Madrid 18:199–206.

———. (1921) Estudio sobre los ganglios sensitivos del hombre en estado normal y patológico. Formas celulares típicas y atípicas. *Trab Lab Invest Biol*, Univ Madrid 19:241–340.

———. (1930) Recherches sur la dégénération et la régénération du système nerveux sympathique. Quelques observations sur la constitution des synapses dans les ganglions. Études anatomiques et physiologiques. *Trav Lab Rech Biol*, Univ Madrid 26:357–456.

DeFelipe, J., and Jones, E. G. (1988) *Cajal on the Cerebral Cortex. An Annotated Translation of the Complete Writings.* New York: Oxford University Press.

Deineka, D. (1912) Der Netzapparat von Golgi in einigen Epithel- und Bindegewebszellen während der Ruhe und während der Teilung derselben. *Anat Anz* 41:289–309.

del Río-Hortega, P. (1914) Alteraciones del sistema nervioso central en un caso de moquillo de forma paralítica. *Trab Lab Invest Biol*, Univ Madrid 12:97–126.

Dogiel, A. S. (1897) Zur Frage über den feineren Bau der Spinalganglien und deren Zellen bei Säugetieren. *Int J Anat* 14:73–116.

———. (1908) *Der Bau der Spinalganglien des Menschen und der Säugethiere.* Jena: Fischer.

Dohrn, A. (1907) Studien zur Urgeschichte des Wirbelthierkörpers. 25. Der Trochlearis. *Mitt Zool*, Station Neapel 18:143–436.

Doinikow, B. (1911) Beiträge zur Histologie und Histopathologie der peripheren Nerven. In: *Histologische und histopathologische Arbeiten über die Grosshirnrinde.* F. Nissl and A. Alzheimer (Eds.). Vol. 4. Jena: Fischer, pp. 445–630.

Donaggio, A., and Fragnito, O. (1905) Lesioni del reticolo fibrillare endocellulare nelle cellule midollari per lo strappo dello sciatico e delle relative radici spinali. *Riv Sper Freniatr*, Reggio-Emilia 31:383–386.

Duesberg, J. (1924) La régénération des ganglions et de leurs connexions médullaires dans la queue des Urodèles. *Compt Rend Soc Biol*, Paris 90:633–634.

Durante, G. (1904) A propos de la théorie du neurone: terminaisons fibrillaires, régénération autogène, différentiation fonctionnelle, et rôle du cylindraxe: sensibilité récurrente et suppléance sensitives; propagation des dégénérescences. *Rev Neurol*, Paris 12:573–585.

Dustin, A. P. (1910) Le rôle des tropismes et de l'odogénèse dans la régénération du système nerveux. *Arch Biol*, Liége 25:269–388.

Eichhorst, H. (1873) Ueber die Nervendegeneration und Nervenregeneration. *Virchows Arch Pathol Anat* 59:1–25.

———, and Naunyn, B. (1874) Ueber die Regeneration und Veränderungen im Rückenmark nach streckenweiser totaler Zerstörung derselben. *Arch Exp Pathol Pharmak* 2:225–253.

Fañanás, J. R. (1913) Alteraciones del aparato reticular de Golgi en las células gigantes y otros elementos del tubérculo. *Trab Lab Invest Biol*, Univ Madrid 11:119–130.

Farrar, C. B. (1908) On the phenomena of repair in the cerebral cortex, a study of mesodermal and ectodermal activities following the introduction of a foreign body. In: *Histologische und histopathologische Arbeiten über die Grosshirnrinde.* F. Nissl (Ed.). Vol. 2. Jena: Fischer, pp. 1–70.

Fickler, A. (1901) Zur Frage der Regeneration des Rückenmarks. *Neurol Centralbl* 20:738–744.

Fleming, R. A. (1902) Review of *The Healing of Nerves*, by C. A. Ballance and P. Stewart. *Edin Med J* (new series) 11:561–563.

Forssman, J. (1898) Ueber die Ursachen welche die Wachsthumsrichtung der peripheren Nervenfasern bei der Regeneration bestimmen. *Beitr Path Anat Allg Path* 24:56–100.

———. (1900) Zur Kenntnis des Neurotropismus. *Beitr Path Anat Allg Path* 27:407–430.

Foster, L. (1911) La degeneración traumática en la médula espinal de las aves. *Trab Lab Invest biol*, Univ Madrid 9:255–268.

García e Izcara, D. (1912) Sobre el diagnóstico de la rabia. *Bol Soc Españ Biol* 1:184–190.

Galeotti, G., and Levi, G. (1895) Ueber die Neubildung der nervösen Elemente in dem wiedererzeugten Muskelgewebe. *Beitr Path Anat Allg Path* 17:369–415.

Gemelli, A. (1906) Ricerche sperimentali sullo sviluppo dei nervi degli arti pelvici di *Bufo vulgaris* innestati in sede anomola; contributo allo studio della rigenerazione autogena dei nervi periferici. *Riv Patol Nerv Ment* 11:328–332.

Golgi, C. (1894) *Untersuchungen über den Feineren Bau des Centralen und Peripherischen Nervensystems.* Translated by R. Teuscher. Text and Atlas, 2 vols. Jena: Fischer.

Halliburton, W. D., and Mott, F. W. (1902) Regeneration of Nerves. Reports of meetings of the British Association for the Advancement of Science, Belfast. Sect. 1:782.

Harrison, R. G. (1906) Further experiments on the development of peripheral nerves. *Am J Anat* 5:121–131.

———. (1910) The outgrowth of the nerve fiber as a model of protoplasmic movement. *J Exp Zool* 9:787–847.

———. (1912) The cultivation of tissues in extraneous media as a method of morphogenetic study. *Anat Rec* 6:181–193.

Hedinger, E. (1921) Die Regeneration im Nervensystem. *Schweiz Arch Neurol Neurochir Psychiatr* 9:1–28.

Heidenhain, M. (1907–1911) *Plasma und Zelle* 2 vols. Vol. 1. *Abteilung: Eine allgemeine Anatomie der lebendigen Masse.* Jena: Fischer.

Held, H. (1905) Die Entstehung der Neurofibrillen. *Neurol Centralbl* 24: 706–710.

———. (1906) Zur Histogenese der Nervenleitung. *Zentralbl Norm Anat Mikrotechn* 3:165.

———. (1907) Kritische Bemerkungen zu der Verteidigung der Neuroblasten und der Neuronentheorie durch R. Cajal. *Anat Anz* 30:369–391.

———. (1909) *Die Entwickelung der Nervengewebe bei den Wirbelthieren.* Leipzig: Barth.

Henneberg, R. (1907) Ueber Nervenfaserregeneration bei totaler traumatischer Querläsion des Rückenmarkes. *Charité-Ann*, Berl 31:161–190.

Hensen, V. (1864) Ueber die Entwickelung des Gewebes und der Nerven im Schwanze der Froschlarve. *Virchows Arch [Pathol Anat]* 31:51–73.

―――. (1868) Ueber die Nerven im Schwanz der Froschlarven. *Arch Mikrosk Anat* 4:111–124.
―――. (1903) *Die Entwickelungsmechanik der Nervenbahnen im Embryo der Säugethiere. Ein Probeversuch.* Kiel and Leipzig: Lipsius and Tischer.
Herxheimer, G., and Gierlich, N. (1907) *Studien über die Neurofibrillen im Zentralnervensystem, Entwickelung und normales Verhalten Veränderunger unter pathologischen Bedingungen.* Wiesbaden: Bergmann.
Herzt, H. (1869) Ueber Degeneration und Regeneration durchschnittener Nerven. *Virchows Arch Pathol Anat* 46:257–285.
His, W. (1889) Die Neuroblasten und deren Enstehung im embryonalen Mark. Abh. Sächs. *Ges Akad Wiss (Math-Physik Kl)* 15:311.
―――. (1890) Histogenese und Zusammenhang der Nervenelemente. *Arch Anat Physiol (Anat Abt Suppl)* 1890:95–119.
―――. (1904) *Die Entwickelung des menschlichen Gehirns während der ersten Monate.* Leipzig: Hirzel.
Hjelt, O. E. A. (1859) *Om nervernas regeneration och dermed sammanhängande förändringar af nervrören.* Helsingfors: Frenckell.
Hofmann, F. B., and Blaas, E. (1908) Untersuchungen über die mechanische Reizbarkeit der quergestreiftensskelettmuskeln. *Arch Gesamte Physiol* 125:137–162.
Homén, E. A. (1885) Experimenteller Beitrag zur Pathologie und pathologischen Anatomie des Rückenmarks (speciell mit Hinsicht auf die secundäre Degeneration). Vorläufige Mittheilung. *Fortschr Med* 3:267–276.
―――. (1890) Veränderungen des Nervensystems nach Amputationen. *Beitr Path Anat Allg Path* 8:304–351.
―――. (1892–1895) Die krankhaften Veränderungen der Nerven nach Amputationen. In: *Atlas der pathologischen Histologie des Nervensystems.* V. Baber and P. Blocq (Eds.). Berlin: Hirschwald.
Hooker, D. (1915) Studies on regeneration of the spinal cord. I. An analysis of the process leading to its reunion after it has been completely severed in frog embryos at the stage of closed neural folds. *J Comp Neurol* 25:469–495.
―――. (1916–1917) Studies on regeneration of the spinal cord. II. The effect of reversal of a portion of the spinal cord at the stage of the closed neural folds on the healing of the cord wounds on the polarity of the elements of the cord and on the behavior of frog embryos. *J Comp Neurol* 27:421–449.
―――. (1922–1923) The nature of the division of neuroblastic cells in the regenerating spinal cords of amphibian larvae. *Anat Rec* 24:377.
Huber, G. C. (1892) Ueber das Verhalten der Kerne der Schwann's Scheide bei Nervendegeneration. *Arch Mikrosk Anat* 40:409–417.
―――, and Guild, S. R. (1913) Observations on the histogenesis of protoplasmic processes and of collaterals terminating in end bulbs, of the neurones of peripheral sensory ganglia. *Anat Rec* 7:331–354.
Jakob, A. (1912) Experimentelle Untersuchungen über die traumatischen Schädigungen des Zentralnervensystems (mit besonderer Berücksichtigung der Commotio cerebri und Kommotionsneurose). In: *Histologische und*

histopathologische Arbeiten über die Grosshirnrinde. F. Nissl and A. Alzheimer (Eds.). Vol. 5. Jena: Fischer, pp. 182–341.

———. (1912–1913) Ueber die feinere Histologie der sekundären Faserdegeneration in der weissen Substanz des Rückenmarks (mit besonderer Berucksichtigung der Abbauvorgange). In: *Histologische und histopathologische Arbeiten über die Grosshirnrinde.* F. Nissl and A. Alzheimer (Eds.). Vol. 5. Jena: Fischer, pp. 1–181.

Kappers, C. U. Ariëns (1908a) Weitere Mitteilungen bezüglich der phylogenetischen Verlagerung der motorischen Hirnnervenkerne. Der Bau des autonomen Systemes. *Folia Neurobiol* 1:157–172.

———. (1908b) Weitere Mitteilungen über Neurobiotaxis. A. Die Selektivitat der Zellenwanderung. Die Bedeutung synchronischer Reizverwandschaft. Verlauf und Endigung der zentralen sogenannten motorischen Bahnen. *Folia Neurobiol* 1:507–521.

———. (1908c) Weitere Mitteilungen über Neurobiotaxis. 2. Die phylogenetische Entwicklung des horizontalen Schenkels des Facialiswurzelknies. *Folia Neurobiol* 2:225–261.

———. (1917) Further contributions on neurobiotaxis. IX. An attempt to compare the phenomena of neurobiotaxis with other phenomena of taxis and tropism. The dynamic polarization of the neuron. *J Comp Neurol* 27:261–298.

———. (1921) On structural laws in the nervous system: the principles of neurobiotaxis. *Brain* 44:125–149.

———. (1922) Dixième contribution à la théorie de la neurobiotaxis. Le tropisme nutritif des dendrites et son rapport avec les phénomènes neurobiotactiques en général. *Encéphale* 17:1–19.

Keresztszeghy, G., and Hannss, [?] (1893) Ueber Degenerations- und Regenerationsvorgänge am Rückenmark des Hundes nach vollständiger Durchschneidung. *Beitr Path Anat Allg Path* 12:35–56.

Kerr, G. (1904) On some points in the early development of motor nerve trunks and myotomes in *Lepidosiren paradoxa. Trans R Soc Edin* 41:119–128.

Key, A., and Retzius, G. (1875–1876) *Studien in der Anatomie des Nervensystems und des Bindegewebes.* 2 vols. Stockholm: Samson and Wallin.

Kimura, O. (1919) Histologische Degenerations- und Regenerationsvorgänge im peripherischen Nervensystem. *Mitt Path Inst Univ Sendai* 1:1–160.

Koch, C. (1876) Ueber die Marksegmente der doppelcontourierten Nervenfasern. No. 49. *Centralb Med Wiss.* [not verified]

Kolster, R. (1893) Zur Kenntniss der Regeneration durchschnittener Nerven; eine experimentelle Studie. *Arch Mikrosk Anat* 41:688–706.

Koltzoff, N. K. (1905) Studien über die Gestalt der Zelle; Untersuchungen über die Spermien der Decapoden, als Einleitung in das Problem der Zellengestalt. *Arch Mikrosk Anat* 67:364–572.

Krassin, P. (1906) Zur Frage der Regeneration der periphoren Nerven. *Anat Anz* 28:449–453.

Kropp, B., and May, R. M. (1924) A study of mitochondria in white blood cells following gaseous inhalation. *Anat Rec* 27:289–292.

Kuhnt, J. H. (1876–1877) Beitrag zur Anatomie der markhaltigen peripheren Nervenfaser. Göttingen, Nachrichten, 1876, pp. 189–192 [*Arch Mikrosk Anat* 13: 427–464.]

Lafora, G. (1913) Beitrag zur Kenntnis der Alzheimerschen Krankheit. Vol. 11. *Ztschr. Gesamte Neurol Psychiatr.* [not verified]

Lafora, G. R. (1914) Neoformaciones dendríticas en las neuronas y alteraciones de la neuroglia en el perro senil. *Trab Lab Invest Biol*, Univ Madrid 12:39–53.

Langley, J. N. (1909) On degenerative changes in the nerve endings in striated muscle, in the nerve plexuses, on arteries, and in the nerve fibres of the frog. *J Physiol*, Lond 38:504–512.

———, and Anderson, H. K. (1903) Observations on the regeneration of nerve-fibres. *J Physiol*, Lond 29:[*Proc Physiol Soc*] iii–v.

Lawrentjew, B. J. (1929) Experimentell-morphologische Studien über der feineren Bau des autonomen Nervensystems. I. Die Beteiligung des Vagus an der Herzinnervation. *Ztschr Mikrosk Anat Forsch* 16:383–411.

Legendre, R., and Minot, H. (1910a) Essais de conservation hors de l'organisme des cellules nerveuses des ganglions spinaux. I. Plan de recherches et dispositif expérimental. *Compt Rend Soc Biol*, Paris 68:795–796.

———. (1910b) Essais de conservation hors de l'organisme des cellules nerveuses des ganglions spinaux. II. Conservation dans le sang défibriné. *Compt Rend Soc Biol*, Paris 68:839–841.

———. (1910c) Essais de conservation hors de l'organisme des cellules nerveuses des ganglions spinaux. III. Influence de la dilution sur la conservation des cellules nerveuses des ganglions spinaux hors de l'organisme. *Compt Rend Soc Biol*, Paris 68:885–887.

———. (1911a) Influence de la température sur la conservation des cellules nerveuses des ganglions spinaux hors de l'organisme. *Compt Rend Soc Biol*, Paris 69:618–620.

———. (1911b) Formation de nouveaux prolongements par certaines cellules nerveuses des ganglions spinaux conservés hors de l'organisme. *Anat Anz* 38:554–560.

Lenhossék, M. von (1891) Zur Kenntnis der ersten Entstehung der Nervenzellen und Nervenfasern beim Vogelembryo. Verhandl. X. Internat. Med. Congr., Berlin, 1890. 2:115–129.

———. (1895) *Der feinere Bau des Nervensystems im Lichte neuester Forschungen*. 2d ed. Berlin: Fischer.

Lent, E. (1855) *De Nervorum Dissectorum Commutationibus ac Regeneratione*. Berlin: Schlesinger.

Leoz, Ortín, G., and Arcaute, L. R. (1913) Procesos regenerativos del nervio óptico y retina con ocasión de ingertos nerviosos. *Trab Lab Invest Biol*, Univ. Madrid 11:239–254.

Levi, G. (1906–1907) Di alcuni problemi reguardanti la struttura del sistema nervoso. *Arch Fisiol* 4:367–396.

———. (1907) Struttura e istogenesi dei gangli cerebro-spinali dei mammiferi. *Anat Anz* 30:154–159.

———. (1908) *I Ganglî Cerebrospinali, Studî di Istologia Comparata e di Istogenesi*. Florence: Niccolai.

———. (1917) Connessioni e struttura degli elementi nervosi sviluppati fuori dell'organismo. Ser. 5. Atti Acad Lincei 12:142.

Lewis, M. R., and Lewis, W. H. (1911) The cultivation of tissues from chick embryos in solutions of NaCl, CaCl$_2$, KCl, and NaHCO$_3$. *Anat Rec* 5:277–293.

Lewis, W. H., and Lewis, M. R. (1912) The cultivation of sympathetic nerves from the intestine of chick embryos, in saline solutions. *Anat Rec* 6:7–17.

Loeb, L (1897) Ueber Transplantation von weisser Haut auf einen Defekt in schwarzer Haut und umgekehrt am Ohr des Meerschweinchens. *Arch Entw Mech Organismen* 6:1–44.

———. (1902) Über das Wachsthum des Epithels. *Arch Entw Mech Organismen* 13:487–506.

———. (1912) Growth of tissues in culture media and its significance for the analysis of growth phenomena. *Anat Rec* 6:109–120.

London, E. S., and Pesker, D. J. (1905) Ueber die Entwicklung des peripheren Nervensystems bei Säugetieren (weissen Mäusen). *Arch Mikrosk Anat* 67:303–318.

Lorente de Nó, R. (1921) La regeneración de la médula espinal en las larvas de batracio. *Trab Lab Invest Biol*, Univ. Madrid 19:147–183.

Lugaro, E. (1904) Allgemeine pathologische Anatomie der Nervenfasern. In: *Handbuch der Pathologische Anatomie des Nervensystems*. E. Flatau; L. Jacobsohn; and L. Minor (Eds.). Vol. 1. Berlin:Karger, pp. 162–187.

———. (1906a) Osservazioni sui "gomitoli" nervosi nella rigenerazione dei nervi. *Riv Patol Nerv Ment* 11:170–179.

———. (1906b) Sul neurotropismo e sui trapianti dei nervi. *Riv Patol Nerv Ment* 11:320–327.

———. (1906c) Sulla presunta rigenerazione autogena delle radici posteriori. *Riv Patol Nerv Ment* 11:337–348.

———. (1906d) Weiteres zur Frage der autogenen Regeneration der Nervenfasern. *Neurol Centralbl* 25:786–792.

———. (1909) La fonction de la cellule nerveuse. 16e Congrès Intern. de Médecine, Budapest, 29 August [not verified].

Marcora, F. (1908) Di una fine alterazione delle cellule nervose del nucleo d'origine del grande ipoglosso consecutiva allo strappamento ed al taglio del nervo. *Boll Soc Med Chir*, Pavia 22:134–137.

Marenghi, G., and Villa, L. (1891) De quelques particularités de structure des fibres nerveuses médullaires. *Arch Ital Biol* 15:404–408.

Marchand, F. (1909) Untersuchungen über die Herkunft der Körnchenzellen des Zentralnervensystems. *Beitr Path Anat Allg Path* 45:161–196.

Marinesco, G. (1892) Ueber Veränderung der Nerven und des Rückenmarks nach Amputationen; ein Beitrag zur Nerventrophik. *Neurol Centralbl* 11:463–467, 505–508, 564–574.

———. (1894) Sur la régénération des centres nerveux. *Compt Rend Soc Biol*, Paris 46:389–391.

———. (1906a) Etudes sur le mécanisme de la régénérescence des fibres nerveuses des nerfs périphériques. *J Psychol Neurol* 7:140–171.

———. (1906b) Annales de l'Académie roumaine. Series 2, vol. 29 [not verified].

———. (1906–1907) Quelques recherches sur la morphologie normale et pathologique des cellules des ganglions spinaux et sympathique de l'homme. *Névraxe* 8:7–38.

———. (1907a) Plasticité et amiboïdisme des cellules des ganglions sensitifs. *Rev Neurol*, Paris 21:1109–1125.

———. (1907b) Quelques mots à propos du travail de M. Nageotte; recherches expérimentales sur la morphologie des ganglions rachidiens. *Rev Neurol*, Paris 15:537–543.

———. (1907c) Le mecanisme de la régénérescence nerveuse, première partie: Dégénérescence et régénérescence des nerfs. *Rev Gén Sci Pures, Appl* 4:145–159.

———. (1907d) Le mécanisme de la régénérescence nerveuse, deuxième partie: Les transplantations nerveuses. *Rev Gén Sci Pures, Appl* 5:190–198.

———. (1908) Sur la neurotisation des foyers de ramollissement et d'hémorragie cérébrale. *Rev Neurol*, Paris 16:1293–1305.

———. (1909) *La Cellule Nerveuse*. 2 vols. Paris: Doin.

———. (1912) Etude anatomique et clinique des plaques dites seniles. *Encéphale* 1:105–132.

———. (1913) Sur la structure colloïdale des cellules nerveuses et ses variations à l'état normal et pathologique. Congrès Intern. de Neurol. et de Psychiatrie, Gand, 2–26 August [not verified].

———. (1920) Recherches anatomo-cliniqes sur les néuromes d'amputations douloureux: nouvelles contributions à l'étude de la régénération nerveuse et du neurotropisme. *Philos Trans R Soc Lond* 209:229–304.

———. (1921) Le rôle des ferments oxidants pendant la croissance et la régénérescence des nerfs. *Rev Gen Sci Pures, Appl* 32:508–512.

———, and Minea, J. (1905) La loi de Waller et la régénérescence autogène. Revistă ştiinţelor medicale, Bucharest. No. 5, September 1905 [quoted by Mott et al., 1906].

———. (1906a) Note sur la régénérescence de la moelle chez l'homme. *Compt Rend Soc Biol*, Paris 60:1027–1028.

———. (1906b) Recherches sur la régénérescence de la moelle. *Nouv Iconographie de la Salpêtrière* 5:417–440.

———. (1906c) Précocité des phénomènes de régénérescence des nerf après leur section. *Compt Rend Soc Biol*, Paris 61:383–385.

———. (1907a) Recherches expérimentales et anatomo-pathologiques sur les lésions consécutives à la compression et à l'écrasement des ganglions sensitifs. *Folia Neurobiol* 1:4–13.

———. (1907b) Changements morphologiques des cellules nerveuses survivant à la transplantation des ganglions nerveux. *Compt Rend Acad Sci*, Paris 144:656–658.

———. (1907c) Nouvelles recherches sur la transplantation des ganglions nerveux (transplantation chez la grenouille). *Compt Rend Acad Sci*, Paris 144:450–452.

———. (1910) Nouvelles contributions à l'étude de la régénérescence des fibres du système nerveux central. I. Neurotisation des lésions en foyer de la moelle et du cervelet. *J Psychol Neurol* 17:116–143.

———. (1911) Sur l'influence exercée par l'ablation totale du corps thyroïdienne sur la dégénérescence et la régénérescence des nerfs sectionnes. *Ann Biol Clin*, Paris 1:17–46.

———. (1912) Essai de culture des ganglions spinaux de mammifères *in vitro*. Contribution à l'étude de la neurogénèse. *Anat Anz* 42:161–176.

———. (1914) Nouvelles recherches sur la culture *in vitro* des ganglions spinaux des mammifères. *Anat Anz* 46:529–547.

May, R. M. (1923–1924) Skin grafts in the lizard *Anolis carolinensis*, Cuv. *Br J Exp Zool* 1:539–555.

———. (1925) The relation of nerves to degenerating and regenerating taste buds. *J Exp Zool* 42:371–410.

———. (1927a) Modifications of nerve centers due to the transplantation of the eye and olfactory organ in anuran embryos. *Proc Natl Acad Sci USA* 13:372–374.

———. (1927b) Modifications des centres nerveux dues à la transplantation de l'oeil et de l'organe olfactif chez les embryons d'anoures. *Arch Biol* 37:335–395.

———. (1957) The possibilities of brephoplastic transplants. *Ann NY Acad Sci* 64:937–949.

———. (1960) The Dormant state in tissue transplantation as exemplified by subscapular grafts of testicles from hypophysectomized mice. *Ann NY Acad Sci* 87:501–511.

———, and Detwiler, S. R. (1926) The relation of transplanted eyes to developing nerve centers. *J Exp Zool* 43:83–103.

———, and Jeanmarie, R. Z. (1963) Positive interracial grafts of embryonic thyroids implanted into the eye of adult mice. *Ann NY Acad Sci* 99:870–881.

Mayer, S. (1876) Die peripherische Nervenzelle und das sympathische Nervensystem. *Arch Psychiat Nervenkrh* 6:353–446.

Medea, E. (1905) L'applicazione del nuovo metodo di Ramón y Cajal allo studio del sistema nervoso periferico (nella neurite parenchimatose degenerativa sperimentale). *Boll Soc Med-Chir*, Pavia 1905:44–47.

Merzbacher, L. (1905) Zur Biologie der Nervendegeneration. Ergebnisse von Transplantationsversuchen. *Neurol Centralbl* 24:150–155.

———. (1910) Untersuchungen über die Morphologie und Biologie der Abraumzellen im Zentralnervensystem. In: *Histologische und histopathologische Arbeiten über die Grosshirnrinde*. F. Nissl and A. Alzheimer (Eds.) Vol. 3. Jena: Fischer, pp. 1–142.

Michailow, S. (1908a) Mikroskopische Struktur der Ganglien des Plexus solaris und anderer Ganglien des Grenzstranges des N. sympathicus. *Anat Anz* 33:581–590.

———. (1908b) Zur Frage über den feineren Bau des intracardialen Nervensystems der Säugethiere. *Int Monatschr Anat Physiol* 25:44–87.

———. (1908c) Zur Frage der Innervation der Blutgefässe. *Arch Mikrosk Anat* 72:540–553.

Minea, J. (1909) *Cercetări experimentale asupra variatiunilor morfologice ale neuronului sensitiu*. Tesis, Bucaresti: Brozer.

Minor, L. (1904) Traumatische Erkrankungen des Rückenmarkes. (Rückenmark-

Zerquetschung, Hämatomyelie, Nekrose etc.) In: *Handbuch der pathologische Anatomie des Nervensystems, in Verbindung mit G. Anton [et al.]*. E. Flatau; L. Jacobsohn; and L. Minor (Eds.). Vol. 2, Berlin: Karger, pp. 1008–1058.

Miskolczy, D. (1925) Ueber die Früveränderungen der Pyramidenzellen nach experimentellen Rindeverletzungen. *Trav Lab Rech Biol*, Univ. Madrid 23:135–156.

Miyake, K. (1908) Zur Frage der Regeneration der Nervenfasern im zentralen Nervensystem. *Arb Neurol Inst Wien Univ* 14:1–15.

Modena, G. (1905) Die Degeneration und Regeneration des peripheren Nerven nach Läsion derselben. *Arb Neurol Inst Wien Univ* 12:243–281.

———. (1910–1911) Régénération des nerfs périphériques. *Arch Ital Biol* 54:419–424.

Mönckeberg, G., and Bethe, A. (1899) Die Degeneration der markhaltigen Nervenfasern der Wirbelthiere unter hauptsächlicher Berücksichtigung des Verhaltens der Primitivfibrillen (Zugleich ein Beitrag zur Kenntnis der normalen Nervenfasern). *Arch Mikrosk Anat* 54:135–183.

Mondino, C. (1884) Sulla struttura delle fibre nervose midollate periferiche. *Arch Sci Med* 8:45–66.

Morgenthaler, W. (1912) Heilungsvorgänge in der Grosshirnrinde des normalen und alkoholisierten Kaninchens nach Einführung eines Fremdkörpers. *Z Neurol Psychiatr* 8:431–462.

Mott, F. W., and Halliburton, W. D. (1901) The chemistry of nerve degeneration. *Philos Trans R Soc Lond* 194:437–466.

———; and Edmunds, A. (1906) Regeneration of Nerves. *Proc R Soc Lond* 78:259–283.

Müller, L. R. (1909) Studien über die Anatomie und Histologie des sympathischen Grenzstranges, insbesondere über seine Beziehungen zu dem spinalen Nervensysteme. Verhandlungen des Kongresses für innere Medizin, 26th Congr., Wiesbaden, pp. 658–681.

———. (1910–1911) Beiträge zur Anat. Histol. und Physiol. des Nervus vagus; zugleich des Herzens der Bronchien und des Mägens. *Dtsch Arch Klin Med* 101:421–481.

———. (1911) Die Darminnervation. *Dtsch Arch Klin Med* 105:1–43.

———, and Dahl, W. (1910) Die Beteiligung des sympathischen Nervensystems an der Kopfinnervation. *Dtsches Arch Klin Med* 99:48–107.

Muñoz-Urra, [?] (1923) Archivos de Oftalmologia [not verified].

Münzer, E. (1902) Giebt es eine autogenetische Regeneration der Nervenfasern? Ein Beitrag zur Lehre vom Neuron. *Neurol Centralb* 21:1090–1098.

Nageotte, J. (1905) Un cas de tabes amyotrophique étudié par la méthode à l'alcool ammoniaque de Ramón y Cajal: régénération de fibres à myéline dans les racines antérieures, de fibres sans myéline dans les racines posterieures. *Compt Rend Soc Biol*, Paris 58:849–851.

———. (1906a) Régénération collatérale des fibres nerveuses terminés par massues de croissance à l'état pathologique et à l'état normal; lésions tabétiques des racines médullaires. *Nouv Iconographie de la Salpêtrière* 19:217–238.

———. (1906b) Note sur le régénération amyélinique des racines postérieures dans le tabes et sur les massues d'accroissement qui terminent les fibres néoformées. *Compt Rend Soc Biol*, Paris 60:477–479.

———. (1906c) Note sur la présence de massues d'accroissement dans la substance grise de la moelle, et particulièrement dans les cornes antérieures, au cours de la paralysie générale et du tabes. *Compt Rend Soc Biol*, Paris 60:811–812.

———. (1906d) Note sur la régénération collatérale des neurones radiculaires postérieurs dans le tabes et sur la signification physiologique des cellules pourvues d'appendices terminés par les boules encapsulées, de Ramón y Cajal. *Compt Rend Soc Biol*, Paris 60:745–747.

———. (1907a) Greffe de ganglions rachidiens, suivie des éléments nobles et transformation des cellules unipolaires en cellule multipolaires. *Compt Rend Soc Biol*, Paris 62:62–64.

———. (1907b) Deuxième note sur la greffe des ganglions rachidiens; types divers des prolongements nerveuses néoformés, comparaison avec certaines dispositions normales ou considérées comme telles; persistance des éléments péricellulaires dans les capsules vides après phagocytose des cellules nerveuses mortes. *Compt Rend Soc Biol*, Paris 62:289–292.

———. (1907c) Troisième note sur la greffe des ganglions rachidiens; mode de destruction des cellules nerveuses mortes. *Compt Rend Soc Biol*, Paris 62:381–384.

———. (1907d) Formations graisseuses dans les cellules satellites des ganglions rachidiens greffés. *Compt Rend Soc Biol*, Paris 62:1147–1149.

———. (1907e) À propos de l'influence de la pression osmotique sur le développement des prolongements nerveux dans les greffés ganglionnaires. *Compt Rend Soc Biol*, Paris 63:71.

———. (1907f) Note sur l'apparition précoce d'arborisations périglomérulaires, formées aux dépens de collatérales des glomérules dans les ganglions rachidiens greffés. *Compt Rend Acad Sci*, Paris 144:580.

———. (1907g) Recherches expérimentales sur la morphologie des cellules et des fibres des ganglions rachidiens. *Rev Neurol*, Paris, 15:357–368.

———. (1907h) Étude sur la greffe des ganglions rachidiens; variations et tropismes du neurone sensitif. *Anat Anz* 31:225–245.

———. (1907i) Neurophagie dans les greffes des ganglions rachidiens. *Rev. Neurol*, Paris 17:933–944.

———. (1910a) Sur une nouvelle formation de la gaîne de myéline; le double bracelet épineux de l'étranglement annulaire. *Compt Rend Acad Sci*, Paris 150:123–126.

———. (1910b) Incisures de Schmidt-Lantermann et protoplasma des cellules de Schwann. *Compt Rend Soc Biol*, Paris 68:39–42.

———. (1910c) Action des métaux et de divers autres facteurs sur la dégénération des nerfs en survie. *Compt Rend Soc Biol*, Paris 69:556–559.

———. (1911) Le syncitium de Schwann et les gaînes de la fibre à myéline dans les phases avancées de la dégénération wallérienne. *Compt Rend Soc Biol*, Paris 70:861–865.

———. (1911) *Notice sur les Travaux Scientifiques de M.J. Nageotte*. Paris: Maretheux.

———. (1914–1915) Le processus de la cicatrisation des nerfs. Généralités et faits particuliers. *Rev Neurol*, Paris, 22:505–521.

———. (1916a) Sur la greffe des tissus morts, et en particulier sur la reparation des pertes de substance des nerfs à l'aide de greffons nerveux conservés dans l'alcool. *Compt Rend Soc Biol*, Paris 79:833, 940, 1031, 1121.

———. (1916b) Substance collàgene et névrologie dans la cicatrisation des nerfs. *Compt Rend Soc Biol*, Paris 79:322–327.

———. (1917a) Sur la greffe des tissues morts et en particulier sur la réparation des pertes de substance des nerfs à l'aide de greffrons nerveux conservés dans l'alcool. *Compt Rend Soc Biol*, Paris 80:459–470.

———. (1917b) Sur l'amoindrissement morphologique des nerfs après cicatrice (Mémoires). *Compt Rend Soc Biol*, Paris 80:597–602.

———. (1917c) Sur la possibilité d'utiliser dans la pratique chirurgicale les greffons des nerfs fixés par l'alcool et sur la technique à employer. *Compt Rend Soc Biol*, Paris 80:925–933.

———. (1918a) Étude expérimentale de la cicatrisation des nerfs. *Lyon Chir* 15:245–292.

———. (1918b) Sur une atrophie musculaire réflexe précoce, après suture des nerfs par affrontement et sur les inconvénients de la greffe nerveuse vivante autoplastique. *Compt Rend Soc Biol*, Paris 81:761–764.

———. (1921) Rapport des neurites avec les tissus dans la cornée. *Compt Rend Acad Sci*, Paris 172:94–96.

———. (1922) *L'Organisation de la Matiere dans ses Rapports avec la Vie; Études d'Anatomie Generale et de Morphologie Experimentale sur le Tissu Conjunctif et le Nerf.* Paris: Alcan.

———, and Guyon, L. (1916) Aptitudes néoplasiques de la névroglie périphérique greffée et non réinnervée; conséquences au point de vue chirurgical. *Compt Rend Soc Biol*, Paris 79:984–991.

———. (1918) Différences physiologiques entre la névroglie des fibres motrices et cells des fibres sensitives, dans les nerfs periphériques mises en évidence par la régénération. *Compt Rend Soc Biol*, Paris 81:571–576.

———, and León-Kindberg, M. (1908a) Nodosités des prolongements protoplasmiques des cellules de Purkinje dans un cas d'idiotie familiale avec atrophie cérébelleux et dégénération des cordons posterieurs, des faisceaux pyramidaux et des faisceaux cérébelleux directs. *Compt Rend Soc Biol*, Paris 65:517–520.

———. (1908b) Lésions fines du cervelet. Tuméfaction fusiforme du cylindraxe des cellules de Purkinje. *Compt Rend Soc Biol*, Paris 65:551–553.

Nemiloff, A. (1908) Einige Beobachtungen über den Bau des Nervengewebes bei Cyanoiden und Knochenfischen. *Arch Mikrosk Anat* 72:575–606.

———. (1910) Ueber die Beziehung der sog. "Zellen der Schwannschen Scheide" zum Myelin in den Nervenfasern von Säugethieren. *Arch Mikrosk Anat* 76:329–348.

Nissl, F. (1899) Ueber einige Beziehungen zwischen Nervenzellenerkrankungen und gliösen Erscheinungen bei verschiedenen Psychosen. *Arch Psychiatr* 32:656–676.

Nothafft, [?] (1892) Neue Untersuchungen ueber die Verlauf der Degeneration— und Regenerationsprozesse an verletzten peripheren Nerven. Thesis, Würzburg [not verified].

Pacheco, A. (1909–1910) Sur les types cellulaires des ganglions spinaux de l'homme à l'état normal et dans quelques états pathologiques. *Arch R Inst Bacteriol*, Camara Pestana, Lisbon 3:59–97.

Pérez de Tudela, M. A. (1983) Publicaciones del Prof. Dr. Santiago Ramón y Cajal existentes en los fondos de la biblioteca del "Instituto de Neurobiología Santiago Ramón y Cajal." *Trab Inst Cajal*, Madrid 74:169–235.

Perrero, E. (1909) Contributo allo studio della rigenerazione delle fibre nervose del sistema nervoso centrale. *Riv. Patol Nerv Ment* 14:193–204.

Perroncito, A. (1905a) La rigenerazione delle fibre nervose. *Boll Soc Med-Chir*, Pavia, pp. 1905:434–444.

———. (1905b) Sulla questione della rigenerazione autogena delle fibre nervose. *Boll Soc Med-Chir,* Pavia, 1905:360–363.

———. (1905–1906) La rigenerazione delle fibre nervose. Preliminary notes II and III. *Boll Soc Med-Chir*, Pavia, 1905:453–462.

———. (1906) La rigenerazione delle fibre nervose. *Boll Soc Med-Chir*, Pavia, 1906:94–105.

———. (1907) Die Regeneration der Nerven. *Beitr Path Anat Allg Path* 42:355–446.

———. (1909) Gli elementi cellulari nel processo di degenerazione dei nervi. *Boll Soc Med-Chir*, Pavia 23:108–117.

———. (1911) Beiträge zur Biologie der Zelle; (Mitochondrien, Chromidien, Golgisches Binnennetz in den Samenzellen). *Arch Mikrosk Anat* 77:311–321.

Pertik, O. (1880–1881) Untersuchungen über Nervenfasern. *Arch Mikrosk Anat*, 19:183–239.

Perusini, G. (1909) Über klinisch und histologisch eigenartige psychische Erkrankungen des späteren Lebensalters. In: *Histologische und histopathologisches Arbeiten über die Grosshirnrinde*. F. Nissl and A. Alzheimer (Eds.). Vol 3. Jena:Fischer, pp. 297–358..

Pfeifer, R. (1908–1909) Ueber die traumatische Degeneration und Regeneration des Gehirns erwachsener Menschen. *J Psychol Neurol* 12:96–123.

Philipeaux, J. M., and Vulpian, A. (1859) Recherches expérimentales sur la régénération des nerfs séparés des centres nerveaux. *Compt Rend Soc Biol*, Paris 1:343–415.

Pick, L., and Bielschowsky, M. (1911) Ueber das System der Neurome und Beobachtungen an einem Ganglioneurome des Gehirns (nebst Untersuchungen über die Genese der Nervenfasern in Neuromen). *Z Gesamte Neurol Psychiatr* 6:391–437.

Pitzorno, M. (1910) Su alcune particolarità delle cellule del cordone simpatico dei cheloni. *Moni Zool Ital*, Firenze 21:111–116.

Poscharisky, J. (1907) Über die histologischen Vorgänge an den peripherischen Nerven nach Kontinuitätstrennung. *Beitr Path Anat Allg Path* 41:52–94.

Purpura, F. (1901) Contributo allo studio della rigenerazione dei nervi periferici.

Communication made in the session of 1 February 1901. *Boll Soc Med-Chir*, Pavia 34:415–419.

Rachmanow, A. (1911) Zur normalen und pathologischen Histologie der peripheren Nerven des Menschen. *J Psychol Neurol* 18:522–545.

Ranson, S. W. (1912) The structure of the spinal ganglia and of the spinal nerves. *J Comp Neurol* 22:159–169.

———. (1914) Transplantation of the spinal ganglion with observations on the significance of the complex types of spinal ganglion cells. *J Comp Neurol* 24:547–558.

Ranvier, L. A. (1872) De la dégénérescence des nerfs après leur section. *Compt Rend Acad Sci*, Paris 75:1831 1835.

———. (1873) De la régénération des nerfs sectionnes. *Compt Rend Acad Sci*, Paris 76:491–495.

———. (1878) *Leçons sur l'Histologie du Système Nerveux*. Compiled by E. Weber. 2 vols. Paris: Savy.

———. (1879) De la régénération des nerfs de l'epithélium antérieur de la cornée et de la théorie du développement continu du système nerveux. *Compt Rend Acad Sci*, Paris 88:979–981.

Raposo, S. L. (1925) La régénération de la moelle épinière et des ganglions rachidiens chez les amphibiens adultes. (*Molge waltlii*, Michah.) *Trav Lab Rech Biol*, Univ. Madrid 23:53–100.

Rebizzi, R. (1904) Sulla struttura de la guaina mielinica. *Riv Patol Nerv Ment* 9:409–430.

Reich, F. (1907) Ueber den zelligen Aufbau der Nervenfaser auf Grund mikrohistochemischer Untersuchungen. *J Psychol Neurol* 8:244–273.

Remak, R. (1862) Ueber die Wiedererzeugung von Nervenfasern. *Virchows Arch Pathol Anat* 23:441–444.

Retzius, G. (1906) Ueber die von Ruffini beschriebene Guaina subsidiaria der Nervenfasern. *Anat Anz* 28:1–4.

Riquier, C. (1913) Sulla fina struttura del ganglio otico. *Riv Patol Nerv Ment* 18:609–628.

Río, E. del (1910) Algunos datos concernientes a la anatomía patológica del leproma. *Trab Lab Invest Biol*, Univ. Madrid 8:157–168.

Río-Hortega. *See* del Río-Hortega.

Rojas, P. (1917) Degeneración y regeneración experimental de los nervios periféricos. *Trab Lab Invest Biol*, Univ. Madrid 15:301–358.

Rossi, O. (1907) Compartamento di alcuni fenomeni riflessi dopo la sezione delle radici posteriori. *Riv Patol Nerv Ment* 12:1–4.

———. (1908a) Processi rigenerativi e degenerativi consequente a ferite assetiche del sistema nervoso centrale; midollo spinale e nervo ottico. *Riv Patol Nerv Ment* 13:481–517.

———. (1908b) Processi rigenerativi e degenerativi consequenti a ferite asettiche del sistema nervoso centrale; midollo spinale e nervo ottico. *Riv Patol Nerv Ment* 13:481–517.

———. (1908–1909) Ueber einige morphologische Besonderheiten der Spinalganglien bei den Säugethieren. *J Psychol Neurol* 11:1–25.

———. (1909a) Sopra ad alcune apparenze morfologiche che si riscontrano nelle cellule nervose del midollo in vicinanza di ferite asettiche sperimentalmente provocate. *Riv Patol Nerv Ment* 14:356–361.

———. (1909b) Sulla rigeneratione del nervo ottico. *Riv Patol Nerv Ment* 14:145–150.

———. (1909c) Anat. Anzeiger, Bd 39, March 26, 1909. [We consider that this refers to: Sala, G. (1909) Ueber die Regenerationserscheinungen im zentralen Nervensystem. *Anat Anz* 34:193–199. This appeared in numbers 9–11 of the journal, published on 26 March 1909, and began a slightly acrimonious correspondence between Sala and Marinesco that continued on pages 443–444 and 583–584 of the same volume.]

———. (1910a) Sull'istologia patologica di una speciale alterazione descritta da Marchiafava nel corpo calloso degli alcoolisti. *Riv Patol Nerv Ment* 15:346–366.

———. (1910b) Nuove ricerche sui fenomeni di rigenerazione che si volgano nel midollo spinale; rigenerazione negli animale ibernanti. *Riv Patol Nerv Ment* 15:201–210.

———. (1911) Sulla rigenerazione del sistema nervoso. *Riv Patol Nerv Ment* 16:193–213.

———. (1913) Klinischer und anatomo-pathologischer Beitrag zur Kenntnis des sogen. Pellagratyphus. *J Psychol Neurol* 20:1–23.

———. (1921) Osservazioni neurologiche sui lesioni del sistema nervoso di trauma di guerra. Sasari [not verified].

Rossi, U. (1908) Per la rigenerazione dei neuroni. *Trav Lab Rech Biol*, Univ Madrid 6:227–241.

———, and Garbini, G. (1912) Intorno a speciali connessioni tra alcuni neuroni cerebellari. Annal. della Facoltà di Medicina di Perugia. Serie 4, vol. 1., fasc. 1 [not verified].

Ruiz de Arcaute, L. (1912) Sobre algunas alteraciones de las células de Purkinje del cerebelo en un caso de sífilis hereditaria. *Bol Soc Españ Biol* 1:190–193.

———. (1913) Tipos morfológicos del gran simpático de los mamíferos de gran talla (buey, caballo, asno, etc.). *Bol Soc Españ Biol*, November [not verified].

Sachs, B., and Strauss, I. (1910) The cell changes in amaurotic family idiocy. *J Exp Med* 12:685–695.

Saito, M. (1908) Zur Frage der Regeneration der peripheren Nerven des erwachsenen Menschen. *Arb Neurol Inst Wien Univ* 24:85–92.

Sala, G. (1900) Beitrag zur Kenntnis der markhaltigen Nervenfasern. *Anat Anz* 18:49–55, 176–178.

———. (1908) Sui fatti che si svolgono in seguito alle ferite asettiche del cervello. *Boll Soc Med-Chir*, Pavia 22:1–7.

———. (1909) Ueber die Regenerationserscheinungen im zentralen Nervensystem. *Anat Anz* 34:193–199.

———. (1910a) A proposito di un caso di sezione trasversa completa del midollo spinale. *Boll Soc Med-Chir*, Pavia 24:424–428.

———. (1910b) Sulla fina struttura del ganglio ciliare. *Boll Soc Med-Chir*, Pavia 24:429.

———. (1913) Sopra un caso di demenzia presenile con sintomi a focolaio. *Boll Soc Med-Chir*, Pavia 27:1–16.

———, and Cortese, G. (1909) Sui fatti che zi svolgono nel midollo spinale in seguito allo strappo delle radici. *Gazz Med Ital*, Torino 60:271.

Saltykow, S. (1905) Versuche über Gehirnreplantation, zugleich ein Beitrag zur Kenntnis reactiver Vorgänge an den zelligen Gehirnelementen. *Arch Psychiatr Nervenkr* 40:329–388.

Schäfer, E. A., and Feiss, H. O. (1915–1916) Notes on the functional regeneration of the cut cervical sympathetic and vagus. *Q J Exp Physiol* 9:329–334.

Schaffer, K. (1910) Ueber Fibrillenbilder tabischer Spinalganglienzellen. *Z Gesamte Neurol Psychiatr* 1:439–468.

———. (1913–1914) Zum normalen und pathologischen Fibrillenbau der Kleinhirnrinde. *Z Gesamte Neurol Psychiatr* 21:1–48.

———. (1922) Tatsächliches und Hypothetisches aus der Histopathologie der infantilamäurotischen Idiotie. *Arch Psychiatr Nervenkr* 64:570–616.

Schob, F. (1912) Zur pathologischen Anatomie der juvenilen Form der amäurotischen Idiotie. *Z Gesamte Neurol Psychiatr* 10:303–324.

Schob, [?] (1922) *Arb Dtsch Forsch-Anstalt Psychiatr*, München. Vol. 5 [not verified].

Schiefferdecker, P. (1887) Beiträge zur Kenntnis des Bau der Nervenfasern. *Arch Mikrosk Anat* 30:435–494.

Schultze, O. (1905) Beiträge zur Histogenese des Nervensystems. I. Über die multizelluläre Entstehung der peripheren sensiblen Nervenfaser und das Vorhandensein eines allgemeinen Endnetzes sensibler Neuroblasten bei Amphibienlarven. *Arch Mikrosk Anat Entw* 36:41–110.

Segale, M. (1903) *Sulla Rigenerazione dei Nerve; Note Critiche Sperimentali Cliniche*. Genoa: Carlini.

Segall, B. (1892) Nouveaux anneaux ou anneaux intercalaires des tubes nerveux, produits par l'imprégnation d'argent. *Compt Rend Acad Sci*, Paris 114:558–559.

———. (1893) Sur des anneaux intercalaires des tubes nerveux produits par imprégnation d'argent. *J Anat*, Paris 29:586–603.

Simchowicz, T. (1910–1911) Histologische Studien über die senile Demenz. In: *Histologische und histopathologische Arbeiten über die Grosshirnrinde*. F. Nissl and A. Alzheimer (Eds.). Vol. 4. Jena: Fischer, 267–444.

Sittig, O. (1911–1912) Anhäufung von polynuclearen Leukocyten um die Ganglienzellen bei epidemischer Cerebrospinal-Meningitis. *Z Gesamte Neurol Psychiatr* 8:14–19.

Spielmeyer, W. (1917) Ueber Regeneration Peripherischer Nerven. *Z Gesamte Neurol Psychiatr* 36:421–430.

———. (1922) *Histopathologie des Nervensystems*. Berlin: Springer.

Stöhr, P., Jr. (1928) Die peripherische Nervenfaser. In: *Handbuch der mikroskopischen Anatomie des Menschen*. W. v. Möllendorff (Ed.). Vol. 4, p 1. Berlin: Springer.

Storch, E. (1899) Ueber die pathologisch-anatomischen Vorgänge am Stützgerüst des Centralnervensystems. *Virchows Arch Pathol Anat* 157:127–171, 197–234.

Strasser, H. (1892–1893) Alte und neue Probleme des entwickelungsgeschichtlichen Forschung auf dem Gebiete des Nervensystems. *Anat Hefte* 1 (1892):721–769; 2 (1893):565–603.

Straussler, E. (1906) Ueber eigenartige Veränderungen der Ganglienzellen und ihrer Fortsätze im Centralnervensystem eines Falles von kongenitaler Kleinhirnatrophie. *Neurol Centralbl* 25:194–205.

Stroebe, H. (1893a) Ueber Degeneration und Regeneration peripherer Nerven nach Verletzungen. *Arch Psychiatr* 25:586–588.

———. (1893b) Experimentelle Untersuchungen über Degeneration und Regeneration peripherer Nerven nach Verletzungen. *Beitr Path Anat Allg Path* 13:160–278.

———. (1894) Experimentelle Untersuchungen über die degenerativen und reparatorischen Vorgänge bei der Heilung von Verletzungen des Rückenmarks nebst Bemerkungen zur Histogenese der secundären Degeneration im Rückenmark. *Beitr Path Anat Allg Path* 15:383–490.

———. (1895) Die allgemeine Histologie der degenerativen und regenerativen Processe im centralen und peripheren Nervensystem nach den neuesten Forschungen. *Centralbl Allg Path Anat* 6:849–960.

Stuart, J. (1906) Proceedings of the Royal Society, vol. 78, 1906. [We believe that this mainly refers to: Mott, F. W.; Halliburton, W. D.; and Edmunds, A. (1906) Regeneration of Nerves. *Proc R Soc Lond* 78:259–283.]

Tello, J. F. (1907a) Dégénération et régénération des plaques motrices après la section des nerfs. *Trav Lab Rech Biol*, Univ. Madrid 5:117–149.

———. (1907b) La régénération dans les fuseaux de Kühne. *Trav Lab Rech Biol*, Univ. Madrid 5:227–236.

———. (1907c) La régénération dans les voies optiques. *Trav Lab Rech Biol*, Univ. Madrid 5:237–248.

———. (1911a) Un experimento sobre la influencia del neurotropismo en la regeneración de la corteza cerebral. *Rev Clin* Madrid 5:292—294.

———. (1911b) La influencia del neurotropismo en la regeneración de los centros nerviosos. *Trab Lab Invest Biol*, Univ. Madrid 9:123–159.

———. (1913a) El retículo de Golgi en las células del granuloma experimental producido por el Kieselgur *Bol Soc Españ Biol* 2:7–12.

———. (1913b) El retículo de Golgi en las células de algunos tumores y en las del granuloma experimental producido por el Kieselgur. *Trab Lab Invest Biol*, Univ Madrid 11:145–161.

———. (1914) Algunas experiencias de ingertos nerviosos con nervios conservados "in vitro." *Trab Lab Invest Biol*, Univ. Madrid 12:273–284.

———. (1917) Génesis de las terminaciones nerviosas motrices y sensitivas. I. En el sistema locomotor de los vertebrados superiores. Histogénesis muscular. *Trab Lab Invest Biol*, Univ Madrid 15:101–199.

———. (1923a) Les différenciations neuronales dans l'embryon du poulet, pendant les premiers jours de l'incubation. *Trav Lab Rech Biol*, Univ Madrid 21:1–93.

———. (1923b) Genèse des terminaisons motrices et sensitives. II. Terminaisons dans les poils de la souris blanche. *Trav Lab Rech Biol*, Univ Madrid 21:259–384.

———. (1923c) Gegenwärtige Anschauungen über den Neurotropismus. Translated by E. Herzog. In: *Vortrage und Aufsätze über Entwicklungsmechanik der Organisen.* W. Roux (Ed.). Vol. 33. Berlin: Springer, pp. 1–73.

———. (1935) *Cajal y su Labor Histológica.* Madrid: Universidad Central.

Ulrich, M. (1910) Beiträge zur Kenntnis der Stäbchenzellen im Zentralnervensystem. *Monatsschr Psychol Neurol* 28:24–79.

Van Gehuchten, A., and Molhant, M. (1910) Les lois de la dégénérescence wallerienne directe. Series 4. *Bull Acad R Med*, Belg 24:576–612.

Vanlair, C. (1882) De la régénération des nerfs périphériques par le procédé de la suture tubulaire. *Compt Rend Acad Sci,* Paris 95:99–101.

———. (1885) Nouvelles recherches expérimentales sur la régénération des nerfs. *Arch Biol* 6:127–235.

———. (1888) Sur la persistance de l'aptitude régénératrice des nerfs. *Bull Acad R Sci, Lett, Beaux-arts,* Belg 16:93–110.

Veratti, E. (1907) Alcune osservazioni sui procesi consecutive alle ferite dei gangli spinali. *Atti Soc Ital Patol* IV[a] reunione, Pavia [not verified].

Vulpian, E. F. A. (1866) Leçons *sur la Physiologie Générale et Comparée du Système Nerveux.* Compiled by E. Bremónd, given at the Musée d'Histoire Natural. Paris: Germer-Bailliere.

Waldeyer, W. (1891) Über einige neuere Forschungen im Gebiete der Anatomie des Centralnervensystems. *Dtsch Med Wochenschr* 17:1213–1218; 1244–1246; 1267–1269; 1331–1332; 1352–1356.

Waller, A. [V.] (1850) Experiments on the section of the glosso-pharyngeal and hypo-glossal nerves of the frog, and observations of the alterations produced thereby in the structure of their primitive fibres. *Philos Trans R Soc, Lond* 140: 423–429.

———. (1852) Sur la reproduction des nerfs et sur la structure et les fonctions des ganglions spinaux. *Arch Anat Physiol Wiss Med* 1852:392–401.

Weissfeiler, J. (1925) Régénération du nerf optique et du chiasma chez le triton. *Compt Rend Soc Biol,* Paris 92:1412.

Wieting, J. (1898) Zur Frage der Regeneration der peripherischen Nerven. *Beitr Path Anat Allg Path* 23: 42–68.

Woollard, H. H. (1927) *Recent Advances in Anatomy.* London: Churchill.

Zalla, M. (1909) I fenomeni cellulari nella degenerazione walleriana dei nervi periferici. *Riv Patol Nerv Ment* 14:7–22.

Ziegler, E. (1892) *Lehrbuch der Allgemeinen und Speciellen Pathologischen Anatomie und Pathogenese. Mit einem Anhange über die Technik der Pathologisch-anatomischen Untersuchung.* 2 vols. Jena: Fischer.

Subject Index

Aberrant
 fibers, 65
 funicular fibers, 51
 motor conductors, 50
Agents. *See* Trophic substances
Agonal
 neurofibrilar colonies, 59
 reaction, 107
 survival, 106
Amoeboidism, 8
 sprouts in phase of, 88
Amputation. *See* Mutilation
Anastomoses, 93, 96, 100
 intracolonial, 98
Apotrophic cells (of Marinesco), 77, 79, 93
Atrophy and degeneration because of disuse, 98
Attractive ferments, 67
Autogenous regeneration, 84, 87
Autogenic regeneration, 103. *See also* Autoregeneration
Autonomy of the neurofibrils, 107
Autoregeneration, 32, 37, 99, 126
 theory of, 91
Autotomy, 60, 116
Avulsion of nerves, 65–66
Axon
 arciform, 55, 56
 distinction of dead from the living, 62, 64
 explorer, of Harrison, 81
 of pyramidal cells sprouting through nerve implants, 46
 stray, 34
 sudden death of, 40

Ball (or club) of retraction, 43, 57, 94, 117
 giant, 67
Basket terminations in the cerebellum
 alterations of, and rabies, 97
 destruction of, in amaurotic idiocy, 96
 hypertrophy and retraction, 97
 maintenance in general paralysis, 95
  after sectioning of Purkinje axons, 95
Bielschowsky method, 97
Brephoplastic transplantation, 13

Büngner, bands of, 34, 79, 86, 89, 103, 105, 119, 120

Catalytic agents, 12, 46, 48
Catenarists, 84
Catenary, theory of. *See* Discontinuity
Cellular colony, 99
Cephalopodic apparatus (or formation), 57, 120
Cerebral cortex, and grafting of sciatic nerve, 120
Chambers method, 99
Chemotactism, theory of, 8, 123
Chemotaxis, 8
Chromaffin cells, 112
Clubs (or boutons)
 of growth, 35, 40, 43, 107, 110, 111
 terminal, 33, 34, 37, 57, 107–9
Compound granular cells, 116
Cones of growth, 49. *See also* Growth cone
Connective tissue as a neurotropic source, 46, 47
Conserved fibers, 62, 64, 107
Continuity
 protoplasmic, rarity of, 99
 theory of (or monogenetic or monogenist hypothesis), 30, 40, 41, 80, 83, 84, 86, 92, 99, 126
Continuous development or monogenesis, 40
Corrosion, point of, 55, 64

Degeneration and limited trauma, 97
Degeneration and intoxication. *See* Intoxication
Degeneration in nerves
 description, 102
 phases of, 105
  fragmentation, 106
  granular disintegration of the neurofibrils, 106
  moniliform state, 105
  reabsorption, 106
 traumatic, 104, 106, 107
 trophic (or Wallerian), 104, 106
Degeneration

Degeneration (Cont.)
  in the gray matter of the nerve centers, 117
  in the white matter of the nerve centers, 115
    traumatic, 115
    trophic (or Wallerian) 116
Dementia
  praecox and alterations of the basket terminations, 97
  senile, 95
Digestive chambers, 104, 105
Discontinuity
  anatomical, of nerve cells, 98
  theory of (or catenary theory), 28, 30, 31, 34, 35, 37, 40, 80, 99
Dogiel, colonial hypothesis of, 98

Experimental transformation of cells with long axon into cells with short axon, 53, 123
  Purkinje cells, 54, 97, 123
  pyramidal cells, 54, 97, 123
Ensheathment
  hypothesis of, 92
  and polygeneticists, 111

Friedreich's disease, 95

General paralysis, 95
  and alterations of basket terminations, 97
Genetic unity, 31
Golgi technique, 5, 31
Grafting (transplantation)
  of ganglia, 65, 79
  of nerve trunks, 67
  of sciatic nerve and photography, 85
Grafts
  dead, 67
  of sciatic nerve into cerebral cortex, 120
  thick and fresh, 67
  thin and very fresh (reimplantation), 67
Growth cone, 34, 51. See also Cones of growth
Growth of nerve fibers independent of cells of the scar, 111
Gudden, method of, 100

Haematoxylin and aniline dyes, 104
Held, chalices of, 97
Henle, sheath of, 82
Hensen-Held, theory of, 7
Heterochronotransplantation, 9
Heterotransplantation, 9
Histopathologic discontinuity, 97. See also Discontinuity, anatomical
Homochronotransplantation, 65

Homotactism. See Stereotropism
Homotransplantation, 65
Hypertrophy, fusiform, 62

Influence of the environment in the morphology of the neuron, 55
Innervation, 14
  factors that affect timing of, 112
  mechanism of, 90
  of the peripheral stump, 83–85, 88, 89
  of the scar, beginning of, 109
Iron haematoxylin, 82
Irregenerability, in central nervous pathways, 43, 118, 120
  refutation of, 47, 48, 94
Intoxication and degenerative processes
  by alcohol, 95
  by lead salts, 95

Key and Retzius, sheath of, 105
Kühne, spindles of, 103

Leitzellen of Held, 93
Lemnoblasts or coleoblasts, 89
Leukocytes, 105, 106, 116, 117
Ligature of nerves, 68–70
Locke's solution, 111, 122
Lycopodium, 111
Laminar membrane of the nerves, rudiment of, 82

Monogenetism. See Continuity, theory of
Monogenists (or monogeneticists), 6, 7, 40
  controversy with polygeneticists, 103
Morphology of the neuron, influence of the environment, 55
Mutilation (or amputation) of axonal segments, 51, 94, 97
Myelin, formation of, 7

Nageotte, theory of (in nerve regeneration), 82
Necrotic foci produced by emboli or thromboses, 95
Neoformation of fibers, types of, 108
Neurocladic catalysts, 52
Neurocladism, 122
Nerve fiber
  new in the peripheral stump, 38
  non-medullated, 33. See also Remak, fibers of
Nerve hemi-section, 84
Nerve ligature, 68–70
Nerve, suture of the distal and proximal segments, 84
Nets, diffuse, 98

SUBJECT INDEX 157

Neural crest, 111
Neurobione, 61
  theory, 9, 40
Neurobiotaxis, 8, 124
Neurofibrillar methods, of Cajal, of Bielschowsky, introduction of, 103
Neuroglial
  chain, 80
  nerve and neuritic nerve, 82
Neuron doctrine, 5, 6, 114
  and His and Forel, 43
  justification of, 93
  return to, 40
  triumph of, 41, 43
  and unity of pathological reaction, 94, 95
Neuronism, 28. *See also* Neuron doctrine
Neuroplasticity, 9
Neurotization, 14, 34, 85, 87, 88, 105, 112, 124
Neurotropic
  action on nerve sprouts, 67
  factors (or susbstances), 12, 46, 47, 51, 65, 67, 70, 112, 120, 123
Neurotropism, 6, 8, 79, 83, 124, 125
  experimental demonstration of, 124, 125
  theory of, 7–9, 45, 46, 67, 72
Nodes of Ranvier, 102, 104
Nodules, residual, 65, 66, 118

Obstacles
  as determinants of axonal ramifications, 70
  collision of sprouts with, 51, 69, 85
  growth of fibers without, 110
  influence of, on dislocations of the sprouts, 51
Odogenesis, theory of, 111
Oily detritus (or drops), 104, 105, 115, 116
Orientation (and emission) of nervous sprouts, hypothesis of the difference of electrical potential, 78
Orienting materials, see catalytic agents
Osmic acid, 104

Paraphytes, 121
Pericellular tangles, 121
Perroncito, apparatus of, 109
Phenomena of compensation, 51
Photography, and degeneration and regeneration, 83, 90
polygeneticists (or polygenists), 6
  controversy with monogeneticists, 103
  theory of. *See* discontinuity, theory of
Polygenetism, 31
Preserved fibers, 117
Pyramidal cell axon sprouting through nerve implants, 46

Rabies, 95
  and alterations of the basket terminations, 97
Ranvier, nodes of. *See* Nodes
Reduced silver nitrate, 5–7, 37, 42, 99, 108, 111, 125
Regeneration
  different interpretation of the same experiment by polygeneticists and monogeneticists, 126
  and monogenetism, 31, 40
  and polygenetism, 31
Regeneration in the gray matter of the nerve centers, 121
  in cerebral and cerebellar cortices, 123
  in retina, 122
  phenomena of, 121
Regeneration in the white matter of the nerve centers, 118
Regeneration of nerves
  main conclusions of Cajal, 32–37
  main conclusions of Perroncito, 37, 38
Regenerative phenomena in central nervous pathways, 118
  in cerebrum and cerebellum, 120
  in dorsal root, 119
  in optic nerve, 119, 120
Reinnervation, 14
Remak, fibers of, 32, 80
Restoration of motor function, 5
Reticularism, revival of, 28, 29
Retraction ball, 10, 59, 65. *See also* Ball of retraction
Retraction club, 53, 60, 115, 116
Ringer's solution, 111, 122
Rosaliform
  degeneration, 97
  metamorphosis, 58

Satellite cells of the sensory ganglia, discovery of, 9
Schmidt-Lantermann clefts, 102, 104
Schwann cell
  in effectiveness of nervous restoration, 41
  mitosis of, 105
  multiplication of, 37
  necessary for regeneration, 43
  neurotropic action, 67
  neurotropic sources, 8, 37, 46, 51
Silver nitrate. *See* Reduced
Sprouts, first in the central stump, 39
Stereotropism (or homotactism)
  phenomena of, 81, 111
  reciprocal, 81, 82
Strangulation, 109
Survival, agonal. *See* Agonal
Syncytial

Syncytial (*Cont.*)
  cells of Schwann, 80
  concept, 77, 80
Syncytium
  cord, 82
  formation of, 82
  orientating, 79
  theory of, 78, 98
  tubes, 81
  tubular, 82

Terminal club or ball, 59. *See also* Retraction ball
Terms, glossary of unusual, 14
Testudinoid apparatus (or formation), 57, 120
Tissue culture and microdissection, 99, 100

Transplantation. *See* Grafting
Traumatic degeneration of the central stump, 60
Trophic center, 6, 30, 40, 102
Trophic substances (or agents), 11
  lack of, and degeneration, 106
  types of, 8
Trophic and neurotropism, Cajal use of terms, 14

Van Gehuchten, method of, 100
vis a tergo, 8, 51

Wallerian degeneration, cause of, 106
Wallerian doctrine, 83, 84, 99. *See also* Continuity, theory of
Weigert-Pal method, 124, 125
Weissmann, fascicles of, 114

Author Index

Albarracín, 13
Anderson, 103
Apáthy, 98
Arcaute, 10, 75, 79, 89, 117, 119, 121, 122
Athias, 31

Ballance, 28, 30
Barbacci, 42
Besta, 31, 105
Bethe, 6, 7, 28–32, 34, 37, 40, 90, 92, 98, 99, 103, 106, 110
Bielschowsky, 96, 100
Boeke, 88, 99 114
Brown-Séquard, 30, 34
Büngner, 28, 30, 32, 37, 103

Cajal, 5–15, 27, 43, 44, 46, 72, 75, 89, 94, 96–107, 109–12, 114, 117–26
Capobianco, 31
Chambers, 99, 100
Coën, 42
Cortese, 40, 60
Craigie, 27, 31, 32, 39, 47, 55, 70

D'Abundo, 119
Da Fano, 110
De Castro, 15, 97–100
De Juan, 97
DeFelipe, 5, 7, 83
Detwiler, 12
Dogiel, 29, 98
Dohrn, 40
Durante, 28
Dustin, 34, 40, 65, 67, 99, 110, 111, 119

Edinger, 31, 41
Edmond, 40
Eichhorst, 42

Forel, 28, 29, 43
Forssmann, 8, 28, 124, 125
Fragnito, 31

Galleotti, 28
García e Izcara, 97, 117

Gerlach, 28
Golgi, 5, 29, 30, 37, 39, 98

Halliburton, 28, 30, 40
Harrison, 28, 30, 41, 75, 88, 89, 110, 111
Heidenhain, 41
Held, 6–8, 29, 43, 80, 81, 96, 98, 99
Hensen, 6, 7
His, 6, 28, 29, 43, 89
Homén, 42
Huber, 28

Jeanmarie, 13
Jones, 5, 7, 83
Joris, 28, 31

Kahler, 42
Kappers, 8, 78, 124
Kerr, 89
Kindberg, 96
Kölliker, 28, 30, 89, 111
Kölster, 111
Krassin, 30
Kropp, 12

Langley, 28, 98, 103
Lenhossék, 28, 31, 41, 89
Leoz. *See* Ortín
Levi, 28, 40, 75
Lorente de Nó, 15, 80
Lowenthal, 42
Lugaro, 28, 30, 31, 40–42, 67, 88, 99, 103

Marchand, 28, 30
Marinesco, 7, 9, 28–30, 32, 34, 40, 41, 65, 67, 75–77, 81, 82, 88, 96, 99, 105, 106, 110, 118, 121
May, 12–14, 102
Medea, 30
Meynert, 28
Minea, 9, 40
Miskolczy, 94, 99
Modena, 40
Mönckeberg, 28, 106
Mott, 28, 30

Müller, 102
Münzer, 28, 30, 103

Nageotte, 30, 34, 40, 42, 65, 75–77, 81, 82, 88, 96, 98, 104, 118, 121
Nissl, 28

Olóriz, 9
Ortín, 10, 75, 79, 89, 117, 119–22

Pérez de Tudela, 5
Perroncito, 7, 30, 34, 37, 39, 41, 44, 81, 88, 99, 103, 106, 109, 110, 112, 119
Philippeaux, 31, 103
Poscharisky, 40
Purpura, 28, 103

Ranvier, 6, 28–30, 88, 92, 102, 107, 125
Renyi, 100
Retzius, 28, 31, 41
Río-Hortega, 96, 99
Rojas, 99
Rossi, 34, 65, 72, 95, 97, 100, 117, 119, 120, 122

Sala, 34, 40, 66
Schaffer, 96, 100
Schiefferdecker, 41, 42, 115
Schob, 96, 99

Schültze, 28
Sedgwig, 28
Segale, 28
Somoza, 96
Spielmeyer, 90, 99
Stewart, 30, 40
Stöhr, 98, 100
Stroebe, 28–30, 42, 102, 111, 125
Stuart, 40

Tello, 8, 9, 10–12, 15, 30, 34, 40, 44, 46, 72, 75, 88, 89, 92, 94, 99, 101, 105, 112, 115, 122, 127

Urra (Muñoz-), 79, 123

Van Gehuchten, 6, 28, 29, 32, 40
Vanlair, 28–30, 88, 92, 102, 125
Verworn, 41
Villaverde, 95
Vulpian, 6, 30, 31, 34, 103

Waldeyer, 5, 28, 29
Waller, 6, 28–30, 88, 92, 102
Weissfeiler, 120
Wietting, 28, 30
Wolff, 96
Woollard, 99, 100

Ziegler, 28, 30, 42

PART II

DEGENERATION AND REGENERATION OF THE NERVOUS SYSTEM

SANTIAGO RAMÓN Y CAJAL

TRANSLATED AND EDITED BY
RAOUL M. MAY

DEGENERATION AND REGENERATION
OF THE NERVOUS SYSTEM

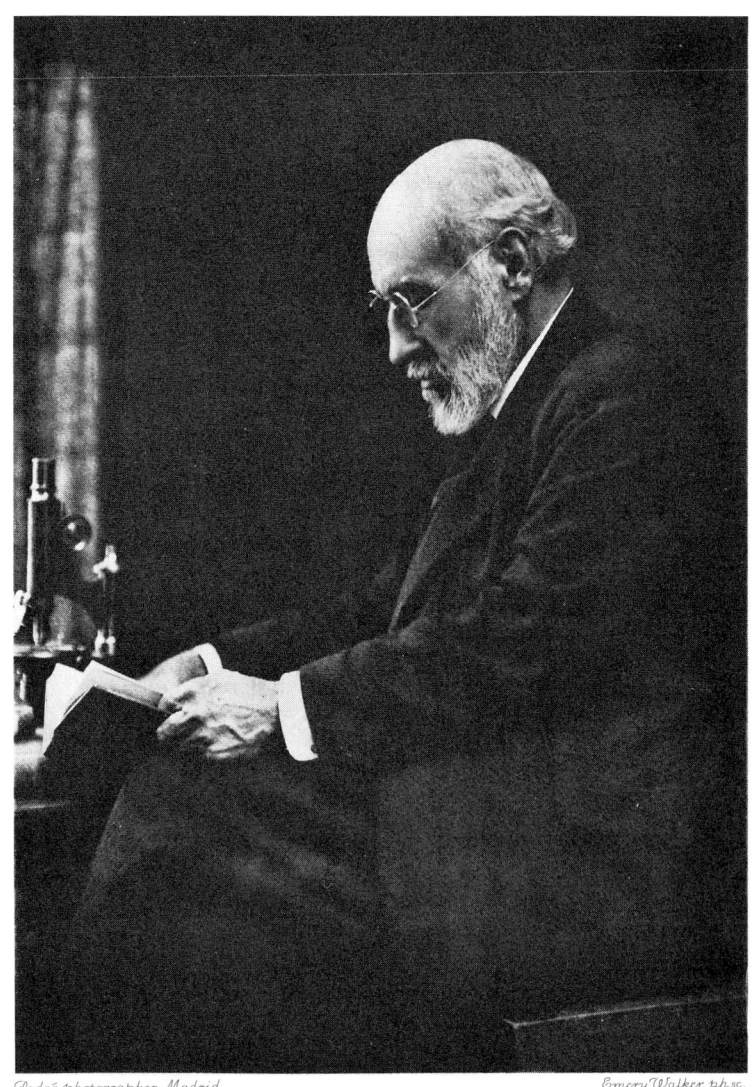

Padró photographer Madrid.   Emery Walker ph.sc.

S. Ramon Cajal.

Degeneration & Regeneration of the Nervous System

BY

S. RAMON Y CAJAL, M.D., F.R.S.
Director of the Instituto Cajal, Madrid
Honorary Professor of Pathology in the University of Madrid

TRANSLATED AND EDITED

BY

RAOUL M. MAY
Ph.D. (Harv.), D.ès Sc. (Paris)
Laboratoires d'Anatomie et Histologie Comparées et de Chimie Biologique
Faculté des Sciences, Paris

VOLUME I

OXFORD UNIVERSITY PRESS
LONDON: HUMPHREY MILFORD
1928

PRINTED IN GREAT BRITAIN BY ROBERT MACLEHOSE AND CO. LTD.
THE UNIVERSITY PRESS, GLASGOW.

AUTHOR'S PREFACE TO THE ENGLISH EDITION

THIS book may be considered, without exaggeration, as unpublished in Europe and North America. Although there appeared, in 1913 and 1914, a Spanish edition which was paid for by the physicians of the Argentine Republic, nearly all the copies were distributed to the South American subscribers. We were getting ready to send the few remaining copies to those European scientists who have specialised in this type of study, when there broke out the dreadful World War which almost completely prevented any scientific interchanges. It is, therefore, not to be wondered at that there are so very few investigators outside Spain who are aware of the existence of this book. The fact that it was written in Spanish, a language rarely known by scientists, is another reason why it is little known.

The present English translation has saved my work from an irremediable loss. To be worthy of the honour of an edition in the land of Waller, the brilliant initiator of these studies, I have attempted to better the text, and to supplement it with some additions which would have been more extensive and detailed had I not feared to add unduly to an already extensive work, which represents the result of eight years of continuous and patient study.

While there exists in any biological investigation a subjective factor which it is difficult to eliminate, a factor which is equivalent to the *personal equation* of the astronomers, I have tried to reduce it to a minimum. To do this I have used for my illustrations only preparations that were transparent, strongly and selectively stained, and moderately thick sections. These alone are appropriate for following the regenerated nerve fibres, which are hardly ever rectilinear.

In order to keep down the number of figures without infringing upon their usefulness, I have used the well-known method of *combined images*. Thus all the degenerated or regenerated nerve fibres depicted in some of the figures are faithfully reproduced from the original specimens, the only artifice employed being the fusion into a single plane of structures taken from two or three successive sections of the object.

While we grant to the facts which are revealed by highly selective methods an unquestionable objective value, we do not extend this confidence to any hypotheses, our own or those of other investigators, no matter how seductive they may appear. Indeed, unpleasant though it be to acknowledge, one has to admit that in biology theories are fragile and ephemeral constructions that are renewed every eight or ten years. Even during this brief lapse of time they never attain unanimous scientific approval. Owing to this relative agnosticism concerning theoretical speculations I present only the *theory of neurotropism* and similar ideas, which the reader will find expounded merely as working hypotheses, useful for the synthesis of facts, and acceptable merely as scientific tools in Weismann's sense. I thus recognise fully that the idea of neurotropism through excitatory chemical actions could be replaced by any other conception, such, for example, as the electrical hypotheses of Strasser, Kappers, or by those of Harrison, Marinesco, and other investigators. At any rate, while hypotheses pass by, facts remain. These constitute the only lasting patrimony of the investigator and the only positive addition to scientific progress.

I conclude by expressing my profound gratitude to my very learned friend and colleague, Dr. Raoul M. May, for undertaking and carrying through the English translation. I am also very grateful to Sir Charles Sherrington, who has interested himself in the publication of this translation, and to the Oxford University Press who have produced it with the proverbial care and elegance of English scientific publications.

S. RAMÓN Y CAJAL.

MADRID, *September* 16*th*, 1927.

AUTHOR'S PREFACE TO THE SPANISH EDITION

THE Nobel Prize with which the Carolinian Institute of Stockholm was pleased to recompense my modest scientific achievements was the signal, among physicians of Spanish race, for patriotic and enthusiastic testimonies of affection and consideration. Among the homages received none did me more honour, because of its delicate and thoughtful nature, than the tribute to the humble man of science from his medical compatriots of the Argentine Republic. They did not deem it sufficient to show their esteem by flattering me with an artistic diploma made the more valuable by their signatures, but, resolved that their noble sentiments should crystallize into something useful and permanent, they decided to print at their cost a book of mine.

Such was the origin of the present work. When I began it I believed that it would perhaps be useful to include in a general treatise the numerous memoirs that my pupils and myself had contributed during the last few years to the arduous problem of the degeneration and regeneration of the nervous system, including also in such a treatise the very valuable contributions by distinguished foreign scientists. When I set to work, however, I saw that if the undertaking were to do justice to the magnitude and dignity of the subject, it could not consist merely of a compilation of published facts. In order, then, to honour as far as possible the disinterested initiative of my colleagues overseas, I set myself the task, at the expense of laboratory work, of revising all the investigations previously published, and also of making a special study of many doubtful or uncertain points. The present book constitutes, then, an extensive monograph, original in large part. The undertaking has required more time and effort than I had expected. The uncertain state of my health has also contributed, with deplorable insistence, to the inevitable delay of publication.

It is a pleasure for me to record here my profound gratitude to my honourable and cultured friends of the Argentine Republic. I hope that the offering which I am sending them in return for their kindness will not be deemed too far below their own generosity. Finally, it is a comfort for me to know that, in spite of all the imperfections and deficiencies of this work, it will always bear witness to the elevating and patriotic example of my countrymen from beyond the seas, and the good will and fraternal affection of the author.

MADRID, *July* 10*th*, 1913.

CONTENTS

Introduction - - - - - - - xix

FIRST SECTION

TRAUMATIC DEGENERATION AND REGENERATION OF THE NERVES

I. Historical Notes concerning Degeneration and Regeneration of the Nerves - - 3

The two opposing schools: the monogenist and the pluralist, polygenist, or catenary.—Investigations of Waller, Vulpian, Brown-Séquard, Büngner, Bethe and Monckeberg.—Histological studies of Ranvier, Vanlair, Stroebe, etc.—Observations of Purpura, Cajal, Perroncito, Marinesco and Minea, Lugaro, Tello, Deineka, Krassin, etc.—Actual state of the problem.—Triumph of the monogenist doctrine of Waller and of His.

II. Technique for the Study of Nervous Degeneration and Regeneration - - - 27

Methods for impregnating the axons.—Methods of Bielschowsky, Cajal, etc.—Methods for staining the myelin (osmic acid, procedures of Marchi, Herxheimer, etc.).—Methods for staining the cells of Schwann (procedures with basic haematoxylin and aniline, procedures of Doinikow, Nageotte, etc.).—Method of Achúcarro for staining neuroglia.—Procedure of Alzheimer.—Animals used for experiments on degeneration and regeneration, and operatory technique.

III. Résumé of the Structure of the Normal Medullated Nerve - - - - - 41

Schwann's membrane.—Nodes of Ranvier.—Nucleus and cytoplasm of the tubular or Schwann's cell.—Its inclusions and reticular apparatus.—Myelin.—Incisures of Schmidt-Lantermann.—Infundibuliform apparatus.—Rings of Segall.—Mauthner's capsule or space.—Axis-cylinder.—Bracelets of Nageotte, etc.

CONTENTS

	PAGE
IV. DEGENERATION OF INTERRUPTED NERVES	66

Wallerian degeneration of the peripheral extremity.—Precocious metamorphoses of the myelin.—Destruction of the soldering disc and of the infundibula.—Modifications occurring in the cells of Schwann: multiplication of these cells and formation of varicose bands.—Apparition of granular elements and resorption of the myelin.

V. DEGENERATION OF THE PERIPHERAL STUMP - 100

Degenerative phenomena occurring in the interrupted axon.—Fragmentation and liquefaction of the axon at a distance from the wound.—Fragmentation and liquefaction of the axon near the lesion.—Agonal neoformation.—Preserved fibres and degenerated fibres.—Degenerative phenomena of the axon *in vitro*.—Experiments of Bethe, Nageotte, and Cajal.—Additional Note.

VI. TRAUMATIC DEGENERATION OF THE CENTRAL STUMP - - - - - - - - 127

Degeneration of the myelin.—Necrosis and liquefaction of the terminal portion of the axon.—Digestive chambers.—Preserved fibres.—Changes occurring in Schwann's cells.—Mode of connection between the necrotic and the active segments.

VII. REGENERATIVE PROCESS OF THE CENTRAL STUMP 141

Preliminary phenomena (formative turgidity) of the axonic neoformation.—Formation of the nervous sprouts.—*Forms of sprouting*: terminal or direct neoformation of the non-medullated fibres of Remak, of the fine medullated tubes; direct sprouting by ravelling.—Indirect terminal neoformation, or at a distance from the wound.—Collateral neoformation.—Various forms of such regeneration.—Apparatus of Perroncito.—Ravelling of the collaterals.—Avalanche of ramification and avalanche of growth.—Sterile nerve tubes.—Course of regeneration in the central stump.—Retrograde fibres, arrested fibres, and spiral structures.

VIII. COURSE OF THE NERVE SPROUTS ACROSS THE SCAR AND FOREIGN TISSUES - - - - - 167

Emergence from the limits of the nerve and entrance into the scar.—Details concerning division of the fibres.—Kinds of terminal buds (clubs of growth, arrested clubs, retraction clubs, and agonistic clubs).—

Comparison between embryonic cones of growth and the clubs of the newly-formed axons.—Structure of the initial scar.—Behaviour of the nerve sprouts in crossing exudates, embryonic connective tissue, muscles, adipose tissue, and foreign bodies.—Segregation and degeneration of the terminal buds.—Relation of the fibroblasts to the newly-formed nerve fibres.—Additional Note.

IX. LATE CONDITIONS SHOWN BY THE NERVE SPROUTS OF THE CENTRAL STUMP AND OF THE SCAR - 198

Fibrillar bundles.—Formation of the protective coverings of bundles and axons.—Formation of the myelin.—Persistent retrograde fibres.—Helicoidal structures or nervous spools.—Motionless degenerating buds and gigantic balls.—Presence of analogous balls in embryos.—Probable fate of the axons and of the aberrant and immovable clubs.

X. INNERVATION OF THE PERIPHERAL STUMP - - 223

Arrival of the nerve sprouts.—Their ramifications and penetration in the distal stump.—Intratubal and extratubal fibres.—Buds of growth and ramifications within the peripheral stump.—Variable velocity of axonal growth in the various situations.—Late, precocious, and extremely rapid neurotisation.—Connections of the sprouts with Schwann's cells of the distal stump.—Schemes for the general course of precocious, difficult, and normal neurotisation.—Formation of the nuclei and medullated sheath of the sprouts.—Additional Note.

XI. ARRIVAL OF THE NERVE FIBRES AT THE END-ORGANS - - - - - - - - 265

Experiments of Tello on the regeneration of motor fibres.—Regeneration of Kühne's spindles and of tactile hairs.—Insufficiency of the regeneration and incongruences of connection between the plates and their terminal regions.—Necessity of admitting, in the end-organs and peripheral stump, specific neurotropic sources.

XII. VARIETIES OF DEGENERATION AND REGENERATION DUE TO TRAUMATIC CAUSES - - - - 281

Degeneration and regeneration of nerves that have been instantaneously crushed.—Degeneration and regeneration following on ligature of nerves.—Compressed or necrotic ligatures (central stump, necrotic segment, and distal stump).—Innervation of the necrotic segment and distal stump (migrating fibres, rows of gigantic balls, and retrograde axons).—Moderately compressed ligatures.

XIII. EXPERIMENTS TO ELUCIDATE THE MECHANISM OF THE GROWTH, RAMIFICATION, AND ORIENTATION OF THE NERVE SPROUTS - - - - - 305

Combined effects of ligature and section.—Topical indifference, etc.—Retrograde neurotisation of neighbouring nerve bundles.—Mechanical obstruction caused by the ligature of the peripheral stump (formation of gigantic balls and of exploratory branches).—Experiments designed to prove the reality of neurotropical phenomena (multiple sections and hemisections, transformation of central infecund axons into fecund sprouts, etc.

XIV. CONTINUATION OF THE STUDY OF REGENERATION UNDER SPECIAL CONDITIONS - - - - 314

Observations showing the indifference, both topical and polar, of nerve sprouts.—Inversion of sequestered nerves.—Union of two central stumps.—Effects of multiple hemisection.—Retrograde penetration of wandering sensory fibres into the posterior roots.—Penetration of sensory fibres into cut anterior roots.—Experiments dealing with the extirpation of nerves.—Experiments designed to place difficulties in the way of neurotisation of the peripheral stump and of the progress of the fibres in their initial direction.

XV. EXPERIMENTS DEALING WITH THE TRANSPLANTATION OF NERVES OR THEIR PRODUCTS, DESIGNED TO PROVE ESPECIALLY AN ATTRACTIVE OR NEUROTROPIC ACTION ON NERVE SPROUTS - - - 329

Experiments of Forssman, Lugaro, Marinesco, Mott and Halliburton, Dustin, O. Rossi, etc.—Indifference of undamaged fibres to grafts.—Effects of live and dead grafts.—Reimplantations of nerves.—Homoiotransplants and heterotransplants.—Subcutaneous intermuscular grafts.—Conclusions.—Are there negative neurotropic actions ?—Action of pus, blood, and mechanical obstacles.—Paralyzing action of the aniline dyes.—Attractive influence of the scar.—Degeneration and regeneration in the lower vertebrates.—Additional Note.

XVI. GENERAL THEORETICAL INTERPRETATION OF THE
PHENOMENA OF NERVOUS REGENERATION   -   362
Reactions caused in the nervous protoplasm by intrinsic or immanent conditions.—Continuous development, growth in a straight line, formative turgidity, growth along the initial direction, formation of the cone of growth, formation of new extensions, etc.—Reactions of the axon that are conditioned by its environment (mechanical, physical, and chemical stimuli).—Trophism and neurotropism.—Hypothesis of the neurobiones.—History of our knowledge of the laws of normal and pathological neurogenesis.—Additional Note.

SECOND SECTION

DEGENERATION AND REGENERATION OF THE NERVE CENTRES

FIRST PART

DEGENERATION AND REGENERATION OF SENSORY AND SYMPATHETIC GANGLIA

I. SUMMARY OF THE NORMAL STRUCTURE OF SENSORY
GANGLIA   -   -   -   -   -   -   -   -   397
Typical forms: morphology, volume, and normal structure of the sensory neurone.—Pericellular capsule and satellite cells.—Atypical forms and dispositions; neurones provided with dendrites, appendices in the shape of balls, ansiform and fenestrated dispositions, frayed cells.—Pericellular and periglomerular nests.—Probable significance of the atypical forms.—Hypotheses of Nageotte and of Levi.—Additional Note.

II. DEGENERATION AND REGENERATION OF THE SENSORY NERVE GANGLIA   -   -   -   -   -   414
Traumatic degeneration of the sensory cells and tubes.—Regenerative acts of the cells and fibres following on wounds, contusions and extirpation of nerves, etc.—Genesis of the pericellular nests.—Additional Note.

III. MORPHOLOGICAL VARIATIONS OBSERVED IN TRANSPLANTED SENSORY GANGLIA - - - - 426

Fundamental experiments of Nageotte.—Confirmations by Marinesco and Minea, Rossi, Dustin, Cardenal and ourselves.—Aberrant nerves.—Neuronophagy.—Experiments of cultivation of ganglia *in vitro* by Cajal, Legendre and Minot, Marinesco, etc.—Theories of Nageotte, Marinesco, and other authors, concerning the mechanism of formation of the neuronal appendices.—Additional Note.

SECOND PART

DEGENERATION AND REGENERATION OF THE SPINAL CORD AND NERVE ROOTS

I. DEGENERATION AND REGENERATION OF THE WHITE MATTER - - - - - - - 484

Technical indications.—Summary of the normal structure of the white matter.—Traumatic degeneration.—Initial phenomena.—Appearance of the granular cells and destruction of the myelin and axon.—Secondary degeneration.—Precocious acts of regeneration.—Late examination of the lesions.—Breakdown of regeneration.—Formation of the scar.—Creation, under special conditions, of very long fibres which abandon the spinal cord.

II. DEGENERATIVE ALTERATIONS OF THE GREY MATTER - - - - - - - 517

Résumé of the structure of the spinal neurones.—Necrotic and degenerative phenomena occurring in them—granular state, chromatolysis, neurofibrillar hypertrophy, hirudiform state, etc.—Perturbations of the endocellular Golgi apparatus.—Regenerative phenomena—regeneration of the dendrites and of the fibres of the grey substance.—Neuroglial and conjunctive scars.

III. DEGENERATION AND REGENERATION OF THE SPINAL ROOTS - - - - - - - 531

Degeneration and regeneration of the anterior roots.—Their invasion by endogenous and exogenous sprouts.—Degeneration and regeneration of the posterior roots.—Invasion of the connective scar by funicular sprouts.—Partial restoration of the posterior fasciculus.

IV. PHENOMENA OF NECROSIS, DEGENERATION, AND REGENERATION BROUGHT ABOUT BY SPINAL CONTUSION AND LACERATION - - - - - 558

Necrotic and degenerative forms of the nerve fibres.—Necrotic and degenerative disorders of the neurones.—Regenerative acts of the axons and dendrites.—Historical notes concerning regeneration of the spinal cord.—Additional Note.

V. TRAUMATIC DEGENERATION AND REGENERATION IN THE OPTIC NERVE AND RETINA - - - 583

Additional Note.

THIRD PART

I. DEGENERATIVE PHENOMENA CONSEQUENT ON CEREBELLAR TRAUMATISMS - - - - - 597

Technical notes.—Degenerative acts in the white matter.—Degeneration of the central stump.—Degeneration of the peripheral stump.—Elimination of the axonic segment beyond the collaterals, and transformation of the cells of Purkinje into elements with a short axon.—Details of this transformation in the pathological human cerebellum.—Absence of regenerative phenomena.

II. CONTINUATION OF THE DEGENERATIVE AND METAMORPHIC PROCESSES CONSEQUENT ON CEREBELLAR TRAUMATISMS - - - - - - 617

Degenerative phenomena occurring in the neurones and their dendrites.—Aneuritic cells and rosaliform, hirudiform, etc., dispositions of the neurofibrillar reticulum.—Swelling of the soma and dendrites.—Destruction of the reticulum.—Creation of aberrant expansions.—Alterations of the basket cells, moss-like fibres, and other elements in the cerebellum.

FOURTH PART

I. TRAUMATIC DEGENERATIVE PROCESSES OF THE CEREBRAL CORTEX - - - - - - 631

Necrotic phenomena consequent on wounds.—Preserved nerve fibres.—Preserved dendrites.—Preserved neurones.—Corrosion and autolysis of the axons and dendrites.—Degenerative metamorphoses of the peripheral stump.—Autotomy of the terminal spheres and their metamorphic phenomena—formation of neurofibrillar plexuses and buckles.

II. STUDY OF TRAUMATIC DEGENERATION IN THE CEREBRAL CORTEX (*continued*) - - - - 656

Degenerative phenomena of the central stump in wounds of the white matter.—Degenerative phenomena of this stump when the interruption is in the grey matter.—Compensatory eliminations.—Transformation of the cerebral pyramidal cells into cells with short axons.—Degenerative phenomena in the nerve collaterals and in some intrinsic fibres of the cerebral cortex.—Additional Note.

III. ALTERATIONS OF THE NERVE CELLS IN CEREBRAL TRAUMATISMS - - - - - - - 678

Neuronal metamorphoses occurring after wounds that entail little or no contusion.—Disorders occasioned by contusions and commotions that are accompanied by traumatisms.—Granular degeneration, chromatolysis, hirudiform state, fusiform hypertrophy and alteration of the neurofibrils, and neurofibrillar pycnosis

IV. PHENOMENA OF ABORTED REGENERATION IN THE CEREBRAL CORTEX - - - - - - 693

Regenerative inefficiency of the central paths.—Internal and external productions of the central stump of the axon.—*Cephalopodic* structures and neurofibrillar spools.—Radial or *testudinoid* formations of the varicosities.—Aspect of these neoformations in the cerebrum of recently-born individuals.—Incongruence and breakdown of these neoformations.

V. ATROPHIC PHENOMENA CONSEQUENT ON CEREBRAL WOUNDS - - - - - - - - 704

Aspect of the traumatized grey cortex in late periods, that is, some weeks and months after the lesion.— Relative immunity of the neurones in the radial wounds.—Late atrophies and necroses in transversal wounds.—Calcified pyramids and residual nodules.

VI. CORTICAL INFLAMMATION CONSEQUENT ON TRAUMATISMS - - - - - - - - 714

Invasion of the grey substance by migratory elements— granular cells, rod-like cells, plasma cells, etc.—

Behaviour of the neuroglia in presence of the inflammation.—Formation of the scar.—Neuroglial and mesodermal scars.—Organization of exudates and haemorrhagic foci.—Gigantic granular cells.

VII. STUDY OF REGENERATIVE PROCESSES OF THE CEREBRUM (*continued*) - - - - - 734

Breakdown of the regeneration of the nerve paths.—Experiments of Tello, showing that regeneration fails owing to the absence in the surroundings of substances that stimulate the growth and orientation of the axonic sprouts.—Theories explanatory of the poverty and incongruence of the natural regeneration.—Historical notes concerning regeneration in the cerebrum of man and the higher mammals.

INDEX - - - - - - - - - - 761

INTRODUCTION

The nerve cell or neurone is a structure which is exquisitely sensitive to normal and pathological stimuli. It is susceptible to many toxins and poisons that do not affect, or only slightly alter, the other histological elements. This great sensibility to pathogenic agents, due, without doubt, to adaptation and heredity, constitutes an acquisition of great utility and efficiency for defensive purposes. If it were permissible to apply such a metaphor where only physical and chemical forces are at work, we might say that, among all the organs, the nervous system, leader and protector of the hive, feels profoundly its responsibility. Docile to the mandates of the latter, it occupies the post of honour and danger, facing bravely the struggle with cosmic forces and pathogenic agents.

Such an exquisite susceptibility to the offences of the mechanical or chemical environment has, however, its reverse side. The neurone, able to co-ordinate for a common purpose the actions of the other elements, sensitive also to whatever changes occur in the normal organism, is peculiarly sensitive to morbid influences. Every organic disorder finds in it a painful reverberation. This reaches its maximum when some segment of its protoplasm is directly affected by the pathogenic agent.

In presence of chemical, thermal, electrical, and traumatic stimuli the neuronal protoplasm responds with interesting intracellular or extracellular metamorphoses. Many scientists have devoted themselves to the analysis and exposition of such structural changes, and the sum of data and observations published in the last few years is already very great. Apart from their intrinsic interest, such observations have an important biological value. As we note below, they reveal some of the fundamental causes of neuronal form and growth, and thereby lay bare some of the mysteries of cellular life.

It is not our purpose to describe the various reactions, as numerous as their causative stimuli. Our aim is more modest. In the present study, largely monographic in its scope, we shall limit ourselves to the connected description of regressive and progressive processes in the nervous fibres and cells, of traumatic origin, and especially of those due to expansional mutilation (section of axons and dendrites).

The present work will give a résumé of our already numerous personal studies on this subject, those of our pupils, and the important discoveries published by scientists such as Bethe and Monckeberg, Marinesco, Nageotte, Lugaro, Perroncito, Levi, O. and H. Rossi, Krassin, G. Sala, Deineka, Bielschowsky, Harrison, etc. Such a synthesis, indispensable after the laborious analysis of the last few years, will nevertheless appear premature and incomplete. It will, however, make clear the actual state of our knowledge, point out the problems, and show the directing principles of future investigations.

The field is vast, and its exposition demands appropriate method. We shall therefore establish two great sections, within which we shall successively study : (1) Traumatic degeneration and regeneration in the nerves or connected neuronal axons. (2) Traumatic degeneration and regeneration of the nerve centres, that is, of the central neurones and nerve paths. To further sub-divide into chapters we shall use the topographic or organic criterion ; that is, each section will be divided into as many chapters as there are differentiated segments or organs in the nerves or centres.

We have especially occupied ourselves, in this book, with the exact and clear descriptions of those facts which are certain and easily verified. This has necessitated a large number of illustrations, some of them semi-schematic representations of unimpeachable preparations. We shall not, however, disdain hypotheses when, as with the theory of neurotropism, they are adequate to explain phenomena or to point the way to new experiments and discoveries.

At first sight it appears that the degenerative processes have nothing in common with regenerative phenomena, and that they should be carefully separated in exposition from the latter. We shall do this whenever possible. There are cases, however, in which degeneration is so interwoven and mixed up with intraneural and extraneural neoformation that demarcation is extremely difficult. In such cases one can only give in the same description the totality of neuronal changes of ambiguous significance, until science can distinguish and ascertain their true meaning.

FIRST SECTION

TRAUMATIC DEGENERATION AND REGENERATION OF THE NERVES

As is well known, the nerves are nothing more than bundles of axis-cylinders, that is, expansional portions of the nerve cells situated within the centres (medulla, spinal cord, sensory and sympathetic ganglia). The fact that they exist far from the centres, submerged in mesoderm and in symbiotic connection with numerous connective elements, gives to such axonal bundles specific anatomical and biological properties, very different from those which are characteristic of the neuronal body.

A similar specialization is seen in the pathological sphere. In presence of toxins, poisons, and traumatic actions, the nerve is much more active than the central cell. Thus, while the neurones themselves (soma and dendrites) possess only slight powers of regeneration, reacting rather by internal or structural metamorphoses, the axis-cylinders of the nerves respond to stimuli not only by structural or intraprotoplasmic metamorphoses, but also by external transformations. Among the latter, that which is represented by the genesis of new expansions possesses a decisive importance, since the development is so powerful and rapid that destroyed peripheral paths are, at times, re-established. An exception to the incapacity for regeneration of the centres is offered by the sensory ganglia, whose cells have retained a notable power of expansive growth.

The general attitude is to attribute the regenerative inefficiency of the centres to the absence of cells of Schwann. It is true that the central nerve cell is an element devoid of nutritive corpuscles and also of neoformative stimuli, while the ganglionic cell, like the axis-cylinder of the nerves, exists in association with certain mesodermic elements from which it receives very valuable help when confronted by pathological dangers, and especially in regeneration.

The contrast between the reactions of the motor neurone and its peripheral axon can thus be seen not to be essential. It does not concern the intimate contexture of the nervous protoplasm, but it derives from external conditions—the presence or absence of auxiliary factors that are indispensable to the regenerative process. This conclusion, suspected by the authors who have observed in the spinal cord and brain ephemeral and frustrated regenerative attempts, has recently received from our studies and those of Tello a decisive confirmation.

I

HISTORICAL NOTES CONCERNING DEGENERATION AND REGENERATION OF THE NERVES

The two opposing schools : the monogenist and the pluralist, polygenist, or catenary. —Investigations of Waller, Vulpian, Brown-Séquard, Büngner, Bethe and Monckeberg.—Histological studies of Ranvier, Vanlair, Stroebe, etc.—Observations of Purpura, Cajal, Perroncito, Marinesco and Minea, Lugaro, Tello, Deineka, Krassin, etc.—Actual state of the problem.—Triumph of the monogenist doctrine of Waller and of His.

Statement of the problem.—It is well known that, when one cuts a nervous cord in a young animal, the peripheral extremity thus severed from its central portion degenerates and dies immediately, resorbing its remnants ; months later the intermediate scar and the peripheral nervous stump show numerous newly-formed fibres ; in the end, totally or partially, the sensibility and motility of the paralyzed member are re-established.

How is regeneration of the distal or peripheral segment effected, and what is the mechanism of junction between the two nervous stumps?

The principal treatises published up to now on this important theme contain two fundamental solutions, around which gravitate all the others : *the theory of continuity or monogenist hypothesis*, and the *theory of discontinuity or polygenist hypothesis* (*catenary theory* of certain authors).

The partisans of the first solution hold that the newly-formed fibres of the peripheral extremity are only the prolongation, by way of budding and growth, of the nervous tubes of the central stump ; while the polygenists or adherents to the second theory hold that such fibres arise from the differentiation and transformation of the ensheathing cells of the old nervous tubes (nucleus and protoplasm of the interannular segment residing under the sheath of Schwann), which constitute a chain whose links ulteriorly unite, forming continuous conductors. Both hypotheses are related to, and are even the logical consequences of, the ideas concerning the origin of nerves in the embryo put forward by the particular neurologist. Thus, those who like His, Forel, Stroebe, Münzer, von Lenhossék, Kölliker, etc., believe that the axon of the neuroblast or embryonic neurone is a simple protoplasmic prolongation, without primitive discontinuities, believe, in neuropathology, in monogenism or the theory of continuity ; on the contrary those who, like Büngner, Ballance, Apathy, Bethe, etc., hold that the embryonic nerve fibres are formed by a fusion of mesodermic cells believe also in polygenism of regenerated axons.

Let us, then, examine the facts adduced by the partisans of each doctrine, as well as the variations of these opinions held by some scientists.

Doctrine of continuity.—Johannes Müller and Longet were the first to prove that any nerve separated from the centres rapidly loses its physiological excitability ; but it was Waller [1] who first advanced a rational theory of degeneration and regeneration of the nerve tubes, based on clear-sighted and well-directed observations. According to this English scientist the fibres of the peripheral stump of the sectioned nerve degenerate and die, being of no value whatever in the process of restorative neoformation ; the production of the new fibres is a function of the central stump, which, because of its substantial continuity and nutritive solidarity with the motor nerve cells of the spinal cord, or *trophic centres*, is able to rebuild the incapacitated distal segment. It thus follows that the death of the fibres of the peripheral stump was due to the fact that the axons were violently separated from such a *trophic centre*, so called from its capacity to excite and promote the nutritive exchanges of the nervous expansions that emanate from it. Such a doctrine found immediate confirmation in the histological studies of Bruch,[2] who nevertheless made the mistake of attributing to the nuclei of Schwann's sheath the genesis of the axons that appeared in the cicatricial tissue.

It is really remarkable that Waller, who was essentially a physiologist, and who lived at a time when histological technique was so

---

[1] Waller : " Sur la reproduction des nerfs et sur la structure et les fonctions des ganglions spinaux," *Müller's Archiv*, 1852.

Idem : " Experiments on the section of the glosso-pharyngeal and hypoglossal nerves of the frog, and observations on the alteration produced thereby in the structure of their primitive fibres," *Philosophical Transactions*, 1850.

[2] Bruch : " Ueber die Regeneration durchschnittener Nerven," *Zeitsch. für wissensch. Zool.*, Bd. 6, 1885.

defective that one was unable to make precise structural observations, was able to formulate, as we shall see below, the true solution of the problem, orienting himself without difficulty in a puzzling field in which even distinguished modern scientists have lost their way. Paradoxical as it may appear, it is certain that in the problem with which we are dealing, contrary to the usual course of science, error is modern while truth is ancient.[1]

There was thus lacking, to the firm establishment of the doctrine of trophic centres, a scrupulous histological observation of the phenomena occurring in the central and distal stumps of the wounded and regenerated nerve. This important work was ably and fitly carried out in part by Bruch, Remak [2] and Eichhorst,[3] and completely by Ranvier,[4] Vanlair,[5] Nothafft,[6] Stroebe,[7] E. Ziegler [8] and many others.

---

[1] Waller's clear-sightedness did not keep him from falling into some errors, due to the defective technique of his time. Thus he believed that the cell of origin or trophic centre of the severed fibre remained perfectly normal, and that all the histological elements of the distal stump disappeared. The truth of the matter is, as shown by the older observations of Dickinson (1868) and by the more modern ones of Gudden, Forel, and Monakow (1882), that there are cases where the neurone whose axon is mutilated or even functionally isolated shows morbid changes, and may even die.

[2] Remak : " Ueber die Wiedererzeugung von Nervenfasern," *Virchow's Archiv*, Bd. 23, 1862.

[3] Eichhorst : " Ueber die Nervendegeneration u. Nervenregeneration," *Virchow's Archiv*, Bd. 59, 1874.

[4] Ranvier : " De la dégénérescence des nerfs après leur section," *Compt. rend.*, 1871.

Idem: " De la régénération des nerfs sectionnés," *Compt. rend.*, t. 76, 1873.

Idem : " Leçons sur l'histologie du système nerveux," vol. ii. Paris, 1878.

[5] Vanlair : " De la régénération des nerfs périphériques par le procédé de la suture tubulaire," *Arch. de Biol.*, vol. iii. 1882.

Idem : " Nouvelles recherches expérimentales sur la régénération des nerfs," *Arch. de Biol.*, vol. vi. 1887.

Idem : " Sur la persistance de l'aptitude régénératrice des nerfs," *Bulletin de l'Acad. Royale des Sciences de Belgique*, t. 16, 1888.

[6] Nothafft : " Neue Untersuchungen ueber die Verlauf der Degeneration und Regenerationsprozesse am verletzten peripheren Nerven," *These*, Würzburg, 1892.

[7] Stroebe : " Ueber Degeneration und Regeneration peripherischer Nerven nach Verletzungen," *Arch. f. Psych.*, Bd. 25, 1893.

Idem: " Experimentelle Untersuchungen ueber Degeneration und Regeneration peripherer Nerven nach Verletzungen," *Beiträge zur pathol. Anat. u. allg. Pathol.*, Bd. 13, 1893, Heft 2.

[8] E. Ziegler : *Lehrbuch des pathol. Anat.*, Band I. 1892.

Ranvier, who studied the problem with particular skill and precision, believes that the phases of degeneration and regeneration of nerves separated from their trophic centres are as follows :

Degeneration : One can perceive as early as the second day that there is a contraction of the myelin, corresponding to the expansion of the incisures of Schmidt-Lantermann, while the cylindro-conic segments become transformed into elongated drops ; at the same time the axon becomes pale and granular, breaks up into irregular, flexuous or spiral pieces, which are well seen in the midst of the fatty droplets. It looks as though the destruction of the conducting filament were the signal for the emancipation of the cells of Schwann [1] from their nutritive function ; their nuclei enlarge and divide, surrounding themselves with a thick cap of protoplasm, which is forced between the blocks of disintegrating myelin. After fifteen or twenty days all remains of the axons have disappeared, and the nerve tube has transformed itself into a solid cord of granular protoplasm. This is provided with central nuclei, developed from the nuclei of Schwann's cells, and is bespattered here and there with fatty droplets which are being resorbed, and with some migrating leucocytes, whose ultimate function appears to be to collect all the detritus of the old nerve and to take this to the circulatory system.

The tubes of the peripheral stump also undergo some modifications in order to receive the new fibres which develop from the central stump, and to harbour them and offer them nutritive protection. These modifications were well studied by Ranvier, Vanlair, and Stroebe. From the twenty-fifth to the thirtieth day, sometimes before, when the fat is almost all done away with by the action of the phagocytes, the old nerve goes through a kind of withering, by means of which the protoplasmic cordon composed of Schwann cells becomes progressively thinner. The nuclei diminish in number and size, become marginal, and a hollow space of varying size is formed ; this is destined to receive the new fibre.

Let us now relate the phenomena occurring in the central stump, according to Ranvier and some of the older monogenist authors. Although it is continuous with the nerve cells, this stump also degenerates. This degeneration is not, however, total, but, unlike that of the peripheral stump, involves only the portion next to the

---

[1] We thus designate, for brevity, the mesodermic corpuscle which is a part of the interannular segment, situated, as is well known, in the centre of the latter and beneath the sheath of Schwann.

traumatic lesion. It is for this reason that it is called *inflammatory* or *traumatic degeneration*, in contradistinction to the so-called *functional degeneration* of the peripheral stump.

Apart from this difference of extent, there is a fundamental difference in the degeneration of the central and peripheral stumps. While in the latter the axon disappears totally from the entire segment that is separated from its trophic centre, in the former the axis-cylinder is retained with only slight modifications. Ranvier believes that the terminal, or rather, pre-terminal portion of this structure becomes somewhat thicker, as though undergoing hypertrophy because of a nutritive hyperactivity.

Regeneration: According to the monogenists (Ranvier, Vanlair, Stroebe, etc.) the young fibres arising from the central stump, like embryonic nerves, are at first very fine and lack a medullated sheath. The rapidity of their appearance in the distal segment is proportional to the nearness of the two cut ends of the nerve and to the way in which they are adjusted in relation to each other. According to Ranvier, they can already be seen on the twenty-eighth day, while other investigators (Kolster, etc.) claim that they are present on the twelfth or sixteenth day. The study of them, however, is really possible only two or three months after the operation, when they nearly all have sheaths which are easily stained with osmic acid. In general, such fine fibres lie under the sheaths of Schwann, within each of which there may be two, three, or even five of them. This was shown by Neumann and Eichhorst, Ranvier, Herzt [1] and Vanlair.

The newly-formed fibres, without sheaths or myelin, are really, as we have said, the continuation of the pre-existent tubes of the central stump. In no case did any such fibres appear discontinuously and independently. This conclusion, upon which Ranvier, Vanlair, and especially Stroebe, laid much stress, is totally opposed to the polygenist theory.

Polygenist or catenary doctrine.—The views that we have just described, founded as they were on exact and concordant observations, were accepted with scarcely a dissentient voice for more than thirty years. We all believed in the doctrine of trophic centres, because we believed it to be based on solid and definitely proved

[1] Herzt: " Ueber Degeneration und durchschnittene Nerven, *Virchow's Archiv*, Bd. 46, 1869.

conclusions. It became generally accepted not only because of its simplicity and unity, but also because it perfectly and clearly explained the totality of physiological and anatomico-pathological facts. As occurs with logical and well-cemented hypotheses, it received brilliant confirmations from various fields of science. Among the most illuminating and decisive of these we may cite the observations of His, ourselves, v. Lenhossék, v. Kölliker, Retzius, etc., showing that during the first stages of the development of the spinal cord the axon of the nerves is produced by amoeboid growth and extracentral ramification of the primordial expansion of the neuroblast or rudimentary nerve cell. It is true that the young axon, once arrived at the mesoderm, is accompanied by connective tissue cells. But these cells of mesodermal origin are entirely unrelated to the formation and growth of the axis-cylinder, forming only a protective covering which isolates and nourishes it. Of no less importance for the monogenist doctrine were the more modern experiments of Harrison, ingeniously conceived and carried out. Using very young amphibian embryos he showed that isolated neuroblasts kept in tissue cultures put out axons ending in clubs of growth. These axons grew by means of an amoeboid motion through the plasma, without the aid of any foreign bodies.[1]

We have just alluded to the importance of the hypothesis of continuity in the fields of neurology and neuropathology, and to its intimate connection with the doctrine of the neurone, established by His for histogenesis, and by Forel and ourselves for histology. It is only fair to say, however, that, in spite of its merits, it was never unanimously accepted. The negative opinions were advanced especially by the physiologists, a group of investigators who, with all the qualities and ability that they display in their particular line, are, we must say, because of the specialization necessitated by the division of labour, little acquainted with the severity and rigour of micrographic observations and with the secrets of histological interpretation. Among such heterodox physiologists we may note Phylippeaux and Vulpian, and also Schiff, and the more modern Alfred Bethe, the spirited and convinced champion of polygenism. We now proceed to set down the facts and theories of this rival

[1] R. G. Harrison : " The Outgrowth of the Nerve Fibre as a Mode of Protoplasmic Movement," *Journal of Experimental Zoology*, vol. 9, No. 4, Dec. 1910.
Idem : " Further Experiments on the Development of Peripheral Nerves," *American Journal of Anatomy*, vol. 5, No. 2, May 1906.

school, which had a few years ago its days of glory, thanks to the propagandist ardour of its adherents, some of them brilliant scientists, and to the polemical ingenuity of the Strasburg physiologist (Bethe). We shall first state the opinion of the precursors of the doctrine of discontinuity or catenary theory.

Among the first authors who attempted to refute the Wallerian doctrine were Phylippeaux and Vulpian,[1] who based themselves on anatomico-pathological experiments on very young mammals and birds (dogs, chicks, guinea-pigs). These physiologists began by cutting out of the young animals large pieces of the sciatic, median, hypoglossal, or other nerves. Months later they exposed the distal stump of the nerve and found it completely regenerated, although anatomically separated from the central stump. When such a distal segment was electrically stimulated, it caused motor reactions of its corresponding muscles, without being accompanied by sensory reactions. Histologically they found numerous newly-formed myelinated fibres. Finally, when this distal segment, regenerated to all appearances, was itself sectioned, the peripheral stump again degenerated. Instead of concluding, as would appear natural, that there existed an anatomical link between the two segments, which was microscopically invisible but which would be revealed by a scrupulous and conscientious micrographic analysis, they supposed that the fibres of the peripheral ends of nerves in young animals are able to regenerate without the help of the cells of origin. They called this strange method of regeneration *autogenous regeneration*. They believed that for adult animals the regeneration of the peripheral stump involves the co-operation of the fibres of the central segment. In a subsequent treatise (1874), however, Vulpian appeared to affirm the doctrine of autogenous regeneration less categorically. He already stated, in harmony with Waller's law, that when the excision of the lingual nerve of the young animals is followed by regeneration of the peripheral stump, this is not due to autogenesis of the latter, but to the penetration into it of new nerve sprouts brought there by neighbouring peripheral nerves.

The refutations of Ranvier, Vanlair, Kolster,[2] Stroebe, etc., had no effect on Phylippeaux and Vulpian. The French physiologists

[1] Phylippeaux et Vulpian: "Recherches expérimentales sur la régénération des nerfs séparés des centres nerveux," *Mém. de la Société de Biol.*, 1859.

[2] Kolster: "Zur Kenntniss der Regeneration durchschnittener Nerven," *Arch. f. mikros. Anat.*, Bd. xli, 1893.

adhered to this doctrine, which, as we shall see below, was taken as a basis, in modern times, by the principal champions of polygenism, Büngner and Bethe.

We must admit that the Wallerian theory does not explain all the facts. There exists a phenomenon in the degeneration of the distal stump which has always been used, especially in these later years, as a ground for questioning the theory of continuity. The cells of Schwann, as can easily be proved, undergo a process of hypernutrition and multiplication while the axons and myelin of both the central and distal stump are degenerating and being resorbed. This fact, along with the presence of longitudinal striations or lines in the protoplasmic cordons formed by such cells in the old tubes, suggested to various histologists and physiologists that such formative phenomena could lead to no other end than the discontinuous production of nerve fibres, as advanced by Vulpian. The most authoritative exponents of this doctrine have been, in modern times, Büngner, Wietting, Ballance and Stewart, Bethe, Galleotti and Levi, Luciani, Cornil, Durante, O. Schultze, Braun, etc.

Lents [1] and Hyelt [2] had already observed in 1861 the division of the cells of Schwann in the peripheral stump, and they attributed to these cells the genesis of the newly-formed fibres. It was Büngner,[3] however, who carefully studied the mitotic phenomena and all the phases of the supposed transition between the cells of Schwann and the nervous fibres. According to this investigator, the newly-formed fibres go through the following phases : as a result of mitotic divisions and protoplasmic growth the cells of Schwann, joining together tip to tip, form cordons or longitudinal bands (*Zellbänder*) which fill in large part the old perimedullar sheath ; then the nuclei which had at first been central, move to the sides until they become marginal. They thus abandon the axial zone, where appears a substance which is longitudinally striated. Finally the axon is differentiated out of this fibrillar material, and the myelin arises around it and under the eccentric nuclei. Such a development is

---

[1] Lents : " De nervorum dissectorum commutationibus ac regeneratione," *Inaug. Diss.*, Berlin, 1855.

[2] O. Hyelt : *Om nervernas regeneration*, Helsingfors, 1859.

[3] Büngner : " Ueber die Regeneration und Degenerationvorgänge am Nerven nach Verletzungen," *Beitr. zur pathol. Anat. u. allg. Pathol.*, Bd. 10, H. 4, 1891.

accelerated near the scar, as Schiff had already noted. The reason for this is that the central stump has an excitatory or trophic action.

In the central stump the same regenerative process takes place. The protoplasm that arises from the nuclei of the pre-existing fibres augments in amount, and the cellular series and protoplasmic bands are formed as stated above. In the interior of the bands the new axons develop by differentiation, and without continuity with the old axons. These new axons can already be seen in the third week. Later the germinative protoplasm decreases gradually in amount, and, with the nuclei, adopts a lateral position under the old sheath of Schwann.

The studies of Huber,[1] Ballance, Wietting,[2] Marchand, Galleotti and Levi,[3] Monckeberg and Bethe,[4] Bethe (A.),[5] Cornil, Durante, O. Schultze, and, finally, v. Gehuchten, were in essential agreement with the conclusions of Büngner.

We need not go in detail over the investigations of these workers, whose conclusions differ only in secondary points. But, in order to form a better idea of the state of the question before the commencement of our own investigations and those of Perroncito and Marinesco, we may give the most essential results of the studies of A. Bethe, the principal and most persistent champion in our day of the hazardous conception of Vulpian and Büngner.

Bethe began his investigations by repeating the experiments of Phylippeaux and Vulpian. He cut out pieces of the sciatic nerve

---

[1] Huber: "Ueber das Verhalten der Kerne der Schwanschen Scheide bei Nervendegeneration," *Arch. f. mikr. Anat.*, Bd. 40, 1892.

[2] Wietting: "Zur Frage der Degeneration der peripherischen Nerven," *Beiträge z. pathol. Anat. u. allg. Pathol.*, Bd. 23, 1898.

[3] Galleotti und Levi: "Ueber die Neubildung der nervösen Elementen in den niederverzeugten Muskelgewebe," *Beiträge z. pathol. Anat. u. allg. Pathol.*, Bd. 17, 1895.

[4] Monckeberg und Bethe: "Die Degeneration der markhaltigen Nerven, etc.," *Arch. f. mikr. Anat.*, Bd. 54, 1899.

[5] A. Bethe: "Ueber die Regeneration peripherischer Nerven," 26 *Wandervers. des Sudwestdeutsch. Neurol. etc., in Baden-Baden*, ann. 8, n. 9, Juni 1901.

Idem: *Arch. f. Psych.*, Bd. 34, 1901.

Idem: "Zur Frage von der autogenen Nervenregeneration," *Neurol. Centralbl.*, Bd. 22, 1903.

Idem: *Allgemeine Anatomie und Physiol. des Nervensystems*, Leipzig, 1903.

in mammals a few days old and arranged the two stumps in such a way that no union, and therefore no physiological continuity, could be possible. In young animals the regenerative process is much faster than in older ones, and so they lend themselves better to study.

Bethe devised various experiments in order to impede the union of central and distal stumps and to eliminate the trophic influences of the central segment of the nerve. He sometimes cut the sciatic nerve as it left the pelvis and folded the distal end back into the poplietal fossa. At other times he tied the superior segment to the gluteal muscles and cut out or folded back the peripheral stump. Again, he would cut the roots and extirpate the spinal ganglia of the sciatic nerve. Finally, he would carefully section the nerve in a muscle, leave the distal portion *in situ*, while he introduced the proximal stump into a muscle and sutured it there. Bethe believed that with such precautions he completely eliminated the objection that the new fibres of the peripheral stump could grow out from the central portion. But this belief is, as we shall see later, a pure illusion.

Under such conditions, Bethe states that in a certain number of cases (not in all, a very significant limitation) a macro-microscopical examination of the scar showed absolute interruption of the two segments, while there was at the same time a more or less complete regeneration of the peripheral end of the nerve, as was well shown by its physiological excitability. These observations, together with the confirmation of all the stages of transition which Büngner had already shown between the cells of Schwann and the young nerve fibres, led Bethe also to suppose that nerves entirely and definitely separated from their trophic centre were capable of autoregeneration. Each axon would thus be the product of many cells of Schwann, in whose matured protoplasm the neurofibrils would differentiate, and would then be the external sign of the reappearance of nervous conductibility.

Bethe founded this radical polygenism much more on the result of physiological experiments than on histological observations. After the above-mentioned nerve sections, when the autoregenerated distal extremity was electrically stimulated the animal would move the muscles of the leg and foot, while it would then be insensitive to any pain, showing thus no sensory communication. If the central stump were stimulated, no contractions would follow.

Bethe explained the exceptions to such results by supposing that, with all his precautions, there had been formed fortuitous connections between the two stumps.

Finally, in order to break down completely the Wallerian conception of trophic centres, Bethe made experiments to prove that, as Brown-Séquard had suggested, there was no essential difference between the *traumatic* degeneration of the central stump and the *functional* degeneration of the distal one. Both, he claimed, were traumatic, and were not concerned with nervous conduction. In the frog, for example, degeneration of the myelin can be caused by compression of the nerve, without a consequent absence of conduction. (He does not state whether the axon also is altered in this type of degeneration.) On the other hand, if a nerve is exposed to vapours of ammonia gas, the conducting action is suspended, while the myelin remains sound. With such experiments he tried to show that degeneration of the nerve is not necessarily associated with the suspension of functional activity, which is really dependent on other conditions. Bethe forgets to explain, however, why the distal extremity of a cut nerve degenerates *in toto* (myelin and axon), including the nervous terminations, while the central stump degenerates only near the wound, and its axons remain entirely unaffected.

Finally, more or less complete concurrence with the ideas of Bethe has been expressed by Ballance and Stewart,[1] who explain the union of the two stumps by a migration towards the scar of cells of the neurilemma or sheath of Schwann, which cells are able to become axons; by A. Modena,[2] who thinks he has shown, using the method of Cox, the discontinuous production of neurofibrils within the cells of Schwann of the distal stump; by Flemming,[3] who has studied regeneration of nerves in the rabbit; by v. Gehuchten, who repeated the physiological experiments of Bethe, without making any histological examination of the nerve segments; finally by

---

[1] Ballance and Stewart: " Le processus de réunion des nerfs," *Travaux de neurologie chirurgicale*, vol. 6, num. 314, Dec. 1901. *Revue neurologique*, 1902.

[2] A. Modena: "Die Degeneration und Regeneration der peripheren Nerven nach Läsion derselber," *Arbeiten aus dem Neurol. Institut*, herausgeb. v. Prof. H. Obersteiner, Bd. 12, 1905.

[3] Flemming: " La théorie périphérique de la régénération des nerfs et la neurite périphérique," *Scottish Medical Journal*, 1902.

Durante,[1] who claims to have proved autoregeneration even in man, and who has devoted to this theme a wealth of theoretical speculations and ingenious generalizations worthy of a better cause.

Such singular conclusions, opposed to the anatomico-pathological facts established by Ranvier, Vanlair, Kolster, Ziegler, and many others, could not fail to arouse a strong antagonism on the part of the surviving representatives of monogenism, from whose ranks death or senility had withdrawn its most distinguished champions—His and Ranvier.

Refutation of the polygenist doctrine.—Even before the application of methods which were much more conclusive than those used by Bethe and the polygenists, serious objections were raised to their views. We shall cite the principal investigators who opposed the ingenious but hazardous opinions of the Strasburg neurologist.

Münzer [2] first showed, that after section of the nerves in young rabbits, the newly-formed fibres of the peripheral segment arise from the 'neuroma,' or nervous tissue of the scar, itself connected with central fibres, or perhaps with neighbouring muscular nerves.

Langley and Anderson [3] came to similar conclusions, noting that if, when the regeneration is completed, one cuts the intermediate scar which bears the uniting fibres, then the peripheral segment again degenerates, showing that its fibres indubitably come from the proximal segment. Halliburton and Mott,[4] working very largely with the method of Marchi, put forward an analogous doctrine.

Lugaro,[5] furthermore, was unable to observe any autoregeneration in young animals when, instead of cutting the sciatic nerve near the muscles, he cut the spinal roots. He believed that the nerve fibres of the peripheral stump, as observed by Bethe, were the result of lengthening and migration of the pre-existing fibres of the central stump. In cases where stimulation of the peripheral segment causes

---

[1] Durante : "A propos de la théorie du Neurone," *Revue neurologique*, 1904.

[2] Münzer : "Giebt es eine autogenetische Regeneration der Nervenfasern," *Neurol. Centralbl.*, 1902.

[3] Langley and Anderson : "Observations on the Regeneration of Nerve Fibres," *Proceedings of the Physiol. Soc.*, Dec. 13, 1902.

[4] Halliburton and Mott : "Regeneration of Nerves," *Rep. of the Brit. Assoc. for the Adv. Science*, Sect. 1, Belfast, 1902.

[5] Lugaro : *Riv. di patol. nerv. e mentale*, 1904.

muscular contractions, although no union with the central segment had been established, Lugaro believed that there was a penetration into the distal stump of collateral fibres arising from neighbouring small nerves, probably attracted by chemotactic substances formed in the distal stump itself. Since in such exceptional cases no axons grow out from the proximal stump to the distal extremity, it is but natural that electrical stimulation of the former causes no contraction of the muscles of the leg.

Segale [1] also held a similar opinion, but he established a distinction between compensation and regeneration, two processes usually associated in functional restoration of cut nerves. Compensation is brought about by the normal nerves and muscles of the member whose main nerve has been cut, while regeneration is due to the growth of axons across the scar, destined to unite the two stumps. Like Langley and Anderson, Segale produced paralysis afresh by cutting across the scar. Where the axons of the central stump find great obstacles in their way collateral paths are formed, whose axons go through tortuous by-ways, deviating little by little and so reaching only in part the peripheral stump.

Using the method of Golgi, Purpura [2] was able to get preparations in which one could see perfectly that the newly-formed fibres come from the central stump, cross the scar, and penetrate the sheaths of the distal stump.

Such was the state of the question in the field of nervous degeneration and regeneration as late as 1905 and 1906. At that time better methods were invented and there were published our observations, those of Perroncito, Marinesco, Tello, Lugaro, Krassin, and Nageotte. All these investigations brought out new facts, gave in greater detail the results previously obtained, and placed the matter under a new aspect.

One may well ask why it is that a problem which is not too difficult of approach, and to whose solution distinguished investigators have applied themselves for half a century, has as yet received no universally accepted solution. Why is it that if, as numerous facts indicate, truth is on the side of the monogenist doctrine, famous anatomico-pathologists and physiologists deny it ?

[1] Segale : *Ueber die Nervenregeneration*, Genoa, 1903.

[2] F. Purpura: " Contributo allo studio della rigenerazione dei nervi periferici. Comun. fatta nella seduta del 1° Febr. 1901," *Boll. della Società medico-chirurgica di Pavia*, 1901.

Leaving aside motives of a psychological nature, unfortunately common enough, such as the feverish thirst for novelty, the suggestion of fashionable theories, and other causes entirely foreign to a calm and disinterested pursuit of the truth, it must be admitted that in the debated question the principal reasons for disagreement are two. One is subjective, the other objective. The first is the generalization in pathology of conjectures and theories that are very hazardous and belong to other fields of science (structure and connections of nerve cells, genesis of embryonic nerve fibres, etc.). The second is the inadequacy of the current technique to present morphological facts with a clearness sufficient to dispel the mist of fancy that envelops them, and thus to exclude all dissension.

As a matter of fact, the technique for showing the genesis, growth, and evolution of the axons is very uncertain. It is only the talent of such men as Waller and Ranvier that has been able to supply the methodological deficiencies which have led astray many modern histologists of no mean capacity. It is hardly necessary to note that the methods of dissociation and section of preparations impregnated with osmic acid show clearly only the old medullated sheaths. As to the ordinary methods, much used by the partisans of polygenism, which consist in staining sections previously fixed in sublimate, osmio-chromic mixtures, formalin, etc., with basic or acid aniline dyes, they show distinctly only the cordons composed of Schwann's cells, within which one can only vaguely see embryonic axons. The method of Bethe for staining the neurofibrils within the new medullated fibres is limited in its use, inefficient, and inconstant. At any rate, the paleness of coloration and the necessary thinness of the sections do not allow one to use this method for tracing out the embryonic fibres. These difficulties forced Bethe himself to adopt usually the osmic acid stain, that is, the traditional inadequate method. The method of Cox, which A. Modena applied with some success, is inconstant, and gives only incomplete and discontinuous impregnations of the cells of Schwann when in process of rejuvenation. As to the method of Golgi, which we have tried, it does not stain medullated fibres and impregnates non-medullated fibres with great irregularity and inconstancy. Nevertheless, Purpura, as we have noted, achieved with this method some valuable results.

Modern investigations of nervous regeneration. The abovementioned technical difficulties, together with the great importance of the problem, led us to try in 1905 the method of impregnation with silver, which had given us (as well as v. Lenhossék, Retzius, Tello, Michotte, v. Gehuchten, Marinesco, Levi, Nageotte, Dogiel, etc.) such good results in the analysis of the neurofibrils in the nerve centres and of peripheral nerve endings. The important investigations concerning the regeneration of nerves by Perroncito, Marinesco and Minea, Medea, Tello, Dustin, O. Rossi, Deineka, etc., were also carried out by this method.

The formula used is that which requires fixation in alcohol to which a few drops of ammonia have been added. In such preparations the axons, medullated or naked, are alone impregnated, and appear brown, coffee-coloured or transparent red, and show up very well on the diaphanous yellow background of the scar. Since it is pieces that are impregnated, one has the advantage of making and studying thick sections, where one can easily follow the fibres. Equally feasible and easy is the observation of the divisions and endings of the young fibres.[1]

The principal results of our observations, whose details we shall give later, may be condensed as follows :

1. When the sciatic nerve of a young animal is cut and the animal is killed at a longer or shorter interval after the operation, one notes in impregnated preparations that a great number of the axons of the central stump are actively in the process of sprouting. This sprouting is effected in two ways : (a) The new fibre or fibres are terminal, and are budded from the enlarged tip of the old axon. (b) The new fibres are collateral, and arise at right or acute angles to the old axon. In both cases the newly-formed shoots have no medullated sheaths, invade the exudate that is present between the two nervous stumps, ramify as they proceed, and, finally, end freely in a terminal club or bud, a kind of battering-ram, which is used to push aside the mesodermal cells and to form a path across the future cicatricial substance.

---

[1] A full exposition of our results, profusely illustrated, appeared under the title " Mecanismo de la degeneración y regeneración de los nervios " in the *Trabajos del Lab. de Investig. biol.*, vol. 4, 1905. These investigations were also given in résumé in the *Boletín del Instituto de Alfonso XIII.*, Nos. 2 and 3, 1905. Finally, two complementary communications of ours on this question were published : " Les métamorphoses précoces des neurofibrilles dans la régénération et la dégénération des nerfs," *Trab. del Lab. de Investig. biol.*, vol. 5, fasc. 2, 1907 ; and " Algunas observaciones favorables á la hipótesis neurotrópica," *Trab. del Lab. de Investig. biol.*, vol. 8, 1911.

The discovery of this terminal excrescence, later confirmed by the investigations of Perroncito, Marinesco, Nageotte, Sala, Tello, Dustin, Rossi, etc., assumes a certain importance for the resolution of the debated question, since with such a terminal protoplasmic bud one can tell in the sections not only the level which the regenerative process has reached, but also the origin and orientation of newly-formed axons.

2. During their initial phases the newly-formed nerve fibres, as well as their terminal buds, lack nuclei or cells of Schwann. From the third or fourth day on, embryonic connective cells are attracted, and around the naked axons and clubs appear marginal nuclei. This important observation of the formative precedence of the regenerated axons over the cells of Schwann singularly compromises the polygenist theory, since it shows that during the first phases of the evolution of the fibres there are absolutely no cellular chains.

3. If one studies the growth of the newly-formed fibres during the first six days after section of the nerve one can easily see that the terminal clubs grow indeterminately along the paths of least resistance. A great many take a reverse direction, in the central stump, where they go back very far, as well as in perinervous tissues. Other fibres, disorientated and wandering, stop before obstacles, follow complicated paths, and lose themselves definitely, as far as the nervous reunion of the peripheral stump is concerned. Such diverted axons, abundantly found where pieces of nerve are taken out or where the two stumps are intentionally pulled apart, are characterized by gigantic encapsulated clubs or spheres, often in process of degeneration. These spheres are nothing else than the so-called *nerve cells*, shown some time ago by S. Mayer of Prague,[1] in the substance of regenerating nerves, and described by Ranvier[2] as enigmatic monstrous formations, situated in the paths of central fibres.

4. After ten or twelve days in adult animals, and six or seven in animals a few weeks old, the young fibres that have not lost their way, wandering in the intercalary cicatricial tissue, approach the sheaths of the peripheral stump, grow into them, and push from their path the remnants of the myelin that are as yet unabsorbed. Before

---

[1] Sigmund Mayer: "Die peripherische Nervenzelle und das sympathische Nervensystem," *Arch. f. Psychiatrie*, 1876.

[2] Ranvier: *Leçons sur l'histologie du système nerveux*, Tome II., page 78, 1878.

obstacles the new fibres subdivide minutely, and the shoots go forward flexibly, and indifferently either through the bands of Büngner or in their interstices.

5. If one repeats the experiment of Vulpian, Brown-Séquard, Bethe, etc., by putting obstacles between the two stumps of a cut nerve, so as to keep them from immediately uniting, one often notes, after two or three months, a well-advanced regeneration of the distal segment. When this is examined by means of our method of staining one can see in its interior numerous young axons which always end, at different levels, with small buds of growth.

An examination of the varied and extensive scar which unites the stumps reveals, not the absence of uniting fibres, as the polygenists arbitrarily claimed, but a complex nerve plexus, formed by small bundles of unmyelinated nerve fibres, which extends uninterruptedly from the central to the peripheral segments.

6. The newly-formed nerve fibres repeatedly subdivide in the scar, especially at the edge of the peripheral stump, where, very often, a large axon reduces itself to a *bouquet* of fine terminal twigs. The branches of a single axon do not go to one old nerve tube, but they distribute themselves to several empty sheaths. From this it follows that a group which is relatively poor in afferent axons can still innervate a good portion of the regenerated nerve. It is to be noted that such branches, always oriented towards the periphery, as well as their free end-clubs, are observed facts irreconcilable with the polygenist theory.

7. When the obstacles to reunion of the nervous fragments are insuperable (suture of the peripheral stump to the skin, insertion of the central segment in the abdominal cavity, etc.), the peripheral segment shows absolutely no regeneration, even months after the operation, and no matter what the age of the animal.

8. The multiplication of the cells of Schwann of the peripheral stump does not occur for the purpose of producing chains of elements which can be transformed by autogeneration, as Büngner and Bethe claimed, but its object is to segregate stimulating substances which are able to attract and direct to the motor and sensory nerve endings the young nerve fibres that are wandering in the scar.

A young Italian investigator, Aldo Perroncito,[1] a pupil of the

[1] A. Perroncito: " Sulla questione della rigenerazione autogena delle fibre nervose. Nota preventiva." *Boll. della Società Medico-chirurgica di Pavia*. Seduta 19 Maggio, 1905. (Published in September, 1905.)

distinguished histologist of Pavia, Golgi, independently of ourselves used the method of reduced silver nitrate to study the regeneration of nerves. We had already in 1904 pointed out the value of this method for anatomico-pathological studies. The principal treatise of Perroncito was published while our extensive monograph on the subject was in the press, and after the publication of our first preliminary note.[1] In this communication he confirmed the existence of terminal clubs, which he saw penetrating into the exudate as early as the second day after the operation ; he showed that the young fibres of the scar and central stump frequently divided ; finally, he was able to follow the branches up to the peripheral stump, where he did not find the least trace of autoregeneration. His conclusions, entirely in accord with the Wallerian conception, are based on unimpeachable preparations and drawings.

Having occupied ourselves with the determination of the origin and evolution of the newly-formed fibres of the peripheral stump, we had somewhat neglected the analysis of the early phenomena in the central stump. The interesting observations of Perroncito, made on dogs on the first, second and third day after the nerve was cut, happily filled in this blank, revealing the three following important facts :

1. The collateral and terminal branchings, observed by us in the central stump, as well as the ramifications of the naked axons growing in the exudate and scar, are produced very early. According to Perroncito, after twenty-four hours, or even earlier, one can perceive in some nodes twigs ending in clubs or spherules and small rings, and early on the second day ramifications of the axons go through the exudate towards the peripheral stump.

2. Besides this method of emission of collateral and terminal branches, nerve fibres are also produced by a process of ravelling or transformation of the old axon into a bundle of independent fibrils, which grow beneath the sheath of Schwann and go to the scar, where they end in clubs, buds, or rings. In honour of its discoverer, or at least of the investigator who first carefully studied it,[2] we

[1] Cajal : *Loc. cit. Boletín del Instituto de Seroterapia*, Nos. of July and September, 1905.

[2] In reality the phenomenon of Perroncito in its late stages was observed at nearly the same time by him, by ourselves, and by Marinesco ; but we must recognize that it is the studies of the Italian investigator that brought out the initial phases and the mechanism by which the process is effected.

have called this curious phenomenon of the multiple production of nervous branches the *phenomenon* or *apparatus* of Perroncito. This singular process, partly pathological, partly normal, is complicated with the intratubal division (that is, division beneath the sheath of Schwann) of some neurofibrils, which frequently grow backwards, describe close loops and spirals, and form such intricate structures that in some cases one cannot attempt to describe or reproduce them.

3. In the days following the operation not only the central stump, but also, though rarely, the wounded end of the distal stump, show clubs and even branchings.

These and other observations of Perroncito, of which we shall speak further at the proper time, were confirmed by us in a special treatise,[1] in which we showed the conditions generative of ravelling of the axon and the significance of the clubs and frustrated divisions of the peripheral stump.

We were fortunate enough to convince Dr. Marinesco,[2] the distinguished anatomico-pathologist, who had believed, up to that time, like many others, in the polygenist hypothesis, owing to the great authority, experimental talent, and polemical ability of the Strasburg physiologist—Bethe. Now, however, no longer hampered by lack of technique, and master of the secrets of the analytical method, Marinesco refuted the premises and inferences of the theory of discontinuity, declaring them to be errors without objective foundation. He confirmed and described very well the clubs of growth and the branching of the central fibres, their continuity with the wandering fibres of the scar, and their entrance into the peripheral stump. He showed the inability of Schwann's cells to form new axons, the presence of ample intercalary nerve plexuses between the two segments that had been pulled apart or separated by obstacles, the formation of nervous spools in the central stump, due to the growth and disorientation of the young axons. He observed the genesis and structural transformations of the gigantic or arrested clubs, and, finally, the nutritive and orienting services rendered to the young axons by the proliferated cells of Schwann of the peripheral stump, which he called *apotrophic corpuscles*.

[1] Cajal: " Les métamorphoses précoces des neurofibrilles dans la régénération et la dégénération des nerfs," *Trav. du Lab. de Recher. biol.*, fasc. 1 et 2, vol. v., 1907.

[2] Marinesco and J. Minea: " La loi de Waller et la régénérescence autogene," *Revista Stüntelor Medicale*, Sept. 5, 1905.

Using a similar technique, Minea, working in Marinesco's laboratory, and G. Sala, who investigated human nerves, both wounded and regenerating, came to identical conclusions.

Lugaro,[1] on his side, using the new process in connection with interesting and well-conducted experiments of excision and ablation of sensory roots and ganglia, showed, as opposed to Bethe, the essential incapacity for regeneration of the sensory roots, if, when the corresponding ganglion had been extirpated, one carefully prevented the intromission of newly-formed fibres from the neighbouring motor root.

Lugaro [2] also showed that if one cuts out the spinal cord and corresponding sensory ganglia of an animal, there is, months later, absolutely no regeneration of the sciatic nerve. The few fibres seen in such a nerve, after staining with silver nitrate, are amyelinated and belong to the sympathetic system exclusively. Their foci of origin, the sympathetic system, had naturally not been involved.

It is interesting and significant in connection with the theory of neurotropism that Lugaro showed that the attractive action of Schwann's cells is not specific, and can cause the growth of surrounding nerves of a different nature. Thus the posterior root, sectioned inside the ganglion, can attract newly-formed fibres of the corresponding motor root.

Levi,[3] another of the most enthusiastic advocates of the heterodox doctrine, who, by using the method of reduced silver nitrate made some important discoveries concerning the morphology of ganglion cells of reptiles and fishes, in a recent treatise pronounced himself against the hypothesis of Vulpian and Bethe.

Almost simultaneously a great number of neuropathologists applied our technique to the study of degeneration and regeneration of the posterior roots and central nervous system with good results. Among those who have made the most numerous discoveries in this

---

[1] Lugaro: "Sul neurotropismo e sui trapianti dei nervi," *Riv. di patol. ner. e mentale*, vol. xi., fasc. 7, 1906.

Idem: "Sulla presunta rigenerazione autogena delle radici posteriori," *Ibid.*, vol. xi., fasc. 8, Aug. 1906.

[2] Lugaro: "Weiteres zur Frage der autogenen Regeneration der Nervenfasern," *Neurol. Centralbl.*, 1906.

[3] Levi: "Di alcuni problemi riguardanti la struttura del sistema nervoso, etc.," *Arch. di Fisiologia*, May, 1907.

field we may cite : Nageotte,[1] who observed the clubs of growth and newly-formed fibres in the ganglia, nerve roots, and spinal cord of tabetics, and who has recently shown the conditions underlying the production of new expansions in transplanted nerve ganglia ; Marinesco and Minea,[2] who have also observed interesting phenomena of regeneration and metamorphosis of the neurones and axons of transplanted ganglia ; O. Rossi [3] and Dustin,[4] who have confirmed a great number of the facts concerning nervous regeneration discovered by ourselves, Perroncito, and Marinesco, and who have formulated suggestive hypotheses regarding the mechanism of genesis and orientation of the newly-formed expansions ; Sala and Cortese,[5] who have observed remarkable phenomena of sprouting in the extirpated anterior roots ; and Tello,[6] who has applied the above-mentioned technique to the muscular nerves and sensory endings, showing for the first time the mechanism of degeneration and regeneration in motor plates and spindles of Kühne. In Tello's beautiful preparations one can clearly see the clubs of growth of the new axons develop along the old sheaths of Schwann of the small muscular nerves, divide when they encounter obstacles, and finally

[1] Nageotte : " Note sur la présence de massues d'accroissement dans la substance grise de la moelle épinière, etc., au cours de la paralyse générale et du tabes," *Soc. de Biol.*, 12 mai, 1906.

Idem: "Étude sur la greffe des ganglions rachidiens," *Anat. Anzeiger*, Bd. 31, Nos. 9 to 20, 1907.

[2] Marinesco et Minea : " Recherches expérimentales, etc., sur les lésions consécutives à la compression et à l'écrasement des ganglions sensitifs," *Folia neurobiologica*, Bd. 1, No. 1, 1907.

See also Marinesco : *Revue neurobiologique*, No. 21, 1907.

[3] O. Rossi : " Processi regenerativi e degenerativi consequente a ferite assetiche del sistema nervoso centrale, etc.," *Rivis. di patol. nerv. e mentale*, Anno 13, fasc. 11, 1908.

Idem: "Nicosi ricerche, etc.," *Riv. di patol. nerv. e mentale*, vol. 15, fasc. 4, 1910.

[4] Dustin : " Le rôle des tropismes et de l'odogénèse dans la régénération du système nerveux," *Arch. de biol.*, Tom. 25, 1910.

[5] G. Sala e Cortese : *Sui fatti che si svolgono nel midollo spinale in seguito allo strappo delle radici*, Padua, 1909.

[6] Tello : " Dégénération et régénération des plaques motrices après la section des nerfs," *Trav. du lab. de rech. biol.*, vol. 5, fasc. 3, 1907.

Idem: " La régénération dans les fuseaux de Kühne," *Trav. du lab. de rech. biol.*, vol. 5, fasc. 4, Dec. 1907.

break up into a new arborization among the remnants of the old plate.

Once the movement of adherence to the classical doctrine of Waller and of Ranvier had begun, and when new morphological facts had been discovered entailing the acceptance of this doctrine as an indisputable postulate, favourable arguments came from all sides. These arguments were not exclusively based on the use of our method of staining, but were founded also on the revelations of other analytical methods, such as Ehrlich's methylene blue, the method of Marchi, and the ordinary histological methods. Thus Krassin [1] of St. Petersburg, using Ehrlich's method of vital staining, saw the process of growth of the central axons, as well as the exodus of the off-shoots across the scar and peripheral stump. Mott, Halliburton, and Edmond,[2] using the method of Marchi, have established these two facts : (*a*) when the obstacles to immediate union are very great, the distal segment is incapable of regeneration, and definitely loses its electrical irritability ; (*b*) if one transplants a piece of nerve to a region that has no nerves, such as the peritoneal cavity, the pretended autoregeneration of nerve fibres is totally absent. Stuart,[3] in an experimental study of the section and transplantation of nerves, reached similar conclusions.

Poscharisky,[4] a pupil of Marchand, in whose laboratory he undertook an investigation of nervous regeneration, used our method and that of Bielschowsky. He was unable to deny the sprouting of the fibres from the central stump, and the possibility of their penetration into the scar, even though he worked under a man who, a few years back, implicitly believed in the polygenist conception.

Finally Modena,[5] a pupil of Donaggio, made use of the latter's method for the study of nervous regeneration. Abandoning the

---

[1] Krassin : " Zur Frage der Degeneration der peripheren Nerven," *Anat. Anz.*, Nos. 17-18, Bd. 28, 1906.

[2] W. Mott, D. Halliburton, and A. Edmond : " Regeneration of Nerves," *Proc. of the Royal Soc.*, vol. 78, 1906.

[3] J. Stuart : *Proc. of the Royal Soc.*, vol. 78, 1906.

[4] Poscharisky : " Über die histologischen Vorgänge an den peripherischen Nerven nach Kontinuitätstrennung," *Beitr. z. pathol. Anat. u. allgem. Pathol.*, Bd. 41, H. 1, 1907.

[5] A. Modena : " Régénération des nerfs périphériques," *Arch. ital. de biol.*, Tom. 74, fasc. 3, 1910.

polygenist doctrine, he has confirmed the essential facts of regeneration as shown by the method of reduced silver nitrate.

As a consequence of these new methods and discoveries, one may say that the polemics which lasted for more than thirty years between the monogenists and the polygenists have now only a historical interest. Everything shows the definite triumph of the Wallerian conception. Some polygenists, like van Gehuchten, kept silence, an attitude that took the place of admission of error. In the neurogenic field, such ardent polygenists as Dohrn [1] and Levi honourably changed their opinions, and Held,[2] the most brilliant representative of the old doctrine of Hensen, made continuous concessions to the winning conception of His. In the field of nervous regeneration, there was only confusion and discouragement among the polygenists. Even Alfred Bethe,[3] who in moments of enthusiasm thought that he had utterly demolished the doctrine of the neurone, later, in his vivacious and somewhat acrimonious answers to Lugaro, Perroncito, ourselves, Marinesco, etc., showed himself progressively less dogmatic and more conciliatory. He did not deny that the sprouts of the central stump enter the scar and at times go to the peripheral stump ; he doubted only that these new growths enter into the centre of the distal segment and that they really constitute the definitive conductors of the regenerated nerve. Finally, such great authorities as Retzius, v. Lenhossék, Schiefferdecker, Heidenhain, Harrison, etc., who were not directly involved, but were interested in the debate between monogenists and polygenists, explicitly or implicitly bowed before the doctrine of continuity, the only one in harmony with the laws of neurogenesis that were put forward some time ago by Kupffer and His, and were corroborated by the histogenic studies of ourselves, v. Lenhossék, Kölliker, Harrison, etc.

Although in moments of impatience one may have deplored the polygenist error, to whose refutation numerous investigators have given years of assiduous and persevering work, still this work and time have not been without profit to science. The criticisms and

[1] Dohrn : " Studien zur Urgeschichte des Wirbelthierkörpers, 25. Der Frochbaris," *Mittheil. aus der Zool. Station von Neapel*, Bd. 18, H. 2 und 3, 1907.

[2] Held: *Die Entwickelung der Nervengewebe bei den Wirbelthieren*. J. A. Barth, edit. Leipzig, 1909.

[3] A. Bethe : " Neue Versuche über die Regeneration der Nervenfasern," *Arch. f. d. ges. Physiol.*, Bd. 116, 1907.

ingenious experiments directed by Bethe and his disciples against the conception of the neurone and the classical doctrine of Waller have given rise to the invention of methods of a higher analytical efficiency and to a general revision of the terms of the problem. The facts that were already known concerning degeneration and regeneration were more scrupulously studied. The conditions of experimentation were varied, and an abundant collection was made of objective data. The real significance of certain phenomena, such as the division of the cells of Schwann of the peripheral stump, was ascertained, after these phenomena had given rise to many doubts. Finally, the Wallerian conception was definitely proved and placed on a firm basis.

The doctrine of the neurone, intimately connected in the pathological field with the theory of continuity, came out of this new crisis strengthened and victorious. Instead of finding, in the field of nervous regeneration, insuperable difficulties, it found, on the contrary, new and peremptory demonstrations, in whose light not a few of the enigmatic phenomena of the morphology and growth of nervous protoplasm are beginning to be understood.

Let us hope that this will be the last ordeal to which the doctrine of continuity will be subjected, and that new investigators, instead of attacking incontestable principles, the common property of modern neurologists, will discard polemics and devote themselves to the enlargement of our knowledge, unravelling the still unknown phases of the growth and orientation of normal and pathological nerve tracts.

II

TECHNIQUE FOR THE STUDY OF NERVOUS DEGENERATION AND REGENERATION

Methods for impregnating the axons.—Methods of Bielschowsky, Cajal, etc.—Methods for staining the myelin (osmic acid, procedures of Marchi, Herxheimer, etc.).—Methods for staining the cells of Schwann (procedures with basic haematoxylin and aniline, procedures of Doinikow Nageotte, etc.).—Method of Achúcarro for staining neuroglia.—Procedure of Alzheimer.—Animals used for experiments on degeneration and regeneration, and operatory technique.

THERE are to-day a great many methods for the study of the changes brought about in the substance of the nerves and their terminations by the regenerative and degenerative processes. The lack of a technique adequate for the problem, that is, of a method for staining selectively the nervous sprouts, so much deplored by those anatomical pathologists who worked before 1903, now no longer exists. Thanks to the new methods the controversial question of the origin of the newly-formed fibres of the peripheral stump has been settled, as we saw above, and the bases have been laid for a rational explanation of the mechanism of regeneration. The technical methods may be classified as follows : 1. Procedures for selectively staining the axons and their sprouts. 2. Procedures for staining the myelin sheath. 3. Procedures for staining the nuclei and the cells of Schwann. 4. Procedures for staining neuroglia and the connective tissue of nerve trunks.

The above methods can be applied, with slight variations, to the peripheral nerves as well as to the white and grey substances of the centres, thus embodying the technique necessary for the study of the nerve tissues generally.

As the reader knows the ordinary methods for staining the nerve tissues, we shall here lay stress only on the more modern procedures, and particularly on those which are favourable for the analysis of the phenomena occurring in wounded nerves.

Procedures for selectively staining the axon and its newly formed branches.—At the head of this list we may cite the *method of reduced* *silver nitrate* which, owing to the ease with which it can be applied, its demonstrative capacity, and its constancy, has been preferred by nearly all the investigators who during the last few years have occupied themselves with the problem of the regeneration of the nerve trunks and centres.

Numerous experiments made by us, in which we varied the fixative and other determining factors of the selective reaction, have led us to the establishment of several formulae, each one of which is applicable to particular cases. For the study of nervous regeneration the following are especially suitable :

A. *Method with ammoniacal alcohol :*

1. Entire nerves of rabbits, dogs, etc., as well as the intermediate scar caused by the wound, are fixed, for twenty-four hours, in :

> 96 per cent. alcohol - - - - 50 c.c.
> Ammonia - - - - - 4 to 6 drops.

2. The pieces are left for a few seconds on blotting paper, to take off the excess fluid. They are then put in the silver nitrate solution :

> Silver nitrate - - - - - 1·5 gms.
> Distilled water - - - - 100 c.c.

One must see that there is an abundance of liquid in relation to the submerged tissues. Thus, for two or three pieces of rabbit's nerve, we would use at least 40 or 50 c.c. of the silver solution.

The flask containing the silver nitrate and the nerve tissues is taken to an incubator which is kept at a temperature of 36° to 38° C., for five days. If the temperature is 40° or 41° C., the pieces are ripe in four days.

3. The tissues are washed for a few seconds (three to six) in distilled water. This washing is to dilute or wash off the silver nitrate on the surface of the pieces. It is the silver nitrate within the tissues which is precipitated as colloidal silver. When one uses very thin nerves, such as those of frogs, guinea-pigs, rats, etc., one does not need to wash them.

4. The pieces are immersed in the following reducing liquid :

> Pyrogallic acid - - - - - 1 grm.
> Water - - - - - - - 100 c.c.
> Formalin - - - - - - 5 to 10 c.c.

They remain in it for twenty-four hours. One may keep this solution with the immersed pieces in the incubator. But the reaction, consisting in the production of colloidal silver at the expense of the warm silver nitrate, is obtained as well at a cold temperature. In presence of the silver salt the neurofibrils of the axon form a combination whose composition is unknown as yet, and which, as a result of the heat, changes state (ripens) and strongly attracts the colloidal silver.

5. After the pieces have been washed for a few minutes in distilled water, they are hardened in 36 per cent. alcohol, then in 40 per cent. alcohol, and they are finally embedded in paraffin or celloidin. As very thin sections are not convenient, we prefer the latter. The sections are cleared in *oil of origanum*. The *oils of bergamot* or of *cloves* are less satisfactory, as they oxidize to some extent the colloidal silver. The sections are finally mounted in balsam or gum dammar. Before mounting one should extract the oil of origanum with xylene.

The effect produced by the deposit of colloidal silver is very interesting. Of all the structural components of the nerve only the axons are impregnated. These take on a greyish-red or a transparent black colour, which contrasts beautifully with the yellow background. Between the old medullated axons and the newly-formed naked axons one can note great differences. While the new shoots and normal unmyelinated fibres are red or dark grey, showing very well their neurofibrils, the adult axons are paler, with a coffee-coloured tint, which sometimes is orange or yellowish. This contrast is greater or less, according to the amount of ammonia in the fixative. In general, the more ammonia is added to the alcohol the paler are the medullated adult axons and the better the contrast with the young fibres. Sometimes the adult axons are not coloured at all.

The method with ammoniacal alcohol has been much used by those authors who have studied nervous regeneration—Nageotte, Lugaro, Perroncito, Marinesco, Tello, G. Sala, O. Rossi, H. Rossi, Deineka, ourselves, etc. As the nuclei are usually not stained, although they occasionally show up very well, one can complete the picture by using a basic aniline dye. Veratti and Perroncito have used saffranin with success ; we use thionin or methylene blue.

The above method has some disadvantages. It stains too deeply the superficial portions of the pieces and the scar tissue, or it may give colorations that are too pale. Finally the old axons may not stain ; this, although useful for analysis in some cases, is often disadvantageous. To suit certain cases of the regenerative process we use other formulae, in which it is only the composition of the fixative and the time in the incubator that vary.

B. *Method with pure alcohol* :

1. The nerves, attached to cork as in the preceding case, remain in 96 per cent. alcohol for twenty-four hours.

2. Immersion in silver nitrate, and ripening in the incubator for six days, at 36° to 38° C.

The further procedure is as in the preceding formula. If one adds to the alcohol a certain quantity of veronal, chloral hydrate, pyridine, etc., one day can be saved in ripening, and the danger of granular impregnations is completely eliminated.

C. *Method with pyridine* :

Introduced into the neurofibrillar technique by Donaggio, pyridine, associated with the method of reduced silver nitrate, has been very much used, these last few years, by Held,[1] who has usually applied it to the coloration of neurofibrils in embryos.

Our observations, which confirm those of Held, lead us to state that pyridine is the most convenient fixative for the first phases of neurogenesis. It vividly stains the neurofibrils and nerve fibres ; they stand out on a transparent yellow background, while the nuclei remain unstained. It greatly augments the penetrative force of the silver nitrate. Other decided advantages are the constancy of impregnation and the evenness of the stain, which is hardly darker on the borders of the nervous organs.

It also gives very good preparations in the study of regeneration. Its effects are similar to those of the method with ammoniacal alcohol, but it never stains the nuclei and it only impregnates the metamorphic portions of the regenerating axons and nerve sprouts. The normal axons of the central stump remain unstained. But the greatest advantages are that the preparations fixed in pyridine show hardly any over-coloration of the superficial zones, and there are never any granular precipitates in the scar and inflammatory exudates.

Thus, when one is dealing with very small pieces, or when one wishes to examine the early phenomena in degeneration and regeneration, pyridine is absolutely necessary, even though it has a propensity to give somewhat pale preparations, in which the old axons are colourless.

[1] Held : " Die Entstehung der Neurofibrillen," *Neurol. Centralbl.*, 1905.

Instead of the pure pyridine, as suggested by Donaggio and Held, we prefer a 50 or 60 per cent. pyridine solution.

The steps are as follows :

1. Small pieces remain for twelve or twenty-four hours in

   Distilled water - - - - - 25 c.c.
   Pyridine - - - - - - - 25 to 30 c.c.

2. The pieces are washed in running water for some hours, until the pyridine is totally eliminated. If there is no running water one should change the water four or five times in six hours.

3. Immersion in 96 per cent. alcohol for twelve to twenty-four hours.

4. The pieces are wiped off with blotting paper, and are then put in the silver nitrate, where they remain four days at 37° or 38° C. If the nerves are small and the temperature is 40° or 41° C., three days will be sufficient.

5. Reduction, as usual, in pyrogallic acid.

D. *Method with chloral hydrate* :

1. The nerve tissues are placed for twenty-four hours in

   Chloral hydrate - - - - - 5 gms.
   Water - - - - - - - 50 c.c.

2. After a rapid wash in distilled water they are put in ammoniacal alcohol.

   96 per cent. alcohol - - - - - 50 gms.
   Ammonia - - - - - - 3 drops.

3. The pieces are wiped off with blotting paper, and they are left for four or five days in the 1·5 per cent. silver nitrate solution, at a temperature of 35° to 38° C.

4. Reduction as usual.

This formula gives very constant results. Besides, it does away with the shrinking of the pieces and therefore with the contraction and deformation of the axons, which appear normal in form and size. After inclusion in celloidin the consistency of the tissues is such that one can cut fine sections very well.

Unlike the preceding formula, it stains nuclei, so that cells are easily seen and one does not need to stain with aniline dyes.[1]

[1] These and other formulæ were given in detail in our paper entitled: *Las fórmulas del proceder del nitrato de plata reducido, etc.*, in the *Trab. del Lab. de Invest. biol.*, vol. 8, fascs. 1 and 2, Sept. 1910.

Observations concerning the preceding formulae. Every nervous organ that is the seat of regenerative phenomena contains two kinds of nerve fibres—the adult fibres and the shoots or newly-formed fibres, generally without myelin. Naturally, the proportion of these two structural elements varies according to the time since the lesion was made and since, therefore, the regenerative process began. Each of these two elements requires, however, a special formula, in order to show up well.

To guide the reader we may cite some examples.

Let us suppose that one wishes to stain the peripheral and central stumps of a nerve one month or more after it is cut, that is to say, during a period when the newly-formed axons are large and partly medullated, and when the inflammatory exudate has been already resorbed. The method with pure alcohol or the method with slightly ammoniacal alcohol (3 drops of ammonia) would be particularly suitable, since they stain both the old and the new fibres, although the latter come out somewhat more strongly than the former.

When the regenerative phenomena are of recent date—nerves from one to ten days after the cut—then the formulae that give the best results are as follows: fixation in alcohol rich in ammonia (6 to 8 drops), or the formula in which pyridine is used as a base. We have already said that the latter stains especially the young fibres and incipient sprouts. The fixation in chloral hydrate gives the most complete results, since both the adult and the newly-formed fibres are stained, as well as the nuclei. But such a complete impregnation is sometimes disadvantageous for analytical study of the sections, because of the insufficient contrast between the background and the nerve sprouts.

One may also fix in formalin instead of in chloral hydrate, as in the method of Bielschowsky. In such a case the pieces are washed in many changes of water in order to take out the formalin, and they have to remain for twenty-four hours in the ammoniacal alcohol before being transferred to the silver nitrate. With this method of fixation the sprouts are well stained, but the background may be too reddish. There are cases, however, in which fixation in formalin is convenient.

Method of Bielschowsky. Bielschowsky has published various formulae for staining the neurofibrils of the cells and axons.

These are of more or less value. One of the best (1908) is the following :

1. Fixation in 20 per cent. formalin.
2. The pieces are washed in water for several hours.
3. Immersion in pure pyridine for twenty-four to forty-eight hours.
4. The pieces are washed in several changes of distilled water, for several hours, until the pyridine odour is gone.
5. Sections are made with a freezing microtome.
6. The sections are left for one day in 3 per cent. silver nitrate.
7. They are washed in distilled water for a short time.
8. Immersion in the ammoniacal silver nitrate solution, made up as follows :

    20 per cent. silver nitrate solution - - 5 c.c.
    Sodium hydroxide - - - - - 5 drops.

The precipitate is dissolved by adding slowly some drops of ammonia. There should be no excess of the latter. The bath is diluted with 20 c.c. of distilled water.

9. The sections are washed for a few seconds in distilled water.
10. Reduction in 20 per cent. formalin, which can be used only one day.
11. Toning with a gold solution—3 drops of 1 per cent. gold chloride ; 10 c.c. of water ; 2 or 3 drops of acetic acid.
12. Fixation in 5 per cent. sodium hyposulphite, to which 1 drop of saturated sodium sulphite solution is added.
13. Abundant washings ; dehydration ; xylene ; canada balsam or gum dammar.

Doinikow, who recently used the method of Bielschowsky in a study of degeneration of nerves, adopts the following procedure :

1. The nerves are fixed in formalin.
2. Slight washing in water, and immersion in pyridine for twenty-four hours.
3. Second washing, in tap water, for twelve hours, to take out the pyridine. The last washings should be done in distilled water.
4. Immersion in 2 or 3 per cent. silver nitrate for three days, in the incubator.
5. Treatment with ammoniacal silver nitrate, as described above, for one to four hours, according to the size of the pieces.

6. Reduction in 20 per cent. formalin for twenty-four hours.

7. Inclusion in paraffin, thin sections, etc., and mounting in balsam.

With this method the axons are stained greyish black and the fibres can be followed pretty well. The omission of the frozen sections is advantageous, since in this way the superficial portions of the piece are not lost. It is well known that when one makes frozen sections, the first sections are broken or otherwise spoilt because of an excessive or defective hardness.

Methods of Golgi and Ehrlich. The results from these are uncertain and are obtained with difficulty. In the hands of Purpura and Krassin respectively, however, these methods have given good impregnations of the newly-formed fibres of the scar. The technique is that described in any book on histological methods.

Methods for staining the myelin. *Procedure with osmic acid.*— Although there are many stains for the fatty sheaths of nerves, the classical *method of M. Schültze*, with osmic acid, is, in nervous degeneration, the best. This method has the advantage, as opposed to the other procedures, of retaining the exact form of the fibres, fixing perfectly the drops of myelin and other liquids. To obtain good results, however, one must use small animals, such as frogs, guinea-pigs, young rabbits, cats and dogs a few days old, etc. This is to ensure thinness of the nerves and a small scar region between the nerve stumps.

The *modus operandi* is as follows:

1. The nerves are immersed for twenty-four hours, or longer, in 1 per cent. osmic acid. In order to prevent folding and contractions, the nerve should be fixed along its length on a cork, with pins. The fixing solution should be plentiful.

2. Washing in many changes of water, for twenty-four hours,

3. Alcohol, celloidin, and moderately fine sections.

4. Staining of the sections with a nuclear stain (saffranin, fuchsin, haematoxylin, etc.).

5. Dehydration, clearing in oil of origanum, and mounting in dammar.

The method with osmic acid is especially useful for the study of the various phases of the process of degeneration and regeneration. At an early stage, that is from the first to the eighth or tenth day after the operation, it enables one to follow with ease the metamorphosis of the medullated sheaths. From the thirtieth or thirty-fifth day on, it is useful for the study of the new myelin sheaths of the young fibres in the scar and of those which penetrate the peripheral stumps. Naturally the amyelinated fibres that develop from the first to the tenth day after the operation cannot be stained with osmic acid; one can use here only those methods which stain the axons.

When the pieces are very thick, we prefer, instead of osmic acid, fixation in potassium bichromate and staining with the methods of Weigert-Pal, Kultschitzky, Nageotte, Benda, etc., all of them based on the production of a lac of haematoxylin. These methods are described in the books on histological technique.

If one wishes to determine the extent of degeneration of the sheaths of the peripheral stump of a nerve or of the white substance of the centres, the best method is that of Marchi.

The fine drops of myelin and various products of disintegration of the medullated sheaths that appear in the peripheral stump of the nerves can best be stained as follows:

Method of Herxheimer. This procedure stains the fats, or, to be precise, the disintegration products of the myelin, red, while the nuclei are dark blue and the cytoplasm is light blue.

1. Fixation for a day in Orth's solution—ten parts of Müller's fluid mixed with one part of formalin. The pieces are then placed for ten days or longer in Müller's fluid.

2. Frozen sections.

3. Staining with *Scarlet R*[1] or *Sudan III.* for a quarter of an hour. Rapid washing.

4. Subsequent staining with Ehrlich's or Delafield's haematoxylin dissolved in distilled water, for ten minutes.

5. Washing in water.

6. Mounting in glycerine.

It is a general rule that when one wants to stain fats or disintegration products of myelin, one should avoid alcohol or other fat solvents. One should fix in formalin, make frozen sections, and mount in glycerine.

---

[1] The solution of Scarlet is prepared as follows: To 70 parts of absolute alcohol add 20 parts of 10 per cent. sodium hydroxide and 10 parts of distilled water. Then add Scarlet R (Scharlach R) in excess. The flask must be only three-quarters full. It is corked, and slowly agitated. After thirty-six hours the solution is ripe, and can be used when it has been filtered.

Methods for staining the cells of Schwann.—Besides the ordinary basic aniline dyes and haematoxylin, all of which stain very well the interannular nuclei, we recommend the following procedures, which we have used with success. They are better than the ordinary nuclear stains, since they stain with fair intensity the cytoplasm which lines the sheath of Schwann, and that which is intercalated between the drops of myelin.

Procedures of Nageotte for staining the cells of Schwann.

(A) 1. Fixation of the nerves in Dominici's fluid—saturated sublimate, 20 c.c ; officinal tincture of iodine, 2 c.c. ; formalin, 2 to 3 c.c.

2. Dissociation of the fibres.

3. Staining with Heidenhain's iron haematoxylin.

4. Alcohol, clove oil, balsam.

With this formula the cytoplasm of the cells of Schwann is well stained. The nuclei are stained dark grey.

(B) 1. Fixation of the nerves in 33 per cent. alcohol.

2. Immersion in 0·1 per cent. nitric acid.

3. Dissociation of the fibres and staining with haematin.

4. Differentiation with Cajal's fluid—indigo carmine, 0·25 ; saturated solution of picric acid, 100 parts.

With this technique Nageotte also stains the cytoplasm of the cells of Schwann and shows the *syncytium* of unmyelinated fibres.

Procedure of Doinikow for cells of Schwann.[1]

1. Fixation of the nerves for one day in Orth's fluid (Müller's fluid, 10 ; formalin, 1). Subsequent hardening for several days in Müller's fluid.

2. Immersion of the sections in the osmio-bichromate fluid of Marchi.

3. Embedding in celloidin.

4. Dissociation of the nerves and immersion for one hour in a saturated solution of phosphomolybdic acid.

5. Washing with water.

6. Staining with Mann's fluid (35 c.c. of 1 per cent. eosin, 35 c.c. of 1 per cent. methylene blue, 100 c.c. of distilled water) for twenty-four hours.

---

[1] Doinikow : " Beiträge zur Histologie und Histopathologie der peripheren Nerven," *Histol. u. histopathol. Arbeiten, etc., von Nissl und Alzheimer*, Bd. 4. 3 N., 1911.

7. After a rapid wash with water, the sections are placed in 96 per cent. alcohol, then in absolute alcohol, and finally in alcohol to which have been added a few drops of a solution of potassium hydroxide in alcohol. In the last fluid the sections are kept until the blue colour changes to red.

8. Washing in absolute alcohol and immersion in alcohol to which have been added a few drops of glacial acetic acid, until the sections have once more a bluish tint.

9. Another washing in absolute alcohol, and after a rapid passage in carbol-xylene, clearing in xylene and mounting in oil of paraffin. The cover-glass is surrounded with gum dammar or any cement.

The sections show intense staining of the cytoplasm of Schwann's cells. The myelin sheath is reddish, the myelin is light red, and its disintegration products are grey, black, or brown (Doinikow). The connecting fibres are blue. This procedure also gives good results without the complementary fixation, with Müller's fluid.

Finally, instructive results are obtained by methods which are useful complements to the impregnation methods for staining the axon, myelin, and cells of Schwann. Such are the *method of Unna*, based on polychrome blue and subsequent differentiation in the *ether-glycerin* mixture; *the method of Unna–Pappenheim for staining the cells of the plasma* (methylene green and pyronine); our *trichromic stain* (basic fuchsin and carmine of picric-indigo); *Mallory's haematoxylin stain*, etc.

Methods which stain the connective tissue of nerves.—One can use for this the acid aniline stains, such as van Gieson's or our trichromic stain. Several formulae of the reduced silver nitrate method also impregnate in dark grey the collagen bundles of nerve tissue. The formulae in question are those in which fixation is by means of a mixture of equal parts of formalin and acetone.

Suitable formulae are:

1. The fresh pieces are fixed for twelve to twenty-four hours in formalin-acetone.

2. Washing in running water for six hours.

3. Immersion in 50 c.c. of 96 per cent. alcohol, to which have been added four drops of ammonia.

4. Silver nitrate (1·5 per cent.) bath at 37° C., for four days.

5. Reduction with the pyrogallic-formalin mixture, etc.

The method proposed by Levaditi for staining the Trepanoma of syphilis, which is a modification of our procedure with silver nitrate, gives also, at times, good staining of the collagen fibres of nerves.

But the best formula of all, because of its constancy and intensity of impregnation, is the method of Achúcarro for staining neuroglia and perivascular collagen bundles of the nerve centres.

Method of Achúcarro.

1. Fix pieces of tissue in 10 per cent. formalin for one or two days or longer. But do not prolong fixation beyond two to three months.

2. Washing in running water for six hours.

3. Frozen sections, 10-20 μ in thickness. One can also use teased preparations.

4. Washing in distilled water.

5. Immersion of the sections in a saturated tannin solution, which is placed for fifteen minutes in an incubator at 50°. One may also simply warm it for a few minutes over a flame. A porcelain dish should be used.

6. Each section, when cold, is put in the ammoniacal silver bath. This bath is the same as that used in Bielschowsky's method. To 5 c.c. of 10 per cent. silver nitrate are added four drops of 40 per cent. sodium hydroxide. Enough ammonia is added to dissolve the precipitate. One takes six drops of this solution and mixes them in a porcelain crucible with 15 to 20 c.c. of distilled water.

The sections thus immersed take on quickly a brownish red colour. They are left for one or two minutes.

7. Rapid washing for a few seconds in distilled water.

8. The sections are placed, for fifteen minutes, in 20 per cent. formalin.

9. Washing, dehydration, clearing, balsam, etc.

This method impregnates the fine intrafascicular connective bundles with a deep black. In some cases it also stains the mitochondria.

Method of Alzheimer for Neuroglia.[1]

1. Hardening in alcohol or Weigert's mordant. If alcohol is used one embeds in celloidin. If Weigert's mordant, one makes frozen sections.

---

[1] Alzheimer: "Beiträge zur Kenntniss der pathol. Neuroglia und ihrer Beziehungen zu den Aufbauvorgängen im Nervengewebe," *Histol. u. histopathologische Arbeiten v. Nissl u. Alzheimer, etc.*, Bd. 3, Heft. 3, 1910.

2. Immersion of the sections, for two to twelve hours, in a saturated solution of phosphomolybdic acid. The celloidin sections remain only one hour.

3. Washing in water for ten minutes or longer.

4. Staining in Mann's fluid, for one hour.

    1 per cent. methylene blue - - - 35 c.c.
    Aqueous 1 per cent. eosin solution - - 35 c.c.
    Water - - - - - - - 100 c.c.

5. Washing in water for ten minutes. When one uses Weigert's mordant, wash only half a minute.

6. Rapid passage in 80 per cent. alcohol, then absolute alcohol, xylene, balsam, etc.

This method, when it succeeds, colours neuroglia and connective bundles red, the axons red, and the blood-vessels blue.

The stains for neuroglia of Weigert, Anglade, Ranke, etc., can only be used with nerve centres.

Animals used for experiments of degeneration and regeneration. Operatory technique.—One should use for experiments on the regenerative process small animals, for several reasons. One can easily, and in a single treatment, impregnate with the reduced silver nitrate method, the method of osmic acid, etc., the whole thickness of the scar and the central and peripheral stumps. The distance between the two stumps, even should they retract considerably, is small. The fibres that have lost their way have shorter distances to travel. Finally osmic acid, alcohol, and pyridine fix best small pieces. Some authors, such as Bethe, who did not take account of the advantage of small nerves, and used large animals, such as adult or almost adult dogs, fell into difficulties of interpretation. We have preferably used guinea-pigs and rabbits one or two months old, and cats and dogs a few weeks old.

Some authors have believed that the regenerative phenomena are different in young and old animals. In reality the process is almost the same, but in new-born and young mammals degeneration and neoformation take place somewhat more actively. There are no essential differences, although we shall subsequently point out slight variations.

All long nerves of a certain thickness, which are isolated from blood-vessels whose lesion is dangerous, can be used. The sciatic nerve of rabbits, dogs, cats, frogs, etc., has these characteristics.

One can also use, with certain operatory precautions, the vagus, hypoglossal, and facial nerves, the brachial plexus, etc. Some authors, like Stroebe, recommend small superficial nerves such as are found in the ear of a rabbit; they cause their degeneration by using methods involving compression. After wounding these fine cutaneous nerves, one can get excellent pictures by using the methods of neurofibrillar impregnation.

Some advice is necessary concerning the method of preparing the pieces for fixation. In general, if the nerves are very thin, one should leave around them some connective or muscular tissue, so as not to lose the superficial zones. In order to prevent shrinkage, which would render it impossible to obtain well oriented longitudinal sections of the nerve, we advise the operator to fix the recently dissected nerves on a flat cork, with pins. One can use fine threads instead of pins. Pieces that are to be impregnated remain on the cork support during all subsequent operations—the silver bath in the incubator, reduction, inclusion, etc. In order that the reagents may penetrate well, one should cut out under the nerve, in the cork, a channel or free space through which the fluids can freely circulate. With fine nerves one need not make a channel; the cork or piece of wood is simply coated with blotting paper. One can take away the cork before inclusion in the alcohol and ether, and, later, celloidin, mixtures. Before hardening the celloidin, however, one should again use the cork support, so that the block may be perfectly even.

III

RÉSUMÉ OF THE STRUCTURE OF THE NORMAL MEDULLATED NERVE

Schwann's membrane.—Nodes of Ranvier.—Nucleus and cytoplasm of the tubular or Schwann's cell.—Its inclusions and reticular apparatus.—Myelin.—Incisures of Schmidt-Lantermann.—Infundibuliform apparatus.—Rings of Segall.—Mauthner's capsule or space.—Axis-cylinder.—Bracelets of Nageotte, etc.

It is well known that the medullated nerve fibre or tube is a complex structure, representing a kind of symbiosis between two elements—the *axon* or *neurite*, which is the prolongation of a neurone present in the centres, and a satellite corpuscle of tubular form, the so-called *cell of Schwann*, so placed that it closely embraces the neuronal expansion. Each axon is surrounded by a great number of cells of Schwann, which are arranged in a longitudinal series. Besides these satellite corpuscles, the nerve tube contains a thick oleaginous sheath, which is placed between the cell of Schwann and the neurite, and which is interrupted, at intervals, to let in more freely the nutritive plasmas. The medullated nerve fibre, then, consists of an *external solid membrane*—sheath of Schwann—of a tubular cell—Schwann's cell—of a *fatty sheath*, and of an *axon*.

We shall now give some details concerning the above components of the nerve fibre or tube.

1. **Membrane of Schwann and nodes of Ranvier.**—The most external layer of the nerve fibre is composed of a thin, transparent sheath, situated outside Schwann's cell, to which it is closely applied, and without any apparent structure. One can clearly see this sheath in transverse sections of the nerve fibre, especially in those preparations in which the myelin had been dissolved out. This is the so-called *sheath of Schwann*.

Nodes of Ranvier.—It is well known, since the classical studies of Ranvier, that Schwann's membrane shows, at intervals that vary with the thickness of the nerve fibre (0·5 to 2 mm.), nodes, that is, certain strangulations which are more or less wide, and at whose level the myelin sheath is interrupted (Fig. 1, *a, b*).

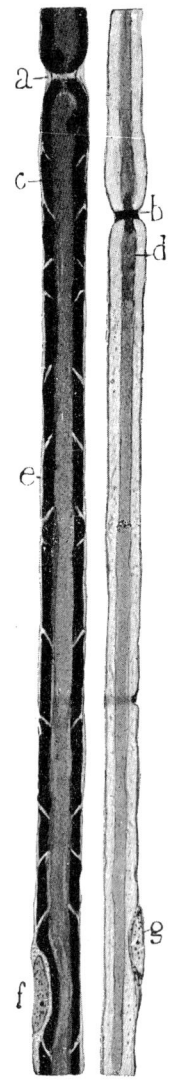

FIG. 1.—Medullated fibres of the sciatic nerve of the rabbit. The one on the left is stained with osmic acid, the one on the right with silver nitrate. *a*, node; *b*, cementing disc; *c*, myelin sheath; *d*, axon; *e*, membrane of Schwann; *f*, *g*, nuclei.

Ranvier believed that at the node not only the myelin sheath but also Schwann's membrane itself was interrupted; he thought that a cementing substance, stainable with silver nitrate (*b*), and arranged as a transversal disc, was there to join the ends of the sheaths and to isolate in that way the various satellite cells. In reality, as our investigations showed long ago,[1] and as modern neurologists such as Schiefferdecker, Nageotte, etc., state, the sheath is not interrupted at the strangulations, but, passing above the cementing substance, it continues along the nerve fibre.

The *disc* or *connecting ring*, described by Ranvier as occurring at the level of the strangulation, is much smaller than he believed (Fig. 1, *b*). The silver reagent is deposited to such an extent on this substance that it doubles or even trebles its thickness. There are some authors, such as Nageotte, who doubt even the pre-existence of such a disc, basing themselves on the fact that it is almost impossible to see, in fresh preparations or in those fixed with certain reagents, a well-defined annular form in the plane of the strangulation. But the presence of such a ring seems to us to be certain. In certain conditions it is demonstrable by other methods, such as by using Ehrlich's methylene blue.

2. **Cell of Schwann.**—Nerve fibres fixed in osmic acid and stained with carmine or haematoxylin show, under the membrane of Schwann, and outside the myelin, a very thin clear zone, finely granular, and which cannot be stained by most reagents.

[1] Cajal: *Manual de Histologia normal y técnica micrográfica*, 1st edition, page 562, Valencia, 1889.

STRUCTURE OF THE MEDULLATED NERVE 43

Towards the interannular centre this protoplasmic layer suddenly thickens and shows an ovoid nucleus. This is composed of a membrane, of a loose chromatic net, poor in stainable granules, and of one or two nucleoli (Fig. 1, *f*, *g*). It lies, with its surrounding cytoplasm, in a small pit of myelin. There is only one nucleus

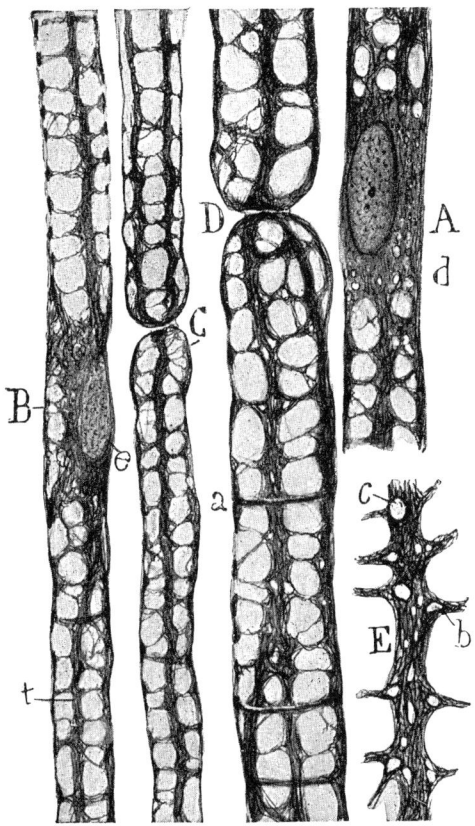

FIG. 2.—Dissociated fibres of the sciatic nerve of an adult cat. Silver impregnation. *A* and *B*, cytoplasmic region near the nucleus; *D*, large fibre at the level of a node; *C* fine fibre; *E*, longitudinal trabecula, very much enlarged; *a*, hoops at the level of the incisures of Schmidt-Lantermann; *b*, vacuoles at the crotch of transverse filaments of the tubular veil; *c*, large vacuole; *e*, nucleus; *t*, longitudinal trabecula.

between two nodes. One cannot determine the true extent of the surrounding cytoplasmic layer in the ordinary preparations, such as those fixed in formalin, Flemming's fluid, osmic acid, potassium bichromate, etc., and stained with carmine, or haematoxylin. It appears as though, after progressively thinning out, it terminates at a short distance from the nucleus. But, as we shall see later, such appearances are deceptive, and are due to the defectiveness of the methods.

Ranvier had an intuition of genius when he put forward the notion of the interannular segment as a vast cellular unit within which are contained the nucleus, myelin, and axon. The modern histologists have confirmed this doctrine in all its essentials. Among those who have contributed very largely to this conception we may cite Nemiloff [1] who, using methylene blue, observed in fishes as well as in mammals a system of protoplasmic trabeculae proceeding from the nuclear periphery and extending to the nodes. We may also name Nageotte,[2] who used the fixative of Dominici and iron haematoxylin, and finally Doinikow,[3] who made very extensive studies of degenerating nerve fibres. By using a special method of impregnation with silver (Fig. 2), we too have been able to confirm [4] the description of these investigators, recognizing, in harmony with the conception of Ranvier, that the cytoplasm of Schwann's cell extends as a tubular veil from the nucleus to the nodes. In this cytoplasm one can see the following structures: the *plaque* or perinuclear protoplasmic mass, the *longitudinal stripes*, the *transverse trabeculae*, the *vacuoles*, the *inclusions*, the *endocellular apparatus of Golgi*, and the *annular system*.

(*a*) *Plaque or perinuclear mass.*—We thus designate that massed

---

[1] Nemiloff: "Einige Beobachtungen ueber den Bau des Nervengewebes bei Ganoiden, etc.," *Arch. f. mikr. Anat.*, Bd. 72, 1908.

See also: "Ueber die Beziehung der sog. Zellen der 'Schwannschen Scheide' zum Myelin in den Nervenfasern von Säugethieren," *Arch. f. mikr. Anat.*, Bd. 76, 1910-1911.

[2] Nageotte: "Incisures de Schmidt-Lantermann et protoplasma des cellules de Schwann," *Compt. rend. des séances de la Soc. de Biol.*, Séance du 15 janvier 1910, vol. 48.

Idem. See also: "Sur une nouvelle formation de la gaîne de myéline; le double bracelet épineux de l'étranglement annulaire," *Compt. rend. de l'Acad. des Sciences*, Paris, 1910.

Idem. See especially: "Notice sur les travaux scientifiques de M. J. Nageotte, Paris, 1911."

[3] Doinikow: "Beiträge zur Histologie und Histopathologie der peripheren Nerven." *Histol. u. histopathol. Arbeiten*, Bd. 4, 3 Pl. ff., 1911.

[4] Cajal: "El aparato endocelular de Golgi de la célula de Schwann y algunas observaciones sobre la estructura de los tubos nerviosos," *Trab. del Lab. de Investig. biol.*, tomo 10, fasc. 4, 1912.

portion of protoplasm which immediately surrounds the nucleus (Fig. 2, *A*, *B*). In it are a few small vacuoles, certain inclusions, and the Golgi apparatus. We shall speak in detail of these structures later on.

(*b*) *Longitudinal stripes and transverse trabeculae.*—To demonstrate this part of Schwann's cell one must use the methods employed by Nageotte (Dominici's fluid with formalin, iron haematoxylin), and by Doinikow (fixation in Orth's fluid, and later in Müller's or Marchi's mixture), then phosphomolybdic acid and staining with Mann's fluid, decoloration in alcohol containing potassium hydroxide, etc. One may also use, as we have stated, a certain formula of staining with silver nitrate, in which one combines fixation in uranium with ammoniacal silver nitrate.[1]

As one can see in Fig. 2, this method of impregnation gives to the cytoplasm of Schwann's cell a dark grey, transparent tint, with shades corresponding to the various thicknesses of it. The perinuclear region appears dark and spattered with clear vacuoles or spaces (*A*, *B*). As to the expansions, that is to say, the cytoplasm situated outside the perinuclear region, one can recognize perfectly the bands and transverse trabeculae and the longitudinal parallel ribs. The *longitudinal bands*, not rigorously parallel to the axon, sometimes bifurcated and with festooned borders, are sometimes three or four in the large fibres, and one or two in the finer ones (Fig. 2, *t*). From their borders issue at right angles the fine *transverse trabeculae*, which, anastomosing among themselves, form around the myelin a very delicate and elegant reticulum. As Nemiloff and Nageotte have observed, the cytoplasm of the longitudinal bands unites, at the level of the incisures of Schmidt-Lantermann, in a strong circular trabecula, which is finely granular and triangular in section

[1] 1. Pieces of adult nerve are fixed for twenty-four hours or longer in

Formalin	15 c.c.
Uranium nitrate	1 gm.
Water	100 c.c.

2. Washing of the pieces in water for an afternoon.

3. Gross dissociation of the stout bundles of the nerve pieces and immersion in Bielschowsky's ammoniacal silver nitrate (1 per cent. silver nitrate +NaOH + enough ammonia to dissolve precipitate).

4. After four or more hours, brief washing in distilled water, and reduction for six hours or longer—formalin, 5 to 8 parts ; hydroquinone, 1. 5 parts ; water, 100 parts ; sodium sulphite, 0·25.

5. Washing in alcohol, fine dissociation or sectioning, etc.

(Fig. 2, *a*). But Nemiloff affirms that this protoplasmic circle does not join with the substance of the incisures of Schmidt-Lantermann, but stops at their external border, as Nageotte has well described and drawn. Nageotte considers very justly the myelin and its accompaniments as a dependence of the axon, and, as such, an apparatus foreign to the constitution of Schwann's cells. Such an opinion, held by various authors, is strongly supported by the fact that in the medullated fibres of the centres there are no Schwann cells.

Careful study of the longitudinal bands reveals in them a network of granular threads, bound into a close net in which are present here and there narrow spaces or coarse vacuoles (Fig. 2, *E*, *b*). These vacuoles, well described by Nemiloff, are often found at the places where the transverse trabeculae emerge. They then take on triangular or ovoid shapes. Here and there on the trabeculae are gigantic round vacuoles (Fig. 2, *c*).

Near the node the net formed by the branches of the longitudinal ribs is somewhat more complicated, justifying the name of *protoplasmic marginal net* given by Nageotte to this segment of the cell of Schwann (Fig. 2, *D*).

In some cases, however, especially in fine fibres and in young animals, the longitudinal bands retain their identity to the end. Usually, once arrived near the region of the node, they converge towards the axon to form the *protoplasmic annulus* of which Nageotte speaks. He believes that from the annulus itself arise expansions which, crossing the node, are continuous with those of the next segment. In this way the cells of Schwann would form a *syncytium* along the entire length of the fibre. We have not been able to see with certainty these protoplasmic bridges across the nodes in our preparations and, for the present, we accept Nemiloff's conception, according to which the cells of Schwann stop completely at the level of the nodes.

The transverse trabeculae are fine granular bridges which are stretched between the longitudinal bands, and which originate at right angles, or nearly at right angles, at the level of a triangular thickening (Fig. 2). The great number of these trabeculae and their numerous branchings lend to the cytoplasm of Schwann's cell the appearance of an elegant tulle or veil, as figure 2 shows. This system of trabeculae does not seem to penetrate into the myelin, nor to form continuations with the infundibula of the incisures of Schmidt-Lantermann. This is opposed to the views of Nemiloff and

Doinikow, for whom the nets in the medullary sheath—the neurokeratin of Ewald and Kühne—as well as the reticula that are sometimes seen in the incisures and are more or less pre-existent, represent expansions of the cells of Schwann.

(c) *Endocellular apparatus of Golgi.*—This structure, first observed by us with the help of a special method of impregnation, is found in all myelinated and amyelinated nerve fibres. As we show

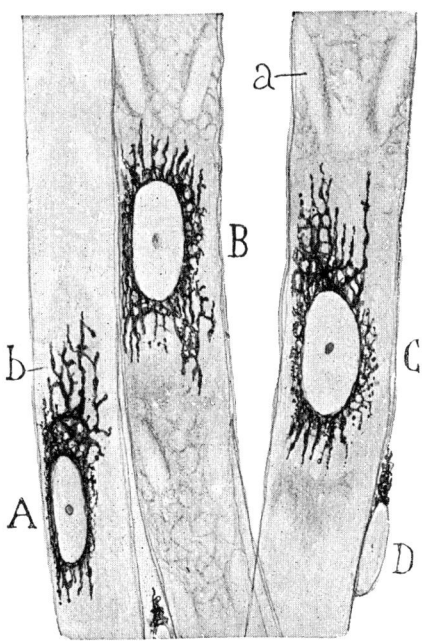

FIG. 3.—Nerve fibres of a three months old rabbit. *A, B, C*, reticular apparatus of Golgi; *a*, incisures of Schmidt-Lantermann; *b*, threads of the endocellular apparatus; *D*, connective interstitial cell with polar endocellular apparatus.

in Fig. 3, it is present around the nucleus, precisely in the position of the perinuclear cytoplasmic thickening. One can best see it in young animals. In these it is formed of a system of relatively thick threads. These are varicose, anastomosed, and arranged in the form of a net whose trabeculae lie usually in a longitudinal direction. The spread and appearance of the endocellular apparatus vary somewhat in the various cells, as can be seen in Fig. 3. In some cells the net takes the form of only two polar wings, below and above the nucleus ; these wings are almost always unequal (Fig. 3, *A, C*) ;

but in the majority of the cells of Schwann the argentophilous threads completely surround the nucleus, although they spread further in the longitudinal than in the transverse direction (Fig. 3, B). One can see the tendency of the longitudinal wings to form two lobules, sometimes made up of only a few threads. Finally, one may note that among the threads there is a certain parallelism and also a divergent orientation, and that the component threads end frequently as free stumps, more or less rounded, at the edges of the cytoplasmic mass. We have not yet seen the penetration of filaments into the protoplasmic bands. Neither do they occur on the

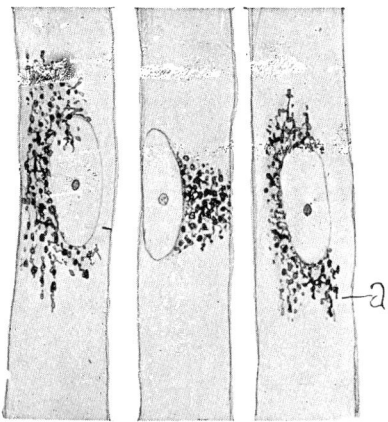

FIG. 4.—Golgi apparatus of nerve fibres in an adult cat.
a, threads and grains impregnated with silver.

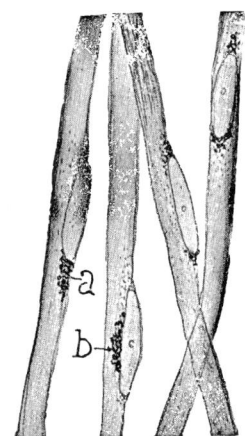

FIG. 5.—Golgi apparatus of unmyelinated fibres.
a, threads polar in position;
b, threads, lateral in position.

top of or beneath the nucleus, that is, between the latter and the myelin, although there are a few exceptions.

In adult animals, as one can see in Fig. 4, the reticular apparatus is finer and more granular. Breaks, due perhaps to imperfection of the method, are much more frequent. In some ways the apparatus resembles an accumulation of dark clots.

The endocellular apparatus is entirely absent in the fibres of the centres, such as the spinal cord, the brain, etc., where there are no cells of Schwann. One can easily see it, however, within the sensory and sympathetic ganglia, where it is very similar to the Golgi apparatus of the peripheral fibres. It is needless to say that in the sympathetic ganglia we are dealing with spinal cord fibres that reach them through the motor roots.

The unmyelinated fibres, or fibres of Remak, also have a rudimentary reticular apparatus. Usually it is merely an accumulation of clots, trabeculae, or moniliform threads, stuck close to the nucleus, in relation to which they may be either lateral (Fig. 5, *b*), or polar (*a*) in position.

(*d*) *Annular apparatus.*—This was observed by Schiefferdecker, Segall, Golgi and his pupils. We have studied it in great detail, by the help of a new technique which is a specific stain for it.[1]

With regard to their position, one divides these rings into two classes : the *fissural rings*, placed in the cytoplasm of Schwann's cell, in front of or at the opening of the incisures of Schmidt-Lantermann, and the *solitary rings*, placed in regions which are far from the incisures, in any portion of the cylindro-conic segment.

The fissural rings are numerous, fine, circular in section, and well rounded. They stain very deeply with the silver stain (fixation in formol-uranium, reduction in hydroquinone), and often attract the deposit of silver to the exclusion of all other portions of the nerve fibre. Nearly always they occur alone. In some cases, however, we have seen two, separated only by a narrow clear space. They lie very superficially inside the cytoplasmic expansion, next to the incisures (Fig. 8, *a*), which, as one can see in Fig. 8, swell very much as a result of the treatment with formalin.

The *solitary rings* have essentially the same characteristics, except that they lie in regions foreign to the incisures. These rings are a somewhat special variant, since, in the preparations where the incisures are intensely and constantly stained, these rings are found far from them (Fig. 7, *c*, *g*, and Fig. 8, *n*).

One also finds *longitudinal filaments* which, coming from one ring, terminate in another more or less remote. Although usually undivided, such trabeculae may be ramified in a complicated way, and connect a great number of rings, fissural as well as solitary. These filaments are found in the cytoplasm of the cells of Schwann, of whose bands or longitudinal striations they appear to be the skeleton.

[1] Cajal : " Fórmula de fijación para la demostración del aparato reticular de Golgi, etc.," *Trab. del Lab. de Invest. biol.*, tomo 10, fasc. 1, 2, and 3, June 1912.

The annular apparatus was observed, although imperfectly, by Boveri,[1] Schiefferdecker,[2] Golgi,[3] Catanni,[4] Mondino,[5] Marenghi and Villa,[6] G. Sala,[7] and, especially, by Segall.[8] But the descriptions of these authors are based on methods that do not sufficiently display the rings. It is because of this that various interpretations were formulated and that doubts have been expressed concerning the pre-existence and natural presence of the rings. For example, Schiefferdecker, criticising the observations of Segall, affirms that the rings are nothing more than the cement of the infundibula (*incisures of Schmidt-Lantermann*), incompletely impregnated by silver nitrate. Golgi and his pupils, Mondino, Catanni, G. Sala, etc., who noted the presence of circular fibres in various positions on the cylindro-conic segments, interpreted them as isolated loops of the spiral apparatus of Rezzonico, which, for unexplained reasons, attracted the silver only partially, that is to say, at its superficial extremity. In reality the rings stained with reduced silver nitrate, after fixation in formol-uranium, are true rings, entirely independent of the spiral apparatus, and they have special morphological and chemical properties. As to the longitudinal filaments, they were perhaps seen by G. Sala; but he found them under the myelin, forming complicated nets and linking, not the superficial rings of

[1] Boveri: "Beiträge zur Kenntniss der Nervenfasern," *Abh. der math. phys. Kl. d. K. bayerischen Akad. v. Wiss.*, XV., Bd. 2, Apr. 1885.

[2] Schiefferdecker: "Beiträge zur Kenntniss des Bau der Nervenfasern," *Arch. f. mikr. Anat.*, Bd. 30, 1887.

[3] Golgi: German translation, "Ueber den Bau der Nervenfasern des Rückenmarks," *Golgi's Untersuchungen über den feineren Bau des zentralen und peripherischen Nervensystems*, Jena, 1899.

[4] Catanni, Josefina: "L'appareil de soutien de la myéline dans les fibres nerveuses periphériques," *Arch. Ital. de Biol.*, tome 7, 1886.

[5] Mondino: "Sulla struttura delle fibre nervose periferiche," *Archivio per le Scienze mediche*, vol. 8, No. 2.

[6] Marenghi and Villa: "Intorno ad alcune particularità di struttura delle fibre nervose midollate," *La Riforma Medica*, 8, vol. 2, No. 99.

[7] Sala, Guido: "Beiträge zur Kenntniss der markhaltigen Nervenfasern," *Anat. Anzeiger*, Bd. 18, Nos. 2 and 3, 1900.

[8] Segall: "Anneaux intercalaires des tubes nerveux," *Compt. rend. de l'Acad. des Sciences*, 7 mars 1892.

Idem: "Sur les anneaux intercalaires des tubes nerveux produits par imprégnation d'argent," *Journal de l'Anat. et de la Physiol.*, tome 29, 1882.

which we have spoken above, but the coils of the spirals of Golgi-Rezzonico. It is thus doubtful that the longitudinal fibrillar plexuses described by him correspond exactly with those which we have pointed out.

As to the physiological significance of the annular apparatus and its longitudinal filaments, one may assume that their function is to maintain the cylindrical form of the nerve fibre. They would thus be a kind of skeleton, differentiated in the cytoplasm of Schwann's cells. The chemical properties of the rings are different from those of the longitudinal filaments, as is shown by the fact that the former are stained by various methods of silver impregnation that fail to colour the latter.

Inclusions of Schwann's cell.—Besides the Golgi apparatus and the rings, several substances are present in the cells of Schwann. These substances are arranged as spheres or granulations, which are usually situated in the perinuclear mass. These granulations have been specially studied by Reich,[1] Rosenheim, Doinikow, etc. Leaving aside those inclusions which are more or less doubtful and which are perhaps due to the precipitating action of the reagents it seems probable that the perinuclear region contains three kinds of granules.

(*a*) *Corpuscles of Erzholz*, fatty droplets, intensely stained with Marchi's method, even more so than myelin itself. These drops, whose number varies from one to three or more, are of various thicknesses, and lie for the most part near the nucleus; sometimes, however, one finds them within the myelin. Although noted long ago by Key and Retzius, they bear Erzholz's name because he described them very well.

(*b*) *Protagonoidal grains* (π grains of Reich).—These grains are arranged as clots, nearly always comma-shaped. They are characterised by the fact that they stain a purple colour with thionin, when previously fixed in Orth's fluid. Rosenheim, who has carefully studied them, using Ehrlich's acid methyl violet, found them not only in the cytoplasm of Schwann's cells, but also outside the sheath, in the connective space.

(*c*) μ *granulations of Reich.*—These are differentiated by their affinity for acid fuchsin and osmic acid. They are composed of a

[1] F. Reich: "Ueber den zelligen Aufbau der Nervenfaser auf Grund mikrohistiochemischer Untersuchungen," *Journ. f. Psych. u. Neurologie*, Bd. 8, 1907.

substance much resembling lecithin. According to Doinikow, who has stained them with Sudan III and Scarlet R, these grains correspond in part to the spherules of Erzholz, and are not a homogeneous product, since they take on with these reagents variable shades of colour.

3. **Myelin sheath.**—When the nerve fibre is quickly fixed in concentrated solutions of osmic acid, the medullary sheath appears homogeneous and interrupted only by the incisures of Schmidt-Lantermann and the nodes of Ranvier. It has this appearance also when alive, When, however, the osmic acid has penetrated slowly, or is weak, as also when the pieces are fixed in formalin, potassium bichromate, alcohol, etc., the medullated sheath shows other more or less artificial structures, on which have been founded several morphological conceptions. Among these are the following:

1. Myelin is composed of a gross skeleton, made up of stout trabeculae which are anastomosed and in whose rounded spaces occurs the myelin proper. These protein nets, observed a long time ago by Lantermann, but better studied by Ewald and Kühne, who used the method of artificial digestion, and who called them "neurokeratin," are generally thought to be the combined result of *post-mortem* decomposition of the myelin and of the extraction of the lipoidal substances of the medullated sheath by alcohol. This interpretation explains very well the great variety of appearance shown by the neurokeratin net, and the impossibility of seeing it in living fibres, or in fibres that have been well fixed in osmic acid.

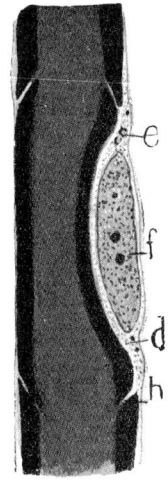
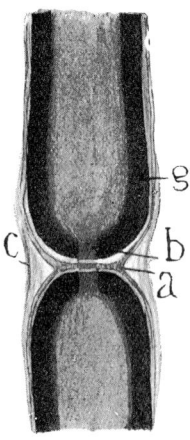

FIG. 6.—Details of the nuclear region and of the node of nerve fibres. Stained in osmic acid and haematoxylin. *a*, colourless cementing disc; *b*, terminal stump of the myelin; *c*, connective sheath of Key and Retzius; *d*, cytoplasm of Schwann's cell; *e*, spherules of Erzholz; *f*, nucleus; *h* incisure of Schmidt-Lantermann.

Ranvier, Gad, Heizmans, Engelmann, Gerlach, Weber, Walstein, Hesse, Boveri, Büngner, Landowsky, Stroebe, Capparelli, Nageotte, etc., all have held that the myelin nets are an artefact. But Chittenden, Leydig, Joseph, Schiefferdecker, Gedoelst, Bolton, Pertik, Kaplan, Hatai, Rebizzi, etc., have stated that they are present in the living fibre. Rebizzi,[1] who has studied myelin with care, bases himself, to show the pre-existence of the nets, on the constancy of their staining with a variety of methods, including a special silver method very much like Fajersztajn's technique, and on the differences between spongioplasm impregnated with silver and the reticulum obtained by extracting the fats.

2. Myelin is composed of two pre-existing factors : (a) A protein spongioplasm which is comparable, if not identical, with the protoplasm of Schwann's cells, with which, at any rate, it is continuous. (b) Rounded hollow spaces within which lies the myelin. The spongioplasm is stainable with thionin and other reagents, after fixation in Orth's fluid, etc., and it is composed of large trabeculae, which converge from Schwann's membrane to the axon into which they are inserted. Inside its meshes, forming one or two series, lie the drops of fatty substance, which are thus a protoplasmic inclusion. Finally, the trabecular system, with its lipoidal inclusions, belongs to the cell of Schwann, with which it is in continuity. If one objects that the spongioplasm is nothing more than the neurokeratin net of Ewald and Kühne, the upholders of the reticular theory reply that the trabeculae of the reticulum described by Lantermann and Ewald and Kühne are much finer and lack a laminar or spongy structure. Kaplan, Dürk, and especially Nemiloff and Doinikow, both of whom published many observations and discussions on this subject, have upheld the above theory, with only slight variations. Doinikow even calls the cells of Schwann *myelin cells*, believing that the lipoid droplets are held in their spongioplasm. Although this theory is based on valuable observations, its partisans have not been able to show that the spongioplasm exists in the living fibre, nor that it is continuous with the cytoplasm of Schwann's cells.

3. Myelin is an organ which is an adjunct of the axon, and as such, it is entirely foreign to Schwann's cells, from which it is perfectly distinct in well fixed and stained preparations. Various

[1] Rebizzi : " Sulla struttura de la guaina mielinica," *Riv. di patol. ner. e mentale*, vol. 9, fasc. 9, 1904.

authors uphold this theory, which has been brilliantly championed by Professor Nageotte. Apart from the results of objective examination, this theory has the advantage of harmonizing with the well known fact that the nerve fibres of the centres are devoid of cells of Schwann.

Nageotte believes that myelin is not a mere secretion of the axon, but that it is a segment of living protoplasm, within which lie various elements possessing different physiological functions : (a) mitochondria, living units, which have been observed by various authors, characterized by their bacillus-like shape and by the fact that they stain with iron haematoxylin after previous fixation in potassium bichromate acidified with acetic acid. These elements are placed radially, crossing each other, and converging toward the axon, in which they are inserted as the spokes of a wheel are inserted in their axle. Peripherally, they end under the cell of Schwann. (b) lipoidal substances which are blackened by osmic acid ; they are assembled in concentric laminae, and lie in the spaces between the mitochondria, which are radially arranged. These substances are a deutoplasm formed by the living units of which we have spoken.

As regards the nets which Lantermann, Ewald and Kühne, Hunger, Joseph, Gedoelst, etc., point out as a constituent of fat-free myelin, according to this theory they are merely the products of abnormal fusion and metamorphosis of the mitochondria. The spherular drops of myelin, and the spongioplasm described by Kaplan, Dürk, Rebizzi, Hatai, Nemiloff, Doinikow, and others, are both artificial. Nageotte believes that the lipoidal laminae that are present in the myelin, alternating with zones of substances of protein nature, are comparable to an electric condenser.

Our studies do not allow us to pass a definite judgment on the preceding hypotheses. All these opinions, based as they are on the results of specific methods of fixation and staining, are somewhat narrow and premature. To understand the mechanism of nervous degeneration, we need to bear in mind only these two ideas :

(1) Myelin is a complex mixture of protein materials and of lipoidal substances, both arranged in concentric laminae ; (2) the combination of these two factors is very unstable. The lipoidal substances separate themselves quickly from the protein materials when the nerve fibre is severed from its cell of origin, or when Schwann's cell is stimulated by physical or chemical causes. In this way

disintegration products are formed which, if they do not necessarily imply, as Nageotte believes, the pre-existence in the myelin of mitochondria or living units that promote chemical changes, nevertheless lead one to believe in the intervention of very active enzymes. Such enzymes are perhaps present in the myelin, perhaps in the axon. If in the latter, under pathological conditions they would act on the myelin sheath to produce coagulations and decompositions. Schwann's cells would have very unimportant functions under such conditions, since it is well known that the fibres of the centres, though they lack a membrane of Schwann, nevertheless degenerate no less rapidly than the peripheral fibres as soon as the axons suffer the slightest injury.

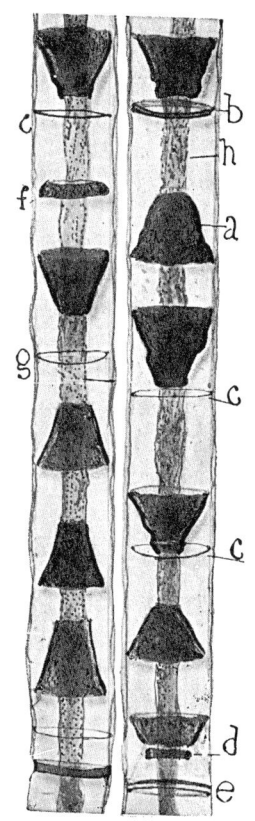

FIG. 7.—Nerve fibres of an adult rabbit fixed in formol-pyridine-manganese, and impregnated with silver. *a* deeply stained infundibular membrane; *b*, annular ribbon; *d*, deeply situated ring; *e*, double solitary rings; *c*, *g* solitary rings outside of the nodes; *h*, axon; *f*, narrow infundibular band.

Incisures of Schmidt-Lantermann.— Besides the interruptions which correspond to the nodes of Ranvier, the myelin is broken up into cylindro-conic segments of variable length by oblique infundibuliform incisions. These incisions begin beneath the protoplasm of the Schwann cells next to the rings, and extend to the axon. Such oblique interruptions (Fig. 6, *h*) are called *incisures of Schmidt-Lantermann*. They can be seen in the fibres of the peripheral nerves as well as in the white matter of the ganglia and spinal cord. Within the incisures are certain differentiated structures, such as the *infundibular membrane*, the *apparatus of Golgi-Rezzonico*, and the *plasmatic chambers*.

(*a*) *Infundibular membrane or cement.*—As is known, in living fibres as well as in preparations made with osmic acid, the incisures are seen as pale interruptions of the myelin, apparently full of plasma, and without any apparent structure. Ranvier believed that they were full of protoplasm, which joined the perimedullar portion of Schwann's cell with its submedullar portion. If one fixes the nerve in osmic acid, or better still, if one uses Boveri's method of fixing in a mixture of osmic acid and silver nitrate, and later stains with silver nitrate, the spaces appear full of a grey substance, finely granular, which extends from the fissural ring to the axon. There are special formulae of the reduced silver nitrate method for impregnating constantly and strongly the entire thickness of the incisures, as we show in Fig. 7, a.[1]

Many opinions have been expressed concerning the nature of the substance found in the fissure.

Kühnt,[2] Boveri,[3] and Pertik,[4] believed that it was a special infundibuliform membrane, characterized by the fact that it was stainable, under certain conditions, with silver nitrate. Koch[5] and Schiefferdecker[6] thought that it was a cement, analogous to that present in the nodes. Johanson, Kaplan, Michotte, Capparelli, Reich, Rebizzi,[7] Nageotte, etc., admit, more or less explicitly, that a special substance, stainable under special conditions with haematoxylin and the aniline dyes, pre-exists in the incisures. But they

---

[1] The technique for demonstrating very well the incisures of Lantermann is as follows:
(1) Pieces of nerve are fixed for twelve to twenty-four hours in
    Formalin - - - - - - - 6 grms.
    Pyridine - - - - - - - 10 ,,
    Manganese nitrate - - - - - 0·5 ,,
    Water - - - - - - - - 40 c.c.
(2) Washing for one day to extract the pyridine and formalin.
(3) 1·5 per cent. silver nitrate, twenty-four to forty-eight hours.
(4) Reduction for a few hours in
    Hydroquinone - - - - - - 1 part
    Formalin - - - - - - - 5 parts
    Water - - - - - - - - 80 ,,
    Anhydrous sodium sulphite - - - - 0·25 ,,

[2] Kühnt: "Die peripherischen markhaltigen Nervenfasern," *Arch. f. mikr. Anat.*, Bd. 13, 1876.

[3] Boveri: "Beiträge zur Kenntniss der Nervenfasern," *Arch. d. math. phys. Klas. v. K. Bayer. Akad. in Wis.*, Bd. 2, 1865.

[4] Pertik: "Untersuchungen über Nervenfasern," *Arch. f. mikr. Anat.*, Bd. 19, 1881.

[5] Koch: "Ueber die Marksegmente der doppeltcontournierten Nervenfasern," *Centralb. f. med. Wissensch.*, No. 49, 1876.

[6] Schiefferdecker: *loc. cit.*   [7] Rebizzi: *loc. cit.*

deny its analogy with the cements, or other known histological substances. Finally, several neurologists have denied that such a membrane or cement, stainable with reduced silver, exists in the living fibre. Among the older investigators who held this opinion we may cite Kölliker, Rawitz, Fürst, Flatau, Chio ; and among the modern investigators, Besta, Nemiloff, and Doinikow. The last two investigators do not absolutely deny the pre-existence of the infundibular substance, but they identify it as part of the neurokeratin net of the medullated sheath. They claim that it represents thickened portions of this net, which are in continuation with the myelin reticulum and with the protoplasmic trabeculae of the cells of Schwann.

We shall not discuss at length these contradictory views. We may say, however, that both the incisures and the infundibuliform substance which takes a silver stain are pre-existent, since one can demonstrate them by a great variety of staining methods.

As to the substance, we may leave aside the discussion as to whether it is a cement or a membrane. We need only state that, unlike the cements, it does not attract silver nitrate when fresh, but only after the action of fixatives. Unlike ordinary cements, it can be stained with haematoxylin and the aniline dyes, and, finally, it is easily impregnated by those silver stains which are based on the action of the reducers—pyrogallic acid or hydroquinone—whereby the ordinary cement is not stained (Figs. 7 and 8, *g*).

This thin wall cannot therefore be mistaken for the cementing disc of the node of Ranvier, nor for the epithelial cements. We have never seen in preparations that had been well fixed in formol-uranium coarse trabeculae such as Nemiloff shows at the level of the incisures.

In preparations thus fixed in formol-uranium and impregnated with reduced silver nitrate one can *sometimes* see bands or striations, which originate at the fissural rings, go forward in the plane of the infundibula, divide here and there, and terminate near the axon (Fig. 8, *f*). We do not know whether these are outgrowths of the ring, thickened portions of the membrane, or superimposed fibres of specific chemical nature. The latter explanation is, with reservations, the most plausible. But such reservations are necessary, since, under certain conditions, the infundibular membrane shows longitudinal folds.

(*b*) *Apparatus of Golgi-Rezzonico.*—This apparatus was first described by Rezzonico as observed in the spinal cord, and by Golgi in the nerve fibres. It consists of an extremely tenuous, spiroidal filament, which begins superficially under Schwann's cell, and loops along the infundibulum in close spirals until it terminates in the axon. According to the Italian investigators, this spiral is the main, and perhaps the only constructive factor of the infundibula, where its function would be to support the myelin and cell of Schwann. Many authors, among them Kölliker, have doubted the pre-existence of this apparatus, which is stainable only with specific and inconstant formulae of silver impregnation. Nevertheless Nageotte has confirmed its presence. He considers it a pre-existent structure. We hold the same view as Nageotte. The apparatus can be more or less seen in osmic acid preparations, and we have also observed it with a certain clearness in preparations stained with reduced silver nitrate after fixation in formol-uranium. As we have shown (Fig. 8, *b*, *j*) its form is very much like that described and drawn by Nageotte, but in our preparations its fibres are thicker and granular.

These filaments are flexuose, circular, apparently anastomosed obliquely, accumulated usually on certain points, and they garnish exteriorly the incisural membrane. Sometimes the filaments are so granular that one perceives them with difficulty. Even when they are best stained, it is difficult to decide whether they are simple spirals, as Rezzonico, Golgi, and the latter's pupils have said, or whether they form a net of transversal meshes, as Nageotte claims.

(*c*) *Vaginal plasmatic chambers.*—The various authors have arrived at different conclusions concerning the structure of the infundibula because they have not, as we believe, sufficiently taken into account the fact that between the myelin and the argentophilous membrane there exist certain potential spaces. These spaces, dilated by the reagents, allow deposits of protein materials and of staining substances to be formed. It is a matter of common observation that the fixatives are able to dilate these spaces. Formalin especially, through its retraction of the myelin, causes the formation of wide plasmatic chambers, in which the infundibulum floats, as Rebizzi and Nageotte have well shown (Fig. 8, *A*, *c*). When one fixes in formalin and then stains with haematoxylin or metallic stains, the same phenomenon takes place. One can see in Fig. 6, *e*, that the infundibulum is separated by an enormous space from the external myelin mantle, although less so from the internal periaxial mantle. These chambers, which may stretch towards the axon, accidentally receive exudates of coagulated protein materials which, thickening the infundibula, lend to them a coarsely reticulated appearance. To this class of artificial deposits belong probably the nets described by Nemiloff as existing in the fissures. On the other hand, he may have mistaken for a pre-existent spongioplasm the artificial net of neurokeratin which is present in the

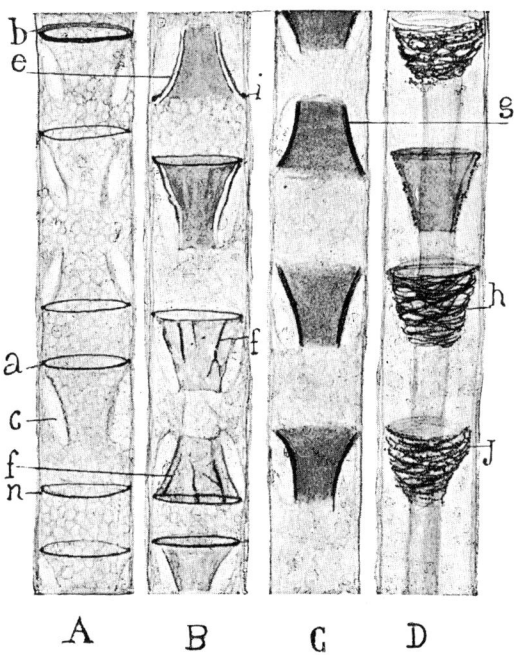

FIG. 8.—Various staining effects produced in nerve fibres by silver impregnation after fixation in formol-uranium. *A*, ordinary reaction showing only the rings; *a*, rings placed opposite the incisures of Schmidt-Lantermann; *b*, thick rings; *c*, incisure of Schmidt-Lantermann; *n*, ring far from the nodes; *B*, less frequent reaction, in which the rings are stained black and the incisures yellow or light grey; *i*, ring in optic section; *e*, infundibular membrane; *f*, dark bands which seem to re-enforce the membrane; *C*, fibres in which only the incisural membranes are stained; *g, j, h*, exclusively impregnated infundibula; *D*, fibres showing more or less clearly the apparatus of Rezzonico. (The nerve was from an adult cat.)

internal mantle of myelin, often adhering to the infundibular membrane.

Boveri, Monckeberg and Bethe have described a membrane which lies under the myelin, between it and the axon, at the level of the nodes. According to these authors, it surrounds the terminal stump of the myelin and it is in continuity with Schwann's membrane (*Innenscheide*). Capparelli [1] also mentions this structure, which he describes as a strong

[1] Capparelli: "La fina struttura delle fibre nervose," *Atti dell Academia Gioenia di scienze naturali in Catania*, Serie 4, vol. 18, 1904.

membrane situated at some distance from the axon, outside the liquid sheath of Mauthner; but, according to him, this lamina is not in continuity with Schwann's sheath, but is inserted in the cement of the node, at the level of the biconic thickening of Ranvier. Our own studies have not allowed us to see with certainty this cover.

Axon or neurite.—The axon, a prolongation of the functional expansion of motor or sensory nerve cells, is the most important organ, both dynamically and anatomically, of the nerve fibre. The axon is cylindrical in form, with a diameter which varies from 3 to 8 μ, and it occupies the centre of the nerve tube, being immersed in a plasmatic chamber (Fig. 1, d), which separates it from the medullated sheath. This liquid or semi-liquid substance, peri-axonic in position, has been the subject of some doubts by Nageotte, who is not certain that it pre-exists; it has been improperly called *Mauthner's sheath*. As one cannot see it in detail in the living nerve, we do not know its real thickness or to what degree it is alterable by fixatives.

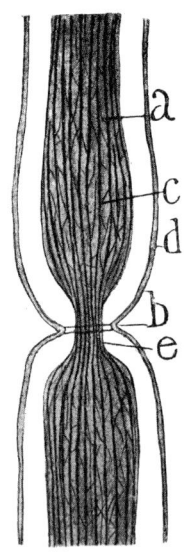

FIG. 9.—Schematic drawing of the nerve fibre at the level of the node. *a*, fine oblique neurofibrils; *b*, cementing discs; *c*, longitudinal stout neurofibril; *d*, neurilemma; *e*, region of the axon which corresponds to the node.

The axon maintains a constant calibre as it takes its course through the inter-annular segment, except at two places: at the level of the node, where it is very much thinned (Figs. 6 and 9), and at a certain distance from the cementing disc, where it forms a fusiform enlargement (Fig. 9). Both of these changes of form pre-exist in the living nerve, for one can see them there, and they can be shown by a great number of methods. Among these Ehrlich's methylene blue brings out very well the changes in calibre. On the other hand, the *biconic thickening* which was described by Ranvier in front of the cementing disc (Fig. 9) is an inconstant detail. It may represent, as Nageotte affirms, a *post-mortem* alteration.

The texture of the axon has been much discussed. Without entering into controversies that lie outside the field of this *résumé*, we may state that the theory which best fits the observed facts is the reticular conception formulated by many authors and defended among the more modern by Retzius, Schiefferdecker, Marinesco, and ourselves.

In harmony with this conception, we recognize in the neurite three principal parts :

(1) The *deutoplasm or neuroplasm,* formed of a transparent material which is probably liquid in nature, unstainable by the neurofibrillar methods, but brought out by carmine, the basic analine dyes, Ehrlich's methylene blue, and Golgi's silver chromate. It has no appreciable structure. This neuroplasm is unequally distributed in the axon. It is very abundant in the terminal arborizations of nerve fibres ; it is scarce, although not entirely absent, as Bethe claims, at the level of the nodes. It is concentrated at the fusiform thickenings which are present near the strangulations. During the degenerative and regenerative phenomena the neuroplasm augments in amount very greatly ; it dissociates the neurofibrils and pulls them apart under such conditions.

(2) The *neurofibrillar apparatus,* a semi-solid skeleton, constituted by longitudinal filaments, which are more or less parallel and arranged in a close bundle. They are characterized by being intensely stained by various methods, such as the neurofibrillar procedure of Bethe, and by those which are based on the use of colloidal silver, such as Bielschowsky's and Cajal's procedures. Among these longitudinal coarse neurofibrils, which might be called *primary neurofibrils,* there are others which are much finer and paler, which are oblique in direction, and whose function is to join and physiologically correlate the former. They are almost invisible at the nodes, where the bundle is condensed, but they are brought out more or less distinctly in the thickened portions of the axon. They are especially prominent at the nerve terminations, where ourselves, Tello, Dogiel, and many other authors have shown with absolute certainty their reticular arrangement. Finally, the neurofibril must be conceived, not as an elemental morphological unit, but as a colony of living ultramicroscopic particles, the *neurobiones,* which are capable of growth, multiplication and progress, as Apathy, ourselves, Heidenhain, etc., have suggested. In the course of this work we shall give ample proof of the existence of these elemental units, which are the seat of a constructive initiative and of a relative functional autonomy within the neuronal tissue.

(3) Finally, the edge of the axon possesses a certain cortical mantle, which is transparent, devoid of neurofibrils, more compact and of a more varied nature than the neuroplasm. It is elastic, very thin, and without any apparent texture. This limiting mantle, a simple continuation of the neuronal membrane, must not be mistaken for the membrane that some authors, such as Boveri, Monckeberg, and Bethe, claim to be present under the myelin and in continuity with the neurilemma. The *Innenscheide* of these investigators appears to us to be a hypothetical conception.

Double bracelet of Nageotte.—In preparations fixed in potassium bichromate for fourteen days, in the oven, then stained with acid

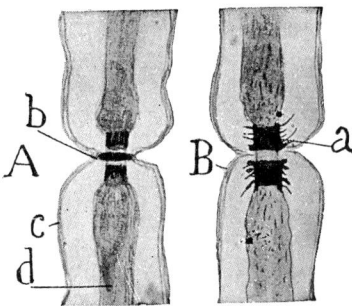

FIG. 10.—Node of nerve fibres. *A*, axonic impregnation often found in diluted and quick-acting silver solutions; *B*, impregnation with silver, after fixation in formol-pyridine-manganese; *a*, spinous bracelets of Nageotte; *b*, disc of Ranvier; *d*, axon; *c*, Schwann's membrane.

fuchsin, Nageotte has observed, above and beneath the node, a *double axonic bracelet*. This is well stained by the fuchsin and is covered with circular spines. In these bracelets he claims that the constitutive laminae of the medullary sheath end perpendicularly. Our observations completely confirm this discovery of Nageotte, on which doubt has been cast by Nemiloff. The preparations in which the bracelets stain best are those which are fixed in formol-pyridine-manganese. In such preparations the axon is not stained at the level of the nodes, and on either side of these structures a small dark grey mantle can be seen, from which issue circularly certain granular crests or laminae. These are denticulated, and penetrate the sheaths of the myelin (Fig. 10, *a*).

Nageotte also describes, under the spinous bracelets, a membrane or sheath which can be stained with methylene blue, and which would represent a sort of re-enforcement of the *Innenscheide* of Monckeberg and Bethe. In the silver preparations one does not differentiate this membrane very well from the bracelets. We do not doubt, however, that it exists. Looking over our old preparations of the posterior roots, spinal cord, and brain, which were stained with Ehrlich's methylene blue, we observed again what we had already noted, that the stain often brings out two cylinders situated on either side of the colourless nodal disc.[1] Such blue sheaths, we believe, correspond to the mantle of Nageotte. Besides, the spinous bracelets do not come out clearly in the preparations of nerve centres.

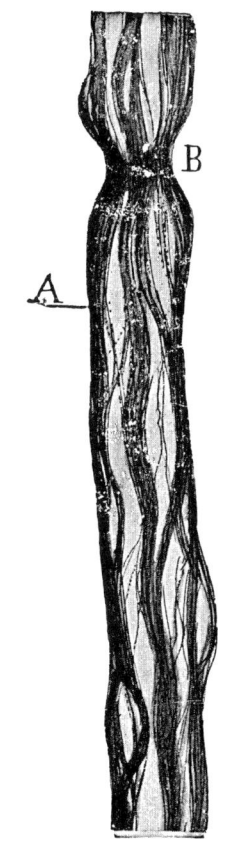

Connective peritubular tunic.—This structure was observed a long time ago by Key and Retzius,[2] who called it *Fibrillenscheide*, and it was well studied by Schiefferdecker, Abreu, Ruffini, etc. It is not a new peritubular sheath, but it is a re-enforcement of the membrane of Schwann. Ruffini called it *subsidiary sheath*. The connective bundles depend on the endoneurium, and are badly stained by the aniline dyes such as v. Gieson's method, Cajal's trichromic procedure, etc. On the other hand, they are well stained, like the *retiform* plexuses

FIG. 11.—Nerve fibre of an adult cat. Silver impregnation after fixation in pyridine-formol. *A*, peritubular bundles; *B*, region of the node.

of the spleen and liver, with reduced silver nitrate. One of the best methods is that based on the use of ammoniacal silver

[1] Cajal: *Histologia del sistema nervioso del hombre*, etc., tom. i, p. 212, 1899.

[2] A. Key and G. Retzius: *Studien in der Anatomie des Nervensystems und des Bindegewebes*, Stockholm, 1876.

Retzius: "Ueber die Ruffini beschriebene *gaina subsidiaria* der Nervenfasern," *Anat. Anz.*, Bd. 28, 1906.

nitrate, with previous fixation in formalin.[1] In such preparations the bundles take on a dark grey colour and a slightly granular appearance. As Fig. 11, A, shows, the connective tunic is well differentiated from the rest of the endonervous tissues. Dissociation of the fibres hardly modifies or disturbs it, and each isolated tube remains covered with its corresponding connective sheath. There doubtless exist connections with the rest of the connective tissue, but such anastomoses are few and of little importance. Usually each bundle follows closely the nerve fibre for very long distances, being straight or flexuous, and closely adhering to the membrane of Schwann. At the level of the nodes the bundles become laminar (Fig. 11, B), widening and adapting themselves to the tubular strangulations, which they follow with some precision. In some nodes, however, the fascicular adaptation is less narrow. The bundles then form surrounding bridges at a certain distance.

Endoneurium, laminar sheath, and neurilemma. — (a) *Endoneurium*. We need only briefly state, to complete this morphological *résumé*, that the nerve fibres are associated among themselves by means of a flexible tissue made up of fine connective bundles. This tissue is only slightly stained by the methods that are selective for the collagenous fascicles. It was called *endoneurium* by Key and Retzius. Its own collagenous bundles, which are relatively scarce in comparison with the peritubular connective re-enforcement, join the *sheaths of Key and Retzius* to each other, and are commonest near the blood vessels and in the periphery of the nerve bundle.

Apart from the interstitial plasma, which fills the spaces between the fascicles, and the numerous capillaries, which are mostly fine and parallel to the nerve fibres, the endoneurium contains certain big flat cells, which are comparable to the sedentary cells of the loose

[1] This is a slight variation of the methods with reduced silver nitrate, as described above. It is as follows:

(1) Fixation of the nerves for twenty-four hours in

Water	40 parts
Pyridine	15 ,,
Formalin	8 ,,

The pieces are then washed in running water.

(2) Immersion of the dissociated nerves in 1 per cent. ammoniacal silver oxide.

(3) Reduction in hydroquinone-formalin, sodium sulphite, etc.

connective tissues. These cells are laminar in shape, with irregular borders which are prolonged into variously elongated appendices. They are composed of a reticulated protoplasm, which has a spongy appearance and contains fine vacuoles and granulations stainable with the basic aniline dyes. These cells are in immediate contact with the nerve fibres which they hug with their laminar prolongations (Fig. 3, *D*). In the endoneurium are also held occasional migrating cells and perivascular cyanophilous cells.

(*b*) *Neurilemma*.—The entire nerve is surrounded by a strong tunic, composed of loose connective tissue, which is in continuity with the *pia mater*. This is the *neurilemma*, a membrane that has an essentially mechanical function in the phenomena of nervous regeneration. In it are fixed cells, Ehrlich cells, and plasma cells.[1]

(*c*) *Laminar sheath or perineurium*.—When a nerve is sectioned one sees that the constituent fibres are arranged in bundles, each of which is surrounded by a delicate and compact membrane. This tunic, which isolates the primary nerve fascicle, contains a concentric succession of very fine and compact connective laminae, among which are present narrow vaginal spaces, bounded by endothelium. Within it are also fixed flat cells, a few migratory elements, mast cells, and clasmatocytes (Doinikow).

[1] The term neurilemma is often used by Anglo-Saxon authors to mean the hyaline sheath of the nerve-fibre—Schwann's membrane. (Translator's note.)

IV

DEGENERATION OF INTERRUPTED NERVES

Wallerian degeneration of the peripheral extremity.—Precocious metamorphoses of the myelin.—Destruction of the soldering disc and of the infundibula.—Modifications occurring in the cells of Schwann : multiplication of these cells and formation of varicose bands.—Apparition of granular elements and resorption of the myelin.

THE degeneration that is brought about in cut nerves is of two kinds, which are physiologically and topographically different : *Wallerian or trophic degeneration*, caused in the peripheral stump when the stimulus from the nerve cell or trophic centre is interrupted ; and *traumatic degeneration*, occurring in the central stump because of traumatism and subsequent phlogosis. Although each nerve stump shows a biological type of regression, one may state that in the peripheral stump both kinds of degeneration really occur. For, as a matter of fact, one can see in that segment, as in the central stump, a real *traumatic degeneration* near the wound. But the rest of the nerve, up to its peripheral termination, shows only Wallerian degeneration.

Wallerian Degeneration of the Peripheral Stump.—When one interrupts the continuity of a nerve by the scalpel or destructive agents, the peripheral stump degenerates rapidly, but all its constituent factors do not disappear. By a process of progressive liquefaction and absorption, the axon, myelin, and a part of the organs that are close to Schwann's cell (soldering disc, rings, infundibula, etc.) are destroyed. But Schwann's cell itself remains and multiplies greatly, as well as the sheath of Schwann and the connective bundles of the mantles of Key and Retzius. The capillaries and all the connective tissues of the nerve also remain. Thus those parts, such as the axon and myelin, which trophically depend on the nerve cell, are destroyed and later restored. Those elements of the nerve which are foreign to the influence of the neurone, instead of being destroyed, undergo formative phenomena which assist in the reconstruction of the mutilated organ, protecting and feeding the young axons which come from the central stump.

In order to make an orderly study of the metamorphoses of all these parts, we shall examine first the changes undergone by the myelin, then those of the cell of Schwann, and finally the phenomena of agony and necrosis of the axon.

Metamorphosis of the medullary sheath.—This was already observed by Waller, and it was well studied by Remak, Ranvier, Eichorst, Vanlair, Nothafft, Stroebe, Ziegler, and later by Monckeberg and Bethe, by Nageotte, etc. The alterations are well known, thanks to the demonstrative capacity of osmic acid, which stains myelin a blue-black, and which brings it out perfectly from the other components of the nerve. As is natural, the metamorphoses are the more accentuated the longer the interval since the nervous mutilation.

Let us take a case in which the sciatic nerve of an adult rabbit was cut, and in which the animal was killed fourteen or sixteen hours after the operation. The peripheral stump, after being fixed in osmic acid and stained in haematoxylin, is examined with a Zeiss 1·30 apochromatic objective.

Most of the nerve fibres, although they are separated from the trophic centre, are still little modified. One can see the nodes, the nucleus of Schwann's cell, and the cylindro-conic segments of the myelin with their normal incisures. But all the fibres do not retain their structure equally well. Besides the fibres which are almost normal, there are others which show clear indications of alterations. The most marked change, although it is not common, is the widening of some nodes, with a longitudinal retraction of the myelin, and the amplification of the infundibula, in whose borders the medullary sheath appears interrupted, ending in irregular stumps. Usually, although all of them are not involved, it is the thick fibres that initiate these changes, which become general only later. In these first changes the initiative seems to be with the myelin, since Schwann's cell, as Nageotte states, shows only the mechanical effects of the contraction of the cylinder-cones.

In Fig. 12 we show a few fibres taken from the peripheral stump of a rabbit killed sixteen hours after its sciatic nerve had been cut. We have chosen only a few fibres, where the changes in the myelin are much accentuated. One can see the slipping of the myelin in a node belonging to a thick fibre (*a*) and the obvious amplification of the incisures of this nerve tube. The axon is, however, still sound.

Against some infundibula one can see a black drop of myelin, coloured by osmic acid, a kind of gigantic spherule of Erzholz (*d*). In some fine and medium-sized fibres certain changes have taken place (Fig. 12, *c*, *e*). But we may repeat that the great majority of the fibres are almost normal (Fig. 12, *f*). The perinuclear region, which later will undergo great changes, is as yet but little altered (*n*).

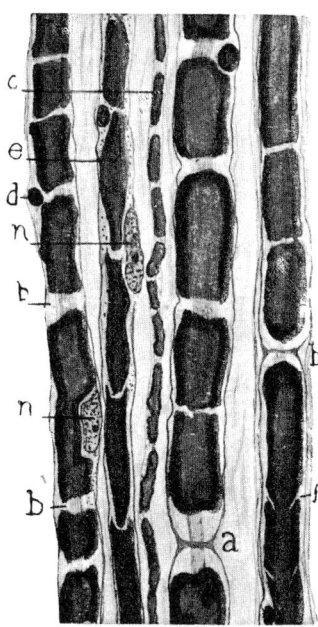

FIG. 12.—Fibres of the peripheral stump of a rabbit, killed sixteen hours after the operation. Osmic acid and carmine. *a*, node ; *b* incisures of Schmidt-Lantermann that have become wider ; *c*. fine fibre broken up into thin ellipsoids ; *d*, drops of myelin ; *f*, normal incisures.

One day after the operation the modifications of the myelin are much more accentuated. Its fragmentation is completed and there are formed between the fatty cylinders wide, transversal, clear, bridges. These extend from the membrane of Schwann to the axon. Some of these interrupting protoplasmic masses may be present opposite the nucleus (Fig. 13, *n*). Others are formed at the level of the infundibula (*m*). Finally, some appear next to the node or within the node itself. This latter structure is then quickly destroyed and replaced by a clear cylinder within which the axon remains, more or less thinned out (Fig. 13, *i*, *e*).

Between the first and the second day these lesions, which hitherto had been present in only a few fibres, appear in all of them, and are much accentuated. The number of interrupting protoplasmic bridges increases. As a consequence the myelin cylinder becomes fragmented into progressively smaller pieces. The perinuclear protoplasmic mass has become much more extensive (Fig. 14, n), pushing the myelin very far apart. On the other hand the clear region next to the node grows, and the strangulation and cementing disc

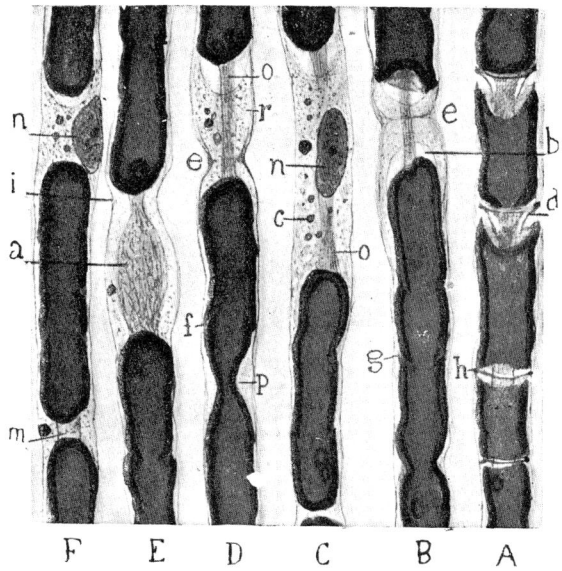

FIG. 13.—Fibres of the peripheral stump of a rabbit killed twenty-four hours after the operation. *a*, fusiform widening of the axon next to a node (I) ; *b*, plasmatic vacuole of the nodes ; *e*, cementing disc ; *f*, normal incisure of Schmidt-Lantermann ; *d*, infundibulum of the incisures ; *h*, fissural rings ; *n*, nuclei ; *c*, spherules of Erzholz ; *m*, protoplasmic bridges being formed at the level of the incisures ; *r*, protoplasm accumulated next to the discs of Ranvier ; *o*, subsistent axon in the protoplasm of Schwann's cell.

completely disappear. When one studies attentively this clear mass one notes that it is not always composed of accumulated protoplasm. It is also formed by the retraction of the myelin. As can be seen in Fig. 13, *b*, there are formed at a certain distance from the cementing disc, when this persists, two wide deposits of plasma crossed by the axon.

In the long myelin cylinders the fissures of Schmidt-Lantermann remain almost normal. Nevertheless many of them appear widened, as though dissected. One can see clearly the membrane of the infundibulum, which lightly attracts the osmic acid and appears to float in the infundibular chambers. In some fissures one can recognize the external ring, which appears with more or less clearness (Fig. 13, h, d).

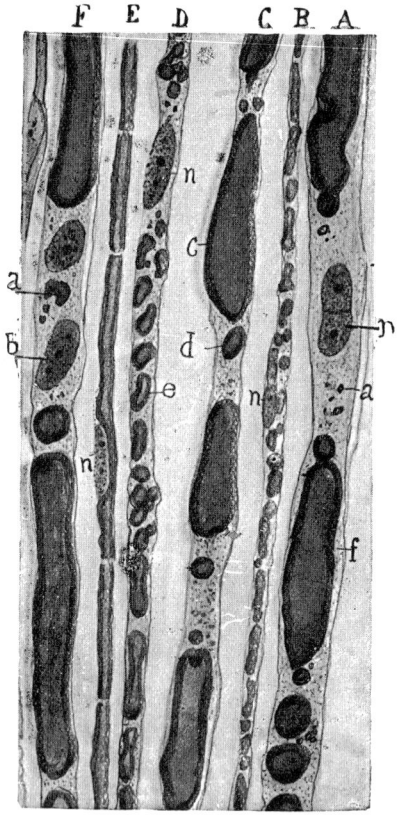

Fig. 14.—Peripheral stump of a dog, killed three days after the operation. Osmic acid and haematoxylin. *a*, spheres of Erzholz; *b*, daughter nuclei; *d*, spheres of myelin; *f*, ellipsoid of myelin with normal incisures; *B*, *D*, fibres in which the medullary fragmentation is well advanced; *n*, dividing nucleus.

Since the investigations of Ranvier, it is generally admitted that the fragmentation of the myelin occurs at the level of the fissures. According to this view, the latter are invaded by the protoplasm of Schwann's cell. The fact is certain, but it is not due to the action of the protoplasm, for the majority of the incisures which are destined to form granular masses are still devoid of this substance. The protoplasm enters only when the infundibulum is much widened and when the stumps of the myelin cylinder retract and round off.

Transitions between the first phase, when the myelin merely retracts, and the second, when there is retraction together with protoplasmic invasion, are seen in Fig. 13. But the myelin may break up also at or towards the centre of a cylinder-cone, and all the gradations of this phenomenon are found (Fig. 13, *p*). The interruption of the myelin next to the nucleus is the most precocious and important of all. It often belongs to that kind of slow fragmentation which always

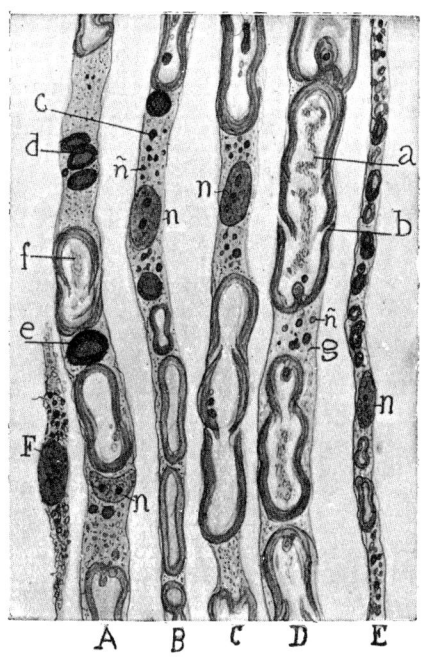

FIG. 15.—Peripheral stump of a dog, killed four days after the operation. Vital staining with Ehrlich's methylene blue. *a*, folded axon within the digestive chamber ; *b*, incisure of Schmidt-Lantermann ; *c*, spheres of Erzholz deeply stained with methylene blue ; *n*, spheres which are but little coloured ; *d*, strongly stained spheres of myelin ; *g*, protoplasmic bridge at the level of an incisure ; *F*, connective tissue cell.

begins by a progressive narrowing of the medullary sheath between two incisures (Fig. 17, *a*, *b*). The disappearing myelin is taken up by the large cylinder-cones nearest to it. These attract it just as a small fatty droplet in suspension in a liquid is attracted by a large drop.

After three days the medullary ruptures can be seen in all the fibres without exception. One can still find long segments with incisures of Schmidt-Lantermann that have retained their form, but there are numerous fibres where almost all the myelin ellipsoids are short, although they vary in length and shape. The protoplasmic mass next to the nucleus is larger, as well as the non-medullated region next to the node, whose cementing disc cannot be seen. The node itself is hardly recognizable.

At this time, from the second to the fourth day, there are found within the myelin large spaces full of plasma, within which one can see the crumpled axon in process of disintegration (Fig. 15, *a*). We shall speak of these spaces, which we have called *digestive chambers*, when we discuss the destruction of the axon. We require to note at present only the fact that the large ellipsoids swell as a consequence of the liberation of a liquid exudate, as Nageotte has observed. This exudate comes from the axonic protoplasm; the medullary ellipsoid rounds itself off, inclosing and folding the axon within the digestive chamber, where it will disintegrate.

From the fourth day onwards the fragmentation of the myelin is progressively accentuated, until the majority of the fibres appear as a transparent mass of protoplasmic aspect, within which drops of myelin of varying thickness detach themselves. Ordinarily this process of fragmentation is more pronounced in the thin fibres. These show series of fatty droplets, some of which are very small and pale (Fig. 15, *E*). In the perinuclear mass may be seen the spherules of Erzholz, which appear to have become more numerous and larger (Fig. 15, *C*). Although the process of breaking up of the myelin has become generalized, there are still left, after four or five days, large belated ellipsoids, with a few more or less altered incisures of Schmidt-Lantermann.

Careful study of the ellipsoids reveals many chemical and morphological changes. Some medullary cylinders are provided with internal fatty droplets or with sacciform invaginations of this substance. Others show exfoliations, and they often terminate in points or are prolonged into appendices shaped like exclamation marks (Fig. 16). At the proper time chemical changes have taken place. This is clearly indicated by the contrasts in staining shown by the ellipsoids according as the preparations have been made with osmic acid, Weigert's haematoxylin, or Ehrlich's methylene blue. This methylene blue stains certain ellipsoids and some fatty droplets (Fig. 15, *e*), while others remain entirely colourless. The shades with Sudan III, or Scarlet R also vary. If one removes the fat from the ellipsoids with alcohol and then stains them with iron haematoxylin, etc., one can see the protein neurokeratin net within them. This, however, is in the form of clots, and of extremely irregular nets and trabeculae. It is very probable that it is such protein materials, products of decomposition of the myelin, that Doinikow and others have taken for prolongations of the protoplasm of Schwann's cell, within which they claimed that the ellipsoids lay. We believe, however, that the ellipsoids always lie in the old channel formed by the cells of Schwann, around the remains of the axon. It is only a few small drops which, by a kind of passive infiltration, are able to penetrate within the protoplasm of these cells.

On the seventh day there are much fewer large ellipsoids. Those which still remain show signs of new fragmentations, that is to say, they show turgid ends and a narrowed intermediate region, where the new interruption is about to occur. The tendency of the fatty accumulations to take on a spheroidal shape seems to be the result of surface tension. In the fine fibres the fatty spherules are very small and are arranged in rows. Many of them have been resorbed and are no longer seen.

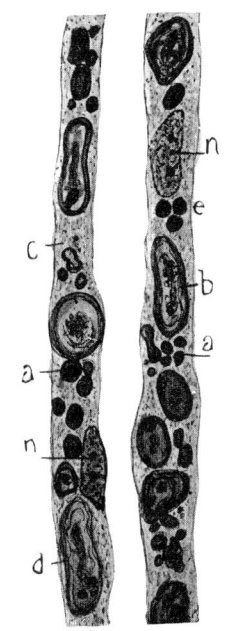

FIG. 16.—Peripheral stump of a rabbit, six days after the operation. Fixation in Flemming's fluid. Iron haematoxylin. *a*, thickened spheres of Erzholz; *b*, *d*, ellipsoids with pale laminar stratifications and axonic remnants in their interior; *e*, fat spheres intensely coloured by osmic acid; *n*, nuclei.

From the tenth day onwards nearly all the large ellipsoids have become very numerous fatty droplets, and in all such conglomerations one sees large and small spheres, closely pressed to each other. At the level of these masses the nerve tube shows fusiform thickenings. These alternate with portions in which there are no droplets and which are very thin. This succession of swollen parts corresponding to those fatty masses which are still present, and of thinned portions in which there is no fat, lends to the fibre a varicose and moniliform appearance which is highly characteristic.

After the second week a considerable portion of the myelin has disappeared through resorption and phagocytosis (Fig. 23). This disappearance is complete or almost complete in the fine and medium-sized medullated fibres. On the other hand the large fibres still show here and there fusiform thickenings with conglomerations of lipoidal drops. The intermediate segment of Schwann's sheath takes on an extreme tenuity. Finally, from thirty to forty days after the operation the majority of the fibres are free from medullary remnants. It is only in a few large fibres that there subsist here and there a few resistant masses of myelin droplets. Three months after the operation even these remnants are entirely or almost entirely gone.

In short, the myelin, after contracting and breaking up, is resorbed, leaving the old cell of Schwann free of debris. The embryonic condition, in which likewise the myelin is arranged in disseminated drops, is thus reproduced.

The process of medullary fragmentation that we have just described occurs simultaneously along the entire length of the peripheral stump. This was observed by Vanlair, Huber, Eichorst, Stroebe, etc. But near the wound the disorganization of the myelin and axon occurs earlier than in the rest of the stump. In the former region the nerve fibres suffer not only the effects of Wallerian degeneration, but also the mechanical effects of the cut and the chemical effects of the inflammatory exudation. One must, however, reject the idea of Bethe, who believes that the degeneration of the peripheral stump progresses centrifugally, that is, from the wound to the nervous terminations. Erb, Tizzoni, Neumann, Büngner, and some others, also adopted this erroneous conception.

One might perhaps suppose that the fact that within a single nerve segment the degeneration of the myelin proceeds faster in some fibres than in others is due to the diverse physiological significance of the various nerve fibres. The motor fibre, separated from its cell of origin, loses immediately its cellulifugal stimulus. But the sensory fibres, receiving the nervous impulse in a cellulipetal direction, may still be able to receive for a time stimuli from the skin or from the muscle spindles (spindles of Kühne) or from those present in the tendons. According to this theory, it is the motor fibres that degenerate rapidly, while the sensory fibres are slower. Bethe holds the opposite view—that it is the sensory fibres which degenerate faster. We have compared, in respect of rapidity of degeneration, the anterior or ventral and the posterior or dorsal roots of the spinal nerves. The fragmentation of the myelin and the destruction of the axon are produced simultaneously or almost simultaneously in the two roots. Besides, Tello has shown that differences in rapidity of degeneration are constantly seen in the axons of nerves within the muscles and even in the motor plates. The causes of unequal rapidity of degeneration appear, therefore, to be independent of the direction of conduction, and cannot be explained in the present state of our knowledge.

While we are thus unable to understand the degenerative precocity of certain fibres, both fine and thick, van Gehuchten and Molhant [1] have proved that the speed with which the myelin passes through its various phases, from fragmentation to resorption, depends on the importance of the medullary sheath, and therefore on the calibre of the fibres. The thinner the nerve tubes the faster do fragmentation and resorption occur. Thus, while the thick tubes still retain some lipoid drops which can be stained by Marchi's method one hundred and twenty days after the nerve is cut, the fibres of medium thickness degenerate in fifteen days and the finest in nine or ten days. Degeneration thus begins simultaneously along the entire length of a fibre, but the evolution of the process is shortened as one proceeds from the fibre to its terminal branches. While this law holds good as regards the rapidity of the process, it is not valid as regards its initiation, since, as we have shown, in each nerve there are often found thick fibres that are precociously degenerated and fine fibres that are relatively resistant.

What are the causes of rupture of the myelin ? The authors who have studied this problem describe the phenomena rather than explain their causes. Nothafft believes that the fragmentation is a passive phenomenon, following upon the initial retraction and rupture of the axon. Büngner, on the contrary, believes that the myelin takes the initiative, and that its rupture causes that of the axon. Howell, Huber, Reich and others correlate this destructive phenomenon with chemical changes in the medullary sheath, such as the production of lecithin, protagon, etc. Marinesco believes that the modifications occurring during Wallerian degeneration in the myelin and axon are the effects of a true digestion, carried out by means of enzymes produced by the cells of Schwann. Such enzymes would normally be inactive, but would quickly ripen under the influence of pathological stimuli. Finally, Nageotte considers myelin, as we have said above, as a living and active material. Its contraction into ellipsoids would occur as a consequence of rupture of the axon, whose pieces would be surrounded by the medullary sheath, which would have become a digestive chamber. He believes that it is an adjustment to the empty space created by the disappearance of the axon ; into this space the myelin would passively penetrate, and when its walls met they would melt and form rounded

---

[1] Van Gehuchten et Molhant : " Les lois de la dégénérescence wallerienne directe," *Le Névraxe*, 1910.

stumps. Nageotte believes that this interruption coincides with the incisures of Schmidt-Lantermann.

None of these theories satisfactorily explains the causative mechanism of the initial retraction of the medullary sheath and its subsequent concentration into ellipsoids and drops. It is evident that a certain relation exists between the size of the axonic fragment and that of the fatty ellipsoid. But the admission of a necessary etiological relation between these two phenomena is inconsistent with some observed facts. One frequently sees, for example, from twenty-four hours after the operation on, axons that are varicose but uninterrupted in nerve fibres within which are many ellipsoids. This is seen by comparison of neurofibrillar preparations with those stained by osmic acid. Sometimes, in

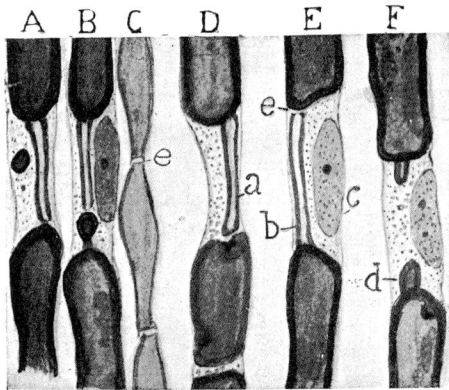

FIG. 17.—Nerve fibres from the peripheral stump of a rabbit, killed two days after the operation. Osmic acid and haematoxylin. Details of the medullary changes at the level of the nuclear region. *a, b*, thinned myelinic segments; *d*, remnants of the thinned myelin; *c*, nucleus; *e*, incisure of Schmidt-Lantermann.

those preparations where the myelin is strangulated and retracted before it breaks (Fig. 32), the axon, enveloped by the myelin, is still present. One sometimes sees the axon, which may be thinned, next to the strangulation and opposite the nucleus, where it is known that the myelin initiates its dislocation (Fig. 13, *o*). Finally, sixteen hours after the operation, as Fig. 12, *b* shows, some ellipsoids are already separated off, while the sound axon is seen at the bottom of the infundibula. The breaking up of the myelin thus occurs before the fragmentation of the axon. But, on the other hand, the rounding off of the segments and their transformation into closed chambers are related to the rupture of the axon.

One may observe two principal modes in the mechanism of retraction of the myelin, in preparations fixed in osmic acid. The first is the abrupt mode shown in nearly all the preceding figures, in which the incisures rapidly widen owing to the longitudinal retraction of the myelin. The second is the slow mode, whose phases are seen in Fig. 17. Here, wherever protoplasmic bridges are to be formed, the corresponding cylinder-cone slowly becomes slender. It is taken in by the neighbouring ellipsoids, which progressively augment in volume, until the fine medullary cylinder breaks at the centre (Fig. 17, F). Later the fatty drops that are pendent at the ends of the thick ellipsoids are absorbed (d). During the phase when the myelinic segment thins out the axon is visible, appearing very slender.

In short, one does not know the causes of the formation of myelinic ellipsoids. All that one may say is that the morphological alterations of the myelin precede those of the axon, and that its fragmentation and degeneration are influenced, like those of the axon, by the suspension of the trophic action of the mutilated neurone. This trophic action is perhaps exercised through some product of catabolism given out by the axon when the trophic current flows. This trophic current, as Heidenhain suggested and as we shall develop later, must not be confused with the ordinary nervous impulse.

The fragmentation of the myelin, as well as the destruction of the axon, do not represent a simple *post-mortem* passive decomposition, but, as Monckeberg and Bethe demonstrated, it is a true living process. These authors were able to see these phenomena in dead animals that had been kept in the incubator for twenty-four hours. Nageotte has recently proved that the fragmentation of the myelin and axon takes place also in nerves removed from the organism and kept in a moist chamber. Under such conditions the process is greatly accelerated. To obtain the survival *in vitro* of nerve fibres, it is necessary to use as a medium, not pure sodium chloride, but a solution in which, besides this salt, are present salts of bivalent metals, such as calcium chloride. We shall speak of these experiments, which we have confirmed, when we deal with the degeneration of the axon.

Alterations of the nodes, infundibula, and annular system.—The study of these alterations, usually neglected, has been the object of certain observations made by us on nerves treated with silver nitrate (fixation in formol-manganese-pyridine, silver nitrate, reduction in hydroquinone). We shall give here a résumé of these observations.

The soldering disc and the node rapidly disappear. After twelve hours one can see them in most fibres, but much altered and only with difficulty revealed by silver nitrate, Boveri's fluid being used.

Twenty-eight hours after the operation nearly all the nodes are unrecognizable, as they do not attract the silver nitrate at all.

In preparations made with osmic acid one can nevertheless see some nodes of Ranvier. These are recognized with difficulty, because of the almost uniform swelling of the terminal region of the interannular segment, whose myelin has broken up (Fig. 13, e). A more or less prominent thin wall marks the position of the cementing disc. In the majority of the fibres, however, it is impossible to find the node, since that region is easily mistaken for the nuclear area, where the myelin also retracts and draws apart. As one can see in Fig. 18, d, the node is sometimes transformed into a fusiform dilatation, which is full of liquid, but without any sign of a transversal disc.

Finally, forty-eight hours after the operation, the cementing disc has disappeared in almost all the fibres. The neighbouring ends of the cells of Schwann come in contact with each other, and a granular cylinder, continuous in appearance, is produced. The bracelets of Nageotte offer greater resistance to degeneration, since they can still be seen two and a half days after the lesion. After twenty-eight hours they are still almost normal, and show their characteristic crests (Fig. 18, d). Through their presence one can easily recognize the place where the node existed before it was destroyed. The disintegration of the bracelets, already much advanced after fifty hours, is completed between the third and the fourth day (Fig. 18, k).

We have observed that the incisures of Schmidt-Lantermann are rather refractory in their degeneration. In preparations made by means of osmic acid one can still observe them three and four days after the operation, at the level of the longer ovoids (Fig. 15, b). In the same way the membrane of the infundibulum is still present for two or three days, and we have found indications of the apparatus of Golgi-Rezzonico forty-eight hours after the operation (Fig. 13, h, i). As can be seen in Fig. 18, b, g, e, the infundibular membrane progressively breaks down, until it finally is composed of a heap of irregular clots (j), which can be stained with silver nitrate after fixation in the formol-pyridine-manganese nitrate mixture. As with the myelin, here also one can see in a single section great irregularities in the rate of degeneration. Next to membranes that are almost normal, others may be seen that are entirely broken up. This disaggregation is accomplished by means of vacuoles, exfoliations, transversal ruptures, dislocations, and the production of granular masses ; finally liquefaction and resorption come about. In Fig. 18, where we reproduce some of these degenerative phenomena, one can see that the infundibulum is often deformed through the pressure of the ellipsoids. It moulds itself to fit their terminal stumps, and it seems to offer some resistance to their retraction and slipping.

Of all the constituent parts of the fissures, the most resistant are the rings. One can still distinguish them four and five days

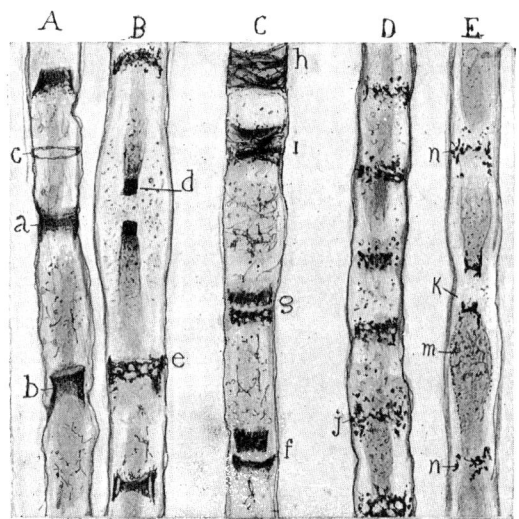

FIG. 18.—Fibres from the peripheral stump of a cat's sciatic nerve. Staining in silver nitrate, fixation in formol-pyridine-manganese. A, B, C, fibres from an animal killed twenty-eight hours after the operation ; a, b, infundibula ; c, extrafissural ring ; d, bracelets of Nageotte ; g, f, infundibula in which degeneration has begun ; h, i, destruction of the apparatus of Golgi-Rezzonico ; e, vacuolization of the infundibular cement ; D, E, fibres from an animal killed three days after the lesion ; j, n, phases of disaggregation of the infundibular cement ; k, node wherein the bracelets of Nageotte are half destroyed ; m, axonic dilatation near the node.

after the operation, although they are more or less deformed and thickened. As is to be expected, they suffer dislocations, often placing themselves in oblique positions, and showing irregular thickenings and indications of liquefaction. In one preparation, stained with iron haematoxylin, we were able to recognize their remnants eight days after the section of the nerve.

Metamorphoses of the cells of Schwann.—While the phenomena that we have just described are taking place in the myelin, while it is undergoing regression and absorption, the cell of Schwann, on the contrary, is the seat of progressive changes, which indicate a great assimilative activity. These phenomena had already been carefully studied by the older investigators, such as Ranvier, Vanlair, Stroebe, and Ziegler. They lead to the multiplication of the cells of Schwann, and to the formation of long cellular chains which are apparently continuous. When these same phenomena were studied later under the influence of theories opposed to the neurone conception, they were the subject of grave errors of interpretation. We shall give the phases of this interesting process of rejuvenescence of the cells in chronological order.

During the first twelve hours the cell of Schwann remains almost passive while it is tolerating the dislocations caused by the retraction of the myelin. From the fourteenth or the sixteenth hour, however, one can see an enlargement of the perinuclear protoplasmic mass. This is especially noticeable in the terminal caps. This protoplasmic excess tends to occupy the space left by the retraction of the myelin, although it does not completely fill it. We have observed that part of this space is filled by plasma which comes from either the myelin or the cell of Schwann, although we do not know from which. As a result of this hypertrophy the longitudinal and transversal bands of the protoplasm swell, as can be seen in preparations made by the methods of Nageotte and Doinikow. Twenty-four or thirty-six hours after the operation this process has gone on to such an extent that the entire fibre appears covered by a continuous granular coat which contains no vacuoles.

On the second day the thickening of the perinuclear protoplasm reaches the axon, which it more or less strangulates. It then takes on an oblong shape (Fig. 13, *n*) with terminal slopes, as was well described by Zalla and other investigators. At a certain moment the granulations of Erzholz hypertrophy and new ones appear. According to Doinikow, this perinuclear mass, which can be stained by Scarlet R and Sudan III, in Herzheimer's method, shows a great number of lipoidal granulations, some of which are arranged in a semi-lunar shape, and which take on a great variety of shades. One can see similar granules by means of Ehrlich's methylene blue, which stains some spheres dark blue and others pale blue; others again remain entirely colourless (Fig. 15, *c*, *n*). It thus appears that the natural granulations of Schwann's cells hypertrophy and multiply under the influence of the physiological rest of the fibre.

As to the terminal protoplasm—the shells of the node—it now

fills all the space up to the region where lay the disc of Ranvier. There is thus constituted a long periaxonic mass which comes in contact with the neighbouring cells of Schwann (Fig. 13, e).

After the fourth day the protoplasm augments still more, and forms new masses between the ellipsoids. The aspect of the nerve fibre is now that of a fatty cell which incloses within itself large drops of lipoidal substances (Fig. 19). Through an apparent or real fusion of their ends, the cells of Schwann constitute a continuous protoplasmic cylinder. Within this cylinder there are parts which are swollen to take in the ellipsoids and small fatty droplets, and parts which are narrowed through contact with the walls of the protoplasmic sheath. While the axon has disappeared at their level, these cordons, which have a compact appearance, always inclose a very fine internal cleft, which is more potential than real, and which is capable of subsequent expansion when the nerve sprouts arrive, or when the longitudinal slipping of the ellipsoids occurs. One can easily demonstrate this fine cleft near the fatty accumulations where the contraction of the walls of Schwann's cell is not so marked (Fig. 20, b).

Mitosis of Schwann's cell.—The nucleus does not remain idle during this process of intensive protoplasmic assimilation. As early as the first to the second day it enlarges and becomes rich in chromatin. On the third day

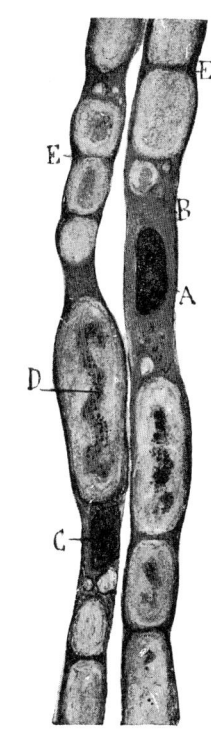

FIG. 19.—Cells of Schwann of the peripheral stump of the sciatic nerve of a rabbit, killed four days after the operation. Fixation in Dominici's fluid. Iron haematoxylin. *A* and *C*, nucleus; *B*, perinuclear protoplasmic region; *E*, thin protoplasmic walls situated between the fatty ellipsoids; *D*, granular axon which has retracted in the centre of an ellipsoid.

it often encloses two, or sometimes three, well-formed nucleoli. Finally, on the fourth day, mitoses begin. These increase very much on the following days, especially from the sixth to the ninth. A week and a half after the operation they are found less frequently, and they are rare in the third week. All modern investigators, such as Büngner, Wietting, Ballance, Bethe, Perroncito, Zalla, Nageotte, etc., agree that this nuclear multiplication is effected through mitosis. We have seen, although rarely, nuclear multiplication on the third, or even the second day, as Stroebe, Durante, Doinikow, and others had already noted (Fig. 14, *b*, *n*). Doinikow observed nuclear multiplication from twenty-four hours after the operation onwards, and considered it an exaggeration of a normal process. But it is very

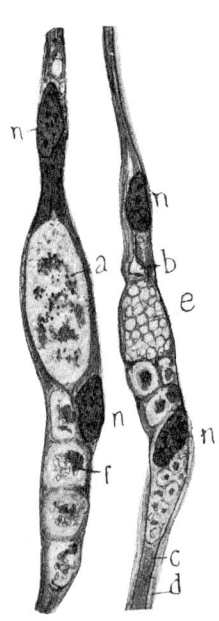
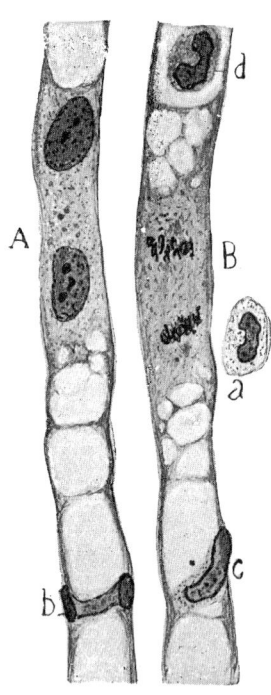

FIG. 20.—Two proliferated cells of Schwann of the peripheral stump of a rabbit, killed seven days after the operation. Iron haematoxylin. *n*, nuclei; *a*, *f*, remnants of the axon; *b*, remnants of the internal hollow space of the nerve fibre; *c*, band of Büngner or protoplasm of Schwann's cell; *d*, connective sheath; *e*, masses of lipoid drops.

FIG. 21.—Cells of Schwann in process of division, taken from the peripheral stump of a rabbit four days after the operation. Fixation in 50 per cent. alcohol. Haematoxylin. *A*, cell with two nuclei; *B*, anaphase; *a*, *b*, *c*, *d*, peritubal leucocytes entering the nerve fibres.

rarely that one sees two nuclei in the normal Schwann's cell. In our preparations one can see that some of these earliest divisions are amitotic (Fig. 14, *n*). It appears that such premature segmentations are commoner in the dog than in the rabbit.

As one can see in Figs. 21 and 22, the prophases, metaphases, anaphases, and telophases are very common. We need not repeat the details of mitosis. These are well known in man and the vertebrates.

We need only note the shortness and thickness of many chromosomes which, at the metaphase and anaphase, appear like elongated granules. Usually, with rare exceptions, the equatorial plane, and therefore the plane of division, is perpendicular to the axis of the fibre. Two ellipsoidal nuclei are thus produced, and they progressively separate along the longitudinal axis (Fig. 21). Cytoplasmic division does not follow nuclear division. The cytoplasm remains undivided, and thus a continuous protoplasmic cordon is formed. This has thickenings which correspond to the accumulations of myelin, and is narrowed down where these masses are lacking. It is at present impossible to determine whether such a *syncytium* is

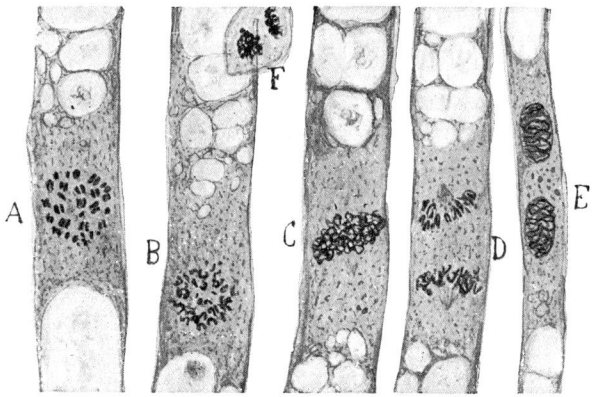

FIG. 22.—Mitotic phases of the cells of Schwann. Peripheral stump of a dog, killed six days after the operation. Fixation in Dominici's fluid. Heidenhain's iron haematoxylin. *A*, splitting of the chromosomes; *C*, prophase; *D*, anaphase; *E*, telophase; *F*, connective tissue cell of the endoneurium undergoing mitosis.

an actual structure or merely an appearance due to the imperfection of the methods. But one may say that the independent cells that make their appearance within the nerve fibre from the eighth to the tenth day are not parts of the old cell of Schwann, but, in reality, migrating leucocytes. We shall speak of these phagocytes later on.

We have observed that the ellipsoids and fatty remnants lie, not within the cell of Schwann, but in the space enclosed by this cell where the axon previously lay; here they undergo a kind of digestion. But, as Doinikow has well shown, Schwann's cell also incloses numerous fine fatty droplets, especially in those regions which are near the nucleus. We are dealing here with a process of absorption that is comparable to the common phenomenon of adiposis or pathological fatty infiltration. As a result the cell of Schwann, which for a long time retains its tubular shape, takes in two kinds of lipoid inclusions—the *large fatty inclusions* which lie in the space where the axon formerly existed, and the *fine lipoid inclusions* which, through absorption, are very largely situated within the protoplasm itself. There are also fine droplets within the sheath, where they are always mixed with the ellipsoids and the large fatty spheres. Mourawieff and Zalla held that the process which we have just described was a degenerative phenomenon of the cell of Schwann, and that the latter was finally destroyed. But we hold the opposite view, namely, that we are here dealing with a progressive act, trophic in a certain sense, and of the same order as the phenomena of fatty absorption that subsequently appears in the fixed cells of the endoneurium and epineurium.

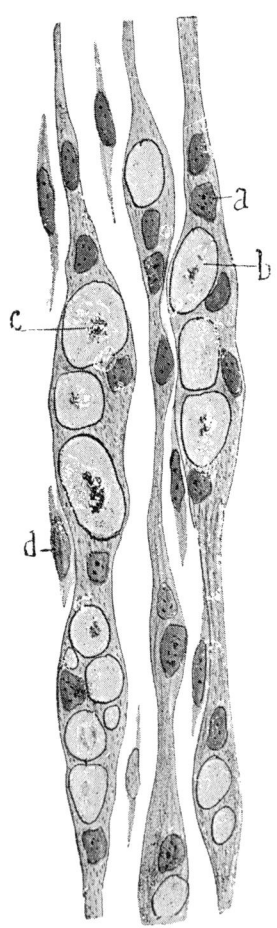

FIG. 23.—Degenerated fibres from the peripheral stump of a nerve, ten days after the operation. Silver nitrate and subsequent staining of the nuclei with thionin. *a*, multiple nuclei of Schwann's sheath; *b*, fatty drops; *c*, remnants of the old axon; *d*, interstitial connective tissue cell.

Ulterior changes in Schwann's cells.—Most of the authors who studied the regenerative process before the period of neurofibrillar stains, described a special late phase as occurring in the cells of Schwann. This phase could be seen from the eighth to the tenth day, and it has been called, following Büngner, the phase of *longitudinal striations* (*Zellenbänder*). Such authors as Herzt, Neumann, Büngner, Wietting, Ballance, Howell and Huber, Bethe, Besta, Durante, etc., influenced by that polygenism which was widespread in the 1890's, believed that such an aspect of longitudinal striations denoted an intraprotoplasmic differentiation. This, according to them, led to the autogenous production, without the help of the central stump, of bundles of new fibres. Our investigations and those of Purpura,

Perroncito, Marinesco, Tello, Nageotte, Krassin, G. Sala, Deineka, Doinikow, etc., have refuted this error, showing conclusively that every new fibre that appears in the peripheral stump represents a sprout from the central stump. But the striated aspect of the sheath of Schwann is a fact that is easily observed.

From the seventh to the tenth day after the operation the nerve tubes already show, as we have stated above, long thin tracts that are devoid of accumulations of fatty droplets (Fig. 23). These fine intercalary cordons lengthen from the eighteenth to the twenty-

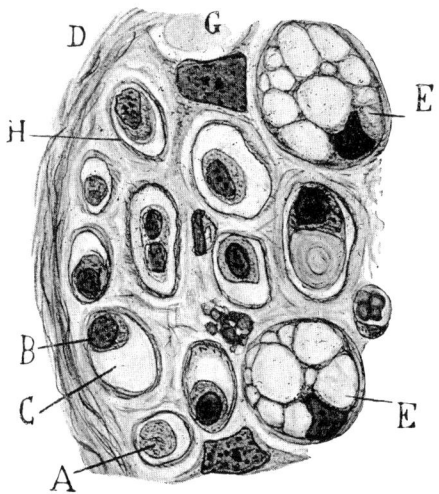

FIG. 24.—Cross-section of the peripheral stump of the sciatic nerve of a rabbit, killed twenty days after the operation. Owing to obstacles placed between the two stumps, the nerve sprouts have not yet invaded the old tubes. A, B, bands of Büngner; c, plasmatic space; H, connective sheath; E, tubes with fatty accumulations.

fourth day, and, after a month, they form almost the totality of the observable fibres. Within the protoplasm appear at variable distances, which may be very long, certain elongated nuclei which derive from the pre-existing nuclei of Schwann's cells. Such nuclei occasionally touch at their ends, forming longitudinal chains. Or two or three of them may be present at almost the same level, and thus increase the diameter of the fibre at that point (Fig. 28, D). In the intervening spaces, outside and at a certain distance from the nuclei, the protoplasm is *finely and delicately striated* longitudinally. A careful examination of these cordons always reveals a clearer axis, which is of varying thickness and finely granular. At the level of the fatty accumulations the fibre shows some interesting structural details. At the poles of tubular swellings one can see certain stout triangular nuclei. These nuclei have level or slightly convex ends, which face the fatty droplets (Fig. 28, *D*). Outside the lipoid masses are seen some long marginal nuclei which are flattened. Finally, around the swollen region one notes a fine striated covering, which appears to be composed of connective tissue.

In the majority of cases this striation is superficial and completely foreign to any process of intraprotoplasmic differentiation. Nageotte was the first to see that the bands of Büngner of the peripheral stump of nerves, twenty-five or more days after the operation, are really composed of two factors which are distinct, but which have been often confounded under the same name. These are : (1) a fine central axis or *syncytial filament*. This is formed by the narrowed portion of Schwann's cell ; and (2) a thick striated portion, composed of the connective bundles of the sheath of Key and Retzius. These condense into a cordon of solid appearance through the withering and progressive paling of the central syncytium. Thus the striated appearance of the bands of Büngner, in those cases in which the peripheral stump has not been invaded by the nerve sprouts which originate centrally, is due, as shown in Fig. 26, *D*, *F*, to their being essentially connective in composition. We shall see later that there are other fibres whose striated aspect is due to other causes.

We must add some details to the description given by Nageotte of sterile or uninnervated tubes. Between the filament or syncytial cordon which he described and the covering of connective tissue there exists a plasmatic space (Figs. 24, *G*, and 26, *K*). The size of the latter is in inverse ratio to the size of the protoplasmic axis. The syncytial cordon, on the other hand, although solid in appearance, is really a potential sheath whose central cavity has disappeared as the result of the contact of the protoplasmic walls. One sees these details with difficulty in dissociated preparations, because the distension that occurs in the nerve tube with such methods blots out the perisyncytial plasmatic space and the internal cleft. Thin cross-sections are more favourable for study. The technique here involves staining in bulk with iron haematoxylin, and inclusion in paraffin. In Fig. 24 we have reproduced the principal types of nerve tubes that are visible in such sections. One can easily see the membrane of Key and Retzius, composed of a more or less regular row of connective fasciculi (*H*), the vaginal space (*G*), and the syncytial cordon, which is more or less excentric, and in which the nuclei are found. Schwann's sheath is not visible; it is only in a few cases that one sees beneath the connective covering a fine circular line which perhaps represents its remnants, which are being resorbed. Finally, the central cleft of the protoplasmic cordon, invisible in the narrow portions of the cordons, can be well observed near the fatty accumulations (Fig. 24, *E*), where one can see that around the latter two concentric fine zones are present. These are the connective and the protoplasmic zones respectively. In such

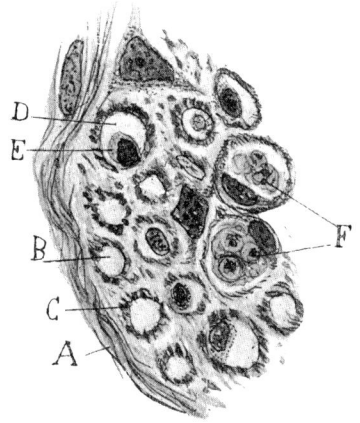

FIG. 25.—Peripheral stump of the tibial nerve of a rabbit thirty-four days after the sciatic nerve was cut near the pelvis. The central stump had been folded back and tied into the skin. Fixation in Flemming's fluid. Staining in fuchsine and picric indigo carmine. Paraffin sections. *A*, perineurium; *B*, *C*, empty old fibres reduced to the membrane of Retzius only; *D*, tubular empty space; *E*, cell of Schwann with its nucleus situated at one side of the empty space; *F*, fibres with lipoidal remnants.

accumulations the dilatation of the fibre has completely obliterated the plasmatic vaginal space. Fig. 25 shows a cross-section which was made at a later stage of degeneration—thirty-four days after the lesion—in which the bands of Büngner begin to atrophy and to disappear. We shall speak of this process more at length below.

One can observe the intracordonal empty space best, according to our observations, when one studies, in longitudinal sections, the polar region of the fatty accumulations. As can be seen in Fig. 28, *d*, this cleft, which is relatively wide near the fatty mass, becomes progressively narrower, until it ceases to be visible with a 1·40 objective in the thinner portions of the fibre.

88 TRAUMATIC DEGENERATION AND REGENERATION OF NERVES

But, to come back to the error of the polygenists, there also exist in the peripheral stump two types of nerve fibres which have a striated aspect, both of which can simulate an intraprotoplasmic fibrillar differentiation even better than the superficial connective fasciculi mentioned above. These fibres are (1) the pre-existent

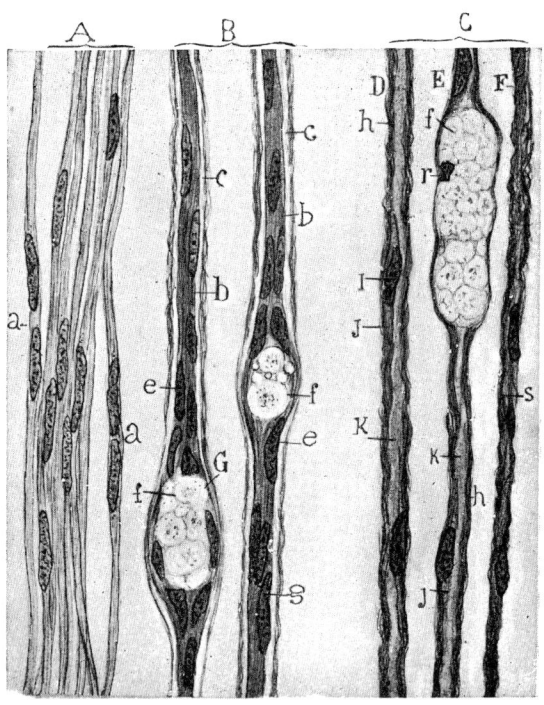

FIG. 26.—Nerve fibres from the peripheral stump of the posterior tibial nerve of a rabbit, two months after the operation. The operation consisted in the section of the sciatic nerve near the pelvis, the suture of the central stump to the skin and the cutting out of a piece of the peripheral stump. Although all precautions were taken to prevent the growth of the nerve sprouts to the peripheral stump, these met with only partial success. Fixation in Orth's fluid. Iron haematoxylin. *A*, intertubal nerve sprouts; *B*, old tubes which are innervated; *C*, sterile old tubes uninvaded by nerve sprouts from the central stump; *a*, non-medullated fibres with proliferated nuclei; *b*, band of Büngner composed principally of nerve sprouts; *c*, connective sheath of Key and Retzius; *G, f*, lipoidal remnants; *g*, nuclei of the intratubal nerve sprouts; *h*, connective sheath of the sterile tubes; *k*, internal space full of plasma; *j*, withered and discontinuous protoplasm of Schwann's cell.

large tubes, containing fatty remains, and within which have arrived very fine nerve sprouts proceeding from the central stump, as we shall describe at greater length below ; (2) fine fibrils which are either separate or else arranged in bundles, surrounded by long nuclei, and which are nothing else than young nerve sprouts which have arrived as early as the sixth or seventh day at the peripheral stump, if no obstacle to such an innervation is present (Fig. 26, A). Perroncito [1] recognized the similarity of such nucleated fibres to the *Zellenbänder* of Büngner. He erroneously thought, however, that they were formed by simple chains of embryonic connective tissue cells. When one uses the ordinary stains, both categories of fibres give the impression of being striated protoplasmic cordons, within which, through successive differentiations, have appeared the nerve fibres or their neurofibrils.

Thus we see that those authors who, following Büngner, have used the term *cellular bands*, have in reality used one term for a heterogeneous mass. They have included at least three factors: (1) the old and sterile sheath of Schwann, which was not innervated by outgrowing nervous sprouts; (2) the bundles of non-medullated fibres, which are fine and independent, and which have separated from the peripheral stump; (3) the bundles of nerve sprouts which have penetrated into the old sheaths of Schwann (Fig. 26, B).

What is the ultimate fate of the narrowed protoplasmic cordon of the syncytium of Schwann? That is a problem which presents arduous difficulties. We have solved it by using various stains on peripheral nerve stumps of animals killed one, two, and three months after the operation. We have always met, however, with a source of error, in spite of all precautions. No matter what measures are taken to prevent the arrival of nerve sprouts from the central stump—such as the cutting out of large pieces of nerve, the tying of the central stump to the skin, the inversion and suture of the central stump into deep muscles, the turning of the nerve into the pelvic cavity—after a month and a half, or sometimes much sooner, the peripheral stump has been invaded by the nerve sprouts. These penetrate into the old sheaths

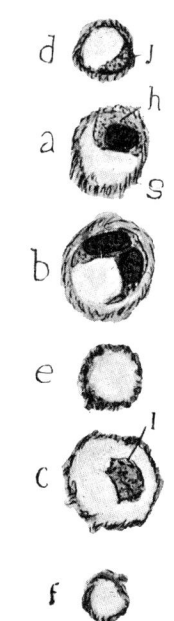

FIG. 27.—Sterile nerve tubes in cross-section. Peripheral stump of a rabbit, two months after the operation, from the same preparation as Fig. 26. *a*, cell of Schwann submerged in a plasmatic space; *l*, floating protoplasmic cordon of a cell of Schwann; *e,f*, sections through regions where there is no protoplasm of the cell of Schwann; *j*, tube with marginal protoplasm; *g*, well differentiated connective tunic.

[1] Perroncito: "Gli elementi cellulari nel processo di degenerazione dei nervi," *Bollet. della Società Medico-Chirurgica di Pavia*, March, 1909.

of Schwann and give new life to its protoplasm, so that it is almost impossible to observe the terminal stages of the evolution of the offshoots from the old cell of Schwann.

Here is the result of our investigations in this domain. We have said that, when the obstacles which are interposed have partially prevented the innervation of the peripheral stump of a rabbit's nerve, two months or longer after the operation, one can easily recognize three kinds of conductors : (1) *new or interstitial free fibres* ; (2) *old sheaths innervated by sprouts from the central stump* ; and finally, more or less numerous according to the cases and the date of the operation, (3) *sterile old tubes*. The last are of special interest in this question.

One can easily recognise the sterile tubes in the dissociated nerves and in the fine sections (fixation in Orth's or Dominici's fluid, staining in iron haematoxylin or mixtures of acid or basic aniline dyes). They have certain characteristics, which are : moderate thickness, somewhat varicose aspect, presence of the thick connective sheath of Retzius, and presence along some portion of their length of lipoid inclusions (Fig. 26, G). As can be seen in Fig. 27, e, g, the vaginal space, which is full of fluid, and of which we have spoken above, subsists and even seems to have enlarged at the expense of the narrowing of the protoplasmic cordon. In some tubes one can see nothing within this space ; all remnants of protoplasm seem to have vanished (Fig. 27, e, f). The tube appears exactly like a normal medullated fibre from which the myelin and axon have been removed. In some other nerve fibres, besides the plasmatic space, one can see a central axis or pale cordon, with or without a nucleus —the remnants of the old *syncytium* of Schwann. The thickness of this protoplasmic mass varies according to the tubes examined. In some it is so thin that it merely covers the nuclear periphery (Fig. 27, j). If the section is through a fatty accumulation, one can see that the protoplasmic perinuclear mantle is dilated and thinned to inclose the lipoid drops (Fig. 26, E). Moreover, in the majority of fibres the plasmatic space is not vaginal but central, as a consequence of the natural or artificial lateralization of the cellular cordon. The sheath of Schwann appears to have been completely resorbed. As Nageotte observed, the tube seems to be protected only by the connective membrane. Finally, even in those cordons which are thickest and rich in nuclei, it is impossible to discover the former cavity of Schwann's cell.

The preparations of dissociated nerves corroborate these histological pictures. Next to tubes in which, as shown in Fig. 26, *E*, there exists a protoplasmic cordon which is more or less atrophied, there are others that are almost completely empty, that are very thin, and whose protoplasm cannot be seen at some distance from the nuclei (Fig. 26, *D*, *F*).

From these observations it seems that the cells of Schwann which are produced through the division of the parent cell do not disappear. They are progressively modified; they break up their syncytial continuity, they narrow down and they flatten in order to apply themselves intimately to the connective membrane (Fig. 26, *J*). As a consequence of this lateralization there is formed in the axis of the old tube a space which enlarges and which is ready to receive the nerve sprouts. As Tello and ourselves have shown, and as Ranvier and other older workers foresaw, one can see this aspect of a wide empty plasmatic space, with marginal nuclei, in silver preparations, a point upon which we shall enlarge below.

The authors have occupied themselves very little with the ultimate fate of the sheath and cell of Schwann of the peripheral stump in those cases where, owing to mechanical obstacles, the nerve sprouts have not grown out to them. This seems natural when we remember that, till recently (1913) investigators have applied themselves to the problem of the regenerative mechanism of the central stump and the innervation of the peripheral segment, preoccupied as they were with the refutation of the polygenist doctrine. For such polygenists as Wietting, Marchand, Büngner, Besta, Durante, Bethe, etc., the question does not exist, since, according to their view, the multiplied old cell of Schwann transforms itself always, or almost always, into a bundle of new fibres, through a process of autogenesis.

Since the theory of a phagocytic action of Schwann's cell and its dissolution into corpuscles containing lipoid matter has been advanced, it is not surprising that various authors have claimed that it disappears, for they regard the above process as a kind of degeneration. With slight variations, both Mourawieff [1] and Zalla [2] have expressed this view. Mourawieff believes that it is especially the excess of newly-formed protoplasm which goes through a fatty degeneration.

Perroncito and Nageotte, who have slightly studied the fate of

[1] Mourawieff: "Die feinere Veranderung durchschnittener Nervenfasern im peripherischen Abschnitt," *Ziegler's Beiträge*, Bd. 29, 1901.

[2] Zalla: "I fenomeni cellulari nella degenerazione walleriana dei nervi periferici," *Riv. di patol. nerv. e mentale*, vol. 14, fasc. 1, 1901.

uninnervated cells of Schwann, believe that these cells are perhaps destroyed after a period of multiplication and phagocytosis. They differ from each other, however, in their interpretation of the part played by the old tube. Perroncito believes that the cells of Schwann are soon destroyed—as early as eighteen days after the operation—and that all remnants of the old nerve fibres disappear. The collagen bundles, or sheath of Retzius, belonging to these old fibres become a part of the endoneural tissues. Nageotte [1] believes that the cells of Schwann perhaps disappear, but that the connective bundles and the empty central space of the old nerve fibre remain, and into these the sprouts from the central stump can penetrate, even in cases of late innervation.

Doinikow,[2] although not precise, also speaks of the destruction of the uninnervated *syncytium* of Schwann, for he describes free masses composed of interstitial or intertubal cells of Schwann which are full of fatty remnants. Thus there would be present in the endoneurial tissue of the degenerated nerve ectodermal phagocytes—the cells of Schwann—besides the leucocytes and fibroblasts that take in lipoid masses.

Phagocytes of the degenerated nerve fibre.—All those who have studied Wallerian degeneration have spoken of certain cells that are present in the interior of disintegrating fibres. These cells are granular, spheroidal, are composed of an alveolar protoplasm, and are entirely analogous to those cells which are characteristic of the degenerating foci of the nerve centres—the granular cells. Such cells have, as a function, the taking up and digestion of the stored lipoidal materials within the old sheath of Schwann. Some of these phagocytes are able to leave the nerve fibre and thus to constitute the numerous free interstitial cells which are full of fatty droplets.

The presence of the intratubal and extratubal granular elements is an ordinary fact, which can be easily seen in the peripheral stump from the seventh day on, at a period when the large ellipsoids are breaking up to form the numerous small droplets (Fig. 28, *A*, *B*). However, doubts are still felt concerning the origin of these cells. Many authors, such as Stroebe, Neumann, Wietting, Lapinsky, Büngner, Zalla, Doinikow, etc., believe that the intratubal phagocytes are an offspring of the cells of Schwann. According to them

---

[1] Nageotte : " Le syncytium de Schwann et les gaînes de la fibre à myéline dans les phases avancées de la dégénération wallerienne," *C.R. de la Soc. de Biol.* tome 70, p. 861, 27 mai 1911.

[2] Doinikow : *loc. cit.*

the leucocytes and other migrating cells are able to invade the endoneurium, even in those parts of the nerve which are far from the wound, but they are unable to penetrate the old fibre. The fragmentation and resorption of the myelin would be only accidentally associated with such migrating elements, but would almost exclusively be connected with the bands of Büngner and their phagocytic descendants.

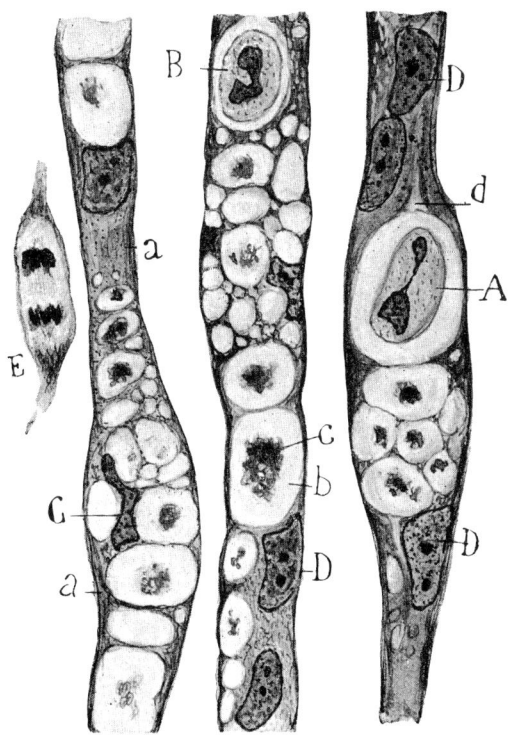

FIG. 28.—Fibres from the peripheral stump of a rabbit, eight days after the operation. Fixation in Orth's fluid. Haematoxylin. *D*, nuclei of Schwann's cell; *A*, *B*, recently arrived intratubal leucocytes; *G*, leucocyte whose cytoplasm contains lipoid masses.

A good many of the modern investigators, however, derive the intratubal granular cells from the blood. They take them to be migrating leucocytes, whose function is to digest the myelin and the remnants of the axon. This is the opinion of Ballance and Stewart, of Monckeberg and Bethe, of Hertl, Tizzoni, Korybalt, Daszkiewicz, Nageotte, etc. Almost all these investigators also recognise the presence in the nerve tube of pre-existing or autochthonous phagocytes. These come from the cells of Schwann which, together with the leucocytes, co-operate in the destruction of the axon and myelin.

The careful examination of many preparations of the peripheral stump, stained by various methods, has convinced us that all the independent spherical cells that are present in the nerve tube and contain fatty droplets are in reality migrated leucocytes. The newly formed cells of Schwann cannot be held to be phagocytes, since the greater part of the lipoid substances with which they are associated is found in the old medullary cleft or cavity. We do not deny the possibility, however, that, within certain limits, the cytoplasm of these cells undergoes a passive fatty infiltration. The arrival of the leucocytes within the degenerating peripheral stump occurs very early after the operation. Ballance and Stewart have seen them after eighteen hours ; and Nageotte after two days, in the interstices of the endoneurium. We have observed them outside the capillaries, wandering between the degenerating fibres, at the end of the second day (Fig. 21, a, b, c). From the third day they increase in number, having up to that time been rather scarce. The greatest quantity of them is found at the beginning of the second week. The size and morphology of these wandering cells are absolutely the same as those of the ordinary large leucocytes, so that their identity is thus established. As can be seen in Figs. 21, a, and 28, A, they are spherical, have abundant cytoplasm, and neutrophile granules are present. Their nucleus is rich in chromatin and takes the basic aniline dyes very strongly ; in shape it appears like a kidney, two connected balls, or else a cordon broken up into rounded lobes. From the third or fourth day on, these phagocytes apply themselves closely to the medullated nerve fibres, migrating and lengthening outside the cell of Schwann, as though they were seeking a weak point which would allow them to enter the central space. One sees very often the disposition shown in Fig. 21, b, where a leucocyte half encircles a degenerated fibre. Apart from these precocious attempts at penetration, the leucocytes are unable to cross the membrane of Schwann until seven or eight days after the lesion. Even then (Fig. 28, B, C) they are very few in comparison with the newly-formed cells of Schwann, and many fibres are seen in which there are no exogenous phagocytes. On the other hand, from the eighteenth day on, when the resorption of the myelin is fairly advanced, nearly all the large masses of fatty droplets inclose one or many wandering cells, which are full of lipoidal masses of varying volume (Fig. 29, *e*, *d*). Finally, after a month the intratubal leucocytes are already rare, and they completely disappear a month and a half after the operation. As Nageotte stated, it is very easy to distinguish the intratubal exogenous phagocytes from the sprouts of Schwann's cells. The greatest differences relate to the nucleus. In Schwann's cell (Fig. 28, *D*) the nucleus is large, ovoid, nearly always oriented in the direction of the tubular axis, and often marginal in position; it encloses one or two large nucleoli and numerous delicate chromatin granules. On the other hand, the nucleus of the leucocytes is small, is irregular in shape (Fig. 28, *B*), is often lobed, lacks a conspicuous nucleolus, and possesses a cortical chromatic skeleton which is heavily stained by the basic aniline dyes and haematoxylin. It is not parallel in position to the axis, like the nucleus in Schwann's cell, but is oblique or transversal (Fig. 29, *f*). Moreover, when the exogenous phagocyte encloses numerous large fatty drops the nucleus shows slopes and angles to accommodate the lipoidal inclusions (Fig. 28, *G*). Finally, as noted above, the cytoplasm of

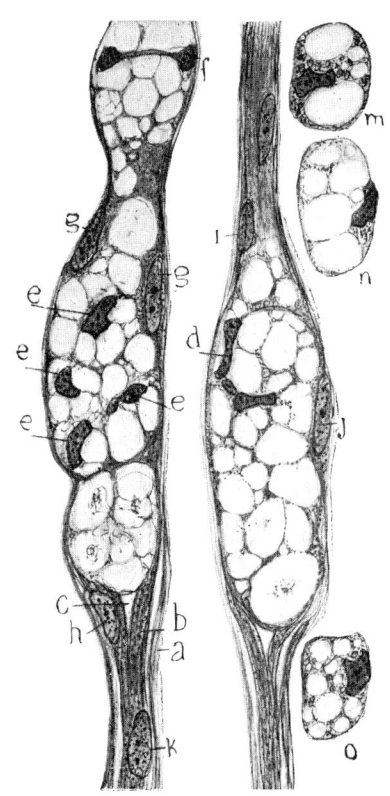

FIG. 29.—Lipoidal masses in nerve fibres from the peripheral stump of a rabbit which died twenty days after the operation. The lipoidal masses are full of leucocytes (*d*, *e*). *j*, *g*, *k*, nuclei of the cells of Schwann; *h*, *i*, triangular nuclei at the ends of the fatty masses; *f*, leucocyte which is pulled out into an arc; *n*, *m*, *o*, free intertubal phagocytes.

the daughter Schwann's cell is never clearly individualized, while in favourable sections one can see that the intratubal leucocyte has a well-defined cytoplasmic edge, which is sharply differentiated from the free lipoid drops present in the cytoplasm of Schwann's cell. Further, one not infrequently sees the leucocytic cell deformed in many ways and showing the nucleus lengthened out and as though applied as a belt to the internal surface of the membrane of Schwann (Fig. 29, *d, f*).

The larger the fatty masses of the old fibres, the more numerous are the included leucocytes. This can be seen in Fig. 29, *e, d,* where we show fibres taken from a rabbit which was killed twenty days after the operation. One may here observe the marginal position of the real nuclei of Schwann, which are elliptical and narrow. Each large agglomeration contains two or three nuclei of that kind, besides the polar or triangular nucleus of which we have spoken (Fig. 29, *h*). The phagocytes, two, three, or more in number, according to the quantity of the fatty accumulation, are usually found in the interstices of the fatty drops. Next to each nucleus one can recognize a wide cytoplasmic area. This is spongy or alveolar, that is, with fine reticular walls and vacuoles of various sizes to take in the fats. The intratubal phagocytes are so compressed that the intercalary spaces are often obliterated, and that, as a result, the edges of these cells can be seen only with the greatest difficulty.

Once full of lipoidal substances, some of the leucocytes leave the degenerating nerve tube and are found in the interstices of the nerve, particularly near the blood vessels (Fig. 29, *m, n, o*). From the tenth or twelfth day on, one can see a few free cells, that is, leucocytes which contain fatty drops and which can be homologized with the granular elements of the nerve centres. They are especially abundant from the twenty-fifth day on, when they are seen under the perineurium, where they tend to congregate, as though they were seeking an exit or attempting to migrate. It seems probable, however, that a good many of the intratubal phagocytes do not abandon the nerve fibre, even though the membrane of Schwann disappears after withering and degenerating *in situ*, and after having brought about in the lipoid masses important changes leading to absorption.

It is difficult to say why the leucocytes congregate in the peripheral stump, far from the wound, where they attack the degenerating fibres. In the absence of a final explanation, we accept as plausible the hypothesis of Ballance and Stewart, who believe that the emigration of the leucocytes and their penetration into Schwann's sheath are due to the influence of chemical changes, which come about in the fibres as these degenerate because of the cessation of function. Translating this opinion into more precise terms, we might conjecture that the decomposition of the axon and myelin liberate positive chemotactic substances capable of attracting the wandering cells. Perhaps these enticing substances are produced by the rejuvenated cells of Schwann. At any rate, this attractive action reaches its maximum from the fifth to the eighth day, at the critical period for the breaking up of the nerve fibre. According to Ballance and Stewart the leucocytic migration ceases at the end of the second week, but we cannot confirm this assertion.

Besides the ordinary polymorphonuclear leucocytes, the lymphocytes are also attracted, according to Doinikow, but it is doubtful whether the latter cells are able to penetrate into the tubes of Schwann. The connective elements of the endoneurium and the mast cells are likewise unable to effect this penetration.

It must be pointed out that probably not all the granular cells which are full of fatty material and which are found from the twenty-fifth day on in the endoneurium and perineurium are leucocytes that have come from the degenerating nerve fibre. It is generally believed that a good many of them are nothing else than fibroblasts from the interstitial connective tissue, which have absorbed lipoid materials derived from the degenerating fibre. This theory fits well with the presence of precocious granular cells in the endoneurium. In some cases we have seen such cells as early as four days after the operation, at a time when the nerve fibres totally lack exogenous phagocytes.

> The above observations confirm the conclusions of Nageotte, who believes that the intratubal phagocytes are in large part of exogenous origin, but they are opposed to the view generally held, that they are an offspring of Schwann's cell. We are even more radical in our belief than the French investigator. Nageotte accepts not only phagocytes derived from the blood, but also isolated intratubal phagocytes derived from the old cells of Schwann. Mourawieff, Zalla, Perroncito, Doinikow, and other modern authors also believe in such endogenous phagocytes. They are supposed to take into their cytoplasm lipoidal matter, which they prepare for absorption. Along with Marinesco and Besta, we have not been able to satisfy ourselves of the reality of this phagocytosis. In our preparations the daughter cells of Schwann are always marginal and *syncytial*, and they have at first a more or less apparent cylindrical form. This form is not easily seen because of the internal empty space and because of the joining of the protoplasmic walls to each other. It is our view, as we have stated above, that the lipoidal accumulations, with the exception of some passive infiltration, are

present in the tubal central space, that is, in the place where the axonic remnants are or have been present. This does not exclude the theory upheld by Marinesco, that the cells of Schwann cause a true digestion to take place in the axonic and fatty masses, and that they thus behave as true phagocytes.

Interstitial cells.—The connective tissue cells of the peripheral stump do not remain idle. The large stellated cells that lie on the tubes are, as many authors have recognized (more recently Zalla, Perroncito, Nageotte, Doinikow), the seat of an active proliferation. These cells first hypertrophy. Their cytoplasm attracts the basic aniline dyes and its spongy structure is less well seen; their expansions retract, become pale, and sometimes disappear. Finally, the cytoplasm takes on an irregularly globular form. From the second to the third day preparations are made for mitosis, and this takes place during the third and fourth days (Figs. 22, F, and 28, E).

As we have stated above, the connective tissue cells of the endoneurium, whether they are newly-formed or pre-existent, absorb fat emanating from the nerve fibres. This fact can easily be demonstrated by staining these cells from the fourth day on with Sudan III or Scarlet R, as Doinikow recommends. Osmic acid also shows lipoid droplets in them.

The fatty inclusions are found as such two or three weeks after the operation in the cells of the perineurium, as well as in those of the neurilemma. The diffusion of lipoidal materials thus goes on radially, that is, from the fibres towards the surfaces of the nerves.

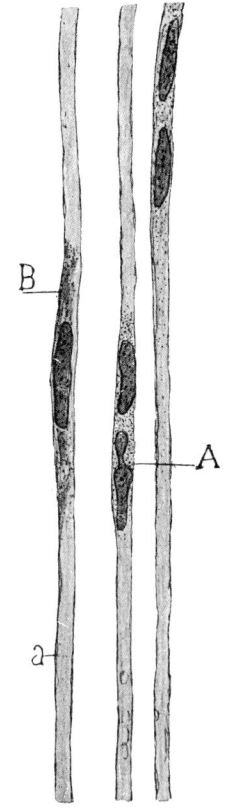

FIG. 30.—Non-medullated fibres of Remak of the peripheral stump of the sciatic nerve of a rabbit, killed four days after the nerve-section. A, recently divided nuclei; B, hypertrophied cytoplasm; a, marginal protoplasmic mantle.

The fatty changes just described must be understood, not as a degeneration of the connective tissue cells, but as a phenomenon of passive infiltration. The lipoid materials then undergo within these cells decompositions which facilitate their absorption.

From the twenty-fifth day on, and sometimes before, one also finds, as the investigators have observed, large spumy elements near the blood vessels. These cells are more or less rounded and are full of fatty droplets, some of which are of a considerable size. We reproduce these granular elements in Fig. 29, *m*, *n*. They probably are transformed leucocytes. The opinion of Ballance and Stewart is thus open to some doubt : they believed that the phagocytes which originate in the blood disappear from the peripheral stump at a relatively early period, to give way to the connective tissue phagocytes. It is doubtful whether the mast cells and cyanophil cells of the plasma become fatty.

Mitosis in the non-medullated fibres of Remak.—The phenomena occurring in those cells which surround non-medullated axons have been very little studied. During the first two days the sympathetic fibres of the peripheral stump show hardly any changes. From the third day on the surrounding cell becomes thicker and more apparent. Its cytoplasm becomes somewhat stained with the basic aniline dyes and haematoxylin (Fig. 30, *B*). It finally proliferates. Numerous cells have two nuclei which are elongated and close to each other. Some of these nuclei show strangulations and thickenings that are not present in normal nuclei. As we shall describe below, the axon becomes pale, granular, and finally is resorbed. Phagocytosis seems to play no part at all in this process.

V

DEGENERATION OF THE PERIPHERAL STUMP

Degenerative phenomena occurring in the interrupted axon.—Fragmentation and liquefaction of the axon at a distance from the wound.—Fragmentation and liquefaction of the axon near the lesion.—Agonistical neoformation.—Preserved fibres and degenerated fibres.—Degenerative phenomena of the axon in vitro.—*Experiments of Bethe, Nageotte, and Cajal.*

Every piece of protoplasm that is severed from a cell and that lacks a nucleus is destined to perish more or less rapidly. This is a law applying equally to Protozoa that have been cut in pieces and to mutilated nerve cells. It is easily proved that the action of the nucleus is absolutely necessary for the nutrition of the cytoplasm in those neurones in which the axon—an expansion of the cellular soma—is cut off. The segregated portion perishes and is resorbed, even though it is far from the trophic centre or cellular body, notwithstanding that it is protected and perhaps nourished by certain satellite cells, the cells of Schwann, and that it lives in a *milieu* of connective tissues rich in plasma and in capillaries. However, we do not wish to deny that the nutrition of the axon is a local process and is to a certain degree autonomous. We shall find a proof of this nutritional autonomy below. But, in order that the nutritional process should be kept up, it is absolutely necessary that some dynamic thing, of whose nature we have no idea, should constantly be radiated from the neuronal soma so as to stimulate the protoplasm and prevent its withering.

We have stated that the amputated axon dies, but this does not occur suddenly, but after a more or less prolonged agony. This agony is quiet, and to a certain extent passive, in that part of the axon which is far from the wound and which is protected, because of the distance, from traumatic irritation. But it is tumultuous, that is, it is accompanied by ephemeral regenerative reactions, in those regions which are close to the lesion, where the protoplasm felt directly the stimulus due to the physical damage. It is thus best to differentiate the degenerative phenomena which occur in these two regions of the cut axon.

DEGENERATION OF THE PERIPHERAL STUMP

Axonic degeneration far from the wound.—This degeneration is entirely Wallerian, and is free from the perturbatory influence of the traumatic inflammation. It takes a course that is nearly always the same. The phases of the process, recognized with difficulty in ordinary preparations, are seen with great clearness and exactness in the sections stained by neurofibrillar methods.

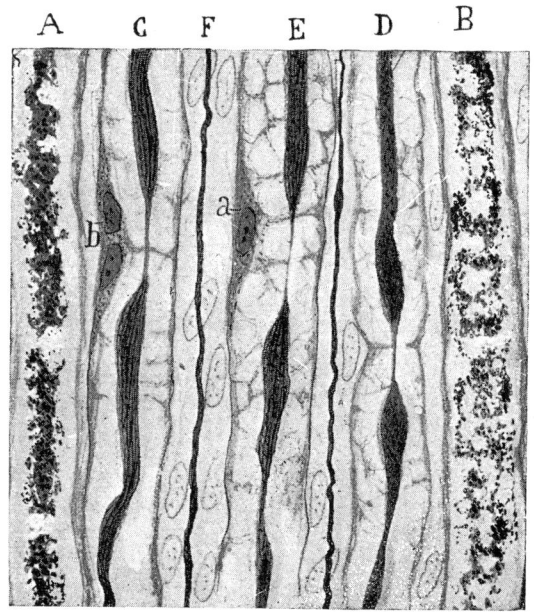

FIG. 31.—Piece of the peripheral stump of the sciatic nerve of a cat, killed forty-eight hours after the operation. Region far from the wound. Reduced silver nitrate. *A, B*, axons that were destroyed at an early stage; *C, E, D*, axons in the varicose phase, relatively resistant; *F*, hardly altered non-medullated fibre.

(*a*) The first perceptible phenomenon in the axon is the *moniliform* or *varicose* appearance, which was observed by all investigators, and which occurs in nerve centres as well as in the nerves. The axonic masses, or rather, the *neurobiones*, are the seat of certain degenerative changes; the living units are dislocated and congregate in certain places, forming colonies or fusiform masses (Fig. 31, *C, E*). Such a phenomenon, which is premonitory of fragmentation, does not depend only on the dislocation of the neurobiones and the movement of the neuroplasm. One must think of it as a mixed process of movement and multiplication of the above-mentioned living units, and therefore of the neurofibrils, since the masses which are formed have a greater volume than can be compensated by the loss of calibre of the thinned portions of the axon. Besides, the colloidal silver stains the varicosities very intensively. The varicosities are found, in some fibres, three or four hours after the section. Usually, however, they begin to be seen from the twelfth hour on. Some axons completely lack such deformations; in these, granular degeneration begins without these preliminaries.

(b) The second phase consists of the *granular disintegration* of the neurofibrils. It was first demonstrated by Monckeberg and Bethe by a special method, and was later confirmed by ourselves, Marinesco, Tello, Perroncito, etc., by the procedure involving reduced silver nitrate. With this method the neurofibrils and their granulations are stained dark brown, while the neuroplasm appears white (Fig. 31, A, B).

The granular degeneration, according to Monckeberg and Bethe,[1] is very rapid in its appearance. They say: "One can already see, after eighteen hours, near the wound, axons in the granular state. This aspect becomes more general during the first twenty-four hours. After thirty-six hours nearly all the fibres which lie within a distance of one centimetre from the wound have become granular. Finally, after four days, the granular state, which spreads from the wound to the periphery has extended along the entire length of the nerve, so that no neurofibrils are recognizable. The granular degeneration goes through various phases. At first the neurofibrils become sinuous in their course, and, at certain places along their length appear thickenings. Later the granulations appear; they are at first large, later they are delicate and hardly perceptible. Finally the disintegration of the axonic protoplasm comes about. The interfibrillar or neuroplasmic substance also degenerates." To all this is added the coagulation and granular disintegration of a special vitreous substance which Bethe shows around the axon—the *perifibrillar substance*. This probably corresponds to the *hyaloplasm*, an exudate described by Nageotte.

The granular degeneration as described by Monckeberg and Bethe is well confirmed in the preparations made with reduced silver nitrate. It appears to begin, however, somewhat later than these investigators supposed, with the exception of some fibres which are precociously disorganized. As is shown in Fig. 33, B, the spherules

[1] Monckeberg und Bethe: "Ueber die Regeneration peripherischer Nerven," *Arch. f. mikros. Anat.*, Bd. 54, 1899.

into which the axon breaks down are dark, round, and are separated by a clear substance which is probably of a semi-liquid nature—the neuroplasm. The granular degeneration begins in most fibres thirty to forty-eight hours after the lesion. There is much variation here, however, as we shall point out later. We have not clearly seen in our preparations the varicose appearance and sinuous course of the neurofibrils as described by Monckeberg and Bethe.

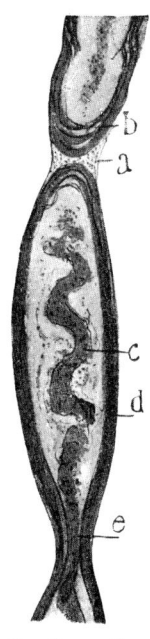 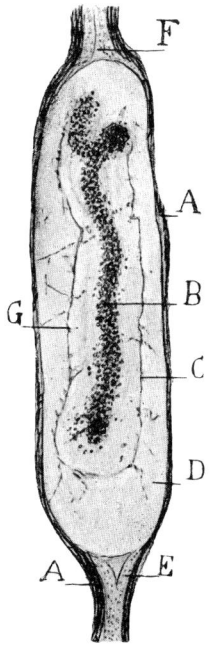

FIG. 32.—Nerve fibre, from the peripheral stump of a nerve, four days after the operation. Osmic acid and haematoxylin. *a*, protoplasmic bridge; *D*, myelin with exfoliations; *c*, axon, flexuous and wrinkled; *e*, axon where it is squeezed at the level of a strangulation of the myelin.

FIG. 33.—Nerve fibre from the peripheral stump of a rabbit's sciatic nerve, four days after the section. Reduced silver nitrate. *A*, sheath of Retzius; *B*, thinned axon; *C*, *G*, limiting membrane of the axon (*Innenscheide* of Bethe); *F*, blank space within the nerve tube.

(*c*) The third phase consists of the axonic fragmentation and longitudinal slipping of the pieces thus formed. The rupture gives birth to flexuous pieces, which are helicoidal and relatively thin. It occurs usually, as noted above, at the level of the nucleus and opposite to the places where the myelin ellipsoids are joined (Fig. 32, *a*).

Once the axonic pieces are formed, the protoplasm that composes them thins out, and its edges, which were very sharp before, become granular, uneven, and appear torn (Fig. 31, *A*). This is because the limiting membrane of the axon has become separated from the protoplasm proper owing to osmotic pressure, and it lies at some distance, dilated by a clear, viscous substance—the hyaloplasm of Nageotte. This cuticle had already been observed by Monckeberg and Bethe, and was well described by Nageotte, who interpreted it as a lipoid substance formed at the edges of the hyaloplasm exudate. Whatever its significance, it appears in silver preparations, as shown in Fig. 33, *C*, as a fine, granular membrane which does not take the stain, and from which originate granular trabeculae which lose themselves in the thickness of the nodular space. The membrane sends to the thick portion of the axon series of delicate granules.

One can also see in preparations made with osmic acid the broken axon, typically convoluted and granular, as in Fig. 32, *c*. The perihyaloplasmic limiting membrane can also be perceived in this figure, although less clearly than in some silver preparations. In the same figure one can also see that each axonic piece resides, as noted above, in a plasmatic chamber, which is surrounded by the myelin sheath.

We have remarked that the axons do not simultaneously undergo granular degeneration, nor do they break up at the same time. As with myelin, great differences are perceptible; these are especially apparent from the second day after the lesion onwards. One can distinguish three kinds of axons in this respect.

(1) *Precociously degenerated axons*. These are thick, few in number, and they already appear granular, vacuolated, and broken into pieces before the second day (Fig. 31, *A*, *B*). Some of them begin to disintegrate long before, from the sixteenth or eighteenth hour. It is probable that such axons do not go through the varicose phase, but immediately suffer granular disorganization and liquefaction. Even the axonic fractures may be absent in such axons as suffer, no one knows why, a process of sudden destruction.

(2) *Resistant axons*, which undergo late pigmentation and an even more tardy neurolysis. Forty-eight hours after the lesion they are still in the varicose stage. They are then striated and their neurofibrils are more or less normal. In Fig. 31, *C*, *D*, we show some of these axons. One can see that the narrowed pieces, which are to be the seat of ruptures, are often formed at the level of the node of Ranvier and opposite the nuclear region of Schwann's cell. In some

of them one can already see a granular degeneration (*D*), which will become more accentuated during the third day and finally pass to the phase of disintegration.

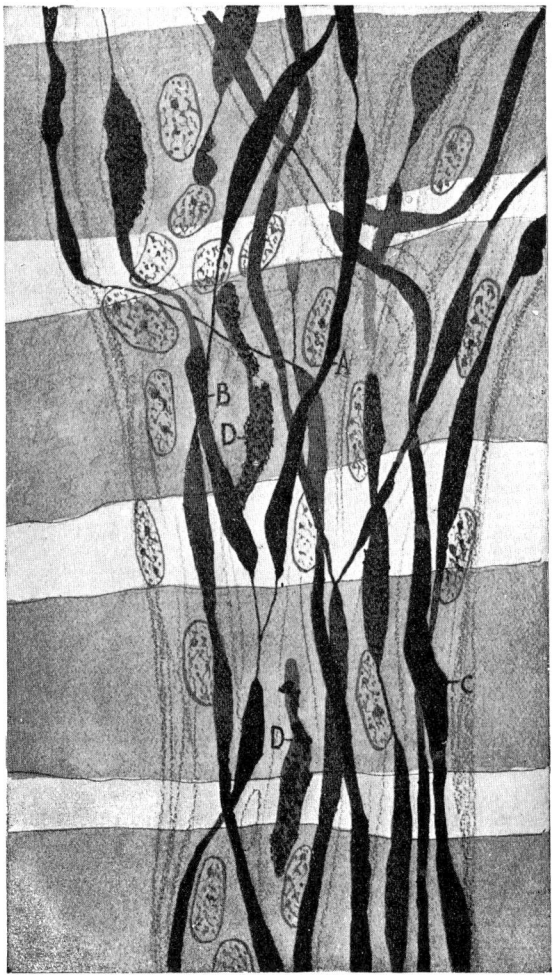

FIG. 34.—Small muscular nerve of a rabbit, killed twenty-one hours after the section of the sciatic nerve. *A, B,* fibres in the varicose phase; *D,* fibres in the phase of granular disintegration and fragmentation.

(3) *Sympathetic or non-medullated fibres* (Fig. 31, *F*). These are the most resistant of all, remaining almost normal forty-eight and fifty-six hours after the section. Finally, that is from the fourth to the seventh day, they too undergo granular degeneration, break up,

and liquefy. Marinesco and Tello also have observed the regenerative resistance of the non-medullated fibres and the unequal speed of this process in the medullated fibres.

(d) *Resorption of the axon.*—Both the wide and the narrow medullated axons are not only destroyed, but also resorbed after the first week, through a digestive process which has been well described by Marinesco and Nageotte. In this respect the interior of the ellipsoids is comparable to a segment of intestine. The enzymes are perhaps produced either by the myelin or by Schwann's cell. This liquefying process is uneven in its action. One can still find, here and there, free axonic grumes and even relatively large

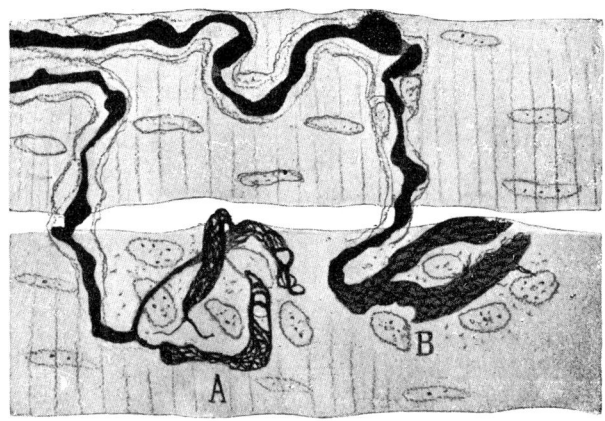

FIG. 35.—Phenomena of hypertrophy and vacuolisation occurring in some motor plates after section of the sciatic nerve. The rabbit was killed twenty-four hours after the operation.

disintegrated pieces belonging to large fibres, in nerves prepared for examination eight days after the section. One can even find in peripheral stumps eighteen or twenty days after the operation granular axonic remnants in the interior of persistent ellipsoids. These remnants are stained black by silver nitrate and more or less dark grey by iron haematoxylin (Fig. 29). On the other hand, the fine medullated fibres are destroyed more rapidly. It thus appears that the law concerning speed of degeneration established by van Gehuchten and Molhant holds good also for degenerating axons.

We may summarise the Wallerian degeneration of the axon as passing through the following phases : (1) the varicose phase, or phase of dislocation of the neurofibrillar substance ; (2) transformation of the neurofibrils into granules ; (3) vacuolisation and fragmentation of the axon ; (4) breaking up of the axonic protoplasm into independent grumes ; (5) resorption of the protein and lipoid substances of the axon.

The bead-like aspect of the axons and the subsequent destructive phases occur simultaneously along the entire length of the nerve. Tello[1] has shown this conclusively in his excellent study of degeneration and regeneration of the motor plates, where he notes that the above-mentioned phenomena begin twenty-four hours after the operation, even in the finest intramuscular nerves. As can be seen in Fig. 34,

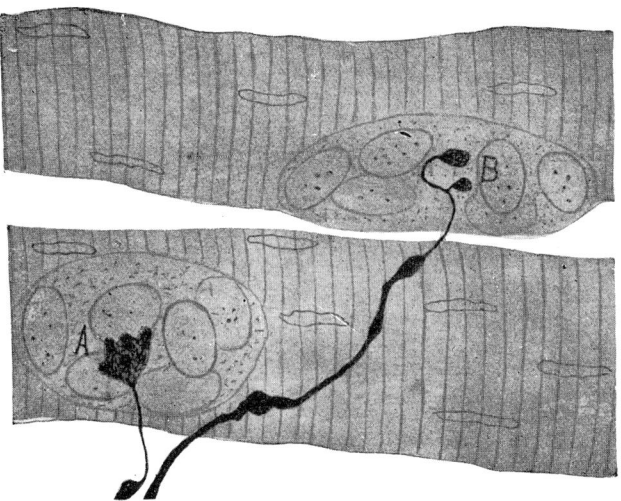

FIG. 36.—Phenomena of retraction of the nervous arborization of the motor plate, forty-eight hours after section of the sciatic nerve of a rabbit. Reduced silver nitrate.

the varicose aspect of the axon and the thinning which is a precursor of rupture are especially prominent where the nerve fibres bifurcate. One can also see in the figure that already after twenty-one hours there are a few axons which are completely fragmented and granular (D).

This difference in the rate of degeneration, already noted above in connection with the fragmentation of the myelin, has been observed by Tello even in motor plates. Thus while one sees after twenty-four hours axonic arborizations which are in a more or less complete stage of granulation and disintegration, there are others which are relatively

[1] F. Tello : " Dégénération et régénération des plaques motrices, etc." *Trav. du Lab. de Recherches biol.*, tome 5, 1907.

well preserved. The latter arborizations sometimes are hypertrophied and show a diffuse staining of the neuroplasm (Fig. 35, B); sometimes they show vacuolisations and local concentrations of the neurofibrillar net, whose threads are thickened and strongly attract the colloidal silver (A). Three or four days after the operation the motor plates are completely disintegrated. Tello also observed that, in some motor plates, the disintegration is preceded by a phenomenon of contraction of the protoplasm of the nervous arborizations. This retracts towards the stem, forming a wide mass which is granular and lobed (Fig. 36, A). All these curious phenomena imply the motility and aggregative capacity of the neurobiones, whose movements perhaps are the result of changes occurring in the chemical composition of the axonic protoplasm, with a consequent modification of the osmotic pressure.

Phenomena occurring in the axon of the peripheral stump, near the wound.—The examination of that portion of the peripheral stump which is near the wound, during the first two or three days after the operation, leads to the observation of three types of phenomena which are perfectly demarcated. These are : (1) The rapid destructive degeneration of the interrupted axons ; (2) the preservation through an instantaneous death and autolytic indifference of the border portions of some axons—our *preserved fibres* ; (3) the phenomena of agonistical transformation and regeneration of the most vigorous fibres.

Very rapid destructive degeneration.—The direct action of the wounding agent causes in certain nerve fibres near the wound, not only Wallerian degeneration, but also a rapid fragmentation and disintegration of the myelin and axon, which occur much more rapidly than in those nerve segments which are far from the traumatism. To this precocious degeneration doubtless contribute the inflammation and the exudates, and especially the migratory leucocytes, which are very abundant in the wound from six or eight hours after the lesion onwards, and which infiltrate between the nerve fibres.

This rapid destruction of the axons near the wound has not been well studied, as it is difficult to distinguish here that which is due to Wallerian degeneration and that which is directly the result of traumatism and of the phlogotic exudate. Since this destructive process occurs to some extent, although very restricted, in the *preserved fibres*, and in those medullated fibres which show agonal reactions, we shall speak of it in great detail below.

Preserved fibres.—Our observations on the effect of traumatisms on the brain, spinal cord and nerves [1] have brought out clearly the fact that near the wound long axonic pieces are present, which, for unknown reasons, retain their normal morphology, are well stained

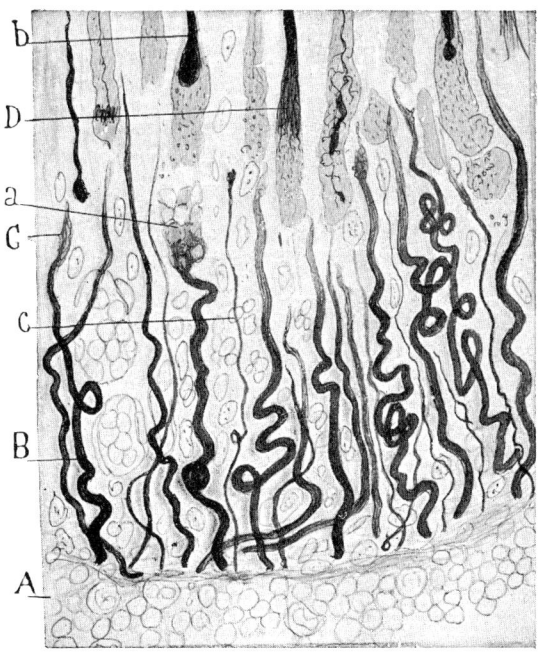

FIG. 37.—Peripheral stump of sciatic nerve of an almost adult cat, fifty hours after the section. *A*, exudate from the wound; *B*, preserved fibre; *C*, point of corrosion of *B*; *D*, terminal segment of the peripheral stump.

by neurofibrillar methods, are sinuous in their course, and stand out from the remnants of the other fibres owing to their resistance to autolysis. These are the fibres that we have named *preserved fibres*.

The *preserved fibres* are abundant near the wound, in cut nerves. As can be seen in Fig. 37, each refractory axon of the peripheral stump shows three distinct regions. These are : (1) the terminal, black, and preserved segment ; (2) the autolytic or disintegrating

[1] S. R. Cajal : " Fibras nerviosas conservadas y fibras nerviosas degeneradas," *Trab. del Lab. de Investig. biol.*, tomo 9, 1911.

segment; (3) the living or metamorphic segment. These three zones can already be seen on the first day after the section and perhaps before. It seems to us, however, that they are best differentiated from forty to seventy hours after the operation.

(a) *Terminal segment.*—This is characterized by its black colour, sinuous and even spiral course, perfect cylindrical shape and absence of vacuoles and of all signs of fragmentation and degeneration. One can see in Fig. 37 that the preserved fibres are both medullated (B) and non-medullated (c). Between them lie leucocytes and remnants of the disintegrated medullary sheaths. Such axons end at the surface of the cut with a cylindrical extremity which is sometimes somewhat thinned and intensely black. Occasionally the terminal portion is seen outside the wound, sometimes folded in a tangential direction, sometimes rounded up in the form of a glomerulus. Within, the axon lies inside Schwann's sheath, sinuous in its course. As it goes inwards its dark colour becomes smoky, grey, and lastly yellow. Finally, at a depth that varies for each fibre, the latter ends abruptly, sometimes in an elongated *point of corrosion*, sometimes in a clot which is granular and more or less broken up (G), sometimes in a wide dilatation which is pale, spongy in texture, and full of vacuoles (Fig. 37, a).

(b) *Zone of disintegration.*—This begins at the level of the above-mentioned point of corrosion, and is characterized by the fact that at its level the nerve tube contains only irregular remnants of the digested axon and detritus from the medullary sheath. It is strange that axolysis should be restricted to the deep portion of the preserved axon, that is, to the neighbourhood of the living or metamorphic segment where lie, more or less altered, the cell of Schwann and the medullary sheath. This fact suggests that in the rapid disintegration of the axon there is present some enzyme derived from the cells of Schwann or from the myelin sheath. We must not forget, however, that in the centres, which lack the cells of Schwann, this phenomenon also occurs.

(c) The *metamorphic segment* of the axon represents the surviving portion of the peripheral stump. We shall speak below of the curious metamorphoses that it undergoes. We need only note here that in the preserved fibre the metamorphic segment is situated farther from the wound than in the ordinary fibres which are not preserved.

The number of preserved fibres in the peripheral stump varies. In some preparations none are to be found; in others they are very abundant—where the animal is killed not later than three or four days after the operation.

There is little doubt concerning the mechanism to which the presence of preserved fibres is due. We believe that this is related to the mechanism of the section of the nerve. When the operation is performed with sharp scissors or scalpels, there are very few such axons; when, however, the operation is complicated by wresting and pulling, as when dull instruments are used, then their number is very much increased. It may be that there are really no preparations which, if they are well studied, within the first few days after the operation, show no preserved fibres at all. The exudates, especially blood, help the preservation of the fibres, but they do not cause it.

We can thus say that the *preserved* fibres are axons which are pulled, compressed, or wrested by the injuring agent. They died suddenly, without degenerating, and they are preserved from autolysis perhaps by some coagulated protein which resists the action of the lysins or enzymes produced either by the myelin or by the cells of Schwann. One must recognize these immune axons in order not to mistake them for regenerating central fibres which are entering the peripheral stump, or for living fibres which are refractory to degeneration. Such errors have been committed frequently, especially in the anatomico-pathological study of the centres, where the preserved fibres are numerous.

Medullated fibres showing an agonal reaction.—Careful study of the peripheral stump during the first eight days after the section shows that, as might easily be presumed, the axons that are violently separated from their trophic centre do not suddenly die, but go through a period of survival and agony which is of variable length. This period is entirely comparable to the phase of languor and weakness which precedes the death of enucleated pieces of cut or artificially fragmented Protozoa.

In the medullated fibres this agony is associated with very curious phenomena of local or intra-axonic mortification and regeneration. In non-medullated fibres, as we shall see below, the dying axon even forms clubs and nervous arborizations. The process in medullated fibres is as follows :

Each nerve fibre shows, beginning from the wound, three successive portions or segments : (1) necrotic or granular segment ;

(2) metamorphic segment or segment of neurofibrillar irritation; (3) indifferent or passive segment. The *preserved fibres* are an exception to this. There, as noted above, the largest portion of the necrotic segment is represented by the terminal portion which is refractory to autolysis.

(a) *Necrotic segment.*—The traumatic agent, acting directly on the nerve, causes the almost instantaneous death of a portion of the

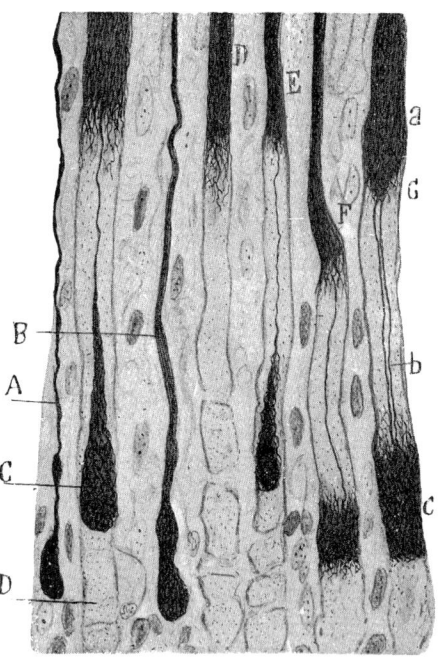

FIG. 38.—Piece of the peripheral stump of the sciatic nerve of a cat, two days after the section. *a*, *b*, non-medullated fibres of Remak; *D, E, G*, metamorphic portion of the medullated axons; *D*, necrotic segment.

axon which, from the first few hours after the operation, appears perfectly well marked off from the metamorphic portion, and has a pale and granular appearance. This segment can be easily distinguished from the living portion, since the latter attracts strongly the colloidal silver, while the former has no affinity for it at all, and appears minutely and transversely fragmented, surrounded by a wrinkled sheath of Schwann (Fig. 28). At the level of the myelin one can see lipoid drops of various sizes and protein detritus of many kinds. This general breaking up of the fibre is completed within twenty-four hours. It begins much earlier, and one can attribute it to the disorganizing action of the traumatic shock and to the subsequent action of autolysis or the lysins from the exudate. In this segment the axon shows, a few hours after the lesion, longitudinal and transversal breaks, extensive vacuolisations, an uneven

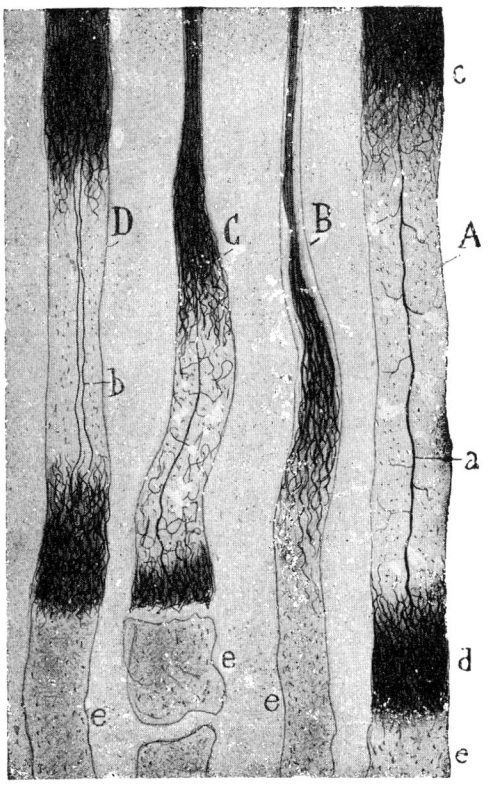

FIG. 39.—A few medullated fibres from the peripheral stump of a cat, forty-eight hours after the operation. *e* necrotic portion ; *c, d* small brushes of hypertrophied neurofibrils of the metamorphic segment ; *a, b*, persistent axial neurofibrils.

margin, and a pale granular aspect which is an indication of advanced autolysis (Figs. 38, *D*, and 39, *e*).

(*b*) *Metamorphic segment*.—Thanks to the affinity of this segment for reduced silver nitrate, one can study the agonal reactions of the neurofibrils, which begin from the eighth to the tenth hour after the lesion. They culminate during the second and third days, they diminish during the fourth, and they totally stop from the fifth to the sixth days.

These changes take on various aspects which, although they show great diversity, may be summed up in the following classes : (1) Type of pyriform thickening. The fibre, progressively thickening, generates a long club which is intensely impregnated and which is full of thick, plexiform neurofibrils (Fig. 38, C, B). Sometimes the neurofibrils of this terminal intumescence hypertrophy and become sinuous, and through resorption or displacement of other fibrils, form clear intercalary spaces. (2) Type of terminal fringe, *preceded by an axial fibre which is surrounded by a necrotic sheath*. This strange arrangement, which is shown in Fig. 39, A, D, demonstrates an interesting fact : that the neurofibrils of the axon are not absolutely dependent on one another, but have a certain autonomy. Thus the central neurofibrils (b), or the single central neurofibrils (a) are able to survive when the peripheral neurofibrils have been destroyed. One can also see that the persistent neurofibrils can ramify and invade the necrotic edges, where they stand out perfectly, thanks to their avidity for colloidal silver (a). This type, apart from the cortical necrotic segment and its living fibrils, is characterized by two regions of neurofibrillar neoformation and hypertrophy. One of these regions is central, that is, it is close to the wound, at the edge of the necrotic portion (Fig. 39, c). The other region is peripheral, fairly prolonged, and from it come the persistent axial fibrils (Fig. 39, d). In both areas the neurofibrils are hypertrophied, sinuous and ravelled like tassels or brushes (Figs. 38, 39). (3) Type in which the axial neurofibrils and the terminal tassel are absent (Fig. 39, B). The metamorphic portion in this type ends, at the necrotic segment, in a large brush of sinuous fibrils. (4) There are, not infrequently, in the course of the metamorphic portion, various necrotic vaginal portions terminated by tassels or brushes. In Fig. 45, A, we show one of these regions of cortical mortification. One can there see a beautiful plexus, formed by collateral branches issuing from the central living neurofibril, which appears to be engaged in repairing the ruins of the neurobional colony.

These curious transformations may also be observed in animals a few days old, as can be seen in Fig. 40. There one may note the great number of fibres in the phase of necrotic sheaths and axial fibrils, and the abundance of terminal clubs preceded by a long peduncle. One may also observe that sometimes in the type of necrotic edge the terminal tassel is continuous with the dilated end of an axial fibril (Fig. 40, A) of which it appears to represent a complicated ramification. In such cases the axial fibril is made up of a growing bundle of straight neurofibrils.

(c) *Zone of transition in the indifferent segment.*—In the majority of the fibres the indifferent segment begins immediately beyond the metamorphic portion. It is characterized by its relative paleness

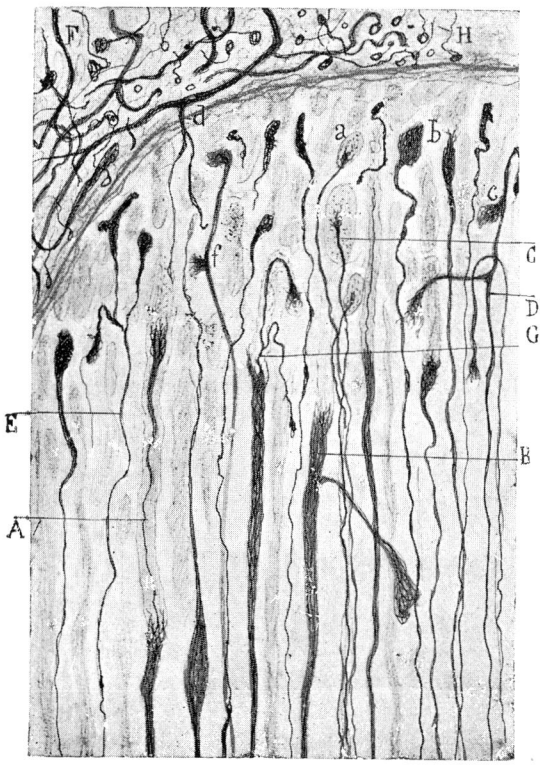

FIG. 40.—Piece of the peripheral stump of the sciatic nerve of a cat one week old, killed two days after the operation. *A, B,* medullated fibres; *E, C, D,* non-medullated fibres of Remak; *H,* exudate which is crossed by nerve sprouts from the central stump.

and its finely granular aspect. It is interesting to note that the neurofibrillar neoformations in question are present only near the wound, in those axons which are powerfully stimulated by external forces. But in some robust fibres one can still observe a transitional region which is relatively extensive and in which, apart from the neurofibrillar hypertrophy, one can see evidence of frustrated neoformations which are agonal in character.

116 TRAUMATIC DEGENERATION AND REGENERATION OF NERVES

These phenomena, which are due to irritation, have been grouped by us in three classes:

(a) *Disposition in the form of a sword-hilt.* This consists of a fusiform thickening formed at the level of the normal axonic dilatations close to the node, limited by two fine narrow regions. Within

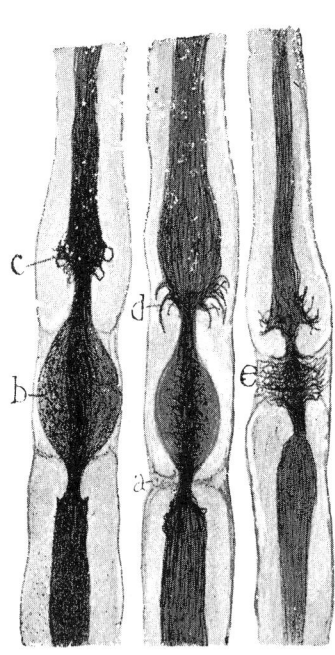

FIG. 41.—Nerve fibres of the peripheral stump of the sciatic nerve of a cat, killed two days after the operation. The alterations shown occurred at some distance from the wound. *a*, remnants of the soldering disc; *b*, axonic thickening next to a node; *c*, *d*, *e*, newly formed neurofibrillar appendices.

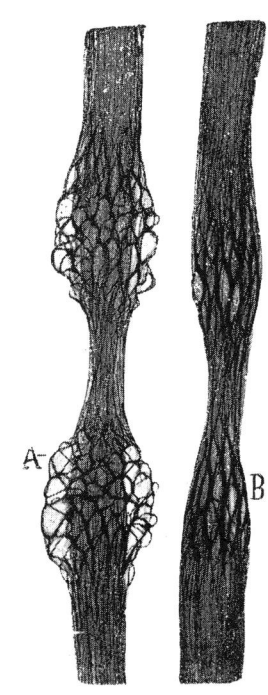

FIG. 42.—Peripheral stump from the sciatic nerve of a cat, killed two days after the operation. *A*, superficial neurofibrillar net situated near a node; *B*, cortical neurofibrillar cordons.

the fusiform intumescence one can distinguish a central bundle of more or less granular neurofibrils, and a peripheral cortex within which are numerous fine particles (Fig. 41, *b*). Farther from the bundle, in a region somewhat removed from the strangulation, that portion of the axon which is relatively normal frequently puts out newly-formed crests, handles, and spines (Fig. 41, *c*). This disposition in the form of a sword-hilt can also be discerned in fibres stained with osmic acid, as we show in Fig. 13, *a*.

(b) *Ansiform disposition, superficially reticulated.* Near the soldering disc the widened axonic regions give rise very often to superficial bundles which are deeply stained. These are analogous to the neurofibrillar spindles of the protein neurones (Fig. 42, B). The widened axonic regions also give rise at times to a complicated system of anastomosing handle-like threads which bulge out and which remind one of the fenestration of sensory cells (Fig. 42, A). These phenomena demonstrate that the region of the axon that is most sensitive and propitious for neoformation is the bundle next to the node, where nervous branches often originate.

(c) *Aborted collateral branches.* These arise at a right angle near the node, and go forward undivided or only somewhat ramified. They terminate within the sheath of Schwann in some bulky mass (Figs. 45, B, and 41, d, e).

Changes in non-medullated fibres.—In general, as noted above, the non-medullated axons resist the destructive process better than the myelinated fibres. One often finds them almost normal five and even seven days after the operation. During the first twenty-four hours after the section the non-medullated fibres become slightly varicose and, as Perroncito[1] was the first to recognize, present an elongated club which takes the colloidal silver very intensely, and ordinarily has no appreciable texture. The position of this club is variable, because of the varying length of the necrotic segment which is thin and seen with difficulty. At any rate, it is very short when compared with the long segment which is precociously destroyed in the medullated fibres.

During the second or third day one can often see that the club has grown towards the scar without having, in most cases, gone past the bounding edge of the peripheral stump, within which it can ramify. Sometimes, as we[2] have previously described in connection with the peripheral stump of young cats, the non-medullated fibre divides completely; it then gives rise to a raceme of fine branchlets, which themselves end in balls or olive-like bodies

[1] Perroncito: " La regenerazione delle fibre nervose," *Bolletino della Società Medico-Chirurgica di Pavia*, 1905.

See also his notes published in the above journal during 1906.

[2] Cajal: " Las metamorfosis de las neurofibrillas en la regeneración y degeneración de los nervios," Cajal, *Revista de Medicina y Cirugía de la Facultad de Medicina de Madrid*, Nos. 2, 3, 4, Nov. 20, 1906.

" Les métamorphoses précoces des neurofibrilles dans la régénération et la dégénération des nerfs," *Trav. du Lab. de Recherches biol.*, tome 5, 1907.

apparently directed towards the wound. In Fig. 43, where such ramifications are reproduced, one may observe that some of the spheres are at the end of thick collateral branches (Fig. 43, *a*), while others are at the end of fine branches (Fig. 43, *C, D*). There are some branchlets which, when they bifurcate, give out two adjacent buds. A detail that has already been pointed out by Perroncito is that each terminal bud consists of two parts—a cortical pale region

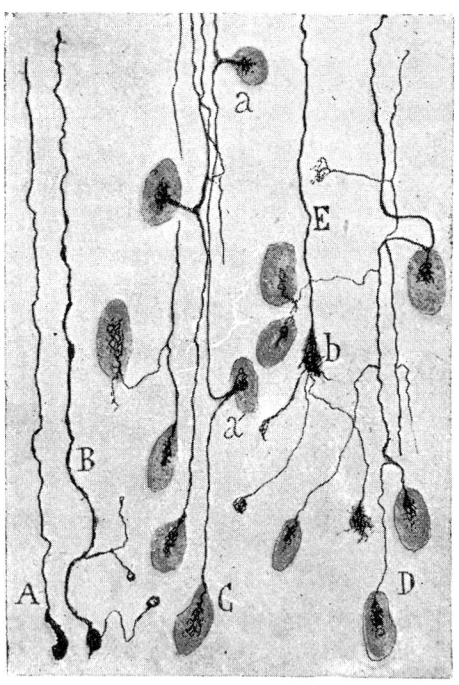

FIG. 43.—Non-medullated fibres of the peripheral stump of a cut nerve. The cat was destroyed fifty hours after the operation. In the figure the most common types of frustrated regeneration of sympathetic fibres have been brought together. *C, D*, terminal clubs; *a*, collateral clubs.

which is finely granular and has no neurofibrils, and a central region, which is composed of a glomerulus, brush or small plexus of neurofibrils in various stages of granular fragmentation. As we shall point out below, this hyaliniation of the cortex of the clubs is evidence of the beginning of a degenerative process which leads to their destruction. Some fibres end in balls or massive neurofibrillar clots, and, sometimes, in fine rings (Fig. 43, *A, B, b*).

The above-described clubs and ramifications of non-medullated fibres are also found in one-week-old cats and dogs, as can be seen in Fig. 40, E, D. There one may observe various axons terminated either by massive buds, or by buds, brushes, and tassels, which are immersed in a spheroidal club whose substance does not take the stain (a, c). Some of these ramifications probably arise from fine medullated fibres which have preserved the same activity as the non-medullated fibres (Fig. 40, G). Some of the fibres have retrograde branchlets (Fig. 40, B).

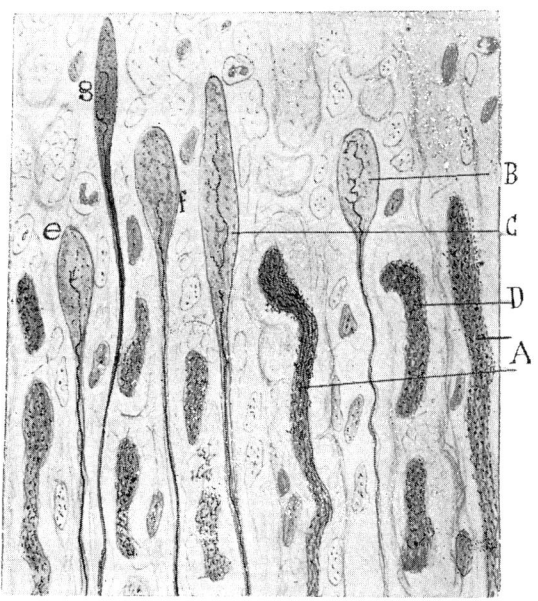

FIG. 44.—Piece of the peripheral stump of the sciatic nerve of an adult rabbit, six and a half days after the operation. A, D, axons from medullated fibres; B, C, granular masses on non-medullated fibres; e, g, clubs in whose interior appear remnants of a disintegrating neurofibril.

It was Perroncito who first pointed out the terminal clubs of non-medullated fibres.[1] He believed they were endings of sprouts, analogous to the terminal buds that we discovered in the central stump and in the scar. He also shows them as forming series along the fibres. As we have already stated, it is evident that such buds are very common especially in the ends of numerous nerve branches.

Perroncito has expressed disagreement with us in regard to these clubs. He is of opinion that their presence in fibres that are evidently

[1] A. Perroncito: "Die Regeneration der Nerven," *Beiträge zur pathol. Anat. und zur allgem. Pathol. v. Ziegler*, Bd. 42, 1907.

separated from their trophic centre and are undergoing Wallerian degeneration militates against our view that the terminal buds from the central stump and from the fibres of the scar represent structures that are homologous to the cones of growth of the embryonic period, and therefore give evidence of growth and progress of the newly-formed fibres. But we believe that the presence of buds and ramifications in the fibres of the peripheral stump, as well as the phenomena of neurofibrillar metamorphoses of the medullated fibres, so far from being opposed to our interpretation, strongly support it. For the formation of terminal buds and ramifications in the fibres of the peripheral stump simply shows that the cut axons did not immediately die, but, before the final withering and destruction, passed through a phase of survival, during which, like the axons of the central stump, they attempted regenerative processes in order to re-establish the continuity of the fibres. It is obvious that such attempts, occurring during the agony of the axons, necessarily fail. According to our observations, which coincide with those of Marinesco and Minea,[1] nearly all the clubs and ramifications of the non-medullated fibres, and all the metamorphic phenomena of the medullated fibres, disappear during the sixth, seventh, and eighth day after section of the nerve. On the tenth day all the remnants of the clubs and branches of the peripheral stump have disintegrated and been absorbed. If at this time one observes buds or fibres that take the stain well, one may be sure that these are nerve sprouts which arise from the central stump and have crossed the scar.

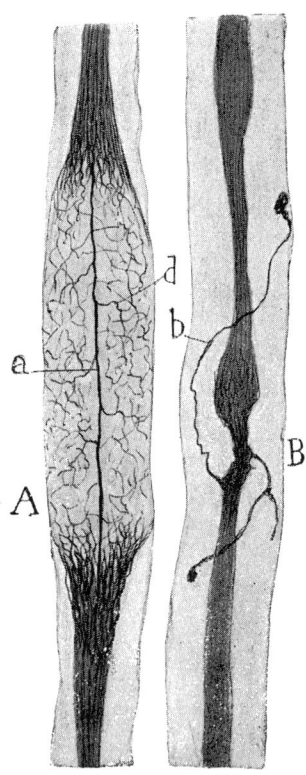

FIG. 45.—Two myelinated fibres from the peripheral stump of an adult cat, taken at a certain distance from the metamorphic portion. A, axon provided with a necrotic discontinuous cortical mantle which is innervated by a beautiful neurofibrillar plexus; B, axon with newly formed collateral branches.

The destruction of the above-mentioned agonal structures occurs through a process of granular degeneration. As may be

---

[1] Marinesco et Minea: " Précocité des phénomènes de régénérescence des nerfs, etc.," *Compt. rend. des Séances de la Soc. de Biol.*, 10 nov. 1906.

observed in Fig. 44, after six days nearly all the thick axons lack neurofibrils, and these have been replaced by a granular magma which later disintegrates (*A*). In the clubs of the non-myelinated fibres the cortical hyaline zone becomes more prominent ; the central neurofibrillar mass is finally resorbed, after having been reduced to a fibrillar axis which is more or less ramified and discontinuous (Fig. 44, *B, c, g*). One may also observe that the cortical hyalinization is often seen in the fibre itself, within which one or two granular neurofibrils appear able to resist disintegration for a certain time.

The agonal reactions of the medullated and non-medullated axons occur only near the wound and especially in the proximal ends of the fibres. One or two millimetres from the wound the axons are unable to put out sprouts, and only display the phenomena of varicosity and final disintegration—changes that are familiar to all who have studied the subject. It may thus be that the direct traumatic excitation, the exudates, or other conditions that are associated with or derived from the phlogotic act, are the cause of the generative action of the *neurobiones*, or neurofibrillar elementary units. Thus is created an environment favourable for sprouting. As we shall develop more fully later, this phenomenon demonstrates once more that the metabolism and growth of the axonic protoplasm are, above all, local processes, which are subordinated to the physical and chemical status of their surroundings.

Degeneration *in vitro* of the axons of the peripheral stump.— When we spoke above of the degeneration of the myelin, we mentioned the experiments of Monckeberg and Bethe on *post-mortem* nervous degeneration, in which they observed nerves in dead animals kept in an incubator. These experiments showed that the degenerative process is a vital act, since it occurs only in living nerve fibres. Once putrefaction begins the process stops.

In these experiments Monckeberg and Bethe observed only the phenomena occurring in the myelin in dead animals which were kept *in toto* at 39° for twenty-four hours. They were unable to see any change in nerves which were cut from the animal and which were kept in a wet chamber and in indifferent fluids, *in vitro*. Nageotte [1] has been more fortunate, in that he has been able to keep alive for many hours pieces from the peripheral stump of cut nerves. He put these nerves on slides and in warm chambers and was able

---

[1] Nageotte : "Action des métaux et de divers autres facteurs sur la dégénération des nerfs en survie," *Compt. rend. des Séances de la Soc. de Biol.*, 17 déc. 1910.

to see evident degenerative changes of the myelin and axon. According to Nageotte, in order that the nerve fibres may remain alive outside of the organism it is necessary to keep them, not in a pure solution of sodium chloride, but in a solution of sodium chloride plus a bivalent metal, such as calcium chloride. Sodium chloride preserves the nerve fibres, and suspends their life without killing them. If, after the nerves have been twenty-four hours in 10 per cent. sodium chloride, they are then put in Locke's solution, they revive and degeneration begins. A temperature of 0° or 45° C. does not allow degeneration *in vitro*. The absence of oxygen is, however, no obstacle to the degenerative process.

The observation of the peripheral stump preserved *in vitro* yields the same results with regard to the axon, as can be obtained by direct examination of dissociated nerves freshly cut from the animal. Within a few hours after the section the axons contract, lose their physiological oedema, and exude a clear liquid which dilates the myelin segments. The calibre of the axon is thus smaller than normally, and appears like that of the normal axon at the level of the strangulations. When the myelin separates from the axon, as a result of the mechanical action of the exudate, certain hyaline threads or protoplasmic trabeculae make their appearance. Nageotte believes that these are normal structures which arise from the axon, cross the myelin, and terminate on the surface of the latter. On the second day the thinned portion of the axon becomes narrower still, and the new plasmatic exudate separates out into two transparent portions which have different viscosities. One of these portions clings to the axon, forming large drops. The other, which is less viscous, diffuses out and remains free under the myelin. In the centre of the more viscous mass the axonic protoplasm undergoes a granular degeneration, which is well seen in fresh preparations.

Between the two fluids occurs the membrane which Monckeberg and Bethe called *Innenscheide*. This is, according to Nageotte, a lipoidal product and a new substance arising from the axonic decomposition. One can at a later stage see the segmentation of the myelin and axon. Thus, all those conditions which have been described in degenerating nerves within the living animal are confirmed in respect of nerves kept *in vitro*. The only difference observed by Nageotte is that in the degeneration *in vitro* and in a warm chamber the metamorphoses of the myelin and axon occur much more rapidly. This is so pronounced that at twenty-four hours the myelin ellipsoids show the characteristics of those in animals three or four days after section of the nerve.

Our own experiments concerning degeneration *in vitro* [1] corroborate the above description by Nageotte. In order to obtain more precise histological pictures, we have fixed nerves, which had been kept in the incubator for twenty-four hours or longer, in pyridine, and have impregnated them with reduced silver nitrate. In such preparations one can see that the axon goes through a granular degeneration beginning from the twelfth hour or even before. At twenty-four hours the axon appears broken up into relatively small vacuolated pieces, which are in great part contracted and corroded. The colloidal silver is attracted only by the solid portion of the axon. The hyaloplasmic exudates which were pointed out by Nageotte remain colourless. One can see already on the first day the formation of myelin ellipsoids, and one may also observe phenomena of turgidity in Schwann's cells, which are preparatory to division. These various phenomena occur even more rapidly in nerves from young animals than in those from adults. Thus fragmentation and granular degeneration of the axon were seen, after eight hours in the oven, in the posterior nerve roots of a dog a few days old. In some nerve tubes the axon was broken up into free clots which lay within small myelin ellipsoids.

As usually occurs with non-myelinated fibres, these, *in vitro*, resist degeneration better than the medullated fibres. One often finds them on the fourth day without any trace of fragmentation.

It is of interest that the degeneration of the nerve fibres outside the organism is produced in a constant way only in those nerves which are isolated and detached from the body of the animal—that is, in nerves that are preserved in a medium somewhat different from that of normal tissues. One can obtain relatively active degenerative phenomena if one keeps the pieces of nerve in a moist chamber within which are air and a certain quantity of Locke's or Ringer's solution. If, instead of an isolated nerve, one puts in the warm chamber a relatively large piece of muscle or other thick tissues, the degeneration in such portions of them as are deep and away from the air is retarded or even completely suspended, whether the tissues be or be not bathed in Locke's solution.

[1] Cajal: "Algunos experimentos de conservación y autolisis del tejido nervioso," Preliminary note Dec. 4, 1910, *Trab. del Lab. de Invest. biol.*, tomo 8, 1910.

We have preparations taken from large pieces of the soleus muscle of adult rabbits which were kept in a warm, humid chamber for five days. The axons are normal and well stained with the colloidal silver. In an eye muscle that had been thus kept in a chamber for four days one could still see the motor plates, in which only the last branchings showed some paleness and granular aspect. Thus nerves which are inclosed in the interior of a muscle and are in that way bathed by the normal muscular plasma remind one, in their characteristics, of the *preserved fibres*. Here, however, the preservation is not limited to the wounded marginal region, but occurs, on the contrary, in the deep portion of the fibres, in the region which is preserved through its very depth from the action of air and of the indifferent salt solution. On the surface of such pieces the fibres show signs of degenerative disintegration. The two types of preservations of fibres, while they appear alike, may be entirely different. This point requires further investigation. One should ascertain whether the unaltered intra-muscular nerves are really dead. The permanent absence of regenerative metamorphoses in peripheral nerves is a sign, but not a certain one, of necrobiosis.

ADDITIONAL NOTE TO CHAPTER V.

Alterations of the Golgi apparatus in secondary and traumatic nerve degeneration.—When one examines the peripheral stump, three or four days after section of the sciatic nerve, using the method of formoluranium, some interesting modifications of the reticular apparatus of the cells of Schwann become apparent, as one may see in Fig. 45A, *a, b*. In general the argentophilous substance has become richer, forming numerous grumes and cordons, which may completely surround the nucleus and are extended through nearly the entire thickness of the nerve fibre. The whole apparatus appears pulled out in an axial direction and its filaments are often arranged in parallel lines. The argentophilous masses are concentrated towards the cellular poles, forming a quadrilateral which is abruptly limited exteriorly by the curve of the neighbouring ellipsoid of myelin. In some cells of Schwann the reticulation appears broken down into a series of grains or small bacillus-like parallel bodies. Finally, when the cell of Schwann is dividing, as is shown in Fig. 45A, *a*, the argentophilous substances becomes disseminated and distributed into three masses : an equatorial mass, which is composed of cordons directed from one nucleus to the other, and two polar masses which are especially dense, and which end where the ellipsoids begin. Where the nuclei are far enough separated the ensemble of the argentophilous masses forms a large

DEGENERATION OF THE PERIPHERAL STUMP

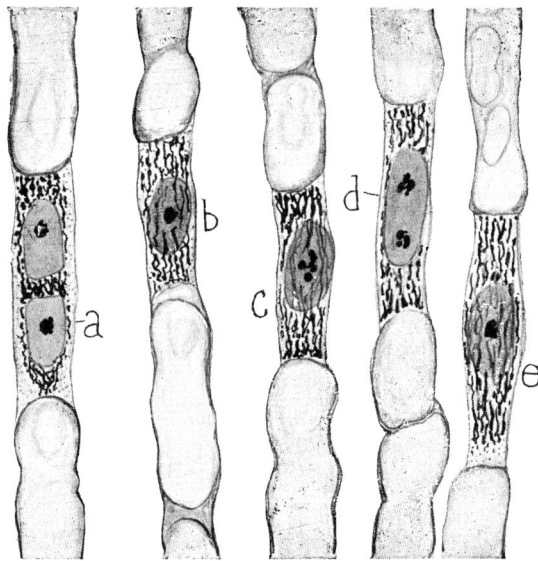

FIG. 45A.—Cells of Schwann of the degenerating peripheral stump of the sciatic nerve of a rabbit one month old, three days after the operation. *b, c, e,* disposition of the Golgi apparatus in resting nuclei; *a, d,* reticulum in cells that are in process of division.

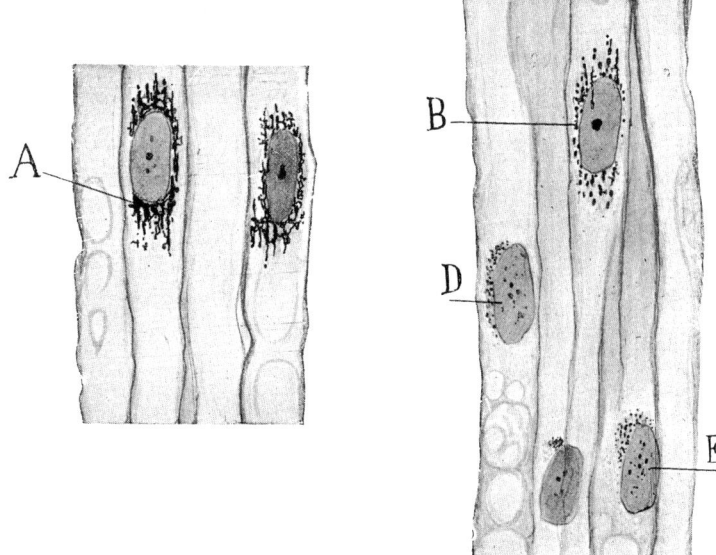

FIG. 45B.—Tubes of the central stump of the sciatic nerve of a rabbit three days after the operation. *A,* normal region far from the wound; *B,* region of the stump next to the interruption; *D, E,* atrophied and pulverized reticula.

fusiform accumulation, the remnants of the apparatus disappearing progressively from the equatorial region. We may observe that during these changes the nucleoli become especially thick, being formed by various robust spheres which join to form a block (Fig. 45A, d).

The Golgi apparatus of the central stump of the cut nerve, at the level of the region next to the wound where traumatic degeneration occurs, behaves quite differently.

The alterations observed here coincide with those observed in the traumatized cerebral cortex, that is, the nearer we come to the wound the more the reticulation disappears, and the trabeculae become converted into free grumes and granules which become successively paler. Near the necrosed region one frequently finds cells in which only one nuclear pole shows a few argentophilous granules, which are delicate and pale (Fig. 45B, E). From this region towards the nervous interruption (territory of fragmentation of the myelin and destruction of the axon) we have been unable to stain the Golgi apparatus. It seems as though its argentophilous substance has completely disappeared. In Fig. 45B we show schematically the degenerative phases of the Golgi apparatus from the wound to the necrosed regions. In regions far from the wound the reticulum of which we speak is always normal.

Thus, after nerve section the Golgi apparatus of the cells of Schwann of the proximal stump, associated to active regenerating axons, and situated far from the wound, suffers no well-defined alteration; while those situated in the attacked zone of traumatic degeneration show an altered reticulum, which is reduced to fine and pale granules.

VI

TRAUMATIC DEGENERATION OF THE CENTRAL STUMP

Degeneration of the myelin.—Necrosis and liquefaction of the terminal portion of the axon.—Digestive chambers.—Preserved fibres.—Changes occurring in Schwann's cells.—Mode of connection between the necrotic and the active segments.

It is well known that the central stump of a cut nerve, remaining as it does in direct continuity with the cell bodies or trophic centres, does not undergo Wallerian degeneration. But there is a region of the nerve—that which borders on the wound—which is the seat of serious alterations. These alterations are variable both in their quality and in their extent, according to the amount of harm done by the vulnerating agent, and according to the dimension and character of the fibres that are involved. Since these changes occur next to the lesion and are the immediate consequence of the physical injury, they have received the name of *traumatic degeneration*. With slight differences this destructive process is the same as that of the proximal portion of the peripheral stump. This is due to the fact that it is caused by the same condition—*external violence*—and that it is influenced by the same functional disorder—the traumatic inflammation.

Myelin.—All the authors, such as Engelmann, Ranvier, Vanlair, Stroebe, Kolster, Wietting, Büngner, Bethe, etc., agree that the medullary sheath of the central stump degenerates in part by breaking up into ellipsoids and fatty drops. They also agree that this degeneration is restricted to a zone near the wound. But they do not agree as to the extent of this region. Thus Engelmann believes that the degeneration extends only to the first node of Ranvier. Ranvier states that the degeneration usually stops at the first soldering disc, but that it may progress into the first or second segment. Büngner advances the view that the degeneration extends to two nodes. Finally, others, like Vanlair, admit much more extensive destructions.

In reality the extent of myelin that is involved varies much within a single nerve, even in those nerves which were sharply cut and where the bruise was reduced to a minimum. In the immense majority of cases the degenerated myelin portion is limited to a few cylinder-cones, thus involving a variable fraction only of the interannular segment. As a proof of this one may point out that in the majority of large medullated fibres an interval between two nodes measures one millimetre, while the degenerated portion of the central stump covers 0·2 to 0·4 millimetre. It may frequently be observed that the degeneration ends, not at the level of a node, but at an incisure of Schmidt-Lantermann. In the fine medullated fibres the degenerated segment is shorter than in the large ones. There are, however, in each section two, three, or more large fibres in which the degeneration extends to two or more millimetres and where myelinic degeneration therefore involves more than a single interannular segment.

While in a single nerve there are such variations in the extent of degeneration, variations are also found in the method and phases of the myelin decomposition. In Fig. 46 we show semi-schematically the principal dispositions that are found three days after the section. These can be classified as follows :

(a) Fine prolonged fibres in which degeneration is absent nearly up to the wound (Fig. 46, A). One may observe that the myelin sheath is normal up to a certain region, where it suddenly ceases. At that point the axon appears naked and disintegrating (a). In earlier stages this naked axonic region shows lipoidal granulations, doubtless rapidly absorbed.

(b) Large fibres that are preserved, almost unaltered, but less so than those described under a, up to a point near the wound. There they are in sudden connection with a granular pale segment, full of small fatty droplets which are very numerous in some places (Fig. 46, B, D).

Nearly all these fatty accumulations have a nucleus and really represent, as Ranvier was the first to note, leucocytes that have migrated within the sheath of Schwann (c). In this type, as in a, there is not so much a degeneration of the myelin as a sudden destruction of the myelin sheath, perhaps through the direct action of the vulnerating agent. The phases of long ellipsoids, short ellipsoids, etc., which are the transitions peculiar to myelin degeneration of the peripheral stump, are here absent.

(c) Large medullated fibres that are the seat of degenerative phenomena comparable to those of the peripheral stump. Here we find : a disintegrated segment with fatty accumulations of droplets near the wound ; a large portion with ellipsoids and large myelin

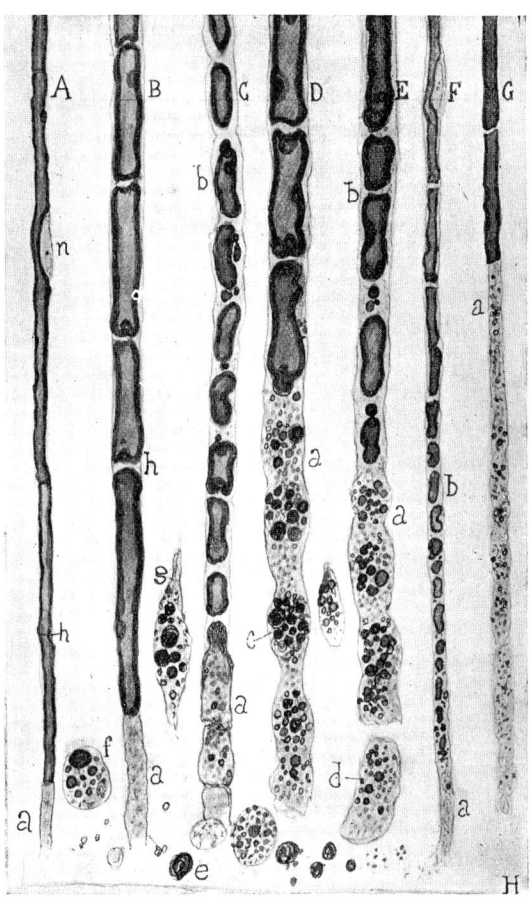

FIG. 46.—Various conditions of the medullated fibres of the central stump of a rabbit, three days after section of the nerve (semi-schematic). Osmic acid. H, level of the cut ; A, B, fibres with a short necrotic segment (a) ; D, E, F, G, fibres with a long necrotic segment ; f, g, free granular bodies ; c, intratubal leucocytes with fatty droplets.

spheres separated by protoplasmic bridges at the level of the incisures of Schmidt-Lantermann and nuclear regions ; and, finally, a normal or almost normal portion.

(d) The last class consists of very large fibres which also have the two above-mentioned segments, but in which the region of the ellipsoids is two or more millimetres long. Perhaps these fibres, which are so sensitive to the traumatism, correspond to the exquisitely vulnerable fibres in the peripheral stump (Fig. 46, C), which undergo a precocious breaking-up, as we have already described.

Many other forms exist. We may mention that in which, near the disintegrated zone, there are large ellipsoids, and, more centripetally, small ellipsoids and a few free droplets.

Finally, there are fine medullated fibres provided with long degenerating segments, in which are strings of small ellipsoids (Fig. 46, F).

At the level of the wound itself there are numerous phagocytized accumulations of myelin drops (f) and free fatty spheres released as the result of the mechanical pressure of the fibres. Between the fibres numerous phagocytes inclose lipoidal masses (g).

Such is the appearance of the medullated fibres of the central stump three days after the lesion. It is obvious that it is different on the preceding days, but, in order not to spend too much time on this analysis, we need give no details. We may point out, however, that from the fifth to the seventh or eighth day a good many of the ellipsoids and phagocytized drops have been resorbed. This work of destruction and absorption falls much more upon the migratory cells than upon the cells of Schwann. Its chemical mechanism is much in need of investigation.

Cell of Schwann.—When the central stump of a nerve is stained with Unna's *polychrome blue* and other aniline dyes, or by the various haematoxylin methods, the nuclei of the cells of Schwann can be well seen. One can then confirm the assertion of nearly all the authors, such as Ranvier, Nothafft, Stroebe, P. Ziegler, Büngner, Wietting, Bethe, etc., that such nuclei proliferate near the wound from the fourth day after the operation or even before. One can also see that, as they state, during the following days the nuclei draw apart, the cytoplasm of Schwann's cells grows, the cells take on a fusiform shape, and finally form a *syncytium* or longitudinal chains. Thus the cells of Schwann of the central stump behave, in its degenerating portion, more or less like the similar cells in the peripheral stump.

In the central stump, however, apart from a regulated regenerative act, there also occurs, as various authors affirm, a sudden disorganization of a more or less extensive portion of the fibre. There are thus in the central stump two segments : the *terminal or disorganized segment*, and the *segment normally degenerated*.

(a) The *terminal or necrotic segment* varies in extent in each fibre. As we pointed out in respect of the degeneration of the myelin, it is the large fibres that show the largest necrotic extent of axon and

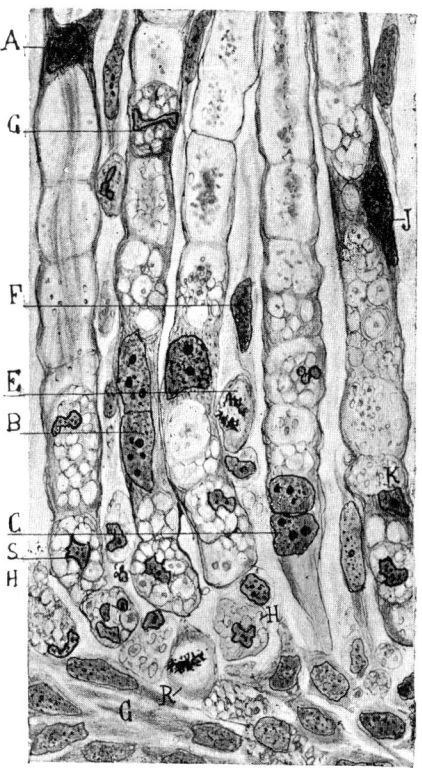

FIG. 47.—Central stump of the sciatic nerve of a cat three days after the section. *A, J*, cells of Schwann of the degenerated portion ; *B, C*, cells of Schwann of the necrotic portion ; *K*, cell of Schwann which is contracted and probably necrotic because of its proximity to the wound ; *G, S*, intratubal leucocytes ; *H*, extratubal leucocytes which are full of fat ; *E, R*, mitoses in connective tissue cells of the endoneurium ; *F*, normal cell of the endoneurium.

Schwann's cell. During the first and second days there are few fibres in whose disorganized region can be found nuclei of Schwann that are alive, that is, that are not broken and that take the stain well. There are, nevertheless, exceptions. In Fig. 47, *B, C*, one can see very near the wound surviving cells of Schwann. This is doubtless due to the fact that the central stump of this nerve was little bruised.

On the other hand, numerous leucocytes appear from the second day on. Ranvier showed that these cells enter the fibres through their amœboid motion, and place themselves among the broken pieces of myelin, which they engulf and digest. Büngner and other polygenists believed that these nuclei belong to cells of Schwann. But such nuclei, which are found precociously in the necrotic portion of the fibre, belong to leucocytes. This can be proved by the fact, shown by Fig. 47, *G*, *S*, that they are relatively small and that they are often lobed. The nucleus of Schwann's cell is ovoid or triangular, is of much larger size than the nucleus of the leucocytes, and contains two or more stout nucleoli (Fig. 47, *J*). From the end of the second day, or during the third day, the phagocytes already contain a large number of fatty spheres. In those preparations which are stained with the aniline dyes no fat is seen, but one observes an abundant protoplasm which is alveolar in structure, that is, full of vacuoles of various sizes (Fig. 47, *S*). Besides the leucocytes and the fatty remnants, the necrotic portion of the fibre contains clots and granulations which belong to the axon and also remnants of the nucleus of Schwann's cell; the latter cell sometimes appears contracted and atrophied (Fig. 47, *K*). The membrane is well preserved, appearing wrinkled and with dilatations which correspond to the fatty accumulations. In many cases the membrane narrows and even closes up at its end, near the wound, forming a *cul-de-sac*— the digestive chamber. Around the membrane the bundles of the *sheath of Key and Retzius* are still found, although they are irregular and contracted. To show them one must use Mann's solution or else the silver methods described above.

Between the fibres that are being destroyed one sees, from the second day on, many migrating leucocytes, some of which are stuffed with lipoid masses, and numerous dividing cells of the endoneurium (*E*). On the third day the edge of the central stump is itself covered and invaded by a multitude of fibroblasts which have come from the matrix (Fig. 47).

(*b*) The *degenerated or living portion of the nerve* is that portion where ellipsoids are formed, and it shows essentially the same structure as the peripheral stump. We need not enter into details concerning the cells of Schwann. It is only necessary to say that their nuclei divide, forming longitudinally-placed pairs (Fig. 47, *B*), and that their cytoplasm grows, filling the spaces between the ellipsoids, and forming thin walls, annular thickenings, and complex reticula. One can see in Fig. 47, where we show Schwann's cells three days after section of the nerve, that the division of the nuclei occurs very early, and that, in part at least, this division is amitotic. One can also conjecture from this figure that the newly-formed elements are able to advance towards the necrotic portion near the wound, where later they will protect the outgrowing axons.

As one follows the nerve in a centripetal direction one can see that the cells of Schwann show less modification. They preserve during the first few days their normal structure and tangential position (Fig. 47, J). They nevertheless have more cytoplasm than normally and they stain more deeply with methylene blue (polychrome blue of Unna) than is usual. Both of these characteristics are also true of dividing cells. Later, from the fourth day on, some of the nuclei at the border of the degenerated region divide, usually mitotically.

As Stroebe, and later many other neurologists have shown, the various modifications of Schwann's cells caused by the traumatic stimulus have nothing to do with the generative process of the new axons. Their accessory function seems to be to prepare the resorption of the fatty and axonic remnants, and their principal function to create a reserve of young cells which will replace those which are destroyed, and also to provide satellite cells to the abundant nerve sprouts which grow out from the central stump.

Degeneration of the axon.—As with the myelin and cell of Schwann, the central stump shows, as regards the axon, two well marked regions—that which borders on the wound and that which is far from it.

In the *border region* the axons undergo many degenerative changes, which it is impossible to reduce to definite classes or types. Nevertheless we shall mention, provisionally, and pending a more careful analysis of them, the most usual dispositions shown in the central stump near the wound.

1. *Axons that break up rapidly.*—A piece of varying length of a medullated fibre shows, from the fourth or sixth hour after the section on, a pale mass, finely granular, irregular in outline, which appears to float in a marginal liquid (Figs. 48, g, and 49, I). This pale substance is not stained by colloidal silver or basic aniline dyes, and is nothing more than the terminal portion of an axon which suddenly becomes necrotic. It is itself undergoing digestion. Sometimes colloidal silver shows, in the thickness of such hyaline

conglomerations, central clots formed by granulations that are somewhat argentophilous. Finally, that is, from the second day on, the remnants of the axon, mixed up with lipoidal drops, become resorbed, thus leaving a clear field to the newly-formed sprouts.

2. *Granular axons that are broken in pieces.*—These are relatively large and are surrounded by myelin ellipsoids. In silver nitrate preparations, these axons present a similar appearance to those in the peripheral stump, that is, forming granular cylinders that are spiral, flexuous, and contracted (Fig. 55). This form of degeneration, which goes on less rapidly than that described in 1, corresponds to the process in those segments which show a true degeneration of the myelin and cells of Schwann. These segments often come very close to the edge of the wound, owing to the small area that is destroyed.

3. *Pale vacuolated axons with neurofibrillar remnants.*—Some medullated fibres show, instead of necrotic masses that are more or less broken down, axons that are neither fragmented nor granular. These axons are weakly stained with colloidal silver and methylene blue (Mann's fluid). They are found abundantly from the sixth to the twenty-fourth hour after the lesion. They show large longitudinal vacuoles and, sometimes, ravellings with more or less apparent neurofibrils (Fig. 48, f, h). At their ends they show a bulb, brush, or irregular pale mass, which is occasionally bifurcated and tangential to the wound. Finally, within some large vacuoles one can see, here and there, necrotic ovoidal clots, or pieces of the axon, surrounded by a protoplasmic cortex which is less broken down.

We believe that these dispositions are evidence of a slow necrosis which is preceded by degenerative phenomena of the neurofibrillar framework. As to certain forms that are somewhat stained by colloidal silver, it is hard to determine whether the axons are dead, or whether they are only diseased, being perhaps able to recover their affinity for silver and to undergo a formative turgidity.

4. *Preserved fibres.*—These are a less frequent, but not exceptional, form of terminal axonic necrosis. As stated above, these axons are flexuous, compact, deeply stained with reduced silver, and they appear normal in structure and size, as though they were entirely refractory to the digestive processes going on in the nerve fibre (Fig. 49, A). As can be seen in Fig. 49, E, the preserved portion ends centrally in a point of corrosion or autolytic point, which is sometimes swollen, vacuolated, or granular. Towards the wound the

axon emerges, terminating in a handle or describing circumflexions (Fig. 49, *A*).

Between the preserved segment and the living portion of the axon there is a piece which undergoes disintegration. This is the autolytic segment. As we shall describe below, the swollen sheath

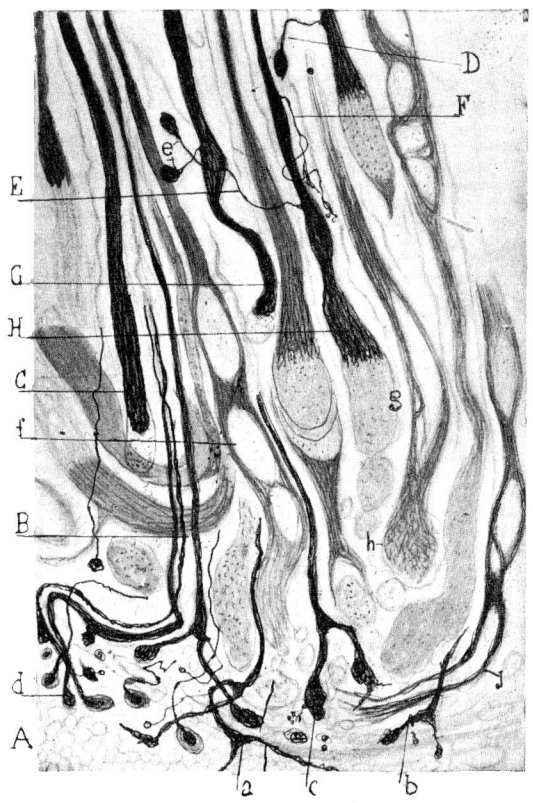

FIG. 48.—Piece of the central stump of the sciatic nerve of a rabbit, six hours after the operation. *A*, wound and blood; *B*, non-medullated sprouting fibres; *f*, necrotic masses within axons; *g, h*, necrotic portion of large axons.

within which lie the preserved axons is ulteriorly invaded by the nerve sprouts.

5. *Non-medullated fibres of Remak.*—These fibres, in a large majority of cases, lack a necrotic segment or have one which is extremely short and can hardly be seen. Thus the region of *formative turgidity* lies next to the lesion, and it is there that later the club of growth will very precociously appear (Fig. 48, *B*).

6. *Thin medullated fibres.*—These behave very much like the non-medullated fibres, showing a necrotic segment that is extremely short and sometimes not recognizable, and, in consequence, they extend toward the wound a long metamorphic portion which shows formative turgidity (Fig. 48, *G*). We shall speak later of their terminal club and ramifications.

It is difficult to understand the cause of the variety of aspects shown by the terminal portion of the medullated fibres. In a single nerve one can see all the forms that we have described and others that we have been unable to study carefully. As to the extent and varieties of the necrotic process there is little doubt that the variety of traumatic actions, such as lacerations, compressions, bruises, etc., have here some influence. One must also take account of the normal physiological differences of the fibres. It is certainly curious that nerve fibres that lie next to one another and that are of equal size show very different aspects and degrees of vulnerability. We know nothing, however, of the correlation between the mechanical mode of action and the degenerative process.

The opinions of investigators with regard to the axonic degeneration of the central stump have been very much divided. Ranvier believed that a more or less elongated piece of the sheath of Schwann degenerated, that the axon did not do so, but that it hypertrophied, took on a longitudinal striation which was more apparent than normally, and prepared to sprout. Others, like Engelmann, Büngner, Wietting, Stroebe, Perroncito, Marinesco, etc., recognized that, besides the corresponding myelin segment, traumatism also involved a more or less extensive axonic segment. Thus the regenerative process takes place not only in the scar and peripheral stump, but also in a considerable portion of the central stump. The two opinions are reconcilable if neither is advanced as a general law. We have already stated that the necrotic portion produced by the mechanical action is very variable in a single nerve, depending on the diameter of the fibres and certain as yet unknown physiological conditions. Thus Ranvier may have been right if his observations related to fibres that were but little wounded, in which the living segment extended to very near the wound. Engelmann, Büngner, etc., also were right when they described axonic portions that had undergone degeneration and necrobiosis. Many of the contradictions are more apparent than real, when they concern the degenerative and regenerative phenomena of the central stump. They can be explained not only by the various effects produced by the same cause, but also by the variability in reaction of individual nerve fibres.

Mode of connection between the necrotic portion of the axon and the metamorphic portion or portion in formative turgidity.—The living portion is at an early stage separated from the dead part by

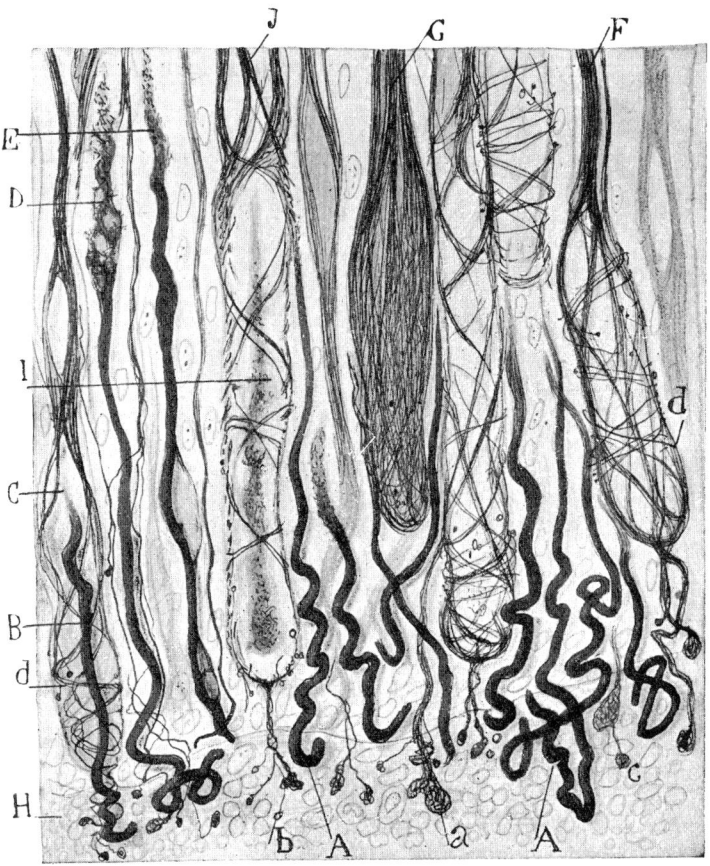

FIG. 49.—Central stump of the cut sciatic nerve of an animal, killed fifty hours after the operation. *A*, preserved fibres partly immersed in the exudate of the wound; *B*, preserved axon surrounded by newly formed fibrils; *C*, point of corrosion or disintegration; *D*, disintegrated and apparently vacuolated piece of a preserved fibre; *G*, living axon which limits the digestive chamber of a mantle of neurofibrils; *d*, typical digestive chamber with sprouts going out to the wound through the inferior opening of the nerve tube; *I*, nerve tube without a preserved axon, whose axon is in full disintegration within a digestive chamber.

a well-marked border. One can already see it from four or six hours after the traumatism. Besides the terminal swelling or club of growth, which appears very early in some fibres, the living segment is differentiated from the dead portion by its homogeneity, absence of granulations, and especially by its avidity for colloidal silver.

138 TRAUMATIC DEGENERATION AND REGENERATION OF NERVES

This avidity not only allows one to distinguish the dead part from the living, but often also hypertrophied neurofibrillar tissue from an indifferent axon.

Another distinguishing characteristic of the living portion is the exaggeration of its striated aspect, a phenomenon that was first noted by Ranvier, and has since been confirmed by Perroncito, ourselves, Marinesco, Tello, etc., with the various neurofibrillar stains.

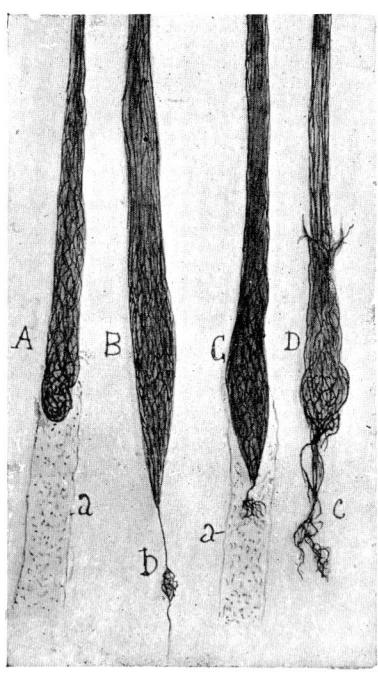

FIG. 50.—Varieties of termination of the axon and of its connection with the necrotic segment thirty hours after the operation. Central stump of the cut sciatic nerve of a cat. a, necrotic segment; b, c, neurofibrillar appendices with neoformations and agonal ravellings present in the interior of the necrotic segment.

Not only are the neurofibrils seen better, but, as Marinesco observes, they are found in full multiplication, although this is less evident here than in the large terminal clubs and balls.

As to the mode of connection between the dead portion and that which is living there are many varieties, which depend on the shape of the dead piece and, especially, on the interval allowed after the operation before the nerve is observed.

During the first six hours there is as yet no separation of the two portions in many axons. In these the dead portion borders on and appears to be substantially a continuation of the living segment (Figs. 48, H, and 51, A). The division is easily recognized, however, since there is at that point a kind of brush or bulb in which one can distinguish the neurofibrils more or less deeply impregnated. From the twelfth to the twenty-fourth hour the autolytic segment has completely separated from the necrosed part. An intercalary plasmatic space is, with some exceptions, now present. During this

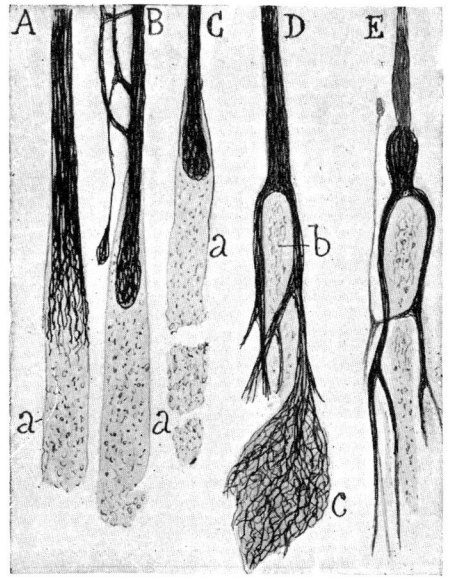

FIG. 51.—Central stump of the sciatic nerve of a cat, fifty hours after the operation. A, uniting point between the living and the dead portions (a), where there are hypertrophied neurofibrils; B, C, axons whose ends are in the form of bulbs immersed in the disintegrated segment; D, E, axons from whose terminal bulb arise newly formed fibrils.

last phase the end of the axon often shows a certain concavity which joins on to the disintegrated part.

After one or two days the living portion becomes wider, often transforming itself into a club or bud, which is strongly differentiated, by its deep colour, from the necrosed mass (Fig. 51, B, C). The forms shown by the living portion vary greatly, according to the fibres and the stage of regeneration. In Fig. 50 we show a few of the dispositions that may be observed in the central stump of the sciatic nerve of a cat killed thirty hours after the operation. One of the most common is the mass that is a little swollen and looks like the end of a probe. This penetrates the axis of the axonic remnants (*A*). Here and there one sees pointed ends with fine appendices terminated by a neurofibrillar clot, as shown in Fig. 50, *a*, *b*, *c*.

These clubs and masses do not all possess a generative capacity. As we shall point out below, some of them, especially those which are pointed, vacuolated, and irregular, are really diseased and abortive.

VII

REGENERATIVE PROCESS OF THE CENTRAL STUMP

Preliminary phenomena (formative turgidity) of the axonic neoformation.—Formation of the nervous sprouts.—Forms of sprouting: *terminal or direct neoformation of the non-medullated fibres of Remak, of the fine medullated fibres; direct sprouting by ravelling.—Indirect terminal neoformation, or at a distance from the wound.—Collateral neoformation.—Various forms of such regeneration.—Apparatus of Perroncito.—Ravelling of the collaterals.—Avalanche of ramification and avalanche of growth.—Sterile nerve tubes.—Course of regeneration in the central stump.—Retrograde fibres, arrested fibres, and spiral structures.*

Preliminary phenomena of axonic regeneration.—We have already said that the living portion of the cut axon rapidly differentiates itself from the necrotic segment by a line which later becomes a fissure or transversal plasmatic space, and that the end of the axon, as Ranvier, Stroebe, and others of the older histologists saw, and as modern investigators have confirmed, exhibits a swelling or thickening of varying form and length. We may note in passing that the swelling described by the older authors represents mostly the weak and degenerating end of the old axon. But besides these weak and sterile end dispositions, of which we shall have more to say below, there are others which are active, capable of sprouting, and to which we have given the name of *bud* or *club of growth*, because of their analogy to the *cone of growth* of embryonic axons.

Our investigations [1] showed that such a terminal bud *is found, not only at the end of active axons, but also at the ends of collateral and terminal outgrowing branches*. The importance of this discovery lies in the fact that the club above mentioned *marks indubitably the true end of the fibres and the orientation of their growth*. Those authors

---

[1] Cajal: "Sobre la degeneración y regeneración de los nervios. First Note." *Boletín del Instituto de Seroterapia, Vacunación y Bacteriología*, June 30, 1905.

who, like Ranvier, Vanlair, Stroebe,[1] Kolster, P. Ziegler, Büngner, Wietting, etc., used preferably the methods with osmic acid or with basic aniline dyes, were never able to see with certainty the true terminus of the non-medullated and young fibres, nor even that of medullated fibres when these end in a naked axon, which it is almost impossible to show in ordinary preparations. The terminal bud or club of growth has been confirmed by all the modern authors such as Lugaro, Marinesco, Minea, Nageotte, Perroncito, Tello, Poscharisky, Deineka, G. Sala, Medea, O. Rossi, Modena, Doinikow, that is, by all those who have used neurofibrillar stains. Krassin and Modena also saw the terminal clubs by using the methods of Ehrlich and of Donaggio. We shall point out below that there are various kinds of clubs and that all have not the same significance nor the same morphology.

Metamorphosis of the terminal swelling of the axon.—This mass changes shape. At first—from the second to the fourth hour—the end of the axon is hardly modified, presenting only the appearance, as we have already stated, of the end of a probe, or of a neurofibrillar brush (Fig. 58, *C*, *G*, *H*). At times, as one can see in Fig. 55, *B*, the above-mentioned end of the axon shows a slight cavity in which is lodged the end of the necrosed segment. From the fifth hour on, however, the enlargement grows and the end of the axon takes on an elongated or olive-like appearance. This disposition is, however, variable, and there are cases in which, twenty-four or forty-eight hours after the operation, the sound-like or brush-like appearance is still to be observed.

Formative turgidity or state of amoeboid division of the axon.—The end of the axon is not the only part of the nervous protoplasm that is affected by the traumatic shock; to a greater or less extent, depending on the fibres, that portion of the fibre which precedes the swelling is also affected. The traumatic shock is propagated centripetally, creating in the protoplasm special chemical, physiological, and morphological modifications. Three characteristic

---

[1] It was Stroebe, among the older investigators, who studied the appearance of the ends of the nerve sprouts with the greatest success. He homologized this end with the *cone of growth* that we had shown in embryonic axons. Unfortunately his method did not permit him to see clearly the ends of the fibres as they grew across the scar and distal stump. Thus, the form that he called *tip of a sound* appears only very exceptionally in the nerve sprouts.

conditions are clearly seen in the irritated portion of the axon, including the terminal bud: (1) A protoplasmic turgidity brought about by absorption of the surrounding plasma ; (2) a strong affinity of the neurofibrils for colloidal silver. According to Perroncito and Marinesco, these appear abnormally large and prominent ; (3) the

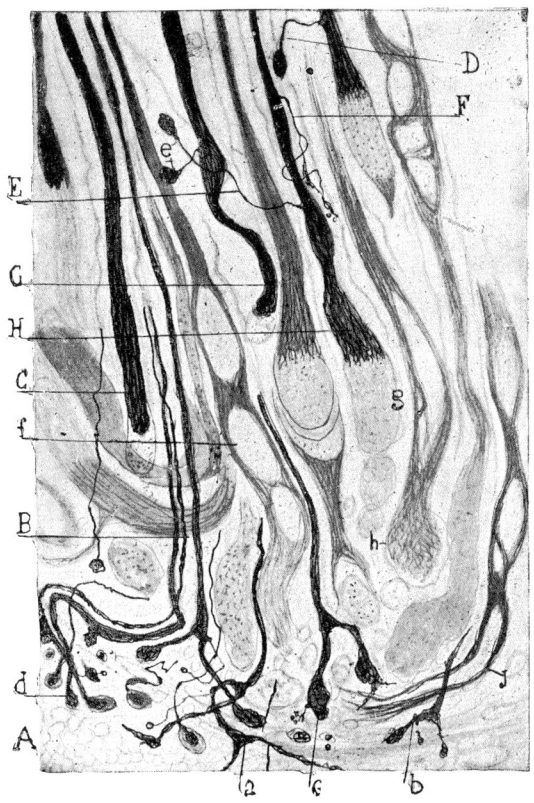

FIG. 52.—Piece of the central stump of the sciatic nerve of a rabbit, six hours after the operation : *A*, wound ; *B*, non-medullated fibres ; *C*, axon ending as the tip of a sound ; *D, F,* newly-formed collateral fibres ; *d*, clubs of non-medullated fibres ; *g*, necrotic segment.

capacity to produce nerve sprouts. It would seem that the entire thickened portion of the axon has gone back to an embryonic state, differentiating itself in its structure from an adult fibre. Its protoplasm is doubtless the seat of an active assimilation and reconstruction of the neurofibrillar tissue. We have called this strange rejuvenescence of the axon, very briefly, the *state of formative turgidity* or of *stimulation to division*. Its extent is very limited in non-medullated fibres, longer in fine medullated fibres, while it involves two or more nodes in large tubes.

As we shall point out below, when we describe the genesis of collateral fibres, besides this continuous *formative turgidity*, which occurs in the pre-terminal regions of the axon, there are also discontinuous segments of *stimulation to division*, which are far from the terminal club, and which appear as muff-like regions near the nodes of Ranvier (Figs. 58 and 59).

FORMS OF THE NERVOUS NEOFORMATION

All the variations of growth that were described or supposed to be present by the older workers, as well as those observed by modern authors, such as Purpura, Cajal, Perroncito, Krassin, Marinesco, etc., may be grouped under two heads : the *terminal axonic neoformation* and the *collateral neoformation*. We shall show that both of these may be found in a single fibre, bringing about very complicated structures and processes.

Terminal axonic neoformation.—This was supposed to be present by such of the older investigators as Notthafft and Ranvier, and it has been well demonstrated by ourselves, thanks to the method of reduced silver nitrate. Marinesco, Deineka, and other authors have also observed it, although in ordinary nervous regeneration (in adult animals, where the section is accompanied by a certain amount of bruising), it is less frequent than collateral neoformation.

In this kind of sprouting there are two varieties :

(1) *Direct or distal sprouting.* This occurs at the end of axons that have almost no necrotic segment or where the necrotic segment is very short and almost indistinguishable.

(2) *Indirect or proximal sprouting.* This occurs in axons of which a certain portion, more or less long, is necrotic. This distinction is not absolute, since all axons lose some protoplasm as a result of a direct traumatism. But the disposition and course of the sprouts in each case permit such a differentiation. The direct or distal sprouting commonly occurs in non-medullated fibres, in fine medullated fibres, and in the majority of fibres of recently-born or a few-days-old animals, where there is as yet no myelin, or only a very thin sheath.

Direct sprouting of non-medullated fibres.—From the sixth hour onwards, or even before, these fibres show a terminal segment that is more or less turgid and is prolonged up to very near the wound. The necrotic portion is very short and is difficult to observe. Sometimes, however, one can see it as a series of pale granulations near the edge of the wound. From the sixth hour the extremities of those axons which have the appearance of the ends of sounds become dilated into terminal clubs. In the following hours one can see the clubs advance towards the wound where sometimes they remain undivided, sometimes divide to give birth to secondary branches.

After twenty-four hours several terminal clubs have gone beyond the limit of the nerve and have penetrated into the exudates. As may be seen in Figs. 52, d, and 55, E, these clubs often form clusters or bundles, and those which are going through the blood coagulum sometimes appear as though they were undergoing a degeneration, in that they show a stainable centre and a granular and colourless cortex. The nerve branches that originate in the terminal buds are often seen in the wound from the twenty-fourth hour onwards. Some of them, when they encounter the exudates or the cicatricial tissues which form an obstacle, turn back and become retrograde. This also occurs with medullated axons. Ordinarily the nerve branches issue from the terminal club itself, and end, after a variable course, in clots or buds of small size. Between the branchlets present in the exudate or the scar one always sees some that end in a curious structure composed, not of massive protoplasm, but of a fine neurofibrillar ring. This was first seen by Perroncito in the outgrowths of medullated fibres. These rings are strongly stained by silver. We shall speak of them in detail below.

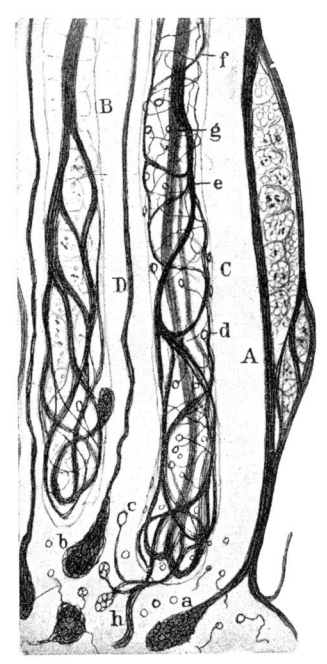

FIG. 53.—Central stump of the sciatic nerve of a cat, killed fifty-two hours after the operation: A, B, axons in which terminal branches arise at some distance from the wound; C, fibre with spiral branches; D, non-medullated fibre; a, b, h, clubs of growth; c, terminal ring.

Direct sprouting of fine medullated fibres and of medium-sized medullated fibres.—This type can be distinguished from indirect or proximal sprouting in that, from the first few hours after the lesion onwards, the terminal club is found near the wound, and the branches that arise from it are free from the beginning, sprouting, not inside, but underneath the interruption of Schwann's sheath. From the second or third day the branches have penetrated into the

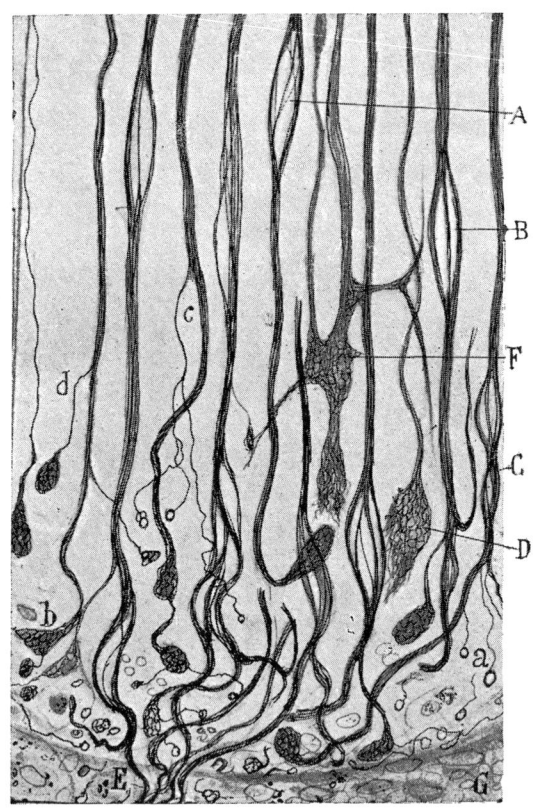

FIG. 54.—Central stump of the sciatic nerve of a fifteen-days-old cat, killed two days after the operation: *A, B, C*, axons with vacuoles and ravelled appearance; *D*, large terminal growth of laminar shape; *E*, axons that go out into the exudate; *F*, thick fibre which gives birth to a retrograde branch; *a*, terminal rings.

scar, producing new outgrowths at a time when the large majority of the branches in those fibres which undergo indirect or proximal sprouting have not yet emerged from Schwann's sheath. They are thus obliged to overcome the obstacle of the axonic clots and the fatty drops. As one may observe in Fig. 61, *C, K*, each branch originating at the principal club also ends in balls or rings. One does find, however, as we shall point out below, terminations in

REGENERATIVE PROCESS OF THE CENTRAL STUMP 147

the wound that have the form of tassels or spindles, more or less ravelled.

Direct sprouting by ravelling.—Sometimes that part of the axon which is near the wound shows longitudinal vacuoles, which separate

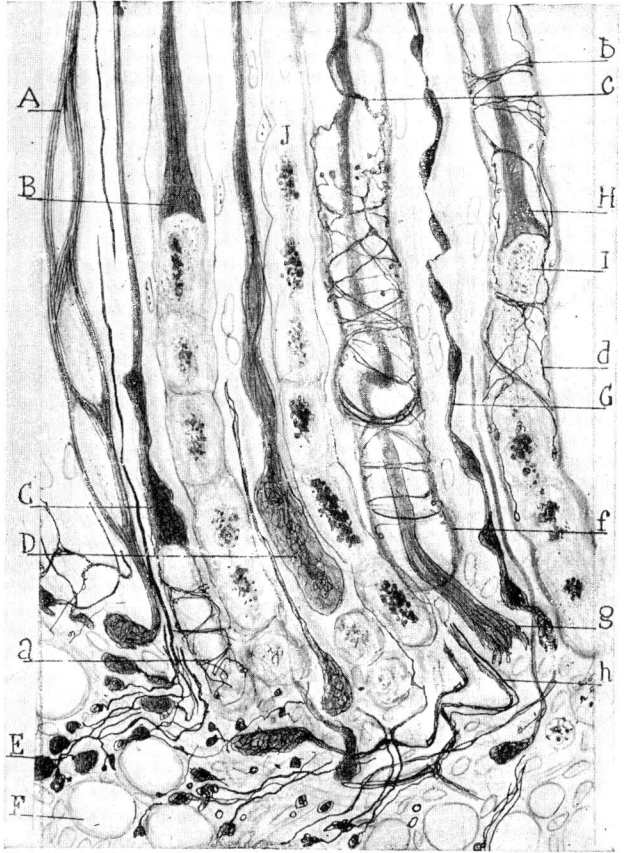

Fig. 55.—Piece of the central stump of the sciatic nerve of a cat, killed twenty-four hours after the operation. *A*, ravelled and vacuolated fibre ; *E*, clubs of non-medullated fibres penetrating into the exudate ; *G*, club terminated by a concave surface ; *B, H*, axonic tips not yet in the form of clubs, in contact with the necrotic portion ; *F*, adipose cells ; *I*, necrotic portion of the axon ; *b, c*, collaterals that give rise to Perroncito's spirals.

bundles of neurofibrils. These bundles come out at an acute angle, their fibrils are dissociated, and they may give birth, once arrived at the wound, to large numbers of branches. We do not know whether all these precocious ravellings are normal phenomena. We believe, however, that those produced in some medullated axons of young animals are normal. We show these in Fig. 54, *B*, *C*. Similar phenomena are found, although less frequently, in the medullated fibres of larger diameter, as can be seen in Fig. 52, *J*.

The older investigators, such as Waller (1852) and Bruch (1862) already spoke of ravelling of the neurofibrils (*primitive fibrils of M. Schültze*) as a method of formation of the bundles of new fibres in the central stump. They attributed such ravellings to the central axons, and not to the branches, where they principally take place, as we shall show below. No matter how they originate, a good many of the daughter branches, having reached the edge of the nerve, turn back and become retrograde, going either inside or outside the sheaths of Schwann (Fig. 56, *e*). Such retrograde projections often bifurcate and end in clubs of various shapes. Naturally, the retrograde branches of the non-medullated fibres are always interstitial or extratubal. We shall speak of these later.

Indirect terminal sprouting, or at a distance from the wound.—As we have already stated, this type involves the necrosis of a long axonic segment, a process associated with the preservation of Schwann's sheath, and the creation of a digestive chamber. It is in this chamber that the axonic and fatty detritus is ulteriorly destroyed. This form of sprouting is common to all the large medullated axons and to a large number of medium-sized ones.

As might be expected, this method of neoformation involves a certain retardation in the growth of the sprouts to the wound. As a matter of fact, the terminal bud, which is in contact with the necrotic masses, may remain as though paralyzed for twenty-four or thirty hours, or even longer. But, in spite of that delay, the terminal bud finally disappears, giving rise to a fork ; the arms of this fork travel under the sheath of Schwann, close to the necrotic segment, whose upper end is at the angle of bifurcation. This can be seen in Fig. 53, *A*, *B*, and in the schematic drawings, *B*, *D*, of Fig. 62.

In Fig. 62, *D*, one can see that the club, which has already disappeared, has given rise to two robust branches, which closely embrace the necrotic piece. In *A*, Fig. 62, the terminal bud has given rise, not to two or more branches, but to a single branch which is placed somewhat laterally, to pass round the axonic *caput mortuum*. In any case, the newly-formed branch or branches run underneath the membrane of Schwann, leaving in the centre the fatty and axonic remnants, up to the free end of the sheath. They then plunge towards the wound. In their intra- and extratubal paths the branches may repeatedly bifurcate, each branch giving

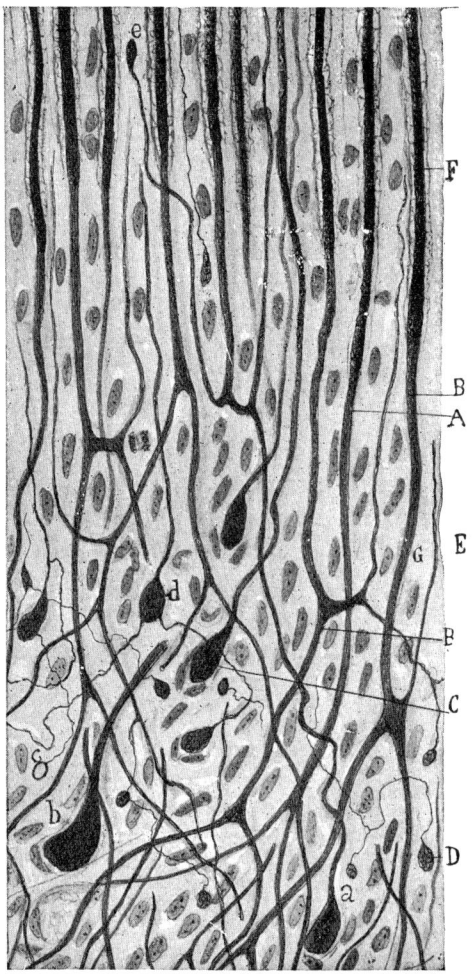

FIG. 56.—Longitudinal section of the central stump of the sciatic nerve of a cat, killed four days after the operation. *A*, newly-formed portion of a central medullated axon; *B*, ramified fibre with retrograde branches; *F*, medullated portion of *A*; *C*, axon undivided as yet and terminating in a club; *a*, small terminal buds; *b*, large clubs; *e*, retrograde club.

origin to a bundle of fibres, which are separated from each other by very acute angles.

This important form of terminal sprouting is shown in several figures (Fig. 53, *A*, *B*). One should especially study the schematic drawings of Fig. 62, where three typical examples are shown ; that is to say, where the axon gives rise to a single robust branch (Fig. 62, *A*), and where two conductors arise at a sharp angle, and are progressively ramified (Fig. 62, *B*, *D*). Retrograde branches, relatively rare in this type of axonic neoformation, are nevertheless seen here and there (Fig. 62, *A*, *f*).

Regeneration through collateral branches.—When the nerve fibres have been much bruised they are liable to show two segments at their ends : a necrotic segment, which is generally long, and a living segment, which, however, is weak, and unable to regenerate. As a result of this the sprouts come, not from the terminal club, but from a turgid region situated above it and more or less remote (Figs. 55, *c*, 62, *C*, and 52, *F*, *D*).

The collateral neoformation had already been observed and drawn by Stroebe, who saw it in the central stump from the seventh to the fifteenth day after section and compression of the nerve. In his drawings the branches in question, which are few in number—usually one—are very long, and they arise at a certain distance above the terminal club or mass of the axon.

Our observations likewise concern late stages of regeneration—from the fifth day on. We have confirmed the presence of these branches and their numerous bifurcations in preparations made with reduced silver nitrate. Already in our first preliminary note [1] on nervous regeneration (June 30, 1905), after mentioning the method of terminal division, we said : " At other times, from the axon arise one, two, three, or more collaterals, which travel underneath Schwann's membrane, sometimes towards the wound, sometimes retrogradely." And we added : " Certain axons give rise, at a right angle, to fine appendices which end at a greater or lesser distance within Schwann's sheath, in reticulated clubs or clots ; some of these daughter fibres trace spirals around the axon of origin." But these descriptions related to animals killed between the fifth and the tenth day. It thus was Perroncito [2] who had the honour of detecting the collaterals and the spiral dispositions from the first moments of their formation—six to twelve hours or more

[1] Cajal: *Boletín del Instituto de Seroterapia, etc., de Alfonso XIII*, June and September, 1905.

[2] Perroncito : " La rigenerazione delle fibre nervose." Preliminary notes II and III published, respectively, Nov. 3, 1905 and Jan. 26, 1906, *Bolletino della Società Medico-Chirurgica di Pavia*, 1905 and 1906.

—and of having given, before anyone else, a detailed description of them, as well as suggestive and beautiful figures. Finally, later observations by ourselves,[1] and simultaneously by Marinesco and Minea [2] have confirmed the precocity of the process and all the curious forms described by Perroncito.

In our preparations of young cats and dogs the above-mentioned collateral branches are easily recognized from the sixth hour on, and

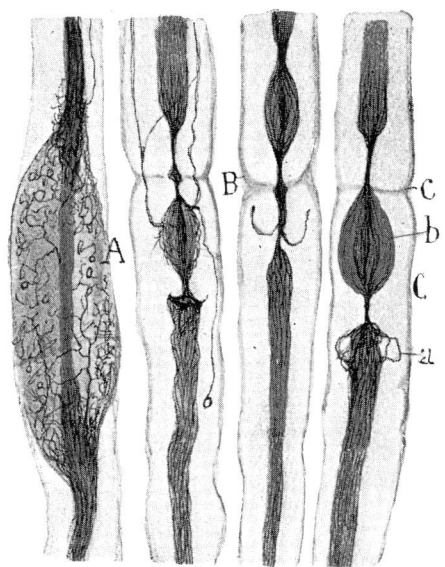

FIG. 57.—Fibres from the central segment of a crushed nerve. Adult cat, killed fifty hours after the operation. The three fibres on the right have collaterals in the region next to the node, or *germinative zone*. *a*, neurofibrillar handles; *b*, fusiform swelling of the axon; *B*, *C*, nodes that have a tendency to disappear.

they are very abundant at the tenth or twelfth hour. Moreover, when one considers that at such a time some of these projections already constitute complicated ramifications (Fig. 52, *F*), an even earlier appearance must be attributed to them.

The above-mentioned branches are not common at first and issue from any region of the turgid segment. They preferably appear, however, in two positions. These are : (1) Near the terminal club

[1] Cajal : " Les phénomènes précoces," etc., *Trav. du Lab. de Rech. biol.*, tome 5, 1907. A previous study was published in the *Revista escolar*, June 20, 1906.

[2] Marinesco et Minea : " Précocité des phénomènes de régénérescence des nerfs après leur section," *C.R. de la Soc. de Biol. de Paris*, 10 nov. 1906.

or brush; this was seen by Stroebe and well demonstrated by Perroncito; (2) they are especially found in more proximal regions corresponding to the axonic swellings near the node. In general, it seems to us that the *collaterals that are nearest to the necrotic segment appear indifferently in any region of the axon; the branches that are distant from the necrotic segment, that is, those which start far up at the beginning of the normal segment, appear exclusively, or almost exclusively, at the dilatation near the cementing disc.* For brevity, we shall designate the above-mentioned impressionable region of the

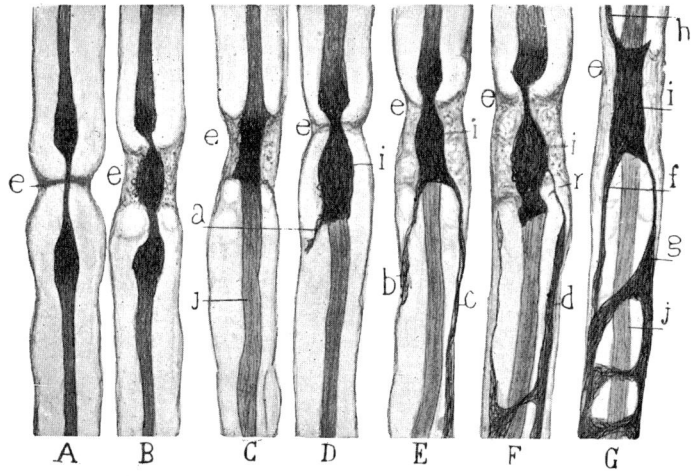

FIG. 58.—Central stump of the sciatic nerve at some distance from the wound. Adult cat, killed fifty hours after the operation. *A*, normal node; *B*, node in which the axon is fusiform; *C*, node about to disappear; *D, E*, germinative muff developed near the node; *F, G*, muffs with thick intratubal branches; *e*, node; *j*, axon; *b, c*, nerve sprouts; *d*, fine branch which becomes thicker; *f, g*, long branches from a germinative muff.

axon the *germinative territory or zone*. This region rapidly—from the twelfth to the twenty-fourth hour—passes into formative turgidity, it thickens considerably, and it takes on the shape of a muff—the *germinative muff*. We shall subsequently give its form in detail, and describe the branches that originate from it.

In Fig. 58 we show the metamorphoses of the nodes of Ranvier and immediately neighbouring regions in the central stump, fifty hours after section of the sciatic nerve, in an adult cat. *A* shows a normal node (*e*), with the axon thinned and relatively pale. The state of turgidity through traumatic excitation sometimes causes the hypertrophy, as in *B* and *C*, of the part of the axon within the node, and the disappearance of the cementing disc; at the sides appears a certain protoplasmic mass which nearly obliterates the nodes of Ranvier. Such fusiform swellings are, in most cases, without branches. Sometimes they give rise to loops and handles and cotton-like accumulations of filaments (Fig. 58, *B*, *e*). Exceptionally we have seen fine branches arise from such spindles, directed towards the wound and situated beneath Schwann's sheath.

On the other hand, the *germinative muffs* situated near the node are nearly always fecund (Fig. 58, *I*). Ordinarily only one of them, that one nearest the wound, becomes unusually thick, is deeply stained with silver, and emits sprouts. One finds, however, fibres that are provided with germinative muffs above and below the node of Ranvier, both of which are fecund. In *F* and *G* the sprouts, thin at the outset, become thicker and longer; they travel under the sheath of Schwann, become more or less ribbon-like and membranous, and often give out branches which come out at, or almost at, a right angle. In such fibres the node is almost unrecognizable at the level of the sheath of Schwann, but the axon sometimes remains (*F*). When, as in *G*, the axon's *germinative zone* gives out ascending and descending branches, all sign of a node has disappeared, and one sees around the stimulated muff a granular mass formed by the protoplasm of Schwann's cell (Fig. 59, *a*).

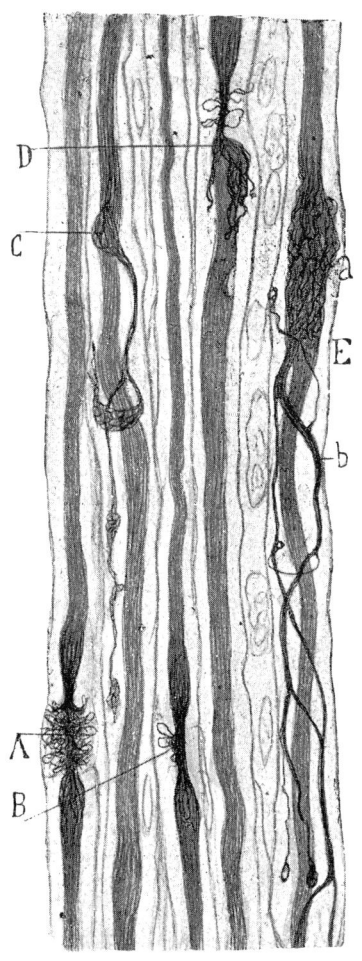

FIG. 59.—Central stump of the sciatic nerve of a rabbit, two days after the operation. Region of the nerve somewhat far from the lesion—almost a millimetre. The nodes have partly disappeared. *a*, germinative zone in the form of a muff, from which arises a collateral fibre which travels toward the wound; *D*, another germinative zone from which arise some incipient collaterals; *A*, *B*, loops and cotton-like projections in regions near the node of Ranvier; *C*, collateral arising from a germinative muff which is little apparent.

It is not always easy to correlate the region of origin of the collaterals with the state and disposition of the myelin sheath. We shall not, however, we think, be far wrong if we say that the majority of the collaterals issue between the degenerated portion of the myelin (region of the ellipsoids) and the normal segment. As the degenerated portion of the myelin sheath is sometimes very short, one understands why the collateral and terminal branches are formed in places very near the wound.

Collateral branches also emerge, although rarely, a little beyond this transitional region, that is, in the indifferent segment. They usually originate at the nodes of Ranvier, where the axon is somewhat thickened, staining deeply with colloidal silver, while the cementing disc is more or less resorbed. Such collaterals, that is those which are far from the wound, have been described by ourselves and others as appearing rather late within the central stump. These distant branches naturally travel along the interstices of the endoneurium. Further, some of these distant collaterals arise from the generative zone. In such cases they immediately perforate the sheath of Schwann and become extratubal.

In general, with some exceptions, the new branch is thin at first and thickens as it proceeds (Fig. 58, *r*), becoming striated, as though its neurofibrils were splitting longitudinally; finally the fibre rapidly elongates and ramifies. This progressive thickening of the collateral we have termed *avalanche of transversal growth*. It has great theoretical importance, for it shows that the assimilative act is principally governed by local conditions.

As to the number of branches and the time of their formation, there are many variations. In some preparations, after twenty-four hours, one sees no collateral branches, while in others they are very numerous from the sixth or twelfth hour after the operation. These differences are visible in a single section, since next to large fibres filled with intratubal branches and plexuses there are others showing no sign of sprouting, or provided only with terminal branches.

After these general remarks, we may now pass on to the description of certain forms of collateral ramification, which we shall separate into *intratubal* and *extratubal*.

Intratubal branches.—It is these which are most abundantly found during the early phases of sprouting, and they take on the following dispositions:

(*a*) *Short collateral loops and efflorescences.* In that portion of the metamorphic region which is farthest from the wound one often sees fine loops arising near the nodes (Fig. 59, *B*), or else delicate appendices arranged in a sort of peri-axonic moss (Fig. 59, *A*); or finally tassels or tufts which cover a piece of the axon, ending in rings (Fig. 59, *D*). Certain axonic thickenings, at whose level the protoplasm shows thick and plexiform neurofibrils (Fig. 59, *E*), are also an indication of the presence of collaterals. This is especially the case with certain local thickenings of the cortical mantle of the axon, arranged in the form of a muff, from which collaterals often arise. We shall speak more in detail of these *neurogenic muffs*, which we have already mentioned, when we describe degeneration following pressure.

We believe that the majority of these appendices represent sprouts or branches in the first moments of their genesis. On the other hand, the ansiform and cotton-like disposition may represent the result of a formative stimulus that was aborted or sterile.

(*b*) *Fine and small collaterals terminating in rings*. Axons may not infrequently be observed from whose surface issue, at an acute angle, one or several fibres. These are placed longitudinally on the axon, and they terminate in clots and rings. They give rise to a delicate inframyelinic plexus by their ramifications and crossings (Fig. 63, *B*, *d*).

(*c*) *Long branches, relatively thick, issuing at an acute angle, and completely ramified under Schwann's sheath*. These arise at any place along the axon. They show conical structures where they encounter Schwann's membrane, and at that point they turn back either towards the wound or in a retrograde path. On their way they bifurcate repeatedly, and their branches, usually ending in clubs or rings, constitute in the cortical region of the fibre a complicated plexus of longitudinal meshes (Figs. 59, *b*, and 55, *b*, *c*). Some clubs, when they encounter Schwann's membrane, instead of continuing in a longitudinal direction, become transversal, and, through stereotropism, of which we shall speak below,[1] they become

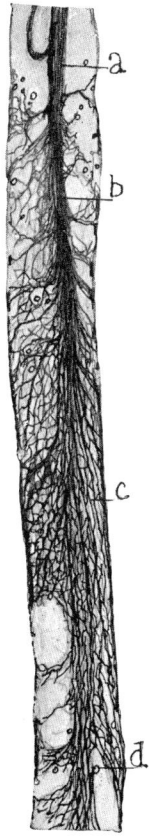

FIG. 60.—Net from a robust collateral branch, more or less extended and vacuolated. Central stump of sciatic nerve of a rabbit, fifty-four hours after the operation. *a*, branch from axon; *c*, membranous neurofibrillar net; *d*, terminal ring.

[1] See p. 186.

intimately applied to the membrane, forming loops and spirals under it. Very naturally the extent and amplitude of this tangential plexus depend on the length of time that has elapsed since the operation. In any case, the presence of these collateral branches occurs very early, since, as can be seen in Fig. 52, *f*, one can already

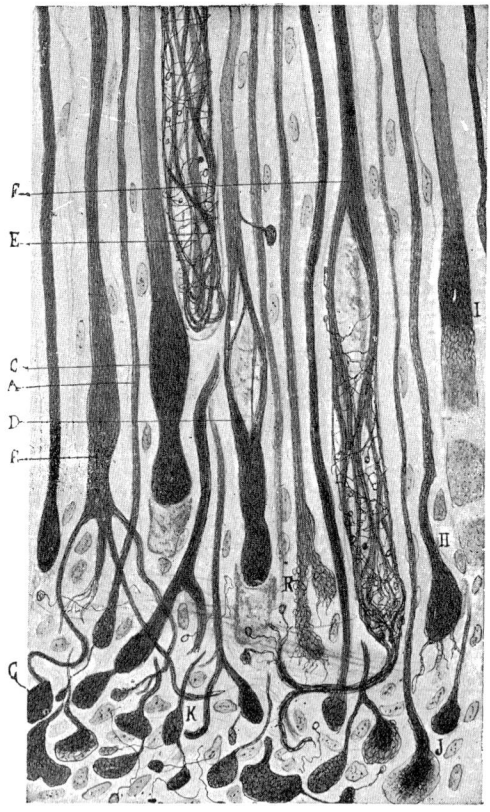

FIG. 61.—Central stump of the sciatic nerve of an adult cat, killed two days after the section. *A*, non-medullated fibre; *B*, medullated axon ending in terminal branches; *E*, *F*, structures of Perroncito.

after six hours detect a few delicate intravaginal branches within some large fibres. It is only from the twelfth to the twenty-fourth hour, however, that such appendices take on a great extension. They sometimes form, through their acute-angled bifurcations, complicated plexuses around the axonic remnants, as can be seen in Fig. 55, *b*, *c*, *d*. In the following two or three days the form, length, and direction of the collateral branches show much variation.

One often sees structures having the form of reticulated ribbons, spades, rackets, etc., which are more or less ravelled towards their tips. Sometimes, as may be observed in Fig. 60, the branches form thin expansions under Schwann's membrane, wide nets of elegant

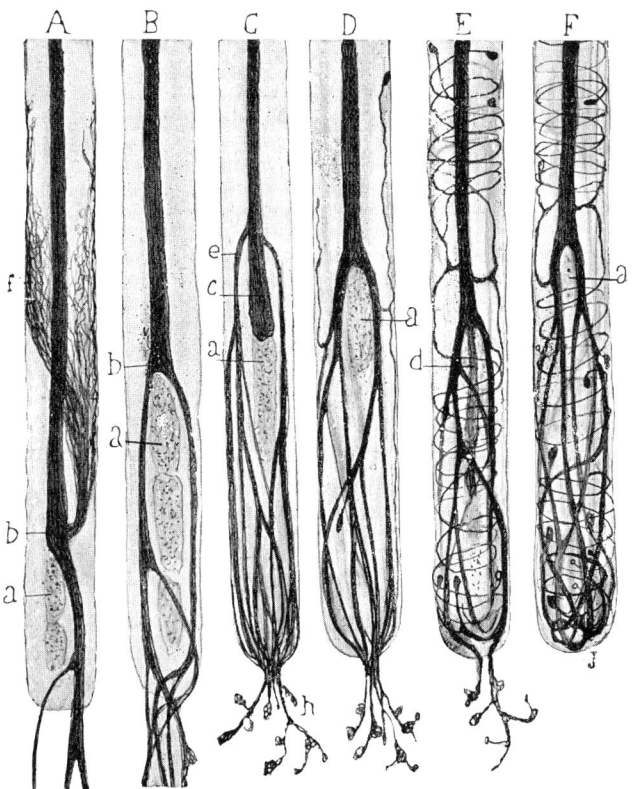

FIG. 62.—Schematic drawings of the form of the nerve branches in medullated fibres, three and a half days after section of the sciatic nerve. *A*, axon that gives rise to an ascending and a descending branch; *B*, axon with two terminal branches; *D*, axon analogous to *B*, but whose branches give rise to intratubal recurrent twigs; *C*, axon with collaterals and a sterile tip (*c*); *E*, helicoidal apparatus of Perroncito, with emergent branches; *F*, sterile apparatus of Perroncito, that is, without emergent branches; *a*, necrotic portion of the axon; *d* sterile segment of the axon in an apparatus of Perroncito.

design. This delicate membrane displays a very clear neurofibrillar reticulum, with primary and secondary filaments, and it has here and there a vacuole. As we show in Fig. 49, *G*, it may extend into true reticulated sheaths, within which appear the remnants of the axon and myelin. Ordinarily the net formation becomes more accentuated the nearer the branch is to its termination; the latter is also often modelled into a brush or membraniform ravelled appendix. From the net often arise fine branchlets which end in rings (Fig. 60, *d*).

Forty-eight or more hours after the operation the intratubal nerve plexus which is formed by the sprouting, growth, and ramifications of the collaterals, is complicated in an extraordinary way, and an apparatus or structure is formed which, because it was first described by Perroncito, is named after him.[1] Its principal components are as follows : Schwann's membrane appears dilated, ending at the side and near the wound as a more or less rounded *cul-de-sac*. There is thus formed a vast longitudinal reservoir in which are found fatty detritus and remnants of the necrotic portion of the axon—the *digestive chamber* (Figs. 49, *b, d,* and 53, *B, G*).

The nervous part shows three variations :

(1) In certain digestive chambers the more or less broken-down old axon subsists. Around it, underneath Schwann's membrane, are found great numbers of oblique, longitudinal, nerve branches, and especially spiral branches, which are extremely long, and of a variable diameter. Each one of these branches divides repeatedly, retrogressing or advancing within the digestive chamber, according to the path of least resistance. The last projections show, according to their size, clubs, buds, or rings (Figs. 55, *c,* and 62, *F, E*).

(2) In other cases the digestive cavity lacks the old axon, containing only the spiral structures, the detritus of the necrotic portion of the axon, and remnants of myelin (Figs. 49, *l, d,* 61, *F,* and 62, *F*).

(3) Finally, there are mixed structures of Perroncito in which, besides the complicated plexus of collateral, longitudinal, and spiral branches, there are present great numbers of terminal branches arranged in longitudinal lines, oblique or parallel, and more or less ravelled. The combinations of these various kinds of fibres—the spiral twigs and the longitudinal nerve plexuses, the helicoidal fibrils emerging along the course of some of the longitudinal shoots, the quantity of more or less voluminous rings and clubs scattered

[1] We have proposed the name of *apparatus of Perroncito* for the spiral and plexiform dispositions precociously found in the medullated fibres (from the twelfth to the forty-eighth hour). But we do not claim that Perroncito was the first to discover the helicoidal structures. As a matter of fact Ranvier, in 1873, saw the spools and spirals of medullated fibres, while those of non-medullated fibres, found from the tenth day after the operation, were described by us in 1905 (*Boletín del Instituto de Seroterapia*, June 1905). Marinesco also described the latter a short time after (November 1906).

throughout the arborization and marking the terminus of the nervous projections, etc.—all these factors lend to the apparatus, from the forty-eighth hour on, a complexity and intricacy not susceptible of precise description. In Figs. 53 and 61, *E*, we show some structures of Perroncito that are relatively simple, taken at a time when the fibrils can still be traced to their origin. But there are some such structures so intricate that it is impossible to give a decipherable picture of them. The schematic drawings of Fig. 62, *E*, *F*, reveal clearly the essential structure of the principal types.

Fate of the apparatus of Perroncito.—Those structures of Perroncito which are little complicated, especially those in which the longitudinal branches begin to appear outside the bottom of the digestive chamber, form regenerative dispositions which are useful for nervous reunion of the scar tissues and peripheral stump (Fig. 53, *C*, *E*). Those structures, however, where the longitudinal branches, once arrived at the bottom of the reservoir, turn back and generate new inextricable spirals and plexuses, represent dispositions that are pathological and sterile (Figs. 53, *B*, *J*, and 62). Later we shall point out that these centres of over-abundant and frustrated neoformation subsequently change into the *spiral structures* of Ranvier, that is, into aberrant nervous dispositions.

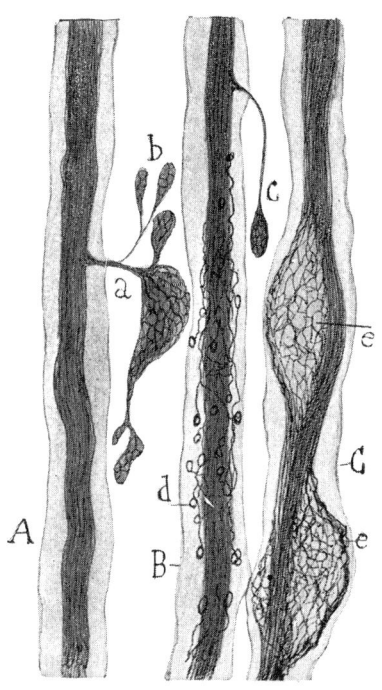

FIG. 63.—Axons in the phase of divisory turgidity. Central stump of a cat, killed fifty hours after the operation. The region seen is somewhat removed from the wound. *A*, axon that gives rise to an extratubal branch ; *B*, axon with an extratubal branch and a multitude of fine longitudinal fibrils which lie on the axon ; *C*, axon with vacuoles surrounded by beautiful neurofibrillar nets.

The existence of the apparatus of Perroncito has been confirmed by ourselves, Marinesco and Minea, Tello, Deineka, Dustin, and by Modena, who used the method of Donaggio to demonstrate it. Poscharisky and Doinikow, using Bielschowsky's method, have also been successful in impregnating the simpler forms of this apparatus, also confirming the presence of the terminal clubs, the rings, and the axonic excrescences.

Extratubal branches.—The large majority of collateral branches arising in the metamorphic portion of the axon represent intratubal collateral projections. In some cases, however, one finds a few extratubal projections. These are robust branches, originating at a right angle, whose pressure on the wall of the fibre finally causes a laceration in Schwann's membrane, and whose terminal bud is then seen in the endoneurium.

We show two typical examples in Fig. 63, A, B, where are reproduced nerve fibres from a cat killed fifty hours after the operation. It can there be seen that the newly-formed branches originate at a right angle and terminate in olive-like excrescences which are clearly reticulated. One of the branches is broken up into a small branchlet of clubs (Fig. 63, a). The formation of extratubal collaterals may occur very precociously. We have found them, at times, six hours after the operation, as is proved by Fig. 52, D, E, where we show two projections of this type. Later, the extratubal branches may grow, turning into bifurcated axons and becoming covered with a medullary sheath. To this type probably belong some of the divisions of medullated fibres seen in late stages in the central stump, of which we shall give examples below.

Progressive disappearance of the weak tip of the axon.—We have stated that in collateral regeneration there necessarily remains below the point of origin of the sprouts a segment of the axon of variable length, whose lack of fertility, numerous vacuoles, and other signs of alteration, show that it is in a pathological state or that there is a grave lack of nutriment. What is the fate of such sterile clubs and segments ? Perroncito believes that this terminal portion of the axon always degenerates and that it finally disappears. He does not give, however, the details of such a degeneration.

Our studies on the central stump of cats and rabbits killed from the sixth to the ninth day after the operation show that in many cases, and perhaps always, the above-mentioned portion of the axon is effectively resorbed. The last collaterals that were formed are thus transformed into terminal branches. In Fig. 64 we show the principal phases in the process of resorption. At first—from the fourth to the fifth day—the segment of which we are speaking retracts and becomes varicose (Fig. 64, A, B). Later the varicosities and terminal club become full of vacuoles, which lend to the neurofibrillar frame a spongy appearance (Fig. 64, *C*). Finally, the point of origin becomes much thinner and then breaks asunder (Fig. 64, *e*). In Fig. 64, *E, g*, we show the remnants of a partly broken-down segment. One can see that, while the weak axon atrophies, the terminal branch or branches become thicker, in such a way as to appear to be the true continuation of the living part of the axon.

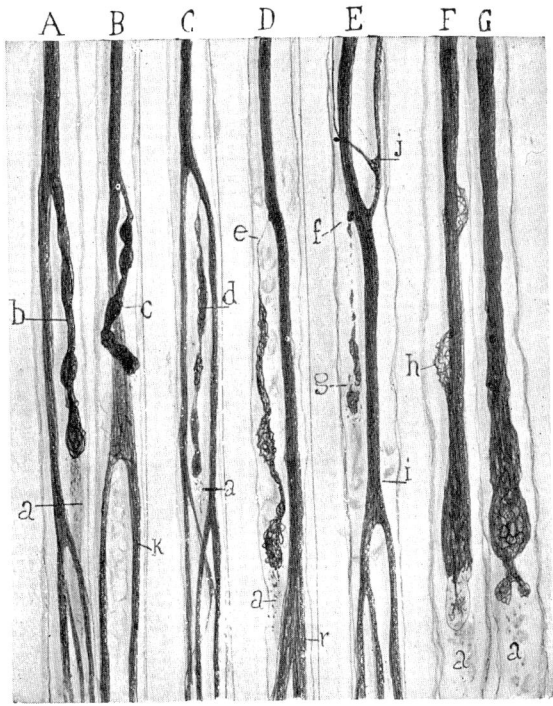

FIG. 64.—Phases of resorption of the sterile axonic tip situated below the collaterals. The sciatic nerve was ligatured and cut below the ligation. The nerve sprouts, after crossing the ligature, invade the scar. Cat killed seven days after the operation. *A, b*, terminal portion of the axon, varicose in appearance; *B, c*, terminal portion of the axon where the point of union of the axon with the collateral is beginning to atrophy; *C, D*, external narrowing of the axonic pedicle (*e*); *E, f*, rupture of the axonic pedicle, and continuity of the branch with the axonic stem; *F, G*, sterile axons; *g*, remnants of the old axon.

When the process is completed, one is unable to recognize the region where the end of the old axon originated. Besides its theoretical importance, the process of absorption has a certain practical importance. An investigator unaware of its existence, and studying the late stages of nervous regeneration, would easily mistake fibres which arose as collaterals for terminal fibres. The existence of sprouts which were originally terminal can only be affirmed with certainty when the examination is made during the first three or four days after the operation.

Ravelling of the newly-formed branches.—In all the methods of sprouting that we have described the newly-formed intratubal fibres, and especially those which travel longitudinally under Schwann's sheath, possess the strange property of dissociating their neurofibrils as they are formed, giving rise, at an acute angle, to very numerous independent branches, which are almost parallel. There are some nerve sprouts that generate by this method, along a short stretch, ten, fifteen, and even more individual projections. Such filaments, which are very delicate, and comparable to neurofibrils at their origin, become progressively thicker, and they appear, some hundredths of a millimetre from the point where they arise, clearly striated, that is, composed themselves of a bundle of neurofibrils.

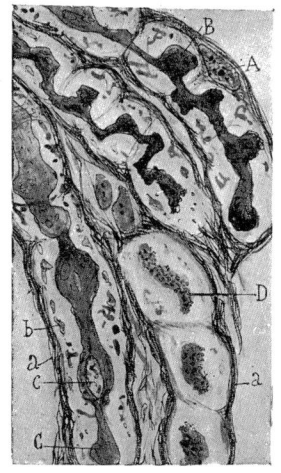

FIG. 65.—Ends of some sterile fibres. Fixation in potassium bichromate-formol. Stained with Mann's fluid. Central stump of a rabbit, killed six days after the operation. *A*, cell of Schwann ; *B*, outgrowths from a sterile axon ; *D*, axonic pieces in granular degeneration ; *a*, connective sheath of the fibres ; *C*, terminal ball of an axon ; *c*, vacuoles.

There are thus, in the process of growth of the collateral and terminal fibres, two avalanche phenomena ; the assimilative avalanche, wherein each branch increases in width, and the avalanche of ramification, where a collateral fibre emits as it advances, and by way of disintegration, great numbers of independent projections. Both phenomena are evidence of a very active nutritive process in the nervous protoplasm, a process which, it is needless to say, draws upon the local fluids and excitatory enzymes. This and other phenomena of neurofibrillar creation oblige one to believe that within the ultramicroscopic units in the protoplasmic skeleton there are present transversal and longitudinal divisions, which cause the formation of new series or linear colonies. We shall speak of this hypothesis below.

When we study the effects of ligatures and sudden pressures on nerves, we shall again occupy ourselves with this curious process of ramification *through dissociation or ravelling*. For the present we shall note only that branches formed in this way are characterized by their almost parallel paths, and by the fact that they follow closely, through a strong stereotropism, the inner surface of Schwann's membrane, accommodating themselves to its widenings and narrowings. As is shown in Fig. 62, C, such fibres surround the necrotic portion of the axon, they touch one another in certain narrow portions, and they finally arrive at the scar, forming independent conductors which end in terminal buds.

The ravelling appears also in many fibres of the apparatus of Perroncito, as we have already stated. Ravellings, more or less like those which we have described,[1] have also been described by Perroncito, Marinesco and Minea,[2] Tello, Dustin, Deineka, and Doinikow.

Sterile axonic tips.—In the cases of regeneration thus far described, we have been dealing with axons whose turgid tips or their pre-terminal regions are at a very early stage the seat of acts of neoformation. There are, however, nerve fibres, generally of large diameter, in which neither the enlarged tip nor the long pre-terminal segment, which appears to be stimulated, show, at least during the first four to six days following the section, active phenomena of sprouting. We do not mean to imply that they are unable to bring about neoformations, but that, once begun, the latter are unable to develop indefinitely. This class may be divided into (1) axons without sprouts, and (2) axons provided with aborted excrescences and shoots.

Both sterile and indifferent axons can be recognized in ordinary preparations, especially in those stained with Mann's fluid or by Stroebe's method. As can be seen in Fig. 65, c, such fibres sometimes are varicose, with thickenings that are either massive or vacuolated; in other cases the axon describes zigzags, all the while showing varicosities and even outgrowths; finally there are fibres whose monolateral thickenings show granular or vacuolated outgrowths (Fig. 65, B).

In preparations made with reduced silver nitrate the sterile fibres appear very deeply stained, with unequal edges which appear festooned, and with large varicosities, the last one of which consti-

[1] Cajal: " Les métamorphoses précoces des neurofibrilles dans la régénération et dégénération des nerfs," *Trav. du Lab. de Recher. biol.*, vol. 5, 1907.

[2] Marinesco et Minea: " Précocité des phénomènes de régénérescence consécutifs à la greffe des ganglions sensitifs chez le chat," *Comptes rendus des Séances de la Soc. de Biol.*, July 22, 1907.

164 TRAUMATIC DEGENERATION AND REGENERATION OF NERVES

tutes a large bud. In some axons one sees that, while the deep zones are indifferent, the superficial layer shows a laminar area, more or less extensive, and formed by a reticulum of strong neurofibrils and of relatively large meshes. In some cases the trabeculae hypertrophy, resembling the robust neuronal cordons of hydrophobia. Sometimes the fungiform lateral protuberances, instead of

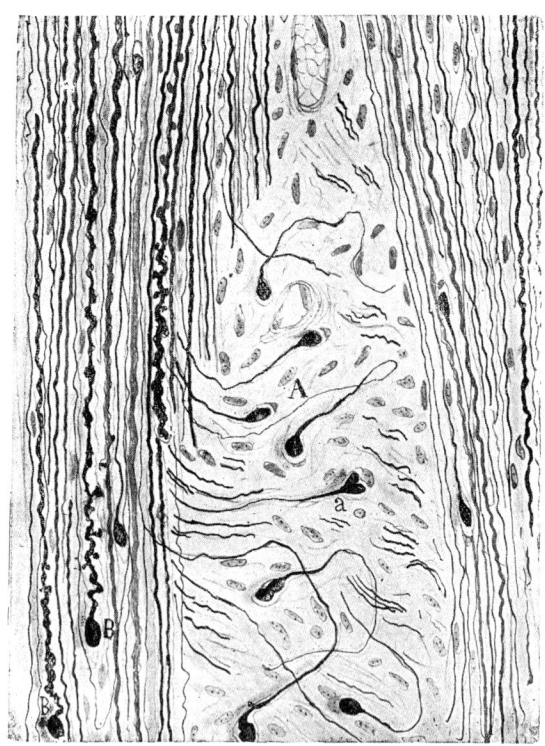

FIG. 66.—Piece of central stump showing many arrested clubs and sterile tubes. Rabbit killed twenty-seven days after the operation. *A*, thin connective wall with clubs which have lost their way and are arrested; *B*, sterile fibres.

a rough vacuolization, show a certain clear central region and a marginal veil, which is more or less wrinkled and composed of a very delicate neurofibrillar net (Figs. 64, *h*, and 67, *d*).

In Figs. 66, *B*, and 67, *A*, *D*, we show some sterile axons in the central stump of a rabbit, killed twenty-seven days after the section. In the schematic drawings of Fig. 64, *F*, *G*, are also shown some examples that are typical, although without protuberances, of these sterile fibres. It can be seen in Fig. 64, *G*, that the terminal club appears covered with a rough meshwork, and that it shows large neurofibrils. In Fig. 67, *d*, appear protuberances with more or less reticulation. In Fig. 67, *c*, one can also see polyp-like appendices, with a relatively long peduncle. It is curious to note that these appendices, although they appear to be in a state of formative

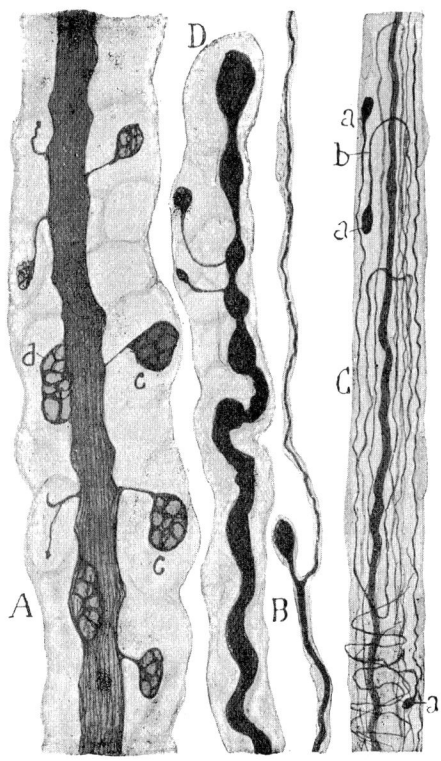

FIG. 67.—Fibres from the central stump of an adult rabbit, killed twenty-seven days after the operation. *A*, *D*, sterile axons with aborted branches; *c*, polyp-like reticulated excrescences; *d*, reticulated protuberances; *B*, axon provided, near the terminal club, with a nucleated collateral which was travelling towards the scar; *C*, helicoidal apparatus.

turgidity, nevertheless remain stationary and become abortive forms. One finds them with the same appearance and length thirty-seven days after the operation. After four months they are totally absent, showing that they have degenerated and been resorbed.

The question presents itself whether the sterile tubes are definitely sterile. Is it not possible that they are really very long terminal segments in continuity with axons that are capable of sprouting at a great distance from the wound?

A priori, such a supposition appears very probable. It does not seem likely that a robust fibre should definitely remain without use because of the weak state of the terminal segment. The sterile tubes might thus be looked upon as apathetic fibres which are delayed in neoformation, as compared with the surrounding fibres. As a matter of fact, we have seen in some medullated axons of medium size, at a great distance from the wound, the emission of a few extratubal collaterals, arising from nodes. But, on the other hand, all the very large sterile fibres with much retracted terminal clubs have been entirely without sprouts ten, twenty, and forty days after the section. This interesting point calls, at any rate, for further investigation.

The older authors doubtless saw some of the dispositions of sterile fibres. Thus Stroebe [1] drew certain festooned axons which were spattered with vacuoles, and which could not be stained with aniline blue. These axons are very much like our sterile tubes. Perroncito,[2] who confirmed our description, believes that the collateral protuberances and polyp-like appendices arising from such fibres are pathological in character. Marinesco [3] likewise recognized and drew polyp-like sprouts and neurofibrillar protuberances on axons from the central stump, as did also Doinikow and Dustin. Marinesco describes them very well, and has seen these appendices up to thirty-eight days after the operation. They then appeared very much as they do twenty and twenty-seven days after the section.

We expressed the opinion, in our first communication, that such appendices were ordinary growing sprouts ; but we are to-day of the same opinion as Perroncito. We hold further that not only the collateral shoots, but also the axons themselves are pathological forms, at least for long distances. In the adult animal, where there are numerous axons provided with wide myelin sheaths, the sterile fibres are in considerable proportion.

[1] Stroebe : " Experimentelle Untersuchungen über Degeneration und Regeneration peripherer Nerven nach Verletzungen," *Beiträge zur pathol. Anat. und zur allgem. Pathol. von E. Ziegler*, Bd. 13, 1893.

[2] Perroncito : loc. cit., *Beiträge zur path. Anat. und zur allg. Pathol. von E. Ziegler*, 1907.

[3] Marinesco : " Etudes sur le mécanisme de la régénérescence des fibres nerveuses des nerfs périphériques," *Journal f. Physiologie u. Neurologie*, Bd. 7, 1906.

VIII

COURSE OF THE NERVE SPROUTS ACROSS THE SCAR AND FOREIGN TISSUES

Emergence from the limits of the nerve and entrance into the scar.—Details concerning division of the fibres.—Kinds of terminal buds (clubs of growth, arrested clubs, retraction clubs, and agonistic clubs).—Comparison between embryonic cones of growth and the clubs of the newly-formed axons.—Structure of the initial scar.—Behaviour of the nerve sprouts in crossing exudates, embryonic connective tissue, muscles, adipose tissue, and foreign bodies.—Segregation and degeneration of the terminal buds.—Relation of the fibroblasts to the newly-formed nerve fibres.

Arrival of the nerve sprouts at the region of the scar.—From the third day on, and sometimes before, the various collateral and terminal branches that issue from the fibres of the central stump have grown so much that they abandon the chambers formed by the membrane of Schwann and penetrate into the scar. As all the sprouts are not equally vigorous, and as they are formed at different times, the invasion of the foreign tissues occurs progressively as if by shifts. As a consequence of this, the examination of the cicatricial border, from the fifteenth to the sixty-fourth hour reveals a mass of fibres of various thicknesses and growing at different speeds. It is frequently not the largest, but the finest fibres that form the vanguard.

One often observes (Fig. 54, *E*) the predilection of the cones of growth, in their growth, for certain determined weak passages in the nerve border. In some of these regions as many as ten or more clubs are grouped and are trying to emerge, all of them of different sizes. At the level of these openings there is a convergence of fibres that have come from regions relatively distant, and are later to radiate out and disperse in the scar itself. It appears that the nerve border is a region difficult to cross and that, once a first gap is made, all the neighbouring fibres take advantage of it in order to economize effort.

Once the border is crossed, the clubs go out into various regions, some of which are more favourable than others. If the migration occurs before the third day, the scar, which is still in the incipient stages of its formation, encloses exudates that are rich in leucocytes. Very often, blood clots form an obstacle to the advancing fibres. Finally, it often occurs that lobules of fat or muscular bundles are present. The nerve sprouts, as though pushed by an energetic and continuous impulse, launch out into the new region, where they try to open a way. Sometimes the terminal club, which acts as a battering-ram against the obstacle, hypertrophies; sometimes there is an abundant ramification of the fibre. Almost every one of the new fibres seems to be, not a compact and perfectly individualized axon, but a bundle of independent fibrils, which are ready to disunite and diminish the volume of the fibre whenever they meet an obstacle which is very difficult to overcome. We shall speak of this dissociation of the new fibres in greater detail below.

All the nerve sprouts that circulate through the scar during the first week are naked fibres in which not only the myelin, but also the cells of Schwann are lacking. The most careful analysis of preparations in which a silver impregnation has been combined with a nuclear strain such as carmine, haematoxylin, or safranin, reveals no satellite nuclei, that is, nuclei that are parallel and adherent to the new axons. This important observation, repeated by Perroncito, Marinesco, and others, is fatal to the polygenist theory, which requires, as a necessary condition of the formation of the nerve fibrils, the pre-existence of protoplasmic chains of cells of Schwann.

After four or five days the scar is almost formed and the axons travel through it with relative ease and speed. Although one observes in it isolated axons, one often finds them in pairs, and, especially, in dense bundles. These bundles contain thick and fine fibres, and they travel in various directions, which are more or less oblique in relation to the axis of the nerve. They cross each other at certain places, forming chiasmas, and together give rise to a complex plexus, which we name the *cicatricial plexus.*

In the places of convergence of the bundles there appear numerous bifurcations; so that each bundle now contains, not only fibres from one bundle as it originated in the central stump, but also shoots from other bundles more or less remote. In Fig. 68 we see the appearance of the bundles and their anastomoses, during the ninth and tenth days after the operation, when the connective tissues are already well formed. Ranvier and Vanlair observed the bifurcations of the fibres in the scar, but only tardily, when the myelin appeared.

Details concerning the divisions of the fibres.—A careful examination of the regions where the sprouts present in the scar bifurcate reveals the fact that very often, though not always, the division occurs before some obstacle, such as a capillary, an accumulation of connective tissue cells, a fat cell, etc., and that the newly-formed branches pass round this obstacle in order to continue on their way.

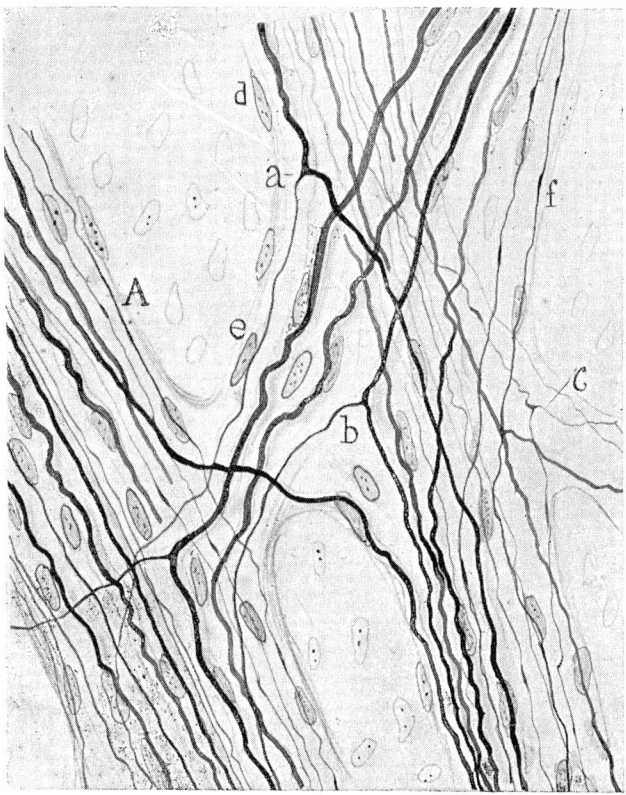

FIG. 68.—Nerve bundles of the intermediate scar. *a* and *b*, division or bifurcation of the nerve fibres; *f*, fine fibres; *d*, nuclei of the laminar sheath; *e*, nuclei of the young axons.

There are usually five methods by which the branches originate: (*a*) The branches arise through dissociation of a bundle of neurofibrils (Fig. 69, *A*). (*b*) The shoots are collateral in character and arise from massive fibres, at the level of a triangular thickening, whose fine texture shows that one or several neurofibrils from the parent axon divide at a right angle. (*c*) The shoots are terminal, arising at an acute or right angle at the end of the axon, where there is a certain triangular thickening, perhaps formed by the anastomoses of the daughter neurofibrils between each other and the parent axon. (*d*) The parent axon is robust and is the seat of active assimilation.

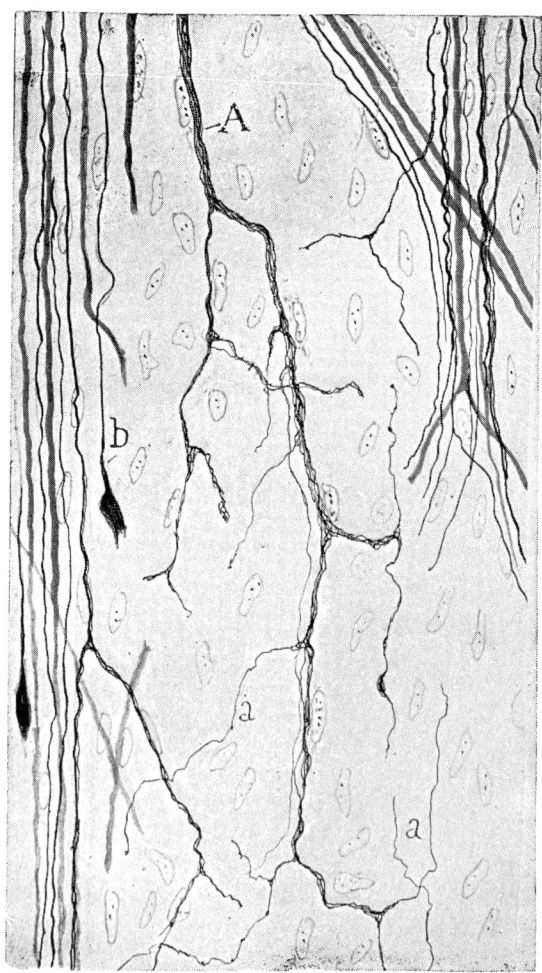

FIG. 69.—Details of the ramification of the fibres in the scar. *A*, fibre ending in an extensive arborization which lies freely within the embryonic connective tissue; *a*, twig composed of a single neurofibril; *b*, terminal club.

It gives rise, in a short region, to a rich and complex terminal and collateral arborization, whose branches end in clots or else in fusiform and very thin stumps. This is the state of division by *amoeboidism* (Fig. 70, *B*). (*e*) The daughter branches are terminal in character and arise from a free club or bud, themselves ending in rings or buds (Fig. 71, *e*). Between the terminal branches that arise from a triangular thickening and those which come from clubs or buds one often sees transitional forms, such as thickenings that are triangular in origin, more or less wide and rounded. We therefore seem justified in stating that the terminal club represents a potential division, in other words that it is a phase of the future bifurcation ; once this occurs, the club disappears progressively (Fig. 72, *H*).

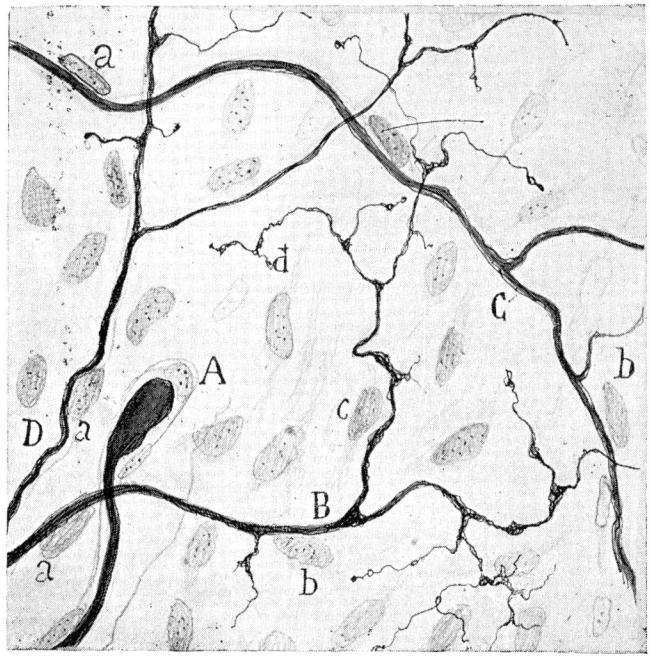

FIG. 70.—Portion of the cicatricial nerve segment displaying fibres that are very much ramified. *A*, large axon terminating in a club ; *D*, bifurcated fibre ; *B*, varicose terminal arborization. Rabbit, ten days after the operation.

We give typical examples of the abrupt ramifications through *division by amoeboidism*, where the terminal stump unfolds into a rich arborization, in Figs. 69, *A*, and 70, *B*. Perroncito and Marinesco, who have confirmed this method of neoformation, also give good descriptions of it.

Thus the neurofibrils, in each method of ramification, appear to result from the division of those in the parent axon, except in those cases of ravelling where they pre-exist, and where they merely segregate.

The dividing capacity of young protoplasm is extraordinary.

It is no exaggeration to suppose that from a simple axonic collateral there arise, through successive divisions within the central stump, scar, and peripheral stump, dozens of branches. These conductors are fine at first, but they become progressively thicker, getting their nutrition *in loco*. This thickening is avalanche-like ; together with the enormous number of conductors that arise from a branch which is relatively thin at its origin in the axon, it constitutes an arborization comparable with a cone whose very broad base is situated in the periphery, and whose very narrow vertex is represented by the shoot of origin, or by the central axon itself.

Variations and structure of the cones of growth.—Some authors have described all the terminal enlargements of the newly-formed fibres as of the same character, an error of interpretation to be avoided. As a matter of fact, there exist four great categories of terminal masses, not all of which have the shape of buds. These are : (*a*) *Clubs and cones of growth* ; (*b*) *spheres, or sterile giant globes* ; (*c*) *retracted or degenerating buds or globes* ; (*d*) *agonistic clubs and balls of the peripheral stump.* Although we have already spoken of some of these, we shall now give fuller details concerning their significance and structure.

Clubs and buds of growth.—Among all the terminal swellings that have been described in embryonic fibres these alone show progressive growth and active neoformation and are comparable to the cone of growth pointed out by ourselves and von Lenhossék in embryonic nerve fibres, and later confirmed by Harrison, through his important experiments *in vitro*, in living nerves of amphibians. These terminal dispositions are not necessarily of the shape of clubs or buds. In embryos, they are often lengthened into cones whose base is peripheral, or appear as fusiform and lance-shaped masses. These lance-shaped forms, as well as the triangular thickenings that give rise to fine appendices, are inherent in the axonic protoplasm. They are also up to a certain point independent of their surroundings, since Harrison, Burrows, W. H. Lewis, and M. Reed Lewis have seen them in embryonic fibres grown in plasma, or even in indifferent salt solutions, in tissue cultures involving embryonic material. The same variety is found in sprouts that invade the cicatricial tissue. Some of them end in buds or olive-shaped structures ; others show triangular or lance-shaped thickenings ; others again are like brushes ; finally, forms that are lobed, verrucose, and with finger-like processes, are not infrequently found.

In Fig. 71 we show some of these singular variations, which have also been well described by Perroncito, Marinesco, Tello, and Deineka. It seems probable that the variable shapes are the result of an

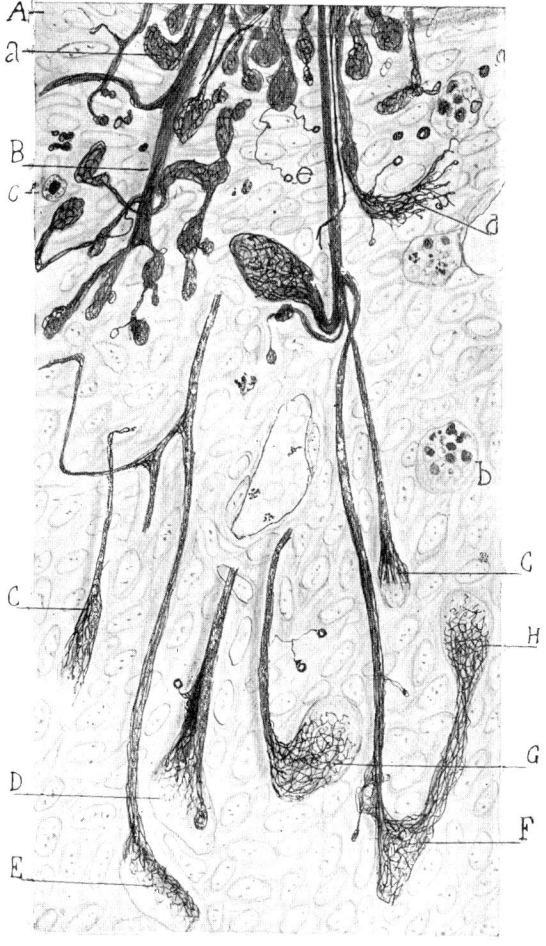

FIG. 71.—Morphological varieties of clubs penetrating the scar. *A*, border of the central stump; *B*, thick fibre terminating in a cluster of clubs; *C*, termination in the form of a brush; *D, E, H*, buds in which the neurofibrillar framework appears contracted and separated from the neuroplasm; *F*, folded clubs; *a*, kidney-shaped clubs; *d*, ravelled club; *c*, segregated clubs; *e*, terminal rings.

accommodation of the club to the shape and extent of the obstacles in its way. The terminal rings, a strange disposition pointed out by Perroncito, are only found in the finer twigs.

We may now say something about the structure of the cones of growth. All living and growing clubs and cones show two constructive factors—a clear interstitial substance, which is sometimes very abundant and especially accumulated at the distal portion of the mass, the neuroplasm ; and a very delicate neurofibrillar reticulum, which, while it is loose and dispersed in the club, is concentrated where it forms the peduncle. The wider and flatter the club the more evident is the silver-impregnated fibrillar tissue (G). Sometimes the periphery of the club is so poor in fibrils or these are so pale that they seem to end freely in the connecting tissue ; thus are found the brush-like forms, so well drawn by Perroncito (Fig. 71, D, G, H). Between these cotton-like neurofibrillar accumulations, which appear free, and the nets of fibrils that are evidently enclosed in a hyaline club, with well-marked borders, all the transitions can be found. It is thus very probable that these two forms are the same thing and have the same significance. The aspect of free and ravelled neurofibrils (Fig. 71, D, H) is thus the result of a polar dislocation of the neuroplasm and of the invisibility of the limiting membrane. In fine, the living and growing club is a pliable and essentially plastic mass, undergoing constant assimilative changes, very unlike the giant forms, which are rigid and stable, and of which we shall speak below.

The power of neoformation and the pressure of growth—the *vis a tergo* of Held—can go so far that the entire club separates itself from the supporting peduncle. There are thus formed free balls and rings, which rapidly fall into necrobiosis (Figs. 71, c, 72, E). We shall speak of them below. We need only say at this point that all free terminal balls show an immediate hyalinization of the cortical region, while the central portion resists for a time, appearing as a plexus or net of more or less granular neurofibrils. This axonic *caput mortuum* is found in greatest abundance where many clubs struggle to open a path concurrently. It is a real corpse, fallen in the struggle for space and food that goes on in the scar or the exudates. Perroncito was the first to draw the free terminal balls, but he did not recognize them as such. The paleness and thinness of certain peduncles led him to suppose that where the buds are clearly isolated there might also be an invisible filament which established continuity of the sphere with a nerve branch. Nevertheless, the noticeable abundance of these free buds, as we shall point out later, in those regions which are unfavourable to nervous nutrition and growth, lead us to believe that they represent eliminated pieces of protoplasm which are degenerating (Fig. 72, E, F).

Gigantic or arrested balls.—We shall speak of these later in detail, when we describe the tardy formations of the central stump and scar. They are large spheres, at times gigantic, immovable, degenerating, and in continuity with thick fibres that have lost their way or are retrograde.

Retraction balls and accumulations.—To this category belong the terminal accumulations that were described above in connec-

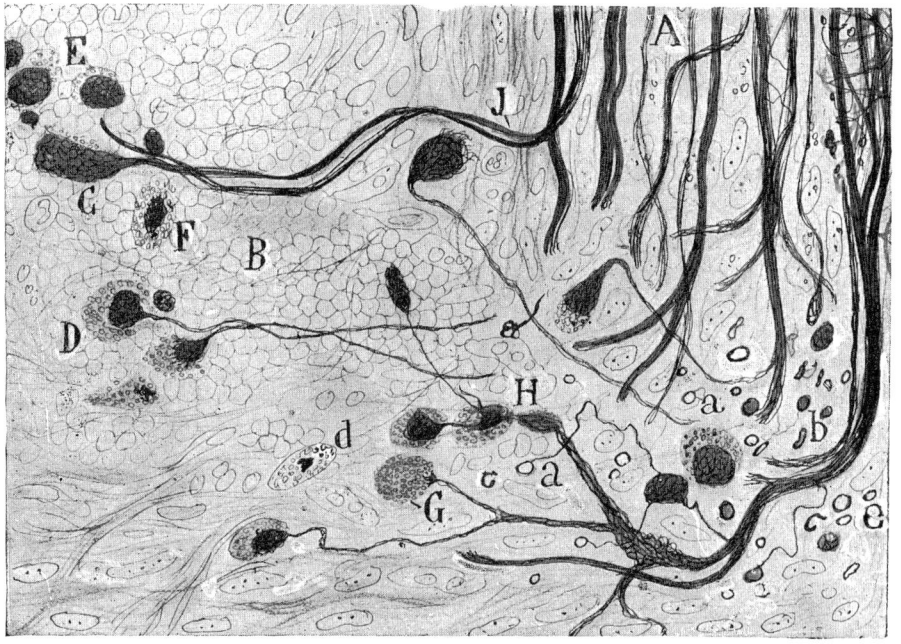

FIG. 72.—Piece of the central stump of a cut nerve of a rabbit, killed fifty-six hours after the operation. The sprouts deviate into the bloody exudate. *A*, central stump; *B*, bloody clot; *C*, more or less immovable terminal clubs; *E, F*, segregated clubs in necrosis; *d*, club in which only a small neurofibrillar central portion remains; *G*, degenerating club; *a*, terminal rings.

tion with the large sterile axons, as well as certain spheres that we discovered in the central nerve fibres and called *balls of retraction*. We shall speak of this important constructive factor of the degenerative foci of nerve centres later on.

Agonistic accumulations and clubs.—We have thus designated the clubs formed in the proximal end of the peripheral segment of a cut nerve. Such forms are also abundantly found in wounded nerve centres, as we shall note later.

Of all these types of terminal accumulations only the first can be considered as a manifestation of the formative erethism of the nervous protoplasm. The first alone is capable of growth and of giving rise to nerve sprouts. One might even sub-divide this type into two classes, according to the relative activity of growth and the capacity for ramification : the intumescences in the shape of lances, brushes, or fine cones with ravelled borders, all of which are forms with very rapid growth ; and the small, massive clubs, with well-marked and sharp borders, rounded at the tip, and nearly always associated with slow-growing nerve branches.

Thus, with some exceptions, the size of the terminal thickening appears to be in an inverse ratio to the speed of growth, and in a direct ratio to the resistance that the surroundings offer to the fibres. It is clear that this formula does not pretend to enunciate an exact relation between values whose real magnitude is unknown. It is merely an approximation and is based on averages. It enables us readily to understand how, in those cases where a club suddenly breaks up into a tuft of branches or gives rise in a short time to numerous projections, these show lance-like ends which are little thickened, or very small clots and rings—our *division through amoeboidism*. For the same reason, the cones are very fine while they grow within the sheaths of the peripheral stump, but they are large when they grow across resistant portions, such as the adipose tissue.

Comparison between the cones of growth of the embryo and those of regenerated axons.—Many years ago we,[1] and also von Lenhossék,[2] saw for the first time the free extremity of a growing fibre, and we pointed out that in the nerve centres, as well as in the midst of mesodermal tissues, the sprouts terminated in a club or cone-shaped thickening, from whose base arose at times spines and fine appendices. We called these structures *cones of growth*. Our further investigations on this subject, carried out by neurofibrillar methods,[3]

[1] Cajal : " A quelle époque apparaissent les expansions des cellules nerveuses," *Anat. Anzeiger*, Bd. 5, 1890.

[2] v. Lenhossék : " Zur Kenntniss der ersten Entstehung der Nervenzellen und Nervenfasern bei Vogelembryo." *Verhandl. d. X. intern. med. Kongress*, Berlin, 1890.

[3] Cajal : " Génesis de las fibras nerviosas en el embrión," *Trab. del Lab. de Inv. biol.*, tomo 4, 1906.

Idem : " Nouvelles observations sur l'évolution des neuroblastes avec quelques remarques sur l'hypothèse neurogénétique de Hensen-Held," *Anat. Anzeiger*, Bd. 32, 1908.

beginning with the third day of incubation, in chick embryos, confirms in principle our first observation and add some details. One can see in good preparations that the neurofibrillar framework does not fill the entire cone, but only part of it, and that it usually takes the shape of the tip of a brush and especially that of a lance-shaped mass (Fig. 73, C). When the growth of the cone is slow, then the buds and olive-shaped forms appear (Fig. 74, C). The motor axons, when they cross the perimedullar connective tissue, take advantage

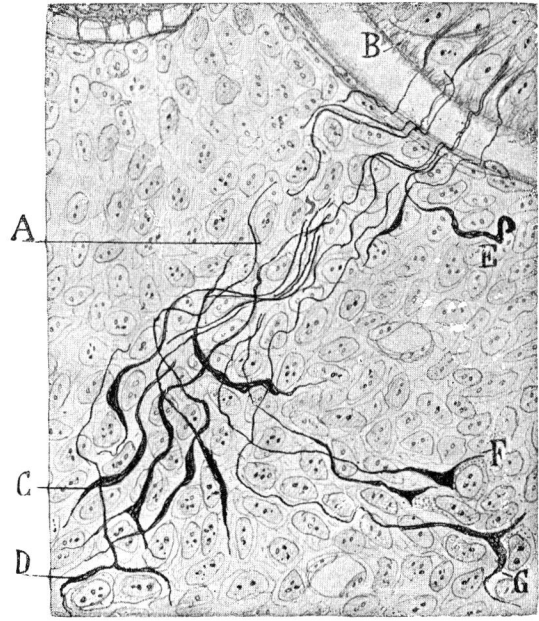

FIG. 73.—Growing fibres from an anterior spinal root. Chick embryo after fifty-eight hours of incubation. A, anterior root; B, spinal cord; E, cone that has lost its way; C, lance-shaped cone; F, G, divisions of the fibres as they encounter obstacles.

of the plasmatic interstices, accommodate themselves to the round edges of the cells, and ramify when they encounter obstacles. When a cone suddenly meets with a cell, a division into two branches occurs (Figs. 73, G, and 74, A). Naturally these appendices, which are rapidly formed, provisionally lack terminal masses. It is only later, when the club of origin disappears and the sprouts acquire a certain vigour, that new terminal cones make their appearance. It is evident, therefore, that the form, connections, and mode of growth of the cones in the embryo correspond essentially with what we have said above with regard to nerve sprouts. We are thus dealing with the same physiological process. Fig. 74 affords good evidence of this remarkable analogy.

As we have already stated, the same dispositions, with slight variations depending on special experimental conditions, have been seen and reproduced by Harrison,[1] Burrows, W. H. Lewis, etc., in their important studies on the growth of pieces of embryonic nerve tissues *in vitro*. In the drawings of these investigators one can see that the fibres, in the lymphatic plasma, grow out in a straight line, and that from the distal end of the terminal club, which is frequently conical, with a peripheral base, there arise two or more short fibres which terminate in a point. It appears certain that if one were able to observe living nerve shoots in mammals, the similarity between the forms described by the American investigators and those pointed out by ourselves would be even greater.

In general, those authors who, like Nageotte, Marinesco, Tello, Deineka, G. Sala, etc., have occupied themselves with the phenomena of nervous regeneration, agree with us that the small club or terminal bud found in ganglia, nerve centres, and peripheral nerves in course of restoration, represents a terminal organ indicative of the path of growth and of the regenerative character of the fibre to which it belongs.

Some authors, however, doubt that such a bud is a constant structure in the end of newly-formed fibres, or that it is, in any case, an unmistakable expression of a regenerative process.

Such is the opinion of Perroncito,[2] who bases it on the following observations : (*a*) From such thickenings, which appear to be terminal, there arise in turn new fibres. (*b*) Clubs are often found along the course of the fibres. (*c*) Analogous thickenings are found in the proximal end of the peripheral stump of nerves, several days after the operative cut, in axons that are evidently degenerating. (*d*) Similar balls and buds are found in the white substance of degenerating nerve centres. Perroncito believes that these facts prove that the terminal buds are not dispositions homologous with the cones of growth of embryonic axons, and that while certain of these buds point to neoformative acts, others have characters that are evidently degenerative. Since some of the largest masses are found in arrested fibres, their

---

[1] Harrison : " The outgrowth of the nerve fibre as a mode of protoplasmic movement," *Journ. Exp. Zool.*, vol. 9, No. 4, Dec. 1910.

[2] Perroncito : " La rigenerazione delle fibre nervose," *Bolletino della Società Medico-Chirurgica di Pavia*, 2nd and 3rd preliminary notes, 1905 and 1906.

formation might be explained by a kind of retrograde amoeboidism, somewhat like the accumulation towards the rear of that protoplasm which is newly formed at the end of the fibres.

Conrado Da Fano,[1] who has studied the terminal buds and the arrested balls in the ganglia and nerve roots of tabetics, believes that these dispositions are the result of degenerative processes. Poscharisky [2] has expressed a similar opinion.

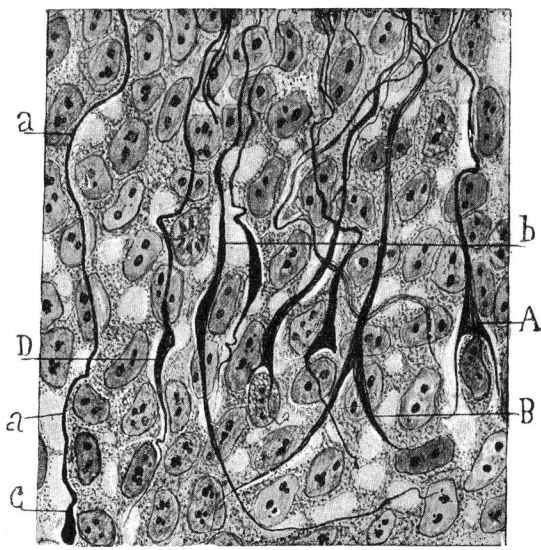

FIG. 74.—Details of the growth of the cones of growth across the mesoderm. Chick embryo fifty-eight hours in the incubator. It can be seen that the cones *A, B, D,* grow between the embryonic connective tissue cells.

Marinesco [3] believes without reservation in the degenerative character of the terminal buds and balls, but he believes that they ordinarily represent a retardment in the growth of the young axon, a retardment related to the diminution of the attractive forces exercised by the cells of Schwann or apotrophic cells of the peripheral stump. On the other hand, he considers the phase of creation of branches—our *phase of*

[1] Da Fano: "A proposito delle nuove dottrine sulle modificazioni della struttura dei gangli spinali nella Tabes," *Boll. della Società Medico-Chirurgica di Pavia,* July 1907.

[2] Poscharisky: "Ueber die histologischen Vorgänge an den peripherischen Nerven nach Kontinuitätstrennung," *Beitr. zur pathol. Anat. u. allg. Pathol. von Ziegler,* Bd. 41, 1907.

[3] Marinesco: "Le mécanisme de la régénérescence nerveuse, 1ère partie," *Revue générale des sciences,* etc., 18ème année, num. 4, Feb. 28th, 1907.

division through amoeboidism—as the true mechanism of active growth of the fibres, a growth caused by the arrival at the axon of powerful currents of alluring substances.

Bethe,[1] under the mistaken impression that we had attributed to the gigantic clubs or spheres the character of cones of growth, states that such forms are arrested at the very place where they are developed, that they are subsequently covered with a sheath of myelin, and that they cannot therefore be cones of growth.

Dustin[2] accepts the opinion of Marinesco, but he exaggerates it very much, for he states that the terminal clubs and balls always belong to newly-formed nerve fibres that are in a state of repose or are arrested by insuperable obstacles. Sometimes, to get round the obstacle, the club emits one or several branches, and the process of growth is reestablished.

The preceding opinions are based on well-observed facts, from which generalizations of too wide a character have been drawn. They involve, however, the erroneous idea that we attach equal value and functional significance to all the terminal masses. It seems to us probable that the investigators alluded to have not carefully analyzed the various kinds of clubs, and that they have not differentiated sufficiently the *balls of retraction* and the *arrested balls* from the true *buds of growth*.

Although what has been said above eliminates the principal sources of confusion with regard to the physiological value and significance of the various categories of terminal masses, it is worth while to summarize here the grounds for thinking that the terminal club is an evident sign of regeneration and a clear index of the normal growth of newly-formed nerve fibres.

(*a*) The terminal accumulations are found as well in the nerve fibres of the embryo as in regenerating nerves. This has been shown by our investigations, those of London and Pesker,[3] and those of Harrison.

(*b*) The terminal accumulations—not the large balls—are constantly seen in the peripheral end of cut nerves, at the extremity of fibres that have penetrated into the old sheaths of Schwann, that is, into the organic region where the growth and progress of the young axons are most rapid and active.

(*c*) From the sixth hour after the lesion onwards there appear in the edge of the wound numerous clubs and buds, whose number and

[1] Bethe: "Neue Versuche über die Regeneration der Nervenfasern," *Arch. f. die ges. Physiol.*, Bd. 126, 1907.

[2] Dustin: "Le rôle des tropismes et de l'odogenèse dans la régénération du système nerveux," *Arch. de Biol.*, tome 25, 1910.

[3] London und Pesker: "Ueber die Entwicklung des peripheren Nervensystems, etc.," *Arch. f. mikros. Anat.*, Bd. 67, 1906.

size increase during the following hours—from the twelfth to the fifty-sixth. The presence of such dispositions during this initial phase of regeneration is so constant that it is impossible not to assign to them a part in the formation of the nerve sprout (Fig. 52, *b*, *c*, *d*).

(*d*) The observations of Tello, confirmed by ourselves, show that there are terminal buds in all the fibres that have recently arrived in the small peripheral nerves and motor plates, in those which have found their way into sheaths of Schwann as well as in those which travel freely along unobstructed paths.

(*e*) The fact that there exist ramifications which start from the outgrowing clubs and buds, as pointed out by Perroncito, far from being opposed to our opinion, confirms it, since we have often stated that to the *club phase* often succeeds the phase *of division through amoeboidism*. It is natural that when, as a consequence of meeting with an obstacle or the sudden irruption of a stimulus to neurocladism, the terminal bud goes through the stage of division by amoeboidism, the protoplasm in it is not immediately absorbed, but remains for a time associated with the branches that grow out from it. This persistence of the bud is especially found in backward and arrested buds. In the small buds that are growing rapidly it is not found, for when a division occurs, the entire substance of the club is distributed among the daughter branches.

(*f*) Marinesco and Dustin generalize too much the phase of division through amoeboidism, forgetting that this process represents only a brief phase of the evolution of the fibres. In general the authors have not distinguished clearly such different phenomena as the growth of the formed fibres and their multiplication. It is true that the act of division implies growth; but it is not less true that once the new branch is formed and oriented, it grows without dividing for long distances, quickly taking on a terminal bud, which it needs in order to remove obstacles from its path.

(*g*) Perroncito, Dustin, etc., state that the *large balls* belong to axons that are arrested, sterile, and useless for regeneration. We have held this view since our earliest investigations,[1] and it is certainly not

[1] In our first treatise on regeneration (*Boletín del Instituto de Bacteriología*, fasc. 2, June, 1905) we already stated: " These outgrowths of the axon (the gigantic buds) often originate from fibres that have been held up by some obstacle, and have been unable to lengthen and grow out towards the periphery."

In our second memoir on the same theme (*Boletín del Instituto de Bacteriología*, fasc. 3, Sept. 1905) we again expressed a similar view: " Certain large axons, which are retrograde or have lost their way inside the central stump, often show at a very late stage—two or three months after the operation—gigantic claviform structures. These structures are more or less pale and

opposed to our conception of the regenerative and physiological significance of the cones and small buds of the free fibres.

(*h*) The fact pointed out by Perroncito, and confirmed by ourselves and Marinesco, that the proximal end of the peripheral stump, two to six days after the section, contains terminal clubs and even ramifications of fibres—*agonistic clubs*—proves only that axons separated from their trophic centre do not die immediately, but attempt, during their long agony, to produce sprouts.

Behaviour of the nerve sprouts in presence of embryonic connective tissue, exudates, and various organic tissues.—As Dustin [1] states, and as we [2] have proved experimentally, young connective tissue, as yet without bundles, in the newly-formed scar is, of all the organic tissues except the nerve tissue itself, that which is most favourable to nutrition and growth of the sprouts. In this it is second only to the special tissue of the peripheral stump, as we shall point out below. Apart from the still unknown chemical conditions that it offers, embryonic connective tissue provides a loose warp comprising interstices and clefts full of plasma and of remnants of exudates, thus allowing the easy passage of the nerve clubs. The sprouts, as they go through the connective tissue, often lean on the connective tissue cells, which act as leaders, as is the case with threads of fibrin in the free growth of axons cultivated in plasma, *in vitro*, as was shown by Harrison.[3]

altered. We believe, as a result of our new experiments, that these structures probably represent ordinary clubs of growth, arrested in their growth and much hypertrophied."

In our study " La génesis de las fibras nerviosas en el embrión " (*Trab. del Lab. de Inv. biol.*, tomo 4, 1905-1906) we once more insisted on the same idea, for the phenomenon of arrest owing to obstacles also occurs in normal embryonic development. We give these bibliographic details because several authors, when they express their opinion concerning gigantic clubs, forget the history of this question.

[1] P. Dustin: " Le rôle des tropismes et de l'odogenèse dans la régénération du système nerveux," *Arch. de Biol.*, tome 25, 1910.

[2] Cajal : " Algunas observaciones favorables a la hipótesis neurotrópica," *Trab. del. Lab. de Investig. biol.*, tomo 8, 1910.

[3] Harrison : " The cultivation of tissues in extraneous media as a method of morphogenetic study," *Anat. Record*, vol. 6, 1912.

This author has shown that when one adds filamentous foreign bodies—such as fibres of fibrin, cotton threads, alveolar tissues, etc.—to a culture of nerve fibres, the sprouts follow these objects and grow more easily. The mesodermic cells perhaps act in a similar way, in the embryo as well as in the regeneration of nerves.

It will be useful to summarize here the histological structure of the scar during the first phases of the formation, that is, from the third to the sixth or seventh day. In it one may observe the following structures:

(a) *Fibroblasts, or embryonic cells of the connective tissue.*—As we show in Figs. 75 and 76, the shape of these cells is at first polyhedral, or else has short and thick outgrowths. The cells soon become fusiform or stellate, with large appendices, some of which

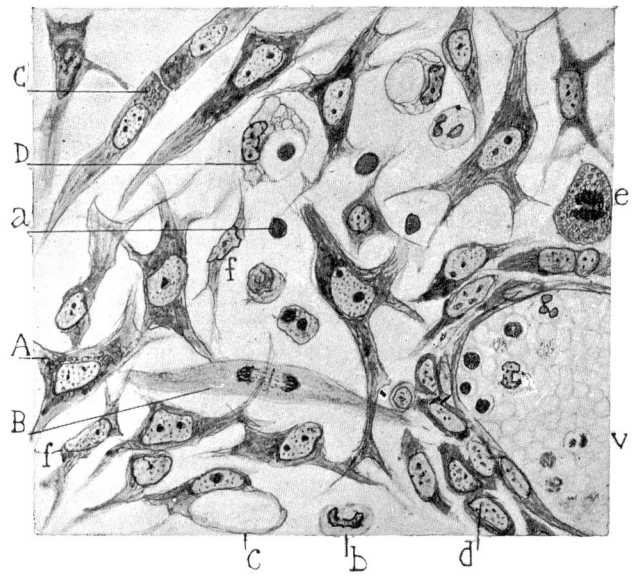

FIG. 75.—Connective elements of the scar three days after section of the sciatic nerve in a rabbit. Unna's polychrome blue stain. *A*, connective cell; *B, C*, fibroblasts in mitosis; *D*, leucocyte with lipoid inclusions and a segregated mass; *V*, blood vessel; *a*, migratory lymphocytes; *b*, free leucocyte; *c*, fibroblast with inclusions; *d*, small perivascular elements; *f*, fibroblasts of small size; *e*, mast cell in mitosis.

are anastomosed, others free. On the third day these mesodermic cells form a net with meshes of variable size, according to the remnants of the exudate that are present. From the third day on, sometimes before, the interstices become narrower, the connective tissue cells come in contact with each other, not only through their appendices, but also bodily, and an even more compact tissue is thus formed (Fig. 76). In general one sees in greatest abundance the elongated cells; these, as though they attracted each other by *homotropism*, are arranged in bundles of various sizes which are often perpendicular to the wound. There are, however, many exceptions.

The connective tissue cells sometimes stain dark grey with reduced silver, after fixation in pure alcohol or ammoniacal alcohol, or else in chloral hydrate. This staining shows not only the protoplasm, but also the nuclei, in which two or three nucleoli stand out, black or grey in colour, and of variable size. Fixation with formoluranium (see above, p. 45) reveals constantly on one side of the cytoplasm an endocellular Golgi apparatus, such as was described by Deineka [1] in ordinary connective tissue cells. One can also confirm the observation of Perroncito [2] and of Deineka that during division the Golgi apparatus breaks up and becomes granular, and that the free clots are distributed to the daughter cells. The cytoplasm of fixed cells can be stained with the basic aniline dyes, and especially well with Unna's polychrome blue, which reveals two protoplasmic regions : an extensive perinuclear zone, which is rich in cyanophil substance and which is net- or sponge-shaped (Fig. 75 A), and the region of the expansions, which is pale and hardly stained by methylene blue (Fig. 75).

We shall not enter here into the much debated question of the origin of the embryonic connective tissue cells, nor is this the place to discuss in detail the genetic theories of Unna, and especially of Maximow. It is sufficient to state our belief that the younger cells come from near the region of pre-existent blood vessels, and that they are perhaps the descendants of certain small spherical or polyhedral germinative elements from which also may come the cyanophil cells—the *plasma* cells of Unna.[3] Such cells, once arrived at a certain stage in their development, augment their cytoplasm, take on two or more expansions and, migrating towards the exudate, form the first rudiment of the scar. From the twenty-fourth hour onwards one finds these cells, not only in the exudate, but in the thickness of the blood coagulum and in the ends of the central and peripheral stumps.

Later, from the second day on, they invade both stumps, and they conglomerate in large masses near them. They divide mitotically. We show two typical examples of this division in Fig. 75, B, C.

[1] Deineka : "Der Netzapparat von Golgi einiger Epithel- und Bindegewebeszellen," etc., *Anat. Anzeiger*, no. 11, May 1912.

[2] Perroncito : "Beiträge zur Biologie der Zelle," etc., *Arch. f. mikros. Anat.*, Bd. 77, 1911.

[3] Cajal : *Manual de Anatomía patológica*, 4th Ed. p. 91. "El estroma de las neoplasias," *Rev. trim. microgr.*, nos. 2 and 3, 1896.

One can see that the stained cytoplasm breaks at the centre, forming two fusiform elements lying in the same direction.

In Fig. 75, moreover, one can see other small connective cells, which are perhaps younger (f), dispersed throughout the exudate, and some cells in which are lipoid remnants (D). Near the newly-formed blood-vessels one perceives an accumulation of young and small connective cells, which are generally polygonal (Fig. 75, d).

(b) *Granular cells.*—These are very numerous near the central stump. They are nothing else than leucocytes that include lipoid particles of various sizes (Fig. 75, D).

(c) *Free nuclei uniformly and intensely stained by the basic aniline dyes* (Fig. 75, a).—As these are homologous to cells found within blood-vessels, we believe that we are dealing here with a variety of lymphocytes. In many of them one can hardly see the cytoplasm; in others it is entirely lacking (Fig. 75, a), but this may be only an appearance.

(d) *Free balls and free fatty clots.*—The former are seen only in preparations made with reduced silver nitrate (Fig. 76, d).

(e) *Capillaries.*—These are formed, from the second day onwards, through the well-known process of germination, in which are present endothelial points of growth, which are solid at first but hollow later. Wherever they arise, each new capillary attracts a great number of young connective tissue cells, which form a kind of discontinuous adventitial membrane (Fig. 75, v).

(f) *Plasmatic spaces.*—Between the cells, as we have already stated, there exist, especially at first, wide spaces or free clefts (Fig. 76). The nerve sprouts travel through them. These spaces later become smaller, and the progress of the clubs is more difficult.

(g) Finally one occasionally sees, when special methods are used, *cells of Ehrlich*, or *mast cells*. In Fig. 75, e, we show one of these in the act of mitosis.

Relations of the nerve fibres with the embryonic connective tissue cells.—Across this favourable region the axons grow out, taking advantage, as noted above, of the intercellular spaces. They curve in their course in order to accommodate themselves to the shapes of the cells, and they ramify when the club encounters obstacles which are difficult to overcome. As we shall point out when we discuss the theories of Held and Dustin, neither the direction of the cells nor the orientation of the plasmatic interstices corresponds, in general, to the common direction of growth of the nerve sprouts. As can be seen in Fig. 76, *a*, *g*, the nerve sprouts, instead of always accommodating themselves to the outlines of the fibroblasts, whose orientation is often transversal to their own, jump from one cell to another across the plasmatic spaces. Such a condition is especially to be seen in those scars (Fig. 76) in which the inflammatory exudate is very slowly resorbed. This does not mean that the clubs avoid the cells. On the contrary one very often sees that, by the process that

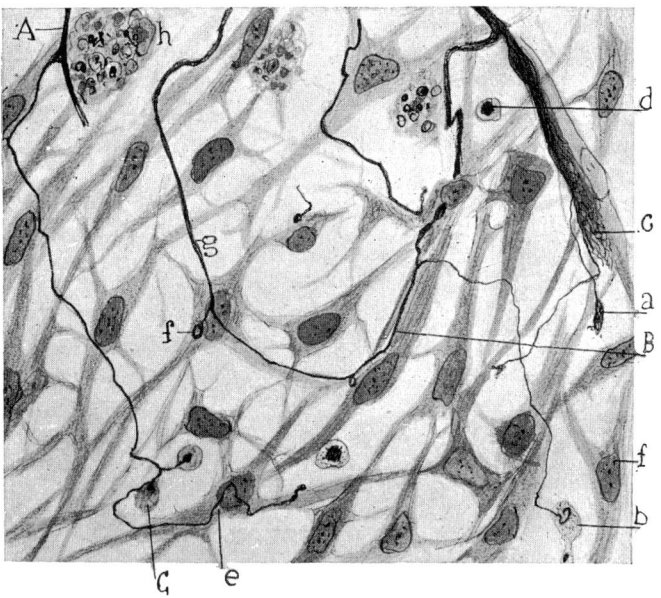

FIG. 76.—Relations of the nerve sprouts with the connective elements of the scar. Rabbit killed three days after section of the sciatic nerve. A remnant of exudate appears between the fibroblasts. *A*, nerve fibre which crosses the fibroblasts; *B*, fibre which follows the outline of the connective tissue cells; *C*, degenerating clubs; *a*, small club; *b*, neurofibrillar loop within a club which is in course of segregation; *c*, cone resting on a cell which it hugs, forming a large neurofibrillar brush; *e*, fibre next to a fibroblast; *d*, segregated club; *h*, leucocyte with lipoid drops; *f*, ring next to a fibroblast.

we have called *tactile adhesion*, and that Leo Loeb [1] and Harrison [2] named *stereotropism*, the nerve sprouts become intimately applied to the cells, and follow their larger outgrowths, if these have in the least the general direction of axonic growth. When, however, the cells stand in the way of the growth of the fibres, the terminal clubs behave differently. Sometimes the terminal thickening is then closely applied to the obstacle, sliding along one side of it, and form-

[1] L. Loeb: *Arch. f. Entw.-mech.*, Bd. 6, 1897, and Bd. 13, 1902.
[2] Harrison: loc. cit., *Anat. Rec.*, vol. 6, 1912.

ing a kind of tassel, capsule, or neurofibrillar veil (Fig. 76, c). At other times, as Dustin noted, the paralyzed club puts out one or two branches which circumvent the obstacle, and a disposition results which is very common in the embryo, where the cones of growth often bifurcate when they encounter cells (C). The club sometimes, as a result of taking the wrong direction, is immobilized and arrested, becoming segregated from the peduncle which, thus freed from the *caput mortuum*, finds a more favourable path (d). One can see these eliminated balls and rings, of which we have already spoken, in Figs. 72 and 76.[1] Finally, if the club encounters a blood-vessel, or

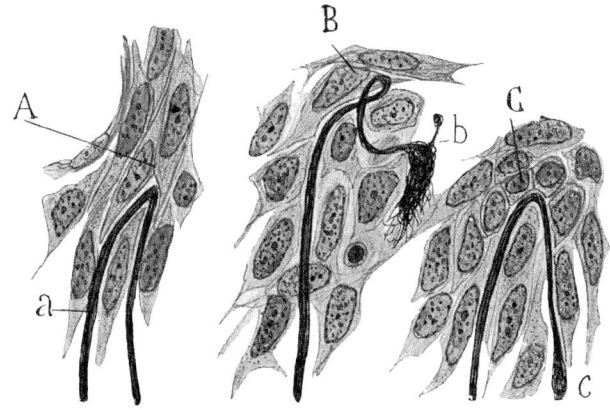

FIG. 77.—Disposition of the connective tissue cells where the fibres turn back. A, interstice which is closing up as a result of pressure from an adjacent blood vessel; B, turning back due to meeting with connective cells placed transversally; C, turning-back owing to the presence in front of the club of a mass of elements without any interstices.

the convex surface of a large connective cell, or if it travels into clefts that progressively narrow owing to the approximation of various cells, the fibre reverses its course, and may, in some cases, return to the nerve. A careful analysis of the region in which such retrogression takes place has convinced us that it is the result entirely of mechanical causes. In Fig. 77 we show some of the more frequent conditions that cause the retrogression and deviation of nerve sprouts. We shall see below that these curious deviated fibres persist indefinitely.

[1] There is a curious analogy between these phenomena of elimination of the clubs and the spontaneous amputations—*autotomy*—of the members of certain crustaceans when one holds the latter tightly.

188 TRAUMATIC DEGENERATION AND REGENERATION OF NERVES

Action of the blood and exudates.—We have stated that the clubs that emerge at an early stage from the central stump, from the twelfth hour onwards, forcibly fall into a pool of coagulated blood which is more or less infiltrated with inflammatory exudate. The *vis a tergo*, that is, the internal impulsion, causes the sprouts to go

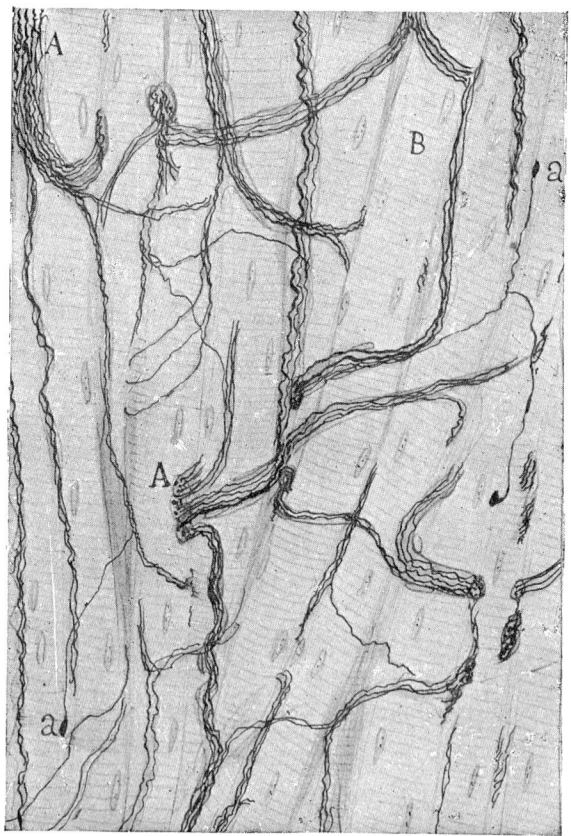

FIG. 78.—Muscle invaded by deviated fibres during their growth towards the periphery. *A*, nerve bundles; *B*, muscular fibre; *a*, clubs of growth seeking for an exit.

out into a region which is very unfavourable to them. Sometimes they cross it during the first and second days, with losses. But the majority of clubs are immobilized and degenerate, unless they take a transversal direction in order to escape from these unfavourable surroundings. This degeneration is seen as a differentiation of a neurofibrillar centre from a colourless and more or less granular cortex (Fig. 72, *D*). Other buds are freed from the peduncles and they degenerate like rotten fruits that have fallen from the tree (Fig. 72, *F*). In some preparations, such as that drawn in Fig. 72, the degenerating clubs are abundant, and they suggest the idea that, among the nerve sprouts which have accidentally arrived in an unfavourable region, there is a kind of struggle or vital competition

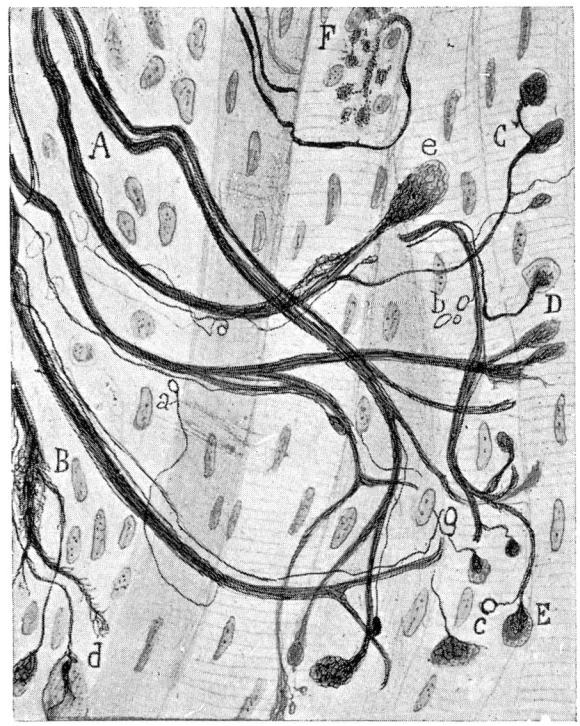

FIG. 79.—Nerve fibres lost in a muscle which is near to the central stump. The animal was killed fifty hours after the operation.

n which the most robust fibres survive or those which, through fortuitous circumstances, have been least exposed to the lethal action of the environment.

Muscular tissue.—Frequently, before the scar is consolidated and completed—from the second to the third day—bundles of neighbouring muscles are interposed in the wound, and offer themselves to invasion by the nerve sprouts. This phenomenon is shown in Fig. 79. Muscular tissue, with its ample interstices full of nutritive juices, constitutes a region that is very favourable to the growth and ramification of the nerve fibres. The fact that the muscle

190 TRAUMATIC DEGENERATION AND REGENERATION OF NERVES

already possesses, more or less complete, its own nerves and motor plates, is immaterial. A multitude of sprouts, arranged in bundles, contribute to its mass. These bundles surround the muscle cells; they follow their outlines and form steps and coils. The fibres ramify abundantly before the obstacle of the muscle cells or of the blood-vessels and an interstitial plexus of great complexity is finally formed.

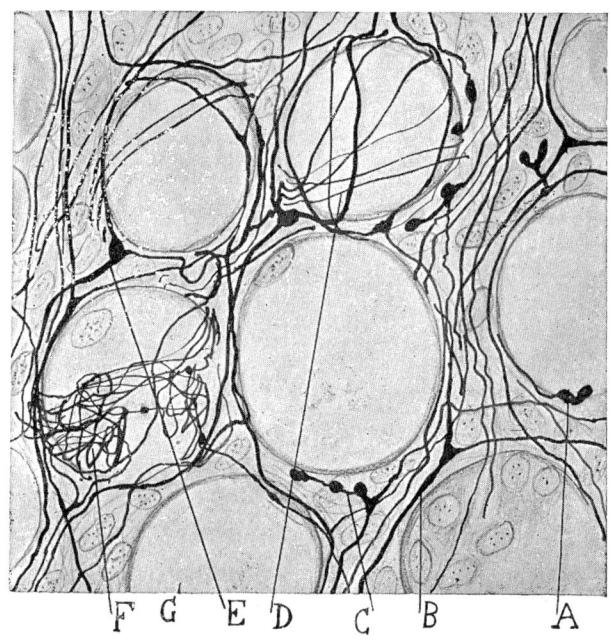

FIG. 80.—Piece of adipose tissue interposed between the two stumps of a cut nerve. Young dog, killed sixteen days after the operation. *A*, terminal clubs; *B*, axonic ramifications; *C*, branch on which several clubs are being resorbed; *D*, periadipose spools; *F*, nervous entanglements; *G*, fat cell; *E*, club from which arise two branches, etc.

In Fig. 78 is shown a later stage—twenty-five days after the operation—in the invasion of a muscle. One can see that the deviated fibres, far from having perished, have multiplied prodigiously, although they have formed no motor plates. Some of them show moderate-sized terminal clubs.

Nerve sprouts in adipose tissue.—Even more frequently than the muscular tissue, the adipose tissue interposes itself, from the first days after the operation, between the nerve stumps. In general, the fat cells are a retarding obstacle to the growth of the axons, which they do not, however, finally arrest.

Fig. 80 shows the innervation of an adipose lobule in a young dog, sixteen days after the operation, that is, at a relatively late stage. At this date the peripheral stump is already innervated. One can see how the axons have taken advantage of the cellular interstices, concentrating in them and closely hugging the membrane of the adipose cells. This growth did not take place without arrests and vacillations. The abundance of terminal clubs, which are relatively rare in the scar at that time, the great number of varicosities along the paths, representing remnants of clubs, the frequent retrograde fibres, etc., all show that the crossing of the obstacle was a laborious undertaking. It will be seen that the majority of the fibres lie closely pressed against the cellular membranes, on which, owing to blind growth, they have described loops and even veritable spools (D). One should especially note the great number of axons that are bifurcated just at the place where they encounter the cell wall. It is also of interest that in some places the bifurcation occurs exactly at the level of a club that has become converted into a more or less triangular varicosity (E). This shows us that the club, detained by a barrier, a kind of dam to amoeboid motion, has emitted two branches to circumvent the obstacle, but that the original arrested club subsists for a certain time, under the shape of a triangular varicosity.

Sprouts before foreign bodies.—Following the example of Vanlair, we have set up artificial obstacles to the growth of the young fibres, and we have confirmed the capacity of the latter to insinuate themselves in the interstices of foreign bodies, provided that the plasmatic exudate and some connective elements have previously penetrated the spaces. Decalcified bone or teeth, small pieces of cork or elder pith, blotting paper, all substances, in brief, that have communicating spaces of a certain width, can be crossed, after a relatively long time (ten to thirty days) by some fibres. These experiments show that the growth of the nerve sprouts does not need, as an essential external condition, anything else than a plasmatic *milieu*. All other factors, such as embryonic connective tissue, capillaries, etc., represent conditions that are favourable to the nutrition and orientation of the axons, but are not absolutely necessary. These results agree perfectly with the interesting experiments of Harrison,[1]

---

[1] Harrison: " Further experiments on the development of peripheral nerves," etc. *Amer. Jour. Anat.*, vol. 5, 1906. " The outgrowth of the nerve fibre as a mode of protoplasmic movement," *Jour. Exp. Zool.*, vol. 9, 1910.

Burrows,[1] and Lewis[2] on growth of embryonic nerve fibres *in vitro*, and with the fact, which we[3] pointed out some time ago, that embryonic neurones and axons which have accidentally fallen into the ventricular fluids grow and continue their morphological differentiation.

ADDITIONAL NOTE ON CHAPTER VIII

During the last ten years many papers have been published concerning the growth of the nerve fibres that penetrate into the scar and the peripheral stump. In consequence of war wounds, entailing great losses of lesioned nerve substance, many experiments of grafting have been performed on men and animals.

Leaving for later consideration the works on grafts and the new theories which aim at replacing the theory of neurotropism, we may resolve all modern interpretations under the three following conceptions :

1. *The fibres of the peripheral stump are supposedly formed within the bands of Büngner without the direct aid of the sprouts from the central stump.*

We have already discussed this theory at length in the first chapters of this book. Out of respect for the great prestige of Bethe and Spielmeyer, almost the only modern advocates of such a doctrine, we shall say a few words on the most recent researches of these investigators:

Spielmeyer[4] studied mostly human material in connection with war wounds. He holds that, for the production of nerve fibres, it is indispensable that, in the scar as well as in the peripheral stump, there be present chains of young cells of Schwann. The neurofibrils appear later through intraprotoplasmic differentiation ; they are never found free between the connective tissue cells. Like Borst, he believes in the pluricellular origin of the axons of the peripheral stump. In a large

---

[1] M. T. Burrows : " The growth of tissues of the chick embryo outside the animal body, with special reference to the nervous system," *Jour. Exp. Zool.*, vol. 10, 1911.

[2] W. H. and M. R. Lewis : " The cultivation of sympathetic nerves from the intestine of chick embryos," etc., *Anat. Rec.*, vol. 6, 1912.

[3] Cajal : " Nouvelles observations sur l'évolution des neuroblastes avec quelques remarques sur l'hypothèse neurogénétique de Hensen-Held," *Trav. du Lab. de Recherch. biol.*, tome 5, 1907.

[4] Spielmeyer : " Ueber Regeneration peripherer Nerven," *Zeitschr. f. die gesamte Neurol.*, etc. Bd. 36, 1917.

and important paper [1] which deals with almost all the lesions of the nervous system, he expresses the same idea.

We may note from the first that his descriptions and microphotographs have to do with very late phases of regeneration, when the axons from the central stump have already penetrated and gone through the peripheral stump almost in its entirety. The Münich scientist, further, offers absolutely no explanation of the difficult problem, how fibres of peripheral and pluricellular origin become joined without any deviations with those of the central stump.

A. Bethe,[2] notwithstanding the arguments of indubitable force that we, as well as Harrison, Perroncito, Marinesco, Tello, Nageotte, and a great number of other authors, have advanced for some time against his theory of autogenous regeneration, returns now to his first point of view, which he bases as much on experiments of nerve section in animals as on the examination of grafts. Like Spielmeyer, he finds newly-formed axons only within cells of Schwann and *bands of Büngner* of the peripheral stump. Nevertheless, Bethe is less exclusive than Spielmeyer, since he recognizes the existence of sprouts originating in the central stump that have penetrated into the scar, although never as free fibres. But this Wallerian regeneration, as well as the balls, tangled spools, and other formations that are found, are without influence on the union of the peripheral stump. They are only abnormal structures.

Later, when we study nerve grafts, we shall speak of other interesting investigations of Bethe.

The fundamental error of both Bethe and Spielmeyer is to have studied preferably the late phenomena of nervous union of the peripheral stump, at a stage when it is already impossible to find clubs of growth, that is, when the process of complete or incomplete regeneration is finished. One is particularly surprised that they should have performed their experiments on dogs in which, owing to the separation of the fragments of nerve, it is very difficult, not to say impossible, to follow efficiently the sprouts in the scar. These two authors have surrounded themselves, for the solution of this problem, with almost insuperable difficulties, when ordinary common sense tells one to use small and young mammals, such as guinea-pigs, cats from fifteen to twenty days old, rabbits from fifteen days to three months old, and to use preferably hemisections, in order further to reduce the distance between the nerve stumps and therefore the size of the scar. Under such conditions one

---

[1] *Idem* : *Histopathologie des Nervensystems*, Springer, 1922.

[2] A. Bethe : *Zur Theorie und Praxis der Verheilung durchstrennter Nerven*. Volume in honour of S. R. Cajal, vol. 2, 1922.

not infrequently sees in the peripheral stump the entrance of a sprout arising from the central stump; and in any case one may clearly see (from the fifth day in the cat) the continuity between the bundles arising from the central and those penetrating into the distal stump, although, owing to the irregularity of their course, one may not always follow each individual fibre. Some days later the new fibres have grown so much within the peripheral stump that it is very rare to find a growing club of growth. In the same scar, ten to twelve days after the section, with the exception of deviated and detained fibres, one is not likely to find anything besides large bundles of axons, surrounded by a covering of enigmatic origin, which could well arise from the cells of Schwann of the central stump, as Marinesco, Nageotte, and many scientists suppose. Neither Bethe nor Spielmeyer seem to know the Spanish edition of this book, which appeared in 1912-1914. This can well be understood, however, since during the war communications with Germany were broken off, and when the war ended the edition was out of print.

2. The opinion which to-day is most in evidence, and which is upheld by the majority of the anatomo-pathologists, is the following: *There is no autogenous regeneration of the peripheral stump, and the sprouts of the central stump, after crossing the scar, alone or in bundles, innervate the peripheral stump, within whose bands of Büngner they grow.* Those who believe in this theory deny that, with some rare exceptions, the sprouts grow freely, either within the central stump, the scar, or the peripheral stump. There always exists, around them, a layer of protoplasm belonging to the more or less transformed cells of Schwann.

This view coincides in its essentials with our own; we differ in our conception only on two points of pure detail. The first of these is that the investigators cited above deny that even in the first phases of nerve-union, from the third to the fourth days, there exist free sprouts growing in the scar. The other point is a conception of the bands of Büngner as solid cordons, while we believe that they are tubes with a central and potential cavity. Some authors hold also that the newly-formed axons not only pass through the protoplasm of the solid bands, but that they also are found in the thin protoplasmic walls which separate the lipoid inclusions and remnants of the old axons.

The most enthusiastic upholders of this theory, which rests, as we have said, very largely on indubitable facts, are, in France, Nageotte [1];

---

[1] Nageotte: *loc. cit.* See also, besides his numerous notes in the *C.R. Soc. Biol. de Paris*, his magnificent book: *L'organisation de la matière dans ses rapports avec la vie*, Paris 1922.

in Germany, Bielschowsky and B. Valentin,[1] Ramanow,[2] Bielschowsky and Unger,[3] Jakob, Hedinger,[4] Berblinger [5]; in America, Ranson; in Holland, Boeke [6]; in Japan, Saito,[7] Kimura.[8] With some exceptions, all these investigators reject the theory of neurotropism. They hold that the inclusion of the axons in the cells of Schwann is sufficient to explain the correct regeneration of the nerves and the orientation of the axons.

If these authors, in accordance with the numerous indubitable facts referred to in this work, were to accept the doctrine put forward by Perroncito, Tello, Dustin, Marinesco, Lugaro, etc., that during the first phases of the invasion of the scar by fibres these are isolated, especially the exploratory fibres, without denying that later they become surrounded by a cellular sheath, and if they admitted that many sprouts during their initial period grow in the peripheral as well as the central stumps outside the cells of Schwann, there would be a perfect conformity between their point of view and ours. Berblinger alone formulates the opinion that, while crossing the scar, some fibres grow naked between connective tissue cells; but later he seems to repent this concession, which is opposed to the prejudices of his school, and he assures us that such free fibres end in granules and are doomed to destruction. As for the theory of neurotropism, far from being for me a dogma, it is simply a working hypothesis which I am willing to correct or even abandon in the presence of better explanations. We shall speak again of this matter when we treat below of the various theories that have been devised to account for the orientation of the sprouts.

[1] Bielschowsky u. B. Valentin: " Die histologischen Veränderungen in durchfrorenen Nervenstrecken," *Journal f. Psychol. u. Neurolog.*, Bd. 29, S. 133, 1922-3.

[2] Ramanow: "Zur normalen und patholog. Histologie der peripheren Nerven des Menschen," *Journal f. Psychol. u. Neurolog.*, Bd. 18, 1912.

[3] Bielschowsky u. Unger: " Die Ueberbrückung grosser Nervenlücken," etc., "Beiträge zur Kenntnis der Degeneration und Regeneration peripherischer Nerven," *Journal f. Psychol. u. Neurol.*, Bd. 22, S. 267, 1916-18.

[4] Hedinger: *Schweizer Archiv f. Neurol. u. Psychiat.*, Bd. 9, 1921.

[5] Berblinger: " Ueber die Regeneration der Achsenzylinder in resezierten Schussnarben peripherer Nerven," *Beiträge zur pathol. Anat. u. allg. Pathol.*, Bd. 64, 1918.

[6] Boeke: " Nervenregeneration und verwandte Innervationsprobleme," *Ergebn. d. Physiol.*, Bd. 19, 1921.

[7] Saito: "Zur Frage der Regeneration der peripheren Nerven des erwachsenen Menschen," *Arbeit aus dem Neurol. Institut Wien*, Bd, 24, 1922.

[8] Onari Kimura: " Histologische Degenerations- und Regenerationsvorgänge im peripherischen Nervensystem," *Aus dem Kaiser. Universität zu Sendai*, Bd. 1, 1919.

We have never denied that the effective innervation of the peripheral stump and motor and sensory terminations is aided by tutor cells (scar). Concerning the origin of the cells that surround the sprouts of the scar from the sixth day after the operation, we must confess that the investigations of the last few years have not dissipated our doubts and that, for us, the ectodermic derivation of those elements is not a demonstrated and irrefutable truth.

3. *The newly-formed fibres grow at first freely through the scar, but they soon become surrounded by a cellular sheath which probably emanates from the cells of Schwann. The penetration into the peripheral stump implies a neurotropic action, or the exercise of electric influences, by the latter.*

We have already defended this third opinion with many facts, and we shall not dwell upon them here. We shall cite only the authors who, during the last ten years, have, with some variations perhaps, accepted this point of view. Among them, and we do not know them all, we may include : P. Rojas,[1] Marinesco,[2] Tello,[3] K. Schaffer, Lorente de Nó, Edinger, Miskolczy, Isuguchi and, in general, all the English and American investigators, among whom the theoretical suggestions of Held and Bielschowsky have been opposed by the essentially positive spirit of the Anglo-Saxon race. Nor have the hazardous theories of these two scientists found much echo in Italy and Spain.

All the authors cited have not, *ex professo*, dealt with the theme of the origin of the newly-formed fibres of cut nerves ; but their figures and descriptions postulate the principle of monogenesis and of the free original growth of the sprouts. Thus, while the interesting investigations of Schaffer and H. O. Feiss,[4] and the more recent work of

---

[1] Rojas : " Degeneración y regeneración experimental de los nervios periféricos," *Trab. del Lab. Investig. biol.* t. 15, 1917.

[2] Already cited above as a partisan of the initial surrounding of the axons by their *apotrophic cells* ; in a private letter, however, he finally rectifies what is exclusive in this idea, accepting the initial nakedness of the sprouts, and attempting to place neurotropism on a physico-chemical footing. We shall speak of his theoretical views below.

[3] Tello: *Discurso de ingreso en la Academia de Medicina. Ideas actuales sobre el neurotropismo*, Madrid 1923. Also " Gegenwärtige Anschauungen über den Neurotropismus," *Vorträge u. Aufsätze über Entw.-mech. d. Organismen*, Heft 33, S. 1-73, 1923.

See also his magnificent studies on neurogenesis : " Genèse des terminaisons motrices et sensitives," *Trab. del Lab. de Invest. biol.*, t. 20 (with 77 figures). See also : t. 21, 1923.

[4] Schaffer and H. O. Feiss : " Notes on the functional regeneration of the cut cervical sympathetic and vagus," *Quart. Jour. of Experiment. Physiology*, vol. 9, pp. 329-334, 1916.

Tsukaguchi [1] have to do with physiological questions, the appearance and growth of the sprouts of the cut and the regenerating vagus and sympathetic nerves imply the initial free growth of the sprouts, and the action of neurotropic or similar impulses in the peripheral segments. The figures of Tsukaguchi are especially suggestive in this respect.

K. Schaffer,[2] of Budapest, describes in the ganglia of persons suffering from *amaurotic idiocy* a large number of naked sprouts arising either from the ganglionic cells or from the axon; many of them appear arranged in pericellular bundles; others grow freely between the altered nerve cells, ending in balls. We may note that Nageotte, who to-day is an enthusiastic partisan of the *entubement theory* of Held, showed some time ago in his beautiful studies of tabes and later in his experiments on grafts of ganglia a multitude of free collaterals lost in the thickness of the ganglion and in the posterior roots.

Miskolczy,[3] who has studied nerve fragments from old war wounds, using the method of Bielschowsky, has not been able to see in the scar any chains of cells of Schwann before the arrival of the axons, and, on the contrary, he has seen nerve fibres isolated within the connective tissue. He also describes certain axonic formations, among others the formation of complicated spirals almost without nuclei, a phenomenon which it is difficult to conciliate with the theory of previous entubement. He has also seen axonic divisions before obstacles, etc.

Lorente de Nó,[4] in his interesting investigations on the healing of wounds in the spinal cord of the amphibian larvae, also found free roots which penetrate naked into the cord, terminal buds of growth, a growth of the regenerated axons across the liquid of the ependyma, and other curious phenomena favourable to the hypothesis of neurotropism. We shall speak of them more at length, as well as of the investigations of Raposo, when we deal with regeneration in the spinal cord. The studies of Edinger,[5] Tello, and other authors, will be given in the chapter on grafts.

[1] Tsukaguchi: "On the regeneration of the cervical sympathetic after section," *Quart. Journ. of Experiment. Physiol.*, vol. 4, No. 4, pp. 281-327, 1916.

[2] Schaffer: "Contributions à l'histopathologie des ganglions rachidiens dans l'idiotie amaurotique," *Travaux du labor. de recherches biol.*, t. 20, 1922.

[3] Miskolczy: "Contribution à l'histopathologie de la régénération du neurone," *Travaux du labor. de recherches biol.*, t. 22, 1924.

[4] Lorente de Nó: "La regeneración de la médula espinal en las larvas de batracio," *Trab. del. Laborat. de Investig. biol.*, t. 19, 1923.

[5] Edinger: *Deutsche Zeitsch. f. Nervenheilkunde*, Bd. 58, 1918.

IX

LATE CONDITIONS SHOWN BY THE NERVE SPROUTS OF THE CENTRAL STUMP AND OF THE SCAR

Fibrillar bundles.—Formation of the protective coverings of bundles and axons.—Formation of the myelin.—Persistent retrograde fibres.—Helicoidal structures or nervous spools.—Motionless degenerating buds and gigantic balls.—Presence of analogous balls in embryos.—Probable fate of the axons and of the aberrant and immovable clubs.

THE structural and dynamic facts concerning the nerve sprouts that we have so far described relate very largely to early phases, that is, to a period of time varying between a few hours and a week. During this period the newly-formed axons remain in a state of formative turgidity and behave like embryonic fibres, since no satellite cells or medullary sheath are found around them. We shall now attempt to set forth the distinctive appearance of fibres regenerated later, and also to study as far as possible the fate of those regenerative dispositions which, like retrograde fibres and the structures of Perroncito, seem to us, from a utilitarian standpoint, to be mistakes or incongruence of the *vis medicatrix*.

Nerve bundles.—Nearly all the older authors, such as Ranvier, Vanlair, Stroebe, Kölster, Neumann, etc., who used osmic acid in their investigations in order to make a histological analysis of the scar and central stump in late stages, from twenty-five to seventy or more days after the operation, described bundles of new fibres, individualized by a common nucleated membrane, and resulting from the successive or simultaneous division of a single axon.

It is very apparent that the older workers did not always succeed, with the stains then in use, in determining precisely the mode of origin of the nerve bundles. To-day, we who have at our disposal much more precise techniques applicable from the first phases of regeneration, at a period when the myelin sheath is not yet formed, marvel at the perspicacity of those scientists. As a matter of fact, it is only to-day, thanks to the techniques above referred to, that we are able to form a just conception of the origin and mechanism of the fasciculated disposition. This fasciculation of the central stump is due to the fact that the immense majority of the nerve sprouts represent collateral or terminal intratubal branches which are forced to run along under the membrane of Schwann. The formidable number of intratubal parallel fibres is the consequence, in many cases, of the neurofibrillar ravelling or successive dissociation of each large intratubal branch. In other cases it is due to the union within the tube of collaterals which may or may not be dissociated, but which arise in different regions along the turgid portion of the axon. Finally, in some cases, although more rarely, it is due to the actual dissociation of the stimulated or irritated axonic stump

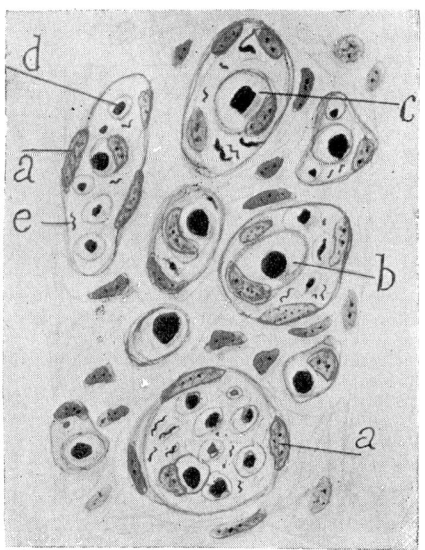

FIG. 81.—Transverse section of the central stump of a nerve near the scar. One can perceive nerve bundles which are individualized by a nucleated membrane. *a*, nucleus of the common sheath of the bundle; *b* and *c*, large medullated tube from the central portion of the bundles; *d*, non-myelinated tube provided with the vitreous sheath of Vanlair; *e*, very fine non-medullated fibres. The nuclei were stained with thionin.

which breaks up into a group or brush of fine conductors. After a while the neurofibrils and fine branches successively thicken, becoming true axons. For all of them the membrane of Schwann acts as a directive force. Owing to its rigidity and narrowness it forces them to unite in a more or less compressed colony. As a consequence, all the nerve bundles, no matter how thick they may be, which are present in the central stump and beginning of the scar, are provided with a nucleated membrane (Fig. 81, *a*).

There is a similar transformation of the old sheath of Schwann into a wide nucleated sheath, in the central stump, during the first week. The newly-formed cells of Schwann are seemingly obliged, perhaps by an impulsion of the nerve sprouts, to become peripheral and to transform themselves into flattened limiting cells. On the other hand the digestive chamber, which had been full of ellipsoids and axonic remnants, becomes progressively freer of detritus, receiving, in compensation, nutritive plasma and a few interstitial cells which are perhaps the progeny of cells from the nerve tube. It seems probable, although precise investigations on this point have not been made, that this old sheath, enormously dilated and perhaps reinforced exteriorly by mesodermal elements, in time becomes the *laminar sheath* or *perineurium* of the new bundle of medullated tubes.

A short time after the old sheath of Schwann of the central stump has become converted into a perifascicular capsule, a membrane surrounding the bundles is also differentiated in the scar. As can be seen in Figs. 82, *e*, and 81, *a*, each nerve fascicle of the scar formed by the union of fine and thick non-medullated axons, is separated from the connective tissue by a granular tunic, which is transparent and bespattered with elongated nuclei immersed in a thin protoplasmic mantle. As we have observed, the nervous fasciculation in the midst of the connective tissue is a phenomenon that occurs very early. One already sees it, at least in some fibres, twenty-four hours after the section. The formation of the nucleated mantle, however, does not occur so early. We believe that this membrane begins to be formed right in the scar, that is, at a certain distance from the central stump, from the fifth to the seventh day after the section. During the eighth and ninth days one can see it perfectly organized, and can perceive that at the level of the anastomoses of the bundles, the sheaths of some of them are in continuity with those of the others. Ranvier, who studied this membrane in late stages, compared it with the membrane of Henle of isolated peripheral fibres, and supposed that it was formed solely of assembled epithelial cells. We believe that, like Henle's membrane, it is composed of an external mantle of connective fibres which are in continuity with the mantle of Key and Retzius of the old, dilated tubes of the central stump, and of flattened cells situated internally.

Formation of the cells of Schwann and of the myelin in the new fibres.—A short while after the perifascicular coverings above referred to have appeared, that is, from the seventh to the ninth day, one can see, within the bundles, fusiform cells, partly free, partly applied to the axons. These cells show an elongation of their nucleus and also of their cytoplasm, which at first is lateral, and they form, as Stroebe already noted, complete protoplasmic sheaths—the *vitreous sheaths* of Vanlair. The appearance of these protected axons

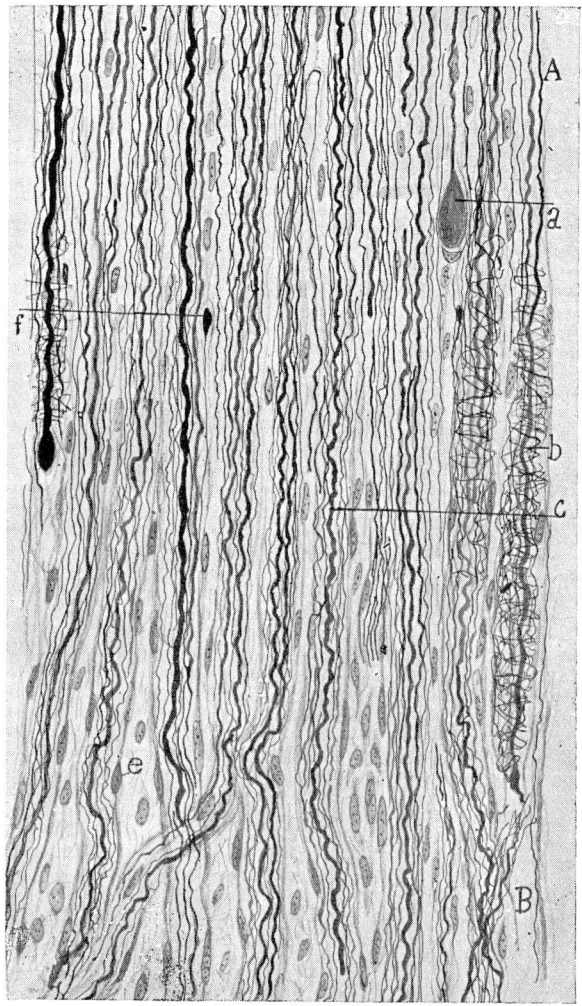

FIG. 82.—Piece of the central stump where the nerve bundles penetrate into the cicatricial segment. One may observe that the fibres are arranged in small parallel bundles, which are covered by a nucleated membrane. *a* gigantic club; *b*, nervous spool; *c*, large fibre of a nerve bundle; *e*, nucleus of the perifascicular sheath.

is exactly like that of adult non-medullated fibres. One can clearly perceive the tubular disposition of the satellite cells in the transverse sections of the bundles, and especially of the separated tubes, in which two concentric tunics can be easily recognized—Henle's membrane and the developing membrane of Schwann (Fig. 81, b, c). Certain axons appear surrounded by two or three successive nuclei, as though they had just been formed in consequence of the mitosis of a parent cell.

Under this tunic, surrounding each axon, there will appear, after a time, the myelin sheath. All the authors, except Leegard and Stroebe, believe that the myelin is formed late, as in embryonic nerves, where the axon is at first naked. The various neurologists differ, however, as to the time of its appearance. Thus Ranvier states that in the scar of the sciatic nerve many medullated fibres are already found on the seventy-second day, while at the same date the similar region of the vagus is composed, almost exclusively, of non-medullated fibres.

Nothafft, Kölster, Büngner, Bethe, etc., also believe that the myelin appears late, and that it grows from the centre to the periphery.

Some of the authors, like Kölster, Kölliker, etc., believe that the recently-formed myelin constitutes continuous mantles, being entirely a product of the axon, without the cellular mantle being at all involved in its formation. The polygenists, on the contrary, believe that it is a segmental discontinuous mantle, elaborated by the neuroblasts or constructive cells of the cellular chain (Büngner, Galeotti and Levi, Wietting, Bethe, etc.). This myelin is thin at first, but it thickens progressively, and, according to Ranvier, the interannular segments become progressively larger also.

Our observations concur, in all essentials, with the general opinions expressed above. In our preparations, the scar begins to show medullated fibres from the twenty-fifth day on, with variations depending on the age of the animal, its species, the calibre of the fibres, etc. The formation, as might be expected, begins centrally and extends peripherally and, as opposed to the view of the polygenists, it is very largely continuous, except at the level of the soldering discs. There are, however, as Ranvier showed, fibres in which a naked portion is followed by a medullated segment. This demonstrates that the production of the medullary sheath is not vigorously centrifugal nor therefore absolutely continuous.

> The formation of the perifascicular membrane of the scar, as well as the appearance within the latter of fusiform cells which ultimately become transformed into cells of Schwann, presents a problem concerning which the opinion of authors is much divided.

Setting aside for the moment the origin of the perifascicular or Henle's sheath, a point as yet little studied, and concentrating our attention on the question of the derivation of the cells of Schwann of the newly-formed axon, we find that two solutions have been put forward, both of them by well-qualified authorities.

They are as follows :

(a) The periaxonic or satellite cells are a direct progeny of the cells of Schwann of the pre-existing nerve tubes in the central stump. A phenomenon of multiplication and migration of the cells of the old nerve tube is supposed to occur. These cells, parenthetically, are considered as legitimate neuroblasts, and therefore of ectodermic origin. All the polygenists (Büngner, Wietting, Galeotti and Levi, Bethe, Howell and Huber) adopt this theory, as do also a number of monogenists, among them the distinguished authors von Lenhossék, Harrison, and Held. The hypothesis of Marinesco, according to which the cells arising from the cells of Schwann of the central stump—the apotrophic cells—migrate to the scar, where they direct and orientate the nerve sprouts, forms part also of the monogenist doctrine, in which it is suggested that these apotrophic cells constitute, after a time, the sheath of Schwann.

(b) The above-mentioned cells, the future cells of Schwann, are of mesodermic origin and they represent embryonic connective tissue elements of the scar or endoneurium. Through a kind of attraction they surround the axon, establishing with it a kind of symbiosis. Kölliker, Kölster, Stroebe, etc., concurred in this opinion. We have ourselves at times upheld it, although without much conviction. To-day we should be still less dogmatic.

We must recognize that the question is a difficult one, and that the arguments advanced by the two schools have almost equal weight. We have already referred to the experimental facts set forth by Harrison,[1] by which he showed that when one eliminates the ectodermic *anlagen*—the ganglionic crests—in amphibian embryos, all the axons that grow out into the mesoderm are without satellite cells ; this gives special cause for hesitation, and suggests that the time has perhaps come to abandon the old hypothesis of Kölliker, although many observed facts appear to support it. The entire difficulty lies in the insufficiency of the technique. We lack a method capable of clearly differentiating the embryonic connective tissue cell, found near the nerve sprouts, from the cells of Schwann that are newly formed, and that have possibly migrated from the central stump to the fibres of the

[1] Harrison : "Further experiments on the development of peripheral nerves," *Amer. Jour. Anat.*, vol. 5, May 1906.

scar. An additional difficulty is that neither in the sheath of the bundles nor along the new fibres are any mitotic phenomena visible. If these existed, one could determine by their appearance and continuity along the nervous paths both the multiplication and the migration of specific elements. One can adduce as an argument for the intratubal origin of the cells of Schwann the centrifugal path of the process, since the marginal cells are continued in a series with those of the central stump, and go from the trunks to the branches. But the upholders of the mesodermic doctrine may answer that this progression is simply the result of the fact that the nerve sprouts must act for a certain time before the surrounding mesodermic elements are attracted and oriented.

We must confess, however, that the unitary theory has, over the rival theory, the advantage of simplicity. Both hypotheses explain the facts very well, but, in the absence of objective proof, the mind is always attracted by the simpler explanation. Let us, then, see how the production of the periaxonic sheaths may be supposed to take place on this hypothesis. At first the cell of Schwann of the parent nerve tube in the central stump gave rise to a great number of daughter cells. Some of these were used to prepare the resorption of the myelin, and perhaps died while accomplishing this function. Others merely augmented the number of cells that formed the interior lining of Schwann's membrane of the old tube, undertaking the task of lining the limiting membrane of the bundle, and, through migration, of the fascicles that were growing into the scar. Others, finally, even greater in number, applied themselves to the nerve sprouts, multiplied rapidly, and, migrating with the axons across the mesodermic formations, became converted into cells of Schwann of the cicatricial fibres. There would thus be two migrations—an *external*, perifascicular migration which would give birth to the sheaths of the bundles in the scar, and an *internal* or intrafascicular migration which would form sheaths around each conductor.

It is evident that other explanations are possible. The facts are equally consistent with the unitary conception set forth above and with a mixed conception such as was upheld by Büngner. He believed that while the cell of Schwann arises from the congenerous cell of the old tube, on the other hand the sheath of Schwann of the new axons, as well as the perifascicular sheath of Henle, originate from cells of the endoneurium.

In the course of this work we shall come upon further facts that support one theory or the other, without enabling us to settle the issue definitely.

Retrograde fibres.—From the first moments of the nervous regeneration a considerable number of branches, detained by chance obstacles and impelled by the energy of growth, suddenly reverse their course, blindly following a centripetal direction. A typical example of the precocity and frequency of the deviations and retrogressions of the collateral fibres is shown by the apparatus of Perroncito ; here most of the spirals are retrograde conductors.

If it were permissible to explain in terms of human behaviour the actions of things that are subject only to unconscious forces, we might compare the phenomenon of growth and progression of the sprouts towards the boundary, that is, their entrance into the peripheral stump and the re-establishment of the terminal structures, to a race by night in which the runners were obliged to run across trackless fields strewn with many obstacles. The strongest among them, that is, the winners. rapidly orient themselves, run without vacillation or flagging, and reach the goal. Others, less well endowed, vacillate, stop at times, and lose themselves in the darkness. While some, the weakest, lacking in vigour and vitality, are arrested by the obstacles or laboriously return to the start.

The existence of retrograde fibres was known to the older authors, but not in all its details. Thus Ranvier [1] in a certain nerve bundle drew a medullated fibre which, after doubling in the form of an arc, returned to its point of origin. It was Vanlair, however, who perceived the importance of the phenomenon of deviation. He stated, with truth, that a great many of the newly-formed fibres fail to fulfil their function. Even this Belgian investigator, however, under-estimated the real importance of the question. As a matter of fact, in an adult animal, and under the best conditions, only a sixth or a seventh of the sprouts formed within the central stump reach their goal. In young animals, on the other hand, the number of sterile tubes and of deviated fibres is much diminished, and as a consequence, the nervous reunion of the peripheral stump is effected much more rapidly and completely. Finally, more recently, ourselves, Marinesco and Minea, Perroncito, Tello, Krassin, Deineka, Rossi, Dustin, etc., have described, from their first phases, the various types of retrograde fibres.

As we shall note below, the deviation of so many sprouts places great difficulties in the way of the functional rehabilitation of the peripheral terminal structures, such as the motor plates, the spindles of Künme, etc.

[1] Ranvier : *Leçons sur l'histologie du système nerveux*, tome 2, 1877.

As Vanlair [1] observed, the deviated fibres turn back, some within the central stump itself, some on reaching the scar ; some, finally, lose their orientation within the scar itself, blindly following the path of least resistance. On the other hand, as we shall show below, those which turn back within the distal stump are extremely rare.

The intratubal retrograde fibres of the central stump are of various diameters, but the fine ones are the most numerous. They follow beneath the membrane of Schwann along the degenerated portion, being usually detained at the level of the healthy or indifferent portion. They often abandon a direct path, and form spirals. Their ends are capped by a bud whose size increases with the time since the fibre was arrested.

The interstitial retrograde fibres of the central stump are very much more numerous and they are usually thicker than those just described. Among them robust terminal branches and even true axons may be seen. Many of them are a continuation of extratubal collaterals or of bifurcating branches of axons that have reached the cicatricial frontier (Figs. 83, C, and 82, f). All these conductors pass through the endoneurium, going back much further than the intratubal sprouts. Among them one often sees fibres which, after having been retrograde, turn back in the right direction, only to become retrograde once more. Such vacillations prove that the clubs grow by chance, without any greater directive force than the path of least resistance, as Vanlair upheld.

Finally, the fibres that have lost their way in the scar do so either at the border or within the first quarter of the scar, taking different paths. Some of them go back to the central stump. The majority, however, choose paths that return less directly. One often sees nerve bundles lost on or under the neurilemma, where they sometimes travel in a direction transversal to the axis of the nerve cordon. Not a few run along the connective tissue walls that separate the fascicles of the nerve. The majority, however, blindly follow muscles, adipose tissue, the aponeuroses, and any organs that lie along the sides of the scar and even on it. There are perineurilemmatic retrograde fibres which, twelve or fourteen days after the lesion, go back more than three millimetres. It is curious to observe that many of those fibres which travel along chance paths across the scar or surrounding tissues are held up by fibrous membranes and

[1] Vanlair : " Nouvelles recherches expérimentales sur la régénération des nerfs," *Arch. de Biol.*, vol. 6, 1885.

blood-vessels that they have followed for long distances. It is only very rarely, however, that they describe spirals around capillaries.

This strange tendency to follow faithfully and passively the outlines of hard and smooth organs is a phenomenon that we [1] had

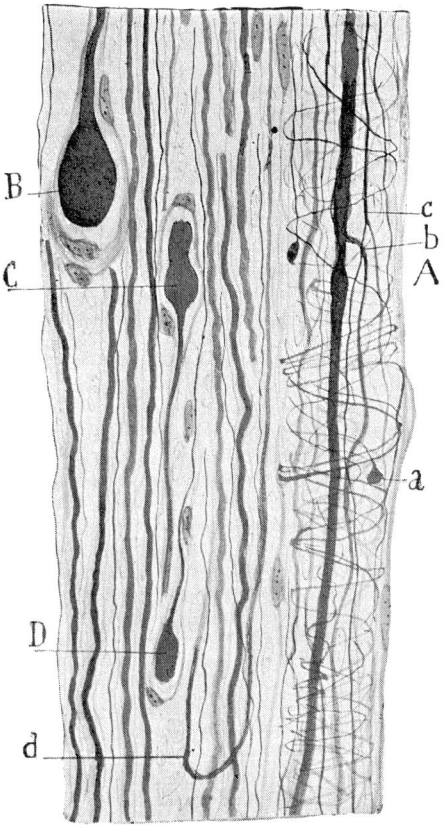

FIG. 83.—Piece of the central stump of a rabbit, twenty-five days after the operation. *A*, nervous spool under a capsule which belongs to a sterile axon; *B*, sphere in continuity with a retrograde fibre; *a*, small clubs of growth; *b*, collateral of a medullated tube; *c*, fine fibres which are ramified within the spool; *d*, loop of a retrograde and deviated fibre.

called *tactile adhesion*, that Dustin called *contact sensibility* and *haptotropism*, and that Loeb [2] and Harrison [3] named *stereotropism*.

[1] Cajal : " Algunas observaciones favorables à la hipótesis neurotrópica," *Trab. del. Lab. de Invest. biol.*, tomo 8, 1910.

[2] L. Loeb : " Growth of tissues in culture media," etc. *Anat. Record*, vol. 6, 1912.

[3] R. G. Harrison : " The cultivation of tissues in extraneous media as a method of morphogenetic study," *Anat. Record*, vol. 6, 1912.

Harrison showed experimentally that embryonic fibres grown *in vitro* follow blindly the paths of threads of fibrin, connective cells, threads of cotton, and even the cover-glass. Dustin [1] has carried out interesting investigations on the tutorial function of the connective tissue cells of the scar, of which we shall speak below.

Naturally, the robust retrograde fibres have large terminal clubs or buds, while the fine fibres are crowned by clubs of lesser size. If they are studied during the first four or five days after the operation, one sees that the retrograde clubs and fibres lack marginal cells. From the eighth day on, the satellite cells appear, and the terminal bud, which has the form of a ball and is more or less immobile, is protected by a nucleated capsule. But of these arrested and capsulated clubs we shall speak at greater length below, as they merit a detailed examination.

Gigantic clubs : their degenerative phenomena.—Very large balls, in size between 10 and 40 or more μ, and residing usually in the thickness of the central stump and beginning of the scar, were doubtless seen by the older investigators. But, as they were working with imperfect methods, they were not able to determine their true relations and physiological significance. Sigmund Mayer,[2] of Prague, who saw them first, declared them to be nerve cells, probably sensory in character. As Ranvier [3] noted, however, such globular formations are without a nucleus and cannot, therefore, be true neurones. Ranvier himself was unable to determine the true relation of the balls to the fibres, and he interpreted them as gigantic masses developed along the course of thick axons, and comparable to the bipolar sensory nerve cells.

Thanks to the new technique, we have been able to definitely determine the morphology and connections of these forms. In our first communications [4] on the degeneration of nerves we noted the relatively late appearance of such spheres, and their character as the terminal masses of fibres that had lost their way, and were arrested and degenerating. We stated : " It is very possible that the retardation of the axons in their course, and an insuperable obstacle between connective bands or nervous bundles, are the conditions of

[1] Dustin : *Arch. de Biol.*, t. 25, 1910.

[2] Sigmund Mayer : " Die peripherische Nervenzelle und das sympathische Nervensystem," *Arch. f. Psychiatrie*, 1876.

[3] Ranvier : *Leçons sur l'histologie du système nerveux*, tome 2, p. 78, 1878.

[4] Cajal : *Boletín del Instituto de Seroterapia de Alfonso XIII.*, no. 3, 1905.

the hypertrophy of such clubs, which show only reticulated neurofibrils and are stained only in their central portion."

This description, which we enlarged and illustrated with numerous drawings in a subsequent treatise,[1] and the interpretation of their origin, were both confirmed by Marinesco. This author made a good analysis of the degenerative phenomena of these balls. He stated that their formation might be the result, not only of the arrest of the fibres by obstacles, but also of nutritive disturbances. Perroncito, Nageotte, Dustin, etc., subsequently gave similar descriptions and interpretations.

Situation and volume of the balls.—The gigantic clubs or balls are found usually within the central stump, in an area that does not extend more than two or three millimetres above the scar. The region where they are commonest is between the scar and the old border of the central stump. In the scar itself, especially in the first quarter, they are rarer, although they are never lacking. Finally, these spheres are relatively little seen in very young animals, either in the central stump or in the scar.

The volume of the ball varies, as we have already stated, within very large limits—6 to 40 μ, with the diameter of the axon or the thickness of the supporting branch. There is, however, no proportion between the diameter of the axon and that of the gigantic sphere. Sometimes, on the adhering pole of the gigantic ball, one sees a delicate peduncle which is continuous with a fine axon or branch. The retrograde character of the axons that bear arrested balls is also inconstant. Although less frequently, one yet finds enormous spheres in continuity with axons whose orientation is normal (Fig. 83, *B*). It is almost certain that in this case the ball represents the end of a sterile axon which is much retarded within the central segment.

Degeneration of the balls.—The arrested ball, after two or three weeks of immobility, has a characteristic structure which we show in Fig. 84, *A, B, C*. It is not naked like the clubs of growth, but is surrounded, as we stated above, by a certain nucleated capsule which is in continuity with Schwann's membrane. This capsule is very probably produced by the multiplication and migration of the satellite cells of the old generative tube. The substance of the sphere shows, according to the date of the arrest and as a result of

[1] Cajal: "Mecanismo de la regeneración de los nervios," *Trab. del. Lab. de Invest. biol.*, tomo 4, 1905-6.

conditions that are as yet unknown, different aspects, which may be considered as phases of a progressive alteration. The principal aspects are as follows :

(a) Those spheres which are least altered show a neurofibrillar network, which is dense, well stained by silver nitrate, and without any signs of a superficial hyalinization (Fig. 85, A).

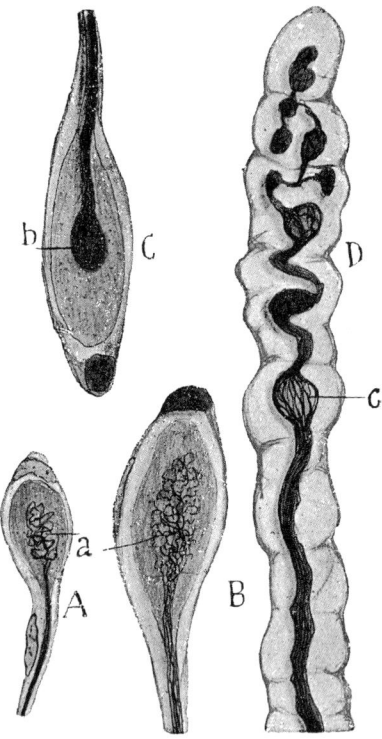

FIG. 84.—Altered clubs, situated at different levels of the central stump. *a*, central network of neurofibrils ; *b*, central mass of argentophilous substance ; *D*, a tube with degenerative forms and tuberose ramifications.

(b) In more advanced periods (Figs. 84 and 85, B) one can distinguish two zones in the protoplasm ; a *cortical* pale zone, furrowed by only a few flexuose neurofibrils, and a central or focal zone, where the neurofibrillar skeleton is dense and, especially, continuous with the axon. Such a degenerative state is very commonly seen from the twentieth and up to the thirtieth or fortieth day after the operation, with many variations. Thus in certain balls the central portion is compact and dark (Fig. 84, *b*), while in others it is loose, rich in neuroplasm, with superficial ravellings (Fig. 84, *a*). In some others, which we reproduce in Fig. 85, *e*, the centre shows a distal pole formed by loose fibrils which are disjoined, like the tip of a brush, and a proximal pole in which the neurofibrils take the form, either of a spool or else of a more or less dense bundle. Finally, the neurofibrillar centre is clearly differentiated from the cortical portion, appearing thickly reticular, as though vacuolated, etc.

(*c*) The ulterior phases consist in the progressive diminution of the neurofibrillar centre, which finally disappears (Fig. 85, *C*, *D*). The fibrils remain only at the place where the axon enters. During this stage the ball, now pale and enormous, takes on a finely granular aspect.

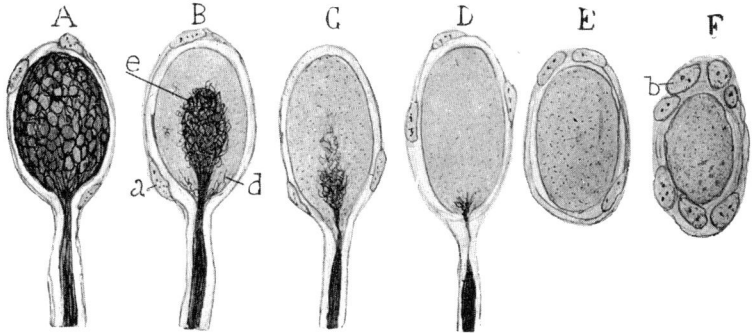

FIG. 85.—Degenerative phases of gigantic arrested balls. Note the progressive hyalinization. *a*, *b*, nuclei of the capsule; *d*, hyaline zone of the ball; *e*, focus of persisting neurofibrils.

(*d*) The axon from which the ball hangs becomes progressively thinner (*D*). Its neurofibrils become first granular and then unstainable; the peduncle is definitely broken, and the sphere remains isolated within its capsule, as though lost in the interstices of the perineurium or in the connective tissue lacunae of the scar (Fig. 85, *E*).

(*e*) Later the ball is digested by the capsular cells. Leucocytes never penetrate within the capsule. The granular mass becomes smaller, becoming uneven in shape, and the capsular cells proliferate and form local conglomerations (Fig. 85, *F*). Finally everything disappears. This process shows great variations in time in each animal and for each fibre. In animals operated on a few days after birth, seventy days after the cut there remains no trace of a ball within the central stump. On the other hand, in adult rabbits and dogs one still finds a few gigantic balls eighty and ninety days after section of the sciatic nerve. These balls are sometimes isolated and in course of being resorbed, sometimes united to a pedicle and showing signs of atrophy.

Groups of arrested balls.—From the twentieth day one can see, here and there, in the central stump near the scar or else at the beginning of the latter, certain capsulated nerve fascicles, within which lie non-medullated fibres of various sizes, all of them arising from the same axon. The perifascicular or Henle's sheath is closed at the distal end, and there is a dilatation, in the shape of a glandular vesicle, reminding one of the capsule of Müller of the uriniferous tubes. Finally, within this reservoir one finds three, four, or more arrested balls, of various sizes (Fig. 86, *a, b*) and forming colonies or accumulations.

The explanation of such a strange disposition is simple if we take into account the tendency, often mentioned in the course of these studies, for the digestive chambers to close up. This impedes or even totally prevents the emergence of the nerve sprouts. In the cases drawn in Fig. 86 the closure was effective and was consolidated by the creation of a robust nucleated capsule which arose from the membrane of Schwann. As a consequence, the buds of growth which crown the bundle of intratubal and isogenous [1] collateral or terminal branches found the path closed, and so remained immobile and, as it were, imprisoned. This, however, does not exclude the possibility that, after a time, some of the branches will be able to perforate the capsule and get to the scar.

Mechanism that produces the gigantic balls.—Two principal causes contribute to the formation of gigantic balls : (1) arrest and definitive immobilization before an insuperable obstacle ; and (2) continuation, at the level of the end of the axon, of the process of assimilation or growth, the *vis a tergo* of Held.

Of the effectiveness of the first condition, apart from the facts upon which we based our opinion in 1905, we now possess direct and indisputable experimental proof. Fig. 87, *b, c*, is a good example of this. In the case here reproduced, ligation of the nerve caused, in the peripheral stump, an insuperable obstacle to the growth of the nerve sprouts. One can see in this figure that as the buds approach the region which is ligated the movement of growth is paralyzed and the delicate terminal cone becomes a more or less voluminous ball. We shall presently speak more at length of this

[1] By " isogenous " we mean " arising from the same axon."

interesting phenomenon. We may note, further, the fact that large balls are found in abundance in the laborious nervous reunions of adipose tissue, elder pith, and, in general, in all cases where the newly-formed axons are caused to grow among almost insuperable obstacles.

The *vis a tergo* of Held, that is, the uninterrupted continuation of the assimilative process, followed by the conditions that we noted

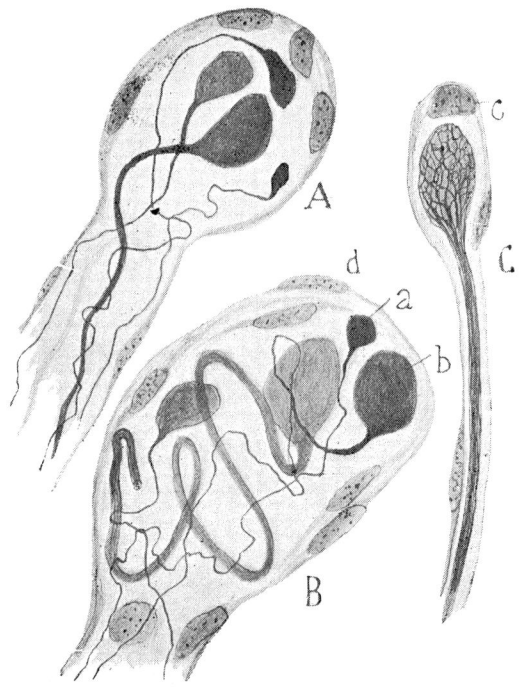

FIG. 86.—Loose balls and nests of balls in the central stump. *A*, a nest of four balls of various sizes; *B*, another and larger nest where the balls are more voluminous; *C*, loose ball in which one can clearly see the reticular texture of the protoplasm and its continuity with the neurofibrils of the axon.

above, seems to be an indubitable joint cause for the enormous protoplasmic accumulation of the sphere and the consecutive neurofibrillar neoformation. It also explains how fine axons sometimes form gigantic balls, and *vice versa*.

Probable cause of degeneration of the balls.—Since, as noted above, the volume of the ball has a limit, and since in time it stops its growth, diminishes in size, and degenerates, one has to invoke some condition which brings about this assimilative suspension and causes the disorganization and death of the end of the axon. This new condition may be functional inactivity, perhaps associated with degeneration of the cell of origin, supposing that the fibre is terminal in character (sterile axons). The nutritive disorders that Marinesco put forward as possible causes of the degeneration must, we believe, be viewed as secondary conditions.

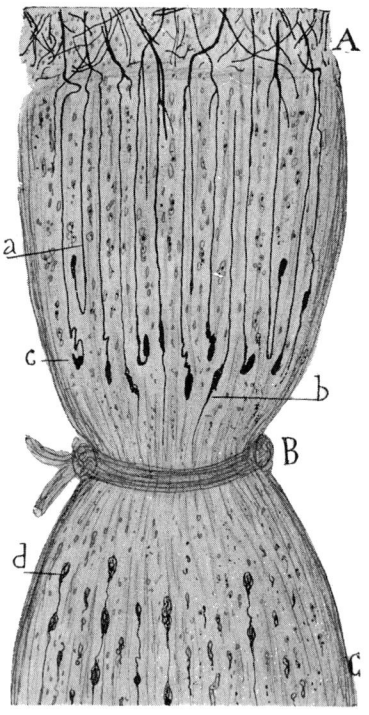

FIG. 87.—Schematic representation of the formative mechanism of large balls and loops of retrogression, within a peripheral stump where a grave mechanical obstacle was put in the way of the newly-formed axons. The peripheral stump of the sciatic nerve was ligated below the cut. Two months-old rabbit, killed eight days after the operation. *A*, scar of the wound ; *B*, thread of the ligation ; *C*, peripheral stump under the ligature—one sees here a few degenerated axons which end in balls ; *a, c*, fibres held up above the ligature ; *b*, arrested ball which sends atenuous fibril toward the compressed region.

Fate of the arrested fibres.—What is the ultimate fate of those fibres which carry a degenerated ball ?

On this point there are no precise and systematic investigations. We are thus reduced to conjecture. If the fibre that carries the degenerated sphere represents a simple axonic branch, it seems probable that with time it would be resorbed from its extremity to its origin in the parent axon.

LATE CONDITIONS OF NERVE SPROUTS 215

On such a theory, if functional activity is maintained in the principal portion of the conductor, the corresponding neurone maintains its normal structure. But if the fibre which is provided with a sphere is of the category of an axon, especially a motor axon, then union with the periphery is entirely frustrated. Under such conditions it appears probable that suspension of function causes not only the retrograde destruction of the axon, but also of the neurone of origin itself. Such destructions and atrophies of the neurone have,

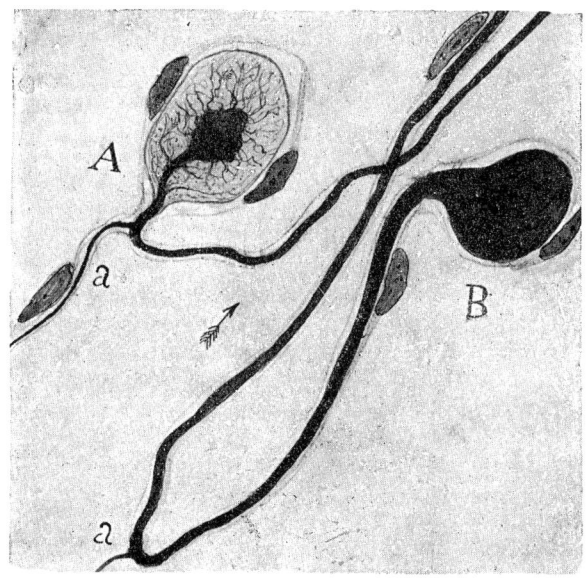

FIG. 88.—*A* and *B*, arrested balls of the central stump; *a*, collateral compensating branches directed towards the scar. Rabbit, killed sixty-eight days after the operation.

as a matter of fact, been described in the ganglia as well as in the spinal cord when nerves were amputated (Marinesco, Lugaro, Klippel and Durante, van Gehuchten, etc.).

It was Marinesco who first formulated this doctrine of atrophy through disuse. He believes that those cells which atrophy are the trophic centres of axons that have definitely gone astray and are totally lost for nervous reunion of the peripheral terminal structures.

Arrested balls which emit compensatory collaterals.—Not all the deviated fibres that carry degenerated balls necessarily perish, compromising their neurone of origin. Some of them attempt, at times successfully, to re-establish the suspended functional connections.

We have several times seen a robust collateral, at various distances from the gigantic ball, which, breaking away from the degenerated sphere, grows actively towards the periphery, taking on the appearance of the axon. We do not know whether such a compensatory phenomenon, of which we show two typical examples in Fig. 88, is widespread enough to make up for the enormous loss of conductors, due to deviations and retrogressions.

Arrested balls and retrograde fibres in the embryo.—One finds with relative frequency, in embryos and foetuses of mammals,[1] sprouts whose terminal cone, arrested by an obstacle which is difficult to cross, becomes notably enlarged and takes the shape of a ball. In Fig. 89, *A*, we show two root bundles of the vagus nerve at its emergence from the medulla in a rabbit embryo 2·5 cms. long. One may observe how, at their exit, where they have struck the perimedullar membranes (*b*), two cones have become arrested, becoming larger. A similar phenomenon is also seen in two afferent or sensory fibres (*a*).

The medullary buttress, where dense fascicles of epithelial cells are placed, constitutes a grave impediment to the progress of the fibres. It is therefore not strange that some of these are temporarily arrested, until, stimulated by the obstacle, they send out an exploratory sprout which rapidly orients itself. The gigantic thickenings which can be seen next to the epithelium represent the remnants of old cones, arrested, thickened, and in course of resorption.

Finally, in the nerve centres not only of foetuses, but also of recently-born animals, one rather frequently finds axons that have lost their orientation, and after describing wide loops, once more find the right path, joining their congeners which had grown out earlier. One often finds disorientations of this kind in the intracellular radicles of nerves whose path is complicated, especially in the N. patheticus and common oculomotor nerves.

It thus appears that the process of normal neurogenesis is subject to the same laws as pathological neurogenesis. Far from being perfect, the regulative mechanisms of the growth and orientation of the axons sometimes break down. Incongruences of a certain importance are thus produced, and, in particular, the number of conductors that are definitely and functionally useful is much reduced. It appears probable that pathological conditions of development result in an even greater increment of loss during these contests, in which only the strongest or

---

[1] Cajal: " Génesis de las fibras nerviosas en el embrión y observaciones contrarias á la teoría catenaria," *Trab. del Lab. de Invest. biol.*, tomo 4, 1905-6.

the most fortunate fibres survive. One can see with what reason we have affirmed—and Heidenhain supports us in this view—that perhaps one of the most powerful causes of physiological diversification of the human brain is the variation, in each individual, in the number of neurones which, having lost their way or formed aberrant connections, have been resorbed. Besides, the surviving fibres are not the same in each individual.

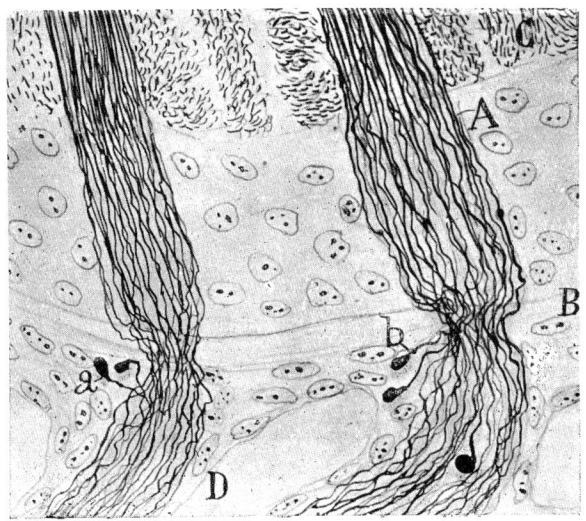

FIG. 89.—Roots of the vagus nerve at their exit from the medulla. Rabbit embryo, 2·5 cms. long. *A*, roots; *B*, pia mater; *C*, white matter of the trigeminus nerve; *D*, neurilemmatic sheath of the nerve cordons; *a*, sensory clubs that are held back; *b*, motor clubs.

Nervous spools.—One of the strangest incongruences of growth in the central stump of cut nerves, as well as in the beginning of the scar, is the spool or helicoidal nervous structure, pointed out as a late formation by Ranvier, Vanlair, and Stroebe, and later described in detail by ourselves, Perroncito, Marinesco and Minea, Dustin, etc. These structures appear to be vivid examples of inadaptation and lack of utility. But they also clearly show to what extent the influence of the environment and the thousand fortuitous incidents that occur around the cone of growth decide the fate of the nerve sprouts and frustrate the most ingenious plans of nature.

The helicoidal structures are seen only in animals that are adult or that were operated on a month or two after being born. This means that they are found almost exclusively in medullated tubes, and especially in the largest ones. One will search in vain for nervous spools in the central stump of cats, dogs, or rabbits that were operated on during the first two weeks after birth.

The nervous spool, as noted above, is in reality nothing more than a persistent apparatus of Perroncito (Fig. 62), whose central and spiral fibres have grown very much in thickness and length, have acquired partially or completely a sheath of Schwann and a medullary sheath, and terminate, either inside or outside the sheath of the old tube, in medium-sized and large capsulated balls.

We can distinguish two principal kinds of helicoidal structures— the sterile type, which has no efferent branches ; and the semifecund type, in which there are some free conductors which are capable of being incorporated into the scar and of joining more or less tardily the early fibres.

(a) We show in Fig. 90, E, D, various examples of the *sterile* type, which is perhaps that most commonly found, and which is especially concentrated at the edge of the central stump.

One can see that the entire fibrillar apparatus is surrounded by the old sheath of Schwann (a), whose nuclei have multiplied. The pocket thus constituted forms a more or less pointed cul-de-sac. Such a sacciform diverticulum is nothing more than the old digestive chamber which has not been perforated. The conductors inside are of two kinds : (1) the central or longitudinal fibres, which are one, two, or three in number, relatively thick, and which, having encountered the end of the sac, turn back by folding upon themselves ; (2) the tangential or helicoidal fibres, which are generally fine, although they vary in thickness, and which describe close spirals under the general capsule and around the central branches. The richness and closeness of the spirals is such, in some cases, that it is impossible to give an exact description or representation of them. Finally, some spiroidal branches, and sometimes the central branches themselves, have bored laterally through the surrounding membrane of the apparatus, showing thick capsulated clubs which are in a phase of paralysis (Fig. 90, b, c).

Cross-sections (Fig. 90, B, C) give one a clear conception of the helicoidal structure. We reproduce three of them in the same figure (A and B). They show that the axial branches and some of the thick spiroidal ones possess sheaths of Schwann and a medullary sheath.

LATE CONDITIONS OF NERVE SPROUTS 219

Concerning the origin of the fibres, there is great diversity. One may say, however, that generally the spiroidal apparatus consists of nervous collaterals, while the thick central fibres represent the continuation of terminal branches. There are cases, on the other hand, where all are transversal.

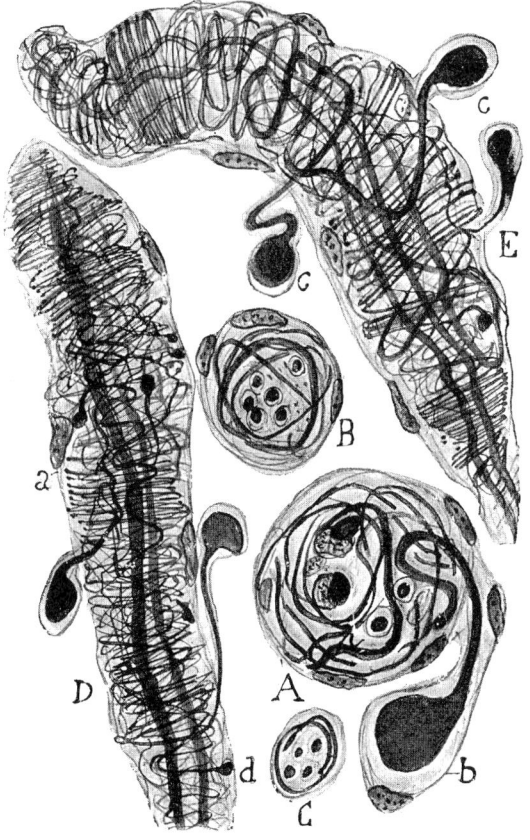

FIG. 90.—Spools of the displaced central stump of an adult rabbit, sixty days after the operation. *A, B, C,* spools of various sizes in cross-section ; *D, E,* large spools seen along their length ; *a,* external membrane ; *b,* covering of a gigantic ball ; *c,* medium-sized balls ; *d,* small internal ball.

(*b*) The semi-fecund spools correspond to the variety of the apparatus of Perroncito that bears the same name. Here again are abundantly found retrograde fibres and helicoidal collateral fibres which terminate in intratubal clubs ; but they also have a characteristic feature, peculiar to them alone. A thick fibre, which usually, but not always, is undivided, travels along the axis in a centrifugal direction, perforates the cul-de-sac of the old tube of Schwann and goes in a straight and direct line to the scar (Fig. 82, *b*). At first sight one thinks that it is the same pre-existent axon. In reality it is nearly always a robust collateral branch that is converted into a terminal one, owing to the resorption of the necrotic segment and the disappearance of the old axonic club, which is more or less sterile. From the twenty-fifth or thirtieth day on, such thick axial conductors have a myelin sheath. The helicoidal fibres, on the other hand, are medullated very late.

What is the fate of the helicoidal structures ? It would be very desirable to investigate this point systematically, keeping alive for three, four, or more months the experimental animals. Those upon which we operated—dogs, cats, rabbits, and guinea-pigs—were almost always killed before the end of four months. Many of them also had the nerve cut during the first few weeks after birth, that is, under conditions very unfavourable to the development of the helicoidal structures. There is evidence, however, that the helicoidal system is finally resorbed, as well as the spiral system of the semifecund structures. In some preparations of cats killed two months after the lesion, we have seen tubes whose spiroidal collateral fibres appeared varicose, retracted, and crowned by pale clubs which were degenerating. Such dispositions are very probably evidence of a slow process of necrobiosis and absorption of the spiral system, without injury to the central fibre or fibres, which would be preserved indefinitely, on condition, of course, of reaching the nerve endings.

Perhaps a similar process of atrophy and destruction befalls the sterile spools. But here we lack precise observations that would permit us to make such an assertion. At any rate, if this conjecture is well founded, the degenerative phenomenon must occur very slowly. Two and a half and three months after the operation in an adult rabbit, one can still see in the central stump some sterile helicoidal structures, which take the stain perfectly, although they show clubs which are more or less hyaline and wrinkled.

Genesis of the helicoidal structures.—Concerning the mechanism that produces the spools the problem is now, fortunately, in a better way of solution than in the days of Ranvier and Vanlair. If we neglect minor causes, four factors are concerned in this process : the *vis a tergo* of growth, the resistance of Schwann's membrane, the closing-up of the digestive chamber or sac, and, finally, the phenomenon of *tactile adhesion—stereotropism* of Loeb and Harrison, *haptotropism* of Dustin.

The first two conditions are well known. We have, at various times, spoken ot their decisive influence in the formation of deviated axons and fasciculation of the sprouts. It is also known, thanks to Perroncito, that the spiral fibres represent intratubal collaterals which have arisen very early in the pre-terminal itinerary of the axon. But neither the influence of the continuous amoeboidism of the sprouts, nor the resistance of Schwann's membrane, nor the fact that the isogenous fibres are forced to grow side by side and to mix with each other intimately, explain the mechanism of this process, nor do they take a principal part in it.

Why is it that, having arrived at the distal pole of the pocket of Schwann, the nerve sprouts turn back ? To what condition is due this strange tendency of the collateral fibres to fold back and to describe close spirals exactly under Schwann's membrane ?

Both of these questions are answered by the two last factors noted above. Thus, the folding back of the central, tangential, or spiroidal fibres, is easily explained, if one admits the idea, which many facts indicate, that the inferior pole of the digestive chamber or terminal sac of the old tube is often obstructed, either through retraction of the membrane or else by the concurrence, under the sac, of the fascicles of Henle's sheath, or, finally, by an accidental grouping of leucocytes, embryonic connective corpuscles, or fatty detritus.

As to the tenacity with which the sprouts apply themselves to Schwann's membrane, describing complicated spirals, it would result simply from the tendency of the cones of growth to seek, like vines and climbing plants, guides or mechanical support. The fact that the spirals are very close, touching each other at many points, may also be explained by a similar need for support. Thus stereotropism and the innate tendency to economy of effort lead an axon to congregate with others which have preceded it, to follow them closely. and thus finally to form bundles and closely-wound spools. Perhaps *reciprocal homotropism*, which we [1] have invoked in another study. also has some influence in causing free axons to join with bundles. as though they attracted each other mutually. As to neurotropism.

[1] Cajal : " Nuevas observaciones sobre la evolución de los neuroblastos," *Trab. del Lab. de Inv. biol.*, tomo 5, 1907.

invoked by Marinesco and Dustin, it has little or no influence in the creation of the helicoidal structure.

In our first communication on nervous regeneration we attributed the production of spiroidal structures to purely mechanical causes, following in this Ranvier's opinion.

Lugaro, who holds very largely the same views, after recognizing the influence of mechanical causes, sees in the spiral phenomenon a clear index of neurotropic disorientation due to the interposition of the scar, which causes irregularity in the flow of attracting substances up to the nerve sprouts of the central stump.

Marinesco propounds, as an explanation, two new ideas : the inertia of amoeboidism in the terminal clubs, and the perturbative action of the intratubal *apotrophic cells*. He believes that a great number of spiroidal structures contain fusiform apotrophic cells capable of attracting the recently-formed sprouts.

Dustin agrees with Lugaro and ourselves that chemotactism is absent in the creation of the helicoidal apparatus. He inclines towards Marinesco's view that, in the spiral disposition, we have the result both of the haptotropism of the sprouts, and of the action of accumulations or glomeruli of satellite cells—the daughter Schwann cells or *apotrophic* cells of Marinesco—situated under the membrane of the common tube.

But this influence of the daughter Schwann cells can no longer be accepted since Perroncito showed that the helicoidal apparatus appears precociously, beginning a few hours after section of the nerve. Besides, as we show in Fig. 55, the helicoidal collaterals appear before the cells of Schwann proliferate, and, as a consequence, before the formation of apotrophic cells. All the spiral fibres, twelve to twenty-four hours after the section, are, of course, completely naked, growing between Schwann's membrane and the myelin sheath. We may add that it is impossible to observe any change of orientation of the sprouts when they travel by the nuclear region of Schwann's cell. The intratubal elements pointed out by Marinesco and Dustin, and seen by us some time ago, are formations that appear late.

Thus everything leads one to believe that in the spiroidal disposition the only extrinsic factors that intervene are mechanical conditions. In order to understand the remarkable growth of the sprouts, one need not, on the other hand, exclude the trophic influence of Schwann's cell and that of the liquid enclosed in the digestive chamber.

X

INNERVATION OF THE PERIPHERAL STUMP

Arrival of the nerve sprouts.—Their ramifications and penetration in the distal stump.—Intratubal and extratubal fibres.—Buds of growth and ramifications within the peripheral stump.—Variable velocity of axonal growth in the various situations.—Late, precocious, and extremely rapid neurotisation.—Connections of the sprouts with Schwann's cells of the distal stump.—Schemes for the general course of precocious, difficult, and normal neurotisation.—Formation of the nuclei and medullated sheath of the sprouts.

THE innervation of the peripheral stump of cut nerves through the growth, across the scar, of nerve sprouts arising in the central stump, is a fact that was long ago demonstrated by Ranvier, Vanlair, Kölster, Nothafft, Ziegler, Stroebe, Münzer, Mott and Halliburton, Stuart, etc. Some of these authors, especially the first two, also noted the bifurcations of the newly-formed axons during their transit through the scar and, especially, when about to enter the peripheral stump and penetrate into the old sheaths of Schwann.

The investigations of these workers, however, were made during late stages of development, at a time when the myelin is formed anew, and the regenerated tubes are thus recognizable in preparations made by means of osmic acid or Weigert's stain. Thus they necessarily missed all that concerns the first phases of the process—the growth of the naked axons in the scar, the mechanism of the divisions, the fate of the buds of growth, and the entrance and growth of the fine nervous projections into the old sheaths of the distal segment. They saw, so to speak, the static, finished product. But they were unable to see its genesis and the thousand early incidents in the process of nervous reunion of the peripheral stump.

In the last few years the work has been to convert that which was static into a dynamic whole, that is, to fill in the histogenetic lacuna. Already Purpura,[1] by means of Golgi's method, was able to see a few non-medullated fibres, from the scar to the distal stump,

[1] F. Purpura: "Contribuzione allo studio della rigenerazione dei nervi periferici. Comunicazione fatta nella seduta del 1 Feb. 1901," *Boll. della Società medico-chirurgica di Pavia*, 1901.

at whose border he described and drew many bifurcations. But the entire process, from the first to the last phases, can be well studied only by means of the method involving reduced silver nitrate. Although we had made some trials in 1904, using this technique with regenerated nerves, it is to Medea [1] that we owe the proof of its applicability for showing non-medullated nerve sprouts.

Our observations [2] on the scar and peripheral stump, from the tenth day after the operation on, gave the essential details of the arrival, ramification, penetration, and growth of the sprouts within the peripheral stump. The important investigations of Perroncito,[3] made by our method, were specially concerned with the analysis of the precocious phenomena of regeneration. His observations, as well as those of Krassin, who used methylene blue, those of Lugaro, Marinesco, Minea, Dustin, Deineka, etc., all of whom used reduced silver nitrate, confirmed our description, clearing up a few undecided points concerning the innervation and functional redintegration of the peripheral stump. We may now describe in order the various phases of the process.

Time required for the nerve sprouts to innervate the peripheral stump.—Nearly all the older authors state that the nerve sprouts arrive at a late epoch at the peripheral stump. But their estimates are very different. Thus while Büngner saw perfectly differentiated amyelinic axons within the peripheral stump (auto-regeneration) at the end of the second week, Stroebe states that an interval of twenty-seven days is required, and Ranvier, more than a month and a half. Naturally, the modern authors, using a much more effective technique for the nerve sprouts, give much shorter times. Thus Marinesco saw the first axons in the peripheral stump fifteen days after the operation; we observed them ten to fifteen days after section of the nerve in young animals; Perroncito described them as occurring in the dog ten days after the nerve was cut and the two stumps sutured. Finally Deineka, accelerating by means of

---

[1] Medea: "L'applicazione del nuovo metodo di R. y Cajal allo studio del sistema nervioso periferico nella neuriti parenchimatosa," *Società medico-chirurgica di Pavia*, Seduta 14 Jennaio 1905.

[2] Cajal: *Boletín del Instituto de Bacteriología y Seroterapia de Alfonso XIII. Fasciculos II. (Junio) y III. (Septiembre)* 1905.

[3] Perroncito : " La rigenerazione delle fibre nervose. Comunicazione fatta nella seduta del 3 Nov. 1905," *Bolletino della Società medico-chirurgica di Pavia*, 1905.

heat the growth of the axons across the scar, and making the latter as small as possible by means of hemisections, was able to see the arrival of the sprouts at the distal stump after the third day, an exceptionally short time, since in rabbits at ordinary temperature the same process requires seven or more days. Nor is this speed found when the fibres have to cross a scar of medium thickness. The time noted is that necessary for the nerve sprouts to penetrate the peripheral stump, not to follow it entirely.

We have studied carefully the question of the time of reunion, both initial and complete, of the distal stump. The initial connection occurs very variably, depending principally on the size of the scar, on the obstacles present in it, and even on the species and age of the animal. There are four main conditions which bring about variations in the time of reunion: (1) degeneration caused by crushing, cold or heat, chemical agents, etc., that is, where there is no interruption of Schwann's sheath; (2) degeneration following upon hemisection, the two stumps remaining near each other; (3) complete section with separation of the stumps; (4) section followed by ablation of a piece of variable length of the peripheral segment, with folding of the central stump, etc.

1. The first case is the most favourable for speedy reunion. Without here going into details concerning the consequences of crushing, we may say that the reunion of the degenerated part occurs with great speed; the nerve sprouts, nearly all of them ravelled, traverse long distances in a few days. One often sees after five days the degenerated portion of the peripheral stump innervated along three or four millimetres. One easily understands so great a speed, since the fibres find in the old tubes of Schwann, not only pre-established routes, but also a very favourable nutritional environment. Besides, they have not to cross any scar, thus avoiding, as we shall show below, great set-backs. This great speed of nervous reunion was noted by Stroebe, who stated that it was accomplished in seventeen days after compression, while it took ten days more—twenty-seven days—after complete section of the sciatic nerve. He very pertinently attributed the rapidity to the absence of a scar. As Stroebe worked with methods which were incapable of staining non-medullated fibres effectively, the time intervals which he observed are far too long.

2. In nervous hemisections the penetration in the peripheral stump occurs much less rapidly. The stumps separate about 0·5 mm.

from each other, sometimes less, and therefore the sprouts have to traverse, not only the central stump, but also an area full of exudate or incipient cicatricial tissue. As a consequence the arrival of the axons at the distal stump and their penetration into it for a few millimetres require seven to eight days. Nevertheless, in some exceptional cases, such as when one operates on cats a few weeks old, in hemisections in which the stumps are very close to each other, etc., the time required is as little as six and a half days.

3. When the section is complete the stumps separate very much. In adult dogs and rabbits this separation exceeds 0·25 cm., and in large dogs may reach 0·50 cm. In one to three weeks-old cats and rabbits, on the other hand, the separation is of about 0·15 to 0·3 cm. At any rate, an extensive scar constitutes a serious cause of retardation, not to mention besides the frequent interposition of foreign tissues, such as adipose tissue, muscle, blood clots, etc., which are even less propitious than young connective tissue to growth of the sprouts. In consequence of such obstacles, one rarely sees nervous reunion extending to 1 or 2 mm. of the peripheral stump before the tenth day. Usually one sees with certainty the axons in the peripheral stump and their growth along the sheaths only from the twelfth to the fifteenth day.

4. Artificial separation of the nerve stumps. When, like Bethe, Münzer, Lugaro, van Gehuchten and others, one cuts off a portion of the central stump to elongate the scar, or when one folds it or sews it to the skin, as we have often done, then the entrance of the fibre into the distal stump may be retarded a month and a half or more. In a rabbit whose central stump was sewed to the skin of the buttock, with resection of the peripheral stump—about 1 cm.— the innervation of the latter required sixty-eight days and was very incomplete. As is to be supposed, there is no nervous reunion of the peripheral stump when, like Lugaro, one cuts out a piece of the lumbar spinal cord with its ganglia.

We may add that cold (Deineka), hydrophobia (Cajal), anaemia, ablation of the thyroid (Marinesco and Minea [1]), anaesthetics (Marinesco), insufficient food (Cajal), and other debilitating conditions, lengthen the process or arrest it completely.

Speed of growth of the nerve sprouts.—This is a problem to which,

---

[1] Marinesco and Minea : " Sur l'influence exercée par l'ablation totale du corps thyroïde et par l'insuffisance thyroïdienne sur la régénération des nerfs sectionnés," *Annales de Biol.*, vol. 1, fasc. 1, 1911.

owing to many disturbing causes difficult to measure, only a roughly approximate solution can be given. A fact that is rather assumed than proved is that *the velocity of growth varies for each region*, such as the central stump, the scar, clots, the peripheral stump. From observation of the facts one easily deduces another law which is no less important, namely : *The vigour of growth—the vis a tergo* of Held, *declines progressively with time, until it becomes nil or almost nil*. This is seen in deviated and arrested fibres, the arrival of the sprouts at peripheral stations, etc. It would be very desirable to know the formula of this retardation, whose quantity must notably alter the figures of axonic growth obtained in different regions, according to the various epochs. To-day, however, we must rest satisfied with a qualitative concept, since greater precision would require a very arduous and fatiguing experimental study.

Putting aside this problem, and confining ourselves to the investigation of the speed of growth during the first two weeks, we find the following causes of error : (1) Inconstancy of the time which it takes for the axons of the central stump to get into a state of formative erethism ; (2) variable extent of the necrosed portion of the pre-existent axons, and therefore variability in the path which the collateral or terminal sprouts must follow in the central stump in order to reach the border of the scar ; (3) inconstant resistance, due to the presence of exudates or the interposition of foreign tissues in cicatricial tissue intercalated between the fragments ; (4) disturbing influence of the obstacles, such as fatty droplets, axonic remnants, etc., which the clubs find in the distal stump.

Taking into account the above causes of error, and insisting that the following data constitute approximate values only, we may give the velocity of growth for the nerve sprouts in various regions. These data are from numerous measurements in rabbits, cats, and dogs, whose sciatic nerve was completely cut across.

As was to be expected, these data show that the speed of growth is much greater for the sprouts in the peripheral stump than for those in the scar. They also show that the phase of dividing turgidity represents a loss of time which, for most fibres, represents about thirty to thirty-six hours. The slowest growth occurs in adipose tissue, and especially in the exudates present between the two stumps. The following data we consider as a mean.

When a necrotic segment exists, the time required for the sprouts to traverse the central stump is about twenty-four to thirty hours, for an intra or extratubal path of 1 mm., more or less. The velocity per hour would thus be about 3 or 4 hundredths of a millimetre. If we add to this the time required for the formation of the state of divisory erethism or formative turgidity, there results about seventy hours, a period which is usually indispensable for the appearance of the sprouts in the border of the scar.

Naturally when there exists hardly any necrosed segment, as when sharp and clean cuts are made in animals a few days old or animals that are just born, then during those thirty hours the sprouts not only have arrived at the border of the scar, but they have also proceeded a few hundredths of a millimetre in it. This occurred in the case shown in Fig. 56, where, after four days, the sprouts had travelled through about 70 hundredths of a millimetre of the scar.

We have stated that growth through the scar is very difficult. Very careful measurements on many animals have given us a velocity of 15 to 24 hundredths of a millimetre for twenty-four hours ; that is, from 0·006 to 0·01 mm. per hour. This figure is subject to great variations. Thus, in a rabbit killed seven days after the operation, the sprouts in the scar had grown only 25 hundredths of a millimetre. Discounting fifty hours for the initial period, we get about 6 hundredths of a millimetre per day. In exceptional cases we have seen velocities of 30 and even 38 hundredths of a millimetre for twenty-four hours.

Such contrasts depend, very probably, upon the constitution of the scar,[1] on the amount of bloody remnants, and especially, on the distance to which the distal stump is removed. Under this aspect, one can distinguish two classes of scars : (1) Those which are directly influenced by the peripheral stump, from whose tubes there probably emanates some stimulating substance, as we shall state below ; (2) scars where, owing to various incidents, histological screens, such as membranes, clots, adipose tissue, threads from the ligature, etc., oppose themselves to the diffusion of this stimulating substance. A great extension of the scar has the same effect.

[1] Often, especially when the central stump remains immersed in blood or remnants of exudate during the third and fourth days, there is a retardation of twenty-four hours or more, owing to the immobility of the clubs which, enlarged through the impulsion of growth, seem to await at the borders of the scar the absorption of the adverse medium and the organization of the embryonic tissue. As a consequence of this suspension of growth, the relative values of the velocity of growth in the scar may be somewhat greater than those noted above.

The velocity of the cones of growth in the peripheral stump is much greater—between 2 and 3 mm. in twenty-four hours. In hemisections and animals killed seven days after the operation, the rate most usually found was of 2·5 mm. per day. In some really exceptional cases the velocity of growth was 4 mm. per day, or about 17 hundredths of a mm. per hour.

With these data before us, we may imagine, in order to conceive approximately the time curve, a typical case—a cat a few weeks old killed twelve hours after the operation. This consisted in a section of the sciatic nerve ; the resulting scar is small and measures only 2 mm. The sprouts had travelled about 4 mm. within the peripheral stump. The time may be divided as follows :

Preparation of the dividing phase and growth of the sprouts within the central stump - - - - -	2·5 days
Growth through the scar at a velocity of 0·25 mm. per day - - - -	8 ,,
Growth of the nerve sprouts within the peripheral stump, at the rate of 2·64 mm. per day - - - -	1·5 ,,
Total - - -	12 days

We may repeat that these data are rough approximations. Heat, proximity of the peripheral stump, the presence or absence of obstacles, the kind of animal, etc., have a decisive influence. It is only necessary for adipose tissue or a hair to be present in the scar, and the time required for the exodus of the sprouts is doubled or trebled.

To sum up : Supposing that the impulsion of the axon (*vis a tergo*) during the first two weeks is constant or almost constant, then the velocity of growth depends on two factors. One is an *accelerating* factor, the presence of stimulating substances. The other is a *retarding* factor, the interposition of tissues whose interstices are narrow or labyrinthine, such as connective tissue, adipose tissue, etc. When, as occurs in the peripheral stump, a maximum of stimulating substances is added to a minimum of mechanical obstacles, the velocity of growth is considerable and much superior to amoeboid motion. We believe that we are not far from the truth when we say that this velocity is fourteen to sixteen times greater in the peripheral stump than in the scar. We shall speak of this result below and we shall try to interpret it in the light of the hypothesis of neurotropism or stimulating ferments.

The velocities that we have recorded above differ somewhat from those mentioned by Harrison, W. H. Lewis and M. R. Lewis, in their interesting experiments of culture of embryonic nerve tissue in the lymph of amphibians and birds. Harrison states that, with many exceptions, the terminal cones may grow 100 μ in six hours, that is, 16·6 μ per hour. In tissue cultures of the intestine of chick embryos, in indifferent salt solution, in the incubator W. H. Lewis and M. R. Lewis have observed a growth of about 1 μ per minute, that is, about 6 hundredths of a mm. per hour. Such velocities exceed those which we found for the growth of the sprouts across the scar—8 to 10 μ per hour. This is not astonishing, since the evaluations of the American neurologists are on embryos, where the velocity of nervous growth is very great. On the other hand, the exceptional speed which we observed in the peripheral stump—83 to 125 μ per hour, notably exceeds that observed by Harrison for free fibres.

Ramification of the fibres on entering the peripheral stump; growth of the branches in it.—The details of the preliminary division, entrance, and growth of the fibres in the distal stump agree in their essentials, no matter what the date of nervous reunion. There are, however, some differences, depending on whether the latter is slow or late, rapid or extremely rapid.

Late nervous reunion.—We may well begin with this, as it is so simple in its evolution that it is easy to analyze. The sprouts within the peripheral stump are few and one can follow them perfectly; their growth is sufficiently slow for one to see relatively frequently the cones of growth. Finally, once the degenerated non-medullated fibres have disappeared, and the lipoid remnants are almost gone, the sprouts stand out with great clearness within the sheaths of the old conductors. We designate *late nervous reunion* that which occurs from the twenty-sixth or thirtieth day after the operation, the tardiness being caused by the great length of the scar and by the artificial creation of obstacles to the union of the stumps.

Such late axons, when they invade the peripheral stump, find the sheaths easily permeable (*sterile tube* phase [1]) and diffusing stimulating substances in the scar. As the neurotropic sources are many and the axons few, one readily understands that the latter,

[1] The description of these empty sheaths of the peripheral stump, at a late date, is given on p. 90.

stimulated from various directions, become ramified owing to this neurocladic stimulus, and fill many sheaths with branches.

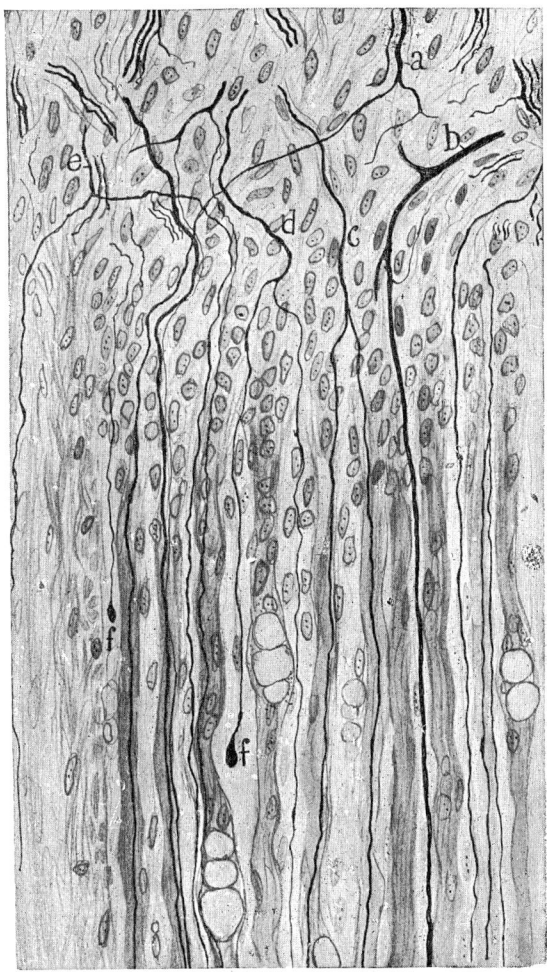

FIG. 91.—Beginning of the peripheral stump of a cut nerve. The rabbit was killed seventy-two days after the operation. *a* and *b*, fibres growing through the scar and arrived from the central stump ; *c* and *d*, fibres that are bifurcated at an acute angle ; *f*, clubs of growth which travel interstitially ; *e*, fibre whose two branches go to different nerve bundles.

These preliminary bifurcations have been confirmed by all the authors, and they have been especially studied by Purpura and ourselves. They are produced, above all, in thick fibres which have the aspect of axons. There are axons which give rise to three, four, and more sprouts, nearly all of which go to different nerve tubes.

The details of this interesting process of ramification are shown somewhat schematically in Fig. 91, where, in order not to complicate the drawing, many branches have been omitted. The nerve in this

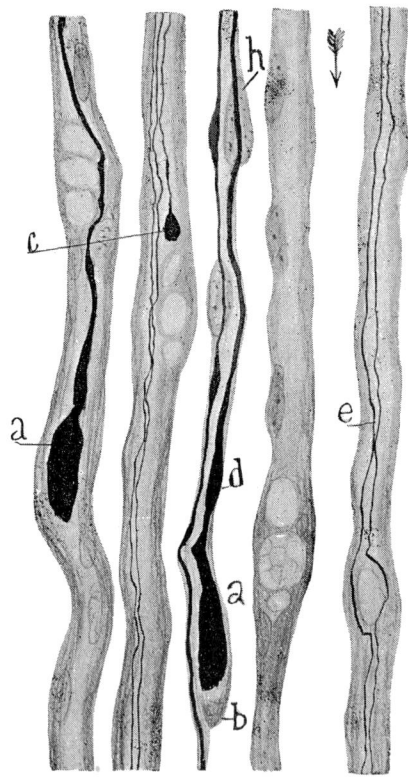

FIG. 92.—Sheaths of the peripheral stump of a nerve seventy-eight days after the section. a, large clubs of growth oriented towards the periphery; b, diverticulum of the sheath which surrounds the club; d, pre-terminal dilatation of the latter; c, fine club; h, nuclei of two fibres which are situated interstitially; e, very fine fibres; the arrow shows the direction of growth.

case was innervated very tardily, owing to obstacles in the path of the sprouts. For this reason, although more than two months had elapsed, the number of fibres that had arrived was small.

The recently arrived axons are of very different diameters. One can classify them as thick, medium-sized, and fine. The last are the most numerous. Some are seen occasionally so very fine as to appear to be formed of a single neurofibril. Ordinarily the thinner branches arriving from the scar go through directly, that is, without dividing within the peripheral stump. A very interesting detail is that while the axons are travelling through the border of the peripheral stump or through the scar near by, they describe complicated loops, as though they were laboriously seeking a path. Once they have penetrated the nerve, however, they grow in an almost straight line.

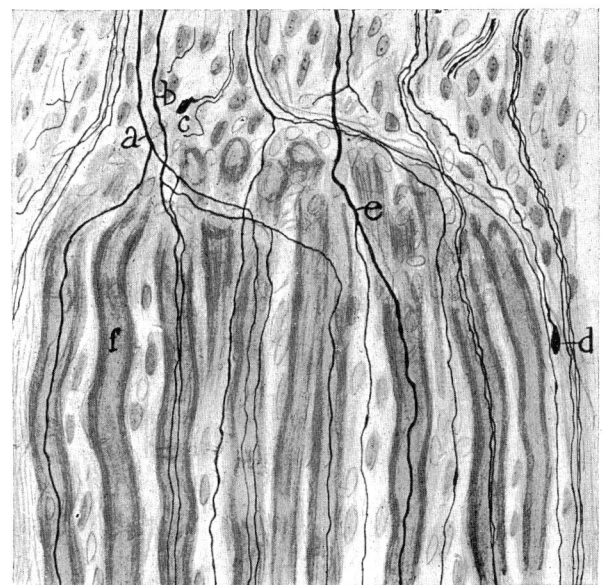

FIG. 93.—Border of a nerve bundle of the peripheral stump. *a* and *b*, nerve fibres of the scar whose branches penetrate into various sheaths of the distal segment; *e*, fibre which bifurcates into a thick and a thin fibre, the latter being interstitial; *d*, club of growth · *f*, empty sheath.

As the authors have noted, the branches in the peripheral stump are either *intratubal* or *extratubal*.

(*a*) The *intratubal* fibres are, without doubt, those most commonly found in late reunions and those of average speed. They are composed of both fine and thick sprouts. We give details concerning their course and connections in Figs. 91 and 93. One can see in Fig. 93, *f*, that there are sheaths in which no fibres are present, a fact which is easily explained by the theory of continuity, but which is very much opposed to the polygenist doctrine.

The innervated sheaths may contain one, two, three, or even a bundle of fibres. These conductors grow between the sheath of the tube and the lipoid and axonic remnants, when these exist, passing round the latter and tracing curves about them. Nerve bundles (Fig. 94, e), when they encounter fatty droplets, become broken up into their component fibrils, which grow side by side.

Although the fibres about which we are speaking are smooth, one often finds, next to the obstacles which they have to cross, accumulations of argentophilous substance which are nothing more, as we showed some time ago, than remnants of cones of growth which are being resorbed. Here and there the intratubal fibres may bifurcate at a variable angle, and the branches take the same direction. Finally, all thick and fine sprouts have at their distal end a thin cone of growth (Fig. 92, c, and 94). This terminal mass is delicate in the finest branches, often taking the shape of a fine grume, or even a ring, but in medium-sized or large branches it is much larger. The cones that are exceptionally large probably belong to fibres which, if they are not completely arrested, at least have a strong tendency to immobilization (Fig. 92, a, b). One also finds fairly often triangular-shaped swellings or cones, ending distally in a brush; these dispositions, as we shall see below, are much more frequent in very rapid reunions than in those which are late.

The growth of the intratubal fibres is so rapid and so uniform that sometimes it is difficult to see the buds of growth. This explains why Perroncito and other authors have not recognized this fact, whose theoretical value is of the greatest importance, since, as we said above, the club or cone of growth marks the end of the axon and the direction of its growth.

Other interesting details can be seen in Fig. 93, a. One of them is the disorder with which reunion is accomplished. Since an axon provides with fibres old sheaths situated far from each other, the initial individuality of the axon is lost, and the distribution of its branches and connections with the terminal structures becomes much disturbed. We shall see below how this fact makes for great difficulty in the interpretation of the mechanism of functional restoration. One must add to these incongruences those which result from the following observations : A single sheath in the peripheral stump sometimes receives branches that originate in several axons (Fig. 93) ; and often a single conductor emits at once intratubal and extratubal projections (Fig. 93, e).

(b) *Extratubal branches.*—These were seen a long time ago by Ranvier, and their existence has been confirmed by nearly all the modern authors. These fibres are most numerous when there are great numbers of sprouts arriving simultaneously at the peripheral stump (Fig. 94, *a*, *f*).

The extratubal conductors are of various sizes. They grow in an almost straight line right in the endoneurium, between the old

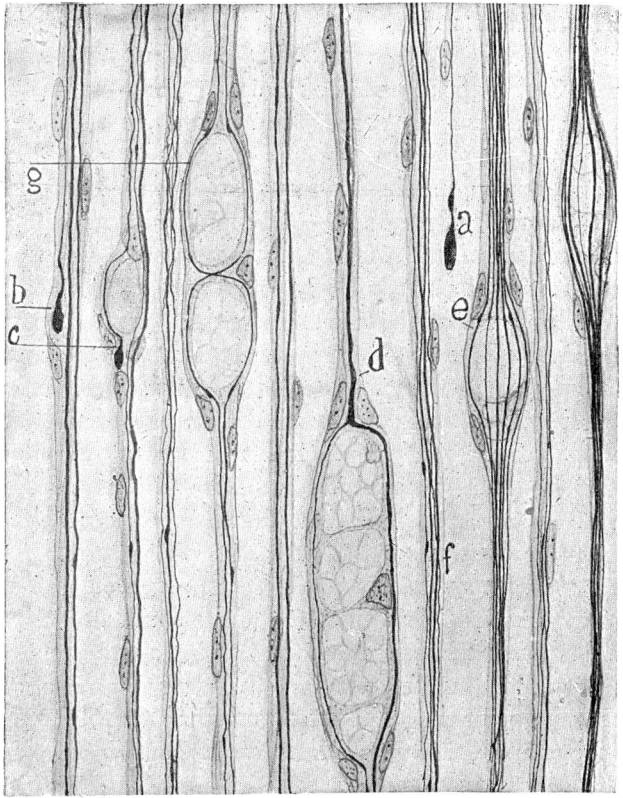

FIG. 94.—Fibres of the peripheral stump of an adult rabbit, which was killed twenty-seven days after the operation. *a*, interstitial club; *b*, club within a cellular cordon; *c*, club which has passed over a fatty droplet; *d*, axon which has divided above a fatty agglomeration; *e*, bundle of axons which surrounds a fatty droplet; *f*, fibrillar fascicle with nuclei; *g*, two fibres which have crossed between two fatty accumulations.

nerve fibres, rarely bifurcating, and ending distally in a club or cone of various shapes, like the intratubal sprouts. These fibres divide here and there when they encounter obstacles, and they show some adaptation to the capillaries and connective tissue bundles by tracing flexuose curves around them. They very rarely become retrograde or definitely arrested. In the latter case they produce large clubs.

Rapid nervous reunion of the peripheral stump.—When the scar is narrow and the peripheral stump is conveniently oriented, the entrance of the nerve sprouts, as stated above, can occur as early as the seventh to the tenth day. In some cases where the phenomenon took place in especially favourable conditions, reunion was already well advanced on the fifth day (Fig. 95, *D*).

Special points in rapid nervous reunion are : the simultaneous arrival of a considerable contingent of fibres of different calibres, which are often congregated in fascicles ; the great number of extratubal conductors, or conductors which are right in the endoneurium ; the presence of fascicles of conductors within the old sheaths ; and, finally, the simultaneous presence of intratubal sprouts with the still abundant remnants of the axon and myelin.

A peculiar fact, which we noted a long time ago, and upon which Perroncito specially insists, is likely to mislead one into believing in an even earlier connection, that is, from the sixth or even third and fourth days. This fact is the conservation, within the peripheral stump, of non-medullated fibres which take the stain perfectly and which are normal to all appearances. As can be seen in Fig. 95, *e*, *d*, and as we stated in another chapter, such resistant axons end at a variable distance from the wound in fusiform clubs of various shapes and sizes. Some of them show, here and there, prolonged dilatations which are paler than the portions of normal diameter, and also neurofibrillar changes which have been well observed by Perroncito. One avoids making the error of taking these conductors for recently arrived sprouts by following them to the above-mentioned terminal thickening and by verifying the fact that they end freely near the scar. Real newly-formed conductors are always prolonged towards the central stump, often arising from an afferent axon.

In Fig. 95 we reproduce a case of especially rapid nervous reunion. Already on the fifth day quite a number of fibres had penetrated into the peripheral stump. Apart from the rapidity of the reunion, this example is very instructive in another way. The sectioned nerve is composed of two large fascicles (*A* and *B*). In front of one of them was resected a piece of the peripheral stump, in order to lengthen the scar. In front of the other, the corresponding distal stump was kept intact, and both stumps remained relatively near to each other owing to the incomplete cutting of the neurilemma. Thanks to this, it was possible to compare easily the speed of growth in the scar of the sprouts arising from the two fascicles of the nerve, and to determine the influence that the substances formed by the sheaths of Schwann of the peripheral stump can exert on the acceleration of the process.

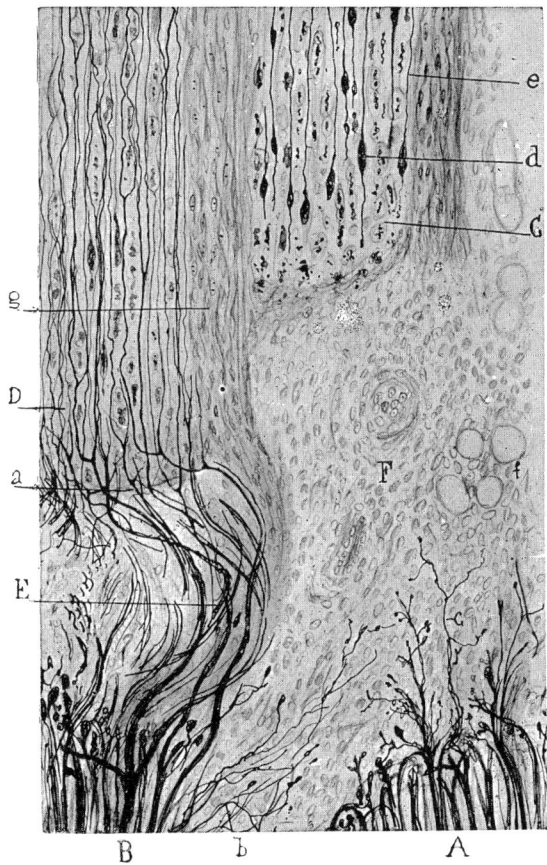

FIG. 95.—Rapid innervation of the peripheral stump. Section of the sciatic nerve of a twenty-days-old cat, killed five days after the operation. From the bundle on the right there was taken out a small piece of the peripheral stump, while the fascicle on the left remained relatively near to the central stump. *A* and *B*, central stumps; *C*, bundle of the resected peripheral stump; *D*, innervated peripheral stump; *F*, scar; *a*, bifurcations of the sprouts at the border of the peripheral stump; *b*, fibres of the central stump lost in the scar, having grown but little because they have not received trophic substances from the corresponding distal stump; *e*, *d*, agonal axons persisting in the peripheral stump; *c*, sprouts destined for the scar; *f*, adipose cells.

One can see in the fascicle on the left (*D*) that there are many sprouts which enter the peripheral stump and the sheaths of Schwann without bifurcating. There are sheaths which contain six or more fine fibres; in others there are only one or two. In some tubes one can see the sprouts passing round the remnants of the old axons and of ellipsoids that are still voluminous.

On the other hand, in the resected distal stump the nerve sprouts have neither penetrated nor even come near. One can see within it the isolated and persistent non-medullated fibres with their agonistic terminal clubs of various forms, frequently lobulated (Fig. 95, d). The extensive intermediate scar is in large part free from fibres. Hardly a third of the extent contains nerve sprouts originating from the central stump (c).

If we compare the sprouts on the right with those on the left we understand the great influence that the proximity of the peripheral stump has on the growth and orientation of the outgrowing newly-formed fibres. We believe it likely that this action is exercised through ferments or stimulating substances formed by the rejuvenated cells of Schwann of the distal stump and poured out by the regions near the scar. We shall give more'attention to this question below. At any rate, Fig. 95, E, suggests that these substances have not only an orienting function, but that they are also trophic in character, since the sprouts which have arrived at the peripheral stump are robust, show a great capacity for ramification, and go straight to their goal without vacillations, as though they were following an irresistible attraction. Those authors who believe that the nervous reunion of the peripheral stump is merely the result of mechanical influences, that is, of axonic growth in the path of least resistance (Ranvier, Vanlair, Stroebe, Dustin, etc.), ought to remember that this path, far from being free and open to the growth of the sprouts, is, on the contrary, full of obstacles. As a matter of fact, the cones have to get by the embryonic connective tissue cells which obstruct the entrance to the tubes of Schwann, and, once they are within the latter, they have to plough their way between the ellipsoids of myelin and the globular masses which completely obstruct the tube. The clefts by which they travel are so narrow that they are invisible under the microscope (Fig. 96). Sometimes the sprouts give the impression that they have created new paths, perforating by force the protoplasm of the bands of Büngner, or separating it from the common membrane. In late connections the disappearance of the ellipsoids diminishes the difficulties.

If one follows the cones of growth along the peripheral stump, one comes to a region, not shown in Fig. 96, about two or two and a half millimetres within the stump, where the cones of growth form steps. When one is dealing with such rapid reunions the terminal thickening no longer appears like a bud, but rather like a spindle with a pointed end, and, even more often, like a more or less ravelled brush. In Fig. 96 we show some of the dispositions of the terminus of axons from various sections of the same preparation. One usually sees the cones in those regions in which the obstacle of the ellipsoids has to be overcome. One can see, in D, two sprouts ending in fusiform pointed structures, which are beginning to slide

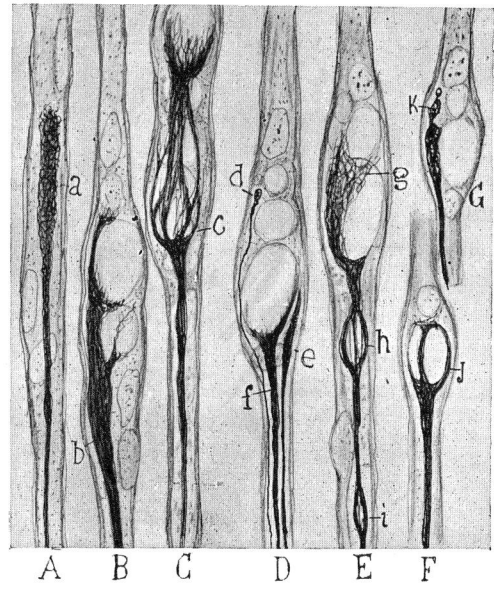

FIG. 96.—Details of the terminus or cone of growth of the sprouts that have penetrated into the old tubes of the peripheral stump during rapid nervous reunions. a, cone in the shape of a boa (fur); e, f, lanceolate cones; B, fusiform ramified cones; g, j, cones in the shape of a chalice; d, terminal bud. Cat killed five days after the operation.

between the membrane of Schwann and a fatty accumulation. In B the end of the axon takes on the shape of a more or less ravelled brush. One also fairly often sees endings in the shape of a fur boa, or a large, loosely reticulated mass which shows signs of ravelling distally (A). When the terminal apparatus encounters a small ellipsoid, it sometimes breaks up, giving rise to an elegant chalice of branches which may join again, once the obstacle has been passed (Fig. 96, g, j). One occasionally finds remnants of this transitory dispersion in the path of some fibres, as we show in h, i. Finally, when the axon takes on a certain thickness and meets with a series of ellipsoids, there are created very complicated dispositions for the accommodation of the end of the axon. The terminus becomes dilated into a membrane or network of more or less dispersed neurofibrils, which surround the fatty droplets (g) ; or else it breaks up, as appears in c, into intricate neurofibrillar plexuses around them. There is a strange tendency on the part of the cones to break up into fibrils which are successively dispersed and concentrated (c). Besides, a considerable portion of the curious forms manifested in those stumps which are rapidly innervated must be considered homologous to the state of divisory stimulus described above, when we spoke of the growth of the sprouts across the scar. A rounded terminal cone, occurring in late nervous reunions—from twenty to twenty-five days on—denotes always a uniform and slow forward growth without any tendency to ramification. Those forms which are broken up represent simply the neurofibrillar skeleton of the terminal swelling. We must not forget that this skeleton is immersed in a plasma which does not take the neurofibrillar stains, and which is itself limited by a thin cuticle. These other elements of the cone are unknown to us to-day in their form and extension. They must lend to the clubs a greater volume than is shown in neurofibrillar preparations, and perhaps somewhat different configurations, as can be seen in the cones of growth that are studied comparatively by Golgi's method and by the method of reduced silver nitrate.

What are the relations of the nerve sprouts with the cells of Schwann of the old tube ? Once they have arrived at the massive portions of the bands of Büngner, how do they cross them ? We have carefully studied these points in rapid nervous reunions of the tenth and twelfth days in adult rabbits, in preparations whose nuclei were subsequently stained with basic aniline dyes. In Fig. 97 we show some details of the connection of the sprouts with the cells of Schwann. At the level of the regions where the fatty ellipsoids are lacking, the cytoplasm and nucleus of the cells of Schwann create a grave obstacle to the growth of the terminal cone. One may note, however, that the bands of Büngner are traversed almost exclusively in two regions. One of these is *axial* or central, very narrow, but easy to dilate, and there many sprouts (Fig. 97, A, a, and D, c), especially thick ones, converge. The other is tangential, situated between the membrane of Schwann or its remains and the protoplasmic mass. When the band of Büngner is very long the majority of the fibres are found in the submembranous path (B, i, j). This preference displayed by the sprouts for travelling under Schwann's sheath shows a loose connection between the latter and its protoplasmic content, or perhaps a weakening or alteration of the membrane, which may become replaced by the sheath of Key and Retzius. Other details are revealed in this figure. One can see a delicate branch (f) arise from the ring formed when a fibre encounters a fatty accumulation. In e one can see the same pheno-

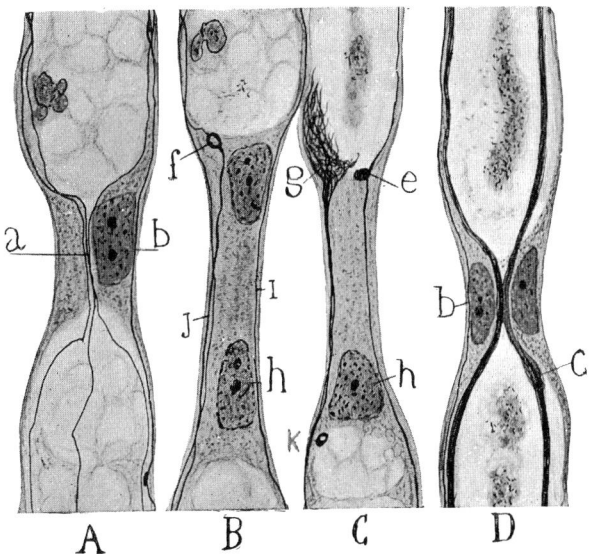

FIG. 97.—Details of the growth of the sprouts among the protoplasmic masses of the cells of Schwann of the peripheral stump. The rabbit was killed twelve days after the nerve section. A, fine sprouts insinuated in the axis of the protoplasmic mass (a); B, fine marginal sprouts; C, other marginal fibres; D, thick axial fibres; b, fibres situated under Schwann's membrane; h, nuclei; e, bud from which arises a fibre; f, ring with filament; g, membraniform terminal cone; k, segregated ring.

menon occurring in a small arrested club. Finally, in K we show a ring which appears to be independent and which has fallen off from some passing sprout. All these phenomena show that the tension of the cones of growth or the impulsive force of nervous amoeboidism is much greater in the peripheral stump than in the scar, since it allows the sprouts to force apart membranes, enlarge obstructed conduits, and perhaps to bore through cells or protoplasmic masses.

Extremely rapid nervous reunion.—This occurs in nerves in which degeneration has been caused by pressure, a ligature, or other means that do not interrupt the continuity of the sheaths of Schwann, and

242 TRAUMATIC DEGENERATION AND REGENERATION OF NERVES

therefore cause the formation of no intermediate cicatricial tissue. Later we shall give the details of this type of reunion, which is also associated with interesting degenerative phenomena. We shall limit ourselves for the present to stating that these reunions have three characteristics : (1) the great speed of growth of the nerve sprouts, which, as we stated above, can in three or four days travel through extensive territories of the degenerated portion ; (2) the formation within the sheaths of bundles constituted by a great number of independent fibres growing out in a straight line ; (3) the almost complete absence of extratubal branches.

To terminate this chapter on the nervous reunion of the peripheral stump we show in Figs. 98, 99, and 100 various schemata. In the first (98) one can see the normal disposition, that is, that which corresponds to the cases in which the stumps are only slightly separated from each other. One may observe that the deviated and recurrent fibres are concentrated in the first fourth of the scar, and especially at the edge of the central stump (*a*). Near the peripheral stump nearly all the conductors are concentrated to enter it (*e*). Once they are within the sheaths of Schwann the fibres go forward in a straight line, and the deviations and retrogressions cease entirely.

In Fig. 99, *B*, we show what nervous reunion would be if it entirely accorded with the mechanical theory of Ranvier and Vanlair. Since the scar is full of obstacles, the deviations and retrogressions would be as numerous at a distance from the central stump as near it. Only a small number of fibres would enter the peripheral stump, within which the obstacles would cause many sprouts to turn back. At the level of the border of the peripheral stump the bowed fibres would predominate, because of their inability to remove the cellular plug which obstructs the entrance to the old sheaths. Under such conditions it is certain that no axon would finally reach the terminal structures. In order to compare this hypothetical mode of nervous reunion with the actual facts, we show in the same figure a normal reunion (*A*).

Finally, in Fig. 100, *A*, we show a scheme of difficult reunions, with folding back of the central stump. A great number of newly-formed axons are lost, and the region of initial disorientation is very extensive. But when the sprouts reach by chance regions of the scar influenced by the peripheral stump, the axons orient themselves and precipitously throw themselves into the old sheaths after a prolific preliminary ramification. One may observe that a considerable portion of the sprouts directed towards the peripheral

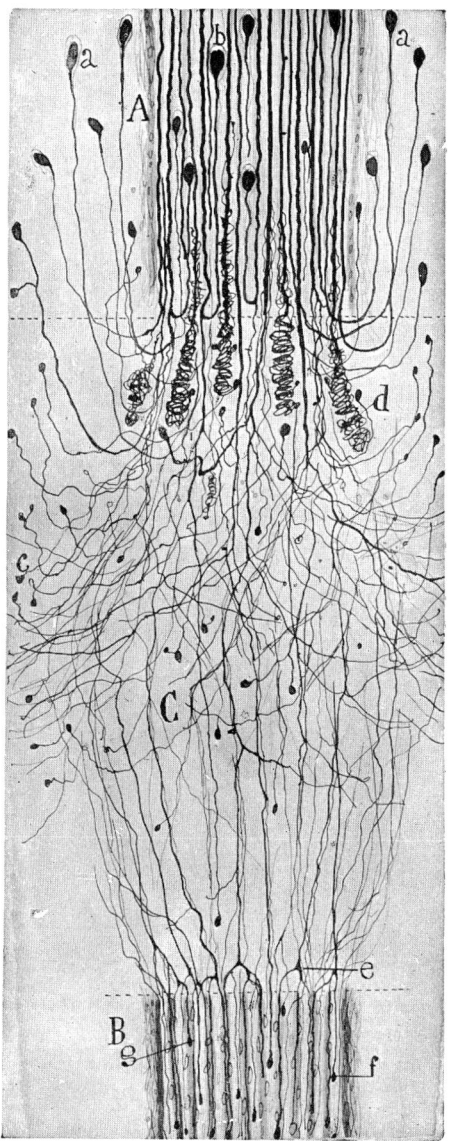

FIG. 98.—Scheme of the general disposition of the fibres in the central stump, scar, and peripheral stump.

stump (*b*), originate from the arch itself of the folded central segment. In *B* we show the effect of a hemisection, as a consequence of which the sprouts, almost without any loss, rapidly innervate the peripheral stump, to whose sheaths, which are still full of ellipsoids, they send, not single fibres, but bundles of branches (b).

Modifications occurring in the fibres of the peripheral stump.— During the three or four weeks following the section, nearly all the

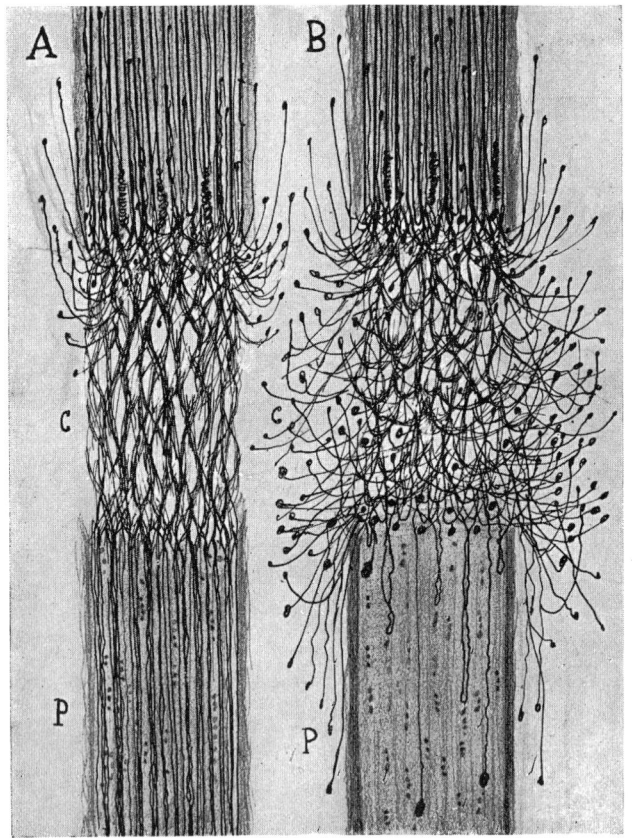

FIG. 99.—Figure to show what the path of the sprouts would be if only mechanical factors were involved. B, central stump; P, peripheral stump. On the left (A) we show schematically the actual disposition.

nerve sprouts present in the peripheral stump are devoid of nuclei and myelin sheath. But from the fourth week on and sometimes before, fusiform cells with an elongated nucleus apply themselves around the fibres. These cells are produced by the proliferation of the old cell of Schwann. We do not know the details of either the proliferation or the attraction of the investing cells by the nerve sprouts. During this period also the extratubal fibres provide themselves with marginal cells. Here the origin of the surrounding cells is difficult to establish. With equal probability, although neither hypothesis is decisive, one might imagine that these cells arise from the mesodermic elements of the endoneurium (Ranvier, Stroebe, etc.),

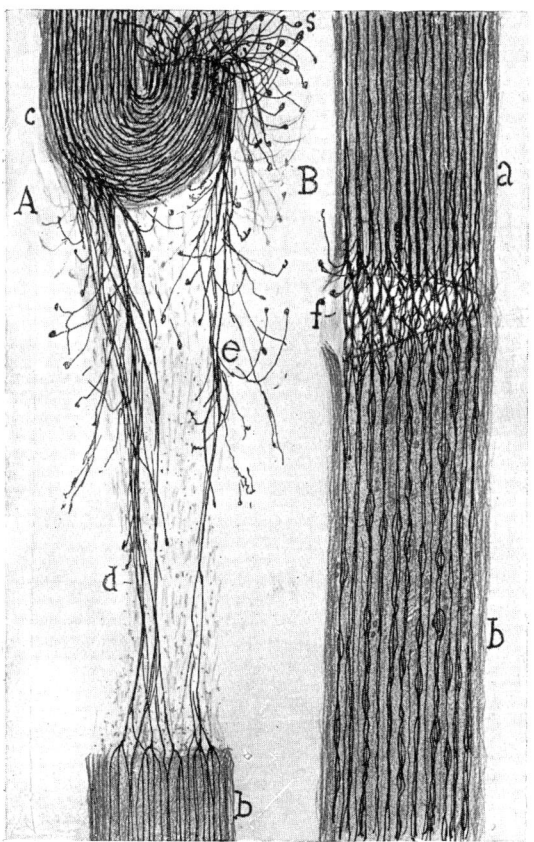

FIG. 100.—Schemata designed to show in *A* a difficult neurotisation and in *B* another which is very easy because of nervous hemisection. *a*, *c*, central stumps; *b*, peripheral stumps; *f*, scar.

or from the cells of Schwann which have migrated for the purpose from the scar or from the old tubes of the distal stump to its connective interstices. One must recognize, however, that as regards the interstitial fibres, the best and most suggestive hypothesis is that of endoneurial origin, which even the polygenist Büngner propounded for the creation of the sheath of Schwann of the old tube.

At any rate, since the majority of the sprouts are intratubal, we see the great importance of the multiplication of Schwann's cells. The old sheath receives a large number of sprouts, and each one of them requires a special investment. The very few pre-existent cells which are in course of rejuvenescence, would certainly not suffice for these needs.

The medullation of the axons is a tardy phenomenon, in regard to whose appearance and mechanism the various authors are not in accord. Stroebe believed that he saw as early as from the second week onwards a thin medullary sheath, stainable by Weigert's method, in the newly-formed fibres of the scar and peripheral stump. Ranvier, on the other hand, saw this covering perfectly formed only from the seventieth day after the operation. Bethe saw it fifty-five days after section of the sciatic nerve in the dog, although he states that he did not examine the peripheral stump a few days before that date. Bethe claims that after three months and twenty-five days the node of Ranvier is perfectly formed. Büngner saw the medullated sheath even earlier than the other authors. He states that there are two successive phases in its formation : the phase in which there is a fine tube, with continuous myelin arranged as a very delicate covering intimately applied to the axon, in the third week ; and the secondary phase of myelin formation, when a thick and discontinuous fatty covering is elaborated, which is in continuity with the covering anterior to it, and which perhaps gets its nutrition from the lipoidal accumulations of the old disintegrated sheath. This large myelin sheath begins to form segmentally, from the thirty-seventh day, in the finely medullated tube. Finally, according to this author, in ligated nerves, there are already in the fourth week nodes of Ranvier in some large tubes.

Another point of discussion concerns the continuous or discontinuous character of the recently-formed myelin sheath. The older authors, like Ranvier, Neumann, Erb, Stroebe, etc., in agreement with the neurogenetic studies of Kölliker, admitted the continuous character of the medullary sheath. The polygenists, such as Howell and Huber, Bruch, Hjelt, Beneke, Büngner, Bethe, etc., considered it discontinuous and thought that it appeared in regions influenced by a cell of Schwann. Thus Bethe affirms that each medullary segment corresponds to a nucleus, and that the naked regions occur always far from the nuclei. In one of the figures of his book [1] he reproduces

---

[1] A. Bethe : *Allgemeine Anatomie und Physiologie des Nervensystems*, p. 202, Leipzig, 1903.

tubes which are medullated segmentally. We need not state that all these assertions of the polygenists are influenced by the concept that the nerve fibres regenerate at the expense of the cells of Schwann.

Our investigations, made on a large number of animals, show that the myelin sheath is a late formation, which begins in a few fibres from the twenty-third to the twenty-fifth day after the section, in those peripheral stumps which are separated from the central stump by a narrow scar. This period may be even shorter, as in guinea-pigs and dogs, when degeneration occurs without a scar, as when the nerve is crushed, when loose ligatures are made, etc. Forty days after the operation the number of medullated tubes becomes larger; one finds four, six, or more in each section of the sciatic nerve in the rabbit. Finally, after two and a half months, a good many of the fibres have a medullated sheath. The majority, however, are still naked and fine. As is to be supposed, the myelin sheath begins to be formed around the thicker axons which are also, although not always, those which first reach the peripheral stump. When the nervous reunion of this stump occurs late, owing to obstacles present in the path of the sprouts, medullated fibres are few even in the third month. This shows that the appearance of the myelin sheath is not related to the age of the sprout, but to the time since the latter has arrived at the peripheral stump, and to its possession, therefore, of surrounding cells. It thus appears that the fatty deposit around the axon implies the settling down and absence of growth of the latter.

Our observations are in accord with those of Kölliker and Stroebe as regards the morphological details of the fibres. In Fig. 101, B, C, which represents a peripheral stump twenty-five days after the section, we show two medullated tubes in the first phase of their formation. One may observe that the myelin sheath is continuous and extremely thin. The osmic acid stain reveals around the axon only a delicate grey line. In some tubes we were able to follow this covering, without interruption, 19 and even up to 25 hundredths of a millimetre. One sees the nucleus, which is relatively large, ellipsoidal, and covered with abundant cytoplasm, towards the intermediate region of such a long segment (a). Finally, there are interruptions of the myelin, which are not extensive, as the polygenists believe, but narrow—6 to 12 μ in length (b). When the myelin reaches these pale regions it becomes thin, and gently ends. Often a few fine fatty droplets (Fig. 101, b) mark this interruption.

Such a cessation of the myelin, whose extent is variable, is nothing else than the node of Ranvier which is being formed, and which has not yet a soldering disc. Later this cement differentiates, the protoplasmic sheath of this non-medullated region narrows, and the node of Ranvier assumes its normal structure.

The evolution that we have just sketched occurs as well in the intratubal as in the interstitial fibres. In Fig. 101, B, one can see an intratubal conductor which, like the precocious sprouts, runs under the external covering of the old sheath, and passes round the fatty droplets of the fusiform accumulations. The great majority of bands of Büngner are lacking in medullated tubes.

Finally, later, the fine medullary sheath thickens, not all at once and as a secondary formation, as Büngner supposed, but slowly, progressively, and, very probably, as a consequence of the formation of new fatty layers between the axon and the first medullary lamina. Like Stroebe, we believe that the formation of the myelin is due to the axon. Those authors who believe that the myelin is a product of the secretory activity of the cells of Schwann ought to remember that the medullated tubes of the nerve centres are lacking, in the embryo as well as in the adult, in marginal cells.

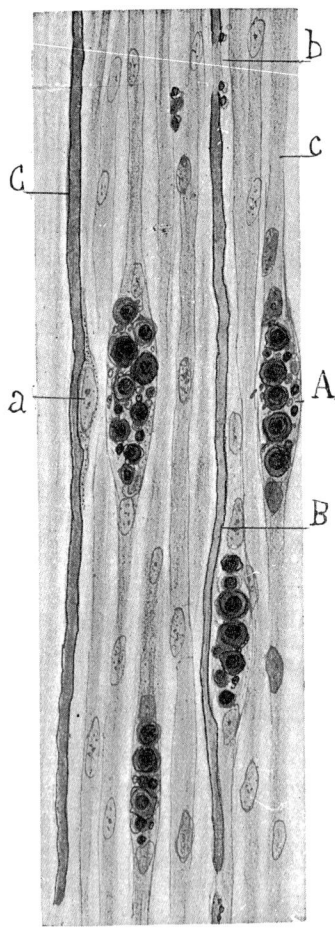

FIG. 101.—Formation of the myelin in the axons of the peripheral stump. Rabbit killed twenty-five days after the operation. A fatty accumulation ; B, intratubal medullated axon ; C, interstitial medullated axon ; a, nucleus of the interannular segment ; b, node of Ranvier ; c, band of Büngner.

Modifications occurring in the central stump many months after section of the nerve.—We have already stated that a portion of the central stump degenerates near the wound, and that the old axons are replaced by new fibres which grow in the old sheaths of Schwann.

We have also stated that these young conductors progressively thicken and become surrounded, after ten days have elapsed since the operation, with a cellular covering developed by the proliferation of the pre-existent cell of Schwann. This phenomenon of protection is seen as well in the intratubal branches, which are both collateral and terminal, as in the extratubal branches, which are almost all collateral, and equally in direct and retrograde fibres.

As time passes new changes supervene. Between the twenty-fifth and forty-fifth days the sprouts become covered with a myelin sheath, and the nodes of Ranvier are formed. Later the collective sheaths that surround all the intratubal sprouts become pale and are resorbed, and the latter remain free in the endoneurium. Finally the extratubal collaterals, which are provided with a myelin sheath, now come out at the level of a node of Ranvier. A general rearrangement has changed the character of the sprouts. The resorption of long tracts of weak axons has transformed many collaterals into terminal fibres, and, at the same time, exiguous collateral or terminal fibres, which have reached the terminal structures, become larger, while other fibres, of the same origin, but which have been immobilized through deviation or retrogression, become thinner and are resorbed. As to the helicoidal structures, we have already expressed the opinion, in concurrence with Lugaro, that spiral fibres, which are not in communication with the terminal structures, very probably are finally resorbed.

In fine, all that is useful remains and becomes more important. All that is superfluous and aberrant undergoes a process of progressive thinning, degeneration, and resorption. In the process of regeneration of peripheral nerves the law of Marinesco [1] doubtless holds. According to this law, function is a necessary condition for the trophism of the neurones and nerve paths. A cell or fibre that does not function sooner or later disappears.

ADDITIONAL NOTE TO CHAPTER X

After the researches carried out during the last fifteen years, with the help of methods that are exquisitely selective of nervous protoplasm, by Purpura, Lugaro, Krassin, ourselves, Perroncito, Marinesco and Minea, Dustin, Tello, Poscharisky, O. and H. Rossi, Deineka, Ruiz, Arcaute and Ortin, Boeke, etc., one may affirm that the problem of the origin, growth, and division of the nerve sprouts that penetrate into the

[1] Marinesco : *La cellule nerveuse*, tome 2, 1909.

peripheral stump of cut or crushed nerves is definitely settled. Notwithstanding the activity shown in fully elucidating all the phases of the regenerative process, there still remain a number of points subject to controversy. We may include among them : the origin of the protecting sheaths of the newly-formed nerve bundles that cross the scar ; the mechanism of production of the new cells of Schwann ; that of the peritubular membrane of Retzius, and of the myelin sheath, etc.

Finally, points that we believed definitely settled, such as : the initial nakedness of the sprouts arising from the central stumps and the orienting action brought about by the liberation of excitatory catalytic agents of nerve growth (neurotropic substances) originating in the peripheral stump, have been revised and discussed during these last few years by such authors as Boeke, Nageotte and Marinesco, Scaffidi, Viale, Bielschowsky, Spielmeyer. Boeke [1] was one of the first investigators who, inspiring himself from the doctrine of the *Leitzellen* and *plasmodesmas* of Held, attempted to give it an objective basis in the field of regeneration. Boeke, however, who is an excellent observer, formulates this idea quite incidentally and without details in one of his interesting memoirs on the experimental union of the peripheral stump of the lingual and the central stump of the hypoglossal nerves. That which interests us now is his affirmation that the sheathed as well as the free sprouts which have gone astray full in the scar always travel within a *syncytium*.

The author who has defended with most zeal, insistence, and conviction the *syncytial* theory is Nageotte,[2] who has made many interesting communications on the problem of nerve regeneration and related problems. All these communications contain a multitude of new facts and points of view which are as ingenious as they are suggestive, and

---

[1] Boeke : " Ueber die Regenerationserscheinungen bei der Nervenheilung von motorischen mit sensiblen Nervenfasern," *Anat. Anzeiger*, p. 366, 1913.

[2] Nageotte : " Le processus de la cicatrisation des nerfs. Généralités et faits particuliers," *Revue neurologique*, No. 19, 1915.

Idem : " Sur la greffe des tissus morts," etc. *C.R. Soc. biol.*, t. 79, pp. 833, 940, 1031, and 1121.

Idem : " Etude expérimentale de la cicatrisation des nerfs," *Lyon Chirurgical*, March-April, 1918.

Idem : " Substance collagène et névroglie dans la cicatrisation des nerfs," *C.R. Soc. biol.*, t. 79, p. 322.

Idem : " Rapport des neurites avec les tissus dans la cornée," *C.R. Acad. Sci.*, t. 172, 1921.

See also Nageotte et Guyon : " Aptitudes néoplasiques de la névroglie périphérique greffée et non réinervée," etc. *C.R. Soc. biol.*, t. 74, 1916.

which we shall resume here in so far as they interest us in our problem :

1. When a nerve is cut, the two stumps separate, as is well known. In the superior stump is formed a *neuroma*, that is, a portion of nervous tissue which is included in a system of neuroglial trabeculae or tracts ; in the inferior stump is formed a *glioma*, another mass of neuroglial tracts which advance until they join those of the superior stump. Later the tract or cordons are inhabited by the nerve sprouts, which never travel freely, but sheathed in the tubular formations.

Such neuroglial tracts are of ectodermal origin, and they are produced by the division of the cells of Schwann of both stumps.

2. If, instead of cutting, one tears out the sciatic nerve of a mammal in order to impede the nervous reunion of the peripheral stump, this develops after a few days a purely neuroglial nerve, which continually advances towards the central stump and whose hollow cells are lacking in neurites. After fifteen days the peripheral glial stump, in which are no axons, and which is formed by tubulose and anastomosed cells, is already 5 millimetres long.

3. One deduces from what has been said above that free progression of the axons is a mere appearance, in the scar as well as in the peripheral stump. The neurogenetic formula which is adopted by Nageotte is categorical : " La névroglie construit le nerf et les neurites s'y logent."

4. In the drawings and descriptions of Nageotte the neuroglial tracts which are stained with iron haematoxylin are thick, tubular, and arranged in longitudinal meshes. They undoubtedly correspond to those shown, of somewhat paler colour, by ordinary or neurofibrillar methods from the seventh or eighth day after the operation. Each neuroglial cordon or tract may contain, in thick intraprotoplasmic tubes, four, five, or more young neurites, as occurs in sympathetic nerve bundles, each one of which, according to Nageotte, is included in a gangue of common protoplasm. Thus the process of growth of the nerve bundles across the scar represents a symbiosis between the neurites and the neuroglial *syncytial* protoplasm.

5. The emerging new fibres from the central stump never come in contact with mesodermal elements, that is, with true fibroblasts, but a neuroglial sheath, which is differentiated at an early stage, is always interposed. This kind of '*horror of mesoderm*' is also seen in the architecture of adult nerves and in all isolated nerve fibres that are travelling towards their termination. The French scientist believes that the neurites are naked only when they penetrate into the ectodermal epithelia ; for example, in the anterior epithelium of the cornea.

6. A corollary of the preceding doctrine is that in the innervation

of the peripheral stump of interrupted nerves there is no neurotropic or chemotactic influence. Since the *neuroglial nerve* necessarily precedes the *neuritic nerve*, and since no sprout can escape from the prison of precocious cordons or from the *syncytium* arising from the migration of the cells of Schwann, the innervation of the peripheral stump becomes an automatic phenomenon. In order to penetrate into it the neurites require only a great power of growth ; in it they advance smoothly like a train on rails, or, better, like water in a tube.

7. For the same reason it is useless to speak of *stereotropism*, which was referred to, under different names, by Harrison, ourselves, Dustin, Marinesco, Tello, etc. At best one might admit an intraneuroglial or intratubal stereotropism.

8. Nageotte [1] invokes the same principles for ontogeny. He states : " Regeneration essentially repeats embryogeny." It is only in the last study of his that we have cited that he makes some restriction : " This law is general except perhaps as regards the emergence of the anterior roots during a very brief period of embryonic development."

The investigations of Marinesco [2] generally confirm the results obtained by Nageotte. He accepts his formula : " Neuroglia first forms the nerve, and later the neurites grow in it."

According to him all newly-formed fibres are enveloped in certain anastomosed cells, which arise from the division of the cells of Schwann and precede the appearance of the nerve sprouts. These elements (Nageotte's *neuroglia*) would be nothing else than the *apotrophic cells* described by Marinesco many years ago. The interstitial paths which, according to Dustin,[3] exist in the scar to orientate the fibres (Dustin's theory of *odogenesis*) must be replaced by intraprotoplasmic spaces of the cells of Schwann, or apotrophic cells, arising from the central stump. Thus, as stated above, neurotropism is superfluous. Marinesco does not absolutely deny, however, the existence of neurotropic sources, but he affirms that in the majority of cases it is the syncytium of Schwann that comes into play essentially, to direct the newly-formed fibres and favour their nutritive exchanges. It is only in the nerve terminations (motor plates, sensory structures, etc.) that neurotropism could play

---

[1] Nageotte : " Rapport des neurites avec les tissus dans la cornée," *C.R. Acad. Sci.*, t. 172, No. 1, 1921.

[2] Marinesco : " Nouvelles contributions à l'étude de la régénération nerveuse et du neurotropisme," *Phil. Trans. Roy. Soc.*, London, Series B, vol. 209, 1919.

See also : *Nouvelle Iconographie de la Salpêtrière*, 1913.

[3] Dustin : " Rôle des tropismes et de l'odogenèse dans la régénération du système nerveux," *Arch. de Biol.*, 1910.

a part. One sees that in this respect Marinesco shares the opinion of Harrison, Heidenhain, and others.[1]

Although he is in principle a partisan of Nageotte's theory, Marinesco does not formulate it in such absolute terms, nor does he generalize it to normal neurogenesis. He says: "Ontogeny is not the same as nerve regeneration." He founds his very prudent reserves on the facts discovered by Tello in regeneration of the retina and cerebrum, where the sprouts grow evidently free, and especially on the experiments of tissue culture of nerves by Harrison and his followers. Marinesco reminds us, in corroboration of this dissimilarity between neurogenesis and regeneration that, in his experiments of culture of ganglia, the new fibres grow freely in the plasma, often adhering to the threads of fibrin or to cells of uncertain origin. He might also have cited, in support of these reserves, the interesting tissue cultures of Levi, done on chick embryos.[2] Levi has seen the neurites growing freely in the plasma with an amoeboid movement, as von Lenhossék and ourselves had many years ago supposed ; these neurites joined each other anastomotically and they emitted collaterals which also grew without any tutor cells.

Marinesco then takes up a series of very interesting questions which constitute what is most original and suggestive in his communication : (1) Concerning the possible difference in electric potential between the central and the peripheral stumps, as a determining condition in the growth and orientation of the sprouts. One may remember in this connection the experiments of Scaffidi and Viale, cited by Marinesco, as well as the suggestions of Ariëns Kappers and his school, to explain the changes in position undergone by medullary centres during phylogeny. (2) Concerning the intimate structure of the neurofibrils and their metamorphoses during the process of regeneration. (3) Finally, on the rôle of the *oxydases* present in the nervous protoplasm and the possible trophic influence of catalytic agents formed by the *syncytium* of Schwann or the neuroglial tracts of Nageotte. All these are extremely interesting matters, into the details of which we shall not enter here.

We shall, to be brief, now summarize the principal assertions of the investigators whom we have cited.

[1] In a personal letter Marinesco recognizes, after reading our "Algunas observaciones contrarias a la hipótesis *syncytial* de la regeneración nerviosa y neurogenesis normal," *Trab. Lab. Inv. biol.*, March 1921, that the axons of regenerated nerves grow *at first* freely across the scar. This is precisely what we hold.

[2] G. Levi: "Connessioni e struttura degli elementi nervosi sviluppati fuori del organismo," *Real. Acad. dei Lincei*, Ser. 5, vol. 12, 1917.

1. *Identification of the proliferated cells of Schwann as neuroglia cells.*—This is perhaps a question of words. But even thòugh the French say " le nom ne fait rien à la chose," still in some cases the excessive generalization of a word may bring about confusion and misunderstanding which it is better to avoid.

It is evident that Nageotte identifies, or at least homologizes, the *cell of Schwann* of normal nerves with the *ectodermal neuroglia* of the nerve centres, and he also believes that the covering of the nerve cordons or bundles arising in the scar are of neuroglial nature. Marinesco calls these surrounding elements *apotrophic cells.*

The differences, both morphological and structural, between the glia cells of nerve centres and the true cells of Schwann are so great and easily seen that we need not enunciate them all here. We may merely note that none of the specific methods that have been developed to stain the neuroglia of the centres (the methods of Weigert, Anglade, Alzheimer, Achucarro, ours with gold and sublimate, Rio-Hortega's carbonate of ammoniacal silver, the modifications of Bielschowsky's process, etc.) stain at all the cells of Schwann or the perifascicular *syncytium* of the scar of cut nerves. We may also note that the glia-cell of the centres, which has a soma that is very poor in protoplasm, has a rudimentary Golgi apparatus, which is visible only in young animals, while the cell of Schwann, as we observed some years ago, has around the nucleus a reticular apparatus, which is very extensive and rich. We omit, for the sake of brevity, many other differences, all of them fundamental.

2. *During the first phases of evolution all isolated sprouts arising from the central stump of a cut or torn nerve grow freely, either across the exudates, or across connective tissue cells or embryonic fibroblasts, by virtue of the well-known phenomenon of stereotropism.*—This assertion is fully confirmed during the precocious phenomena of regeneration (studied by Perroncito, ourselves, and Marinesco) that occur before the formation of the *syncytial tracts* of which Nageotte speaks. In Fig. 101A we show a nerve whose neurilemma was triturated with forceps. The pieces were fixed in pyridin two days after the operation. The exudate formed through the perinervous inflammation is still present. Many leucocytes, granular cells (*a*), and a few embryonic fibroblasts (*c*) are to be seen in it. There is not the least vestige of a syncytium. A multitude of exploratory fibres and some bundles of neurites, issuing from the stimulated axons of the central stump or proximal portion of the nerve, precipitate themselves outside the nerve through a gap or cleft in the neurilemma. One can see that all the precocious neurites, without exception, grow freely across the inflammatory exudate, some of them terminating in small clubs (*d*). This figure also shows that many buds of growth have

broken off while crossing the neurilemma and outside it, reproducing the phenomenon of *nervous autotomy*, of which we have had much to say above. Two days after the operation the cells of Schwann have not divided, and there are consequently none of those colossal neuroglial

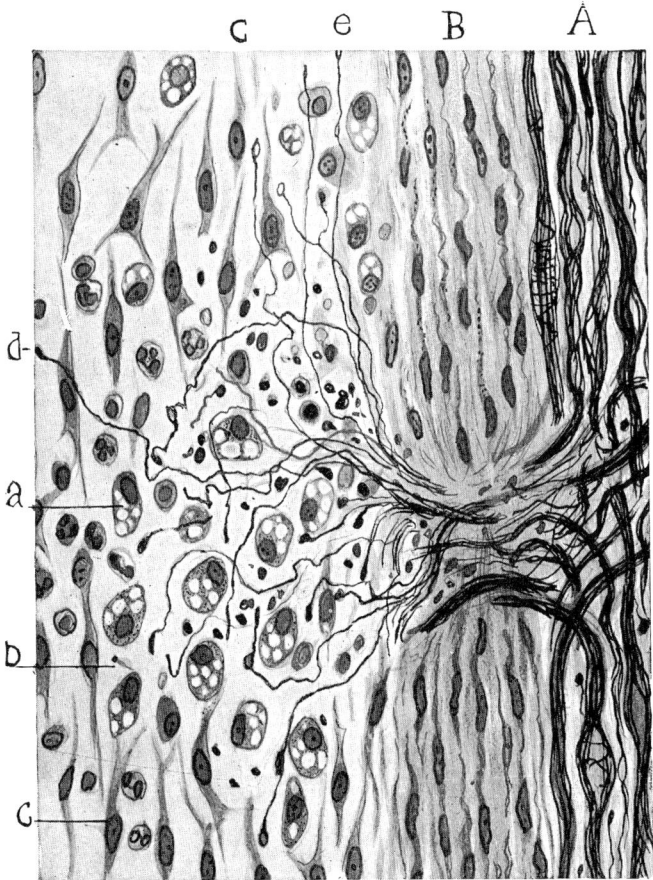

Fig. 101A.—Peripheral portion of a nerve that had been pinched with a pair of forceps. Young cat, killed two days after the operation. *A*, tangential axons of the nerve in a productive phase; *B*, neurilemma; *C*, perinervous exudate through which grow many axonic sprouts; *a*, granular cell; *b*, neurite seen as a point; *c*, fibroblast.

sheaths described by Nageotte; we therefore consider it certain that the sprouts travel freely around the lesioned nerve. If one looks at a fibre endwise (*b*) no syncytial protoplasm is to be seen around it.

Fig. 101B is also highly suggestive. This is the case of a rabbit whose sciatic nerve was completely cut after having been loosely ligatured a short distance above the lesion. This ligature did not impede the production of sprouts, which circulated in the scar ; it only retarded a little the projection of the first exploratory fibres. The animal was killed four and a half days after the operation, that is, before the appearance of the large orienting sheaths of Nageotte. A remnant of inflammatory exudate, separating the young fibroblasts (*A*), which are stained dark grey by the silver, greatly facilitates the search for the sprouts growing in the mesoderm (*b, c, e*). With Zeiss 1·3, 1·4, and 2 mm. apochromatic

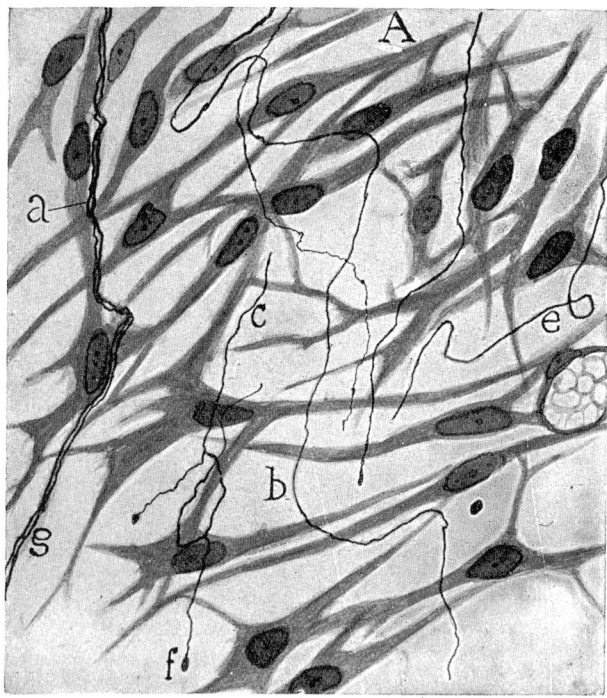

FIG. 101B.—Scar near the central stump of a nerve which was cut and ligatured a short distance from the section. The animal was killed four and a half days after the operation. *A*, fibroblasts ; *a*, neurites growing on the fibroblasts ; *b, c, e*, other neurites growing naked across the plasma ; *f*, fibre ending in a small club.

objectives, it is impossible to see any protoplasmic sheath round the exploratory axons ; the result is the same if one uses no diaphragm or a very narrow one. In general the fibres grow normally in the direction of the fibroblasts, jumping frequently across the large plasmatic spaces (*b*). One sees, however, here and there, some phenomena of stereotropism (Fig. 101B, *a, g*). There are also cases of autoneurotomy.

There are regions, like that shown in Fig. 101c, in which stereotropism is much more frequent, and where one finds some neurites lying on both sides of a fibroblast or pair of fibroblasts (*a, c*). In *f, b*, one sees a fibre which, after accompanying a connective tissue cell, has gone back to follow another one, growing in a reverse direction. In its course it shows a detention ball. Finally, in *e*, one sees a neurite with a ball of degeneration.

In the two preceding preparations there appears, it is true, a more or less complete cicatricial *syncytium*; but, we repeat, this syncytium is exclusively composed of ordinary fibroblasts. It is impossible to see any continuity of such fusiform or stellate cells with the cells of Schwann of both nerve stumps. We think it very probable that all these cells, within which there is absolutely no empty space, are proliferated connective tissue cells, and not the progeny of migrated neuroglial cells of Schwann.

3. *The neuroglial sheaths of Nageotte and other investigators are late in their formation, appearing only from the sixth to the eighth day after section of the nerves, when the scar has been invaded, not only by exploratory fibres, but also by thick bundles of neurites, a product, as we have shown, of ravelling of the nerve branches arising from a cut axon. Thus the sheaths do not precede the bundles but, on the contrary, are a consequence of their formation.*

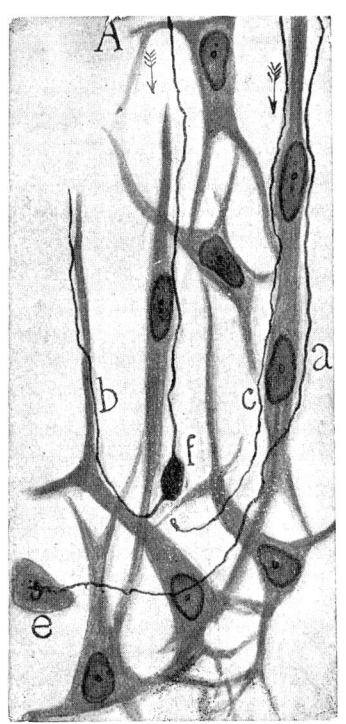

FIG. 101C.—Part of the scar in which stereotropism is evident. *A*, direction of the central stump: *a, b, e*, neurites supported on fibroblasts *e*, a delayed club; *f*, thickening of a fibre.

4. *Once the bundles of fibres, and therefore the sheaths, have begun to be formed, the neurites increase as a result of the penetration into the latter of new fibres from the central stump.*—The late neurites become incorporated with the pre-existing bundle, either because they originate from the same axon and are covered by the same sheath, or through ramification of the pre-existing intrafascicular fibres, or else through a kind of attraction exercised by all axons on those which are not very far off, a phenomenon that we have called reciprocal neurotropism, which perhaps is only a variety of stereotropism.

But even in these late periods when the immense majority of fibres, sheathed or not, have arranged themselves into bundles protected by a membrane, one finds naked wandering axons, which are in the state of *divisory* turgidity or irritation ; we have drawn many cases of these in our first monograph on nervous regeneration.

5. *In embryos, the initial exploratory fibres also grow without sheath in the mesoderm. It is only later, when a number of neurites become aggregated as a result of reciprocal stereotropism that the sheath becomes differentiated, as has been described by von Lenhossék, Held, and others.*— In proof of this assertion we might cite almost all our neurogenic observations on the chick embryo from the second to the fourth days of incubation. Readers interested in this point should consult the figures and descriptions contained in the publication in which we combated the Hensen-Held theory,[1] the admirable neurogenic investigations of Tello[2] on the differentiation of the sensory nerve terminations in incipient muscles, tendons, and Pacinian corpuscles, and, finally, our more recent observations concerning the genesis of intraepithelial, sensory, and sensitive ramifications.[3] Of great value also are the memoirs, no longer recent, of His, Kölliker, Lugaro, Graham Kerr, von Lenhossék, etc.

A careful examination of the preparations used in these researches shows that all fibres that are searching for a terminal region grow absolutely naked between the mesodermal interstices. It is only when one examines late stages in the development that the neurite appears, even when travelling alone, surrounded by a protecting nucleated sheath of enigmatic origin, and which is, in any case, very much anterior to the differentiation of the cells of Schwann and of the myelin sheath (*vitreous sheath of Vanlair*).

In order not to repeat, in this connection, observations already published in earlier papers, we shall give here only two new demonstrations. But we must first speak of some points of technique.

In general, as is well known, sections impregnated by reduced silver nitrate, especially if, like Held, one uses pyridin as a fixative, without subsequently using alcohol, are difficult to interpret. One often obtains

---

[1] Cajal : "Nouvelles observations sur l'évolution des neuroblastes," etc., *Anat. Anzeiger*, Bd. 32, 1908.

Idem : "Génesis de las fibras nerviosas del embrión," etc., *Trab. del Lab. de Investig. biol.*, t. 4, 1905-1906.

[2] Tello : "Génesis de las terminaciones nerviosas motrices y sensitivas," etc., *Trab. del Lab. de Invest. biol.*, t. 15, 1917.

[3] Cajal : "Acción neurotrópica de los epitelios (Detalles sobre el mecanismo genetico de las ramificaciones nerviosas intraepiteliales sensitivas y sensoriales), *Trab. del Lab. de Investig. biol.*, t. 17, 1919.

sections in which the neurites stand out very deeply stained on a background of fibroblasts which are pale, and of perinervous sheaths which are hardly perceptible. On the other hand, when one uses, as was done in the time of His and the catenary hypothesis, sections that are intensely stained by haematoxylin or the aniline dyes (also with iron haematoxylin, after fixation in Laguesse's fluid), one sees the syncytial sheaths more or less well; but one either does not see the neurites at all, or else very vaguely. Thus, neither the former nor the latter procedure gives, under ordinary conditions, absolutely clear images which are not subject to false interpretations.

There are cases, fortunately, when reduced silver nitrate stains at once and with sufficient vigour both elements : neurites and perinervous tissue. These are the only preparations that are fit to elucidate the problem, especially if the nuclear and cytoplasmic stain of the fibroblasts and perifascicular cells is reinforced in a bath of strongly selective haematoxylin.[1]

Another circumstance which is favourable to observation, and of which we have taken advantage, is the looseness of the connective tissue across which the sprouts travel. In most regions this tissue, made up of fibroblasts, is so compact and coheres so intimately with the wandering neurites that it is difficult to determine the true relation of the latter to the former, or to the supposed migrating ectodermal cells (*lemmoblasts*) of von Lenhossék. There are, fortunately, regions where the fibroblasts and *lemmoblasts* are separated by wide spaces which are full of plasma and where, as a result, it is easy to see precisely the connections of the young neurites. Such privileged regions are especially found in the places where later the cavity of the arachnoid is to form, or where non-cartilaginous bones will be developed (region of emergence of the facial, trigeminal, ophthalmic, and suborbital nerves).

The above-mentioned propitious conditions occurred in the sections drawn in Figs. 101D and 101E. Fig. 101D shows a section of the head of a chick embryo on the third day of incubation, at the level of the terminal region of the trigeminal. One sees that the embryonic connective tissue with its anastomoses (*Leitzellen* and *plasmodesmas* of Held) are very well stained; between them occur hollow spaces full of plasma (*a, b*). One can see that the nerve trunks of a certain calibre (*A*) undoubtedly possess a cellular covering, homologous perhaps to that

---

[1] A good nuclear and cytoplasmic stain is often obtained in pieces that are exclusively fixed in alcohol or chloral hydrate. But we also possess sections whose mesodermal cells are beautifully stained even after fixation in pyridin; the important thing here is to deal with regions whose connective tissue is loose and soaked in an abundant interstitial plasma.

which Nageotte calls *neuroglial tract*; on the other hand, all the isolated fibres are lacking in a cellular sheath and are independent of the neighbouring syncytium (*B*, *C*, of Fig. 101D). It is especially important to note in this figure two points : As we have stated above in connection with the regenerative process, it is impossible, even using the best objectives and a very narrow aperture in the diaphragm,

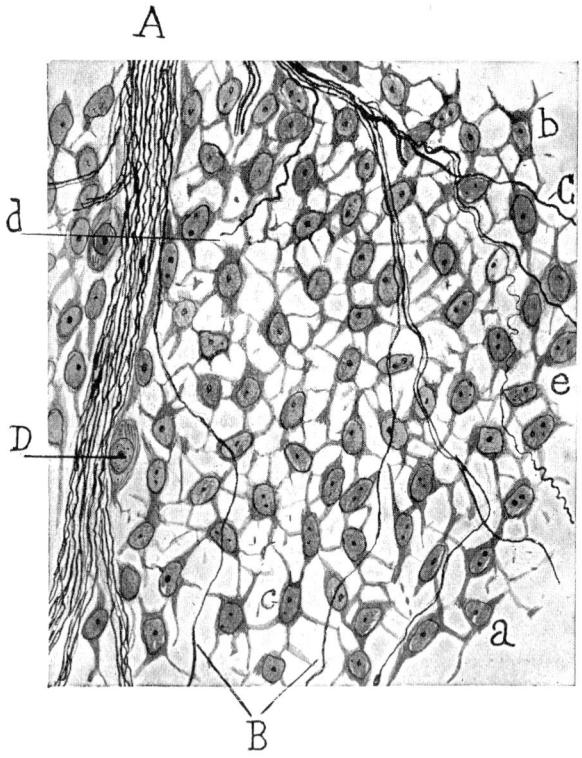

FIG. 101D.—Section of the region of the trigeminal, where the ophthalmic nerve is developing. Chick embryo on the third day of incubation. *A*, voluminous bundle ; *B*, isolated nerve fibres which are growing through the plasmatic interstices ; *C*, *e*, anastomosed fibroblasts.

ever to see next to the independent neurites the least sign of a marginal nucleus, or of a protoplasmic sheath, even though the cells surrounding the nerve bundles are well impregnated ; (2) the path of the fibres, which are largely free within the plasmatic spaces, is rectilinear or slightly curved, instead of being sinuous or zigzag, which it would inevitably be if the fibres grew within the thickness of the *plasmodesmas*. We may finally observe how improbable it appears, *a priori*, that the fine expansions of the fibroblasts, some of them as fine as the young neurites themselves, contain an interior conduit, of which, moreover, the best objectives do not allow one to see the least sign.

Fig. 101E is even more instructive; it is taken from a cat embryo 2 cms. long, at the level of the plane of emergence of the fibres of the *oculomotor* nerve. One can clearly see in it the path of the neurites and the relative position of the mesodermal syncytium. As in the preceding figure the bundles that are rich in fibres formed precociously, have some marginal nuclei, although it is impossible to determine

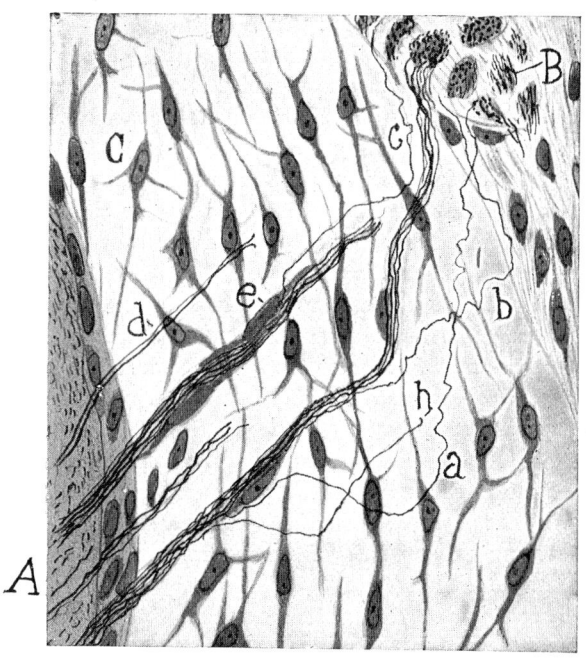

FIG. 101E.—Region of emergence of the fibres of the oculomotor nerve in a cat embryo 2 cms. long. *A*, protuberance which is surrounded by a rudiment of *pia mater*; *e*, surrounding cells or lemnoblasts; *B*, transversal section of the bundles of the oculomotor nerve; *C*, fibroblasts; *a, b, c, d*, fibres which grow naked and isolated from the medulla to become incorporated in the nerve.

whether they form a continuous or a discontinuous tube. On the other hand, all the neurites that are detached from the bundles (*a, b, c*) and that grow isolated along the perimedullar tissue up to the point where they become incorporated with the principal portion of the nerve, are absolutely naked. It is important to note here that we are dealing, not with deviated or lost fibres, but with solitary neurites which, although they are separate from the main bundles, finally become correctly oriented, since nearly all of them become incorporated in the nerve trunk. Finally, it is important to note in Fig. 101E that there is no parallelism between the direction of the connective tissue cells and that of the travelling neurites; these grow preferably in a direction normal to the expansions of the fibroblasts; we do not, therefore, deny the existence of some cases of stereotropism.[1]

6. *The nerve centres, especially the spinal cord, when they are traumatized, often emit fibres which arise from the white matter and which, without the assistance of Nageotte's neuroglia (proliferated cells of Schwann) or of the apotrophic cells of Marinesco, grow for long distances outside the pia or inside the ependyma.*—We have already cited many cases of these acts of growth and axonic dislocation which are absolutely free, at least in their initial phases, from the immediate orienting influences of the cells of Schwann. These facts are so significant and conclusive that it is not without surprise and some disillusionment that we have seen how the new school of catenarists disregards or overlooks them. We prefer to believe that these investigators have not read our papers, or the admirable experiments of Tello who, for the first time, has achieved the feat, which seemed impossible, of giving an enormous regenerative power to the apathetic and inert cerebral neurites. This neglect is, of course, to be understood, since the Spanish language is not very familiar to investigators. Marinesco alone, so far as we know, has paid some attention to these facts, of which we shall speak more anon.

7. *Within the peripheral stump of cut nerves a large number of the penetrating sprouts travel freely between the tubes of Schwann, as we showed some years ago* (1905).—The same occurs with the neurites that invade the grafts placed in the nerve scar, and that not only with fresh grafts,[2] but also with those preserved *in vitro* for many days, as Tello [3] showed in his interesting experiments of nerve grafting, which confirmed in principle that made long ago by Nageotte.[4] This fact refutes the arbitrary hypothesis of Held, Bielschowsky, Spielmeyer, and others, for whom growth within the protoplasm of the cells of Schwann is an

---

[1] Nageotte, in his book, *L'organisation de la matière dans ses rapports avec la vie*, Paris 1922, has sought to contest this fact by suggesting that in the preparation of the sections the neurites had been pushed out of their sheaths. To this we shall only reply that these free fibres are constant in their apparent origin (mesodermal growth) in the oculomotor nerve of the cat and other animals, being revealed through the quantity of interstitial plasma that lies between the connective tissue cells. We are probably dealing here with late neurites which, although they grow freely, finally become oriented.

[2] Cajal: See this volume, I. p. 347.

[3] Tello: "Algunas experiencias de injertos nerviosos conservados *in vitro*," *Trab. Lab. Investig. biol.*, t. 12, 1914.

[4] Nageotte: *C.R. Soc. biol.*, t. 69, p. 556, 1910.

indispensable condition for the progress and orientation of the young axons.

8. *The young axons are able to grow and ramify across nutritive plasma without the assistance of any kind of satellite cell.*—All the tissue culture experiments made by Harrison and his pupils, as well as by Marinesco, Levi, and others, show indisputably this specific property of the neurites of growing and ramifying within the blood plasma. Their growth across coagula and exudates was demonstrated some time ago by Perroncito and ourselves.

As to the neuritic growth within the ependymal liquid, we need only note that whenever, during ontogenetic development, a neuroblast or axon happens to fall within the central cavity of the cord and medulla, the functional expansion becomes oriented, not without some vacillations, towards its destination. One may refer, in proof of this assertion, to Figs. 9 and 10 of our polemical memoir directed against the views of Held.[1] We may note also that the same occurs, as was shown by Lorente de Nó [2] in my laboratory, in the larvae of amphibians, when, after a partial or total section of the spinal cord, great ependymal dilatations are formed.

9. *In the nerve centres and during the first phases of ontogenetic development the axons grow and become admirably orientated in the white and grey matter without the help of the cells of Schwann or of neuroglial elements. These cells and elements all become differentiated after the fundamental architectonic plan of the nerve paths and the principal interneuronal connections have been realized.*—It thus appears very improbable that the congruent growth of the central neurites occurs without the help of *Leitzellen* or of *a syncytium* of Schwann; the peripheral axons which, even in the adult state, have an extraordinary capacity for growth and neurocladism, may need, in order to reach their destination, mechanical supports. The proof of this doctrine will be found in all the neurogenic investigations carried out by precise methods since the time of Golgi, Kölliker, ourselves, von Lenhossék, van Gehuchten, Lugaro, Retzius, Athias, etc. (Golgi method), down to those carried out by neurofibrillar methods.

We may thus say that the theory of Held, which was adopted by Nageotte, Boeke, Bielschowsky, Spielmeyer, and many others, is based on insufficient attention to the precocious phenomena of regeneration in the central stump, studied years ago by Perroncito, ourselves, and

[1] Cajal: " Nouvelles observations sur l'évolution des neuroblastes," etc., *Anat. Anz.*, Bd. 32, pp. 21 and 23, 1908.

[2] Lorente de Nó: " La regeneración de la médula espinal en las larvas de batracio," *Trab. Lab. Investig. biol.*, t. 19, 1921.

Marinesco. As a matter of fact, in favourable circumstances, there penetrate into the exudate, as noted above, no later than the day after the lesion, naked exploratory neurites (and even isolated bundles) which are crowned by fusiform clubs or masses; this occurs before any possible migration of the cells of Schwann. And if these early phases of regeneration have been seen by Nageotte (which does not appear to be the case according to his communications) may he not, like Held and some German and Dutch neuropathologists, have taken a simple phenomenon of stereotropism for the intraprotoplasmic or intrasyncytial position of the young neurites ? This would, of course, be impossible when, from the seventh day after the nerve section onwards, the enormous syncytial tubes or perifascicular sheaths have become formed.

XI

ARRIVAL OF THE NERVE FIBRES AT THE END-ORGANS

Experiments of Tello on the regeneration of motor fibres.—Regeneration of Kühne's spindles and of tactile hairs.—Insufficiency of the regeneration and incongruences of connection between the plates and their terminal regions.—Necessity of admitting, in the end-organs and peripheral stump, specific neurotropic sources.

AFTER a long journey through the peripheral stump and its derivatives, the nerve sprouts, now much reduced in number, attack the small terminal sensory and motor nerves, travelling almost constantly under the sheaths of Schwann, which discharge a tutorial function.

When a nerve trunk bifurcates or emits small collateral branches many axons also divide, and the new branches penetrate into the recently-formed cordons. This fact, interesting from a theoretical point of view, has been drawn attention to by Tello,[1] from whom we copy a few suggestive figures (Figs. 102 and 103). One can perceive that at the level of each bifurcation there exists a certain triangular enlargement, the remnant of an old club, and that the new branches take on an equal or unequal thickness, becoming collateral or terminal. Ordinarily, if the new nerve cordon represents a thin collateral projection from the trunk, it receives preferably collateral axonic branches (*B*). If the trunk bifurcates, the axons bifurcate also and the new nerve trunks receive terminal branches, which come out at a right or acute angle (Fig. 102, *A*). Besides these newly-formed branches, each small nerve contains a greater or lesser number of axons that are simply separated or loosened from the nerve bundle (Fig. 102, *C*). Tello affirms that, as the nerve becomes thinner and approaches the muscles, more of its axons represent fibres that have divided. In many of these divisions the ramification of the axon is forced by the pre-existent division of Schwann's sheath. One nevertheless finds some places where the

[1] F. Tello: "Dégénération et régénération des plaques motrices," etc., *Trav. du Lab. de Recher. biol.*, tome 5, 1907.

sheaths have divided at an acute angle, but where the clubs of growth have not divided, entering instead into one of the pre-established paths (Fig. 104). One also finds at times nerve branches which, perforating the membrane of Schwann which served as a directing path, become free or penetrate into small collateral nerves.

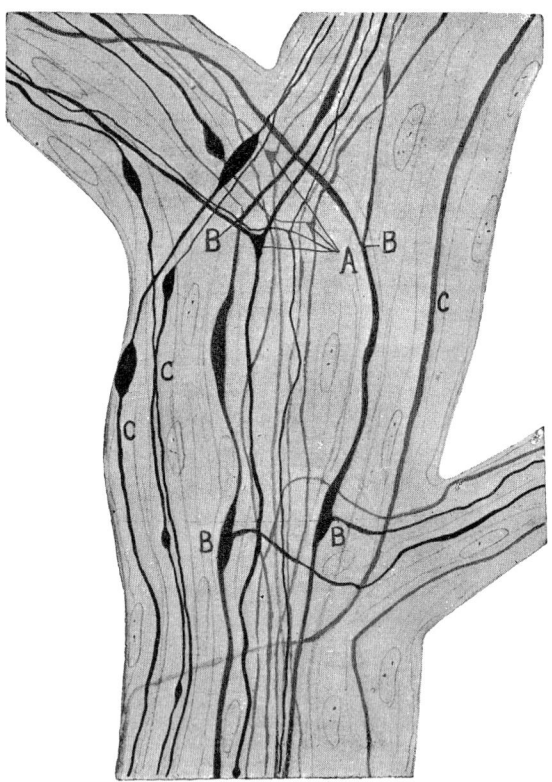

FIG. 102.—Divisions of a small regenerated muscular nerve. *A*, bifurcation of sprouts; *B*, emission of collaterals; *C*, fibres that cross the nerve without dividing. (After Tello.)

After many divisions the muscular nerves, as is well known, are reduced to isolated tubes, protected by a double membrane: the *external* or *Henle's membrane*, and the *internal* or *Schwann's membrane*. The sprouts reach these solitary sheaths, sometimes isolated (Fig. 103), sometimes united in bundles. One often sees the cone of growth advancing freely through the protoplasmic gap of the nerve tube. One must remember that while the axons are reaching the muscles— a period of a month and a half and more—the medullary sheaths have disappeared, the cells of Schwann have become more or less marginal, and a free space full of liquid is formed, into which the sprouts will enter. One can see these details in Fig. 104, *A*, where one notices that if the fibres are thin, they grow free and naked; but if they are of some size, which means an early arrival, there lies next to them, and as though surrounding them, a fusiform cell with an

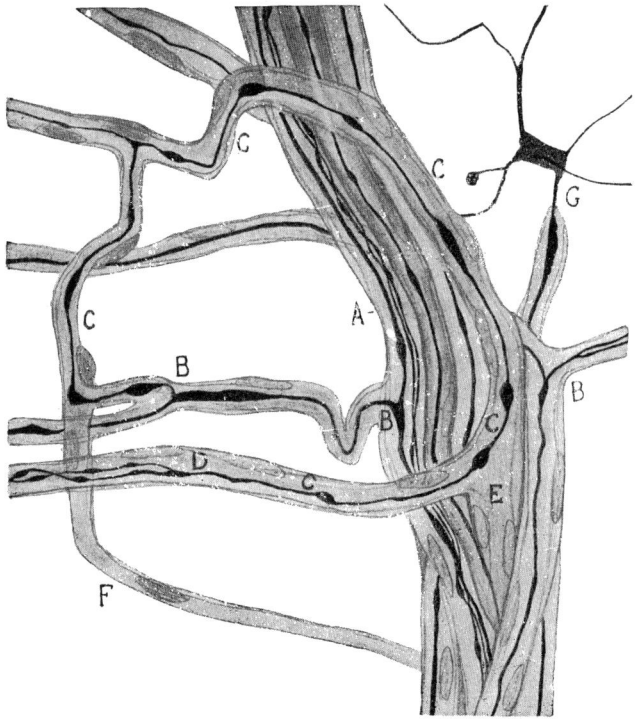

FIG. 103.—Small regenerated muscular nerve. Rabbit killed three months after section of the sciatic nerve. (After Tello.)

elongated nucleus. These elements, the future cells of Schwann of the new axon, very probably are descendants of the cells of the old sheath. Retrograde paths, although they are rare, can be seen sometimes in axons that are arrested for a time by obstacles.

Degeneration and disappearance of the motor arborization.—When we spoke of the degeneration of the peripheral stump we referred to the observations of Tello on the degeneration of the motor plates as a result of section of the sciatic nerve (see p. 107). We may state here that three or four days after the operation in the rabbit, the branches of the motor arborization are in full granular disintegration. After eight days the nerve branches of the plate have been completely resorbed. Later, the region where the plate had existed can be recognized by the presence of an accumulation of nuclei, which is more or less rounded, and by the increase in the granular material. The membrane of the plate persists, although it seemed to us that it had changed, having perhaps become softer and weaker. As is to be expected, in cold-blooded animals such as the frog the degenerative disorganization of the plate following section of the nerve is much slower. Langley,[1] who has used Ehrlich's methylene blue, states that the hypolemmal branches of the arborization become granular, presenting the appearance of intensely coloured granules, after three weeks, and disappearing within two and a half months. Hofmann and Blass [2] believe that such arborizations are resorbed between forty and sixty days after section of the nerve.

Arrival of the axons at the muscles and regeneration of the motor plate.—When do the newly-formed fibres arrive at the muscles, there to form motor plates ? It is evident, *a priori*, that this period is very variable, since the age of the animal, the temperature, and, especially, the size of the scar, have an influence in this respect. Tello affirms that, under normal circumstances, the nervous reunion of the muscle fibres in an adult rabbit begins in the gastrocnemius about two months and a half after section of the sciatic nerve, and it is at its height three months after the operation. As may be supposed, when circumstances are favourable, the muscular connection occurs very much earlier. In our observations on guinea-pigs and cats a few days old, after section of the sciatic nerve the gastrocnemius muscle often shows regenerated plates within forty days. In a young guinea-pig, whose sciatic nerve was cut very high up in order to include in the peripheral stump certain small nerves distributed in the muscles of the thigh, we saw in these muscles motor plates that were almost perfect on the twenty-fifth day. In this case the speed is easily explained, since the muscles were very close to the central stump and the small muscular nerves had to travel only a short distance. Tello has given us the details of the production of the plate. The older observers, like

[1] J. N. Langley : " On degenerative changes in the nerve endings in striated muscle, etc., of the frog," *Journ. of Physiol.*, vol. 38, July 2, 1909.

[2] Hofmann and Blass : *Arch. f. das gesamt. Physiol.*, Bd. 125, 1908.

Cipollone,[1] Galeotti and Levi,[2] and others, owing to the lack of a proper technique, were able to study only completed plates, when the afferent fibres were provided with a medullary sheath. The muscle fibre, more or less altered by degeneration due to inactivity, retains its motor plate, of whose constructive factors only the nervous ramifications have disappeared, as a result of a process of fragmentation and resorption similar to that described in the peripheral stump. One also observes, at the plate, an increase in the quantity of granular material and a certain turgidity of this material. Perhaps the nuclei proliferate somewhat.

The nerve sprouts coming out of the ends of the solitary sheaths or old intermuscular nerve tubes are attracted towards these persistent motor plates. In order to explain this attraction Tello supposes that there is elaborated in the plate a positively chemotactic substance capable of acting on the cones of growth. Otherwise one cannot understand why, since the ends of the old solitary tubes are open, the terminal cone chooses immediately the granular substance of the plate and no other region of the muscle bundle. Exceptionally, however, the recently arrived sprouts miss their mark and, taking the agglomerations of newly-formed protoplasm and the multiplied nuclei of the degenerated muscle fibre for legitimate terminal plates, are furnished with collateral arborizations which probably are resorbed later. These tendencies

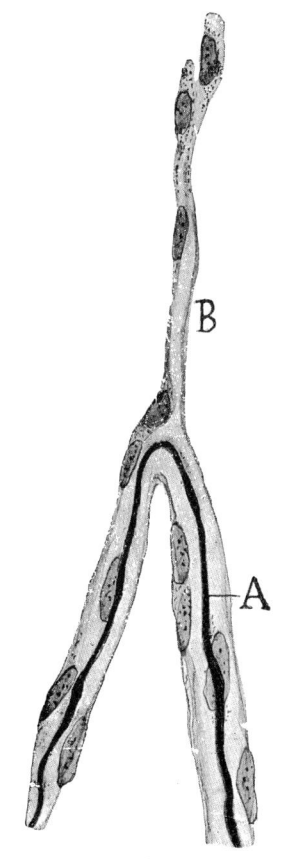

FIG. 104.—Free muscular nerve tube within which is a sprout. *A* axon; *B*, empty tube.

---

[1] L. T. Cipollone: " Ricerche sull anatomia normale e patologica delle terminazioni nervosi nei muscoli striati," *Supplemento agli Annali di Medicina navale*, 1887.

[2] Galeotti und Levi: " Ueber die Neubildung der nervösen Elemente in der wiedererzeugten Muskelgewebe," *Beitr. zur pathol. Anat. und allgem. Pathol.* 1894.

270 TRAUMATIC DEGENERATION AND REGENERATION OF NERVES

show that not only the legitimate plate, but all nuclear accumulations of the contractile fibre have a neurotropic influence. We do not know, however, whether this orienting influence is exercised by

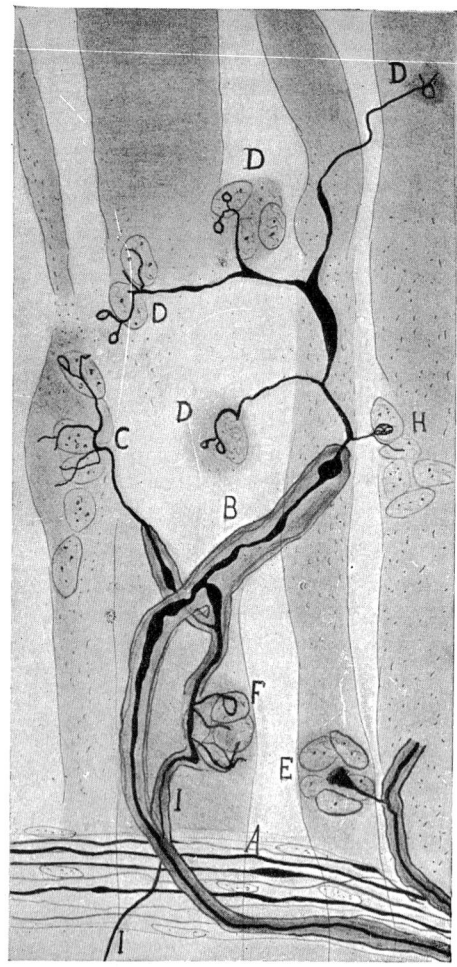

FIG. 105.—Motor plates in different stages of restoration. *A*, nerve; *B*, fibre that gives rise to several plates; *E*, *H*, plates as yet without ramification; *C*, *F*, plates with a well-developed arborization. (After Tello.)

the nuclei alone, by the newly-formed muscular protoplasm, or by both factors at once.

Once the fibre has arrived at the nuclear accumulation of the plate, the terminal cone flattens out and becomes more or less triangular. From it, in various directions, arise several projections. These are at first short and undivided, afterwards longer, and often bifurcated. The last fibrils, whose thickness varies, end freely in rings, grumes, or bulbs, or else in brush-like tips or flattened clubs that are clearly reticulated. These projections grow out among the nuclei, touching them at many points, and never get beyond the edges of the granular material. A single afferent fibre may give rise, as can be seen in Fig. 105, to many motor plates. One can see that the fibre which gives rise to the motor arborization is, at times, a simple collateral branch, while it may also be the terminal branch

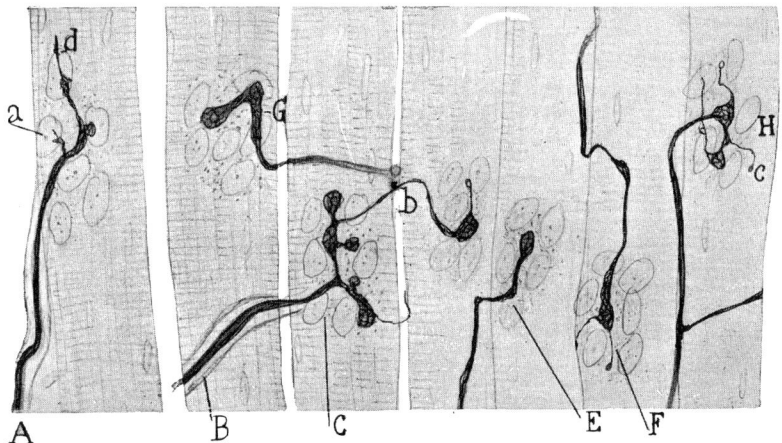

FIG. 106.—Muscle of a guinea-pig which was killed twenty-five days after section of the sciatic nerve. Regenerating plates taken from a small section of the muscle. *A*, *B*, afferent tubes; *E*, *G*, sprouts, as yet unramified, which have arrived at the plate; *F*, *H*, beginning of the final ramification; *C*, plate innervated by collateral branches.

(Fig. 105, *F*). The attractive power of the plate is sufficiently strong to cause passing fibres, which are protected by the double sheath of Henle and the remnants of Schwann's sheath, to form axonic projections and terminal arborizations. Sometimes the fibre, taken away from its sheath, completely misses its original path and fate, since, instead of following the path of the old sheath, it pierces through the latter and comes out entire into the plate that attracts it (Fig. 105). Many other curious dispositions may be seen in Tello's interesting paper, and especially in the drawings that accompany the text.

Our own observations concerning regeneration of the motor plates fully confirm those of Tello. In the rabbit and cat, twenty-five, thirty, and forty-five days after the operation, the gastrocnemius muscle is still lacking in afferent sprouts. On the other hand, as we stated above, in the adductor muscles of the guinea-pig, and in general, whenever the region to be innervated is near the wound, the terminal arborizations are formed earlier. In Fig. 106 we show various motor plates of a young guinea-pig, killed twenty-five days after the operation. One can see that, as stated by Tello, the afferent fibre of the plate makes use of the old sheath, terminating, generally, within the granular material in a more or less flattened and reticulated club (Fig. 106, E). Later the club stretches out, becoming folded in various ways (Fig. 106, G, b); it takes on, at times, a beaded aspect and it shows an elegant neurofibrillar framework (Fig. 106, a, G). Finally, from the end and sides of the club emerge fine sprouts, terminating in rings or delicate grumes, which subsequently become the end branches of the terminal motor arborization (c, d).

The innervation of the plate requires, as an almost absolute condition, the arrival of the sprouts by the channel of the small muscular nerves. In our numerous preparations one often finds around the scar, from the twelfth day on, a great many small nerve bundles, which are newly formed and deviated from the normal path, and which are ramified in a complicated way between the contractile muscle fibres. It appears natural, *a priori*, that from such bundles should arise fibres destined for the degenerated motor plates. This, however, does not occur; nearly all these newly-formed conductors wander about, and their terminal ramifications lie, not in the plates, but in the interstices of the muscles. Thus the sprouts that are destined to restore the terminal structures are always, or almost always, axons enclosed by the old sheath of Henle and in continuity with the membrane of the muscle cell of the corresponding sensory organ. We do not wish, however, to exclude the possibility that, where the fibre arrives at the muscle along its natural path, it may emit, outside its route, free collateral branches capable of eventually innervating other plates. But such occurrences, of which Tello has reproduced beautiful examples, while they are frequent in the terminal portion of covered sprouts, and while there are normally many of them near a plate, are seen rarely when one is dealing with conductors that are blindly dispersed through a muscle suffering from traumatic paralysis. One must remember, in order to understand this difficulty, how hard it is for even a trained histologist to discern in the very long muscle fibres the region—relatively extensive—in which is situated the normal nervous arborization.

Regeneration of sensory structures.—There have been few precise investigations in this field. The attempts made by Ranvier, Galeotti and Levi, etc., at a time that is already remote, were carried out with inadequate methods, and say nothing of the first phases of the process, which are the most interesting.

Concerning the regeneration of the *spindles of Kühne*, however, there is a very exact paper by Tello,[1] from which we shall extract here the essential facts.

After section of the sciatic nerve in the rabbit, the two classes of terminations of the *bundle of Kühne* or *Weismann*, degenerate simultaneously. Both arborizations, the *sensory* and the *motor*, go through the well-known phases of destruction—formation of varicosities, neurofibrillar hypertrophy, granular degeneration of the neurofibrils, rupture of the axon into helicoidal pieces, formation of granular grumes, etc. The resulting detritus appears to be digested by the nuclei of the terminal structures, since one never sees the penetration

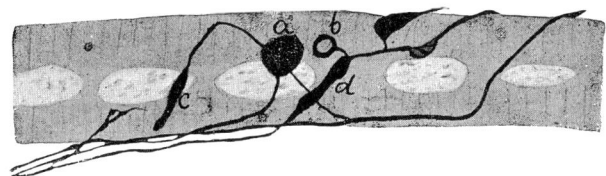

FIG. 107.—Piece of a spindle of Kühne in which the motor nervous termination is regenerating. *a*, terminal ball; *b*, terminal ring; *d*, thickenings along the course of a sprout. (After Tello.)

into the latter of exogenous phagocytes. Ordinarily the degeneration begins earlier in the sensory than in the motor arborizations. On the third day all axonic vestiges have disappeared.

Motor arborization of the spindles.—The arrival of the newly-formed fibres occurs two and a half months after the operation, a period which is shorter in the case of muscles close to the scar, or when, instead of complete interruptions, one makes hemisections. It is only after three months that many spindles show sufficiently regenerated motor plates. Moreover, once the regenerated fibre has arrived at the plate, it forms the arborization, repeating the phases that we have described : a primary final bulb from which appendices ending in rings or reticulated grumes subsequently issue at right angles (Fig. 107).

Regeneration of the sensory termination of the muscular spindle.—It is well known that this structure, the sensory termination, is present

[1] F. Tello: "La régénération dans les fuseaux de Kühne," *Trav. du Lab. de Rech. biol.*, tome 5, fasc. 4, 1907.

under a complicated and extensive capsular apparatus, which lends to the muscle fibre the appearance of a spindle. We may also note that in the region where the terminal arborization, of a very varicose character, extends, there is lacking the striation of the contractile cell and there is present a granular substance containing many nuclei. The sensory fibres arrive in the same nerve bundles as the motor fibres. When, however, they reach the capsule, and sometimes before, the two classes of conductors separate out. It appears as though the sensory fibres are attracted by a chemotactic substance which cannot act on the motor fibres.

Later they divide, giving rise to branches which are successively finer though each of the same diameter throughout. These branches are arranged in the form of tassels or small bundles and are terminated by buds or rings. Some of these small nerve brushes, composed of almost parallel branches, travel towards the granular material of the spindle, while others take various and even contrary paths.

In Fig. 108 we show two spindles of Kühne in different phases of nervous reunion. In A the motor arborization is very much developed, while the sensory branches are still growing under the capsule in search of the terminal region (b), tracing a few exploratory loops, as though scenting the specific chemotactic fount. In Fig. 108, B, the process of sensory nervous reunion is very much advanced. One can see that the fibre c, which has arrived through the old sheath, directs itself at first towards a region remote from the sensory plate ; later, when the sheath of Henle is lost, it gives rise to four branches, which divide and sub-divide and which, changing their course, cover a good part of the muscle fibre. After a few trials, the majority of the thin branches at last reach the region where the granular material and the nuclei of the sensory apparatus are situated.

In the fine work from which we extract the above details, Tello reveals to us a multitude of other interesting facts, such as the retrograde movement of axons beneath the capsule, the deviation of motor fibres that have accidentally entered the afferent tube of the sensory apparatus and later turn to more appropriate paths, etc. These phenomena show that if the orienting action of the sensory and motor structures has a specific character, it has it only for a short distance, and that if the pre-established path which is accidentally innervated by a conductor is a guide in the right direction, it may also cause deviations and useless wanderings.

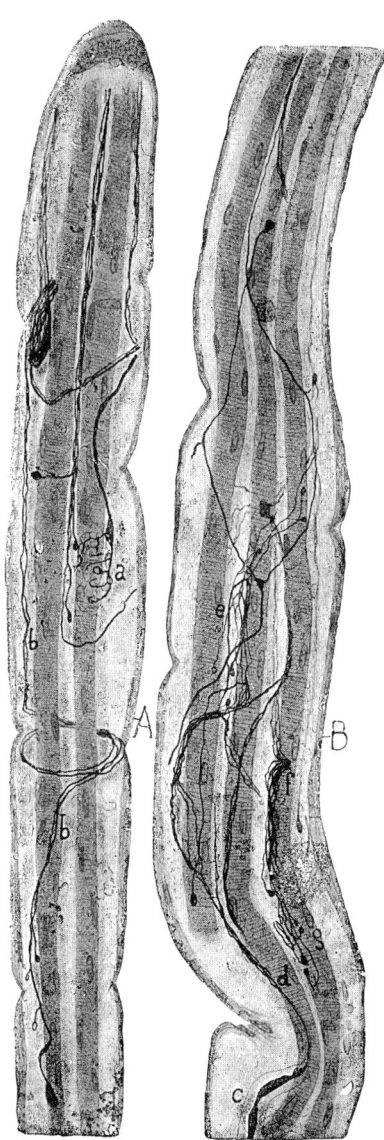

Fig. 108.—Two bundles of Weismann in course of regeneration. Rabbit killed three months after section of the sciatic nerve. Gastrocnemius. *a*, regenerated motor plate ; *b*, fibre directed towards the sensory plate ; *c*, large sprout which, after a long tortuous path enters the region of the sensory arborization ; *f*, fine sensory fibres arriving from another direction and ending in clubs or rings.

Regeneration of the sensory nervous apparatus of tactile hairs.—
An investigation by Dr. Tello makes known to us that in these structures regeneration begins early, twenty or twenty-five days after section of the nerve in the snout of a rabbit one month old. The newly-formed fibres, few in number, reach the hair by the old sheaths, where there still subsist the remnants of the degenerated axons. In Fig. 109 we show a preparation in which a few sprouts, resulting from the division of a single afferent tube, grow towards the region of the rings and tactile menisci, which they have not reached as yet. The complete differentiation of the terminal apparatus requires more time.[1]

Insufficiencies and incongruences of the peripheral regeneration.—
A conclusion supported by physiological and clinical observations is that the restoration of the sensory and motor innervation of the terminal regions of sectioned nerves is never perfect. Even when one experiments on recently born mammals one sees that, three or four months after the operation, the movements of the operated leg are not as precise and vigorous as those of a healthy leg. One also observes more or less extensive lacunae in the tactile and pain senses of the skin.

Such imperfections are explained completely when one remembers the mechanism of penetration of the sprouts into the peripheral stump. One must remember that a great many of the conductors which are newly-formed in the central stump are retrograde or deviated fibres. Many tubes also have sterile clubs or become useless in the helicoidal structures. Finally, those sprouts which reach the peripheral stump enter it in great disorder ; some sheaths have no sprouts, and the great majority, if not all, of the sheaths, instead of receiving the outgrowth of the same axon which was present in them before the operation, are invaded by sprouts that have come from axons in other regions of the central stump. Thus the observed facts compel us to reject the supposition of those authors who believe that the newly-formed fibre infallibly ends in the old sheath of the peripheral stump and unerringly restores the old terminal arborization, thus preserving the anatomical and physiological individuality of the pre-existent conductor. On the contrary, the errors and incongruences are so many that one wonders whether the whole

[1] For the case of taste buds see: R. M. May: "The relation of nerves to degenerating and regenerating taste buds," *Jour. Exp. Zool.*, vol. 42, 1925, pp. 371-410.

mass of sprouts which penetrate into the peripheral stump is not entirely superfluous, seeing that the connections between the central neurones and the peripheral structures which formed, since the embryonic period, such an intimate anatomical and dynamic whole,

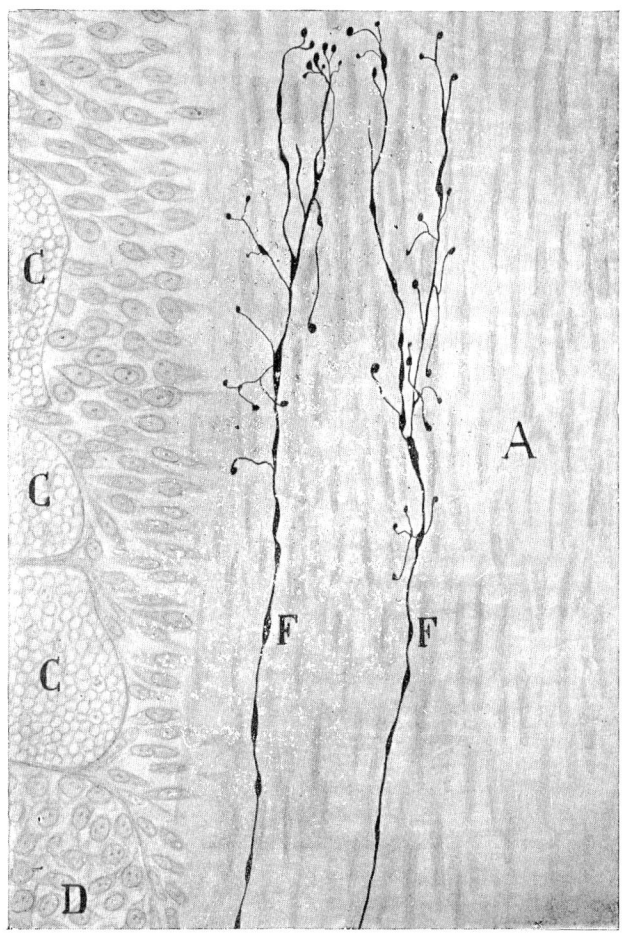

FIG. 109.—Tactile hair of the snout of a rabbit, killed thirty days after the operation. *A*, epithelial sheath which is cut tangentially; *D*, annular bolster; *C*, vascular spaces; *F*, regenerated nerve fibres.

are now so disturbed and confused. Moreover, in the cases of rapid nervous reunion after hemisection or complete sections with a small scar, sensibility and movement are only more or less imperfectly restored.

To what is due this relative success or lack of success in the reunion of the terminal structures ? Ranvier and Vanlair believe that it is the result of chance. The sprouts, growing in the path of least resistance, enter first the old sheaths and later reach the terminal structures.

Without going into too many details at present, it seems necessary to postulate the existence of *alluring* or *attracting substances*, both in the peripheral stump and in the terminal structures. These substances have the faculty of orienting or facilitating the growth of the axons in determined paths. We believe, and Lugaro, Marinesco, and other neurologists share our opinion, that the action exercised by the peripheral stump—the proliferated cells of Schwann, etc., on the growth of the young fibres is not *individual* and *specific*, that is, from tube to tube, but is general and collective, summarily directing the new axons towards the periphery. But once the axons are near the terminal structures, no matter what their position in the distal segment, the terminal clubs are influenced by another neurotropic influence which now has an *individual* and *specific* character, and by means of it each group of epithelial or muscle cells gets into intimate and exclusive contact with the terminal arborization of the old axon. In order that this connection may re-establish the old symbiosis it is only necessary that a single sprout from the many which arise from the old conductor should be attracted. The projections from other axons which by chance have reached the same region ulteriorly atrophy through disuse and disappear, as was supposed by Heidenhain to occur in the case of the excess of pre-terminal fibres and nerve plexuses formed in the skin and muscles during embryonic growth.[1]

Among the specific orienting substances, those which appear especially necessary are those elaborated by the spindles of Kühne and the musculo-tendinous structures of Golgi, and those also which

[1] This hypothesis is in accordance with the observations made long ago by us on the excessive formation of dendrites and nervous collaterals in many embryonic neurones. Thus the Purkinje cells of the cerebellum possess during the first phases of their evolution incongruent expansions which have an exploratory character, and which later disappear. It is only those expansions which are able to establish useful relations with afferent nerve fibres which survive in this contest for space and connections. In nervous regeneration this process of hyperformation is repeated.

See Cajal: *Textura del sistema nervioso del hombre y vertebrados*, vol. 2, p. 395, 1904.

are produced by the various categories of sensory organs of the skin and mucous membranes.

There is no doubt that, at first, many imperfect connections are formed, and that many duplications and errors of distribution occur. But these incongruences are progressively corrected, up to a certain point, by two parallel methods of rectification. One of these occurs in the periphery, and is the atrophy through disuse of superfluous and parasitic ramifications, in combination with the growth of congruent sprouts. The other occurs in the ganglia and spinal centres; by this there would be a selection, due to the atrophy of certain collaterals and the progressive disappearance of disconnected or useless neurones, of the sensory-motor fibres capable of being useful. Concerning the restoration of central connections, it would be still more satisfactory to admit the re-arrangement or re-organization of pyramidal and sensory-reflex collaterals destined to rectify the aberrations of connection that have occurred in the periphery. But the dogma of the irregenerability of the central paths prohibits us from putting forth such a hypothesis.

Such explanations seem complicated. To-day, however, one cannot assume a simpler and more plausible conception of the anatomical and functional restoration of the sensory and motor structures. At any rate, this re-establishment is not more perfect in recently born and young animals. It is generally admitted that important changes occur in the nerve centres after nerve sections. Such modifications, which are marked and constant, were first observed tardily in the spinal cord after amputation. As early as 1869 Dickson observed atrophic phenomena in motor neurones that were trophic centres for mutilated axons. Dickson also observed, at the same time, that the central stump of the nerves after amputation becomes smaller, and that its fibres progressively disappear. Similar facts were noted by Darschewitsch,[1] and especially by Marinesco,[2] who observed important changes in the central stump and trophic centres after amputation. The authors have repeatedly observed atrophies and degenerations in sensory ganglia. Marinesco[3]

---

[1] Darschewitsch: "Ueber die Veränderungen in centralen Stumpf eines motorischen Nerven," etc. *Neurol. Centralbl.*, 1892.

[2] Marinesco: "Ueber Veränderungen des Nerven und des Rückenmarks nach Amputationen," *Neurol. Centralbl.*, 1892.

[3] Marinesco: See his memoirs on nervous regeneration and especially his book, *La cellule nerveuse*, vol. 2, p. 153 *et seq.* 1909.

believes that the sensory and motor cells that atrophy and disappear correspond principally to those axons which are deviated and arrested during the process of regeneration. In other works he notes that these atrophies, occurring years after the amputation, begin at the cells and progress towards the nerve, thus having the character of a Wallerian degeneration. Lugaro [1] upholds a similar doctrine; he believes that all the retrograde fibres and spiroidal dispositions of the structures of Perroncito are condemned to resorption. We believe that such a tardy *central* regressive process may perhaps extend also to all the neurones whose axons have been unable to establish congruent connections with the periphery, such as motor fibres that have arrived accidentally at the skin, sensory fibres for the skin that have arrived in positions normally occupied by motor fibres, etc.

[1] Lugaro: " Osservazioni sui gomitoli nervosi nella rigenerazione dei nervi," *Riv. di Patol. ner. e mentale,* vol. 11, 1906.

XII

VARIETIES OF DEGENERATION AND REGENERATION DUE TO TRAUMATIC CAUSES

Degeneration and regeneration of nerves that have been instantaneously crushed.—Degeneration and regeneration following on ligature of nerves.—Compressed or necrotic ligatures (central stump, necrotic segment, and distal stump).—Innervation of the necrotic segment and distal stump (migrating fibres, rows of gigantic balls, and retrograde axons).—Moderately compressed ligatures.

Degeneration and regeneration following on instantaneous pressure.—This traumatic process, utilized equally with ligatures by various authors to cause degeneration, was especially studied by Stroebe in his interesting experiments on permanent or slow compression of the nerves of the rabbit's ear. Our own observations show that the results obtained are much more interesting and richer in theoretical teaching when the compression is made instantaneously, and is limited to a short segment of the nerve cordon. When one operates in this manner one simplifies the etiologic process, reducing it to the simple mechanical excitation of the conductor. One understands easily that if the nerve compression is permanent, with the mechanical influence are mixed various other derived conditions, among them a grave anaemia of the nerve, with a consequent perturbation of the regenerative process. Of all the procedures of rapid compression, the simplest and most convenient employed by us is as follows. The sciatic nerve is exposed and rapidly squeezed with the tips of a forceps. The forceps must not be too fine in order to avoid wounding or cutting the nerve. The animal is killed two, three, or more days after the operation. In order easily to recognize the compressed region, we put a little carbon black on the tips of the forceps.

While bringing about curious degenerative acts which we shall describe below, this method of traumatic excitation has the inestimable advantage of maintaining the normal circulation of the nerve and of *leaving uninterrupted the sheaths of Schwann*. Thus, in the absence of haemorrhage, a wound, and a real scar, one avoids all retardations of nervous reunion of the peripheral stump, since the sprouts can immediately invade the degenerated portion, travelling, as though on rails, inside the uninterrupted sheaths of Schwann, and finding nourishment in an exceptionally favourable region. Stroebe observed the special speed of this kind of regeneration, and he rightly attributed it to the absence of a scar and to the continuity of the tubular sheaths.

Between the simple traumatic excitation, which merely promotes regenerative acts, and an energetic compression which causes axonic necrosis and myelinic degeneration, there exist all possible transitions. One readily understands that in the same nerve which has been vigorously crushed there appear, according to the region under examination, effects of mere formative excitation, without necrosis, and an almost instantaneous destruction of the axons. In general it is the superficial zones that are attacked with the greatest violence by the traumatic injury. For this reason we often find, in nerves that have been moderately compressed, a superficial region rapidly necrosed, and a deep region where the axons survive in a phase of formative excitation or turgidity.

Although one cannot microscopically determine, as in sectioned nerves, a central and a peripheral stump, nevertheless one sees two equivalent regions microscopically : a *central segment* or living portion of the axon in the state of divisory turgidity, and a *peripheral stump*, corresponding to the degenerated segment. The two segments, anatomically continuous, thanks to the fact that the neurilemma, endoneurium, and the sheaths of Schwann and Retzius are uninterrupted, are connected by an intermediate region which is especially affected by the traumatic violence, and which corresponds to the *necrotic segment* of the central stump of cut nerves.

Peripheral stump.—This is represented, as stated above, by the entire nerve segment between the necrosed region and the periphery. Its conductors degenerate rapidly, passing through the well-known phases of secondary or Wallerian degeneration—formation of myelinic ellipsoids, metamorphosis and division of the cells of Schwann, fragmentation and resorption of the axon, etc. Since this degeneration offers no special characteristic, we shall pass forthwith to the analysis of the necrosed segment.

Necrosed portion.—This is the region of the nerve directly attacked by the traumatic agent. From the twenty-fourth hour after the operation one sees that in it the majority of the medullated axons, large and medium-sized, have fallen into a state of necrobiosis, showing, according to the region studied, various grades of hyalinity, fragmentation, and disintegration of the axons. On the other hand, the non-medullated fibres remain intact, unless the pressure has been so great that it has caused the complete disorganization of the nerve. In the same way the cells of Schwann and the cells of the endoneurium and perineurium very largely persist.

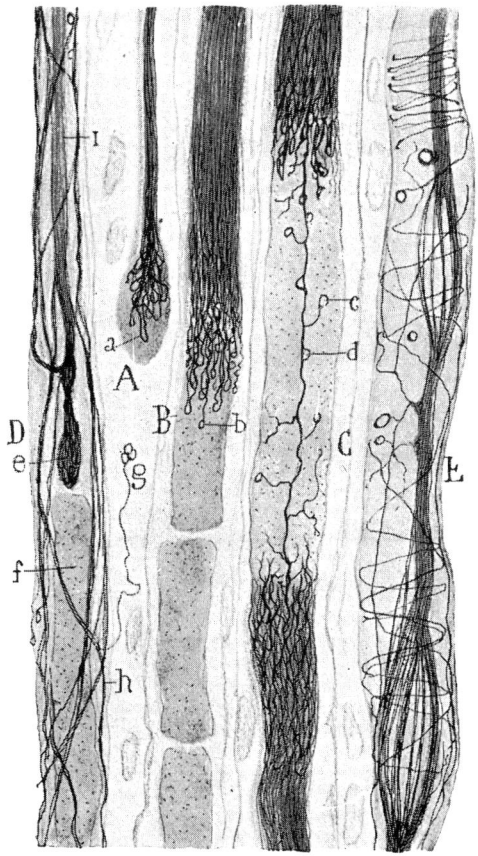

FIG. 109A.—Crushed portion—necrotic segment—of a nerve compressed by a forceps. Cat killed fifty-two hours after the operation. *A* and *B*, end of the living portion of the axon; *C*, necrotic segment with a newly-formed central fibril; *D*, *E*, tubes with nerve sprouts.

We shall not repeat here what has been already said concerning the changes occurring in necrosed axons. We shall merely note, because of their theoretical interest, a few interesting dispositions observed in the tubes where the axonic necrobiosis was initiated.

As we show in Fig. 110, *A*, this necrobiosis is not always total nor does it occur instantaneously. In fibres that are moderately compressed there exists an agonistic period during which, as occurs at the edge of the peripheral stump of cut nerves, there are attempts at intra-axonic regeneration. One can see in Fig. 109A, C, a certain axon whose necrosed portion, pale and granular in aspect, shows a thick central neurofibril, which is somewhat hypertrophied and intensely stained. As early as the fifty-second hour after the operation this axon shows evident signs of neoformation, since there issue from it, at an almost right angle, various collateral branchlets which are likewise constituted by a single filament. These twigs bifurcate here and there, and they end in the peripheral region of the necrotic mass in a ring which takes the colloidal silver very strongly. This central filament also has a few intercalated rings (d), a circumstance which suggests that even the axial neurofibril is an effect of the intraaxonic sprouting, since the rings and buds along the axis of the fibre represent cones of growth in process of resorption.

Fig. 110, A, shows another curious variety of cortical segmental necrosis. The axonic segment that is dying appears swollen and has the shape of a spindle, with a central region where there persists, almost unaltered, an axial neurofibrillar bundle, and a cortex full of liquid and granular detritus, in which a great number of newly-formed filaments ramify and terminate in rings. Some of them issue at a right angle, as in the last case, from the neurofibrillar bundle, while others are separated from the cortical portions of the undamaged axons, although they are in a state of formative turgidity.

Finally, phenomena analogous to neurofibrillar axonic regeneration occur also in the brush with which many axons effect contact with the necrosed segment (Fig. 109A, B, b). The end of such fibrils, which penetrate into the granular material, often shows terminal buds and loops.

These interesting phenomena of intra-axonic sprouting show the relative autonomy of the neurobiones or ultra-microscopic units of the neurofibrils. Apart from the total axonic regeneration, we see here a partial or elemental regeneration, thanks to which an axon which is wounded in its cortex can restore the full number of its neurofibrils. It follows that what we call sprouting of the axon is not a function of the axon working *in toto*, as a single physiological unit, but the sum and co-ordination of the divisory neoformations of the living units of the argentophilous substance—the neurobiones.

The same neurofibril represents a unit of the second order, or a complicated colony of neurobiones—the *histomeres* of Heidenhain.

Central stump.—We include in this all the living portions of the nerve present above the necrosed portion, and in a state of formative turgidity. In their union with the mortified segment these living portions, far from limiting themselves along a transversal plane, end at very different levels. Ordinarily, the more robust the nerve tubes, the further are the terminal clubs removed from the wounded region.

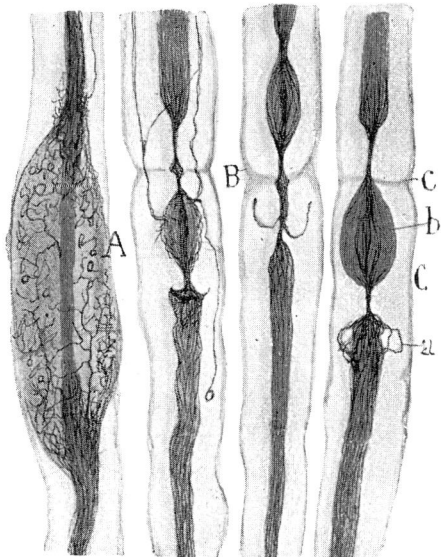

FIG. 110.—Fibres from the central portion of a crushed nerve. Adult cat killed fifty hours after the operation. *A*, necrosed portion of the axon; *B*, *C*, axons that have germinal muffs in a state of formative excitation.

There is nothing new to state concerning the form of the terminal mass and the junction of this thickening with the necrotic mass. We see repeated here, with slight variations, the gradations of shape of the terminal club and the forms of separation between the living and the dead portions that we have already described in another chapter.

In Fig. 111, *A*, we show the end of a thick axon from which arise, at a distance from the terminal sterile ball, various fine sprouts, which penetrate into the necrotic segment. One can see the elegant neurofibrillar net of the terminal sphere, whose central region is vacuolated. In regeneration, as in sectioned nerves, one can

286 TRAUMATIC DEGENERATION AND REGENERATION OF NERVES

distinguish two modalities : *pre-terminal sprouting*, or that which occurs near the final axonic intumescence, and *distal sprouting*, or that which occurs in regions far from the above-mentioned mass. The pre-terminal sprouting, of which we show a good example in Fig. 109A, D, shows no special points. The distal neoformation

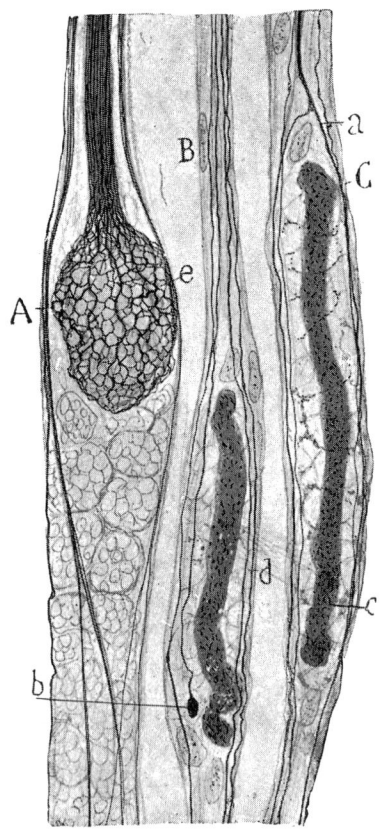

FIG. 111.—Three fibres from the degenerated portion of a crushed nerve. Rabbit killed four days after the operation. *A*, sterile axonic tip ; *e*, superficial sprouts which arise at some distance from the ball ; *c*, pieces of dead axon.

occurs almost exclusively in the germinal zones, which hypertrophy into a muff, giving rise later to intratubal branches which grow towards the mortified region and the peripheral stump. This neoformative tendency of the axons near the soldering disc is perhaps influenced by purely mechanical conditions. Thus the waves caused in the myelin and periaxonic fluid by pressure of the forceps, when they are propagated in a longitudinal direction, impinge violently on the soldering disc and neighbouring axonic intumescence, causing in the latter the state of formative turgidity. One thus explains not only the above-mentioned preference, but also the fact that it is almost always the germinal region directed towards the wound that gives rise to sprouts. One infers from this that the germinative

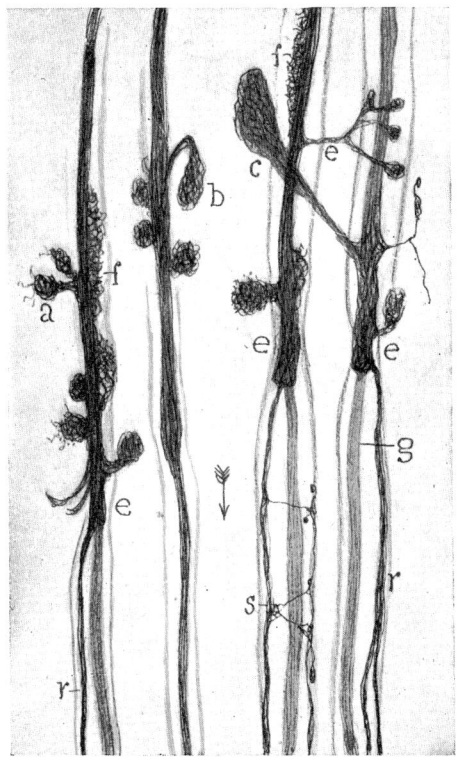

FIG. 112.—Central stump of a nerve crushed by a forceps. Region where the axon is in formative turgidity. Twenty-days-old cat, killed two days after the operation. *e*, node of Ranvier; *a*, fungiform excrescences; *b*, *c*, *e*, various types of newly-formed appendices; *f*, cotton-like axonic thickenings.

region does not possess a structure which is especially formed for the regenerative process ; it represents simply the region of maximum action of the mechanical stimulus.

Regeneration of the necrotic portion and peripheral stump.—This is brought about by the two methods of collateral and terminal neoformation which we have already described. The *collateral neoformation* occurs at a variable distance from the necrosed region, and it occurs at the level of long germinative muffs. Nearly all the sprouts are intratubal.

In young animals, such as cats and dogs from eight to twenty days old, the intratubal branches are less numerous, and there is a preponderance of collaterals and free terminal branches, due to the absence of a medullary sheath in many conductors. In the largest tubes there are often present, as shown in Fig. 112, e, c, long germinative regions, from which arise certain fungiform collateral excrescences which have a fine reticular structure, and which rapidly become extratubal. Some of these appendices ramify, giving rise to bouquets of terminal bulbs (e). The long collateral branches come out usually from the inferior end of the germinative muff and travel under Schwann's membrane.

But the characteristic facts about regeneration of crushed nerves are not connected with the manner in which the sprouts are formed, but with the speed of their formation and invasion of the peripheral stump, and with their invincible tendency to ravel immediately, giving rise to a multitude of parallel intratubal branches, which are first fine, and progressively thicker.

We have already spoken of the speed of nervous reunion in Chapter X. We need here only record the fact that four or five days after the nerve is crushed the sprouts not only have crossed the necrotic segment, but have advanced many millimetres within the peripheral stump, in which they always occupy a submembranous position, following the sides of the remnants of the dead axon, and conforming themselves to the contours of the myelinic ellipsoids.

Figs. 109A, E, 111, and 113 give an idea of the rapid ravelling and of the luxuriance of secondary ramification of the sprouts. In Fig. 113, E, one can see various tubes within which stand out a multitude of fine parallel fibres situated beneath Schwann's membrane, which quickly separate to surround the ellipsoids, and again join and are concentrated in the fine protoplasmic regions of the bands of Büngner.

All, or nearly all, of these independent fibrils *represent the result of the neurofibrillar disintegration of a collateral or terminal branch of the axon*. The sprout is thin at its origin but becomes progressively thicker; its neurofibrillar texture is accentuated; those secondary filaments which unite its primary neurofibrils disappear, and there remains, at last, a band of robust fibrils, which surrounds like a thin veil the axonic remnants of the necrotic region. Subsequently each neurofibril, converted into an independent branch, becomes thicker, and there results a thick skein or fascicle of parallel fibres. As we noted some time ago,[1] *the abundance, straightness, and parallelism of these branches constitute the characteristics of crushed nerves.* Owing to the fact that the sheaths of Schwann are uninterrupted, there is a great facility for nutrition, growth, and orientation of the axons, and the phenomenon of Perroncito, as well as arrested fibres, are almost completely lacking. As an exception, we show in Fig. 109A, *E*, a tube where the nerve sprout which is ravelling gives rise to a few spiral branchlets which terminate in rings.

This almost complete absence of helicoidal formations, no matter what the age of the animal, corroborates the opinion, which we expressed above, that in the production of the phenomenon of Perroncito, the decisive influence is exercised on one side by the obstruction of the nerve tube—the *digestive chamber*—of the necrosed portion, near the scar, and on the other by the absence of orienting substances. In crushed nerves, where the sheath is continuous, the peripheral stump is able to act directly on the central stump, sending by diffusion, along the tubes, chemotactic substances.

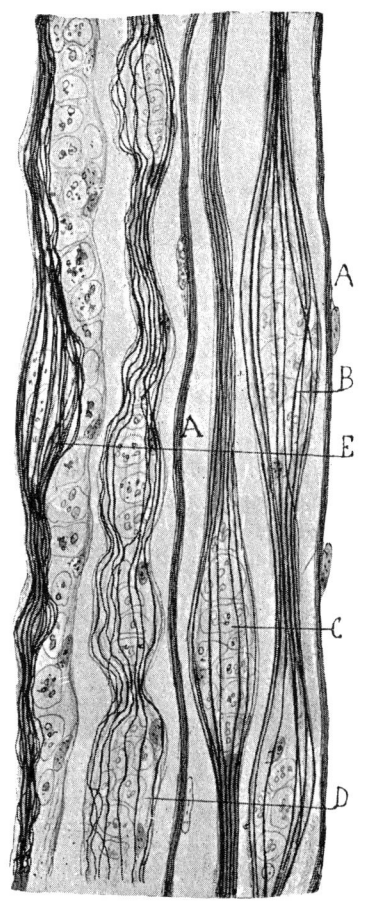

FIG. 113.—Peripheral segment of a nerve bruised with a forceps. Rabbit killed six days after the operation. *A*, non-medullated fibre which is undamaged; *B, C, D*, ravelled sprouts. In *E*, the skein of fibres occupied a lateral position; in *B, C, D*, the skein was under the membrane, surrounding the axonic remnants.

In our first paper on the effects of compression of the nerves we had supposed that the mechanical stimulus is the direct cause of the

[1] Cajal: " Les métamorphoses précoces des neurofibrilles dans la régénération et la dégénération des nerfs." *Trav. du Lab. de Rech. biol.*, fasc. 1 et 2, avril 1907. See also *Revista escolar*, 1906.

neurofibrillar disintegration of the axon, and, therefore, of its breaking-up into a bundle of branches. The same interpretation was adopted first by Marinesco and Minea, and later by Dustin, who have studied this phenomenon in the sensory ganglia as well as in the nerves. But our later and more careful observations on bruised nerves have led us to modify this opinion in part. Ravelling exists, *not in the old axon, but in its sprouts.* In order to make certain of this it is only necessary to examine the process in its early phases, twenty-four to sixty hours after the operation. One then sees that the majority of the axons have a dead segment, and that at the level of the living portion of the same axons arise proximal or distal collaterals. Many axons end in sickly balls, which are at times vacuolated and elegantly reticulated. Even in preparations made six days after the operation one sees in the peripheral stump, next to the ravelled sprouts, remnants of ellipsoids and axonic grumes (Fig. 113, *C*). The appearance of neurofibrillar ravelling of the axon, which sometimes impresses itself forcibly on the observer in late preparations, is due to two causes, which are difficult to suspect : (*a*) in crushed nerves the end of the sick axon, as well as the necrosed portion that lies below the region of sprouting, disappear rapidly ; (*b*) the persistent collateral branches thicken so much and so quickly that as early as the third day they appear to be the continuation of the axon. Owing to the combination of these effects and the precocious neurofibrillar dissociation of the sprouts, all preparations made from the fourth day on give us a picture of axons that open and disintegrate to become bundles of independent fibres. Our doubts were completely dissipated when we observed the remnants of a dead or sickly axon remaining constantly visible during the first two or three days in the very bifurcation that gave rise to the apparent axonic ravelling.

Degenerative and regenerative phenomena following ligature of the nerve.—Ranvier, Vanlair, Büngner, Stroebe, and other authors, have made frequent use of ligation to produce degeneration of the nerves. Some employed horse-hair, some catgut, others, finally, ordinary thread, tied round nerves exposed with aseptic precautions. We have used the ordinary suture thread on the sciatic nerve of young cats and rabbits. We carried out the examination of the lesions from the third to the tenth days after the operation.

The effects obtained vary according to the amount of constriction caused. A nerve that is very much constricted becomes rapidly necrosed throughout its thickness, and the degeneration and regeneration obtained do not differ essentially, with the exception of the absence of a microscopic interruption, from the same phenomena following sections of the nerve. A ligature which is moderately loose causes the necrosis and degeneration of the cortical region of the nerve while the central portion remains unchanged. Finally a thread so arranged that it lightly compresses the surface of the nerve, does not cause necrosis. It only brings about the creation of axonic sprouts in the germinative zones. In order to investigate the vitality and sprouting capacity of compressed axons we have often combined a ligature with a nerve section performed a short distance distally along the nerve. In other cases, which are still more instructive the ligature compressed only half of the nerve, the rest serving as a control, both halves being cut lower down. Finally, in a few experiments, the ligature was applied below a total or partial section.

We shall now set forth the effects of the ligature itself, excluding those caused by a light compression, which are very little or not at all different from those resulting from instantaneous crushing.

Like sectioned nerves, those which have been tied show: a *central stump*, situated above and at a certain distance from the ligature; a *necrotic segment*, placed under the thread itself and in neighbouring portions of the nerve; and a *peripheral* or *degenerative stump*, which extends from near the ligature to the periphery.

Central stump.—This differs little from the corresponding portion of instantaneously crushed nerves. We shall note only that this central stump is formed at a certain distance above the ligature and that one sees in it the two types of regeneration of which we have so often spoken—*collateral* and *terminal*. In the same way, in the cases of collateral sprouting, one sees the two varieties of which we have spoken: the *distal*, in which the sprouts appear near a sterile axonic mass or end, and the *proximal*, occurring near the nodes.

In Fig. 114 we show various examples of the most common variety, that is, the distal kind, as it appears two days after the operation. The morphological details which one can see in this figure dispense us from giving descriptive details. These details were, moreover, set forth in part when we dealt with the study of ordinary regeneration. We need note here only the abundance of thick germinative muffs; the circumstance that these muffs nearly always lie in the axonic thickening which is oriented towards the lesion; the fact that the neighbouring node is usually fairly well preserved; and finally, that exceptionally, when the node is obliterated, the germinative zone emits direct and retrograde branches. We shall not insist, either, on the phenomenon of neurofibrillar dissociation, nor on the avalanche of growth, which takes on in this type of central stump an unusual importance, so much so that a few hundredths of a millimetre from their point of origin the collateral as well as the terminal fibres become transformed into bundles of parallel branches which are situated under the membrane of Schwann (Fig. 114, C, D, E).

As may be expected, in the following days, from the third to the seventh, the fibres created through dissociation of the collaterals grow in length and thickness, and travel in a straight line towards the ligature, accommodating themselves on their path to the ellipsoids of myelin and the axonic remnants. Besides these parallel fibres one finds, although less frequently, small transversal or oblique branches and band-like dilatations or delicate neurofibrillar tubes. In general the membranous sprouts and the delicate veils are due to precocious phenomena. Nearly always, before the sixth day, all the membranes that are composed of parallel neurofibrils have become intratubal bundles. The apparatus of Perroncito is completely lacking. We may add that a great number of large tubes become sterile and degenerate retrogressively over long stretches, showing a large terminal club, excrescences on the outlines, etc.

Necrotic segment.—This embraces the region of the ligature and two margins, a proximal and a distal, of a variable extent. It is curious to note that *under the ligature and in the immediate neighbourhood the axons have not been autolyzed*. They are very much thinner, and appear straight, homogeneous or lightly granular, slightly stained by colloidal silver and without the slightest appearance of sprouting. Around them lies the sheath of Schwann, which is hardly visible. The myelin and periaxonic fluid have disappeared, pushed in a proximal and distal direction by the pressure of the thread, as the older authors, especially Büngner, had already noted. For this reason the sheaths of Schwann of the central stump are exceptionally dilated, as though they had to enclose a considerable supplement of dislocated myelin. The cells of Schwann and cells of the endoneurium have fallen into necrobiosis. One sees their granular remnants among the axons only with difficulty. Finally, the capillaries are obstructed, and it is almost impossible for any exudative infiltration to occur across the compressed region.

It follows from what we have here stated that not only the

phenomenon of degeneration, but axonic autolysis also, require the survival of the cell of Schwann, or, at least, the collaboration of living migratory cells. Without vascular ferments or enzymes elaborated by living cells the axon behaves like the *preserved fibres*.

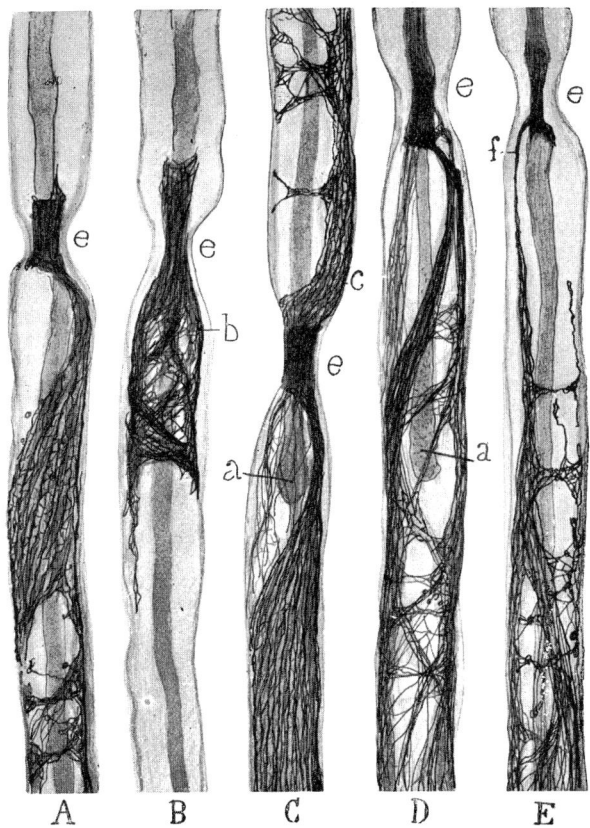

FIG. 114.—Region of the central stump far from the ligature and in a state of divisory excitation. Adult rabbit killed two days after the lesion. Formation of germinative muffs near the nodes. *e*, node; *b*, neoformation in the form of a membranous net; *a*, club of a pre-existent axon.

Peripheral stump.—This shows phenomena of axonic fragmentation, a transformation of the myelin, and a multiplication of the cells of Schwann. Since all these are characteristic of the Wallerian degeneration, we need not repeat their description here.

Nervous reunion of the necrosed region and peripheral stump.—The interesting point concerning ligature of the nerve is that by means of it we can exercise a direct influence on the process of growth and orientation of the nerve sprouts, opposing three hindrances to nervous reunion of the peripheral stump : a *mechanical hindrance*, due to the narrowing of the intratubal and extratubal interstices ; a *nutritive hindrance*, due to the more or less accentuated vascular obstruction ; and a *dynamic* or *trophic hindrance*, due to the narrowness of the path through which the neurone of origin can influence the outgrowing sprouts.

The energy of these three inhibitory conditions depends, naturally, on the amount of constriction of the ligature. If it is much constricted the current of growth is repelled and nervous reunion is paralyzed ; if the ligature is moderately constricted, the current of nervous reunion becomes parsimonious and, accommodating itself to the circumstances, shows curious and instructive adaptations. We shall study both cases.

Extreme compression.—After a strong pressure the trophic influence of the centres subsists integrally, but the mechanical and nutritive inhibitions, especially the mechanical, render impossible both the nervous reunion of the peripheral stump and the crossing of the necrosed portion which was directly compressed by the ligature. In such circumstances the intratubal bundles formed by ravelling of the sprouts advance towards the lesion. Being unable to cross it, however, they do one of three things. They may escape under the neurilemma or towards the interfascicular partitions ; they may become arrested, creating balls of a variable size ; or they may become retrograde, producing retrograde clubs and branches.

(a) *Migrating fibres.*—The tension of growth under the sheaths of Schwann and the obstacles accumulated in an axial direction cause the mass migration of many sprouts. These, after they have broken through the tubal sheath, travel in various directions, especially transversally, between the neurilemma and the nerve bundles, or between the latter and the large connective tissue membranes. Such sprouts, which are particularly robust, bifurcate repeatedly and appear crowned with cones of various shapes ; the discoidal, membranous, net-like, and hederiform shapes predominate, however, among these cones (Fig. 115, *E*). Indeed, this phenomenon of migration can be seen in ordinary sections of the nerve ; it assumes considerable proportions, however, only in cases where the nerve is ligated. The migration of the sprouts occurs at variable distances from the ligature, often at the level of the zone of divisory turgidity.

(b) *Arrested fibres.*—These are reproduced in Fig. 116, *G*, *I*. One may there observe the loop which precedes the immobile club, the ellipsoidal or elongated shape of the latter, and especially the formation of the very fine exploratory filament sent out by some of the clubs in the direction of the ligature, as though determined at any cost to force a path.

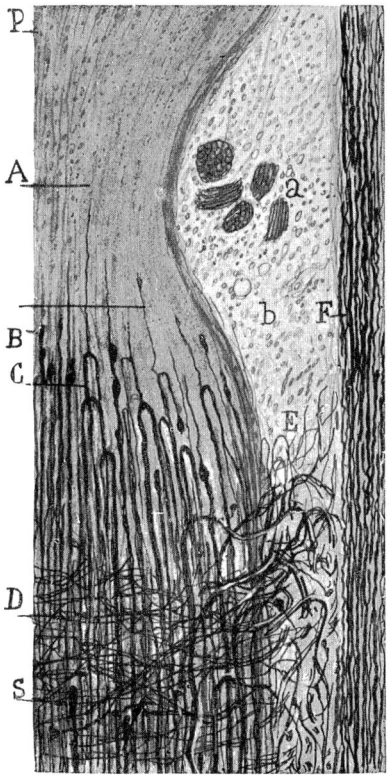

FIG. 115.—Sciatic nerve of a young rabbit. Partial ligature. The animal was killed three days after the operation. *a*, threads of the ligature; *A*, compressed region of the nerve; *D*, *E*, migrating fibres; *C*, retrograde fibres; *B*, arrested fibres; *P*, peripheral stump; *F*, nerve bundle which was not included in the ligature.

Fig. 117 shows various arrested fibres, examined in late phases, from the thirteenth to the eighteenth day after the operation. The sprouts have become notably thicker. Their clubs, which are immobile, have reached enormous proportions. Some of them show voluminous lobulations. All, or nearly all of them, have fallen into partial or total hyaline degeneration. As might be expected, the ball, immobilized in a region poor in nutritive juices, and constantly

296 TRAUMATIC DEGENERATION AND REGENERATION OF NERVES

urged on by the internal impulsion to growth, wears out and becomes degenerated. For this reason one frequently finds nests of dead balls or balls with a few remnants of a neurofibrillar net (Fig. 117, c).

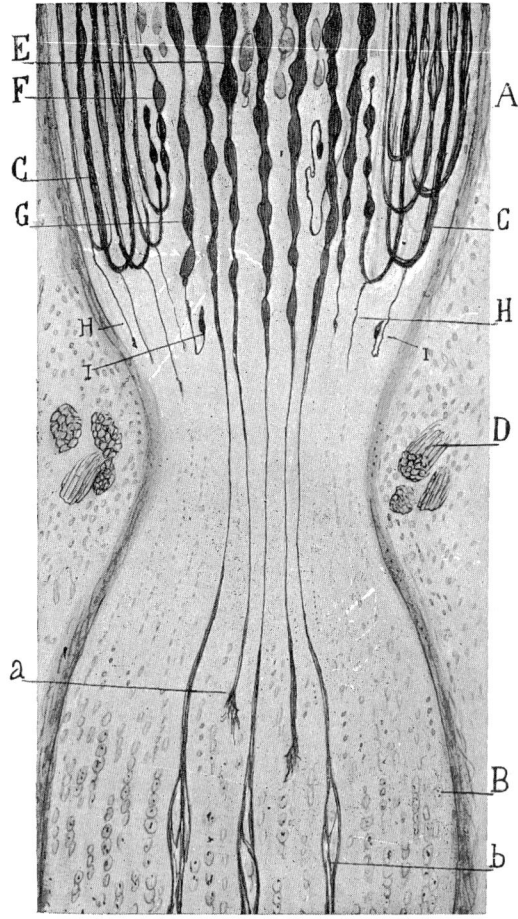

FIG. 116.—Ligature of the sciatic nerve of a rabbit. Semi-schematic. Central stump thirteen days after the lesion. A, central stump; D, ligature; B, peripheral stump; C, superficial retrograde fibres; F, arrested fibres; E, fibres in the shape of a string of beads with an exploratory branch which penetrates into the compressed region; H, fine exploratory fibres; a, terminal cone; b, nervous reunion of the peripheral stump.

But the most characteristic feature in the late stage of arrested fibres consists in the exhibition of chains of balls, that is, of a series of thick fusiform prominences which alternate with thinned segments (Fig. 116, E). Each varicosity along the path corresponds to a phase of immobilization. One thus sees that the balls translate in space *a phenomenon occurring in time.* It appears as though the fibres travelled by stages, impulsive efforts alternating with more or less prolonged resting periods. There is here a static-dynamic rhythm, whose irregular periodicity is objectively seen in the string of balls. All the incidents along the path, all the conflicts occurring

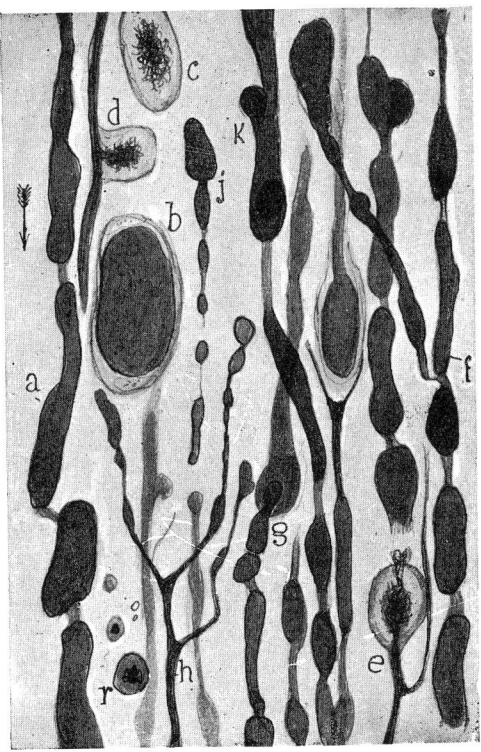

FIG. 117.—Details of the region of the central stump where the bead-like fibres are situated; *a*, fusiform masses; *b*, segregated balls; *c*, degenerated ball; *d, e*, balls with an exploratory fibre; *g, k*, excrescences of the masses; *h*, ramified retrograde fibre.

in the struggle for space, remain as though photographed in these long strings of beads. One might thus compare the latter to a cinematographic film, examined at rest, one picture after the other. In Fig. 117, *a, g,* we reproduce these strings of balls very much enlarged. One may note the narrowness of the thread that separates each enlargement, and the frequent changes in axial position. Finally, one can see balls segregated through autotomy and others that are about to separate (Fig. 117, *e, r*).

Not all the arrested axons fail completely. As one can see in Fig. 116, *E*, many of them, examined during late stages, show, beyond the last varicosity, an appendage of variable size, which is straight and that has gone boldly forward into the narrows of the compressed portion. If one follows these exploratory fibres one sees them occasionally within the peripheral stump, where they end at various distances in more or less dilated cones (*a*). Those which have grown furthest break up under Schwann's sheath into bundles of fibres (*b*). Ordinarily the fibres that behave in this way are the deepest, that is, those situated in a region where the pressure is felt less than in the cortical portion. We have drawn some of these details in Fig. 116.

(*c*) *Retrograde fibres.*—These are very numerous, of various sizes, and they are present throughout the thickness of the central stump. They are especially abundant, however, in the cortex of the nerve segment. This is easily understood, since the narrowing of the tubes brought about by the ligature is much greater in the cortex of the nerve than in its centre. These superficial conductors are easily recognized by the bends which they make in order to turn back, these bends being situated nearly all at the same distance from the ligature (Fig. 116, *C*), and by their fasciculated structure. Twelve days after the lesion they have grown so much in a retrograde path that it is difficult to see their terminal cones. In their retrograde paths the majority of these sprouts travel through the interstices of the endoneurium. When they turn back, some of them also show strings of clubs, showing that there are obstacles to progression and places hard to cross in a fairly large area round the ligated points. There are certain regions where the balls belonging to the retrograde fibres constitute a formidable agglomeration. Next to immobile fibres provided with colossal balls, other fibres are found growing and emitting retrograde branches which bifurcate repeatedly (Fig. 117, *h*). Some of the branches of this class are occasionally seen to abandon the sheaths of Schwann, and to wander without any special direction among interstices of the nerve.

When the cortex, although it has been compressed, retains some narrow clefts, delicate exploratory sprouts issue from the bend of the retrograde fibre. These sprouts are directed towards the ligature, but they hardly ever reach its level. To accommodate themselves to the narrowness of the interstitial paths such sprouts have a thin point, which is more or less lanceolate and never ends in a ring (Fig. 116, *H*).

We may mention finally the fact that certain recurrent branches thrown out by the retrograde sprouts sometimes attain a great length, forming a connexion in a cellulipetal direction to a great number of myelinic ellipsoids, around which they ramify intricately. As we show in Fig. 118, *a, c*, one sees fibres of this kind arranged in glomeruli and forming intricate turns within the very large intratubal chambers created by the reflux of the myelin ; these chambers are full of liquid and axonic detritus.

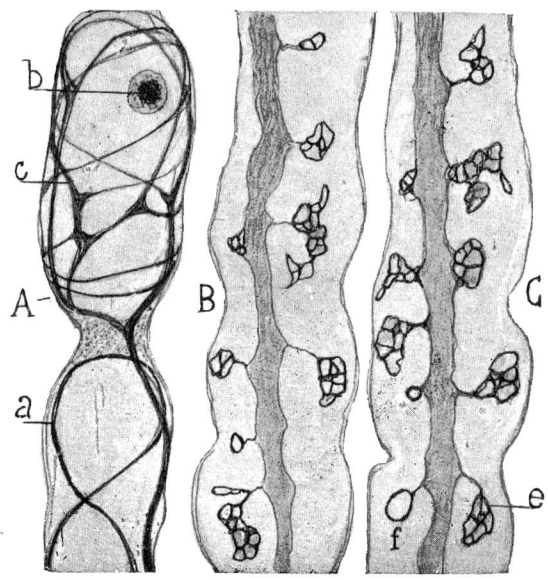

FIG. 118.—Details of the central stump some distance from the ligature. Rabbit killed fifteen days after the operation. *A*, degenerated tube with enormous dilatations innervated by retrograde fibres (*a*), which ramify (*c*) and form plexuses ; *b*, segregated mass ; *e*, reticulated appendices in sterile axons.

Sterile tubes are very common in the central stump of ligated nerves. One sees them often, as shown in Fig. 118, *e*, within enormous dilatations of Schwann's sheath, pale in appearance and provided with abortive collateral appendices. The excrescence which crowns such growths shows vacuoles and a thick and intensely stained neurofibrillar net.

Moderately tight ligatures.—In the previous case the obstruction to the growth of the fibres almost completely impeded the nervous reunion of the necrotic portion and peripheral stump. When, however, the ligature compresses the nerve moderately, the pressure can only somewhat retard the arrival of the sprouts at the distal stump, and cause inequalities due to the more or less superficial position of the fibres. It is important to note that the effects obtained with moderately tight ligatures are very variable, owing to the impossibility of regulating the energy of compression. For this reason one sees in some cases almost the entire thickness of the nerve degenerated, while in others necrosis occurs only in the cortex, the axial tubes remaining unharmed or only slightly damaged. We shall describe this last effect, which is relatively frequent in our experiments.

As shown in the scheme of Fig. 119, a moderately tight ligature divides the nerve into two concentric regions—a central and a peripheral.

Peripheral region.—All or nearly all its fibres fall into necrobiosis, and must be renewed owing to the compression and stimulus of the thread. Under ordinary circumstances only a few non-medullated fibres remain undamaged. Such a mortification is propagated in a centripetal direction, to a certain distance from the ligature. The sprouting of the central stump occurs very much above the ligature, collateral and terminal sprouts being formed as described before. Each axon gives rise in this way to an intratubal bundle which, from the second to the fourth day after the section, grows toward the region of the ligature (Fig. 119, *a, b, c*).

The behaviour of these bundles in the compressed region is very interesting. An essential feature is that the diameter of the newly-formed conductors becomes much thinner, and when they cross the compressed region, they are very much less stained by the colloidal silver (*e*). Once the obstacle is crossed, however, these sprouts thicken, their susceptibility to the stain is restored, and their branches bifurcate repeatedly, giving rise within the sheaths of the peripheral stump to robust and beautiful bundles of conductors (*h, m*). To get an idea of the diminution in diameter of the sprouts at the level of the obstruction, we have made a few measurements of typical cases. The extratubal branches lose half or two-thirds of their thickness. Thus robust fibres 4 μ thick were reduced to 2 and $1\frac{1}{2}$ μ, resuming, once the ligature was crossed, their normal diameter. The transversal reduction of each intratubal bundle of fine fibres is even more marked; thus a bundle of 8 μ dropped to less than 2 μ, returning beyond the obstruction to 8 or 10 μ. At the level of the ligature each integrating fibre of the fascicle hardly exceeds the diameter of the neurofibrils. Although their close approximation within the bundle is such that any numerical determination is almost impossible, it has seemed to us that not a few of them stop before

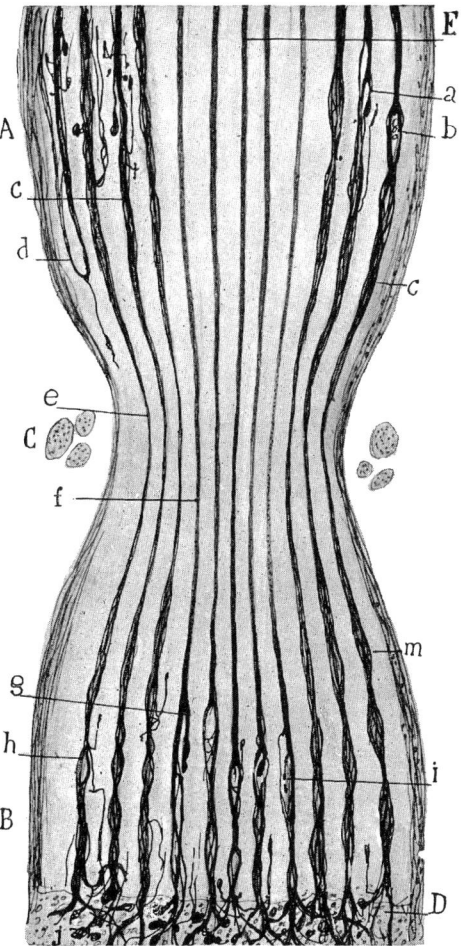

FIG. 119.—Regenerative effects of moderately compressed ligatures. Young rabbit, killed eight days after the ligature. *A*, central stump; *B*, peripheral stump; *D*, region of the nerve section; *C*, ligature; *E*, undamaged fibres of the central region; *b, c*, fibres of the peripheral region in formative turgidity; *g, i*, fibres of the central region of the nerve whose state of divisory excitation can be seen near the wound. The nerve was cut at a certain distance from the ligature.

reaching the obstruction. A certain portion of those fibres which are present below the ligature thus perhaps originate through ravelling of the pale fibres that have succeeded in crossing the obstacle (Fig. 119, *e*).

In order to find out whether those sprouts which have crossed the obstacle have lost in so doing, in consequence of their notable thinning, their energy of growth and neoformation, we have several times combined a ligature with a section of the nerve at a short distance. It results from these experiments, as shown by the schemata in Figs. 119 and 120, that the *vigour of growth is as great as that of axons in the axial region which were very little or not at all compressed*. Near the wound the sprouts undergo a process of rapid multiplication, creating very complicated bundles of nerve filaments. We may add that, once they have reached the scar, these fibres, after nine days, have grown out as much as companion fibres arising from deep axons. What is even more important, *they are as long and as well able to cross the cicatricial connective tissue as fibres from nerves which were not ligated but which were cut at the same level* (see Fig. 120, a, b).

These observations make it seem probable, in accordance with Heidenhain's suggestion, that the *trophic influence exercised by the central neurones is of a dynamic and not of a material nature*, since a sprout can diminish to less than a third of its calibre, without suffering, once the narrowed region is past, the least retardation or impediment in the phenomena of assimilation and growth. The thesis, so often put forward, that *assimilation and growth of the axons are purely local processes*, that is, that they are not influenced by materials or chemical reserves of the soma or nucleus of the neurones, also harmonizes with these results. We shall speak more at length of these important points in the chapter on the theoretical interpretation of regeneration.

Central regions.—These are characterized by the fact that their axons are undamaged or only slightly altered, that they have retained their normal structure and their medullary sheath. Nevertheless, one can often see that on crossing the obstruction they have diminished from $\frac{1}{4}$ to $\frac{1}{3}$ in diameter, they have taken on a flexuous course, and they show granular spots which alternate with portions less well stained.

Where a section has been associated with the ligature (Fig. 119, f, g), one can see that the fibres have not been much altered, since they are still able to give rise, at variable distances from the wound, to collateral and terminal fibres which invade the scar. The details of the schematic Fig. 119 dispense us from giving any further description. We need only note that in the operations of hemisection, in which it is possible to compare the growth of central

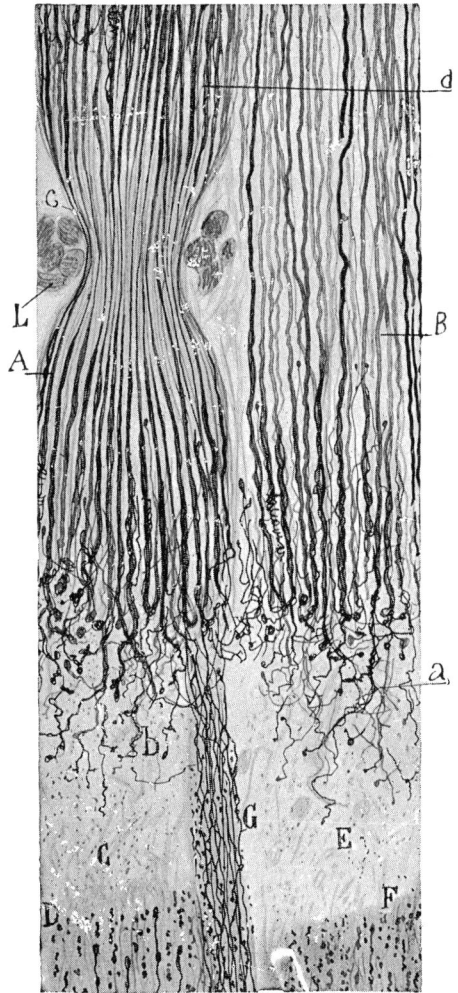

FIG. 120.—Semiligature of the sciatic nerve in a rabbit, killed eight days after the operation. Total section of the nerve near the ligature, in order to compare the sprouting capacity of the two portions. *A* peripheral stump of the ligated nerve; *d*, central stump of the same; *L*, ligature; *B*, central stump of the non-ligated fascicle; *C*, *E*, scars; *D*, *F*, degenerated stumps. In the ligated nerve are represented only the fibres of the cortical region, all of them in the phase of ravelling.

axons that are little compressed, with cortical axons that have sprouted and are narrowed at the level of the obstruction, and with free axons or those belonging to cut nerve bundles which were not ligated, we can see that the three classes of conductors have the same or a similar extension in the scar. Sometimes, nevertheless, the cortical axons, in ligated nerves, appear retarded, a fact which is natural, since it is they that have the longest way to go before reaching the scar. When this delay does not occur, however, as shown in Fig. 120, one must suppose that the force of growth has a greater energy in those fibres which were stimulated by pressure of the ligature than in those which were free from any stimulus or permanent constriction.

XIII

EXPERIMENTS TO ELUCIDATE THE MECHANISM OF THE GROWTH, RAMIFICATION, AND ORIENTATION OF THE NERVE SPROUTS

Combined effects of ligature and section.—Topical indifference, etc.—Retrograde nervous reunion of neighbouring nerve bundles.—Mechanical obstruction caused by the ligature of the peripheral stump (formation of gigantic balls and of exploratory branches).—Experiments designed to prove the reality of neurotropical phenomena (multiple sections and hemisections, transformation of central infecund axons into fecund sprouts, etc.).

THE observation of the phenomena that follow a section is highly instructive. But one learns even more when one sees a regenerative process carried out in extraordinary circumstances, when one opposes experimentally a diversity of obstacles to the growth of the sprouts and sets up unusual perturbatory conditions. Such experiments shed a flood of light on the mechanism of ramification, the production of large balls, the act of retrogression, and, finally, even on the trophic action of the centres and the chemical orientation (neurotropism) of the growing sprouts.

We have conducted numerous experiments of this kind during the last few years.[1] We shall here refer only to those which are most important and of the greatest theoretical value.

Experiments with sections combined with semiligatures.—We have stated that sections made below a semiligature afford us a simple method of comparing the regenerative power of compressed and of free fibres. This amounts to investigating whether the diminution of the path through which the trophic impulse comes from the centres (after compression of the axons) manifests itself in a variation of the sprouting capacity of the axons or their branches.

These experiments bring about, at times, phenomena of nervous reunion of great theoretical significance. This is shown by Figs. 121 and 122. Frequently the sprouts arising in a macroscopic nerve

---

[1] Cajal: " Influencia de las condiciones mecánicas sobre la regeneración de los nervios," *Trab. del Lab. de Investig. biol.*, tomo 9, fasc. 4, 1912.

fascicle, when they reach the cicatricial masses, seem to divide into two currents. One of these, the principal one, laboriously crosses the connective tissue in order to reach the peripheral stump (Fig. 121, C). The other is marginal and contains much longer sprouts. It becomes suddenly retrograde and innervates with unexpected energy a neighbouring nerve cordon—the macroscopic *tertiary fascicle* (c).

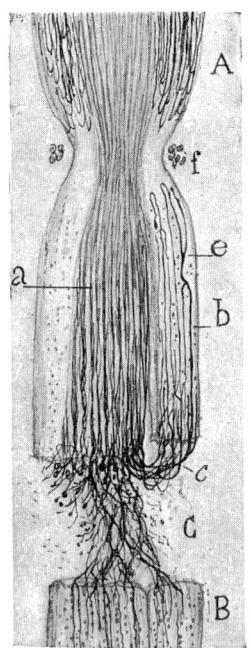

FIG. 121.—Nerve from a cat fifteen days old, killed seven days after the operation. Section of the peripheral stump (B); A, central stump; f, ligature; C, scar; c, retrograde fibres which innervate a degenerated bundle included in the ligature. The ligature was compressed enough to cause necrosis of the cortical region of the nerve, but not of the central region, from which arise the retrograde sprouts.

Among these dislocated fibres there are some robust ones which, once arrived at the edge of the cordon, suddenly break up into various branches, which in their turn insinuate themselves either within the tubes of Schwann, where they have to work their way among the fatty ellipsoids, or else into the interstices of the endoneurium. The power of growth of such sprouts is so great that we have seen them, at times (Fig. 121, e), assaulting the ligature, and before that obstacle, becoming retrograde a second time and going back to the end of the stump.

In those cases in which the ligature is moderately compressed, so that the cortical regions of the peripheral stump which were primitively degenerated are innervated by exploratory filaments arising from retrograde fibres, one finds within the marginal portion two classes of sprouts—ascending and descending. The scheme of Fig. 122, b, c, shows this interesting detail. The current of fibres coming from the scar originated from axons of the central region that were stimulated by the wound, but were not degenerated by the ligature.

One can see the details of the process of retrograde penetration of the sprouts that have come from the wound in Fig. 123. There one sees the luxuriance of neoformation that occurs in the fibres when they reach the end of the degenerated tubes. Within a short distance fibre C has broken up into six very long branches, besides several short appendices ending in spheres. Most of these sprouts are intratubal, but some of them are interstitial.

Experiments of semi-ligature combined with total section.—A curious variation of the phenomenon of retrograde nervous reunion above described appears in the schematic Fig. 124, C, where the fibres that effected the reunion arose from a neighbouring non-ligated cordon, in an experiment involving a semi-ligature. The retrograde sprouts which were bound to assault the degenerated cordon travelled an enormous distance across the scar after ligature and section (experiment on a cat fifteen days old). More than one sprout became retrograde on reaching the ligated region (a). Since, in this case the ligature was very tight, all the fibres of the ligated bundle became degenerated, and the sprouts which migrated from the non-ligated fascicle did not have to contend with those which arose from its proximal segment.

That which most impresses one in these phenomena of retrograde nervous reunion is the extraordinary vegetative energy of the newly-formed fibres, shown not only within the innervated cordon, but also within the interposed scar, across which they travel a much greater distance than direct or ordinary sprouts (Fig. 124, D). One is also surprised by the fact that various fibres situated at a certain distance from each other usually combine to form the new path, as though all alike they felt the attractive force. Finally, the sudden breaking up of these fibres into parallel branches, once they have arrived at the edge of the neighbouring cordon, in order to innervate simultaneously various sheaths of Schwann, is a phenomenon worthy of attention. We believe

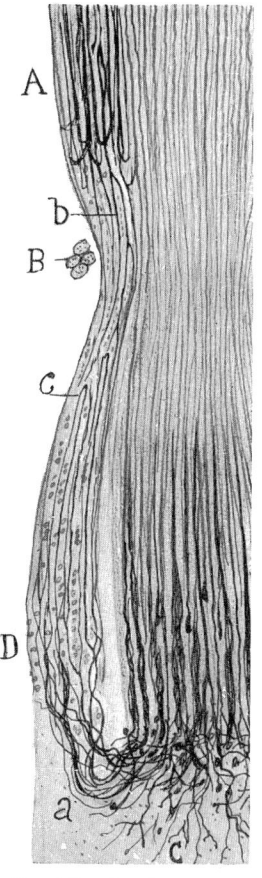

FIG. 122.—Cat fifteen days old killed six days after ligature of its sciatic nerve. Section of the peripheral stump. The degenerated cortical region is innervated by the sprouts of the central region originating not far from the wound. A, central stump; B, ligature; D, bundle innervated by retrograde fibres; C, scar; b, exploratory fibres which pass over the compressed region and mix with the fibres coming from the wound. Semi-schematic figure.

that these facts of *sudden inveiglement of a current of sprouts by a neighbouring nerve, and the penetration of the former along a retrograde path within the sheaths of Schwann* involve three necessary conditions, one of which is positive, the other two negative : (1) The degenerated nerves of the peripheral stump give out into the scar some substance—an enzyme, nutritive substance, or

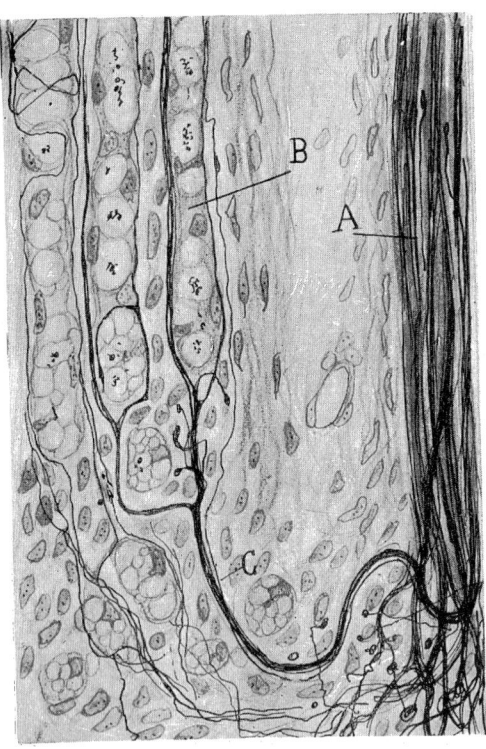

FIG. 123.—Details of the retrograde nervous reunion shown in Fig. 122. *A*, central stump, stimulated near the section; *C*, migrating sprouts; *B*, ramification of the migrating sprouts within a large degenerated nerve tube.

other material—which stimulates the assimilation and growth of the sprouts in an opposite direction from the diffused current. (2) The nerve sprouts innervate indifferently any cortical or axial region of the nerve or any fascicle of the peripheral stump. There is thus a *topographic indifference*. (3) As opposed to the views of Bethe and other authors, the degenerated nerves lack a neurotropic polarization, that is, the sprouts that they attract are indifferently influenced by the proximal or distal side of the peripheral stump.

We shall cite below further examples of this polar indifference, already imperfectly observed by Forssman and other authors, though up to now it has been insufficiently studied.

Effects of ligature of the peripheral stump.—We have already spoken of this when we discussed the significance of the large arrested balls. In Fig. 125 we show schematically the growth of the sprouts across the scar and ligated peripheral stump, in a rabbit two months

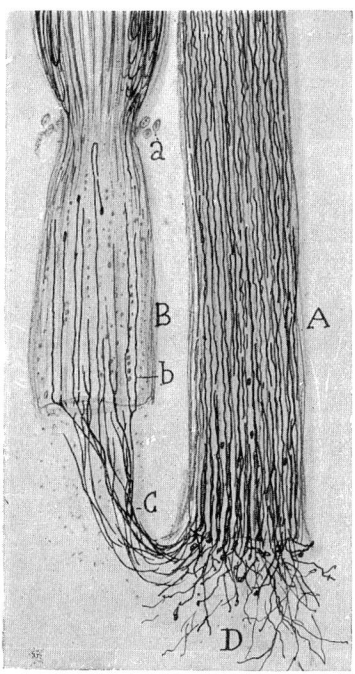

FIG. 124.—Very tight semiligature with complete section at different points for each nerve bundle. Young rabbit, killed eight days after the operation. *A*, central stump of the non-ligated fascicle; *B*, degenerated stump of the ligated bundle; *D*, fibres dispersed in the scar; *c*, migrating fascicles which grow out to the degenerated and ligated fascicle. Semi-schematic figure.

old, killed eight days after the operation. One can see how the fibres produce large balls (*c*) on being arrested near the ligature, and how the more or less elliptical buds are preceded by a flexuose pedicle which reveals the vacillations of growth. One can also see that the very few exploratory fibres (*b*), which arise from the clubs and cross the obstacle assume extreme thinness in order to accommodate themselves to the exceptional narrowness of the interstices. Lastly, one may observe how a few clubs have moved back, only to be arrested afresh at various distances from the ligated region (*a*).

Thus this experiment, which we have repeated in various ways, shows once more that the formation of large balls as well as the retrograde courses depend exclusively on the presence of obstacles.

Effects of the ligature of the branches of a nerve after they are converted into a peripheral stump by a previous section of the trunk.—This experiment, which we show in Fig. 126, once more

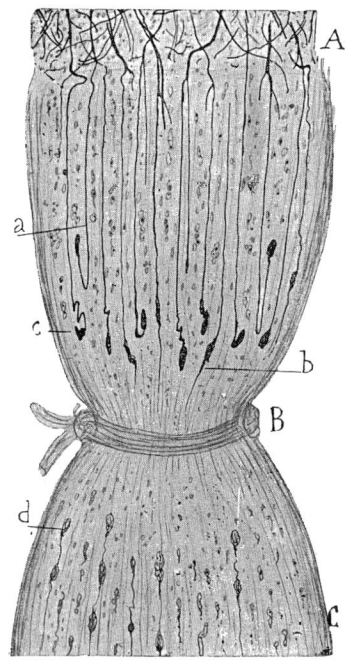

FIG. 125.—Schematic representation of the mechanism of formation of the large clubs and arches of retrogression within a peripheral stump where a grave mechanical obstacle to the growth of the newly-formed axons had been set up. The peripheral stump of the sciatic nerve was ligated below the section. Two months old rabbit, killed eight days after the operation. A, scar of the wound; B, thread of the ligature; C, peripheral stump situated below the ligature, where one can see a few degenerated axons ending in balls; a, c, fibres arrested above the ligature; b, arrested fibre which sends a tenuous fibril towards the compressed region.

corroborates the doctrine of the topographic indifference of the nerve sprouts. It also distinctly shows that the sprouts arising from a cut nerve trunk can innervate indifferently any of the latter's branches. In this actual case—a rabbit killed fourteen days after the lesion—the fibres originating from the cut in the tibial nerve innervate the peripheral stumps of both branches, the tibial and the peroneal. Owing to the ligature which was put there in order to keep the two nerves together, and to the fact that the neurilemma was not cut on one side, the respective distances between the two central stumps and the common peripheral stump have become unequal, and the central segment which is nearer to the peripheral portion has prevailed over the other in the process of reunion.

Thus, when there is no intromission of adipose tissue or of foreign tissues such as hairs, cotton threads, etc., the peripheral stump which is nearest to the scar is always innervated, whatever may be the origin and physiological category of its fibres. A grave cause of

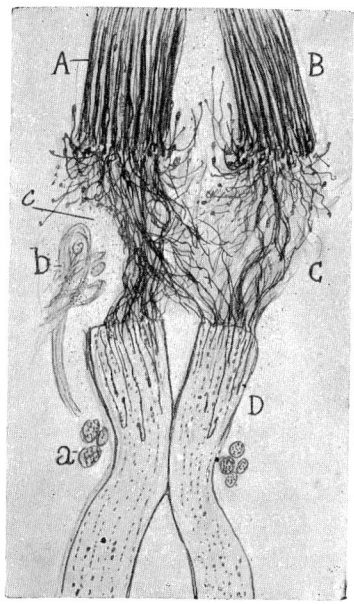

FIG. 126.—Section of the peroneal and tibial branches of the sciatic nerve; they are ligated below the lesion. Young rabbit, killed fourteen days after the operation. *A, B,* central stumps; *C,* scar; *D,* peripheral stumps; *a,* ligature; *b.* threads of the ligature, surrounded by connective tissue which the nerve sprouts avoid.

retardation and perturbation in the growth of the sprouts is the fortuitous presence in the scar of adipose lobules or of blood clots that have not been resorbed, as we have noted above. But the greatest obstacle is the accidental presence in the scar of foreign bodies. Hairs, filaments of silk, wool, or cotton, threads of the ligature, etc., bring about the formation of a close connective tissue wall whose cells only rarely let the sprouts through (Fig. 126). We shall speak below at greater length of this peculiar disturbing influence of the phagocytes that encyst foreign bodies, and of the repulsive action of pus.

Experiments of multiple sections, with or without ligature of the central stump.—This operation is especially useful for determining the conditions that bring about bifurcation of the nerves.

We have already stated that divisions of the sprouts are often caused by striking against obstacles of the cicatricial tissue that are difficult to surmount.

In Fig. 127 we show schematically a new proof of this assertion. The peripheral stump of a nerve was completely cut in three successive regions, so that the nerve sprouts arriving from the main scar and insinuated in the old sheaths of Schwann had to cross on their way various interruptions of these sheaths, in other words, three small scars. One can see that while the axons are growing within the sheaths of Schwann or along the interstices, that is, across a region that is evenly saturated with trophic substances, their path is rectilinear and without bifurcations. When they reach the small scars, however, the axons lose their orientation (Fig. 127, b), they describe loops and form branches, some of which are insinuated in the immediate peripheral stump, others of which go back towards that portion which acts as an immediate central stump.

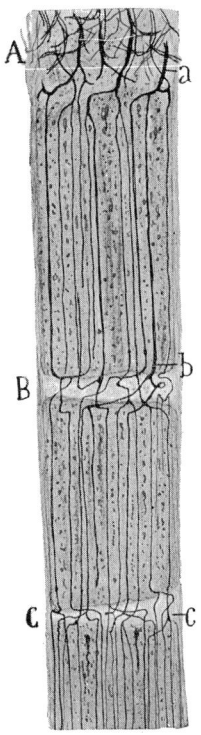

FIG. 127.—Sciatic nerve of a cat one month old, killed nine days after the section. Schematic representation of the aspect presented by a peripheral stump which is cut into three portions and invaded by nerve sprouts. A, principal scar through which grow the axons that have come from the central stump; B and C, small scars corresponding to incomplete sections of the peripheral stump; b, fibres that have lost their orientation and have ramified in the first scar; c, fibres that have ramified in the second scar; a, large ramified fibre that has come from the central stump.

There is no doubt, as Dustin observes, that the obstacles present in the intercalary scars contribute to the disorientation of the fibres, and cause turns, retrogressions, and bifurcations. Is it not possible, however, that in the production of these multiple divisions, which are never so abundant in ordinary scars, the multiple neighbouring neurotropic sources also exert an influence ? The presence in the scar of inert cells, of capillaries, etc., perhaps multiplies and breaks up, through the creation of irregular interstices, the current of neurotropic substances liberated by the immediate peripheral stump.

There is also great significance, from the point of view of the attractive action of the sheaths of Schwann, in the force of growth and neurocladism of the sprouts, and especially in the fact that the latter never lose themselves beneath the neurilemma, nor come to a stop among the embryonic connective tissue cells, even though they form complicated turns and ramify abundantly on crossing the intercalary scars. The retrogression of newly-formed fibres, which is frequent in such preparations, is easily explained by the simultaneous, equal, and opposite action of two neighbouring chemotactic sources.

XIV

CONTINUATION OF THE STUDY OF REGENERATION UNDER SPECIAL CONDITIONS

Observations showing the indifference, both topical and polar, of nerve sprouts.—Inversion of sequestered nerves.—Union of two central stumps.—Effects of multiple hemisection.—Retrograde penetration of wandering sensory fibres into the posterior roots.—Penetration of sensory fibres into cut anterior roots.—Experiments dealing with the extirpation of nerves.—Experiments designed to place difficulties in the way of nervous reunion of the peripheral stump and of the progress of the fibres in their initial direction.

Observations demonstrating the polar indifference of the nerve sprouts.—In the preceding chapter we set forth certain facts that prove the capacity possessed by the axons of innervating in a retrograde direction, along any plane, a degenerated nerve segment.

The following experiments once more corroborate the theory of the topical and directive indifference of the sprouts that have penetrated into the nerve. They show besides the trophic influence of the border of any nerve or nerve fascicle that is undergoing degeneration. Before describing them, however, let us glance at the concept of polarization, as it was understood by Bethe and accepted by Lugaro.

Bethe [1] states, as a result of his numerous experiments of union between nerves belonging to different physiological categories, that all the nerve fibres possess a certain polarity, which does not depend on the direction of the nerve impulse, but on its orientation in relation to the ganglion cell with which they are connected. It is well known that in a mixed nerve the motor and sensory fibres carry impulses in opposite directions. But their polarity is the same, because their position in relation to the soma—the sensory and motor cells—is the same. One thus understands how a central motor stump can innervate a sensory peripheral stump, or again a peripheral stump belonging to another motor nerve. On the con-

---

[1] A. Bethe: " Ueber Nervenheilung und polare Wachstumserscheinungen aus Nerven," *Münchener med. Wochensch.*, No. 25, 1905.
See also: *Allgemeine Anatomie und Physiologie des Nervensystems*, 1903.

trary, this union or nervous reunion becomes impossible when one places the cells of origin in the artificially united fibres in opposite positions. Thus, Bethe joined the stump of the superior maxillary nerve with the cut optic nerve (the portion connected with the retina) and observed that there was no fusion of the fibres, because the cells of origin of the visual fibres reside in the periphery—the retina —while those of the sensory fibres reside in a centre, the Gasserian ganglion. For the same reason one cannot bring about the penetration of sensory fibres into the central stump of a motor nerve, nor, reciprocally, that of motor fibres into the central stump of a sensory nerve. The union of two central stumps, whether they be sensory or motor, remains sterile, as was shown some time ago by Stefani, and as Bethe [1] recognized. Finally, Bethe affirms that when one cuts a nerve in two places and the intermediate piece is inverted, its auto-regenerated fibres are unable to join with those either of the central or of the peripheral stumps. This experiment, interpreted in the light of the monogenist doctrine, implies the impossibility of a sequestered piece of nerve being innervated in a retrograde direction.

Lugaro,[2] in his interesting experiments on ablation of the ganglia and regeneration of the nerve roots has often seen fibres originating from the anterior or motor root which, after crossing the scar, penetrate into the sensory root, in that portion situated between the ganglion and the spinal cord, and grow in it up to near the posterior cordon. Once they have reached that point they stop suddenly and they disperse themselves under the *pia mater* without reaching the spinal cord, perhaps in consequence of a negative chemotropic action exercised by the latter centre on afferent nervous sprouts. In this interesting experiment it is shown that the law of polarization remains the rule whenever the axons that come from the anterior root retain the same position in relation to the cell of origin (posterior root united with the medulla) as the normal axons arising from the corresponding sensory ganglion.

[1] We show the doctrine of Bethe on polarization according to the interpretation that Lugaro gave to it, that is, from the point of view of the doctrine of the neurone. But we must not forget that when Bethe speaks of impossibility of union of two peripheral or two central stumps he alludes especially to the problem of the union of auto-regenerated fibres, either among themselves or else with the normal fibres of the central stump.

[2] Lugaro: " Sui neurotropismo e sui trapianti dei nervi," *Riv. di patol. ner. e mentale*, vol. 11, 1906.

The principle of polarity can be applied with certainty only to the distant consequences of the incongruent unions above quoted. But it is then involved in a more general law—that of the atrophy and resorption through disuse, so often mentioned. All deviated fibres disappear through resorption—that is, all the axons that travel along foreign paths and are unable to fulfil their function, in other words, to invade the terminal region, in view of which the connections of the neurone of origin were co-ordinated. But if one applies the above quoted principle of polarity to precocious unions, it is radically false. No matter what is the position of the trophic centre of the recently arrived sprout, every nerve receives the latter in its sheaths, even though it should later become insensitive and degenerate through physiological uselessness. Besides the case, so often referred to, of retrograde fibres within the central stump, we shall now give a few observations that are contrary to the hypothesis of polarization of Bethe.

Inversion of a sequestered piece of nerve.—In our experiments in nerve transplantation on the resected sciatic nerve, we have often inverted the portion between the two stumps, It was always innervated. We shall give details of these experiments below.

Union of two central stumps.—This experiment, verified some time ago by Schiff (1858) and repeated by Stefani and Bethe, was effected by ourselves on the two branches of the sciatic nerve. After thirteen days the two stumps have exchanged fibres. These grow in a retrograde direction, both in the interstices of the endoneurium and in the degenerated sheaths of Schwann. Each nerve stump receives a number of sprouts which is greater in proportion as its own necrosed and degenerated region is more extensive. Nevertheless the majority of the sprouts become dispersed through the intermediate scar, the surface of the neurilemma and the neighbouring tissues. One must suppose that after a time all the fibres that penetrate into the central stumps become atrophied.

This experiment only reproduces on a larger scale the well-known phenomenon of retrograde nervous reunion occurring in all central stumps, especially those of adult animals.

Effects of multiple hemisection.—This experiment is rich in theoretical value. We show it in Fig. 128, where we reproduce schematically the regenerative phenomena following a single section of one half of the sciatic nerve, associated with the multiple interruption of the other half. The animal was a cat fifteen days old, killed six days after the operation. As occurs in this species, the regenerative phenomena took place with great speed. Apart from less important details, the most instructive thing in this case is that, within the peripheral stump, represented by the half of the nerve

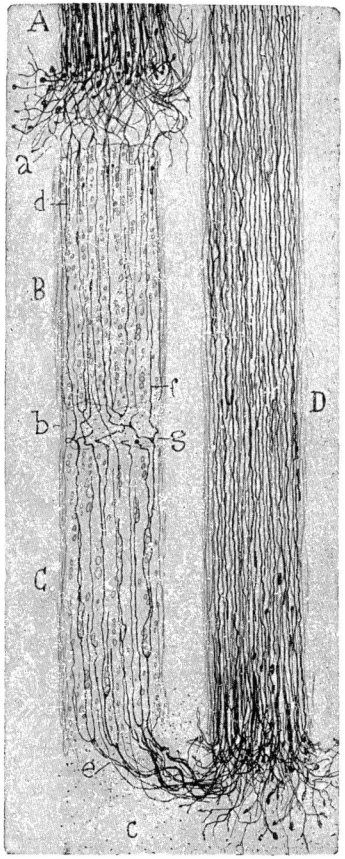

FIG. 128.—Experiment of multiple hemisection. Young cat, killed six days after the operation. *A*, central stump of the half which was multisected; *B*, first peripheral stump; *C*, second peripheral stump; *D*, half of the cordon that was cut only once; *a*, first scar; *b*, second scar; *c*, third scar; *d, f*, sprouts that have penetrated into the first peripheral stump; *g*, bifurcations in the second scar.

that was cut into three portions, two currents of sprouts join, a *direct* and a *retrograde* current. The *direct* fibres arise from the corresponding central stump (Fig. 128, *d*), and, after crossing two scars, where they bifurcate abundantly, they debouch in part in the general or comprehensive scar of both nerve halves. The retrograde current, which is very powerful, arises from the central stump of the other half of the nerve (*e*), and, tracing arcs, it eagerly invades the last portion of the contiguous peripheral stump. *One thus finds within the latter, and often within the same sheaths, both ascending and descending conductors*, which show no bad results from being present together, and which manifest exactly the same energy of growth and neurocladic capacity. We may add that in this actual case the impulse of growth of the retrograde sprouts within the peripheral stump of the contiguous degenerated half was as powerful as in the general scar (simultaneous section of both halves). The turn taken across the scar by such recurrent fibres seems so determined and along such a distinct path that one is led to think that the degenerated stump not only elaborates trophic substances but diffuses them in a relatively extensive region, which in certain cases may reach about a millimetre in radius. It is clear that such an influence is especially felt by the sprouts which are closest to the central stump. One might designate these areas of the scar which are full of the emanations of the peripheral stump *regions of influence*. It is also significant, from the neurotropic point of view, that there is an absence of such currents in very long fibres, and in those which are bent back in a bow on the opposite side from the central stump.

Retrograde nervous reunion of a posterior root.—In Fig. 129, *C*, we show a typical case of these retrograde neurotisations, frequently observed by us in experiments of section and especially of inflammation of extirpated spinal roots. We are here dealing with a ten-day old cat whose lumbar spinal cord was almost completely sectioned at the level of the *cauda equina*. The animal was killed five days later, and one recognized the fact that several posterior roots near the wound in the spinal cord had also been cut. One single bundle, coming from a long distance, reached the central stump of one of these posterior roots (Fig. 129, *C*). This bundle was formed of sprouts arising in another central stump—the portion of the root united to the ganglion ; these sprouts, when they approached the degenerated posterior root, that portion which was united to the cord, suddenly broke up into an elegant tuft of branches destined for various bands of Büngner.

This observation is an additional proof of the doctrine of neurotropism. The fact that the bundle is single, that it travels a long way before reaching the degenerated radicular bundles, the orientation of the terminal branches, the absence of perinervous or deviated appendices, and especially the formative excitation of the branches on their arrival at the root, as though they received some stimulus to their divisory capacity, all lead one to believe in a neurotropic

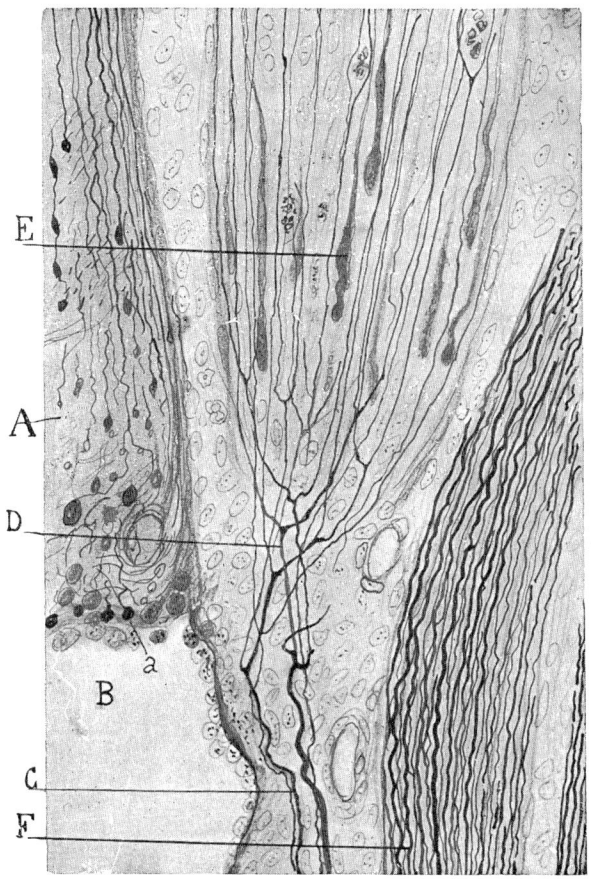

FIG. 129.—Synchronous section of the spinal cord and of a posterior root in a young cat which was killed five days after the operation. *A*, posterior cordon of the spinal cord; *B*, cyst formed in the wound; *C*, nerve fibres of the scar which have penetrated into the central stump of a sectioned posterior root; *E*, old axons of the posterior root; *D*, branches produced at the border of the root; *F*, undamaged sensory root.
The posterior root was cut between the spinal cord and the ganglion.

and even neurocladic action exercised by the stump of the root on the young wandering fibres.

Penetration of sensory fibres into degenerated anterior or motor roots.—Another instructive case of neurotropism and heteromorphic nervous reunion is shown in Fig. 130. It was a wound of the spinal cord involving also the destruction of the base of an anterior or motor root. The fibres that wandered in the scar, probably sensory in origin, precipitated themselves resolutely into the degenerated anterior root, as though they were attracted by something given out through the opening of the degenerated anterior root. They ramified luxuriantly within the bands of Büngner and in the interstices between the latter, always travelling in a centrifugal direction, as though they were true motor fibres.

In this example the law of polarization is not infringed, since the sprouts follow in the anterior root the same direction as the normal fibres. It is transgressed, however, in other cases of section of the anterior roots, in which we have seen numerous sensory or motor sprouts that were wandering across the scar penetrate through the edge of the central stump. We shall give other examples of retrograde motor nervous reunion when we discuss traumatic regeneration in the spinal cord. The cases of extirpation of nerves, of which we shall now speak briefly, also give new arguments against the conception of polarity.

Experiments in extirpation of nerves.—It is generally admitted that when nerves are extirpated near their origin, such as the hypoglossus near its emergence from the foramen, or the motor nerve roots near their cells of origin, they atrophy, and since the trophic centre is thus abolished, the regeneration of the peripheral stump is impeded. When this extirpation is done in recently-born or very young animals, the atrophy of the corresponding motor focus is sufficiently marked, months later, to serve as the basis of an excellent method of investigation of the origin of motor nerves. This is the *method of atrophy*, named also the method of Gudden and Forel.

Several authors, among them Bethe, Marinesco, and Sala and Cortese,[1] have carried out experiments of extirpation. Bethe and Marinesco had in view the investigation of nervous reunion of the peripheral stump. Sala and Cortese wished to investigate the regenerative phenomena of the central stump. Marinesco, in opposition to current theories, deduced from his studies that not all the cells of the corresponding trophic centre succumb. According to him, a few persistent axons of the central stump are able to innervate the scar and even to reach the peripheral stump. Sala and Cortese have seen indisputable phenomena of sprouting and even real bundles

[1] G. Sala e Cortese : *Sui fatti che si svolgono nel midollo spinale in seguito allo strappo delle radici*, Pavia, 1909.

and spools of newly-formed fibres, even in those motor roots which were extirpated from the white matter.

Our experiments on extirpation of the hypoglossus and of the roots of origin of the sciatic nerve of cats a few days old confirm the observations of Sala and Cortese that the trauma acts very differently on different axons. Ordinarily, even if the nerves are torn out near the *dura mater*, the sensory roots persist, often showing a

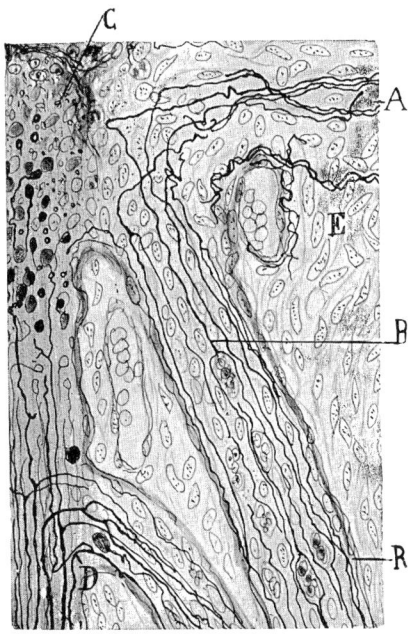

FIG. 130.—Longitudinal section of the anterior roots of a cat which had been cut in the spinal cord. *A*, sensory fibres of scar invading a degenerated anterior root; *B*, invading fibres ramifying at a fatty agglomeration; *C*, necrosed portion of the anterior cordon near the wound; *D*, *E*, cordonal fibres penetrating into a motor radicular bundle.

central stump in the segment which is external to the ganglion; this is seen in full sprouting, and from it issue branches that travel to the scar, as well as retrograde sprouts dispersed about in the ganglion itself.

The mechanical violence involves a much greater area of the motor roots. One often sees in the anterior roots of the extirpated sciatic nerve tubes in which, six days after the operation, the axon has disappeared up to the cell of origin. In other tubes appear granular remnants of the axons, which take the colloidal silver stain.

A few end in balls in the intraspinal portion of the root, or give rise to bundles and spirals which are strewn with clubs, such as were described by Sala and Cortese. Nevertheless, the majority of the radicular motor fibres persist, and one can follow them across the anterior spinal bundle, up to near the grey matter. Many of them appear absolutely normal, that is, they are free from growths and excrescences.[1]

If one follows these axons, which are more or less entire, along the subdural space and outside of the spinal membranes, one always, at a point different for each conductor, comes upon the segment that is stimulated or in the phase of formative turgidity. This examination allows one to see (besides the sprouts that emerge in the scar, arranged in bundles which wander through the contiguous extra and subdural spaces and give rise to plexuses of great complexity) a great number of nerve collaterals, originating within the tubes and fibres, which, ravelling and becoming retrograde, invade the subdural portion of the root and, without stopping at the borders of the cord, assault the anterior spinal bundle. These retrograde fibres behave like those which arise along the course of degenerated anterior roots owing to grave traumatic inflammations, or as a consequence of being crushed and lacerated, as described above.

We reproduce in Fig. 131 the appearance of some motor roots which were pulled out in a cat killed ten days after the operation. The neoformation of sprouts was enormous, as can be seen by the internal plexus of the roots (Fig. 131, C, D). One should note the retrograde fibres, which form a crown around the normal axon. There are tubes under whose membrane one sees sixteen or more fibres. Apart from the intratubal, one sees also interstitial sprouts, although they are not so numerous (Fig. 131, G). Finally, a fact which is of particular interest is the penetration of these newly-formed and retrograde fibres into the intraspinal portion of the roots, with which they grow, constituting complicated plexuses even up to the grey matter (a). It would be interesting to investigate the mode of termination and the ultimate fate of these curious retrograde conductors, lost in the intramedullar plexuses. Unfortunately, the abundance of fibrils in the grey substance does not allow one to follow such deviated sprouts to their termination. There are, moreover, retrograde conductors which, deviating from the plane of the

[1] We shall describe in detail below the alterations in the spinal cells and roots, as well as those occurring in the ganglia, in extirpation experiments.

radicular sprouts, take oblique or more or less longitudinal directions, reaching the interior of the antero-lateral bundle (Fig. 131, b). Others, deviating in a lateral direction, beneath the basal bundle, give rise to a complicated perispinal plexus (Fig. 131, c).

These facts show, not only the polar indifference of the sprouts, but also the absence of a negative chemotaxis in the tissues of the

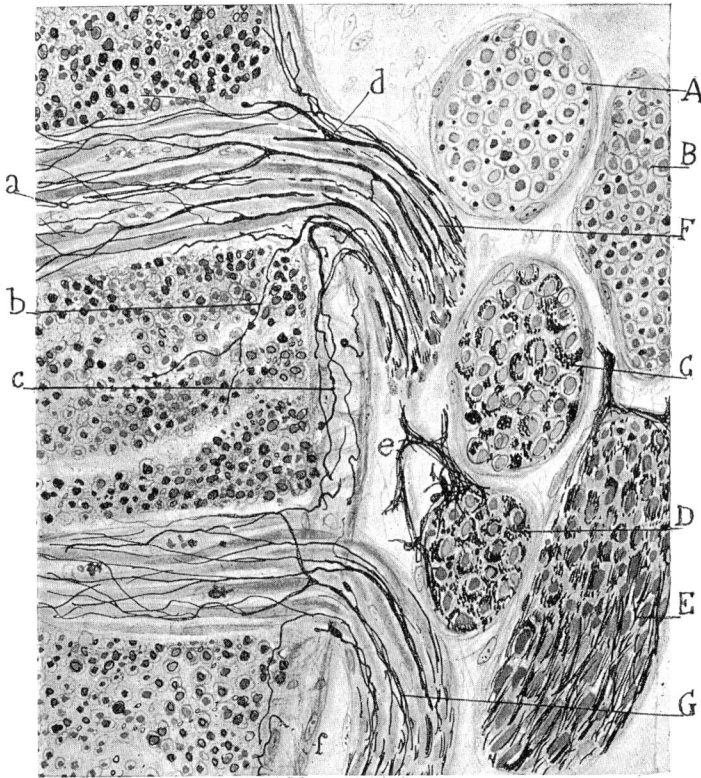

FIG. 131.—Transversal section of the antero-lateral bundle and anterior roots. Young cat, killed ten days after the extirpation of the sciatic nerve. A, B, undamaged radicular fascicles; C, D, E, roots that include retrograde sprouts; F, G, anterior roots invaded by newly-formed fibres; a, sprouts that penetrate into the root; c, perispinal plexus.

spinal cord. They also show that when the impulse to growth is great the sprouts are able, with the aid of suitable guides and taking the path of least resistance, to penetrate into dense tissues and regions that are full of obstacles.

Operations designed to place difficulties in the way of nervous reunion of the peripheral stump and of the progress of fibres along their

initial direction.—Many authors have carried out experiments with a view to impeding or preventing nervous reunion of the peripheral stump by the sprouts originating in the central stump. Among them we may cite Phylippeaux and Vulpian, Ranvier, Vanlair, Forssman, Bethe, ourselves, Lugaro, Marinesco, Münzer, Perroncito, Langley, Mott and Halliburton, etc. These experiments were especially abundant during the memorable controversy between auto-regenerationists and monogenists. We have referred to some of these experiments in the *Introduction* to this book. Now that the polygenist error is definitely refuted, these experiments, apart from their critical value, have lost much of their interest. To-day no one can doubt that the newly-formed axons in a peripheral stump that has been violently separated from the central stump, cut out over great distances, hidden in collodion tubes, or folded back between muscles, really proceed from the central stump, although the difficulties put in their way retard for a few months the arrival of the fibres. It is not doubtful either, that if, following the example of Lugaro, one cuts out pieces of the spinal cord with its sensory ganglia, the corresponding nerves are never regenerated. When in such cases, one exceptionally sees in the peripheral stump a few living nerve fibres, these originate, either from a sympathetic nerve, or from small muscular nerves that were accidentally cut during the operation.

Experiments of this type are also instructive from other points of view. When one hides both stumps under the skin or the muscles, one elongates the scar, the sprouts have to grow along a very extended path, and there are created nutritive modifications in the nerves. These, far from their normal vascular channels, have to establish new ones, and they remain, in the interim, as 'auto-inserts.' In order to gain some light concerning the changes that such nervous displacements induce in the mode of origination of the sprouts of the central stump and in the velocity of such tardy growth, we have repeated some experiments of this type. We had made many such during the great controversy of 1905-1906. Here is a typical case.

The sciatic nerve of a cat one month old was cut, and a piece 1 cm. long was removed. The central stump, thus shortened, was folded back and sewn to the skin of the gluteal region. The inferior stump was pushed out of its normal position and inserted between the muscles of the thigh. The animal was killed after forty-eight days.

The peripheral stump had gone back almost to its normal position ; but the central stump was under the skin, ending in a voluminous neuroma ; at first sight the distal stump appeared grey and somewhat atrophied. A long scar or connective interstice, apparently free of medullated bundles, joined the two nerve segments.

Nevertheless, a careful examination under a lens showed that fine and pale small bundles arose, not from the neuroma of the central stump, but from the course of the latter before it was folded back. These bundles grew between the muscles and connective tissue tracts of the scar, and then precipitated themselves into the distal stump. A microscopical examination after staining with reduced silver nitrate revealed the fact that some of these bundles had really reached the peripheral stump and penetrated some distance within it. A certain portion of the sprouts, however, had not yet reached their destination, and had deviated into muscular bundles and had even wandered some distance in an oblique and transverse direction. It was interesting to note that the bundles in the scar, along the axis of the segment that had disappeared, took an almost straight direction, that is, the meshes of the plexus formed by them tended

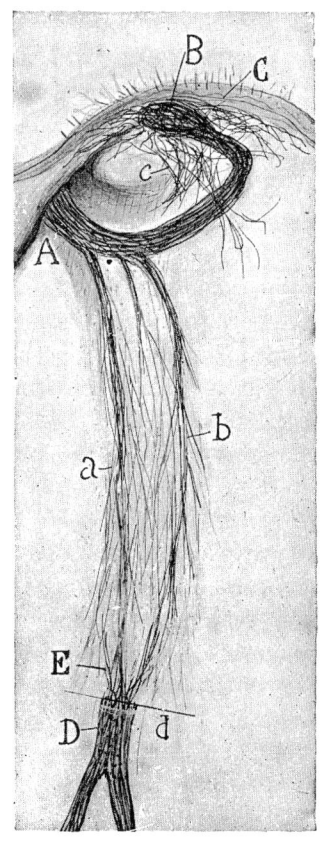

FIG. 132.—Section of the sciatic nerve of the cat, with resection of a large piece of nerve, and folding back of the central stump beneath the skin of the gluteal region. *A*, trunk of the central stump ; *B*, subcutaneous neuroma; *C*, skin ; *D* peripheral stump ; *a, b, tractus* of fibres that broke away along the central stump and entered into the peripheral stump.

more and more to become parallel interstices. Another notable feature was the fineness of the fibres next to the border of the peripheral stump, in comparison with those next to the central stump.

As was to be expected, a good many of the tubes of the central stump that were folded back had degenerated before the bend.

Other conductors, ordinarily deeper than in this case, were undamaged, but in a phase of divisory excitation. As a consequence of this numerous sprouts had been produced in many axons, before the nerve flexion; these, having first broken into the sheaths and then into the neurilemma, were attacking the scar. The two fibrillar *tractus*, which can be seen in the scheme of Fig. 132, *a*, *b*, were principally constituted of such migrating fibres. The tubes of the neuroma of the central stump lost themselves under the skin and between the muscles of the thigh without a definite orientation (*c*). None of them were incorporated in the nervous currents referred to above, and nearly all the sprouts of the central stump lost themselves in the creation of sterile helicoidal structures and retrograde and deviated conductors. Finally, in the region situated between the bend and the cutaneous neuroma, along a path several millimetres long, were found tubes that were degenerated and had been invaded by terminal and collateral branches originating at a great distance in a proximal direction. This circumstance shows that the flexion and separation of the nerve, with the consequent nutritive perturbations, bring about an intense retrograde degeneration.

We were unable to determine with certainty the velocity of tardy growth. It would be necessary to carry out many experiments of this type, killing animals at various stages, in order to get fairly certain results. We need only note that in this case the scar between the point where the innervating sprouts originated and the peripheral stump was about three centimetres long, and that the average velocity per day, deducting the first three days for the creation of the state of divisory turgidity and penetration of the sprouts into the scar, was 0·60 mm., much higher than that obtained for early sprouts growing across short scars.

All these experiments of difficult nervous reunion show that:
(1) The nerve sprouts, in order to avoid circuits, are able to leave the neurilemma and travel by shorter paths to the peripheral stump.
(2) The principle of *initial direction*, considered by Vanlair, Held, Harrison, Heidenhain, Dustin, etc., as an important factor in the orientation and ulterior position of young axons, does not play the principal role in nervous regeneration, since the tubes from which the sprouts issue may, without grave consequences, take a retrograde direction. (3) The arrival of the sprouts within the peripheral stump from long distances and across many obstacles indicates, as we have

said many times, the nutritive or orienting collaboration of something arising from that segment. Without this we cannot explain the arrival of the fibres at their destination.

Regeneration in the nerves of amputated members.—Dr. Cardenal, under our direction, performed several experiments of amputation of the posterior extremities. This operation is difficult in small laboratory animals. It was only dogs that were able to survive the operation for several months. Homen [1] also used dogs for his investigations of the changes in the central stump in the nerves of amputated limbs.

In one case where the dog was killed two months after the operation the scar showed, at its union with the central stump, a typical neuroma, whose nerve bundles, dispersed in all directions, folded back and lost themselves under the skin of the stump of the amputated limb, ending in balls of various sizes.

In the central stump, what was especially noticeable was the presence of enormous helicoidal structures, much more voluminous and complicated than those produced after a simple nerve section. In certain spools the spiral fibres, instead of constituting a single file, formed three, four, and even more strata of revolutions. In such structures there are numerous colossal internal clubs which are often wrinkled and degenerating. In the centre of the structures one often finds thick bundles of robust axial sprouts, partly folded back upon themselves, partly free, that is, having emerged from the bottom of the sac formed by the helicoidal structure. Nearly all the axial or spiroidal conductors appear surrounded by cells of Schwann, and in the most robust among them one sees a vaginal space, an index to the presence of a myelin sheath. Finally, the capsular membrane has undergone, without breaking, a notable dilatation, and it appears to be formed by a fine fibrillar mantle and internal nuclei.

Besides the large spiroidal structures, one finds some that are medium-sized and small, and, especially, a large number of gigantic clubs belonging to deviated and retrograde fibres. Not a few voluminous balls are contracted and provided with a thick capsule which is rich in fusiform elements.

Dogs killed eight and twelve days after the section showed no

[1] Homen : *Zieglers Beiträge*, Bd. 8, 1894.
See also : *Atlas der pathologischen Histologie des Nervensystems*, H. II., Liefer. *Regeneration der Nerven*, etc., Berlin, 1894.

points of special interest. In the central stump and scar one saw the well-known regenerative and degenerative dispositions. Concerning the changes in the myelin and nuclei, the investigations of Cardenal are in accord with those of Homen.

It can be deduced from these observations that the absence of the peripheral stump, and therefore of the trophic influence of the cells of Schwann, does not stop the process of neoformation and growth of the central axons. On the other hand, the lack of space for the lengthening of the sprouts and the total absence of orienting substances cause an enormous multiplication in the number of retrograde fibres and gigantic arrested balls, and bring about in the central stump and beginning of the scar the production of helicoidal structures of unusual dimensions and complexity.

XV

EXPERIMENTS DEALING WITH THE TRANSPLANTATION OF NERVES OR THEIR PRODUCTS, DESIGNED TO PROVE ESPECIALLY AN ATTRACTIVE OR NEUROTROPIC ACTION ON NERVE SPROUTS

Experiments of Forssman, Lugaro, Marinesco, Mott and Halliburton, Dustin, O. Rossi, etc.—Indifference of undamaged fibres to grafts.—Effect of live and dead grafts.—Reimplantations of nerves.—Homoiotransplants and heterotransplants.—Subcutaneous and intermuscular grafts.—Conclusions.—Are there negative neurotropic actions?—Action of pus, blood, and mechanical obstacles. —Paralyzing action of the aniline dyes.—Attractive influence of the scar.— Degeneration and regeneration in the lower vertebrates.

Since we [1] formulated in 1892 the hypothesis of chemotactism, that is, of the amoeboidism of young axons brought about by an orienting stimulus from attracting or neurotropic substances, in connection with our studies of neurogenesis, many experiments have been undertaken with a view to supplying an objective basis for this conception. As is natural, these experiments have dealt with nervous regeneration; in young or adult animals artificial intervention by means of chemical or traumatic agents, during embryonic neurogenesis, is too difficult and delicate for experimental proof of the type wanted.

The first author who tested this hypothesis was Forssman,[2] who described in two interesting memoranda the results that he obtained in a long series of experiments on cut nerves.

Forssman carried out varied experiments. In some cases he rendered nervous reunion difficult by enclosing in tubes the central as well as the peripheral stumps. In others he tested the attractive actions of various organic substances which he placed near the

[1] Cajal: "La rétine des vertébrés," *La Cellule*, 1892.

[2] Forssman: "Ueber die Ursachen welche die Wachsthumsrichtung der peripheren Nervenfasern bei der Regeneration bestimmen." *Zieglers Beiträge*, Bd. 24, 1898.

See also: "Zur Kenntniss des Neurotropismus," *Beiträge zur pathol. Anat., etc., von Ziegler*, Bd. 27, 1900.

central stump. In other cases, again, he used grafts of nerves of the same or other mammals—homoiotransplants and heterotransplants. He killed the animal several months later, and used the method of Pal-Weigert and osmic acid to observe the newly-formed fibres. Let us set out briefly some of these experiments.

(a) Section in a rabbit of the tibial and peroneal nerves, into which the sciatic nerve breaks up. To separate them from the central stump he put the peripheral segment of each of these nerves in a tube of collodion. Months later he observed that, notwithstanding the obstacle which appeared insurmountable, the axons of the central stump had reached both the peripheral segments and had innervated them indifferently. The sprouts, therefore, did not follow the path of least resistance, as Ranvier and Vanlair believed, but, after surmounting a great obstacle and describing very complicated turns, they threw themselves on the degenerated sheaths of the peripheral stump.

(b) Which are the substances of the distal segment that attract the sprouts ? Forssman answered this by devising various experiments. In one of them he left near the central stump two tubes, one of them full of pieces of liver, the other of brain substance. He showed that the newly-formed fibres avoid the glandular remnants while they precipitate themselves into the tube containing the grey substance. Instead of brain matter he also used pieces of the spinal cord, likewise with a positive result. On the other hand, the spleen and other parenchymas exercise no influence whatever.

(c) Repeating experiments of nervous transplantations done by Gluck, Johnson, Nothafft, Stroebe, Assaky, etc., Forssman cut the sciatic nerve of rabbits and guinea-pigs. He then cut out a piece of the nerve and in its place he placed a piece of nerve taken sometimes from an animal of the same species (homoiotransplantation) or from another species (heterotransplantation). The central stump, graft, and peripheral stump were joined and protected by a tube of collodion. When the graft was from another species, such as dogs and chickens, no new fibres penetrated into it. It constitutes in such cases a foreign body which is finally resorbed. It does not become vascularised, and only a few leucocytes are present on its surface. When the living nerve was taken from an animal of the same species, however, the graft was conserved, and at the end of a certain time one saw in it newly-formed fibres. Moreover, the peripheral stump situated distally to the graft was also innervated.

From his various experiments Forssman concluded, in opposition to Ranvier and Vanlair, that the mechanical action is a secondary factor in the growth of the sprouts and their arrival at the terminal structures. The principal factor in the nervous reunion of the peripheral stump is to be attributed to some soluble substance which has a neurotropic action, and which is produced by the disintegration of the myelin sheath. This substance is contained as well in the nerve grafts as in the remnants of the white substance of the brain and spinal cord.

The experiments of Merzbacher [1] concerning nerve grafts, should be mentioned, even though they are foreign to the problem of neurotropism. In accordance with the conclusions of Forssman, he states that when the nerve graft comes from an animal of the same species, it undergoes a typical Wallerian degeneration ; when it comes from an animal of a different species, however, the graft undergoes a necrobiosis without degenerating, retaining its histological character for a shorter or a longer time. Merzbacher used mostly methods that stain the myelin.

In principle, the conclusions formulated by Forssman are admissible ; but his neurotropic formula needs an essential correction. Our investigations [2] showed that the most powerful chemotactic sources, those which act in ordinary regeneration, cannot be the remnants of the myelin and axon. It is during the second and third week after the nerve section, when the myelin ellipsoids have largely disappeared, that the attractive activity of the peripheral stump reaches its maximum. Moreover, in the cases in which nervous reunion is difficult, owing to the cutting out of large pieces of nerve or the folding back of the stumps, etc., the sprouts from the central stump are able, several months after the operation, to orient themselves and to assault the bands of Büngner, even though the great majority of the latter are totally devoid of fatty remnants. Even in early reunions it is impossible to detect a marked difference, as regards their number and thickness, between the sprouts in sheaths that are full of myelinic remnants, and those in sheaths that are almost free of all fatty and axonic detritus.

The experiments of grafting cerebral, spinal, and other substances

[1] Merzbacher: " Zur Biologie der Nervendegeneration. Ergebnisse von Transplantationsversuche," *Neurol. Centralbl.*, 15 Feb. 1905.

[2] Cajal : " Mecanismo de la regeneración de los nervios," *Trab. del Lab. de Invest. biol.*, tomo 4, 1905-06.

have but little value, since Dustin and Rossi have shown, and we have ourselves recently confirmed, that the tissues of the centres are rapidly resorbed, and that when sprouts are attracted among their remnants, this is simply explained by virtue of the nutritive or attractive action of the cicatricial tissue (*odogenesis* of Dustin) which replaces the disappeared graft.

As a result of these and other observations we were led to the conclusion that the neurotropic or attractive substance is present in the old tubes, under the form of a soluble, non-lipoidal substance, and that its elaboration is brought about by the cells of Schwann, especially during the phase in which the latter, multiplying and transforming themselves, become the *bands of Büngner*.

Lugaro,[1] independently of ourselves, had the same idea, and after our observations had appeared he made some interesting experiments on grafting. We may mention, among others, the following :

(*a*) Suture of the anterior with the posterior root. The animal was killed some months later, and Lugaro observed the penetration of nervous motor sprouts in the sensory root. Such fibres become dispersed before reaching the spinal cord. In this and other experiments this Florentine scientist, interpreting the pretended auto-regeneration of the posterior root (without ganglia) described by Bethe, calls attention to the structural complexity of this root. In it, besides ordinary sensory axons, are contained : fine centrifugal fibres arising in the spinal cord, aberrant fibres coming from adjacent sensory roots, and sympathetic axons, centrifugal in character ; none of these conductors, of course, can degenerate when the section of the root is made between the ganglion and the spinal cord.

(*b*) Nerve graft on the cerebrum. In two young dogs he transplanted on the cerebrum, beneath the *dura mater*, a large piece of sciatic nerve from the same animal. Examination of the cerebral cortex and meninges, eighteen and twenty days respectively after the operation, showed that the grafted nerve does not attract the

---

[1] In a chapter of the book entitled *Handbuch des pathol. Anat. des Nervensystems von Jacobsohn, Flatau und Minor*, Lugaro, after assenting to the neurotropism of Forssman, notes that this orienting influence might as well be a function of the cellular chains of the degenerated peripheral stump.

See also Lugaro : " Sul Neurotropismo e sui Trapianti dei Nervi," *Riv. di Patol. nervosa e mentale*, vol. 11, fasc. 7, 1906.

" La fonction de la cellule nerveuse," 16ᵉ *Congrès intern. de Médecine*, Budapest, Aug. 29, 1909.

fibres of the cerebrum, although some of them are regenerating. Within the graft one recognizes characteristic bands of Büngner. We shall show below that if the nerve had been placed, not outside the cerebrum, but full in the white matter, as Tello did, the results would have been very different.

(c) Graft of a nerve on a healthy sciatic nerve. A piece of sciatic nerve from one side of a dog or rabbit was cut out and superposed on its mate of the other leg. Lugaro saw that, after twenty-five days, the normal nerve has not become modified in the least. He concluded from this, and rightly so, that the cells of Schwann of a degenerating nerve do not attract the axons of another healthy nerve nor do they cause in them the creation of collaterals. If by chance a few fibres penetrate into the degenerated nerve, they originate from the small muscular nerves wounded in the course of the operation, which circulate in the scar.

(d) Apposition of two nerve roots, one of which is cut and the other is not. Lugaro affirms with reason that the ideal experiment to demonstrate the possible neurotropic action of a degenerated on a healthy nerve consists in the extirpation in the lumbar region of the ganglion of a sensory root. As a consequence of this the peripheral stump of the cut root remains in intimate contact with the undamaged accompanying motor root. Nevertheless the closeness of the neurotropic source does not provoke in the healthy root the least regenerative effort. A similar negative result is obtained when one cuts a root of origin of the sciatic nerve, etc.

Lugaro infers from these and other experiments that neurotropism is a complex process, whose influence is felt only by the nerve sprouts created after the interruption or grave lesion of the nerves ; this amounts to the recognition that the organs which are exclusively sensitive to the substances evolved by the cells of Schwann are the cones and clubs of growth, or the recently-formed conductors.

Marinesco,[1] shortly after the publication of Lugaro's results, also undertook experiments of grafting in order to contrast the results of Merzbacher, Forssman, and Lugaro. He used the method of reduced silver nitrate, also eventually used by Lugaro. Here are the principal results :

In the space created by the resection of a sciatic nerve Marinesco

[1] Marinesco : " Le mécanisme de la régénérescence nerveuse, 2e partie. Les transplantations nerveuses," *Rev. gén. des Sciences*, 15 mars 1907.

grafted a piece of dead nerve taken either from an animal of the same species (*homoiotransplant*) or from an animal of a different species (*heterotransplant*). At other times he used living grafts, both homoiotransplants and heterotransplants. Finally, he transplanted into the wound living sensory and sympathetic ganglia.

When the graft, whether it be dead or alive, comes from an animal of a different species, its nervous reunion is impossible, as Forssman and Merzbacher had already observed. The cells of Schwann die quickly, without giving rise to apotrophic cells. The axon remains unaltered for a few days, and then disappears through autolysis. The nerve sprouts that issue from the central stump keep away from the graft, as though influenced by some negative chemotactic substance, avoiding it and making circuits, in order finally to assault the peripheral stump. Marinesco believes that the death and destruction of these grafts occurs, in accordance with the antibody theory of Ehrlich, by means of some neurotoxic substance.

On the contrary, when the living graft is from the same animal or from an animal of the same species, its tubes undergo Wallerian degeneration and its apotrophic cells attract the sprouts of the central stump, giving out to the surrounding tissues positive chemotactic substances.

If instead of wounding the nerve and transplanting the graft into the wound, one places the latter on an undamaged nerve, as Lugaro had done, the axons remain indifferent, the transplanted nerve falls into necrobiosis and is absorbed, no matter what may be the state of the sheaths of Schwann of the graft. At any rate the union of the connective tissue of the graft with that of the old nerve occurs rapidly and effectively.

Marinesco cautiously distinguishes between circatrisation and nervous reunion of the grafts. The transplantation of the living nerve brings about the union of the neurilemmatic connective tissue, as well as that of the apotrophic cells of the graft with those of the old nerve. But if the apotrophic cells—the proliferated cells of Schwann—of the transplanted segment have lost their vitality, the reunion of the latter does not occur, even though a cicatrisation or connective fusion occurs.

Mott and Halliburton,[1] without having in mind the theory of neurotropism, carried out interesting experiments of nerve grafting.

[1] Mott and Halliburton: "Regeneration of nerves," *Proc. of the Roy. Soc. B.*, vol. 78.

Repeating old attempts of Vulpian and Phylippeaux and of Kennedy, they transplanted pieces of sciatic nerve under the skin or in the peritoneum. The animals were killed one hundred or one hundred and fifty days after the operation. Examination by means of osmic acid showed that the pieces of nerve were well rooted, except in one case in which there was total resorption. While there were a few regenerated tubes in the cutaneous grafts none were found in the peritoneal transplants. This result is decisively opposed to the theory of auto-regeneration defended by Kennedy, Huber, Bethe, etc. It was interpreted by English authors as meaning that, in accordance with Lugaro's views, there was a partial innervation in the first case, because there was a penetration of sprouts from wounded sensory cutaneous nerves, while since there were no interrupted peritoneal nerves, there was no innervation in those cases.

Dustin,[1] with a view to elucidating the mechanism of the growth and orientation of the axons, repeated the experiments of Forssman, Lugaro, and Marinesco, and made some new ones which are very instructive. (*a*) He fixed at times on an undamaged nerve of a rabbit a segment taken from the peripheral stump of another animal, and containing the bands of Büngner. (*b*) At other times he placed within the two ends of a resected nerve wound a piece of degenerated nerve, from another animal, which was giving out neurotropic substances. (*c*) He sometimes grafted next to nerves which were lacerated by pressure from a forceps, but without interruption of the neurilemma, a piece of nerve whose degeneration had begun ten days previously. In no case was Dustin convinced that the bands of Büngner attract especially the axons of the central stump, either normal or sprouting, and in the *phase of formative turgidity*. No doubt, in the experiments of intercalary grafting of the degenerated stump, there occurred nervous reunions of the bands of Büngner. But this was due to the conducting action of the intercalated connective tissue cells and of those which penetrated into the transplanted piece, without these cells exerting a stronger influence on the growth and orientation of the sprouts than is exercised by ordinary scars in reunion after nerve section. Thus the penetration of the sprouts into the nerve grafts is a function of the *odogenesis* of the connective tissue; that is, it is merely the effect of the disposition of the recently-formed mesodermal cells which provide interstices

[1] Dustin: "Le rôle des tropismes et de l'odogenèse dans la régénération du système nerveux," *Arch. de Biol.*, tome 25, 1910.

or orienting paths from the central stump up to the transplanted nerve.

O. Rossi [1] reached similar results in some experiments of suture of roots and grafts of nerves as well as of pieces of spinal cord, etc., on the cut sciatic nerve. Like Dustin, he recognizes that in the process of orientation of the sprouts the newly-formed connective tissue plays an important rôle. But he does not specify by what method the mesodermal cells create paths. He nevertheless seems inclined to look upon the newly-formed connective tissue as a system of guides which mechanically orient the nerve sprouts. We shall speak more in detail of O. Rossi's studies when we describe regeneration of the spinal cord and transplantation of the ganglia.

From the experiments that we have cited it might be concluded that nerve grafts do not confirm or only weakly support the hypothesis of neurotropism. We may say, however, that even if the interpretation given by Dustin to the above facts were correct, they could not shake the basis of the conception of Forssman. There is little doubt that conditions are not the same in the normal nervous reunion of the peripheral stump and that of a graft whose cells are gravely altered, if not dead, and, at any rate, badly nourished. It would not be surprising if the catalytic substances or stimulating agents elaborated by the cells of Schwann and capable of influencing the growth and orientation of the nerve sprouts should, under such conditions, be weakened or absent.

Here are a few experiments undertaken in order to appraise the conditions determining the penetration and growth of the nerve fibres in the grafts:

Simple hemisection of a nerve.—In order to ascertain the insensibility of normal axons, which are not stimulated by traumatisms or chemical agents, to the substances given out by degenerated nerves, we have performed various experiments of hemisection of the sciatic, of the posterior spinal roots, of the hypoglossus, etc.

The result, as can be seen in Fig. 133, confirmed the conclusions of Lugaro. A normal nerve which is not stretched, bruised, or wounded never initiates processes of neurocladism or of collateral neoformation, no matter how near are the nerve tubes that have degenerated or are in process of transformation of the sheath of Schwann.

[1] O. Rossi: "Sulla rigenerazione del sistema nervoso," *Riv. di Patol. nervosa e mentale*, vol. 16, fasc. 4, 1911.

On the other hand, the slightest lesion of the axons, when these are near a degenerated nerve trunk, determines a formidable production of sprouts.

In Fig. 134 we reproduce a case of nerve hemisection in which the scissors had lightly scratched the otherwise undamaged half of the nerve. One can see how from the deteriorated region there arise a great number of collateral and terminal branches which, taking advantage of an adjacent scar, precipitate themselves into the

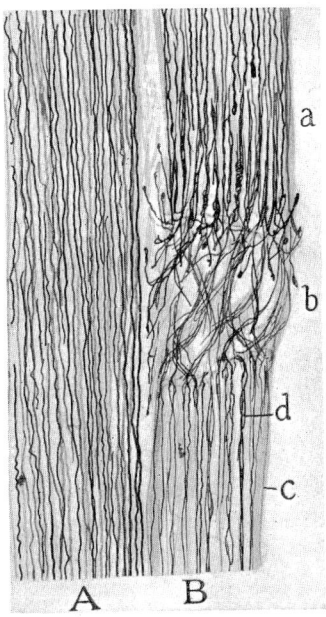

FIG. 133.—Hemisection of the sciatic nerve of a twenty days old cat. Semischematic. The animal was killed nine days after the operation.

degenerated nerve and innervate it in both an ascending and a descending direction. In this case the degenerated segment had been cut in three parts.

Graft of a degenerated nerve on a healthy one (Fig. 135).—Like Lugaro, Marinesco, and Dustin, we attached, by a ligature, a piece of nerve ten days after its section, when the bands of Büngner had been formed, on the sciatic nerve. At a certain distance, in a distal direction, a total section of this nerve was effected. The animal was killed twelve days after the operation.

As was to be expected, and in accordance with the conclusions of the authorities above cited, the soluble products that are poured out by a ripe graft during the twelve days following the operation do not induce in the neighbouring axons any phenomena of neurocladism. Neither do they attract sprouts arising in a nerve wound situated at a great distance. It is a fact, however, that pieces of degenerated nerve, when they are very near the wound in the nerve, often receive young axons which are able, as noted above, to describe complicated retrograde courses to reach their goal. It thus seems probable that in this actual case the absence of neurotropic phenomena is due to the great distance between the graft and the nerve wound. It is very probable that, given a longer interval of time—fifteen to twenty-five days—the preparation would have shown some retrograde sprouts penetrating into the graft.

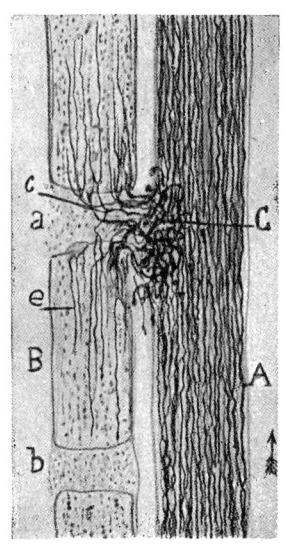

FIG. 134.—Experiment in which half of the nerve was cut in three pieces, while the other half was slightly scratched with the scissors. A, healthy portion; B, degenerated pieces of the nerve; C, axons in the state of divisory excitation; a, scar invaded by the sprouts; e, fibres that have penetrated into the degenerated nerve segments; c, fibre that has branched into two pieces of nerve. Semi-schematic. Young cat, killed five days after the operation.

Experiments of grafting of dead nerves.—(a) *Nerve immersed for half-an-hour in chloroform.* A piece of sciatic nerve killed in this way was transplanted in the hollow space formed by the wound of the sciatic of a young cat. The animal was killed after twelve days (Fig. 136).

The nerve was stained with reduced silver nitrate. Examination revealed that the graft had deviated somewhat from the axis of the scar (B). It was blackish in colour and without any trace of nervous reunion. A considerable portion of its axons were *conserved*, that is, they were spiroidal, black, sometimes varicose. As was to be expected, these *conserved* conductors were seen especially at both ends and in the cortex of the graft, that is, where the chloroform acted directly. In the central regions the medullated fibres have had their myelin and axon altered through a process of autolysis.

As to the nerve sprouts, few of them reach the region of the graft and, instead of penetrating into it, they turn aside to grow towards the peripheral stump (Fig. 136, C).

Grafts of nerves killed in boiling water, formalin, chloral hydrate, by desiccation, etc., have given similar results. The fibres are preserved more or less well, being finally, after a time, phagocytized and autolyzed. It is only when the graft which is being resorbed is replaced partially or completely by a connective scar that the space which it occupied becomes full of sprouts. At any rate the dead cells of Schwann are unable to attract the newly-formed fibres. It thus appears that the process of attraction and penetration of the new fibres into the peripheral stump is closely related to the vitality of the cells of Schwann. In the following experiments we shall see fresh proofs of this fact already noted by Marinesco.

(*b*) *Graft of a nerve that is in seminecrosis through crushing.*—A piece of sciatic nerve, repeatedly crushed by a wide forceps, was intercalated in the wound made by resection of the sciatic of an adult rabbit. The animal was killed after seventeen days (Fig. 137).

The transplanted piece (*B*) had doubled up in the shape of a letter C, becoming somewhat separated from the axis of the scar. Notwithstanding the mechanical violence, not all the cells of Schwann had succumbed. Those in the centre, especially, appeared disintegrated and the remnants were phagocytized by migrating leucocytes. But in some points of the periphery a few cellular bands were preserved with their normal orientation. Neither the neurilemma nor the endoneurium had perished, as could be seen in fine sections stained with thionin or haematoxylin. Here one saw that many of their connective elements were multiplying.

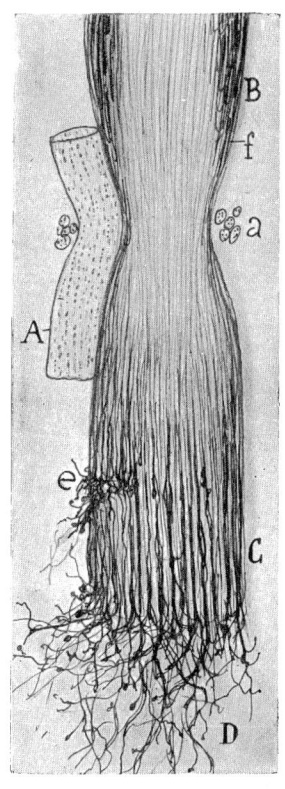

FIG. 135.—Graft of a degenerated nerve on another nerve which is cut at some distance. *A*, graft; *a*, ligature to hold it; *D*, scar through which sprouts grow. Schematic.

On examination of the central stump, one discerns, among other currents of sprouts directed towards the region of the graft, these two : one very rich in fibres which, tracing a curve, precipitated itself towards the proximal end of the transplanted nerve and penetrated into its interior (Fig. 137, *e*) ; another, less important, after proceeding through the scar at a distance from the graft, turned back in part to invade the latter by its distal end (Fig. 137, *f*). Once arrived in the interior, the sprouts seem to choose the un-

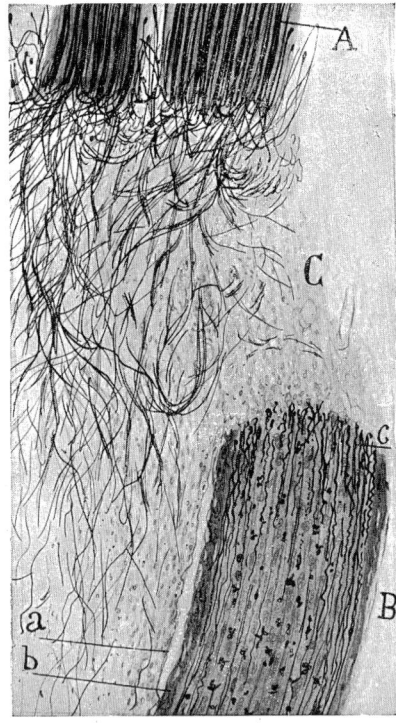

FIG. 136.—Graft of a nerve killed by chloroform into the wound of the sciatic. Young cat, killed twelve days after the operation. *A*, central stump ; *B*, dead graft ; *C*, scar ; *a*, connective tissue of the graft ; *b*, neurilemma with dead elements ; *c*, dead axons stained by the silver. Semi-schematic figure.

damaged or only slightly altered bands, avoiding or abandoning the lacerated central region, where no bands of Büngner are present, and where enormous accumulations of phagocytes full of fat are to be found. The axons run, not only in the bands of Büngner, but also in the interstices between them. The few fibres that are lost in the disintegrated portions are large, travel without orientation, trace complicated circuits, and are often ramified (Fig. 138, *B*). Those which are insinuated in the old sheaths of Schwann, on the other hand, are fine (showing rapid growth), are arranged in parallel bundles, and follow straight paths (Fig. 138, *A*).

This experiment, besides corroborating the statement that the growth and penetration of nerve sprouts in the peripheral stump

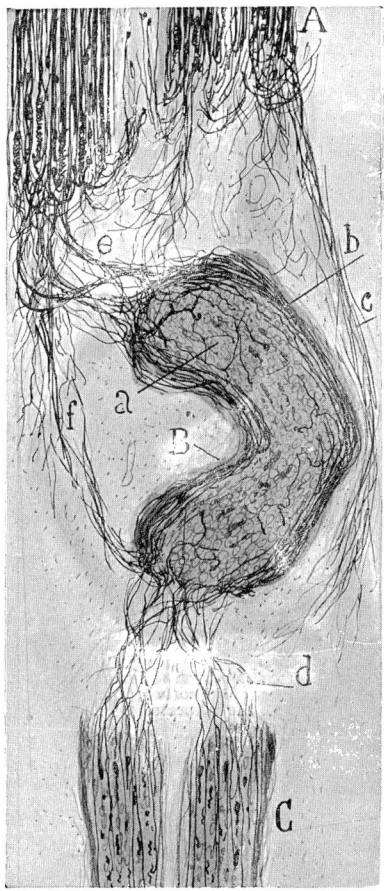

FIG. 137.—Graft of a crushed and lacerated piece of nerve in the wound of the sciatic nerve of an adult rabbit. The animal was killed seventeen days after the operation. *A*, central stump; *B*, graft; *C*, peripheral stump; *a*, lacerated central portion; *b*, peripheral cortex, rich in sprouts; *e, f*, currents of axons going towards the graft; *d*, fibres which, after leaving the graft, innervate the peripheral stump. Semi-schematic figure.

are functions of the living nerve, reveals to us that the soluble products liberated by destroyed cells of Schwann do not attract, or attract only very feebly the clubs of growth. This is shown by the fact that at the level of the lacerated zones, whose cells of Schwann

342 TRAUMATIC DEGENERATION AND REGENERATION OF NERVES

have been replaced by numerous gigantic granular cells, the sprouts grow badly and seem to follow the path of least resistance. But even these few fibres which have arrived in that region have perhaps been influenced by the attractive action of the cells of the endoneurium, some of which have survived the ruin of the nerve tubes.

Similar results were obtained in experiments of re-implantation of crushed pieces of nerve in young rabbits, although here the number of sprouts that penetrated was greater.

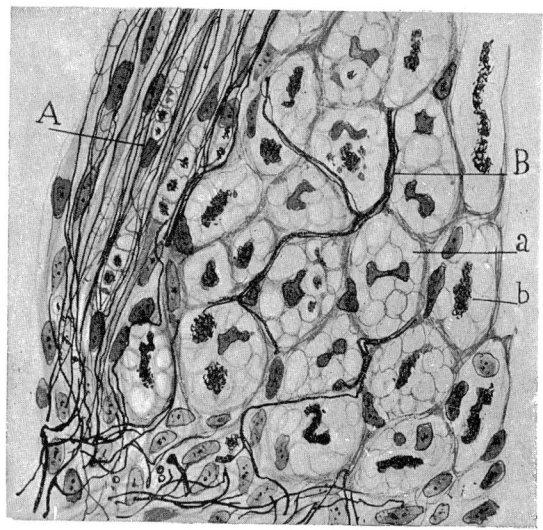

FIG. 138.—Details of the lacerated central region of the crushed graft. *A*, fibres insinuated in the bands of Büngner of the cortex ; *B*, scanty fibres, irregular in their course, which have ventured into the triturated region ; *a*, exogenous phagocyte ; *b*, piece of a cell of Schwann.

(c) *Graft of a piece of degenerated nerve that had been exposed to the air during four hours* (Fig. 139).—In a young cat the sciatic nerve was cut, and a piece of it was taken out in order to retard the arrival of the sprouts at the peripheral stump. Nine days later the animal was killed by chloroform ; a piece of the degenerated peripheral stump was cut out and implanted in the wound of the sciatic nerve of another cat. This latter animal was examined at autopsy twelve days later. The graft had taken perfectly, being in connection with the endoneurium of both stumps. The connective tissue of the scar had become perfectly united with the neurilemma.

The graft being stained by the method of reduced silver nitrate, the good condition of vitality of the bands of Büngner, neurilemma, and endoneurium was manifest. Thus, in accordance with the results obtained by other authors, it appears that neither four hours' exposure to a cold of 14° C. nor the fact that the animal was killed

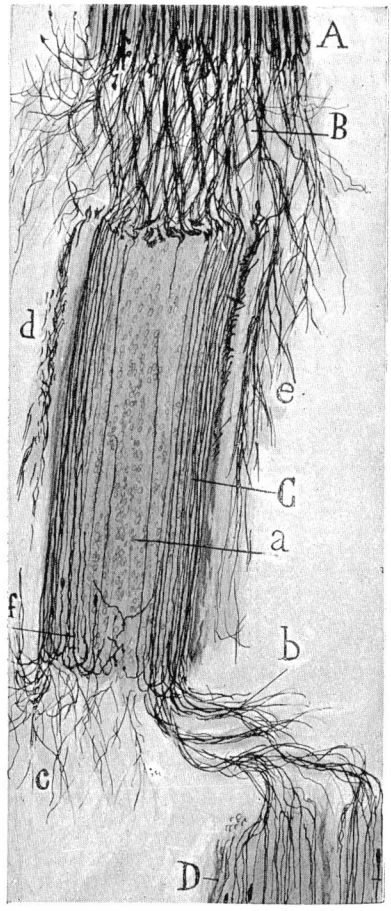

FIG. 139.—Graft of a piece of nerve in the phase of bands of Büngner, which had been exposed to the air for four hours at the ordinary temperature. Young cat, killed twelve days after the transplantation. *A*, central stump; *B*, first scar; *C*, graft; *D*, peripheral stump; *a*, central region of the graft, poor in fibres; *d*, *e*, sprouts growing outside the neurilemma of the graft; *f*, retrograde fibres of the distal extremity of the graft; *b*, sprouts that turn to reach the peripheral stump. Semi-schematic figure.

by chloroform, nor even the fact that the nerve had begun to dry, lessened the vitality of these elements. It was only the central region of the graft that showed evidence of necrobiosis, due, no doubt, to nutritive and respiratory deficiencies, since one must not forget that there are no blood-vessels in the graft, and that it is nourished by imbibition from the surrounding plasma. It is thus not surprising that while the cortex (Fig. 141) contains typical bands of Büngner that are almost free from fat, through a rapid absorption, the central regions are invaded by a great number of phagocytes (Fig. 140, c), which are full of fatty drops derived from the disintegrated nerve tubes.

The sprouts of the central stump, notwithstanding the fact that only twelve days had elapsed, had already crossed the scar, which

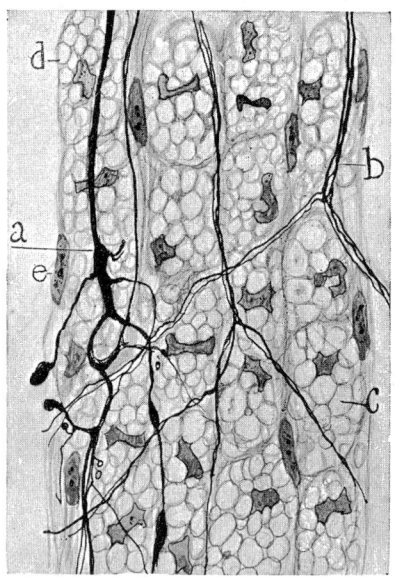

FIG. 140.—Details of the paths of the fibres in the central regions of the graft shown in the last figure. a, axon with arrested branches; b, disoriented fibres; c, d, exogenous phagocytes—leucocytes full of lipoid masses.

was not very extensive, and had penetrated into the graft, which they followed along its whole 3·5 millimetres. Nearly all the sprouts grow along the cortical region of the graft, preferably within the bands of Büngner, and show all the dispositions of mechanical adjustment to their surroundings, such as ramification, etc., that were described for the cases of normal nervous reunion of the peripheral stump (Figs. 139, C, and 141, e, d).

As was to be expected, few sprouts enter the central region, which is badly nourished and poor in oxygen, and those that do show signs of lost orientation. As may be seen in Fig. 140, b, there are numerous axons that divide into diverging branches and cross these central regions obliquely or transversely between the granular cells ; one also fairly often finds retrograde fibres and fibres terminating in large clubs or rings (*a*).

Even in the peripheral regions, where close and perfectly oriented bundles (Fig. 141, *a*, *c*) are seen within the bands of Büngner, one

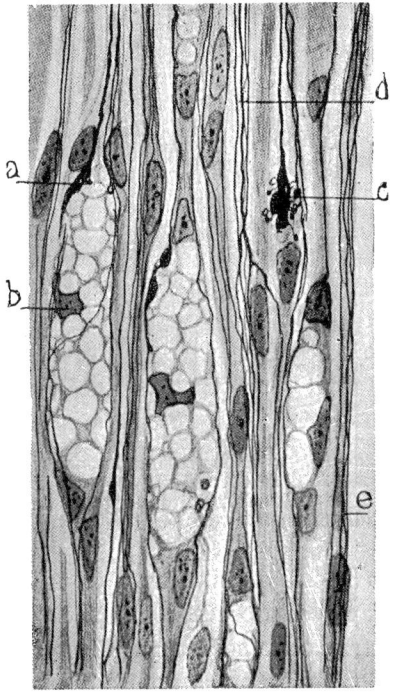

FIG. 141.—Details of the cortical region of the same graft as in Fig. 140. *a*, intratubal cones of growth ; *b*, nucleus of a phagocyte ; *c*, free club with appendices ending in rings and excrescences ; *e*, intratubal bundle ; *d*, interstitial fibres.

finds sprouts whose exodus is difficult, as one can judge by the thickenings that they exhibit where they assault the ellipsoids, by their complicated ramifications, retrograde clubs, and, finally, by the presence of strings of balls, a disposition which, as is well known, is typical of sprouts that advance intermittently across difficult regions. In Fig. 141 we show some of these dispositions which indicate these arrests, common in grafts, but unusual in a normal peripheral stump.

Besides the rich current of newly-formed fibres on its way to the graft, one can see another almost as strong, which runs along the graft outside the neurilemma and which describes complex perinervous plexuses. Some of these bundles take a transversal direction and trace circles and spirals (Fig. 139, *d, e*).

We have said that those sprouts which penetrate into the graft pass through its entire length and then appear in the second scar. Such fibres, on reaching the second scar, do one of two things. Either they abruptly describe a semi-circle and return within the graft (Fig. 139, *f*); or else, and this occurs in the majority of cases, they grow out into the scar and reach the peripheral stump (Fig. 139, *b*). Such conductors, weakened by the long exodus, are very fine, and they grow within the peripheral stump for about 1 millimetre, joining with other axons that have arrived independently along the scar without going through the graft (Fig. 139, *D*).

Quite apart from the resistance of grafts to cold and chloroform, the preceding observations show that pieces of nerve which are altered but not dead still attract the sprouts and are able to nourish them. But they do not greatly favour the growth of the sprouts, as compared with the scar, since the fibrillar current within the graft and the current growing freely through the connective tissue reach the peripheral stump almost at the same time.

Nerve grafts in a healthy state.—Many experiments of this type were performed on adult as well as on young animals. In general, the results which were obtained confirm the descriptions of Forssman, Lugaro, Marinesco, Dustin, and O. Rossi. In order to avoid repetitions we shall give only a few typical cases.

(*a*) *Reimplantation of a piece of nerve recently cut from the sciatic nerve of a young cat. The animal was killed thirteen days later* (Fig. 142). —This is the ideal graft, from the point of view of the good conservation of the cells. As a matter of fact, when one operates in this manner, the transplanted piece has not had time to become cold, and if one proceeds with speed and avoids haemorrhage, the piece cut out and reimplanted will occupy exactly its normal position. The only important change that has occurred is the rupture of the surrounding blood-vessels, and when the little nerves are thin and are from young mammals, such as cats, dogs, and rabbits from ten to fifteen days old, this lack of vascularization has hardly any effect on the nutrition of the graft. Days later the central as well as the peripheral zones are perfectly healthy and show real bands of Büngner. It was to be expected that the graft would be fully and quickly innervated. This actually occurred, as we show in Fig. 142, B, where one can see that it is full of small parallel bundles of fibres, which are partly intratubal, partly interstitial. There are bands of Büngner which enclose twenty or more parallel fibres. The sprouts accommodate themselves to the ellipsoids and lipoid masses just as the normal sprouts in the peripheral stump. The large clubs are rare and are often absent, as are retrograde and disoriented fibres such as were noted in the preceding case. In fine, it appeared as though we were dealing with a legitimate peripheral stump, innervated in normal physiological conditions.

If one follows the fibres along the graft one sees that not only do they run through its entire length but that, crossing the second scar, they invade the peripheral stump in great numbers (*E*). Some of the sprouts have advanced more than one millimetre within the latter.

Other fibres, on emerging from the graft, lose themselves in the scar. Finally, when the graft is made up of several nerve bundles, one often finds conductors which, after having reached the scar, innervate retrogradely another fascicle of the same transplant (Fig. 142, *d*). It is also curious to see, among those sprouts which do not penetrate into the graft (*b*), small bundles arranged in close spirals around its border, as though they were looking in vain for a favourable region.

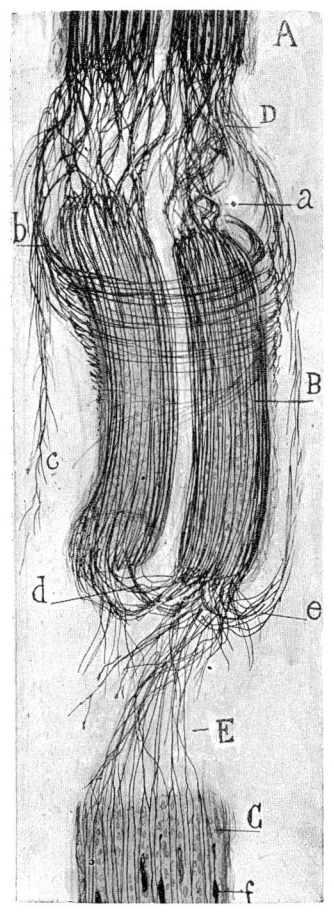

FIG. 142.—Semi-schematic drawing of the innervation of a reimplanted piece of nerve, in the sciatic nerve of a young cat killed thirteen days after the operation. *A*, central stump; *B*, completely innervated graft; *D*, first scar; *E*, second scar; *C*, peripheral stump; *a*, fibres that penetrate into the graft; *b*, sprouts that follow exteriorly the neurilemma of the graft; *d*, sprouts which, after issuing from one fascicle of the graft, are attracted by a neighbouring fascicle of the same; *f*, remnants of the old axons of the peripheral stump.

Thus the innervation of a thin reimplanted nerve occurs under the same conditions of speed and perfection as that of a normal peripheral stump. Since the graft is living along its whole extent it has the maximum neurotropic power. Three facts are particularly important for the theory of neurotropism: (1) the bundle of retrograde fibres that innervate the external fascicle of the graft (Fig. 142, *d*); (2) the rapid concentration of the sprouts in the proximal edge of the graft; (3) the small number of fibres in the region of the scar, that is, outside the axis of the transplanted nerve.

(*b*) *Reimplantation of a piece of sciatic nerve, which was well isolated, in the same region of the nerve that it had previously occupied. The adult rabbit was killed sixteen days after the operation.*— The result, coincident with that obtained in the preceding case, was less striking because of two new conditions: relatively large thickness of the nerve and adult state of the nerve tubes. Nevertheless the graft became perfectly united with the ends of the sciatic nerve, and the sprouts innervated the old sheaths of Schwann, which had become converted into bands of Büngner. This innervation, which was rather precarious, was confined, owing to the reasons stated above, almost exclusively to the cortex of the graft. In the badly nourished centre, which was undergoing an intense phagocytosis, the sprouts were rare and more or less disoriented.

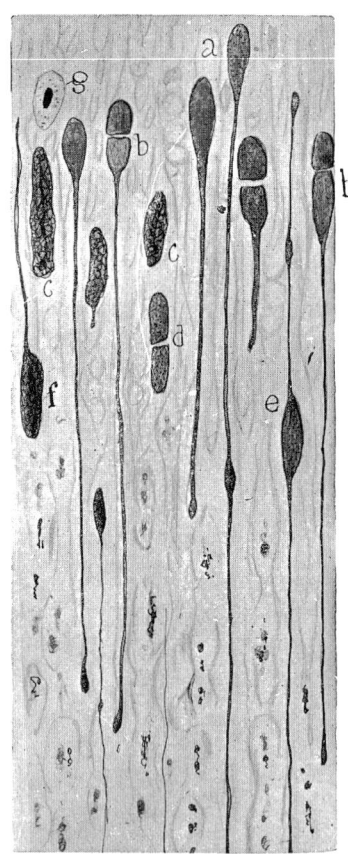

FIG. 143.—Appearance of the proximal ends of the surviving fibres of Remak in the peripheral stump. Young cat, killed after ten days. Owing to the width of the scar and of the grafts, no sprouts had penetrated into the peripheral stump. *a*, clubs; *b*, segmented forms; *e*, spindles; *f*, spermatozooid-like form; *C*, isolated and reticulated colony; *g*, last phase of a free ball which is undergoing hyaline degeneration.

This and similar experiments show that large and adult grafts are innervated with greater difficulty than thin grafts belonging to young animals.

In some cases in which during the days following the operation the graft becomes spontaneously dislocated, one would think that the distinction between the graft and the real peripheral stump would be difficult. Even without examining the connections of the graft and its frequent foldings there are certain histological facts that determine it at first sight. There are no permeable capillaries in the graft. There is another negative character which is absolutely constant, at least from the fourth day on. There is an absence in the graft of the large clubs, sometimes in process of ramification, that are characteristic of all genuine peripheral stumps. Such living clubs, noted by Perroncito and described in detail by ourselves (see p. 118) belong to the peripheral portion of non-medullated axons. They are rapidly resorbed in adult animals, but subsist under various forms in young cats, dogs, and rabbits, eight, ten, and twelve days after the operation [1] (Fig. 143).

Another structural feature serves to distinguish a graft from a true peripheral stump. While, after the same lapse of time, in the latter the fatty ellipsoids are rapidly resorbed and the tissues appear mostly composed of parallel bands of Büngner in which are scattered a few fatty droplets, in the grafts this process of resorption takes place very slowly; the fatty agglomerations of the tubes of Schwann are retained for two or more weeks and a great number of thick granular cells appear in the interstices. We may add that reduced silver nitrate has a tendency to stain the graft deeper than normal nerves (see Fig. 140, c, d).

(c) *Experiments wherein pieces of nerve of one rabbit were grafted on the wound of the sciatic nerve of another rabbit. The animal was killed sixteen days after the operation.*—When the operation is

[1] Some recent observations made by us on the living clubs of the peripheral stump have convinced us that their formation is a process of reaction of the portion of the axon which is in continuation with the nervous terminations. When one cuts a nerve in three or four successive pieces, it is only the long piece—the piece connected with the terminations—which shows clubs eight, ten, and even fourteen days after the operation, in young animals. This axonic reaction is not absolutely lacking in the intermediate pieces, but there it is very ephemeral. The grafts belong to this category of segments, where the clubs rapidly disappear. The smaller the number of axons that penetrate into the peripheral stumps, the greater is the persistence of the clubs. It seems as though the reactional phenomena of the isolated axon take place at the expense of some substance which is rapidly consumed when the sprouts arrive. We shall speak again of these phenomena below.

rapidly performed and when one avoids crushing the transplanted nerve the results are almost the same as those obtained by reimplantation. The connective tissue of the host joins with the neurilemma of the graft and the ends of the latter are invaded by migrating connective tissue cells which come from the scar. Nervous reunion may, however, be much retarded, especially in the central regions, where the nerve tubes appear to have died through asphyxia. We shall not repeat here details given in connection with reimplantations.

One must attribute the negative or poor results obtained by Dustin in his experiments of nerve transplantation, as regards the attractive influence of the graft, to this defective nutrition of adult grafts and consequent weakening of the neurotropic action. This had already been noted by O. Rossi. As a matter of fact, in consequence of the rupture of the vascular links, the tubes of the graft are in an inferior position relatively to the degenerated sheaths of the peripheral stump and the sheaths of Schwann of the central stump. It follows from this that the attractive power of the graft is weak or precarious and, at any rate, unable to counteract the powerful retrograde neurotropic actions of the proximal segment and the slightly less energetic, but none the less important, action of the cicatricial tissue. Another grave disturbance to the nervous reunion of the graft may also be due to haemorrhage or the presence of large quantities of serous exudates ; these liquids, when they surround the transplanted nerve, constitute insuperable screens to neurotropic influences, which no sprout of the central stump can pass through. Once the exudate is resorbed, the situation is different. But the sprouts, in their growth, may already have passed over the plane of the graft and be decisively attracted by the peripheral stump. The nervous reunion of the graft is thus frustrated. As a result of all these *contretemps* and deficiencies, even in the most favourable circumstances no graft is ever innervated as rapidly and completely as the degenerated fascicles of a cut nerve ; this is shown by experiments of total section combined with various partial hemisections of the same nerve.

(*d*) *Graft of nerve roots, with or without ganglia, on wounds created by resection of the sciatic nerve. Two weeks old cats, killed nine to fourteen days after the operation.*—As was to be expected, there was a rapid innervation of the graft (Fig. 144). The roots, sensory or motor, are penetrated by the sprouts emanating from the central stump, all the more easily as the thinness of its bundles—in cats a few days old—and the tenuity of the neurilemma lend to the graft special facilities for its nutrition *in toto*. When the animals are killed after sufficient interval one always sees that the sprouts, after having crossed the graft, copiously innervate the peripheral stump (Fig. 144, *e*).

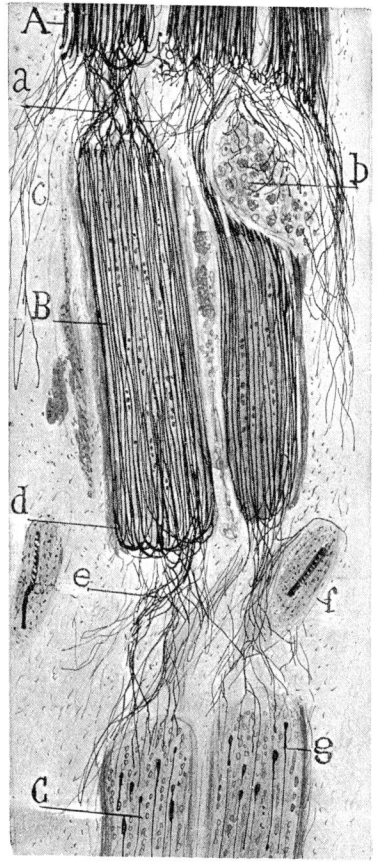

FIG. 144.—Graft of spinal roots on the wound of the sciatic. Young cat, killed fourteen days after the operation. *A*, central stump; *B*, living roots; *C*, peripheral stump; *a*, bundles penetrating into the graft; *b*, remnants of a small ganglion which is largely destroyed; *c*, nerve current that accompanies the graft at a distance; *d*, retrograde sprouts in the distal end of the graft; *e*, current that reaches the peripheral stump after passing through the graft; *f*, connective tissue surrounding a hair, which is refractory to invasion by the sprouts. Semi-schematic figure.

We shall not dwell further on this and other experiments, as our results are in perfect accord with those of the other authors.

Free grafts on to the skin and muscles.—Several authors, among them Phylippeaux and Vulpian, Kennedy, Mott and Halliburton, have observed nervous reunions in nerves left under the skin and in other positions. We have repeated these experiments, transplanting living nerves either into muscles or else into subcutaneous connective tissue. The animals were killed twenty and twenty-eight days after the operation.

Although not invariably, one can yet fairly frequently see, by the method of reduced silver nitrate, the arrival in the graft of a few young fibres. These fibres originate, as Mott and Halliburton have shown, from small muscular or cutaneous nerves which were accidentally wounded or sectioned in the course of the operation. Sometimes the sprouts come from long distances, tracing complicated paths, to reach the tubes of the transplanted nerve. This fact is very significant from the point of view of neurotropism.

Grafts of entire limbs on amphibian larvae.—The nervous reunion of entire limbs, obtained by Braus and Bianchi in various species of amphibians, belong to this same category of phenomena. As these ingenious experiments have been much discussed, we need here give only a short résumé.

Braus [1] took a pelvic extremity of a larva of *Bombinator* and grafted it on any region of the skin of a larva of the same species. After a time the transplanted limb contained newly-formed nerves which, according to Braus and Bianchi,[2] are not derived from the host, but are the result of an autoformation of axons by cellular chains or ectodermal cells—the future cells of Schwann, present in this limb at a period anterior to its ablation. As was to be expected, this experiment of Braus was claimed to furnish a decisive argument against the monogenist doctrine of regeneration. But Gemelli [3] was able to recognize, by the method of reduced silver nitrate, that in *Bufo vulgaris* the regenerated nerves of the graft constantly originate from the nerve trunks of the host, thus demolishing the idea of auto-regeneration. Harrison, in his critical studies of the experiments of Braus and Bianchi, has come to the same conclusion.

Experiments of nervous heterotransplantation. *On the wound of the sciatic of an adult rabbit was grafted a piece of nerve from a young*

---

[1] Braus: " Experimentelle Beiträge zur Frage nach der Entwicklung periph. Nerven," *Anat. Anz.*, Bd. 26, no. 17-18.

[2] Bianchi: " Sullo sviluppo dei nervi periferici," etc. *Anat. Anz.*, Bd. 28, no. 7-8, 1906.

[3] A. Gemelli: " Ricerche sperimentali sullo sviluppo dei nervi degli arti pelvici di *Bufo vulgaris*, innestati in sede anomala," *Rendiconti del R. Instituto Lomb. di scien. e lett.*, serie 2, vol. 39, 1906.

cat. The rabbit was killed after sixteen days.—In accordance with the above cited experiments of Forssman, Merzbacher, and Marinesco, it was manifest that the transplant did not become united with the connective tissue of the host. A well-marked border limited the graft, whose neurilemma enclosed cells which were shrunk, granular, and obscurely stained with silver, contrasting with the clear colour, large volume, and proliferative state of the surrounding connective tissue cells.

Within the graft, which was dark, one could distinguish a granular mass in which stood out, not genuine ellipsoids, but black and irregular precipitates, and brown relics or granular series which were axons in course of autolysis. The irregular aspect of the tissue, which was full of vacuoles with fatty remnants, nowise resembled the degenerative process of ordinary grafts. On the edges of the graft, as well as in some of its superficial portions, one found granular cells which were replete with lipoid material. We were here doubtless dealing with migratory leucocytes, arising from the host and destined to destroy the graft. Finally, although a few sprouts arising from the central stump came near the region of the transplant, none seemed to be attracted by it.

From the preceding experiments in grafting, and from many others which we cannot describe here, an important conclusion may be deduced : the trophic, attractive action, or whatever the action may be that the cells of Schwann of the graft or peripheral stump exercise, is closely associated with the vitality of these cells. This influence is increased in young and well nourished cells, as shown by experiments of reimplantation in young animals, and it diminishes and even disappears when one hinders nutritive metabolism or reduces the amount of available oxygen, as in the internal portions of the graft, etc. Accordingly, if from the bands of Büngner or endoneurium arises some trophic or neurotropic ferment, its action is felt only within a small radius, and it is promptly dissipated. It must, therefore, be constantly renewed. It is only on this condition that it can accumulate in the scar and in the paths which are preferred by the sprouts, in sufficient quantity to stimulate effectively the assimilation and growth of the newly-formed axons.

Another result, also very important, of the experiments in grafting, is the proof that under favourable conditions the graft exercises a neurotropic action which is almost as efficient as that of the peripheral stump of cut nerves. Thanks to this influence, the transplanted nerve is advantageously substituted for the long scar, and it thus markedly reduces the time required before the sprouts attack the stump in question. The hypothesis of Ranvier-Vanlair—growth of the sprouts in the path of least resistance—cannot explain these facts. For instance, one cannot understand, with their hypothesis, the rapid concentration of sprouts at the edge of the graft, the presence of curves of orientation to reach it when it becomes pushed out of place, and, finally, the frequent retrograde nervous reunions (Fig. 137, *f*).

Supposed negative neurotropic substances. (*a*) *Paralyzing action of the bacteria of pus.*—In connection with the study of the degeneration and regeneration of the spinal cord we shall examine in detail the question of the existence of negative neurotropic stimuli as accepted by Lugaro. We may say here, however, that, in the nervous reunion of the peripheral stump, nothing indicated the intervention of negative neurotropic substances, that is, of substances able to repel the clubs of growth or to cause them to take another direction. As a matter of fact, all the phenomena of paralysis, autotomy, retrogression, arrest, etc., of the axons are explicable, either by mechanical action or by the absence or diminution of the trophic and orienting substances, or else by the paralyzing influence of toxic substances.

A typical case of the lack of this stimulative action of the immediate environment of the clubs of growth is shown in infected wounds. Sometimes negligence in aseptic precautions during the operation of section of the sciatic nerve, especially in the rabbit, brings about contamination by the bacteria of pus (*Staphilococcus pyogenes aureus*, *Streptococcus pyogenes*, etc.). An abscess is thus formed near the scar, or in the scar itself. Its pus thickens and hardens for weeks, and is very slowly resorbed. Examination of the intercalary connective tissue of the scar between the two stumps often reveals, twelve, sixteen, and even twenty days after the operation, deteriorated sprouts of a pale colour, which seem to have been paralyzed in their growth. Those which are nearest to the abscess are always at a certain distance from it, as though they shrank from coming into contact with the bacteria or cells of the pus. The absence of gigantic clubs and of constant retrograde paths, seems to show that the sprouts do not grow away from the pus, but that they stop growing towards it, whether because we have here a region which is unfavourable from a nutritive point of view, or because of the lethal influence of toxic substances. We are thus dealing with a pathological state which arrests the push of growth and the ramification of the sprouts. On the other hand, one sees vigorous axons at a distance from the abscess, which are well grown and ready to attack the peripheral stump.

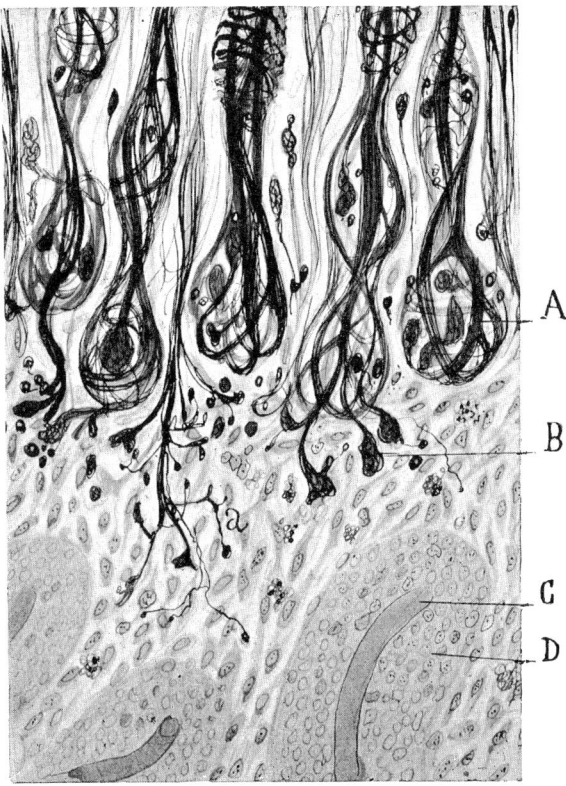

FIG. 145.—Piece of the central stump and scar of an almost adult rabbit in whose nerve wound had been placed a piece of cotton, saturated with concentrated methylene blue and then dried. The animal was killed ten days after the operation. Note the sparse growth of the sprouts and the swelling and enormous hypertrophy of the intratubal fibres. *A*, closed digestive chamber; *B*, emergent axons with large clubs; *D*, connective tissue closely pressed next to a cotton filament.

(*b*) *Influence of blood and of plasmatic exudates.*—We have already spoken on page 188 of the degeneration undergone by clubs that have accidentally fallen into a pool of blood. In general, the coagula and abundant serous exudates do not always destroy the sprouts; but they often paralyze their growth towards the peripheral stump. Coagulated blood or serofibrinous plasma undoubtedly are poor regions for the nutrition of the nerve fibres. When the coagulum, after a time, begins to be resorbed and is invaded by the fibroblasts, the sprouts grow out between the remnants of the blood clot. In this late growth the clubs rest upon the fibroblasts or escort the newly-formed capillaries. This seems to show that the embryonic fibroblast adds to the plasma some substance favourable to assimilation and growth of the sprouts issuing from the central stump. The leucocytes do not seem to attract the sprouts. In our very numerous preparations of nervous regeneration we have never observed a living cone of growth surrounded by leucocytes. It seems as though the latter gave out some substance that is unpropitious to axonic assimilation and growth.

(c) *Perturbatory action of the aniline dyes and of various substances of organic origin.*—Our experiments with various dyes such as neutral red, methylene blue, eosin, safranin, etc., and with analgesic substances, such as cocaine, chloral hydrate, morphine, etc., undertaken to show whether there exists some agent that energetically stimulates axonal growth, have given negative results. In general, the aniline dyes notably moderate or entirely suspend the growth of the axons which, twelve days after the section, have hardly crossed the borders of the central stump. Within this stump one can see large digestive chambers, bead-like in shape, in which has accumulated the entire protoplasmic mass of the sprouts which should have been used up in making ramifications and clubs. Fig. 145, A, shows this characteristically. In this case a piece of cotton saturated with methylene blue had been placed in the scar. One should repeat these experiments, however, and determine to what extent it is the cotton or gelatin used, and to what extent the soluble dye, that bring about the arrest and thickening of the fibres.

Experiments of section with interposition of indifferent foreign bodies in the wound.—We have already referred to the retarding effect of the interposition in the nerve wound of nodules of elder pith, hairs, etc. The same occurs with cotton, silk, small pieces of sponge, etc. In general, any foreign body is immediately surrounded by a colony of giant cells and of ordinary fibroblasts, arranged in a close wall which is almost impenetrable to the nerve clubs. It seems to us probable that this more or less perfect impenetrability does not depend only on the compactness of the tissues. It is to be expected that the fibroblasts differentiated around foreign bodies elaborate enzymes which, while they are favourable to the dissolution of certain organic products, are perhaps noxious to the nutrition of the axons. At any rate, the cellular walls around the foreign filaments notably narrow down the regions occupied by loose connective tissue, a tissue which is especially permeable to the sprouts. Under such conditions the nervous reunion of the peripheral stump is considerably

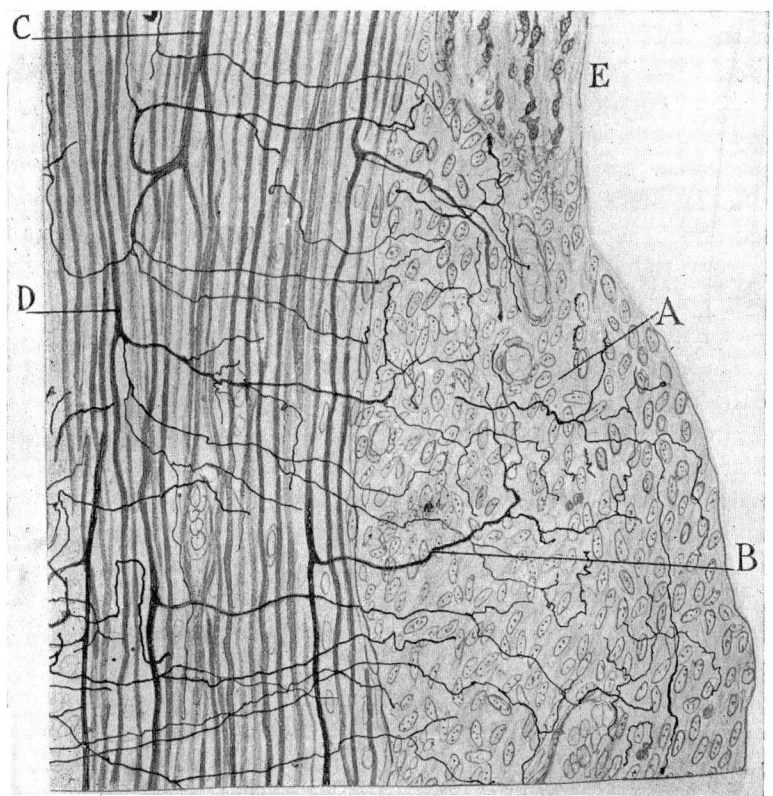

FIG. 146.—Sensory root of the lumbar spinal cord of an eight-day old cat. *A*, scar; *B*, collateral from a healthy axon; *E*, dura mater; *D*, axon which gives out thick branches ramified in a complicated way; *C*, large interstitial branch.

retarded. Thus in a cat fifteen days old, whose wound in the sciatic nerve contained a minute bundle of cotton full of plasma, the young fibres had not yet, after eighteen days, reached the peripheral stump, whereas, under ordinary conditions, and with a small scar, this stump is richly innervated after six or eight days.

Attractive effects of the scar.—We have alluded, in various passages of this work, to the facility that the newly-formed nerve fibres find for their growth and ramification in the scar itself. Is this facility the result of purely mechanical causes—*stereotropism* of Loeb, *odogenesis* of Dustin—or does it imply some trophic and stimulative action of the scar on the axon, comparable, although on a lower scale, to the influence of the peripheral stump on the sprouts ?

Without pretending to offer a final solution of this question, we shall cite an example that tells in favour of the latter hypothesis.

The animal in question was a cat eight days old, upon whose spinal cord, in a longitudinal direction, had been inflicted three wounds. These wounds were entirely separate from the roots ; the three connective scars touched the latter only very slightly. The animal was autopsied four days after the operation.

Under a low power one saw that each scar had a neuroma which arose from the nearest healthy sensory root, and this neuroma appeared to be exclusively constituted of collaterals originating from sensory fibres in a state of formative turgidity. Here and there a few ramified terminal conductors might be discerned.

The branches issue nearly at right angles and penetrate into the cicatricial tissue, where they ramify abundantly (Fig. 146, *D*). The terminal arborization is exclusively distributed in the embryonic tissue. This and many other examples which we have not the space to give in detail here show that the chemical stimuli which arise in the embryonic connective tissue act on the axons, which are more or less excited by the adjacent contusions or wounds, and provoke in them the formation of collaterals that are capable of boring through the sheath of Schwann and the peri-radicular arachnoidal endothelium.

At first we had believed that a similar action could be brought to bear on perfectly normal fibres.[1] To-day we admit that the neurocladic stimuli act only on axons that are excited by mechanical commotions, compressions, wounds, and various chemical agents.

Bethe already had propounded the idea that the connective tissue cells are able to attract the nerve sprouts. But he believed, with his theory of auto-regeneration, that the neurotropic action operated to attract the fibres both of the central and of the peripheral stump. Dustin and O. Rossi, while adopting other points of view, also insisted on the favourable character of the cicatricial region for the arrival and growth of the sprouts.

[1] Cajal : " Algunos experimentos favorables á la hipótesis neurotrópica," *Trab. del Lab. de Invest. biol.*, tomo 8, 1910.

ADDITIONAL NOTE ON CHAPTER XVI

Since the above experiments were published, there have been many attempts at grafting on animals, almost always with the object of replacing in men wounded in the war, the pieces of nerve that had been destroyed, and of facilitating the nervous reunion of the peripheral stump. At the same time surgeons have carried out experiments in which tubular organs, or sutures, are placed between the central and peripheral stumps, with the object of excluding the deviated fibres arising from the former, and of guiding the principal current of sprouts towards its destination.

It was therefore important to determine whether pieces of nerve preserved *in vitro* or completely dead are still able to attract the newly-formed fibres of the central stump, in the same way as fresh nerves. With this object, Tello[1] made various experiments from which it appears that pieces of nerve preserved in the incubator at 37° C. and in an indifferent salt solution retain their vitality for three weeks, and may be reunited when they are inserted between the proximal and distal segments of a cut and resected sciatic nerve. Like Nageotte, Tello shows also that pieces of nerve preserved *in vitro* degenerate if they are placed in liquids containing some bivalent metal (Ringer's and Locke's solutions, etc.,) but do not do so if placed in a simple salt solution of 0·9 %. When the grafts are of living and fresh nerves, they may be functionally reunited, even if mortised, within the cerebral cortex.

Tello distinguishes, like Marinesco, between *cicatrisation* and *nervous reunion*. A graft may become united cicatricially to the tissues of the host, and yet not become functionally united. The most interesting point in these experiments is the proof that, after conservation for twenty-one days in the incubator, in a salt solution, the grafts still have their cells of Schwann alive, and are therefore able to attract the sprouts, subject to the condition that an end of the transplanted nerve be placed near the central stump of the host, and that there be no flexions or irregularities in the former. Suture favours the innervation of the graft. Tello explains the orientation of the sprouts as due to neurotropic influxes.

Nageotte[2] has made many experiments of grafting in the rabbit and other animals. The most important point in the numerous studies

[1] Tello: "Algunas experiencias de injertos nerviosos con nervios conservados *in vitro*," *Trab. del. Lab. de Invest. biol.*, t. 12, 1914.

[2] Nageotte: "Sur la possibilité d'utiliser dans la pratique chirurgicale les greffons de nerfs fixés par l'alcool; technique à employer," *C.R. Soc. biol.*, t. 80, décembre 1917.

See also his various communications to the *Société de Biologie de Paris* (1917-1918), where are given in detail the results of his numerous experiments, some of them done in collaboration with Mlle. Guyon.

of this investigator is that, paradoxical as it may seem, grafts that have been killed by preservation in alcohol can still be inervated. Thus, if one examines the grafts in the host after thirty-seven days one sees that the dead nerve fibres have disappeared and are replaced in part by *granular bodies*. The connective sheaths do *not disappear to be replaced*, but are repeopled by the cells of the host.

Dead grafts, made according to Nageotte's technique, have given good results in war wounds. Long believes that the intercalation of a nerve that has been sterilized in alcohol is the best procedure in treating great losses of substance in nerves.

As to Nageotte's theories concerning the origin of the orienting bands of the scar (central *neuroma* and peripheral *glioma*), which he supposes arise from both stumps, migrating until they touch, and also concerning the neuroglial character that he attributes to the cells of Schwann, and other no less transcendental theoretical suggestions, we lack the personal experience necessary to judge them.

Inspired by Harrison's studies, Edinger joins the ends of interrupted nerves by means of a cow's artery which is full of agar ; he notes that after a short time the axons from the central stump grow very much and terminate in balls within the tube. To ascertain the penetration of the fibres he used with advantage our technique of impregnation with reduced silver nitrate. Edinger believes that the intercalation of the arterial tube avoids the formation of large scars, which are the principal obstacle to the growth and orientation of the nerve sprouts. We may note that many years ago a similar method with various substances was already used by Vanlair.

Spielmeyer, and also Bielschowsky and Unger, have not observed great benefits from using Edinger's method. According to them the innervation of the peripheral stump fails owing to the difficulty of invasion of the agar by the orienting cells of Schwann. On the other hand, they obtain good results in man and animals by grafting human nerves preserved in a solution of boric acid with a few drops of formaldehyde. In order to encase the fibres they use a tube formed by the perispinal *dura mater* ; they thus arrange that the interval between the stumps becomes filled with newly-formed cells of Schwann, and that the new axons which are guided by them reach the peripheral segment. In a dog, whose sciatic nerve was cut and resected, movement in the posterior extremity was already partly re-established after five weeks. The large balls that were observed by ourselves, Perroncito, Marinesco, Edinger, etc., in young axons appear covered by cells of Schwann. Bielschowsky and Unger, in their experiments on grafting and the tube method in man also obtained good results.

On the other hand other authors, such for example as Quervain, show little enthusiasm about the suture method and grafting, when dealing with repair of the innervation in war wounds.

Many descriptions have been published of nervous trauma, from a clinical point of view, in man. One of the most interesting and documented is that of Ottorino Rossi.[1] We do not give a full bibliography of the literature that has appeared during the last ten years, in order not to depart from the essentially histopathological character of this work. We may, however, summarize the results obtained in man as well as in animals, with regard to nerve wounds and grafts, in the following propositions, which reflect the opinion of the majority of the investigators :

(*a*) The nearer together the nerve stumps and the smaller the scar (suture), the more rapidly does the innervation of the peripheral stump take place. The scar is always a source of deviation and disorientation of the sprouts.

(*b*) Homoiotransplantations give better results than heterotransplantations.

(*c*) Nerves killed by agents that alter them but little can be innervated, although tardily ; this is dependent upon their penetration by connective cells and an invasion by capillaries.

(*d*) The ideal graft is the peripheral stump, with bands of Büngner, newly taken from an operated animal, eight to fifteen days after the operation. The newly-formed fibres travel through it with an extraordinary speed, deviations and retrogressions being very much diminished. In order of effectiveness there then follow grafts of fresh nerves without bands of Büngner, and, finally, normal nerve segments which are preserved in a physiological salt solution under aseptic conditions (Tello).

(*e*) For a graft to be effective, a necessary condition is that it should be accepted by the host, forming one body with it. It is for this reason that nervous connexion does not occur in grafts killed by certain antiseptic substances, such as chloroform or sublimate, or by heat.

[1] Ottorino Rossi : *Osservazioni neurologiche sui lesioni del sistema nervoso di trauma di guerra*, Sasari, 1921.

XVI

GENERAL THEORETICAL INTERPRETATION OF THE PHENOMENA OF NERVOUS REGENERATION

Reactions caused in the nervous protoplasm by intrinsic or immanent conditions. —Continuous development, growth in a straight line, formative turgidity, growth along the initial direction, formation of the cone of growth, formation of new extensions, etc.—Reactions of the axon that are conditioned by its environment (mechanical, physical, and chemical stimuli).—Trophism and neurotropism.— Hypothesis of the neurobiones.—History of our knowledge of the laws of normal and pathological neurogenesis.

WE have shown at various times, in a fragmentary way, the mechanism by which the growth, orientation, and multiplication of the nerve sprouts are accomplished. We shall here collect all these various theories into a single doctrine. We shall include in this all the legitimate inferences that may be drawn from the study of normal neurogenesis and of pathological regeneration. This is permissible because the regenerative process of the nerves and central tracts interrupted by traumatic or toxic violence represents merely a repetition, under somewhat special environmental conditions, of the creative act of the embryonic neuronal appendices and nerve trunks. Nature favours unity and economy of procedure, and it repeats itself, always choosing identical means for the same ends.

The laws of neurogenesis are the convergent work of many investigators who laboured in the domain of normal development— Kupffer, His, Kölliker, ourselves, von Lenhossék, Retzius, Harrison, Held, etc.—and of many others who studied pathological degeneration and regeneration—Waller, Ranvier, Vanlair, Münzer, Stroebe, Bethe, Perroncito, ourselves, Marinesco, Nageotte, Tello, O. Rossi, Dustin, etc. We hope here to collect their achievements into an organic whole. We shall follow each law or empirical induction with a brief commentary or a critical allusion. At the end of this chapter, in connection with the historical review, we shall state and discuss the most outstanding theories concerning the mechanism of neurogenesis.

If we consider the character of the notions that we have acquired concerning nervous regeneration, we may note that they can be classified into two categories : (1) those which have to do with internal, immanent properties or tendencies of the neuronal protoplasm, acting in relative independence of their surroundings ; and (2) those which have to do with reactions of this protoplasm brought about by the mechanical or chemical conditions of the region traversed. As an abbreviation we shall designate these two groups of manifestations respectively : *intrinsic* and *extrinsic phenomena*.

Intrinsic or immanent phenomena of regeneration.—1. *Law of continuous growth*.—This law, formulated by His and other authors, has been called by Held *vis a tergo* and by Dustin *axonal turgescence*. It expresses the tendency of the axon to grow constantly in a longitudinal direction, through an incessant assimilation of protoplasmic material. This impulsion towards longitudinal growth is maintained with a certain constancy, as long as the surrounding conditions remain normal.

2. *Law of virtual growth in a straight line*.—Every recently-formed axon or branch tends to grow in a straight line and retains its initial direction, as long as it does not encounter mechanical obstacles or does not receive neurotropic or neurocladic impulses. This initial direction is marked in the neuroblasts by the position and orientation of the cone of growth, and in regenerating nerves by the direction of the axon itself and sheath of Schwann.

This law was formulated, with more or less precision, by His, Harrison, ourselves, and Held, and it constitutes a postulate which is comparable to the physical principle of inertia. To affirm that the axon tends to grow in a straight line amounts to saying that the material that is newly-assimilated by the terminal bud and axonic cortex—the neurobiones, neuroplasma, limiting or cortical mantle, etc.—indefinitely maintains the initial geometrical and architectural plan of the original nervous sprout. A necessary corollary of this law is to attribute to an external perturbatory action any change that has occurred in the path or in the individuality—ramification—of the axon.

3. *The longitudinal growth of nerve fibres is especially localized in their free ends, where the cone of growth is situated, a constant organ of the axon in embryos as well as in nerves undergoing pathological regeneration.*—This terminal intumescence, whose form varies to fit the interstices of the mesodermal elements, constitutes a protoplasmic segment, which is differentiated in a special way to facilitate the

assimilative process, create exploratory sprouts, and orient them suitably in space. To accomplish such functions the *cone of growth* enjoys a certain autonomy in the matter of nutrition, possesses great softness and plasticity, and is extremely sensitive to mechanical and chemical variations of its surroundings. The concept of amoeboidism of the embryonic axon, suggested some time ago by von Lenhossék and ourselves, and later developed by Harrison, is accurately applied only to this portion of the neurone, which is specially organized in view of the process of neoformation and growth. On this hypothesis the appendices that arise from the *cone* are comparable to the pseudopods of a leucocyte.

4. *Besides the potentiality of creating terminal cones, every stimulated axon also has the capacity to evolve along its path new branches, which arise at the level of a turgescent region, comparable, dynamically, to a cone of growth.*—Any stimulated region of non-medullated fibres gives rise to collateral sprouts ; but in medullated fibres the region that is particularly adapted to give rise to sprouts is that which coincides with the axonal widening near the discs of Ranvier. This region, especially open to irritation by the mechanical vibrations of the wounded or contused tube, has been designated by ourselves the *germinative zone* or *germinative muff*. Once the sprout has arisen in this turgescent region, it becomes crowned with a cone of growth of various shapes, such as a ring, a brush, a club, etc.

5. *The cone of growth possesses two important functions : to lengthen the conductor (longitudinal growth), and to create new nerve paths.*—These two functions alternate like the two phases of a rhythmic movement. The first phase, that of axonic lengthening, occurs in more or less straight fibres which are crowned by a fine bud, club, or lanceolate thickening, which circulates through regions that are free from serious obstacles, such as soft scars, the peripheral stump, etc. The second phase, which we have designated the *state of divisory irritation* or *turgescence,* and during which the new sprouts emerge, is characterized at first by the hypertrophy and irregularity of the terminal intumescence from which subsequently arise triangular, pale, and divergent pseudopods or appendices. Such exploratory prolongations, which are comparable to the basal spines of embryonic cones, lack terminal thickenings, seek out, as it were, the practicable regions, and are converted, once they are definitely oriented, into stable conductors. On the other hand, incipient conductors that have taken wrong paths are rapidly resorbed. During

this process of stimulation the *cone* is thus the seat of a double phenomenon of appendicular creation and atrophy, entirely similar to the double movement of expansion and retraction of the pseudopods of a leucocyte. The lengthening of the new fibres, the disappearance of the cone or protoplasmic germinal accumulation and, finally, the formation of fine clubs or terminal cones in each new outgrowth, marks the end of the phase of creation and the beginning of the phase of simple growth.

From the utilitarian point of view the appearance of small cones that are compact, bud-shaped, and as it were rounded by friction—axons growing slowly—seems to answer to three requirements : to slide easily over the resistant surfaces of the mesoderm ; to augment the mechanical efficiency of the end of the axon ; finally, to offer a large surface susceptible to stimulating and neurotropic substances. It is clear that these last inferences are merely more or less plausible conjectures.

6. *There is a constant relation, leaving out of account the initial calibre of the fibres, between the volume of the terminal bud and the speed of growth.*—As a general thesis one may affirm that the slower the growth of the sprouts the larger is the terminal intumescence. When the axon is paralyzed or arrested the club takes on a very large dimension, and ellipsoidal or rounded shapes.

7. *Other conditions being equal, the fibres are thinnest when they grow most rapidly.*—The fibres are fine while they grow in the peripheral stump, where growth is very rapid, but they are relatively thick when they grow across the scar. This law has some exceptions.

8. *The increase of calibre of the axon is a function of the entire fibre.*—While longitudinal growth seems to be specially localized in the terminal cone, which lengthens like the pseudopod of an amoeba, the transversal increment, or thickening, occurs simultaneously along the entire newly-formed axon. This growth in diameter continues long after the appearance of the medullary sheath.

9. *The rapidity of growth of the sprouts depends on the physical and chemical conditions of the region traversed.*—The growth is very rapid in the central and peripheral stumps—90 to 125 μ per hour—but it is slow in the scar—8 to 12 μ per hour, and almost *nil* in blood and inflammatory exudates. The speed of growth is greater in animals a few days old than in adults. In chick embryos of three days' incubation it approaches 10 μ per hour.

10. *The assimilation of materials that are indispensable to*

transversal and longitudinal growth constitutes a local process which is independent, up to a certain point, of the cells of origin.—The formation of the cone, its neurocladic process, the outgrowth of exploratory appendices, the neurofibrillar metamorphoses are primitive phenomena which occur as well in the central as in the peripheral stumps of cut nerves. But for these formations to become consolidated and to progress, the action of the trophic centre or nerve cell is indispensable from every point of view. For this reason the neoformations of the peripheral stump are ephemeral, while those of the central stump are stable. For a similar reason clubs that are segregated from the axonic sprouts rapidly perish, while retrograde and deviated fibres are conserved fairly well.

11. *The cell of Schwann is not necessary for the genesis and growth of the axons.*—This results from our neurogenic studies and the experiments of Harrison. It is only very late that the symbiotic relation is established between the *lemmoblast* (v. Lenhossék) and the new axon, a relation connected, it appears, with nutrition and protection.

12. *Dynamic character of the trophic influence.*—Although in the present state of knowledge one is unable to define the mechanism of the trophic action, the opinion of Heidenhain appears to tally with the facts. According to him the neuronal mass that carries the nuclei and the sheaths of Nissl acts on the sprouts, not by sending out a material substance or soluble enzyme, but by the propagation of a special impulse, different from the functional motor or sensory current, which he called the *histodynamic impulse.* Indications that this hypothesis is correct are found in our experiments of nerve ligature and section.

Heidenhain justly notes that if this dynamic influence were the same as the ordinary physiological current, one could not understand why nerves at rest do not degenerate, and why in embryos, before the conductive function is present, the peripheral stump degenerates after nerve interruptions.

Concerning the reality of this prefunctional degeneration there is much significance in the results of our experiments of section and traumatic inflammation of the cerebellum of recently born mammals— degeneration of the cells of Purkinje, pericellular baskets, axons of the white matter, etc.—as also in the results obtained by L. Forster after traumatism of the ganglia and spinal cord of pigeons a few days old. Like adult nerves, the peripheral stump of all embryonic axons fragments and is resorbed. The same occurs, as is well known, when one cuts the peripheral stump of a regenerated nerve, even though the young axons do not as yet reach the terminal regions, and so lack a normal physiological activity. We must also remember that in the central stump of a cut nerve the sensor fibres sprout as well as the motor, even though in the former the nervous impulse from the periphery is wanting, as the functional current is centripetal in sensory nerves, but centrifugal in motor nerves.

Finally, if the trophic action depended on the diffusion of some soluble substance, capable of circulating along the axon, the absence of this substance in the peripheral stump would manifest itself in the centrifugal degeneration of the latter. But, as we have stated, this degeneration is simultaneous along the entire course of the conductor, with a relative survival of the axonic protoplasm near the wound (agonal clubs sprouting from the edge of the peripheral stump).

It is very possible that from the point of view of the rôle of the soma there are differences between the embryonic and the adult nerve cells. Thus in normal neurogenesis the initial development of the axon occurs, as Harrison and Lewis believe, at the expense of the internal or immanent energy of the system, that is, of the energy in the body of the neuroblast—*auto-differentiation* of W. Roux—deriving little or no energy from the immediate environment. Under this aspect the embryonic nerve cell may be considered as a store-house of nutritional and histo-dynamic reserves.

Once the neuronal evolution is completed—in post-fetal regeneration —the growth and ramification of the axon would occur very largely at the expense, chemically, of the region traversed, the soma then limiting itself to its function as a histo-dynamic centre.

13. *Law of atrophy through disuse.*—Besides the trophism through the conservation of the continuity of the axon with the cell of origin, there exists another which depends on functional exercise. This trophic law, suggested by Marinesco and Lugaro, can be formulated as follows : Any newly-formed axon which, having reached the end of its evolution—medullation, etc.—has not been able to establish congruent anatomico-physiological relations with the terminal structures, such as sensory cutaneous organs, motor plates, etc., degenerates and is finally resorbed. In this way all the conductors that go outside the regenerative area disappear, that is, the arrested, deviated, and retrograde axons. A similar fate befalls the fibres that have reached their terminal points very late, when these terminal districts are completely innervated, or when, after a long

time, the cells with which these conductors should have established dynamic connections atrophy and die.

14. *The various acts of multiplication, degeneration, ravelling, dispersion and segregation or autotomy of the neurofibrils, described so far in this treatise, and many others that will be described in connection with the degeneration of axons of nerve centres, lead us to believe that in the neurofibrils of the nerve cells there are ultra-microscopical units, i.e., invisible granules, which have the fundamental attributes of living protoplasm.*—The principal physiological attributes of these units, which we have named *neurobiones*, would be : the capacity to reproduce by equal divisions and to form lineal chains and colonies ; the aptitude to migrate by changing histomeres (neurofibrils) or by creating new histomeres ; an extreme sensitiveness to physical agents, especially mechanical shocks and vibrations ; and, finally, a certain polarity, already assumed by Herbert Spencer for his hypothetical *physiological units*, and by means of which these corpuscles would attract each other reciprocally, forming groups of different dimensions and morphology. In order not to disturb the nerve wave, which probably travels along the interstitial liquid, and to facilitate the nutritive exchanges, the neurobional colonies form fibrils, reserving, in the axons as well as in the soma, continuous spaces full of neuroplasma. Finally, even though the *neurobione* is nourished *in loco* and multiplies independently of the cells of origin, the well-being of its colonies requires the co-operation of dynamic stimuli originating in the soma.

Later on, when we study the transformations of the reticulum of nerve cells in the cerebrum, cerebellum, and spinal cord, as well as the process of autotomy of the central axons, we shall adduce other facts tending to prove the theory of the *neurobiones*—the *protomeres* of Heidenhain.

Reactional phenomena caused by extrinsic conditions, that is to say, conditions of the regions traversed by the nerve sprouts.—The reactions of the axonic protoplasm due to mechanical and chemical variations of its environment are very numerous. We have referred to all of them, so that we shall simply briefly summarize the principal categories.

1. *In presence of a mechanical obstacle or a neurotropic stimulus the nerve fibre does not deviate abruptly, forming, for example, a right or obtuse angle, but it adopts a parabolic direction.*—This direction is a kind of diagonal between the initial rectilinear impulse and the

direction of resistance of the disturbing agent. A similar law holds for the emission of branches. Before adopting their definitive orientation all nerve branches describe parabolic diagonals between the line of internal impulsion of the shoot and that of the external trophic or mechanical influence.

2. *The newly-formed nerve fibres have a tendency to adhere to obstacles*, and especially to those which have smooth surfaces, along which they slide rapidly, and around which they sometimes trace complicated turns. This *adhesive attraction*, noted by ourselves and Dustin, is nothing else than *stereotropism*, observed some time ago by L. Loeb in the growth of transplanted pathological cells, and by Harrison and his pupils in the growing nerve fibres of embryos in tissue cultures.

This strange propensity of the nerve sprouts to adhere to supports or pre-established paths constitutes in many cases a serious resistance to the trophic and orienting influences and is a frequent cause of arrests and deviations.

3. *Law of reciprocal homotropism.*[1]—We have given this name to the property that nerve sprouts possess of congregating in bundles, as though they attracted each other, in order to pass, with the greatest economy of effort through the mesodermal tissue and to insinuate themselves in the sheaths of the peripheral stump. This tendency to fibrillar symbiosis or aggregation also explains the fasciculated disposition adopted by the spinal roots from the moment of their first appearance. This longitudinal adhesion is not, however, very vigorous, since it is easily overcome in presence of mechanical obstacles or strong neurotropic resources.

4. *The neurocladic process, or process of production of collateral or terminal branches is always caused by external mechanical or chemical conditions.*—These stimuli, in adult medullated axons of the central stump, act ordinarily on the *germinal zones* or *muffs*. In non-medullated sprouts the neurocladic stimulus acts on the terminal cone and neighbouring regions.

As a general thesis, but with exceptions, one can affirm that ramification due to mechanical causes preponderates in the central stump and scar, and neurocladism due to chemical stimuli at the edge and within the peripheral stump, and in the terminal nervous structures. In some cases stereotropism seems also to play a part,

[1] Cajal: "Nouvelles observations sur l'évolution des neuroblastes," etc. *Anat. Anzeiger*, Bd. 32, 1908.

as in the ravelling of the fibrils of the sprout and their adherence to the membrane of Schwann, the clinging of a cone to some supporting structure while it is receiving neurotropic impulses from another side, etc.

5. *The act of axonic growth and the emission of branches imply complex processes of organization of the membrane, the neuroplasma, and the neurofibrillar framework.*—The neuroplasma must be conceived, not as an inert liquid, but as a complex protoplasmic organ, full of special invisible physiological units.

The part played, in the production of the sprouts, by *osmotic pressure* (Nageotte) or the local lowering of surface tension, has not as yet been determined. It nevertheless appears that these physical changes, together with the chemical phenomena on which they depend, such as the oxidizing action of the environment, etc., are the initial conditions that bring about the phenomenon of co-ordinated organization of all the axonic factors, which essentially constitutes the act of neoformation.

6. *When the mechanical obstacle that presents itself before a club of growth is insuperable, the axon often reacts by segregating or eliminating the club (nerve autotomy).*—In presence of an obstacle the axon may behave in one of three ways : it may create a large club, which becomes definitely arrested ; it may emit one or several exploratory branches which surmount the obstacle, and the ball or ring is then after a time resorbed ; finally, it may segregate or autotomize the club, which rapidly degenerates. By analogy with the well-known phenomenon of *autotomy* of the legs of certain Crustaceans, we have designated this curious protoplasmic elimination *neurofibrillar autotomy*. The production of free balls shows, we may add, that when the neurone is in conflict with its environment, it makes a purely utilitarian choice : between frustrating its destiny and sacrificing a piece of its own substance it chooses, naturally, the lesser of the two evils. Autotomy, as we shall show in the second volume of this work, is a very frequent phenomenon in both stumps of the interrupted nerve fibres of the cerebrum and cerebellum.[1]

7. *The detentions that occur during the growth of the sprouts are shown by the presence along them of varicosities or swollen portions, that is, by remnants of clubs in process of resorption.*—The number of

[1] Cajal : " Los fenómenos precoces de la degeneración traumática de los cilindrosejes del cerebro," etc., *Trab. del Lab. de Invest. biol.*, tomo 9, 1911.

forced arrests and of periods of easy progression correspond, respectively, to the number of varicosities and their intervals.

8. *All gigantic clubs that are definitely arrested or autotomized degenerate.*—This process of necrosis begins at the periphery of the club and progressively gains the centre, whose neurobiones persist for a shorter or longer time.

9. *The nervous reunion of the peripheral stump and restoration, without physiological errors, of the terminal nerve structures, are the combined effect of three conditions: the neurotropic action of the sheaths of Schwann and terminal structures; the mechanical guidance of the sprouts along the old sheaths; and, finally, the superproduction of fibres, in order to insure the arrival of some of them at the peripheral motor or sensory regions.*—Of all these conditions the most essential, especially as regards the reconstruction of the terminal apparatus, is the *trophism* or *neurotropism* of the peripheral stump, motor plates, and sensory structures.

10. *The orienting chemical stimuli are probably, so far as their selective power is concerned, both generic and specific.*—The attractive substance elaborated by the embryonic connective cells and by the cells of Schwann of the peripheral stump—the *apotrophic* cells of Marinesco—have a generic character, acting without distinction on all sprouts; while the attractive substances given out by the *spindles of Kühne, motor plates, cutaneous sensory structures*, etc., have a specific character, acting only on certain functional categories of regenerated axons. These specific stimuli are both neurotropic and neurocladic. The terminal arborization of the motor plate and the final bundle of Meissner's corpuscle represent, in normal ontogeny as well as in pathological regeneration, the last neurocladic effect of specific stimuli.

The specific stimuli of the orientation of sprouts are very numerous in the embryonic period. At that period the most active appear to be those elaborated by the cells of the myotome, by primordial connective elements, and by sensory epithelia and neurones that are forming dendrites.

Once the ontogenetic evolution is ended, the trophic and neurotropic sources appear to be especially localized in the *cells of Schwann* of the nerves—the *apotrophic* cells of Marinesco, and the *lemmoblasts* of v. Lenhossék, in the substance of degenerated motor plates, in the *satellite cells* of the sensory ganglion cells, in the elements of the *terminal sensory structures* such as the sheaths of Kühne, the cells of Meissner, etc., and, finally, in the *embryonic connective tissue.*

11. *The neurotropic stimulus acts as a ferment or enzyme, provoking protoplasmic assimilation.*—While in the present state of knowledge we cannot penetrate the mechanism of the neurotropic action, an analysis of all the facts of nervous reunion known to us suggests the hypothesis that the orienting agent of the sprouts does not operate through attraction, as many have supposed, but by creating a region that is favourable, eminently trophic, and stimulative of the assimilation and growth of the newly-formed axons. No doubt the axons do not need, in order to grow longitudinally and transversely, to be stimulated by these agents. But without them this growth has not the intensity shown by fibres that are stimulated, and at last it definitely ceases, as in the degeneration of arrested and deviated fibres.

To this new conception of the neurotropic agent must be added a few complementary hypotheses in order to explain all or the majority of the facts of regeneration.

12. From the point of view of their action on the nerve sprouts the substances diffused in the interstices of the mesoderm may be distinguished as follows : (1) Those which are *active* or *stimulating,* that is, those which stimulate the process of assimilation, growth, and ramification of the nervous protoplasm ; (2) *moderating substances*; (3) *indifferent substances*; (4) *toxic or paralyzing substances.*

As stated above, the *active substances* are elaborated by the cells of Schwann, terminal nervous structures, etc. The embryonic connective elements seem to elaborate them on a lesser scale. Tello believes that the fusiform cells of the endoneurium have a similar activity.

One of the attributes of these *active enzymes* is their rapid change once they are liberated in the interstitial plasmas. As a consequence of the instability of these substances, their existence is intimately associated with the life and activity of the secretory cell, the cell of Schwann.

The *indifferent substances* are probably the majority of colloids found in the plasmas, the blood, and the aseptic inflammatory exudates. On this point, however, we lack sufficient data.

The *paralyzing substances* accompany pus. Microbial toxins and various aniline dyes act perhaps in a similar way, although we know nothing precise concerning the mechanism of the action of these products.

The *moderating substances* are perhaps the product of the same nerve fibres and the result of oxidations or other chemical reactions occurring in the axonic protoplasm during the process of growth and ramification. Under ordinary conditions these moderating substances—products of catabolism—are perhaps rapidly eliminated and therefore do not hinder the axonic growth and ramification. But when the neoformation is very active, assuming a very impetuous character (the phase of divisory amoeboidism), these substances are not quickly eliminated, and one might thus explain the state of relative rest that follows neurocladic super-activity. This relative inhibition of growth may perhaps also be compared to the moderation or cessation of ordinary fermentations when there is an excess of the end-products.

The preceding hypotheses explain fairly satisfactorily the main difficulties of the theory of neurotropism. Among them we may mention the following :

(a) *Rapid growth of the axon through the peripheral stump.*—The progression of the axons in the bands of Büngner is somewhat difficult to understand on the chemotropic hypothesis, according to which, when an axon finds attractive substances, it combines with them, creating bodies that are without stimulative action. Dustin states : " If the cells of Schwann give out neurotropic principles, the young axon, on reaching each one of them, should be detained, since the attracting substance or material would rapidly be saturated." According to the old neurotropic conception, the stimuli given out by the bands of Büngner may serve only to attract the axons ; the latter, once saturated, then grow within the sheaths by virtue of the assimilative *vis a tergo*. Leaving aside this possible explanation of the continuity of axonic growth, there is no doubt that, with the enzyme hypothesis, the above difficulty disappears, since the fibres that penetrate into the bands or their interstices live in a region rich in agents that stimulate assimilation and growth, agents that do not combine with, and therefore are not neutralized by, the receptor substances of the nervous protoplasm.

(b) *Difficulties experienced by the nerve fibres in crossing membranes.* —We have seen that all degenerated nerves are innervated through their end, and not through the neurilemma. Mechanical factors doubtless are involved in this ; but there are cases in which this lack of capacity seems to depend on the retention of stimuli. We may remember the negative results in attempted nervous reunion of pieces of nerve that were placed on undamaged nerves (Lugaro, Marinesco, Dustin). This resistance is easily understood if the neurocladic agents are enzymes, which, as is well known, are little or not at all dialysable.

(c) *Temperature, when it rises, lends more activity to regeneration* (Deineka).—This is a very natural fact if the substance that activates the growth of the sprouts is an enzyme.

(d) *Neurotropic incapacity or weakness of sick or dead cells of Schwann.* The reader will recall the difficulty with which the nervous reunion of crushed and dead nerves is effected. This fact bears out the view that the neurotropic material is an enzyme segregated by the living cells, instead of a product of the decomposition or disintegration of the nervous tissue.

(e) *Difficulty experienced by the axons in orienting themselves at a distance from the peripheral stump or living grafts.*—This observation suggests the idea that either the orienting enzymes have only a small diffusive power, or else that a short time after they are given out they are broken down and dissipated by the action of the environment.

(f) *Extreme velocity of growth of the sprouts within the sheaths*, which appear like inexhaustible trophic regions.

(g) *Exceptional capacity of the bands of Büngner to attract, lodge, and feed numerous sprouts* (20 or more), which rapidly thicken, and acquire nuclei and a medullary sheath.

13. *It is doubtful whether there exists a negative neurotropism* as Lugaro, Nageotte, and Marinesco have supposed for certain special cases. The examples of relative incapacity of the new nerve fibres to invade the spinal cord (Lugaro); the repulse of the nerve sprouts by the sensory neurones (Nageotte), and, in general, by their cell of origin—negative autotropism; their paralysis in the presence of blood and serous exudates, etc., etc., can be explained simply by assuming the absence in such regions of positive neurotropic substances or the presence of paralyzing materials. The sudden retrogressions of young sensory fibres at the edges of transplanted ganglia or in the stump of interrupted sensory roots may be accounted for in the same way. This point requires further investigation.

14. *Several neurotropic currents may act simultaneously on the same cone of growth.*—The axon is then always deflected in the direction of the most powerful current. The frequent retrogressions of new intratubal fibres on reaching the scar; the predilection shown by wandering fibres for the peripheral stump, even though they are in

the scar, which has a great neurotropic activity; etc., are phenomena that may be explained by the influence of embryonic cells of Schwann predominating over that of connective tissue cells.

15. *The membranes or tissues of indifferent neurotropism have a positive influence on the growth and orientation of young axons.*—Some sheaths, like that of Schwann, the neurilemma, the laminose sheath of nerve fascicles, the perimedullar membrane, are screens that are almost entirely impermeable to neurotropic and neurocladic currents. It is owing to them that, when a source of neurotropic substances is at hand, adult fibres or fibres in the phase of erethism are retained in the corresponding nerve or centre. It is they also that segregate the neurotropic substances, more or less impeding or moderating their diffusion and creating something akin to isolated regions of cultivation of the nerve sprouts. In some cases the mechanical obstacles, like the pillars of a bridge or the prow of a vessel, have the effect of dividing the neurotropic currents. The cone, solicited in two different directions, divides. This would explain the bifurcations that occur in front of superable mechanical obstacles such as fat cells, accumulations of disintegrated myelin of the peripheral stump, muscle fibres, etc.

HISTORY OF THE EXPLANATORY THEORIES OF NORMAL AND PATHOLOGICAL NEUROGENESIS.—The mechanism of normal growth (neurogenesis) and pathological growth (regeneration) of the nerves has been the subject, since the time of Kupffer, Hensen, Kölliker, and His, of numerous observations and speculations.

As we have described in the preceding paragraphs the well determined laws and the probable hypotheses relating to neurogenesis, it remains for us here to set out, in chronological order, the chief theories that lead to the explanation on physico-chemical grounds of this very important process. Nearly all the hypotheses that have been put forward concern both normal and pathological regeneration. There are some, however, like that of Forssman, which are easily applicable only to pathological conditions.

The explanations offered by the various authors revolve around four conceptions which we shall briefly designate as: (1) *Theory of pre-established paths.* (2) *Mechanical theory—or theory of growth along the path of least resistance.* (3) *Chain or catenary theory of the polygenists.* (4) *Theory of neurotropism, or the growth by virtue of the orienting action of chemical stimuli.* Each of these theories contains a variable number of explanatory principles.

1. *Theory of pre-established paths.*—This theory has two principal

variations, according to whether the paths are conceived as intercellular spaces or interstices, or as intracellular conduits.

(a) *Theory of His concerning pre-established intercellular paths.*— Leaving aside the highly speculative conception of Held, we may say that the first explanation of the normal neurogenic process, based on precise objective facts, is due to His.[1] This famous embryologist, to whom the science of ontogeny owes so much, subordinated the growth and orientation of the axons in the embryo, and therefore the formation of the nerves, to these two conditions : (1) *Continuous growth* by the internal impulsion of the nervous protoplasm ; this is immanent and depends on the intimate organization of the cell. (2) *The pre-existence in the mesoderm of established interstitial paths*, such as the perimedullar membrane, mesodermal fibrous structures, interstices between the connective tissue cells, etc. ; this is an extrinsic condition. In the latter condition the paths are so established that they conduct the axons, without error or deviation, from their origin in the spinal cord and sensory ganglia to the terminal structures.

(b) *Held's hypothesis of intracellular paths.*—According to Held,[2] who has published important studies on normal neurogenesis (made by the method of reduced silver nitrate, with fixation in pyridine), the embryonic axons result from the growth of a special zone, called *fibrillogenous* zone, of the neuroblast or primordial nerve cell. Once the medullar membrane is crossed, the growth of the fibres towards the terminal structures is determined mainly by two principles : the *vis a tergo*, that is, the internal impulsion and incessant growth of the neurofibrils of the nerve sprout (His and Ranvier) ; and the existence in the mesoderm, along the entire path which the fibres must follow, of a system of conducting cells (*Leitzellen*), in the interior of which the neurofibrils grow with no possible loss or deviation. Differing thus from His, and reviving an old idea of Hensen, Held believes that the sprout does not progress freely, but is ensheathed in a system of mesodermal tubes, which are organized at an early stage, by virtue of the orientation and anastomosis of embryonic connective tissue cells. Held mentions besides two accessory principles : that of the *lengthening of the paths* (*Wegstrecke*) and the *elective capacity of the axon* (*Auswahl*).

[1] W. His : " Die Neuroblasten und deren Entstehung im embryonalen Mark," *Abhand. d. math. phys. Klass. des König. Gesellsch. d. Wissensch.*, Bd. XV, 1889-90.

[2] Held : " Die Entstehung der Neurofibrillen," *Neurol. Centralbl.*, Aug., 1905.
Idem : " Zur Histogenese der Nervenleitung," *Verhandl. d. Anat. Gesellsch.*, *X Versamml. zu Rostock*, 1-5 Juni, 1906.
Idem : " Die Entwicklung des Nervengewebes bei den Wirbelthieren," J. A. Barth, Ed. Leipzig, 1909.

(c) *Dustin's hypothesis of odogenesis.*—The theory of Held, refuted by the investigations of Harrison, ourselves, and many other authors, has found little favour among anatomo-pathologists. Dustin,[1] however, in his studies on nervous regeneration, seems to be inspired by Held's doctrine, although with reserves and modifications that make his theory akin to that of the pre-established intercellular paths of His. According to Dustin, in pathological regeneration the embryonic connective tissue cells become oriented in such a way that the cones of growth which are insinuated in their interstices necessarily reach the sheaths of the peripheral stump. Dustin has called this property, by which embryonic connective tissue cells reserve orienting spaces and easy paths between the two stumps, central and peripheral, *odogenesis*. He believes that the process of orientation has in large part, if not exclusively, a mechanical character, the mere result of the growth of the axon in the path of least resistance.

The theory of Dustin is completed by his belief in the *turgescence* of the terminal bud and nerve sprout, in combination with *tactile adhesion* (stereotropism of Loeb and Harrison) that is, with the tendency possessed by the fibres to adhere to and grow on solid bodies, such as connective tissue cells, blood-vessels, and membranes. The combination of these facts form the neurogenetic theory of Dustin, and explains, according to him, all the phenomena shown by regenerating nerves.

In the hypotheses of His, Held, and Dustin there are certain positive elements explanatory of the mechanism of axonic growth, of which we have made frequent use. Such are : *Continuous growth* (law of His and Ranvier, named *vis a tergo* by Held), the *mechanical influence* of the region traversed, the *stereotropism* of Loeb or *tactile adhesion*, etc. But these theories also comprise suppositions that are devoid of objective verification or directly in conflict with observed facts. Although we have already refuted these suppositions in various chapters of this work, we may record here some of the arguments against them : (1) The intracellular conduits of Held are visible neither in the mesoderm of the embryo nor in the intermediate cicatricial tissue of cut nerves. (2) The tissue cultures *in vitro*, in a medium of plasma, made by Harrison and his pupils, show the superfluity and uselessness of such conduits, since the cones of growth advance with perfect sureness across the plasma. (3) As we have observed, in chick embryos the axons can travel freely across the interstitial plasma, and in certain pathological cases they can cross the ependymal liquid without perishing. (4) The observations of Perroncito and our own have shown the capacity

---

[1] Dustin : " Le rôle des tropismes et de l'odogenèse dans la régénération du système nerveux," *Arch. de. Biol.*, tome 25, 1910.

possessed by newly-formed axons of crossing exudates and blood itself. (5) It is not true that the connective tissue cells of the scar reserve interstices that are constantly oriented towards the peripheral stump; these cells extend their branches in all directions, and the sprouts often cross them perpendicularly. (6) The sheaths and interstices of the peripheral stump, far from being, as Dustin and Stroebe believe, an easy path for the sprouts, offer mechanical obstacles greater than those of the scar—such as the complete obstruction of the bands of Büngner, both at their entrance and along their length; nevertheless the cones of growth easily penetrate them and travel in them with great rapidity. (7) The above-cited theories do not explain all the strange facts of nervous reunion that suggest the neurotropic process (see the three preceding chapters). (8) There exist cicatricial masses which join the intermediate region between cut nerves and the skin, but in this region of embryonic tissues the axons rarely lose themselves. (9) Finally, in the theoretical domain, one can make the same objection to Dustin as to Held, that instead of resolving the problem, they displace it and transform it into a much harder one, as follows: In virtue of what conditions do the embryonic connective tissue cells and the cells of the bands of Büngner at the edge of the peripheral stump so arrange themselves that their interstices are precisely the most convenient paths for the orientation of the new fibres and for their arrival without error at the peripheral terminal structures?

2. *Mechanical theory, or theory of growth along the path of least resistance.*—This was first put forward by Ranvier,[1] and it has been adopted by several authors, especially by Vanlair and Stroebe. Ranvier in a communication to the *Académie des Sciences* in 1879, stated, as a conclusion from his investigations on regeneration that "the nerve branches, following a plan imposed by their organization, have a tendency continually to grow towards the periphery without being detained in their growth except by the obstacles in the way, much like the roots of plants in the earth." Vanlair [2] also professed similar ideas. He believed that the nerve sprouts grow blindly across the scar and peripheral stump, taking advantage of the interstices of the cells and membranes. He stated: "The direction of the newly-formed fibres is determined solely by the physical state of the region traversed" ... "it is not the organic conditions, but the mechanical influences that regulate the growth of the peripheral nervous tissue." Stroebe also

[1] Ranvier: *Compt. Rend. Acad. Sciences*, 1879.
 Idem: *Leçons sur l'histologie du système nerveux*, vol. 2, Paris, 1878.

[2] Vanlair: "Nouvelles recherches expérimentales sur la régénération des nerfs," *Archiv. de Biol.*, 1885.

defends this conception of Ranvier-Vanlair of growth along the path of least resistance. According to this doctrine the terminal structures are invaded by the sprouts, thanks to the special organization of the peripheral stump, in whose interior exist empty tubes, that is, paths of least resistance, from the scar to the muscles and skin. Since arrival from the central stump is merely a question of chance, most of the fibres lose themselves on the way, taking various, and even retrograde, paths (Vanlair). As a compensation superfluous conductors are created in great abundance.

The *mechanical theory* was refuted a long time ago by Forssman.[1] He carried out ingenious experiments of flexion or concealment of nerves in celloidin tubes, in order to impede the arrival of the sprouts at the peripheral stump, the latter becoming transformed into the path of greatest resistance. Nevertheless the new axons constantly reached their goal.

Apart from these experiments on difficult nervous reunion, repeated by Bethe, Lugaro, Marinesco, ourselves, etc., the theory in question is insufficient to explain, among other phenomena, the following : (*a*) The seemingly intentional turns of sprouts to reach the edge of transplanted nerves or the degenerated fascicles of the same nerve ; (*b*) the retrograde nervous reunion of medullary roots by wandering motor or sensory roots ; (*c*) the normal innervation of the peripheral stump which, as we have often stated, constitutes for the sprouts, especially during the first two weeks, the path of greatest resistance ; (*d*) the nervous reunion of nerves transplanted under the skin ; (*e*) the unerring innervation of degenerated motor plates ; (*f*) the facts of stimulation of central axons in the brain and spinal cord, and their penetration into grafted nerve segments, in Tello's experiments, etc.

Among the recent partisans of the mechanical theory, subject to important additions and reserves, one may include Harrison and Heidenhain.

(*a*) *Theory of Harrison.*—This American scientist,[2] whose interesting experiments on neurogenesis *in vitro* of embryonic amphibian tissues afford an absolute refutation not only of the polygenist doctrine, but

[1] Forssman : " Zur Kenntniss des Neurotropismus," *Ziegler's Beit. zur pathol. Anat.*, etc., Bd. 27, 1900.

[2] Harrison : " Further experiments on the development of peripheral nerves," *Amer. Journ. of Anat.*, vol. 5, 1906.

See especially : "The outgrowth of the nerve fibre as a mode of protoplasmic movement," *Jour. Exp. Zool.*, vol. 9, 1910.

" The cultivation of tissues in extraneous media as a method of morphogenetic study," *Anat. Record*, vol. 6, 1912.

also of that of pre-established paths, attributes normal neurogenesis to the following factors :

1. Initial orientation of the neuroblast and growth in the direction of the shortest path towards the periphery.

2. Continuous growth (His and Ranvier), that is, constant increment by virtue of the impulsion of forces immanent in the cell, independently of the environment, and without external stimuli.

3. Internal tendency, notwithstanding the accidental or natural difficulties of the path, to grow in a special direction and to reach determined organs.

4. Stereotropism of L. Loeb,[1] that is, the property of the sprouts to adapt themselves to the compact cells, fibres, or septa found along their path. Without mechanical supports the fibres are incapable of growing, except for very short distances.

A similar condition, studied by Dustin and ourselves in pathological regeneration, has been analyzed *in vivo* by Harrison, thanks to his method of growing the nervous tissue in lymph, *in vitro*. In the cultures the supports are the fibrin threads. Marinesco has confirmed this in his cultures of mammalian ganglia in plasma.[2]

5. Harrison also indicates, as a condition of neurogenesis, *neurotropism*. But he believes that this factor is of value only in the last stage of growth of the sprouts. He thus believes in the specific materials segregated by the tissues in which the terminal structures are differentiated. He does not speak, *nominatim*, of a neurotropic action, but of *specific reactions* between the axons and the tissues, somewhat like that of the egg on the spermatozoön.

6. The innervation of the mesoderm and of other regions of the embryo passes through two phases : at first isolated, irresolute fibres arise from the spinal cord ; these were designated by Harrison *exploratory fibres*—literally path-finders ; later these are joined by the rearguard of the sprouts which, owing to the growth of the tissues, have to traverse a larger space.

7. Finally, he mentions yet another neurogenetic factor represented

---

[1] L. Loeb : *Archiv. f. Entwick.-mech.*, Bd. 6, 1897, and Bd. 13, 1902.

Idem : "Growth of tissues in culture media," etc., *Anat. Record*, vol. 6, 1912.

[2] Mar. Lewis has seen sympathetic fibres grow freely in pure salt solutions. This seems to contradict the absolute value of stereotropism. There nevertheless remains the possibility that the cones of growth advance by applying themselves to the surface of the cover-glass.

See M. Lewis and W. H. Lewis : "The cultivation of tissues from chick embryos in solutions of Na Cl, Ca Cl_2, K Cl, and Na H CO_3," *Anat. Record*, vol. 5, 1911.

by certain complicated nerve plexuses, which are situated in the peripheral regions, such as the skin of amphibians and fishes, etc. From these plexuses, which arise in amphibians from the *dorsal cells* or *Rohon-Beard cells*, are differentiated the branches that give rise to the terminal sensory arborization.

The ideas of Harrison agree for the greater part with the observed facts, and are perfectly applicable to normal neurogenesis as well as to nervous regeneration. In the course of this work, along with the general theoretical interpretation described in the preceding pages, we have noted the decisive influence exerted, among other conditions, in the nervous reunion of the peripheral stump, by continuous growth in a straight line, stereotropism, the formation of exploratory fibres, the organization of pre-terminal plexuses, etc.

Some of these principles are formulated by Harrison in terms that are too absolute, as in the case of growth in a straight line, which must be estimated as a theoretical postulate, somewhat like an ideal condition which is never realized. A very brief examination of a section of the spinal cord of very young embryos, such as chick embryos from the second to the third day, shows that the exploratory axons fold back before emerging from the base of the spinal cord, and that once they have reached the mesoderm they follow flexuose courses, often describing complicated turns. Once the region of the future ganglia is crossed, many fibres bend abruptly backwards to form the posterior branch of the rachideal pair. After three and a half days, the majority of these precursory axons fold back, sliding in an antero-posterior direction along the *muscular plate*. The assertions of Harrison must be attributed to the technique that he used. We must not forget that his experiments are essentially analytical. In them the natural medium is suppressed, or, to put it better, another is substituted which is homogeneous and devoid of neurotropic influence. Naturally, under such conditions, there is no reason why growing fibres should deviate from the straight line and the shortest path.

Some of the neurogenic factors mentioned by Harrison seem to us highly doubtful; for instance, neuronal morphological pre-determination and axonic growth along pre-established directions to reach the peripheral tissues. Such principles are relegated to the category of untenable hypotheses by the experiments of ganglionar transplantation of Nageotte, Marinesco and Minea, ourselves, etc., by the observations concerning the transformation of neuronal morphology in traumatized centres (Cajal, H. Rossi, Marinesco), and by the infinite varieties in quantity and orientation that the least obstacle provokes in cut nerves. Besides, the admission of morphological pre-determinations and of internal tendencies destined to create, without the concurrent aid of the immediate environment, congruent connections between axons and tissues, is opposed to the mechanistic spirit of modern science, according to which any explanation consists in subordinating the facts to physico-chemical conditions. It leads us, without any advantage for the comprehension of the phenomena, to the dangerous position of metaphysical entities. We find more useful and plausible, for scientific comprehension, these two other neurogenetic factors, of which Harrison made ingenious use : the intervention of exploratory fibres and that of pre-terminal nerve plexuses. The *exploratory fibres* actually exist. We had seen them [1] some time ago in developing nerve centres, although we attributed to them no special physiological function ; v. Lenhossék and Held also had seen them but gave them no special designation. These conductors are, of course, very common in pathological regeneration. We have often mentioned them when speaking of the neoformative reactions of deviated or arrested clubs.

The name of *exploratory fibres* or *path-finders* has such an anthropomorphic and teleological connotation that it would be desirable to use another word—*precursors*, for example. As a matter of fact, in the embryo as well as in the scar of cut nerves these conductors are nothing else than precociously formed sprouts which grow out singly right into the mesoderm. The rest of the axons join them, so far as their position and orientation are fixed by the reception of neurotropic stimuli, by virtue of stereotropism or of the property that we have called reciprocal neurotropism.

The pre-terminal plexuses of the embryo also constitute an actual entity, discovered by ourselves [2] and Bardeen in the muscles, and seen in the skin by O. Schültze [3] and Harrison.[4] Heidenhain believes that their function is of great importance for the methodical and serial organization of nerve terminations; this is a good interpretation. Thanks to these plexuses there remains stored up near the terminal structures a considerable deposit or reserve of young fibres, largely superfluous, which, as the structure of the muscular and cutaneous

---

[1] Cajal : *Textura del sistema nervioso del hombre y vertebrados*. tomo 2, page 395, 1904.

See also : *Anat. Anzeiger*, Bd. 5, 1890.

[2] Cajal : " Génesis de la fibras nerviosas en el embrión," etc., *Trab. del Lab. de Inv. biol.*, tomo 4, 1906.

Idem : "Die histogenetischen Beweise der Neurontheorie von His und Forel," *Anat. Anzeiger*, Bd. 30, n. 5 u. 6, 1907.

[3] O. Schültze : " Beiträge zur Histogenese des Nervensystems," etc., *Arch. f. mikros, Anat. u. Entwick.*, Bd. 46, 1905.

[4] Harrison : loc. cit., *Journ. Exp. Zool.*, vol. 9, 1910.

elements becomes perfected, proceed in an orderly fashion, and according to the physiological necessities of the moment, to establish the final nervous arborizations. In regenerating nerves these plexuses are constantly found, in the scar as well as near the terminal structures, where Tello has seen large numbers of superfluous conductors.

(b) *Theory of Heidenhain*.[1]—Although Heidenhain has not personally analyzed neurogenesis experimentally, he has reflected on the rich harvest of observations in the domain of normal and pathological formation of nerves, and he has deduced some important truths. The theory of Heidenhain, like that of Harrison, has a syncretic character. Nevertheless, owing to the decisive value that Heidenhain attaches to mechanical factors, it seems to us that it can be associated with the old conception of Ranvier and Vanlair.

He believes that in the neurogenetic process the following factors come into play : (a) axonic turgescence or continuous development ; (b) growth along the shortest path ; (c) initial orientation of the neuroblast and cone of growth ; (d) the stereotropism of Loeb and Harrison ; (e) proximity of the terminal regions, such as the myotomes, skin, etc., to the centres from which arise fibres ; (f) the contralateral separation of the nerve roots and fascicles into well-defined physiological categories—sensory, motor, sympathetic fibres, etc. ; (g) the super-production of sprouts by their successive divisions, in order to facilitate their arrival at the organs ; (h) the creation of pre-terminal plexuses which surround the organs and which are a fibrillar deposit for later differentiation of the terminal districts ; (i) the entrance and successive growth of new axons into the nervous paths already formed, while these grow with the growth of the embryo ; (j) *syngenesis* or simultaneous development of nerves and organs and systems of organs for which the axons are destined, a process that begins in relatively early stages, etc.

Heidenhain holds as unfounded conjectures the supposed pre-established paths of Hensen and Held. Apart from our own arguments against this highly conjectural opinion, he mentions this further consideration : The tissues and organs where the nerve fibres end are differentiated late. Far from being pre-established in the embryo, the terminal districts and structures are organized and perfected later than the principal nerve paths. Thus, the limbs are lacking or are but little differentiated when the sensory, sympathetic, and motor nerve cordons are well organized. Under such conditions, how can the rudiment of the extremities offer congruent paths to the sprouts ? What can be the significance of a path pre-established towards a muscle or tendon which has not yet appeared ?

[1] Heidenhain : *Plasma und Zelle*, Bd. 2, p. 587, 1911.

The central idea of Heidenhain's theory is the admission that the development of the peripheral portion of the nervous system is the result of a double and successive differentiation and co-ordination : on one hand appear and are progressively differentiated the terminal organs and districts ; and on the other the nerve plexuses are progressively formed in them ; from these plexuses, according to the physiological needs, arise the last arborizations. The super-production of branches is a means of guaranteeing the arrival, in sufficient numbers, of conductors to the terminal regions in question ; many of these conductors are destined to lose themselves, owing to their travelling along the path of least resistance. Finally, once the differentiation and nervous reunion of the peripheral structures is ended, all the superfluous fibres, which failed to reach their destined end, owing to various incidents, become atrophied and are resorbed.[1]

Heidenhain's theory, and especially the idea of super-production, and of the survival of certain more fit or fortunate fibres, is very attractive, and it fits in with well established facts of normal neurogenesis and pathological regeneration. We may note, among other facts, the formidable super-production of sprouts in the central stump ; the number of useless and deviated fibres that are lost in the scar ; the genesis of superfluous branches in the terminal structures. However, for the adequate explanation of the known phenomena of nervous reunion of the peripheral stump and terminal organs, the fruitful idea of super-production and of resorption through disuse must be combined with the principle of neurotropism. Heidenhain does not reject this neurogenic factor in the process of regeneration, since he expressly mentions the neurotropic capacity of products of catabolism in the peripheral stump. But he does not, in our judgment, attach to it its true importance in the process of orientation of the sprouts. Neither does he speak of neurotropism as an explanatory element in the formation of nerves in the embryo.

On the other hand, the neurogenetic principles pointed out by His, ourselves, v. Lenhossék, Harrison, Held, Heidenhain, etc., are not sufficient to render clear all the facts known to-day concerning the evolution of the nervous system. A scrupulous analysis of this process

---

[1] We demonstrated, for the first time, many years ago, that many dendrites and nervous ramifications which appear during the differentiation of the grey matter, in foetuses and young mammals, are superfluous productions, destined to be resorbed. It is only the fibres that have reached their terminus and are able to establish useful functional connections which remain and develop completely.

See Cajal : *Textura del sistema nervioso del hombre y vertebrados*, tomo 2, p. 395, 1904.

in the chick embryo from the second to the sixth day of incubation easily convinces one that the process of formation of the nerves and central nerve tracts is an operation whose intimate causes as yet remain obscure. In reality this problem is a particular case of the arduous problem of ontogeny. In the development of the embryo, as well as in the differentiation of the nervous organs, the aforementioned principles doubtless come into play; there also intervene, however, enigmatic causes, ultimate conditions which are as yet inaccessible. The very list of the principles invoked by the abovementioned neurologists needs to be revised and enlarged. Our own recent investigations allow us to add yet other secondary factors which, if they are not new, have been incompletely enunciated by the embryologists. We may mention the following :

i. *Principle of primitive cellular migrations.*—From the thirtieth to the fiftieth hour of incubation in the chick embryo there escape, from the primitive canal as well as from the immediate regions of the ectoderm (v. Lenhossék), germinative cells in a phase of amoeboidism, perhaps attracted by chemotactic substances. Thus are formed the sympathetic ganglionic conglomerations of the vertebral chain and visceral masses, and the sensory ganglia. The tracks which are thus opened in the mesoderm constitute, for the future radicular axons, regions of least resistance.

ii. *Principle of successive neuroblastic differentiation.*—Once the germinative phase is passed the neuroblasts become progressively differentiated and enter into action according to a rigorously pre-established plan. This order, whose physical causes are unknown, unquestionably is the principal means of nervous ontogeny.

Without pretending to determine at present all the successive series or batches of neuroblasts which from hour to hour enter into action, we may record here that there exists a cellular category, that of precocious motor neuroblasts, whose activity is of the greatest importance. As a matter of fact, it is the incipient cones of these cells that penetrate the basal membrane of the spinal cord and open a way into the mesoderm. In allusion to this property they might be called *hymenoclastocytes*. These effects may be due as much to the tension of growth as to the secretion and diffusion of peptonizing enzymes.

We may cite two typical examples. A small group of motor neuroblasts, whose clubs are inserted perpendicularly in the lateral wall of the primitive canal, open a path through which the first exploratory fibres grow out. Later, attracted by a reciprocal homotropism or else led by the path of least resistance, the congenerous axons of successive batches use this tunnel, converging in it. The same occurs with the posterior root : a bundle of precocious bipolar cells strikes with its cones, like battering-rams, on the posterior basal membrane and opens a narrow breach in it. Other sensory fibres, differentiated later, make use of this opening, and assault the interior of the spinal cord along its dorsal portion.

iii. *Principle of dominating direction.*—We have stated that the principle of growth in a straight line is an ideal tendency, which is comparable to the physical law of inertia, but which cannot be realized under natural conditions. One must recognize, however, that, in spite of the innumerable flexuosities and turns described by the axon across the mesoderm, there prevails a general direction, as though there were an axis around which the cones oscillate in the positions alternately occupied by them, as in the propagation of a transversal vibratory movement. This law, as well as some exceptions,[1] might come within the theory of neurotropism.

iv. *Principle of the transportation of the axon by the growth of the surroundings.*[2]—One must not think of the cone as a projectile that advances freely across an immobile and resistant medium, but rather as a vessel which sometimes goes with, and sometimes against, the current of the tide. In reality, while the axon grows, the surrounding *terrain* also expands in virtue of a double phenomenon of cellular multiplication and differentiation. Hence the pressures, lengthenings, and transportations experienced by the axons, which explain many peculiarities of direction and position of the fibres. Perhaps this growing pressure of the *terrain* influences the transformation of the loose primitive nerves into compact cordons.

v. *Principle of growing velocity of the cones.*—Although our investigations on this point lack precision, it has seemed to us that the velocity of axonic growth is in accord, in principle, with the incessant movement of expansion of the '*terrain*,' increasing along with the latter. The rate of this increase is not exactly known ; but, during the first days, from the second to the seventh, of incubation of the chick embryo, it seems to approach a geometric progression.

vi. *Principle of evolutive preference of the nerves.*—Much before the skin, glands, muscles and tendons are organized, the nerves that are destined for them are formed. This gives rise to *expectant plexuses and cordons*, that is, to a local system of nerves which is relatively paralyzed in its differentiation while waiting for the maturing of the terminal organs. This expectant situation is so much prolonged that in a rabbit

[1] For example : the curve that the sensory roots of the vagus-glossopharyngeus nerves trace as they enter the medulla, the turn of the pathetic nerve, etc.

[2] This principle has also been formulated in somewhat different terms and with somewhat different significance, by Held and Heidenhain.

embryo 3 cms. long, where the majority of muscle fibres are already formed, there is not as yet a single motor plate. In general the terminal arborizations appear, according of course to the animals, between the last days of foetal life and the first days after birth, as in the chick, rabbit, cat, dog, etc.

vii. *At first only the primordial connective tissue possesses nerves.*—During the first days of embryonic evolution, from the second to the sixth day or more, the nerve bundles are exclusively limited to the masses of primitive connective tissue cells.

viii. *Principle of innervation by steps.*—As Heidenhain states, the innervation, general at first, becomes progressively more individual and specific. Our observations allow us to distinguish three principal steps in this process : (*a*) at first, from the second to the ninth or tenth day, the fibres approach the organ or tissue for which they are destined, without penetrating into it ; (*b*) once the specific cells of the organ have appeared, such as embryonic muscle fibres, papillar dermoid tissue, etc., the nerve bundles arise through fibrillar multiplication and growth, and the plexuses that we have mentioned so often then become organized ; (*c*) finally, once the structural differentiation of the tissue is terminated or almost terminated, the connections become specific and individualized, and the definitive terminal arborization is formed.

2. *Chain or polygenist theory.*—Founded on purely physiological inductions or on an insufficient objective study of nervous regeneration, this conception has been definitely disproved by the use of neurofibrillar stains. Almost all the facts of the preceding chapters militate against it. We shall not discuss it here, since we have done so fully in Chap. I. of this book. Here we need only remind the reader that the nerve fibres of the embryo as well as regenerated nerves are not produced by a discontinuous differentiation in the protoplasm of a chain of neuroblasts, but simply by the continuous growth of the axon or principal expansion of a motor or sensory neurone [Küpffer, His, Kölliker, Kerr, ourselves, v. Lenhossék, Stroebe, Ranvier, Harrison, Held, etc.[1]]

---

[1] Those who wish to acquaint themselves with the polemics concerning embryonic neurogenesis that took place some years ago between the polygenists and those who upheld the monogenist theory of His may consult, among other papers, these two :

Cajal : " Die histogenetischen Beweise der Neurontheorie von His und Forel," *Anat. Anzeiger*, Bd. 30, Nos. 5 u. 6, 1907. *Trav. du Lab. de Recherches biol.*, tome 5, 1907.

Idem : " Nouvelles observations sur l'évolution des neuroblastes avec quelques remarques sur l'hypothèse neurogénétique de Hensen-Held," *Anat. Anzeiger*, Bd. 32, 1908.

3. *Hypothesis of neurotropism.*—The partisans of this explanatory principle admit also, as the reader has seen, all the positive neurogenetic conditions pointed out by His, v. Lenhossék, Ranvier, Vanlair, Harrison, Held, etc., such as : *continuous protoplasmic growth, growth in a straight line, Loeb's stereotropism, the super-production of sprouts, atrophy of superfluous or deviated sprouts, mechanical influences of the terrain,* etc. ; but these factors involve, besides, a complementary condition—*neurotropism,* or *chemotactism,* that is, the intervention of certain trophic or orienting substances, of various natures, which are given out in the path in which the sprouts grow, and especially concentrated in the bands of Büngner of the peripheral stump, and in degenerating terminal nervous structures.

This theory has been explained in detail, in various chapters of this work, especially in the last. But it is worth while insisting once more on its range and explanatory value. We shall here give the history of this conception of neurotropism and show how it was proved and perfected by Lugaro, Nageotte, Marinesco, and Tello.

The chemotactic or neurotropic hypothesis was, as we have already stated, devised by us in 1892 in order to obtain a comprehensible picture of the formation of nerves and of the constancy and congruence of their connections. Von Lenhossék,[1] who approved this conception, and who moreover confirmed our discovery of the *cone of growth*, had prepared the way by pertinently comparing the metamorphoses of the cone of growth with the amoeboid movement of leucocytes. Harrison, especially, has insisted on this similarity in his studies on the growth of the cones in amphibian larvae, directly in lymph. If the appendices of the cones are similar to the pseudopods of the leucocytes, it seems natural to attribute their production and orientation to chemotactic influences, that is, to the action of chemical substances given out in the medium ; this is supported by the fact that bacteriologists such as Pfeiffer, Massart and Bordet, Gabrichewsky, Metchnikoff, etc., hold that the presence of attractive or positively chemotactic substances given out by the bacteria is a necessary condition of the growth and orientation of the leucocytes towards the bacteria that they are to attack. At first we applied the principle of neurotropism to the comprehension of certain phenomena of dislocation and connection of the cells of the embryonic retina [2] and of other nervous organs. Later we generalized the hypothesis for the entire field of neurogenesis.[3]

[1] v. Lenhossék : *Der feinere Bau des Nervensystems*, etc., 2 Auf. 1895.

[2] Cajal : " La rétine des vertébrés," *La Cellule*, tome 9, 1892.

[3] *Idem* : " Mecanismo de la degeneración y regeneración de los nervios," *Trab. del Lab. de Invest. biol.*, tomo 4, 1905-06.

We owe to Forssman [1] the application of this theory to nervous regeneration. We have already stated that this scientist, who worked in ignorance of our own investigations, carried out many experiments to place the chemotactic hypothesis on a solid foundation. He invented the word neurotropism (from νεῦρον, nerve, and τροπή, attraction). As to the origin and nature of the attractive substance, Forssman believed that it was a product of disintegration of the nervous tissue, and particularly of the myelin.

When in 1905 we studied [2] the phenomena occurring in nervous regeneration, and established the correctness of the monogenist conception, we invoked as an explanatory idea the hypothesis of neurotropism. But the formula of Forssman called for important rectifications. The products of disintegration of the myelin and the materials of decomposition of the grey substance are in reality without any attractive action. If they had, as Forssman claims, such an influence, one would expect that any wound of the spinal cord, causing disorganization of the white or grey substance, would bring about the innervation of the spinal detritus, by an invasion of sprouts arising in the sensory roots; but this phenomenon never occurs. Neither do grafts of grey or white substance attract the sprouts, when they are placed near the central stump of the sciatic nerve. As O. Rossi notes, young fibres do not innervate the nervous tissue, but the embryonic connective tissue which gradually takes its place. On the other hand, it is a fact of observation that the greatest neurotropic influence of the peripheral stump coincides precisely with the phase of the *bands of Büngner*, at a time when most of the myelin has been resorbed. Moreover, the majority of the sprouts choose the interior of these bands, often crowding within them in considerable numbers. For this and other reasons it was necessary to rectify the hypothesis of Forssman, localizing the neurotropic action in the rejuvenated or proliferated cell of Schwann—the *bands of Büngner*.

In this way the attractive and selecting substance, far from being a product of the breaking-down of the myelin, becomes a substance segregated by living cells, which are in a phase of proliferative rejuvenescence.

Such was the new form of neurotropism which we described in our treatise of 1905. It was fortunate enough to persuade such noted

[1] Forssman: " Zur Kenntniss des Neurotropismus," *Ziegler's Beiträge zur pathol. Anat.*, etc., Bd. 27, 1900.

[2] Cajal: " Mecanismo de la degeneración y regeneración de los nervios," *Trab. del Lab. de Invest. biol.*, tomo 4, 1905-06.

neurologists as Lugaro,[1] Marinesco, and Nageotte. Marinesco,[2] above all, ingeniously developed the theory, attributing to the young cells of Schwann, which he named *apotrophic cells*, not only a nutritive and orienting function, but also the capacity to migrate within the scar in order to act directly on the sprouts. He also explained, by means of the apotrophic cells, many strange phenomena of arrest and retrogradation of the sprouts within the central stump. Tello,[3] for his part, not only confirmed the neurotropism of degenerated nerves and motor plates, but he stated that the stimulating agent is present not only in the cells of Schwann, but also in the fusiform cells of the endoneurium. This conception, besides harmonizing with the fact that the sprouts of the peripheral stump are often found interstitially, suggests the idea that the cells of the endoneurium are a reserve of cells of Schwann, in an embryonic state, and that they are destined to surround those sprouts which have migrated out of the sheaths, or those, both in the central and peripheral stumps, which are travelling between the nerve tubes. Nageotte,[4] without especially alluding to the theme of regeneration of the nerves, has collected in his studies concerning tubes, and especially in his beautiful experiments of transplantation of ganglia, various facts which reinforce the chemotactic hypothesis. Among them we may note the energetic attraction that the pericellular satellite cells of the sensory ganglia exert on the sprouts emerging from the initial portion of the axon.

Finally, to complete our review of the neurotropic theory, we may add that Ariens Kappers [5], calling it *neurobiotaxis*, has used it, with

[1] It appears that Lugaro, independently of ourselves, had also, when commenting on the works of Forssman, the intuition that the cells of Schwann of the peripheral stump perhaps enter into the neurotropic process.

See Lugaro in " Jacobsohn, Flatau, u. Minot," *Handbuch der pathol. Anat. des Nervensystems*. Also : " Sul neurotropismo e sui trapianti dei nervi," *Riv. di patol. ner. e mentale*, vol. 11, fasc. 7, 1906.

[2] Marinesco : " Le mécanisme de la régénérescence nerveuse," 1ᵉ partie, *Rev. gen. des. Sciences*, etc., 18ᵉ année, No. 4, février 1907.

[3] Tello : " La influencia del neurotropismo en la regeneración de los centros nerviosos," *Trab. del Lab. de Invest. biol.*, tomo 9, 1911.

[4] Nageotte : *C.R. de la Soc. de Biol.*, 19 janvier, 23 février, 3 mars, 13 avril, 22 juin, 13 juillet, 1907.

Idem : "Recherches expérimentales sur la morphologie des cellules et des ganglions rachidiens," *Revue neurol.*, No. 8, 1907.

Idem : "Note sur l'apparition précoce d'arborisations péricellulaires," etc., *Compt. rend. de la Soc. de Biol.*, 13 avril, 1907.

[5] A. Kappers : " Weitere Mitteilungen bezüglich der phylogenetischen

some variations, to explain the phylogenetic modifications of position and form, shown by the motor and sensory nuclei of the medulla in the animal series. According to him, under the influence of the nervous discharges, with their concomitant neurotropic phenomena, the dendrites lengthen in the direction of the greatest action, and even the cell bodies migrate to come nearer to the foci where the afferent paths of the dominating influxes terminate. We may also add that this author, inspired by the facts of galvanotropism discovered by Verworn, suggests the idea that perhaps there occur in this process electromotor phenomena, an idea which is akin to the old electrical conception of Strasser [1] concerning the growth of embryonic nerve fibres.

On the other hand, the nutritive and tutorial functions of the cells of Schwann had already been recognized by the embryologists, many of whom believed that the successive thickening of young fibres and the development of the medullary sheath were the principal functions of these cells. We may especially cite Graham Kerr,[2] who studied the behaviour of these cells in the normal development of nerves, and Mott and Halliburton,[3] who attributed to the bands of Büngner of the peri-

Verlagerung der motorischen Hirnnervkerne," etc., *Folia neuro-biologica*, No. 2, 1908.

Idem: "Weitere Mitteilungen ueber Neurobiotaxis," etc., *Folia neurobiologica*, Bd. 3, 1909.

We had already expressed the idea, in connection with spinal ganglion cells and cerebellar cells, that there is a possibility that the nerve cells are able to migrate, under the influence of chemical actions arising in afferent fibres. Our explanation naturally concerns ontogeny, and not phylogeny, with which the interesting investigations of Kappers are concerned. See : *Textura del sistema nervioso del hombre*, etc., tomo 2, p. 560, 1899. (*Histologie du système nerveux*, 1909-11, Maloine, Paris.)

Recently, evidence of neurotropic influences, as shown in experimental embryology in amphibians, has been given by May and Detwiler: "The relation of transplanted eyes to developing nerve centers," *Jour. Exp. Zool.*, vol. 43, p. 83-103, 1925, and by R. M. May: "Modifications des centres nerveux dues à la transplantation de l'œil et de l'organe olfactif chez les embryons d'Anoures," *Arch. de Biol.*, t. 37, fasc. 3, pp. 335-395, 1927.

The entire question of neurotropism has been reviewed by F. Tello: "Gegenwärtige Anschauungen über den Neurotropismus," *Vorträge und Aufsätze über Entwicklungsmechanik der Organismen*, Springer, Berlin, 1923.

[1] Strasser : " Alte und neue Probleme der entwickelungsgeschichtlichen Forschung auf den Gebiete der Nervensystems," *Ergebn. der Anat. u. Entwickelungsgesch.*, Bd. 1, 1892.

[2] Graham Kerr : " On some points in the early development of motor nerve trunks, etc., in Lepidosiren," *Roy. Soc. Edin. Trans.*, vol. 41, 1904.

[3] Mott and W. D. Halliburton : " The chemistry of nerve degeneration," *Phil. Trans.*, vol. 194, 1901.

See also: "Regeneration of nerves," *Proc. of the Royal Society*, vol. 78, 1906.

pheral stump of cut nerves the function of feeding and protecting recently arrived sprouts. There is only a step between the recognition of these cells as a nutritive placenta and the admission in them of secretions capable of stimulating and orienting the sprouts that are wandering in the scar.

We may thus say that the cell of Schwann has multiple functions. Normally it protects and regulates the nutritive exchanges of the axon and myelin with their surroundings. Under pathological conditions it digests the remnants of the axon and myelin and it elaborates substances capable of stimulating the assimilation and amoeboidism of the nerve sprouts.

It is difficult, in the present state of knowledge, to imagine what is the nature of the stimulating substance. As a tentative hypothesis we [1] have supposed that the substance contained in the sheaths of Schwann of the peripheral stump should be conceived, not as a fixed, quiescent principle, capable of being neutralized like an alkali by some acid substance within the cone of growth, but as a ferment or catalytic agent which stimulates the assimilation of the axonic protoplasm and which does not become used up while acting on the nervous protoplasm. The substances of the cone and the neurotropic enzymes are perhaps comparable, respectively, to the antigens and antibodies put forward by bacteriologists.

It is evident that the theory of neurotropism is still wanting in the precision and clarity that are characteristic of good scientific hypotheses. In order to lend to it the factors that it lacks and to elevate it to the rank of a scientific doctrine, it would be necessary to have a more precise knowledge of the elements or sources of neurotropic action; to isolate the attracting substances, or at least to determine their nature and mode of action, as the bacteriologists have done with the various kinds of antibodies; to discover the laws which regulate their production and extinction; to explain, finally, the mechanism of chemical reactions and equilibria provoked in the receptor substances present in the young axon and terminal club, by the stimulating enzymes contained in the active cells, equilibria that are variable for each phase of the regenerative process. All this, however, seems to us still far off, and an ideal difficult of realization.

[1] Cajal: " Algunas observaciones favorables á la hipótesis neurotrópica," *Trab. del Lab. de Invest. biol.*, tomo 8, 1910.

ADDITIONAL NOTE ON CHAPTER XVI

Marinesco [1] has attempted, during these last few years, to place the hypothesis of neurotropism on an exact footing. He supposes, along with Scott, that, in embryonic nerve cells the iron is found in the chromatin and, as development proceeds, it becomes concentrated in the Nissl *bodies*. It is also abundantly found in the neurones of amputated individuals, as may be seen by using Perls' reaction or the stain with Berlin blue ; it is very abundant, besides, in the nuclei of the syncytium of Schwann, and even in the fibroblasts of the epineuron and perineuron. It is absent, however, in old fibres. As the volume of the nuclei is greater in the regenerating bundles of the central stump than in the pre-existing ones, one must admit that the metabolism of the iron is much more active in the former. In adult neurones the iron diminishes in quantity ; but when the phenomenon of growth of the axons begins the syncytium of the sheaths of Schwann forms an oxydase and a peroxydase represented by the colloidal iron which acts as a catalytic agent.

In another paper,[2] which deals only with oxydases, Marinesco observes that these enzymes become concentrated near the central stump of cut nerves ; they are found within certain cells which he calls *oxydasophore cells* and which are placed, some within the blood-vessels and others outside them. In the syncytium of the scar also (*apotrophic cells*) there exist oxydases which may be demonstrated by the Winkler-Schultze reaction as blue granules. These granules are present in the cytoplasm, but not in the nuclei, nor in the newly-formed nerve fibres. The rôle of the oxydases would consist in accelerating the assimilative function of the newly-formed nerve fibres, bringing about their growth.

It thus appears that in the growth of nerves in the embryo and in that of the sprouts during the process of regeneration iron collaborates as well as the oxydases. This view, while it represents an advance in the conception of neurotropism, is unfortunately not a complete explanation.

As a matter of fact, it is difficult to adjust exactly all these ideas to the various complex and variable singularities of the process of nerve regeneration.

[1] Marinesco : " Nouvelles contributions à l'étude de la régénération nerveuse," *Philos. Trans. of the Royal Society of London*, Series B, vol. 209, 1919.

[2] *Idem* : " Recherches anatomocliniques sur les neurones des amputés," *Phil. Trans. Roy. Soc.*, London, Series B, vol. 209, 1920.

Following a different path, other authors to-day attempt to rejuvenate and perfect Strasser's electrical theory. In this connection, and even though there is no strict relation with the problem of growth and orientation of regenerated nerve fibres, we may cite the investigations of Scaffidi, who many years ago showed that the central stump of cut nerves in process of regeneration is positively electrified. He calls this a *regeneration current* (Kappers' *growth current*).

In this line of thought one may also cite the very interesting experiments of Ingvar performed on tissue cultures of neuroblasts, according to Harrison's technique.

Ingvar states that when neuroblasts are submitted to weak galvanic currents, expansions are produced on them which grow parallel to the lines of force; some expansions become directed towards the anode and others towards the cathode.

Other partisans of electrical influences as forces in the process of normal neurogenesis are Ariëns Kappers,[1] who has published a large number of monographs on this point, Bok,[2] Child,[3] and others. In this work, which is devoted to traumatic degeneration and regeneration, we cannot, without digressing excessively, give all the details of the hypotheses of these investigators, which are not always concordant and fail to explain why in ontogeny and phylogeny the dendrites grow in one direction, that is, towards the entering functional stimuli, as we suggested many years ago, and why the axons grow in the opposite direction (*stimulofugal*, according to Kappers' nomenclature).

Kappers' more recent studies notably alter his first ideas. Thus to-day Kappers adheres to the idea of galvanotropism and believes that the axon grows along the course of the stimulus, that is, towards the anode, while the dendrites grow towards the cathode (*stimulopetal growth*); one thus infers that the dendrites are attracted by the stimulating centres, while the axons flee from them.

[1] See Ariëns Kappers: " Further contributions on neurobiotaxis, IX. An attempt to compare the phenomena of neurobiotaxis with other phenomena of taxis and tropism. The dynamic polarization of the neurone," *Jour. Comp. Neurol.* vol. 27, p. 261, 1917.

Idem : " On structural laws in the nervous system ; the principles of neurobiotaxis," *Brain*, vol. 44, 1921.

Idem : " Dixième contribution à la théorie de la neurobiotaxis. Le tropisme nutritif des dendrites et son rapport avec les phénomènes neurobiotactiques en général. *L'encéphale.* 1922.

[2] S. T. Bok : " Die Entwicklung der Hirnnerven und ihrer centralen Bahnen. Die stimulogene Fibrillation." *Folia Neurobiologica*, Bd. 9, 1915.

[3] Child : " The origin and development of the nervous system from a physiological viewpoint," Chicago, 1921.

In these electrolytic phenomena intervene substances capable of changing the positive galvanotropism into a negative one. Thus the potassium compounds which Macdonald, Macallum, and Menten have shown to be present in the axon would force the soma and dendrites to grow towards the negative pole, that is, towards the stimulating nerve tracts ; the Nissl bodies, where acids are present, as well as in the nuclei, etc., would attract the axons in their growth. All these ideas are still evolving, and we can but hope for new investigations which may corroborate or correct the hypothesis of galvanotropism and explain all the cases that are difficult to interpret by means of it.

Tello,[1] who has devoted several papers to the problem of neurotropism, as we have said before, states, in a long and well documented monograph concerning the orientation of the axons in the embryo and nerve regenerations, that at first (in the embryo) bioelectric phenomena are at work to bring about the emergence of the nerve roots, bioelectric influences whose radius of diffusion is very large. Later, however, when the nervous terminations—sensory, motor, gustatory, acoustic, etc.—are formed, neurotropism would in turn come into play. Physical action thus forms the principal nerve paths ; while ulterior chemical actions would explain why each epidermal or mesodermal cell or group of cells becomes joined only with one or several nerve fibres. Neurotropism thus acts only at a short distance ; electrical influences, on the other hand, act from far and between nervous organs and regions, some of which are very distant from each other.

The principal cause of the orientation of the nerve sprouts in the innervation of the *peripheral stump* of cut nerves would be neurotropism (attraction of the peripheral stump). According to Tello, the mesodermal cells of the scar, and even the connective tissue cells present in the perifascicular tissue of nerves, also collaborate, as we have stated, in the innervation of this distal stump.

He agrees with Hermann, Marchand, Landacre, etc., concerning the close relation which exists between developing nerves and gustator papillae,[2] and he attributes a decisive importance, in the tropism and orientation of the sprouts, to the stereotropism of Loeb and Harrison. He recognises also that so long as, in the foetus, the terminal organs—

[1] Tello : " Ideas actuales sobre el neurotropismo," *Discurso leido en la Academia de Medicina de Madrid*, January 1923. Also " Gegenwärtige Anschauungen über den Neurotropismus," *Vorträge und Aufsätze über Entwicklungsmechanik der Organismen*, Springer, Berlin, 1923.

[2] Concerning this point see May, R. M. : " The relation of nerves to degenerating and regenerating taste buds." *Jour. Exp. Zool.*, vol. 42, pp. 371-410, 1925.

tactile hairs, spindles of Kühne, etc.—are not formed the definite nervous arborizations do not differentiate. Moreover, the idea of a reciprocal co-operation of the terminal regions and of the young nerve fibres has already been put forward by Heidenhain,[1] and warmly defended, during these last few years, by Boeke and his school of investigators. We ourselves have brought to notice some facts favourable to this conception, of which we have already spoken above, in our communications on the attractive power of epithelia—sensory nerve terminations [2]—and on the definite modelling of the *horizontal cells* of the retina.[3]

[1] Heidenhain : *Plasma und Zelle*, Bd. 2, 1911.

[2] Cajal : " Acción neurotrópica de los epitelios. Algunos detalles sobre el mecanismo genético de las ramificaciones nerviosas intraepiteliales sensitivas y sensoriales," *Trab. Lab. de Investig. biol.* t. 17, 1919.

[3] *Idem* : " La desorientación inicial de las neuronas retinianas de axon corto," *Trab. del Lab. de Investig. biol.* t. 17, 1919.

END OF VOLUME I

DEGENERATION AND REGENERATION
OF THE NERVOUS SYSTEM

Degeneration & Regeneration of the Nervous System

BY

S. RAMÓN Y CAJAL, M.D., F.R.S.

Director of the Instituto Cajal, Madrid
Honorary Professor of Pathology in the University of Madrid

TRANSLATED AND EDITED

BY

RAOUL M. MAY

PH.D. (HARV.), D.ÈS SC. (PARIS)

Laboratoires d'Anatomie et Histologie Comparées et de Chimie Biologique
Faculté des Sciences, Paris

VOLUME II

OXFORD UNIVERSITY PRESS
LONDON: HUMPHREY MILFORD
1928

PRINTED IN GREAT BRITAIN BY ROBERT MACLEHOSE AND CO. LTD.
THE UNIVERSITY PRESS, GLASGOW.

CONTENTS

SECOND SECTION

DEGENERATION AND REGENERATION OF THE NERVE CENTRES

FIRST PART

DEGENERATION AND REGENERATION OF SENSORY AND SYMPATHETIC GANGLIA

                                                                                                 PAGE

I. SUMMARY OF THE NORMAL STRUCTURE OF SENSORY GANGLIA - - - - - - - - 397

Typical forms: morphology, volume, and normal structure of the sensory neurone.—Pericellular capsule and satellite cells.—Atypical forms and dispositions; neurones provided with dendrites, appendices in the shape of balls, ansiform and fenestrated dispositions, frayed cells.—Pericellular and periglomerular nests.—Probable significance of the atypical forms.—Hypotheses of Nageotte and of Levi.—Additional Note.

II. DEGENERATION AND REGENERATION OF THE SENSORY NERVE GANGLIA - - - - - 414

Traumatic degeneration of the sensory cells and tubes.—Regenerative acts of the cells and fibres following on wounds, contusions and extirpation of nerves, etc.—Genesis of the pericellular nests.—Additional Note.

III. MORPHOLOGICAL VARIATIONS OBSERVED IN TRANSPLANTED SENSORY GANGLIA - - - - 426

Fundamental experiments of Nageotte.—Confirmations by Marinesco and Minea, Rossi, Dustin, Cardenal and ourselves.—Aberrant nerves.—Neuronophagy.—Experiments of cultivation of ganglia *in vitro* by Cajal, Legendre and Minot, Marinesco, etc.—Theories of Nageotte, Marinesco, and other authors, concerning the mechanism of formation of the neuronal appendices.—Additional Note.

SECOND PART

DEGENERATION AND REGENERATION OF THE SPINAL CORD AND NERVE ROOTS

PAGE

I. DEGENERATION AND REGENERATION OF THE WHITE MATTER - - - - - - - - 484

Technical indications.—Summary of the normal structure of the white matter.—Traumatic degeneration.—Initial phenomena.—Appearance of the granular cells and destruction of the myelin and axon.—Secondary degeneration.—Precocious acts of regeneration.—Late examination of the lesions.—Breakdown of regeneration.—Formation of the scar.—Creation, under special conditions, of very long fibres which abandon the spinal cord.

II. DEGENERATIVE ALTERATIONS OF THE GREY MATTER - - - - - - - - 517

Résumé of the structure of the spinal neurones.—Necrotic and degenerative phenomena occurring in them—granular state, chromatolysis, neurofibrillar hypertrophy, hirudiform state, etc.—Perturbations of the endocellular Golgi apparatus.—Regenerative phenomena—regeneration of the dendrites and of the fibres of the grey substance.—Neuroglial and conjunctive scars.

III. DEGENERATION AND REGENERATION OF THE SPINAL ROOTS - - - - - - - - 531

Degeneration and regeneration of the anterior roots.—Their invasion by endogenous and exogenous sprouts.—Degeneration and regeneration of the posterior roots.—Invasion of the connective scar by funicular sprouts.—Partial restoration of the posterior fasciculus.

IV. PHENOMENA OF NECROSIS, DEGENERATION, AND REGENERATION BROUGHT ABOUT BY SPINAL CONTUSION AND LACERATION - - - - - 558

Necrotic and degenerative forms of the nerve fibres.—Necrotic and degenerative disorders of the neurones.—Regenerative acts of the axons and dendrites.—Historical notes concerning regeneration of the spinal cord.—Additional Note.

V. TRAUMATIC DEGENERATION AND REGENERATION IN THE OPTIC NERVE AND RETINA - - - 583

Additional Note.

THIRD PART

I. Degenerative Phenomena consequent on Cerebellar Traumatisms - - - - - 597

Technical notes.—Degenerative acts in the white matter.—Degeneration of the central stump.—Degeneration of the peripheral stump.—Elimination of the axonic segment beyond the collaterals, and transformation of the cells of Purkinje into elements with a short axon.—Details of this transformation in the pathological human cerebellum.—Absence of regenerative phenomena.

II. Continuation of the Degenerative and Metamorphic Processes consequent on Cerebellar Traumatisms - - - - - - - 617

Degenerative phenomena occurring in the neurones and their dendrites.—Aneuritic cells and rosaliform, hirudiform, etc., dispositions of the neurofibrillar reticulum.—Swelling of the soma and dendrites.—Destruction of the reticulum.—Creation of aberrant expansions.—Alterations of the basket cells, moss-like fibres, and other elements in the cerebellum.

FOURTH PART

I. Traumatic Degenerative Processes of the Cerebral Cortex - - - - - - 631

Necrotic phenomena consequent on wounds.—Preserved nerve fibres.—Preserved dendrites.—Preserved neurones.—Corrosion and autolysis of the axons and dendrites.—Degenerative metamorphoses of the peripheral stump.—Autotomy of the terminal spheres and their metamorphic phenomena—formation of neurofibrillar plexuses and buckles.

II. Study of Traumatic Degeneration in the Cerebral Cortex (*continued*) - - - - 656

Degenerative phenomena of the central stump in wounds of the white matter.—Degenerative phenomena of this stump when the interruption is in the grey matter.—Compensatory eliminations.—Transformation of the cerebral pyramidal cells into cells with short axons.—Degenerative phenomena in the nerve collaterals and in some intrinsic fibres of the cerebral cortex.—Additional Note.

		PAGE
III.	ALTERATIONS OF THE NERVE CELLS IN CEREBRAL TRAUMATISMS	678

Neuronal metamorphoses occurring after wounds that entail little or no contusion.—Disorders occasioned by contusions and commotions that are accompanied by traumatisms.—Granular degeneration, chromatolysis, hirudiform state, fusiform hypertrophy and alteration of the neurofibrils, and neurofibrillar pycnosis

IV. PHENOMENA OF ABORTED REGENERATION IN THE CEREBRAL CORTEX - - - - - - 693

Regenerative inefficiency of the central paths.—Internal and external productions of the central stump of the axon.—*Cephalopodic* structures and neurofibrillar spools.—Radial or *testudinoid* formations of the varicosities.—Aspect of these neoformations in the cerebrum of recently-born individuals.—Incongruence and breakdown of these neoformations.

V. ATROPHIC PHENOMENA CONSEQUENT ON CEREBRAL WOUNDS - - - - - - - 704

Aspect of the traumatized grey cortex in late periods, that is, some weeks and months after the lesion.—Relative immunity of the neurones in the radial wounds.—Late atrophies and necroses in transversal wounds.—Calcified pyramids and residual nodules.

VI. CORTICAL INFLAMMATION CONSEQUENT ON TRAUMATISMS - - - - - - - 714

Invasion of the grey substance by migratory elements—granular cells, rod-like cells, plasma cells, etc.—Behaviour of the neuroglia in presence of the inflammation.—Formation of the scar.—Neuroglial and mesodermal scars.—Organization of exudates and haemorrhagic foci.—Gigantic granular cells.

VII. STUDY OF REGENERATIVE PROCESSES OF THE CEREBRUM (*continued*) - - - - - 734

Breakdown of the regeneration of the nerve paths.—Experiments of Tello, showing that regeneration fails owing to the absence in the surroundings of substances that stimulate the growth and orientation of the axonic sprouts.—Theories explanatory of the poverty and incongruence of the natural regeneration.—Historical notes concerning regeneration in the cerebrum of man and the higher mammals.

INDEX - - - - - - - - - - 761

SECOND SECTION

DEGENERATION AND REGENERATION OF THE NERVE CENTRES

In this section of our work we shall study the degenerative lesions and regenerative phenomena produced in the nerve centres as the consequence of wounds, commotions, crushing, the action of cold and of certain infections. We shall treat the following points: 1. Degeneration and regeneration of the sensory and sympathetic ganglia. 2. Degeneration and regeneration of the spinal cord and nerve roots. 3. Degeneration and regeneration of the retina and optic paths. 4. Degeneration and regeneration of the cerebellum. 5. Degeneration and regeneration of the cerebral cortex. 6. General interpretation of the results obtained.

FIRST PART

DEGENERATION AND REGENERATION OF THE SENSORY AND SYMPATHETIC GANGLIA

I

SUMMARY OF THE NORMAL STRUCTURE OF SENSORY GANGLIA.

Typical forms : Morphology, volume, and normal structure of the sensory neurone.—Pericellular capsule and satellite cells.—Atypical forms and dispositions : Neurones provided with dendrites, appendices in the shape of balls, ansiform and fenestrated dispositions, frayed cells.—Pericellular and periglomerular nests.—Probable significance of the atypical forms.—Hypotheses of Nageotte and of Levi.

Normal morphology of the sensory cells.—As is well known, the *spinal* or cerebro-spinal *ganglia* are situated on the course of the posterior or sensory roots of the spinal nerve pairs, and on all the sensory cranial nerves.

If one examines a section of a spinal ganglion, one notes two zones: one zone is cortical, greyish, and rich in nerve cells; the other zone is central, and is constituted principally by medullary tubes. This zone, which is almost free from cells in the lower vertebrates, is constituted in mammals by neuronal islands separated by

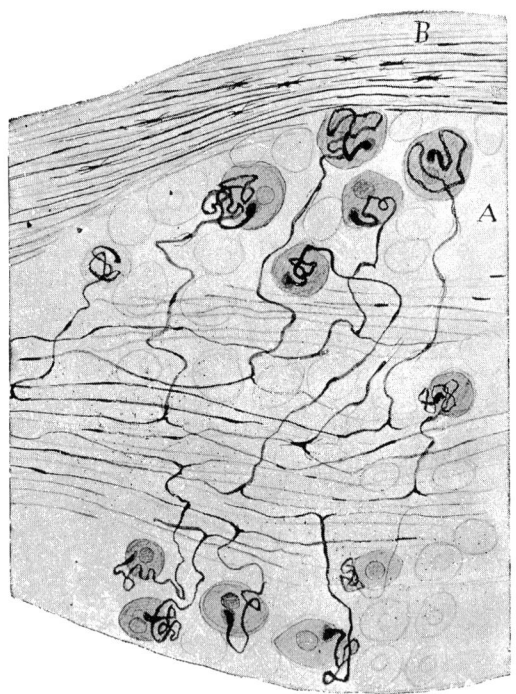

FIG. 147.—Piece of a sensory ganglion, stained with methylene blue. *A*, sensory cells; *B*, bundles of nerve fibres.

bundles of white matter. The ganglion is surrounded by a connective covering, a kind of capsule which is in continuity with the neurilemma.

The *nerve cells* are voluminous—from 20 to 50 μ—rounded or slightly polyhedral. They are not all of the same thickness, and one can differentiate them into large cells—from 50 to 60 μ—and small cells—from 20 to 26 μ. As we shall point out below, the smaller elements have a somewhat different morphology from the larger ones.

Each neurone has : a covering or protective capsule of a fibrous nature, invested interiorly with an endothelium ; abundant cytoplasm, strongly granular and marked, on one of its sides, by an accumulation of melanic grains ; and a spheroid nucleus. This last is voluminous and provided with a large nucleolus, which is easily stained with carmine and the basic aniline dyes (Fig. 152). By using Nissl's method one can recognize in the protoplasm a great number of large grumes which are finer and more closely set than the corresponding grumes in the motor cells. The aspect and fineness of these grumes vary in the different ganglionic cells. Finally, the cytoplasm also shows a very fine and close neurofibrillar net,

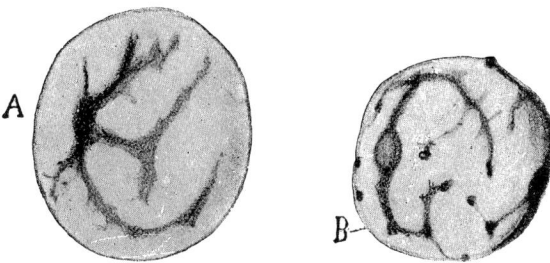

FIG. 148.—Satellite or endocapsular cells of the spinal ganglia of the cat.

whose fibrils are condensed and diminish in number at the pole of the single expansion, where they are in continuity with the fibrillar bundle of the axon.

Besides the fibrous cover garnished with endothelial cells which were well described by von Lenhossék, there exists around the protoplasm, in a plasmatic subcapsular space, certain elements which were first pointed out by ourselves and Olóriz. We discovered them by the methods of Ehrlich (methylene blue) and of Golgi. They were later confirmed by numerous authors—Nageotte, Marinesco, von Lenhossék, Dogiel, etc. These cells, which we called *satellite cells* or *endocapsular elements*, are small, fusiform or star-shaped, and provided with expansions which are sometimes short and hardly ramified, sometimes large and curvilinear, and intimately applied (Fig. 148) to the outlines of the sensory cell. In the ordinary cells, the satellite cells are few in number ; but, as we shall point out below, in fenestrated, frayed, and regenerating neurones they constitute thick masses around the cytoplasm (Fig. 154).

The satellite cells, as will be noted below, seem to play an important part in the trophism of the neurones. While these remain normal the number of satellite cells is small; when the neurones decline through age or are the seat of degenerative lesions the satellite cells multiply and seem to corrode, through neurolysis, the sensory soma.

The sensory cells, both large and small, are monopolar. This was seen by Ranvier, von Lenhossék, Retzius, etc. The single thick expansion, after a variable course within the ganglion, bifurcates, giving rise to (1) a *fine branch* destined for the spinal cord, into which

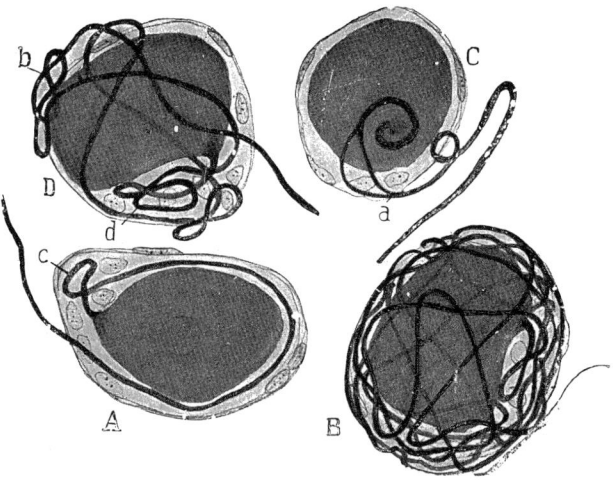

FIG. 149.—Sensory cells of man. Reduced silver nitrate. Various types of glomerular cells.

it penetrates, thus constituting the posterior or sensory root of the spinal nerves; and (2) a *thick branch* which is directed towards the periphery, entering into the corresponding spinal pair, and ramifying in the skin or else ending in a sensory terminal structure—corpuscles of Pacini, Meissner, etc. The single axon, as well as its two branches, is surrounded by a myelin sheath. The dichotomous division occurs at the level of a node.

The investigations of Dogiel, confirmed by ourselves and by Olóriz, show that the single expansion forms, on its exit from the cell, and underneath the capsule, a glomerulus or spool of complicated turns which is absent in embryos and recently-born animals. This glomerulus lacks a medullary sheath and is in relation with

NORMAL STRUCTURE OF SENSORY GANGLIA 401

the satellite or endocapsular cells. The complexity of the glomerulus varies much within the same ganglion and in the various species. In man it is composed sometimes of a single loop or initial turn (Fig. 149, *A*), while in certain cells it takes the form of a complicated nest which entirely surrounds the soma underneath the capsule (Figs. 149, *B*, and 149, *D*). Near the place where the axon emerges the cytoplasm shows a pit or flat surface in relation with satellite cells (Fig. 149, *D*).

As will be pointed out below, the monopolar disposition does not originate as such, but appears late in birds and mammals. The

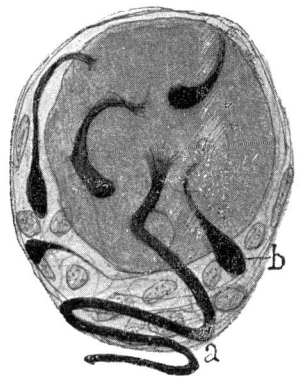
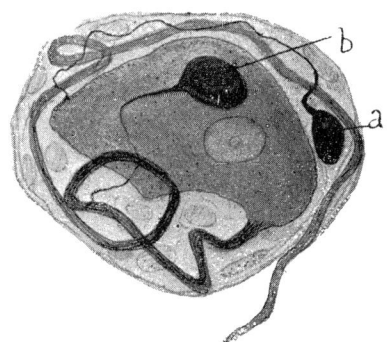

FIG. 150.—Human ganglion cell provided with protoplasmic appendices. *a*, axon.

FIG. 151.—Cell whose filiform expansions end in balls (twenty-five year old woman). Ganglion of the vagus.

primitive form is bipolar, a type of morphology which is retained in the adult in invertebrates and some species of fishes. Exceptionally in mammals one sees in some cranial ganglia, such as the plexiform ganglion of the vagus, some bipolar cells (Fig. 153, *B*).

Atypical forms.—The monopolar ganglionic type that we have just described is the most abundant and, frequently, the only one found. For that reason we consider it to-day as the normal neurone, that is, a neurone exempt from phenomena of decadence and regeneration. From time to time, however, one sees, especially in the adult and the old, other cellular types. We have been able to stain these for some years, by the use of reduced silver nitrate, in man as well as in dogs, donkeys, horses, and cats. The principal types are as follows:

1. Multipolar cells, which remind one of those described by Disse, Spirlas, von Lenhossék, and ourselves. These cells are provided with short and thick dendrites, which are widened at their tip and end under the capsule; these elements also possess a common glomerulated axon. These strange cells, which are rare in spinal ganglia,

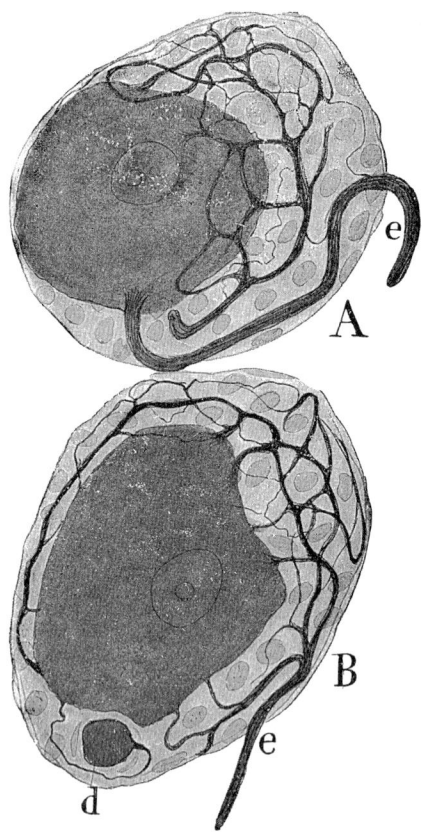

FIG. 152.—Cells of the spinal ganglia of the sheep. They show a fenestrated system. *e*, axon.

are found in some abundance in cranial ganglia, especially in the plexiform ganglion of the vagus, and must be considered as the first phase of those types which are provided with long dendrites ending in a club (Fig. 150, *b*).

2. Multipolar cells provided with very fine expansions starting either from the border of the soma or from the initial portion of the

axon and which, thickening successively, end in colossal spheres surrounded by a concentric system of nucleated capsules. Sometimes these appendices bifurcate, giving rise to two or more terminal globes (Fig. 151, a, b); not infrequently one sees fibres that terminate

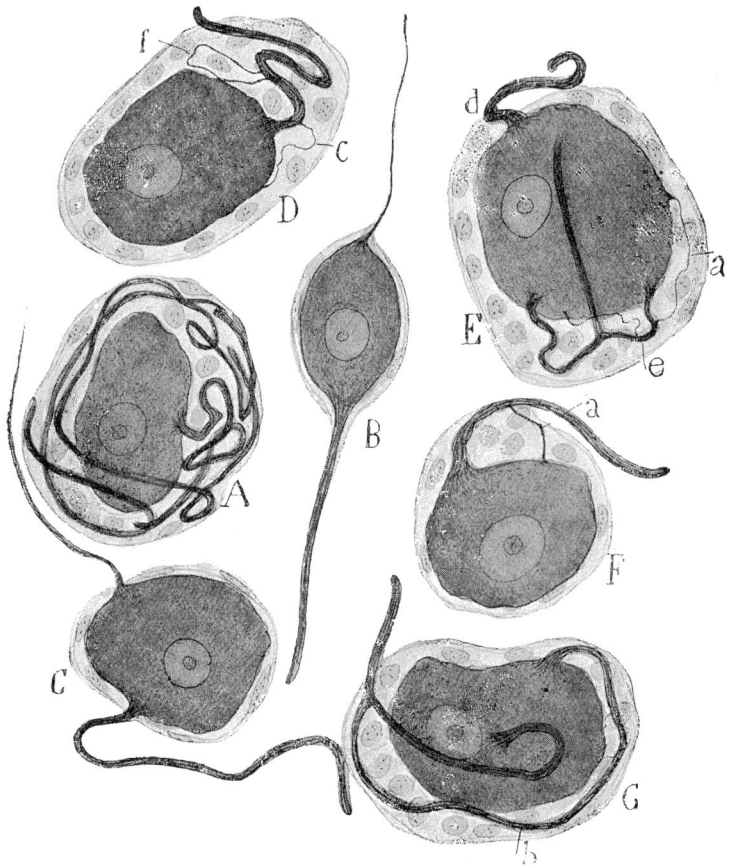

FIG. 153.—Sensory cells of the plexiform ganglion of the vagus of an adult man. A, glomerular cell; B, bipolar cell; D, E, neurones with fibrillar bundles in the periphery of the cytoplasm.

in a series of spheres or masses in very close proximity to each other. When the ball or mass is a recent one, the nucleated capsule is lacking.

Among the varieties of this strange cellular type, which reminds one somewhat of a type described many years ago by Huber, as found in an American frog, one may note these two: cells whose terminal spheres reside and end beneath the capsule of the cell of origin (Fig. 151, a), forming connections with the pericellular nerve nests of Dogiel; and cells whose very fine dendrites, which issue either from the cell or from the axon, send their terminal globes into the intercellular spaces, sometimes at a great distance from the original cell. Such strange elements are relatively common in man, donkeys, and horses, less common in dogs and cats.

3. *Fenestrated cells*, that is, cells that are perforated in the region of origin of the axon by two, three, or more openings, which are full of intracapsular neuroglial elements (Figs. 152 and 153, *E*).

These interesting cells, which were noted some time ago by H. Daae in the ganglia of horses, were thought to be an error of

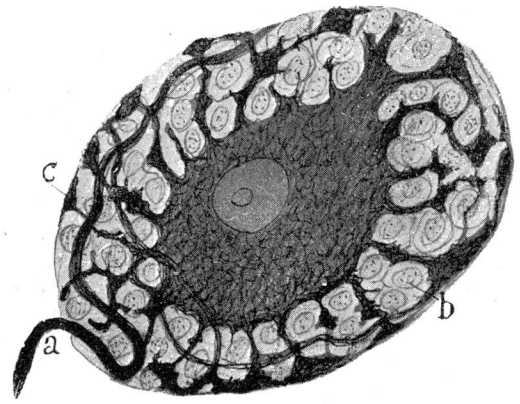

FIG. 154.—Sensory cell of an aged man. The peripheral portion of the protoplasm has been invaded by the satellite cells. *a*, axon; *b*, satellite cells; *c*, cellular appendices.

interpretation of the glomerulus, and were forgotten for many years. They were rediscovered by ourselves in numerous vertebrates, thanks to the method of reduced silver nitrate, which stains them very well. The appearance of the fenestrations varies much in different animal species. Thus in the sheep the fenestrated protoplasm assumes the form of a delicate mesh-work, whose hollow spaces are full of satellite cells. There are some extremely fine cordons and some that seem to be constituted by a single neurofibril. This fenestrated system lies sometimes in the region of origin of the axon, and the latter appears to result from the convergence of various protoplasmic arches or cordons; but in many cases the fenestrations are situated in cortical regions of the cell which are entirely foreign to the axon (Fig. 152, *A*). In the dog the fenestrations are simple and the uniting cordons are thick and short. In man they are still simpler. There they take the form of large holes or of a single opening surrounded by an arch or loop of great length (Fig. 153, *D, E*).

Levi (1908), using our method on fishes, found that in these animals the fenestrations, which are sometimes very complicated and arranged as a very delicate mesh-work, are situated exclusively in the voluminous cells.

4. Finally, in aged men, another cellular category is found, which we have called frayed cell, since it shows a frayed and festooned

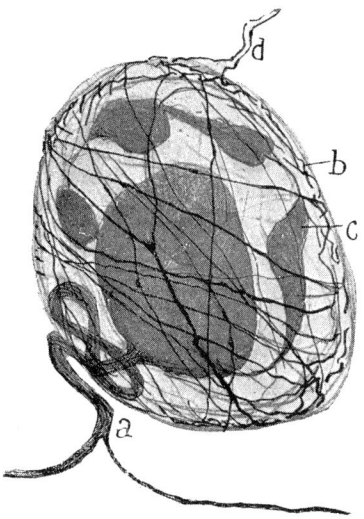

FIG. 155.—Pericellular nerve nest of a sensory cell of the gangliform plexus of the vagus in man. *a*, axon and its bifurcation ; *d*, afferent nerve fibres ; *b*, nerve nest ; *c*, bead-like dendrites.

outline which is full of pits and short expansions (Fig. 154). Each expansion, which reminds one of the teeth of a gear-wheel, is apt to end under the capsule in a thickening, or again in short branches which widen at their tips. Between such appendices there are present numerous satellite cells ; the axon appears normal. Various authors have confirmed the existence of this cellular type, not only in old men, but also in adult animals and in animals suffering from various pathological states (Levi, Rossi, Schaffer, Marinesco, Pacheco, etc.). They are, however, present more often in very old than in young mammals.

Spools and pericellular nervous arborizations.—Underneath the endothelial and connective capsule are found some fine varicose nervous ramifications, intimately applied to the protoplasm, and arranged in the form of a pericellular basket. These ramifications were first seen by Ehrlich in the frog, by ourselves in female mice, and somewhat later by Dogiel in the cat (Fig. 155).

The *pericellular baskets* or *nests* have been confirmed by ourselves in human sensory ganglia, where they are particularly abundant, especially in the ganglia of sensory cranial nerves. We called attention to the fact that they are not present in all the cells, but only in a small number of elements that are usually of the glomerular type. These arborizations are generally situated in the thickness of the capsule itself, outside the satellite cells (Fig. 155, *b*) and at a certain distance from the cell.

When one compares these pericellular arborizations with one another, one sees that they fall into three classes, according to their arrangement : (1) Type of pericellular spool in which one or several fibres, which retain their individuality, describe turns and loops round the soma, producing a complicated spool. These are the *spools* of Dogiel. One sometimes observes bifurcations. (2) Arborization type. The afferent fibres ramify around the cell, giving rise to varicose branches which end in terminal intumescences. (3) Periglomerular type. The afferent fibres, after going round the axon spirally, continue tracing turns around the glomerulus, producing a special plexus which is in contact with this portion of the axon. In many cases the fibres, after forming this periglomerular spool, advance towards the soma and form a perisomatic ramification. This latter type of nerve nest is known by the name of *mixed type*. We shall see that there are reasons for thinking that all these complicated arborizations are pathological dispositions.

Probable significance of the atypical forms.—The interpretation of those unusual forms which we have just noted and which have been confirmed in man as well as in many animals by various neurologists (Nageotte, Marinesco, Levi, Dogiel, O. Rossi, von Lenhossék, etc.), constitutes an arduous problem. The undertaking would be simple were such multipolar cells, nerve nests, etc., present only in pathological states or in very aged men and mammals. But many such dispositions have been observed in adult and healthy mammals. We discovered them for the first time in young men and women who died through accident. Levi has seen them even in embryos and in large numbers of perfectly normal vertebrates—fishes, reptiles, and mammals.

As is natural, such forms were at first taken for physiological dispositions. We all supposed that, besides the classical monopolar type of cell, the sensory ganglia contained a few multipolar neurones and certain nerve nests, which were considered as the terminal apparatus either of exogenous fibres (Cajal) or of ramified axons belonging to autochthonic neurones (Dogiel). But later investigations imposed a change of opinion. To-day it seems indubitable that these multipolar cellular types, as well as the pericellular nests, represent structures of a pathological and more or less ephemeral character.

The grounds on which this opinion is based are as follows :

1. The almost complete absence of these forms in recently born and young animals and their notable frequency in old age.

2. The extraordinary number of atypical elements, nests, and plexuses, that are found in various morbid states. They have been seen by Marinesco and Minea in crushed ganglia ; by Nageotte, Marinesco, Rossi, in transplanted ganglia ; by Nageotte, C. da Fano, and Schaffer, in tabes ; by Esposito and Rossi in various pathological states, such as dementia precox, progressive paralysis, senility, etc. ; by Pacheco in the ganglia of amputated individuals ; by Bielschowsky, in tabes and multiple sclerosis ; by ourselves, in wounded and excited ganglia, etc., etc.

3. The irregularity of their presence in the same individual. There are ganglia in which they are present in relative abundance, while in other ganglia of the same animal they are totally lacking.

4. Finally, nearly all the atypical cases can be produced, as we shall see below, by experimental means, such as ganglionic wounds, transplantations, excitations, crushing, etc.

The preceding facts suggest a certain point of view which is perhaps too much neglected by pathologists and anatomists, that of the *organic normal*. What must we understand by a normal organ or tissue ?

In an organ, as in a society, the *normal* always expresses a dominant type. The physiological organs and tissues are not those the whole of whose cells retain excellence of form, structure, and physiology, but those the great majority of whose components show these characteristics. But such healthy tissues or organs also contain decadent, fatigued, or degenerating elements, or even elements that are entirely destroyed. Finally, some of them, capable of restoration, are the seat of compensatory reactional processes—the renovation of expansions.

It is thus natural to think that the number of strong and active cells diminishes with age and with the various diseases of the animal. It cannot be otherwise, when one recalls the law of specific chemical activity of the nerve cells and that of functional localizations. Indeed, one cannot suppose, in view of the social principle of the division of labour, that at the end of a long life, full of vicissitudes, those neurones which acted and suffered most should be as normal as those which functioned slackly or from time to time.

A special property of all suffering cells seems to be, as Nageotte notes, the quick emission of new and multiple expansions, as though, in the sick and dying cell, the instinct of compensatory reproduction reappeared through atavism. This instinct is frustrated, since, as is well known, the neurones do not multiply. But if these cells have lost their power of reproduction and if neither the nucleus nor the soma can divide, there still remains in the cells a capacity to sprout. The cortical zone of the cytoplasm is able to put out expansions, as is also the axon along its entire length, the axon being itself a functional expansion. Thus the neurofibrils or living units of the neurofibrils, as other ultramicroscopic elements of the neuroplasma, have retained unaltered the privilege of multiplication, subject to the condition that the resulting mass be modelled in the shape of thin and ramified prolongations.

Theories of Nageotte on the significance of atypical ganglionar dispositions.—In view of the frequency of these forms in various pathological processes, and especially in the spinal ganglia of tabetics, and in view of their constant association with indisputable phenomena of degeneration and nervous sprouting, etc., Nageotte has been the first to propose[1] that we should consider all the dispositions referred to—including the nests, cells with dendrites, frayed cells, etc.—as resulting from pathological regenerative processes. He believes that already in the normal state some tubes degenerate and that the neurone prepares to restore the nervous expansion that is necrosed or gravely compromised, either by direct emissions from the soma, or by collaterals developed along the initial course of the axon.

It is only under pathological conditions, however, that the neoformative and degenerative processes of the axon assume extraordinary proportions, enormous quantities of free axons and bundles of newly-formed fibres (as in tabes) being then produced between the ganglion cells and in the roots. Since the majority of the newly-formed axons originate as collaterals from the axis-cylinder or the soma of the sensory neurone, Nageotte calls this form of sprouting, *collateral regeneration* to distinguish it from the *ordinary* or *terminal regeneration* that is produced, as is well known, at a great distance from the soma, in the interrupted or wounded axonic stump.

[1] Nageotte : " Régénération collatérale des fibres nerveuses terminées par des massues de croissance à l'état pathologique et à l'état normal," etc. *Nouvelle Iconographie de la Salpêtrière*, No. 3, mai, juin, 1906.

In connection with the interesting experiments of ganglionic transplantation of which we shall speak below, Nageotte [1] has amplified his theory of normal and pathological collateral regeneration, making it more precise, and enriching it with some very ingenious and suggestive hypotheses. Such especially is the distinction that he makes, in all nerve cells, and particularly in the sensory ganglion cells, between two kinds of appendices; the *orthophytes* or normal prolongations—the axon and dendrites—which have a constant morphology and connections, and whose function is the propagation of the nerve impulse; and the *paraphytes* or superfluous appendices, which are foreign to the conduction of currents and are not in connection with other neurones. Their function would be essentially trophic, since they are attracted by the subcapsular or satellite elements, whose nutritive mission seems to be certain.

Not all the *paraphytes* have the same fate nor have they the same significance. According to Nageotte, besides the paraphytes of a purely trophic character in relation with the satellite cells, there exist others, which ordinarily are larger, and which issue either from the soma or from the axon. They are characterized as follows: they show a terminal club or ball, they have a great capacity for growth, and, finally, they tend to reach those regions where there exist nervous lesions or interruptions that are in need of repair. These *regenerative paraphytes* might thus, after a time, be converted into legitimate *orthophytes*, re-establishing the interrupted nervous connections. Nageotte places in the category of *trophic paraphytes*—the first kind—the nests of Dogiel, our periglomerular plexuses, the appendices of the frayed cells, and many expansions described by us in the normal ganglia of man and in those of animals affected with hydrophobia. The second kind of paraphytes are especially the fibres that terminate in capsulated balls, whether issuing from the soma or from the axon.

The theory of Nageotte is tempting and exact in principle. After some hesitation we have accepted without reserve, as stated above, that the multipolar cells and those which are provided with balls, as well as the nerve nests, etc., represent abnormal dispositions. We think it certain that the majority, if not all, of the atypical expansions—*orthophytes* and *paraphytes*—have a regenerative character and may be compared to the sprouts of the central stump of an interrupted nerve.

There is something, however, in the conception of the French scientist, which leaves us with some doubts. Inspired by the principle of utilitarian adaptation, which is basically plausible, Nageotte seems

[1] Nageotte: " Etude sur la greffe des ganglions rachidiens," etc. *Anat. Anz.*, Nos. 9 and 10, Bd. 31, 1907.

preoccupied with giving to each atypical expansion its adequate function. This, no doubt, accounts for the somewhat artificial distinction among the expansions between *orthophytes* and *paraphytes*. But are the paraphytes anything else than the young or aborted forms of the orthophytes ? We are accustomed to see nature produce superabundantly in order to make sure of attaining once the goal, as when an enormous number of sprouts are created and frustrated in the regeneration of nerves.

In our opinion the neoformative act—the multiplication of the neurofibrils, etc.—does not necessarily imply a congruent nervous restoration. The arrival of the sprouts at the peripheral stump and the re-establishment of interrupted connections constitute secondary, and, to a certain extent, fortuitous phenomena, which have nothing to do with the essential act of production. This arrival occurs when the newly-formed appendices succeed in orienting themselves and possess enough energy of growth to reach their goal ; it fails if these requisite conditions are lacking. It is, moreover, recognized by Nageotte that the orthophytes and paraphytes, which are very abundant in tabes and other pathological states where the axons suffer, are also present in neurones whose axon is entire and apparently in a good physiological state. Their production cannot therefore always be the result of the necessity of restoring or regenerating communications that are destroyed or impaired.

We believe, upon a survey of these phenomena, that one should lay aside all teleological conceptions and consider the phenomena as reactional manifestations of the axon or of the neuronal soma in presence of mechanical, physical, or chemical stimuli ; a doctrine which, in its essentials, has been defended by Levi and other authors.

Theory of Levi.—The theoretical inductions of Nageotte have been opposed by Levi,[1] who based himself on anatomico-pathological studies of the ganglia of man and on the comparative histology of many vertebrates.

Levi is of opinion that the fenestrations and appendices that we pointed out in mammals, the analogous dispositions that he found in fishes and reptiles, and those shown by Nageotte in his masterly analysis of tabetic lesions, all lack any regenerative purpose. Their production would, in his view, be a mere effect of the multiplication of the neurofibrils and consequent augmentation of the nervous protoplasm, under the influence of normal or pathological stimuli. But,

---

[1] G. Levi : " Struttura e istogenesi dei gangli cerebro-spinali dei mammiferi," *Anat. Anz.*, Bd. 30, 1907.
See also : *Gangli cerebro-spinali*, Firenze, 1908.

owing to the exigencies of nutritive metabolism, this augmentation of the soma cannot take place as a whole, through the apposition of mantles, but the excess has to be distributed in fine appendices. Thus when, as occurs in tabes, the pathological stimulus brings about neurofibrillar multiplication, the reticulum, through a compensatory reaction, distributes itself in loops, fenestrated systems, and especially in protoplasmic and axonic prolongations. According to this view all the newly-formed fibres possess a trophic character, since they all tend to amplify and stimulate the chemical exchanges with the environment ; but, not even in tabes, where the nests and other newly-formed appendices are found very abundantly, as Nageotte has discovered, can one ever see the re-establishment of interrupted paths.

Levi's theory contains also, like Nageotte's, an element of truth, but it errs by its exclusiveness. It appears certain that the cell, stimulated by certain chemical influences, creates appendices which are superfluous or unable—perhaps *per accidens*—to restore lesioned paths ; but it is not less certain, as Nageotte observed, that many fibres have anatomically and dynamically all the properties of regenerating fibres, and travel towards the lesioned parts.

Besides, the theory of *protoplasmic unfolding* is not easily applicable to all the cases of neurofibrillar neoformation. In our opinion, only the fenestrated system of sensory neurones answers fully to Levi's conception. Laying aside for the moment the formative mechanism, it is indubitable that the fenestrated dispositions are constant systems that are almost exclusively localized in sensory neurones of large size. They appear necessary to guarantee the nutrition of the superabundant protoplasmic material. But the appendices of the frayed cells, the sub- and extracapsular fibres terminating in a ball, and, finally, the fine appendices issuing from the axon, are formations that have an unquestionable regenerative significance.

We cannot here discuss in detail Levi's hypothesis. We must be content to cite here a few facts which it is difficult to reconcile with that theory.

1. The nests of Dogiel, often produced by retrograde fibres coming from the wound of the cut sensory root, are evidently regenerated fibres ; to suppose that they are the effect of a protoplasmic unfurling of a trophic nature would be equivalent to attributing the same character to the innumerable sprouts of the central stump of a regenerated nerve. 2. The majority of cells provided with appendices are smaller in size than their congeners in the same ganglion. 3. In frayed cells the soma has become smaller. 4. As we shall see below, in wounds and contusions of the ganglia a mere traumatic excitation or the

resulting nutritional perturbations cause the formation of somatic appendices which are capable of growth, without there being appreciable alterations of size or structure in the soma. 5. Finally, many appendices, especially those arising from the axon, grow towards the white substance of the ganglion and reach the roots, or even traverse the ganglionar capsule to emerge from the ganglion, behaving entirely like the newly-formed fibres of the central stump of interrupted nerves.

In fine, without prejudice to a further discussion of this important problem, it appears to us certain that, by virtue of conditions which as yet are enigmatic, any sensory neurone can temporarily, and in the absence of destructive axonic processes, enter into *neurocladism* (*divisory turgescence*), emitting appendices that are nervous in character, since they all grow, ramify, and terminate like true axons. Obeying a law that is very evident in the central stump of interrupted nerves, the stimulated cell, as though it foresaw possible injuries and desired better to insure the act of restoration, gives rise to a great number of sprouts. When the stimulus is due to chemical agents incapable of seriously altering the neurone, the resulting neoformation is incongruent and superfluous. It represents, as it were, a purposeless pathological atavism, a vicious functional habit, comparable in principle to the emission of the polar bodies from the egg. When, on the other hand, the neoformation is due to grave pathological causes, such as toxins, traumatic agents, etc., some fortunate sprouts are able to reach the lesion and to repair, more or less imperfectly, the interrupted paths. Any paraphyte would thus be capable, if circumstances favour it, of conversion into an orthophyte. Ordinarily, however, the paraphytes, detained by various obstacles and transformed into abortive formations, rarely reach their goal.

ADDITIONAL NOTE TO CHAPTER I.

F. de Castro [1] has made an extensive and very careful study of the interpretation of the atypical forms of the ganglion cells of man, their development, and their relation with various pathological states. This study contains many observations of new dispositions, both normal and pathological. We cannot enter here into the details of this lengthy and conscientious monograph. Suffice it to say that Castro adds many new types to those previously known, and that his observations, relating to a considerable number of cases, constitute to-day the most

[1] F. de Castro: " Estudio sobre los ganglios sensitivos del hombre en estado normal y patológico." *Trab. del Lab. de Investig. biol.*, t. 19, 1921.

complete picture of the morphology and development in man of the ganglion cells.

The work of Agduhr,[1] also very interesting, has to do with the post-foetal development of the spinal ganglion of mammals. According to him young animals have, besides the formed cells of almost the adult type, other small cells arranged as zoogloea, maintained in the embryonic phase, and capable of dividing directly and indirectly. From these two polar expansions emerge at a late stage. Lorente de Nó has seen something of this in the ganglia of tadpoles, where, by the side of fully-formed cells, there are others whose central branch, crowned by a ball of growth, has not yet perforated the *pia mater*. He has not seen in these tadpoles, however, either the embryonic types of Buehler or mitotic figures.

[1] Agduhr: "Studien über die postembryonale Entwicklung der Neuronen." *Journ. f. Psychol. u. Neurol.*, Bd. 25, 1920.

II

DEGENERATION AND REGENERATION OF THE SENSORY NERVE GANGLIA

Traumatic degeneration of the sensory cells and tubes.—Regenerative acts of the cells and fibres following on wounds, contusions, and extirpation of nerves, etc.— Genesis of the pericellular nests.

PHENOMENA FOLLOWING ON GANGLIONAR TRAUMATISMS

THESE phenomena must be distinguished into primary or *degenerative* and secondary or *regenerative*. Ordinarily the primary phenomena precede the secondary. But in certain cells regeneration is so precocious that both processes occur simultaneously and become mixed up.

1. **Degeneration of the sensory cells and tubes**—When one produces a wound or contusion on a spinal ganglion, all the cells that are situated near the lesion, as well as those which are reached indirectly by the mechanical agent, fall into necrobiosis, appearing two or three days later as granular masses in the process of being resorbed. The remnants of the cellular protoplasm disappear progressively, and in their place is established a nest of polyhedral cells which are mingled with leucocytes ; these are the *residual nodules* of Nageotte. The polyhedral cells indubitably arise through the proliferation of satellite or subcapsular cells; these resist traumatic violence much more than nerve cells. The leucocytes come from the blood. We shall speak of both these kinds of phagocytes, especially when we study *neuronophagy*.

Similar phenomena of degeneration and necrobiosis occur in contused or interrupted nerves. In the immediate vicinity of the wound the necrosis of the axon and the cell of Schwann occur rapidly, and the *detritus* is resorbed. At some distance from the lesion the tubes degenerate, passing through the well-known phases of axonic and myelinic fragmentation. In the ganglion three types of degeneration are mixed up, which it is difficult to discern in each tube : *primary centrifugal degeneration*, brought about in the two branches of the sensory cell by granular destruction or by a grave lesion of the soma ; *traumatic degeneration*, which occurs in the central stump—the segment which is united to the unharmed neurone— of interrupted fibres ; finally *secondary* or *Wallerian degeneration*, brought about in the peripheral stump of the aforementioned branches consecutively to the interruption between them and the normal soma.

For degeneration of the tubes and sensory cells to take place it is not necessary to operate on the ganglion itself ; it is sufficient for the traumatism to act on the nerves at a distance, subject to the condition that the mechanical commotion is propagated, like an oscillatory movement, to the neurone of origin. In this way the extirpation of the sciatic nerve at some distance from the ganglia brings about the mortification of some cells, as well as the primary retrograde degeneration of their expansions. Five days after the extirpation, in young cats, one already finds half resorbed neurones, and even true residual nodules similar to those described by Nageotte in transplanted ganglia, as we shall point out below.

Between the region of the dead cells and those which remain apparently unharmed every wounded ganglion shows, as we have noted,[1] certain cells that are still living, and possessing either no axon or else an axon that is more or less altered and in whose soma have occurred metamorphoses of a degenerative character.

The principal types found are as follows :

(*a*) *Frayed cell or cell in the shape of a toothed wheel.*—This is similar to the special cell that we found in senile ganglia, and it is characterized by the fact that in its periphery are certain divergent appendices terminating under the capsule, which they never cross. Between them the latent cells have proliferated abundantly. (Fig. 156, *K*).

(*b*) *Hirudiform cell.*—We have thus named certain elements whose protoplasm has lost the neurofibrillar skeleton ; this has occurred least near the nucleus, where one can see a network of neurofibrils, sometimes replaced by bundles of fibres, which are intensely stained by colloidal silver and in continuity with the nervous expansion. We call them *hirudiform* because they remind one of the neurofibrillar disposition described by Apathy as his *type I* in the ganglia of leeches (Fig. 156, *P*).

[1] Cajal : " Algunas observaciones favorables à la hipótesis neurotrópica," *Trab. del Lab. de Investig. biol.*, tomo 8, 1911.

(c) *Angular cell.*—Around this type of cell the satellite cells have grown in a marked degree, submerging the cortical region of the sensory neuronal protoplasm and creating in it small pits which lend to the soma an angular and irregular aspect (Fig. 156, *R*). Ordinarily this lesion is combined with a partial or general hypertrophy of the superficial neurofibrils, which sometimes take on the disposition of anastomosed cordons separated by large meshes of neuroplasm. In other cases the neurofibrils merely unite as anastomotic bundles which are separated by vacuoles. The transitions between this fasciculated disposition and that of thick anastomotic cordons show that we are dealing with phases of the same process. Nageotte and Marinesco have seen a similar superficial reticulation of hypertrophied neurofibrils in transplanted ganglia.

(d) *Retracted cell, whose periphery bristles with neurofibrillar arches and loops,* reproducing something like the first phase of the fenestrated state of certain normal sensory cells.

(e) *Deformed cell,* pulled out, and sometimes strangulated in its centre, with irregular lobulations and excrescences which remind one of certain ganglionic cells of turtles.

All these transformations show that the sensory neurone is attacked and gravely perturbed by the adjacent section of the axon, and perhaps by the mechanical action of the vulnerating agent. At any rate, ten and fifteen days after the operation the majority of these altered cells are still present. But we do not know whether they ultimately become normal, the piece of axon or the mutilated and regenerated branches being restored, or whether, on the contrary, they finally atrophy and die. We think it probable that the abovementioned perturbations are of varying importance for the biology of the cell. Thus, the *hirudiform* elements and, in general, those in which no axon is present, seem more gravely compromised than the frayed cells and those which retain their functional expansion.

2. **Regenerative phenomena.**—These occur in the cells as well as in interrupted ganglionic nerve tubes.

(a) *Production of expansions in the sensory cells.*—These appendices, the *paraphytes* of Nageotte, arise, like those in transplanted ganglia, both from the soma and from the initial glomerulus. They are usually fine, they travel beneath the capsule, and they contribute to the complexity of the plexuses or pericellular nests. As we shall note below, the *paraphytes* or atypical expansions are seen less frequently in wounded than in transplanted ganglia.

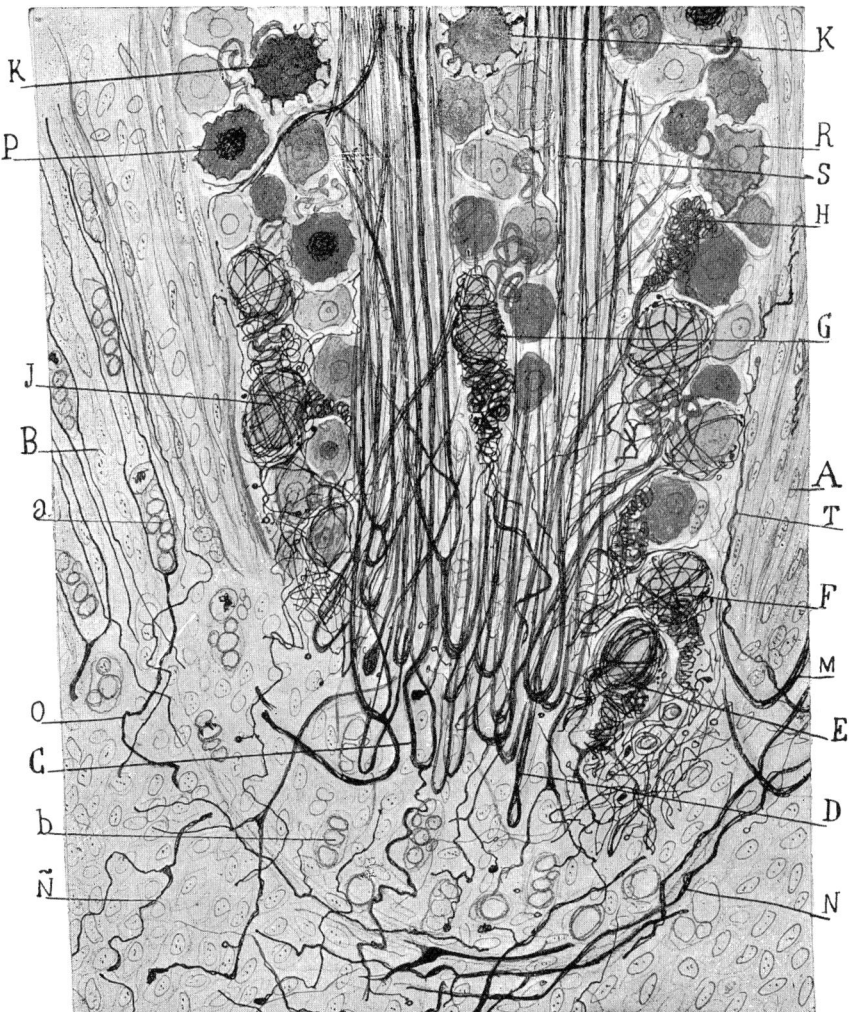

FIG. 156.—Axial section of a sensory ganglion of the sacral region, cut transversely. Young cat, killed six days after the operation. *A*, connective tissue capsule of the ganglion; *B*, neighbouring sensory root which was cut and is in full degeneration; *C, D*, curves described by bundles of fibres on reaching the scar—ravelled and growing fibres; *E, F, G, J*, pericellular nests; *H*, periglomerular nest; *K*, frayed cells; *R*, angular cells; *P*, hirudiform cells; *M*, fibres coming from another neighbouring root; *S*, axons with ravelled collaterals; *N, Ñ*, sensory fibres ramified in the scar.

(b) *Cells from whose soma arise appendices that do not divide or do so rarely, and end in more or less voluminous balls.*—These elements also are relatively rare in ganglionic wounds.

(c) *Pericellular spools.*—These were first seen by Veratti [1] in traumatised ganglia, and they constitute an almost constant factor in them. We may note that they occur whenever there is, near the ganglion or within it, a source of retrograde nerve sprouts. In wounded ganglia such nests occur preferably in cells that are close to the lesion. As the distance from the lesion increases they progressively diminish, until they fail completely (Fig. 156, *J*).

There are also numerous periglomerular spools and loops of newly-formed fibres around the extracapsular portion of the axons (Fig. 156, *F, H*). There are some spools which are so extensive that they enclose, within their circles, two and three neighbouring cells, as we shall see below. We shall speak more in detail of these and other pericellular nests when we describe ganglionic grafts.

Regeneration of cut tubes.—As in the nerves, the sensory axons that are interrupted either in the ganglion or near it—the nerve roots—show: a *peripheral stump* which has degenerated, and a *central stump* which is regenerating. Between these two stumps lies the scar, composed of embryonic connective tissue.

Neither the degeneration of the peripheral stump nor the regeneration of the central stump presents anything of particular interest. We need only note that the collateral and terminal branches of the axons of the central stump become ravelled, and in each one of them is formed a close bundle which, on arriving at the scar, rapidly turns back to the ganglion. It is from these retrograde fibres, which we reproduce in Fig. 156, *C, D*, that are very largely formed the pericellular and periglomerular nests. The frequency and relative ease with which the fibres adopt this retrograde path, and their arrival at the perineuronal capsule, are well explained by stereotropism. The sprouts lean on the sheaths of Schwann, either within or outside them, and guided in that way they reach the ganglion cells. We need not exclude neurotropism, which possibly acts preferentially on the intratubal sprouts. We may add that a great many conductors that contribute to the formation of the pericellular spools or bundles do not come from the scar, but arise

---

[1] Veratti: "Alcune osservazioni sui procesi consecutive alle ferite dei gangli spinali," *Atti della Soc. ital. di Patol.* IVa reunione, Pavia, 1907.

along the intraganglionar path of axons which are stimulated by the vicinity of the wound (Fig. 156).

Veratti,[1] who has seen these pericellular spools following on wounds of the ganglia, does not venture definitely to consider them as newly formed, but he supposes that they are pre-existent and limits himself to saying that they *take the stain better than in the normal*

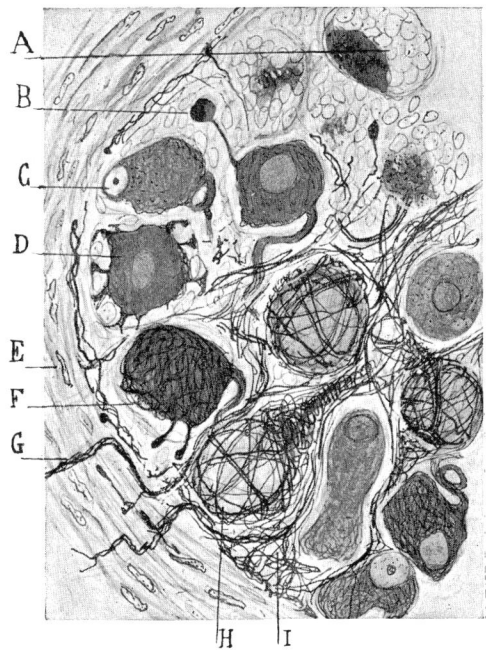

FIG. 157.—Piece of a ganglion of a young cat, which was killed five days after the extirpation of the sciatic nerve.—*A*, necrosed cell; *B*, cell from which arise appendices ending in balls; *C*, cell with a marginal nucleus; *D*, cell of the frayed type; *H*, pericellular spools; *G*, newly formed fibres which cross the capsule of the ganglion.

state, and that they possess a greater richness and complication of fibres. O. Rossi,[2] on the contrary, when making a résumé of this paper by Veratti, is led to think that these nests may, in pathological ganglia, be more numerous than usual.[3]

Phenomena of degeneration and regeneration occurring in the

[1] He states: "Non è possibile però asserire con sicurezza se questo insolito modo di presentarsi degli apparati pericellulari sia da considerare como espressione di un processo degenerativo o rigenerativo."

[2] O. Rossi: *Rivista di pat. ner. e mentale*, vol. 12, fasc. 8, 1907.

[3] See additional note on p. 425.

ganglia as a result of the extirpation of the sensory roots.—When one extirpates the sciatic of a rabbit or young cat in such a way that the nerve rupture occurs about half a centimetre below the ganglia, the examination of the latter generally shows alterations that are fairly similar to those caused by wounds. The phenomena observed are both degenerative and regenerative.

Degenerative processes.—As in the case of ganglionic wounds, certain sensory neurones become necrobiosed and their remnants progressively disappear (Fig. 157, *A*). In their place are concentrated a great number of polyhedral cells, doubtless arising through a proliferation of the subcapsular elements. At the same time all the nerve tubes in continuity with these susceptible neurones also degenerate.

Besides these mortified elements, the interior of the ganglion exhibits others which have preserved their vitality, although they show evident signs of degeneration. The analogy between these surviving cells and those which were described in the case of ganglionic wounds dispenses us from describing them in detail. We need merely mention that the following types, shown in Figs. 157 and 158, are frequently present : (*a*) the *frayed cells* (Fig. 157, *D*) ; (*b*) the *lobulated* or *deformed cells* ; (*c*) elements whose cortical region is sprinkled with *vacuoles* and *neurofibrillar cordons* ; (*d*) cells that have *nerve loops*, etc. Such diseased elements may not be present in the entire ganglion, but only in some special region, that is, the territory from which arise the nerve tubes most affected by the extirpation.

Regenerative phenomena.—These are interesting, and may be studied in Figs. 157 and 158, where, among other cells, can be seen the following : (*a*) elements provided with extracapsular appendices ending in prolonged clubs (Figs. 157, *F*, and 158, *C*) ; (*b*) neurones from whose soma arise thin fibrils ending outside the capsule in voluminous clubs (Fig. 157, *B*) ; (*c*) cells undergoing chromatolysis, as can be seen in preparations stained with the aniline dyes, with a tangential nucleus (Fig. 157, *C*) ; (*d*) cells from whose soma or axon, but at a short distance from the former, arise long and ramified fibres ending in a point and wandering in the intercellular spaces. In Fig. 158, *A*, *B*, we show two typical cells of this type, whose expansions, five days after the operation, in a young cat, were already very long. One of them (*B*) showed two thick branches issuing from a warty axonic stump ; the rest of the axon had doubtless disappeared through degeneration. In the neurones *C* and *D* the sprouts leave the healthy axon at some distance from the soma.

The phenomenon that is most interesting, because of its intensity and general occurrence, is the production of *pericellular nests* and of *interstitial nerve plexuses* (Figs. 157, *H*, and 158, *g*).

The *spools* or *nests* can be distinguished into two categories, in respect of the origin of their elements. Some represent the point of

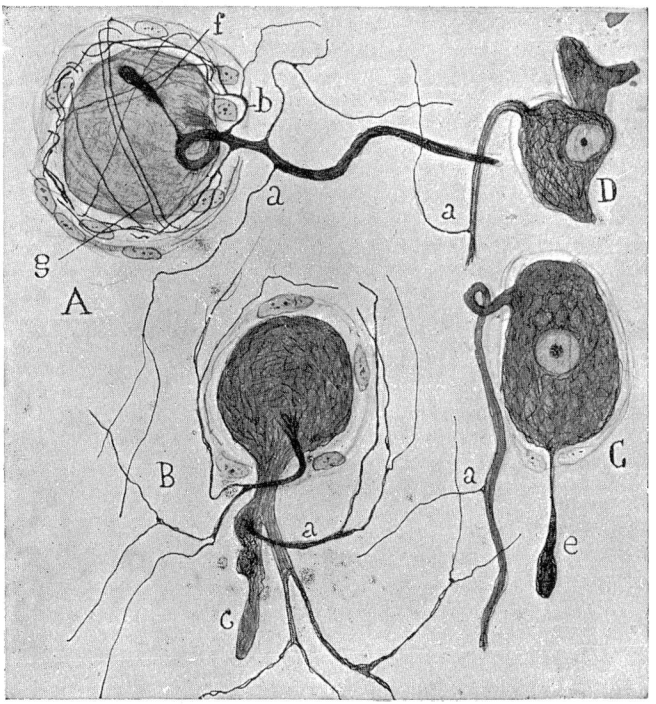

FIG. 158.—A few types of ganglionic sprouting taken from the ganglion of a cat, which was killed five days after extirpation of the sciatic nerve. *A*, cell with pericellular plexus and branches arising from the axon; *B*, cell provided with long newly-formed fibres proceeding from the soma and remnants of the broken axon (*c*); *D*, lobulated cell; *C*, cell with an appendix ending in a club.

concurrence and unfolding of appendices originating in the initial portion of neighbouring axons or of the axon of the neurone that carries the nest; others, doubtless the great majority, issue from retrograde nerve fibres that have come from a great distance, that is, from the central stump of the wounded nerve tubes—the scar.

The *interstitial plexuses* also are composed of these retrograde fibres. They form, in certain portions of the ganglion, very complicated skeins and spools, which insinuate themselves irregularly between the neurones and extend up to the periganglionic capsule (Fig. 157, *I*). A few bundles, which appear precociously, do not

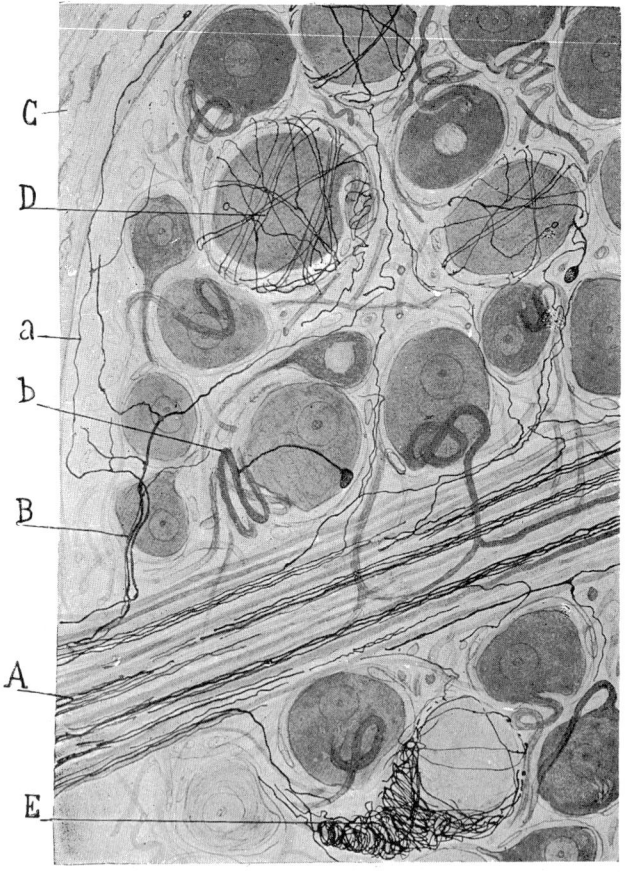

FIG. 159.—Section of a lumbar ganglion of a cat a few days old, whose corresponding root was lesioned. *A*, bundles of new fibres penetrating into the white substance of the ganglion; *B*, fibres lost beneath the ganglionic capsule; *C*, capsule; *D*, spool of Dogiel; *E*, periglomerular bundle; *b*, glomerulus which has produced a branch terminating in a club.

stay within the connective capsules, but, as though scenting out its clefts, they traverse it, tracing stair-like paths, emerging finally on the opposite side and losing themselves in the surrounding plasmatic spaces (Fig. 157, *G*).

Many of the above-mentioned lesions have also been observed

by Marinesco and Minea [1] in ganglia which were momentarily crushed by a forceps. When the compression is moderate the majority of the cells survive, but the medullated tubes fall into neurolysis. According to these scientists the lesioned axons of the central stump give rise, through a collateral or terminal branch, or through a simple neurofibrillar dissociation, to a multitude of sprouts which, travelling with the nerve tube up to the neurone of origin, form complicated pericellular spools or bundles. When the compression is vigorous many sensory cells die, and those which survive show, among other alterations, the following : appendices ending in subcapsular clubs, marginal ravelling of the soma, which becomes covered with loops and meshes or clear spaces, etc. Finally, after a time—eighteen days after the compression—the white matter becomes full of newly formed bundles.

As to the origin and significance of the pericellular nests, normal as well as pathological, we have already given the opinion of Nageotte [2] which we have adopted without reserve. It is certainly not shared by all the neurologists, however. Thus Dogiel [3] in his investigations of the ganglionic nests of the horse, is inclined to hold the old doctrine which regards them as normal forms, foreign to any regenerative acts. We have already spoken of the views of Levi [4] which differ from those of both Nageotte and Dogiel. On the other hand the neuropathologists, *mutatis mutandis*, incline towards the views of Nageotte, especially in conceding a neoformative and pathological character to the interstitial nerve plexuses. Among such scientists one may include Marinesco and Minea,[5] O. Rossi,[5] Pacheco,[5] Schaffer,[5] Bielschowsky,[5] etc., who have studied these structures, especially in various diseases of man.

[1] Marinesco et Minea : " Recherches expérimentales et anatomo-pathologiques sur les lésions consécutives à la compression et à l'écrasement des ganglions sensitifs," *Folia neurobiologica*, Bd. 1, No. 1, Nov. 1907.

[2] Nageotte : " Etude sur la greffe des ganglions rachidiens," etc. *Anat. Anzeiger*, Bd. 31, Nos. 9 and 20, 1907.

[3] Dogiel : " Zur Frage des feinere Bau der Spinalganglien beim Säugethieren," *Inter. Monatschr. f. Anat. u. Physiol.*, Bd. 14, 1897.
Der Bau der Spinalganglien der Menschen und der Säugethieren, Jena 1908.

[4] Levi : *I Gangli Cerebrospinali*, Firenze, 1908.

[5] Marinesco et Minea : " Quelques recherches sur la transplantation des ganglions nerveux," *Revue neurologique*, No. 6, 1907. " Nouvelles recherches sur la transplantation des ganglions nerveux " (transplantation chez la grenouille), *Compt. rend. de la Soc. de Biol. de Paris*, 25 février 1907. " Plasticité et amiboïdisme des cellules des ganglions sensitifs," *Revue neurologique*, No. 21, 25 nov. 1907.

[5] O. Rossi : " Ueber einige morphologische Besonderheiten der Spinal-

Apart from the suggestive arguments of Nageotte, Marinesco has proved that the nests appear also on ganglia transplanted on a cut nerve, developing at the expense of the newly-formed fibres of the central stump. Ottorino Rossi, for his part, has repeated this interesting experiment with the same result. Finally, the observation by Marinesco and Minea of complicated pericellular nests in ganglia stimulated by crushing, and the presence of such forms in wounded ganglia (Veratti and Cajal), or in ganglia whose roots have been extirpated (Cajal), do not leave the least doubt as to the regenerative character of the nests. This is a special phase of the incongruent exodus of the sprouts which are influenced by stereotropism and the mechanical conditions of the environment.

Naturally, in wounded ganglia and nerves, the sprouts have their origin in the interrupted tubes; but when the spools or nests appear in normal animals (Dogiel, Cajal and Olóriz, etc.), we can only invoke, as stated above, the stimulating action of some agent of catabolism, toxic substances of digestive origin, etc.

Although all that has been stated above elucidates sufficiently the origin of the spools, we cannot resist the temptation of making known a decisive proof obtained by us when carrying out an experiment of crushing and cutting the sensory roots, away from the ganglion, in young cats (Fig. 159).

When one examines the central stump of the roots five or six days after the operation, one can see that the axons in course of divisory turgescence have generated a multitude of retrograde fibres, some of which are intertubal, others intratubal, and which, after a very long itinerary, reach the completely normal ganglion. There the small retrograde bundles abandon, along different planes, the sheaths of Schwann of the old tubes, and make for the cortical region of the ganglion, where they become definitely lost. A comparative study of the intra and extraganglionic portions of the posterior root shows that all or nearly all the above-mentioned fibres end in the ganglion. While the intraganglionic portion is furrowed by numerous newly-formed bundles, in the extraganglionic portion one sees only a few

ganglien bei den Säugethiere," etc. *Journ. f. Psychol. und Neurol.*, Bd. 11, 1908.

[5] Pacheco : " Sur les types cellulaires des ganglions spinaux de l'homme à l'état normal et dans quelques états pathologiques," *Arch. du Real Institute Bacteriol. Camara-Pestana*, vol. 3, fasc. 1, 1910.

[5] Schaffer : " Ueber Fibrillenbilder tabischer Spinalganglienzellen," etc. *Zeitschr. f. die gesamte Neuropat. u. Psychiatrie*, Bd. 1, H. 4, 1910.

[5] Bielschowsky : " Ueber den Bau der Spinalganglien in der normal und pathol. Verhältnissen," *Journ. f. Psychol. u. Neurol.*, Bd. 2, 1908.

rare fibres which have been unable to leave the bundles of the central ganglionic region.

Once they have ventured among the sensory roots, the fate of these wandering fibres is very diverse. A considerable number lose their way among the bundles of sensory tubes and in the interstices of the ganglionic grey matter, where they repeatedly divide, ending in very small clubs. Others reach the capsule, above which they travel along parallel paths, giving rise to ample arborizations (Fig. 159, a). Finally the majority, after having reached the ganglionic grey cortex, become resolved into pericellular or periglomerular nests or spools. The disposition of these spools is shown in Fig. 159, C, D, where one can see how the number of their afferent fibres varies. Some neurones receive two or three fibres which, having reached the capsule, describe numerous turns around it. Others show only a single afferent fibre which is reeled up into little complicated spools. One often sees in these nests bifurcations and fine spherules or terminal rings (Fig. 159, D). One sometimes sees next to pericellular spools periglomerular spools; in Fig. 159, E, we show one of these, which is very complicated in design. There the afferent fibril or fibrils first trace spirals, outside the membrane of Schwann, around the extracapsular portion of the nerve tube; they finally penetrate beneath the capsule and circle about the flexuosities of the glomerulus. Moreover, Nageotte, and also Marinesco and Minea, have seen periglomerular spools in transplanted ganglia.

Thus the facts of experimental pathology that we have adduced leave definitely established the opinion of Nageotte as to the regenerative and abnormal character of the fibres that produce the spools or bundles found in normal as well as in pathological ganglia.

ADDITIONAL NOTE TO CHAPTER II.

An important confirmation of the lesions described above is due to F. de Castro.[1] In a man who underwent an operation in the neck, the surgical intervention produced a section of the vagus next to the *plexiform ganglion*. This was examined six days after the operation, when all the cells of the ganglion were found transformed into multipolar cells, displaying handles, numerous fenestrations, appendices ramified either within or without the capsule. There were seen, besides, a large quantity of *bundles* or *spools* of nerve collaterals, arising from their intra and extra-capsular path in the ganglion. These bundles, devoid of nuclei, which have nothing to do with Nageotte's residual nodules, are another proof of the free growth of the newly-formed fibres.

[1] F. de Castro: "Estudio sobre los ganglios sensitivos del hombre en estado normal y patológico." *Trab. del Lab. de Investig. biol.*, t. 19, 1921.

III

MORPHOLOGICAL VARIATIONS OBSERVED IN TRANSPLANTED SENSORY GANGLIA

Fundamental experiments of Nageotte.—Confirmations by Marinesco and Minea, Rossi, Dustin, Cardenal and ourselves.—Aberrant nerves.—Neuronophagy.— Experiments of cultivation of ganglia " in vitro " by Cajal, Legendre and Minot, Marinesco, etc.—Theories of Nageotte, Marinesco, and other authors, concerning the mechanism of formation of the neuronal appendices.

Experiments of transplantation of sensory ganglia.—The transplantation of sensory ganglia had been attempted by various authors, especially by Marinesco,[1] who observed, besides a necrosis and absorption of the sensory elements, the proliferation of the satellite cells around the cellular cadaver, and *neuronophagy* by migratory leucocytes.

It was only Nageotte,[2] however, who was able to show the survival of the sensory neurones in the grafts, and who revealed, along with curious modifications brought about in the soma, the important fact of the sprouting of new expansions. He says : " In the course of experiments designed for the investigation of the form of sprouting of the axons, I have been led to try the grafting of spinal ganglia. The resistance of these organs to temporary anaemia in Stenon's experiment had led me to suppose that one should be able to effect their survival in grafts. On the other hand, I presumed that the

---

[1] Marinesco : *Annales de l'Académie roumaine*, Série II. tome 29, et *Moniteur officiel* du 16 mai, 1906.

See also : *Revue générale des Sciences*, 15 mars, 1907.

[2] These facts are taken from the excellent résumé made by Nageotte in his *Notice sur les travaux scientifiques de M. J. Nageotte*, Paris, 1911.

See also the notes of this author in the *Compt. Rend. de la Soc. de Biol. de Paris*, of Jan. 19, Feb. 23, Mar. 9, and April 13, 1907, and especially the two following studies.

Idem: " Neurophagie dans les greffes des ganglions rachidiens," *Revue neurologique*, no. 17, 15 sept. 1907.

Idem : " Etude sur la greffe des ganglions rachidiens, variations et tropismes du neurone sensitif," *Anat. Anzeiger*, No. 9-10, 1907.

abnormal state brought about by transplantation would provoke modifications in the cells, and especially the appearance of new fibres which would arise through collateral regeneration at the expense of the preserved cells. My hopes were not disappointed. Not only have I obtained the survival of a great number of cells in the grafted ganglia, and the appearance of numerous new expansions, but also considerable modifications in the cell body, which, from being unipolar, becomes multipolar, taking on complicated and even monstrous shapes. . . . In these experiments we must consider the appearance of new fibres as the result of the perturbation brought about in the nutrition of the cells during the dangerous phase of the rooting and accommodation of the graft. A great number of neurones die at that moment, in particular all those in the centre of the ganglion; the rare cells that have resisted, which are those situated beneath the ganglionic capsule, have had their vitality gravely impaired for a time. . . . We know, indeed, that in states of suffering one observes in organized beings phenomena of hastened reproduction or attempts at regeneration. Pruning is a method designed to cause suffering systematically in such plants as are required to give an abundant and precocious flowering. It seems to me probable that in the grafts of ganglia the intense plastic activity of the cells, following a danger of imminent death, is a fact in the same category, being due in part at least to the stimulus brought about by physiological suffering. . . . Doubtless the variations of the osmotic pressure are also factors in this phenomenon."

We have quoted this long passage in order to show the inspiring ideas that led Nageotte to the interesting discovery of artificial multipolar cells.

The technique of transplantation is very simple. Nageotte takes out, with antiseptic precautions, a sensory ganglion of a rabbit recently born or a few days old, and transplants it under the skin of the ear of an adult rabbit. The interesting phenomena begin from the fifth or sixth day on, and the cells die between the second and the third week. The ganglia to be examined were fixed in ammoniacal alcohol, and stained by our method of reduced silver nitrate. Fixation in pyridine, as used by us, is even better.

The facts observed by Nageotte may be summarized as follows:

1. A few surviving marginal cells give rise to one, two, or more fine expansions, which are dendritic in appearance, ramified in a complex way, and have branches that often terminate within the

capsule, and less frequently outside it (Figs. 163 and 169). Certain elements of this category, richly provided with expansions, take on the appearance of sympathetic cells, closely resembling the cells with a dendritic crown described by us in the sympathetic system of aged men.

2. Other neurones, which are also multipolar, instead of having long and fine expansions, show thick, nodular appendices, covered, that is, with tubercles and fungiform eminences and ending in clubs which are usually situated outside the capsule, right in the connective interstices. Some dendrites break up into tufts of appendices crowned with balls. Nageotte says : " We are doubtless dealing here with forms of involution indicative of the senility of the cell ; and indeed, these elements die, for after the third week the grafts are generally free of any nerve cells " (Fig. 162).

3. Lobulated cells, that is, cells whose protoplasm appears fragmented into divergent lobules, which remind one of those forms with gulf-like indentations described in Chelonia by Pugnat and J. Levi.

4. More rarely one sees among the living elements some whose neurofibrils are united into close bundles, simulating anastomotic cordons such as were described by ourselves and García in rabies. In some elements which have lost their axon these thick anastomotic cordons constitute a perinuclear net.

5. Nageotte points out a curious phenomenon of neuronophagy in the centre of the ganglion, where the cells rapidly fall into necrobiosis. This phagocytic process may be due to polymorphonuclear leucocytes. But it usually is due to certain specific macrophages, which actively multiply around the soma, avidly attack the protoplasm, in which they cut out wide anastomotic galleries, and give to the whole the aspect of a tubular net communicating with the exterior. A short while after, the soma, corroded and liquefied in many places, breaks up and disappears through resorption. A voluminous phagocyte takes in the neuronal nucleus. Finally, when the macrophages have accomplished their mission and the ganglionic cell has been resorbed, the satellite or subcapsular elements proliferate and form in the region formerly occupied by the ganglionic cell a persistent cellular accumulation, called by Nageotte the *residual nodule*. The satellite cells are incapable of phagocytic action, although they are able to carry fatty granulations and other remnants of the neuronal cadaver. The system of hollows

formed in the cellular body perhaps pre-exists, resulting from the swelling of the conduits of Holmgren—the *neurospongium*.

6. Pericellular nests formed of fine sprouts issuing from the glomerulus or subcapsular portion of the axon and moderately ramified. Analogous fibres sometimes also give rise to periglomerular bundles.

7. Some sprouts originating from axonic glomeruli cross the capsule, circulate through the interstitial spaces of the ganglion and reach the residual nodules, in which they form very complicated arborizations and spools. Nageotte rightly attributes this strange concentration of fibres round the satellite elements to the orienting influence of some neurotropic substance which these liberate. He believes that, thanks to this association, when it occurs, the nerve sprouts become more vigorous and the glomeruli from which they issue develop luxuriantly.

8. Finally, a careful study of the paths preferably followed by the axonic sprouts leads Nageotte to state that the appendices which branch off within the subcapsular portion of the axon and soma always direct themselves towards the satellite cells, while those which branch off outside the capsule direct themselves towards the nerve tubes of the central ganglionic portion ; the latter are attracted by the bands of Büngner, or rather by the regenerating cells of Schwann. The former appendices, which are related to the atypical appendices of normal ganglia, lack a restoratory tendency. They join with the pericellular capsule, or its remnants—the *residual nodules*—only for trophic or nutritional purposes. It is for this reason that Nageotte called them *trophoparaphytes*. The second kind of expansions are crowned with a club or capsulated ball, and are entirely similar to the newly-formed fibres of the central stump of cut nerves. Their purpose, which in this case is frustrated, is to restore the *orthophyte* or degenerated axon ; they are the *neuroparaphytes*.

Leaving out some points of secondary importance, the interesting discoveries of Nageotte in his experiments of ganglionic grafts have been fully confirmed by Marinesco and Minea, Cardenal, Dustin, ourselves, O. Rossi, and other authors.

Of all these studies of confirmatory and contrasting phenomena, those by Marinesco are worthy of special mention. A short time after the publication of Nageotte's investigations, Marinesco undertook numerous experiments of ganglionar grafting—*homoio*- and *heterotransplantations* in nerves, skin, liver, etc.—not only in rabbits, but also in other animals, especially young cats, a species of mammal that is very appropriate for this type of research. Besides corroborating the transformation of monopolar into multipolar cells, the formation of the pericellular and perinodular nerve nests, neuronophagy, etc., he also found in transplanted ganglia morphological types which are entirely comparable to our frayed or *senile cells*, as well as cells whose neurofibrillar cortex was ravelled and covered with loose loops and nets.

This Rumanian neurologist does not, however, interpret certain dispositions in the same way as Nageotte. Thus, he believes that the nerve nests emanate, at times, not from fibres originating in the glomerulus, but from recurrent sprouts originating in the extracapsular portion of the axon and even in the white matter. He also excludes from any destructive neuronophagy the satellite cells; Nageotte, in his first notes, had attributed to this element a phagocytic role. Marinesco believes that the function of the satellite cells is to model the cellular morphology and to regulate the formation of expansions. Neither does he believe that the macrophages merely swell pre-existent conduits of the neurospongium of Holmgren. He believes that they make entirely new paths.

The studies of Marinesco [1] have been confirmed by his pupil Minea [2] who, in his doctor's thesis, gave a good representation of the totality of the metamorphic phenomena of the sensory neurone, which he called *plasticity*, provoked by the compression and transplantation of ganglia into various organs.

Dustin [3] also made confirmatory experiments. He saw many of the phenomena of neuronal plasticity referred to by Nageotte and Marinesco, in ganglia grafted in the vicinity of a cut nerve. Like Marinesco he notes that the sprouts of the central stump of the cut nerve are able to penetrate into the white matter, and there ramify abundantly and even form pericellular nests.

O. Rossi,[4] although he considered especially the problem of the

---

[1] Marinesco : " Quelques recherches sur la transplantation des ganglions nerveux," *Revue neurologique*, No. 6, 30 mars, 1907.

[2] Minea : " Cercetari experimentale asupra Variatiunilor morfologice ab Neuronului sensitiv," *Thesis*, Bucaresti, 1909.

[3] Dustin : *Arch. Biol.*, t. 25, 1910.

[4] O. Rossi : " Sulla rigenerazione del sistema nervoso," etc. *Rivista di pat. ner. e mentale*, vol. 16, fasc. 4, 1911.

regenerative mechanism of the nerves, also undertook experiments of ganglionic transplantation. Usually, like Marinesco, he grafted ganglia with their roots in wounds of the sciatic nerve. He

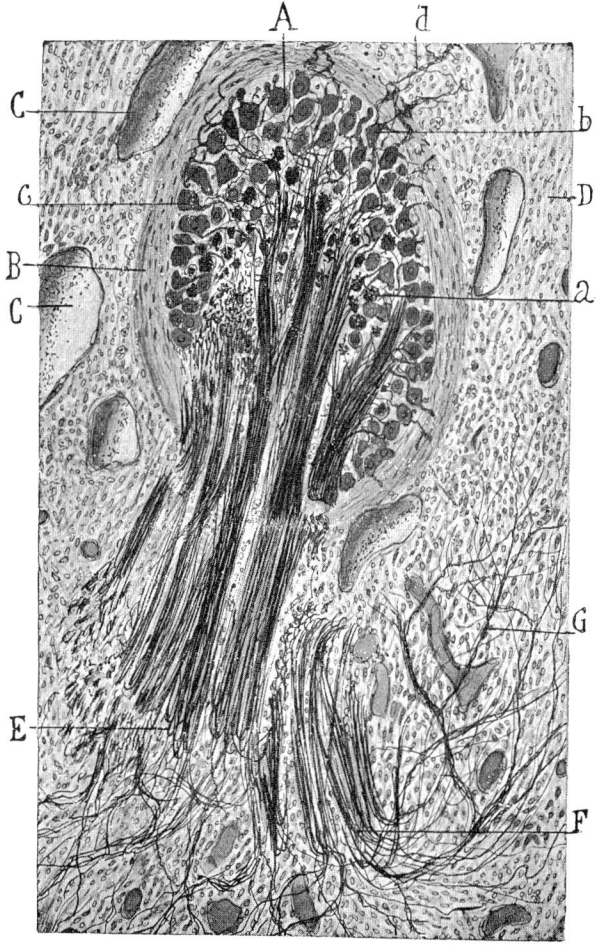

FIG. 160.—Small ganglion of the *cauda equina* of a cat a few days old, which was grafted into an animal of the same age. This second animal was killed nine days after the operation. *A*, ganglion; *B*, its fibrous capsule; *C*, periganglionic sanguineous cavities; *D*, embryonic connective tissue of the host; *E, F*, section of the peripheral branch of the ganglion, where numerous sprouts are seen innervating the newly-formed connective tissue.

observed the phenomena of sprouting discovered by Nageotte, and he also confirmed the assertion of Marinesco and Dustin concerning the penetration of exogenous fibres, from the sciatic nerve, into the ganglion itself, where they produce pericellular nests. We have already referred to these studies when we dealt with nervous regeneration.

We,[1] too, have made experimental studies on the attractive theme of ganglionic grafts, and we shall here give a brief account of them, since they are almost entirely limited to the confirmation of the results obtained by Nageotte and other investigators named above. Like Nageotte and Marinesco, we have made both *homoio-* and *heterotransplantations* of ganglia ; but instead of using as hosts adult rabbits and as grafts ganglia of recently-born rabbits, we have used brother animals, for example cats and dogs from eight to fifteen days old. Ordinarily we have used very small ganglia taken from the *cauda equina* and transplanted beneath the skin of the back of another animal of the same age. In order to distinguish this type of graft from one generally used by Nageotte and Marinesco (*heterochronotransplantation*) we shall call our type *homochronotransplantation*. The animals were killed from the third to the tenth day. In some cases we have also made *autotransplantations*, like Marinesco, that is, we grafted the ganglion under the skin of the animal from which it was taken.

All large transplanted ganglia die nearly in their entirety ; there survives only, as Nageotte discovered, a peripheral continuous or discontinuous row of sensory neurones which are directly soaked in the plasma of the host and which are vivified by the surrounding oxygen. When, however, the ganglion is very small, one often obtains the survival of the majority of the cells. The host forms around the graft an embryonic connective tissue which is sprinkled with leucocytes (Fig. 160, *D*). The ganglion is not penetrated by new capillaries ; on the other hand, the newly-formed connective tissue shows voluminous vessels, often dilated in the form of cavities. These *capillary cavities*, so called because their walls show only the endothelium of capillaries, sometimes surround the ganglion with extensive sanguineous lakes (Fig. 160, *C*).

We may begin by saying something of the phenomena of necrobiosis.

Necrobiosis and neuronophagy.—The death of the central cells of large ganglia occurs rapidly and probably as the consequence of asphyxia. Twenty-four hours after the operation, and even earlier,

---

[1] Cajal: "Algunas observaciones favorables á la hipótesis neurotrópica," *Trab. del Lab. de Investig. biol.*, t. 8, 1910.

the sensory soma is very much altered; the neurones become granular and are difficult to stain; the chromatic grumes disappear after crumbling up; finally, from the first to the second day onwards, migratory leucocytes, coming from the tissues of the host, penetrate into the interstices of the ganglion (Fig. 161, *a*), aiding the destructive action of autolysis. From the third to the sixth day the phenomena of neuronophagy, pointed out by Nageotte and Marinesco, are seen at their climax. Large sensory cells are then visible, perforated by anastomotic galleries within which lie the macrophages, that is, amoeboid cells whose nucleus is frequently lobulated and whose cytoplasm is almost invisible. It is difficult to give an opinion concerning the origin of these cells. Nageotte believed them at first [1] to be a progeny of the satellite cells; to-day, however, he

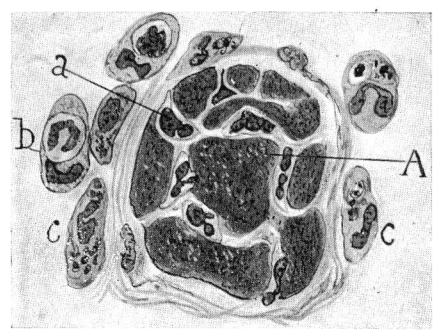

FIG. 161.—Dead ganglionic cell which is perforated and run over by leucocytes. *A*, dead protoplasm; *a*, nucleus of a phagocyte; *c*, leucocyte with fatty drops; *b*, leucocytes with axonic remnants.

takes them to be a particular kind of migratory leucocyte of enigmatic caste. Marinesco [2] believes that they are polymorphonuclear leucocytes whose function it is to devour and digest the nervous protoplasm; the satellite cells only passively penetrate into the hollow spaces of the dead neurone. K. Schaffer,[3] in his study of human neuronophagy in tabes and other pathological processes, advances a similar opinion. He believes that the capsular cells possess a real cytolytic property, but not the property of piercing

[1] Nageotte: "Neuronophagie dans les greffes des ganglions rachidiens," *Revue neurologique*, sept. 1907.

[2] Marinesco: "Quelques mots à propos du travail de M. Nageotte," etc. *Revue neurologique*, juin 1907.

[3] K. Schaffer: "Ueber Fibrillenbilder tabischer Spinalganglienzellen," *Zeitsch. f. die gesamte Neurol. u. Psychiatrie*, Bd. 1, H. 4, 1910.

and devouring the cytoplasm. We hold similar views, and we believe also that the phagocytes—our *traumatocytes* [1]—which have penetrated into the neuronal cadaver positively represent large leucocytes with a lobulated nucleus, which have come from the host's blood. Certain smaller elements, provided with an ovoid nucleus and sometimes present in the galleries above referred to, perhaps belong to the category of mononuclear cells.

This leucocytic invasion of the dead neurones is not surprising. It is a general law that any mortified portion, no matter what is its character, becomes a pasture-ground for phagocytes. We believe that the protagonists of all acts of neuronophagy are nothing else than the *granular corpuscles* which accumulate so prodigiously in the necrotic foci of the centres and in the peripheral stump of degenerated nerves. Besides their perforating activity, they have the property of becoming laden with fats and protein remnants. In the cells of transplanted ganglia, as Nageotte observed, are numerous intra-protoplasmic phagocytes which are charged with lipoid materials; there are also satellite cells which are swollen with materials that take the osmic acid stain intensely (Nageotte).

The process of neuronophagy is suspended in many necrosed cells in consequence of the calcareous infiltration of the neuronal protoplasm. In the ganglia of young cats it is very common to observe calcification, manifested in preparations made with reduced silver nitrate—the formula with dilute pyridine—by a deposit of particles and irregular blocks that are stained a deep black.[2] This calcareous

---

[1] We gave this name some time ago to the migratory cells of carcinomas and epitheliomas which are capable of perforating the epithelial cells and of cutting out hollows in living or dead protoplasm.

See: "Las defensas orgánicas en el epitelioma y carcinoma," *Boletín Oficial del Colegio de Médicos de Madrid*, Jan. 1896.

[2] This reaction, which was pointed out by Kossa (1901), consists in the formation of silver phosphate at the level of the deposits of calcium phosphate. Owing to the action of the reducing agent, pyrogallol, the silver phosphate is reduced and black grains of metallic silver are deposited. We may say, in parenthesis, that the method of reduced silver nitrate constitutes an excellent means of demonstrating the phosphate precipitates of dead or living tissues, as we have satisfied ourselves by analyzing the calcareous infiltration of pathological tissues and the process of normal ossification. We think it very probable that the black grains shown by the platelets in silver preparations are formed by salts of calcium. In grafted ganglia the calcareous infiltration that follows on necrosis may be so extensive as to render almost the whole of the focus opaque, owing to the black metallic precipitate.

precipitate sometimes is present throughout the protoplasm, sometimes only in the central region (Fig. 160, *a*).

From the fifth day on one finds abundant *residual nodules*, which are nothing else, as Nageotte showed, than the accumulation of satellite cells that have proliferated where the destroyed neurone used to be. One can see in Fig. 170, *F*, the phases of this process of resorption of the sensory neurone and the filling up of the space

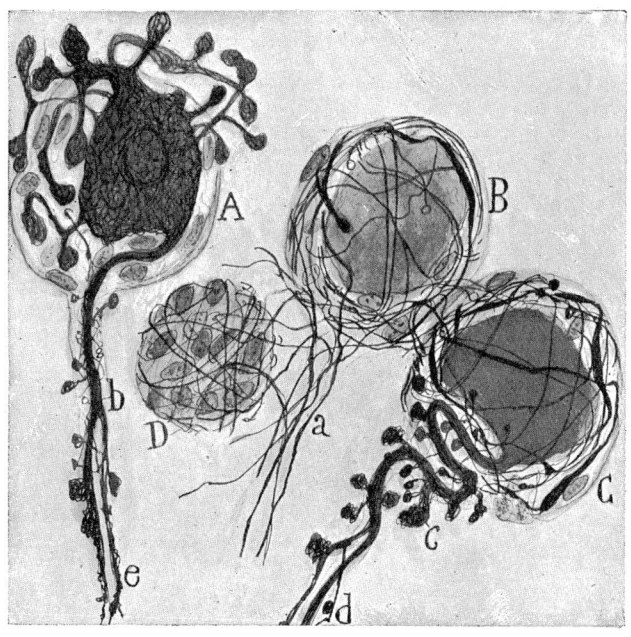

FIG. 162.—Various cells seen in the cortex of a grafted ganglion, taken from a rabbit one week old. The host of the graft was killed six days after the operation. *A*, cell with intra and extracapsular thick dendrites ending in clubs and balls; *B*, cells surrounded by a nervous spool; *C*, cell also provided with a spool and from whose glomerulus issue appendices ending in balls; *D*, residual nodule.

which it occupied. Among the very numerous satellite cells the leucocytes are almost totally lacking. Once the destruction of the neurone is complete, the macrophages migrate, with their load of protoplasmic remnants (Fig. 162, *D*). In the cat one often finds residual nodules around calcified neuronal remnants.

The nerve tubes and neuroglial cells of the centre of large and adult ganglia also succumb to asphyxia, and become white with phagocytic leucocytes. Some fibres, which are relatively near to the surrounding plasma of the host, retain some vitality and undergo a degenerative process which is similar to that of the peripheral nerves in the large ganglia. We shall see below that survival is much greater in the small ganglia.

Creation of atypical appendices (*Trophoparaphytes of Nageotte*).—On this point the descriptions of Nageotte and Marinesco are very full. We confine ourselves, therefore, to confirming their observations in all respects. In Fig. 162 and the following figures we show the main types of these neuronal transformations of the large ganglia. We will merely note that the transplanted neurones reproduce with

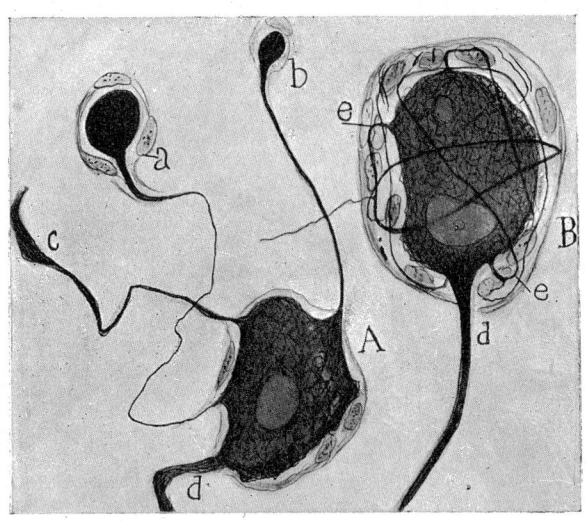

FIG. 163.—Cells from a grafted ganglion of a young cat. Homochronotransplantation. The animal was sacrificed nine days after the operation. *A*, cell with long appendices ending in capsulated balls; *B*, neurone provided with appendices which are folded back around the cell.

surprising fidelity all the atypical expansional forms described by ourselves in normal men and animals, as well as those observed in tabes by Nageotte, and by Marinesco, Levi, Schaffer, Pacheco, O. Rossi, Expósito, Bielschowsky, etc., in other pathological processes. We may enumerate a few kinds:

(*a*) Large and varicose appendices which emerge from the soma, curve beneath the capsule, ramify richly and end in stout clubs and thickenings of various shapes.

In Fig. 162, *A*, we show a cell with appendices of this type in the rabbit. One may note the remarkable robustness and almost monstrous appearance of such appendices, some of which invade a good part of the interstitial connective tissue, often coming to a stop beneath the ganglionic capsule, where they end in enormous balls or terminal clubs (Fig. 166, B).

(b) Cells with long and fine prolongations, either sub- or ultra-capsular—the *sympathicoid neurones* of Nageotte—ending in points and rings or in thin cones of growth.

In some cells of this type that were studied late—nine days after the graft—one can see the paralysis of the growth of the appendices, which end in thick capsulated balls (Fig. 163, A). The capsulated spheres are found both in the coverings of the ganglions and in its interior (Fig. 166, g).

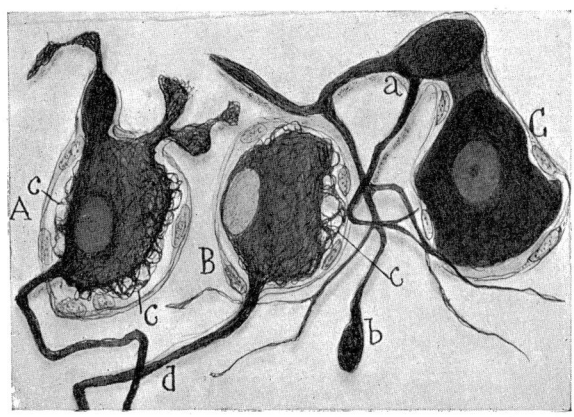

FIG. 164.—Cells from a grafted ganglion of a cat a few days old. Homochronotransplantation. A, cell with lobulated appendices and cortical loops; B, cell with loops; C, cell whose axon is lobulated.

(c) Neurones provided on their peripheral side with thick, ramified, sinuous trunks which pass through the capsule and end in flattened and monstrous masses (Fig. 167, A). This type is a curious variant of the lobulated type well described by Nageotte and Marinesco. In the small ganglia of the cat this last type predominates (Figs. 164, A, and 165), and one may note that the majority of the excrescences in question arise at the peripheral side of the neuronal soma, sometimes perforating the pericellular capsule and even the periganglionar capsule. The push of growth can be so strong in such lobules that one not infrequently sees extensive hollows or pits in the periganglionic connective covering which they have made in order to place themselves therein (Fig. 165, B). From each lobule sometimes arise branches which end in thickenings (Fig. 164, a). Some of these long appendices which have penetrated into the periganglionic capsule are bead-like, showing that they have been repeatedly detained by obstacles (Fig. 166, B). Finally, in these elements the nucleus is often dislocated, either becoming peripheral or approaching the lobulations, as though marking the centre of the figure.

(d) Neurones whose appendices, fine or of medium thickness, form nests around the soma from which they arise (Fig. 163, B, e).

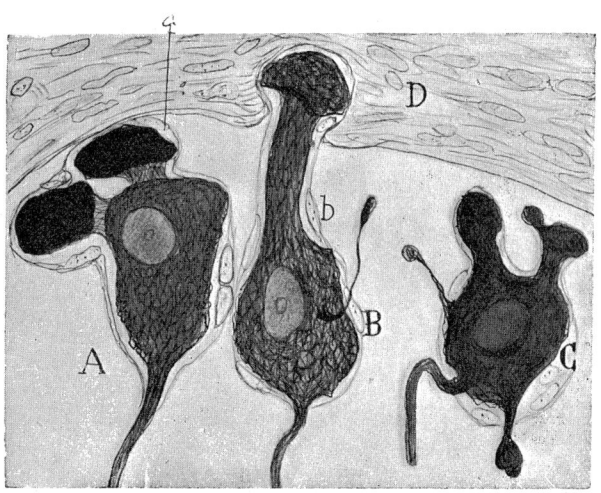

FIG. 165.—Various types of lobulated neurones. D, capsule of the ganglion. Three days old graft in a young cat.

(e) Neurones that are angular, tuberose, lozenge-shaped through amoeboid movement of the protoplasm. These varieties have been well shown by Nageotte and Marinesco.

In some types of this kind the ganglionic cortex is cut up into pits owing to the proliferation and consequent pressure of the satellite cells. Between the excavations sometimes arise mound-like excrescences, tubercles, and even appendices ending in excrescences (Fig. 168).

(f) Cells covered with fine loops or superficial plexuses of neurofibrils, like those described by Marinesco. In these elements the nucleus is eccentric and even tangential (Fig. 164, A, B).

(g) Cells of the hirudiform type, characterized by the fact that they show a net confined to the region of the nucleus and to the axis of the principal expansion, with more or less extensive hyalinization of the cortical region of the protoplasm (Nageotte).

Branches issuing from the axon. (*a*) *Glomerular or subcapsular appendices.*—We have already stated that in large ganglia, especially when the host is an adult animal, nearly all the axonic path is destroyed, including the cells of Schwann. There are cases, nevertheless, (Fig. 162, *C*), as Nageotte showed, in which the glomerulus, and even a more or less extensive part of the ultracapsular course of the axon are preserved. In such elements the subcapsular portion of

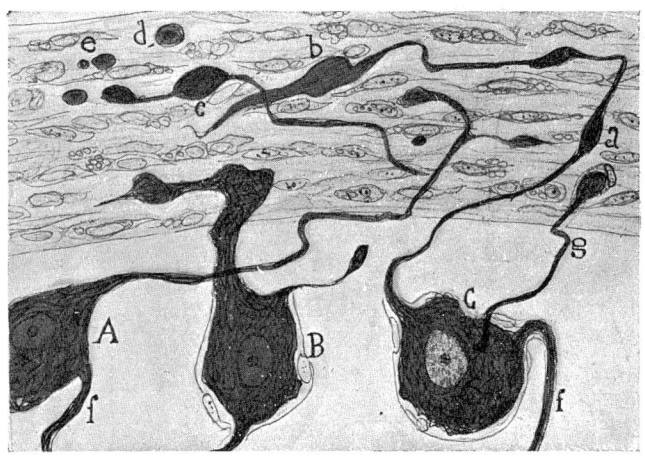

FIG. 166.—Cells whose long appendices penetrate into the capsule of the ganglion, where they show varicosities due to arrests, and free spheres, produced through autotomy. Nine day old graft in a young cat.

the axon gives rise frequently to fine projections which are ramified, produce nests or plexuses, and are concentrated, sometimes round the neurone of origin, sometimes round the immediately adjacent neurones. We think it probable, as Nageotte admits, that the source of the substances that attract the glomerular sprouts lies, not in the neurones, but in the satellite cells, upon which, in order to augment the surface of influence, the terminal branches spread out and trace complicated turns. This chemotactic influence appears especially evident in the case of the ultracapsular elements which are disposed round neighbouring neurones or residual nodules. In the unfolding of the spools or bundles under the capsule (*autobundles*) stereotropism also perhaps plays an important part.

Nageotte affirms that every nest represents the terminal unfolding of paraphytes of the soma or glomerulus of the axon. This derivation is exact in the majority of cases, especially when one is dealing with voluminous ganglia. When the grafts are made on recently-born cats and dogs, however, one can well see that a good number of the pericellular plexuses arise from the extraglomerular portion of the neurite, and sometimes from recurrent fibres that start from its bifurcations, that is, right in the white matter. In Fig. 170, C, G, we show several of these ascendant fibres which have their origin in regions very far from the sensory axon. One occasionally, though infrequently, finds appendices issuing from the starting-point of the

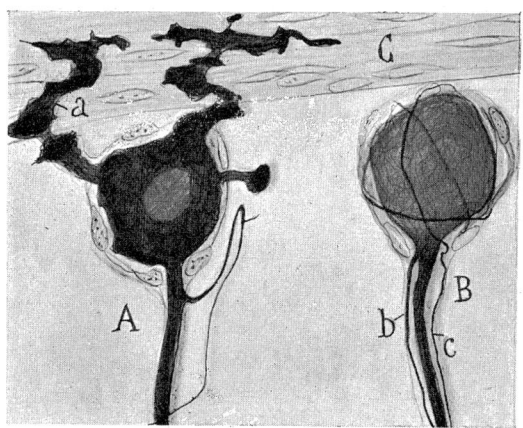

axon, which travel towards the periphery beneath the sheath of Schwann (Fig. 167, b), instead of proceeding towards the capsular apparatus.

(b) *Fibres originating in the ultraglomerular course of the axon.*— These usually follow a descending path, travelling beneath Schwann's membrane towards the white matter, where they degenerate and die through lack of oxygen or food. When, as often occurs, the entire central region of the axon rapidly succumbs, these appendices, on nearing the necrosed portion, become varicose and even form voluminous balls, suddenly ceasing to grow. The collateral fibres of such sprouts, often issuing at a right angle, break through the membrane of Schwann and end in thick masses whose presence denotes that mechanical or chemical obstacles have been encountered (Fig.

162, *b*, *d*, *e*). Finally, not a few branches become retrograde, leaving the sheath of Schwann to lose themselves in the cortical regions of the ganglion where they often dispose themselves, as we have already stated, in pericellular nests (Fig. 167, *c*).

(*c*) *Perinodular bundles.*—These dispositions, which were perfectly described by Nageotte, also appear in our preparations from the fifth to the seventh day. They are less frequent in young cats than in the rabbit (Fig. 162, *D*), and they are sometimes completely absent in the former animal.

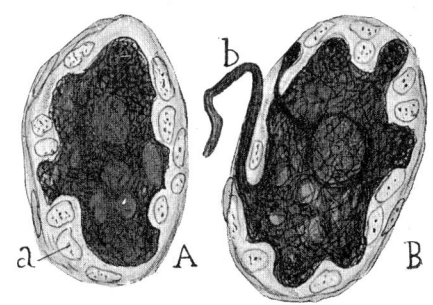

FIG. 168.—Proliferation of satellite cells into two tuberose bodies. Nine days old graft in a cat.

The residual nodules and the perinodular nests that were discovered by Nageotte in transplanted ganglia seem to us to correspond to those which we observed some time ago in the sensory ganglia of old individuals, although we did not ascertain their generative mechanism.[1] Entirely similar structures have been found by G. Sala [2] in the ganglia of wounded men, by O. Rossi [3] in the sensory foci of old individuals, by Marinesco and by K. Schaffer [4] in those of tabetics, and by ourselves [5] in wounded ganglia or those which had been stimulated by extirpation of roots.

[1] Cajal: "Tipos celulares de los ganglios sensitivos del hombre y mamíferos," *Revista de la Real Academia de Ciencias*, tomo 2, Marzo 1905.

See also: "Die Struktur der sensiblen Ganglien des Menschen und der Tiere," *Ergebnisse der Anat. u. Entwickelungsgeschichte v. Merkel u. Bonnet*, Bd. 16, 1906.

[2] G. Sala: "A proposito di un caso di sezione transversa completa del midollo spinale," *Boll. della Soc. med. chirur. di Pavia*, Giugno, 1910.

[3] O. Rossi: "Ueber einige morphologische Besonderheiten der Spinalganglien bei den Säugethiere," *Journ. f. Psychologie und Neurologie*, Bd. 11, 1908.

[4] K. Schaffer: "Ueber Fibrillenbilder tabischer Spinalganglienzellen," *Zeitsch. f. die gesamte Neurol. u. Psychiatrie*, Bd. 1, H. 4, 1910.

[5] Cajal: "Fenómenos de excitación neurocládica en los ganglios y raíces nerviosas consecutivamente al arrancamiento del ciático," *Trab. del Lab. de Invest. biol.*, tomo 11, fasc. 2, 1913.

It thus appears that the *residual nodule* is not a specific lesion of grafted ganglia. It appears in all the pathological processes of the ganglia where neuronal necrobioses occur. Our recent researches concerning the sensory and sympathetic ganglia of old individuals, in which these nodules are found almost constantly, force one to admit the reality of a normal atrophic and destructive process affecting nerve cells which have perhaps previously been impaired through fatigue, poisoning, or other lethal influences. The persistent and numerous satellite cells mark, like an epitaph, the precise place occupied by the neurone that has since died and been resorbed. This place is easily recognized, thanks to the fidelity with which the nerve bundles maintain their symbiosis with the colony of satellite cells.

We do not know the destiny of the nerve bundles and their associated cells. One may believe that after a time they are all resorbed. We lack sufficient data, however, on which to base a confident opinion as to their ultimate fate.

Phenomena observed in cases of homochronotransplantations.— We have said above that if the ganglia are small and if the animal is recently born or only a few days old, the ganglionic graft is sometimes characterized by the survival of the majority of the cells including their axons.[1] Such a case is that of the small terminal ganglia of the *cauda equina* (Fig. 160). Under such favourable conditions of nutrition, many cells remain entirely normal, emitting axonic expansions exclusively at the level of the radicular wounds, where there is an interruption of the bifurcations of the axon when the ganglion is taken out, or in the regions near to the lesion. Other cells, violently shaken by the traumatism, form new appendices, not only at the level of the axon (both from its main trunk and from its bifurcations), but also at the level of the soma. Finally, a few elements, ordinarily central in position, and which are the more numerous the larger the ganglion, show degenerative phenomena which may end in neuronal atrophy and destruction.

[1] A phenomenon also visible in small ganglia that are homochronotransplanted is the disappearance or attenuation, through neurofibrillar retraction or other mechanisms, of the axonic glomerulus. This absence of the initial spool is perhaps also partly due to the suspension of the normal process of axonic bundling, which, as is well known, becomes notably accentuated in young cats and dogs from birth up to the second week. There is thus perhaps something like a return of the axon and neurone to the embryonic period (See Fig. 170).

Aberrant nerves.—In small homochronotransplanted ganglia the regenerative acts attain a greater activity than that observable in adult ganglia, as may be seen in Figs. 169 and 170 ; these show

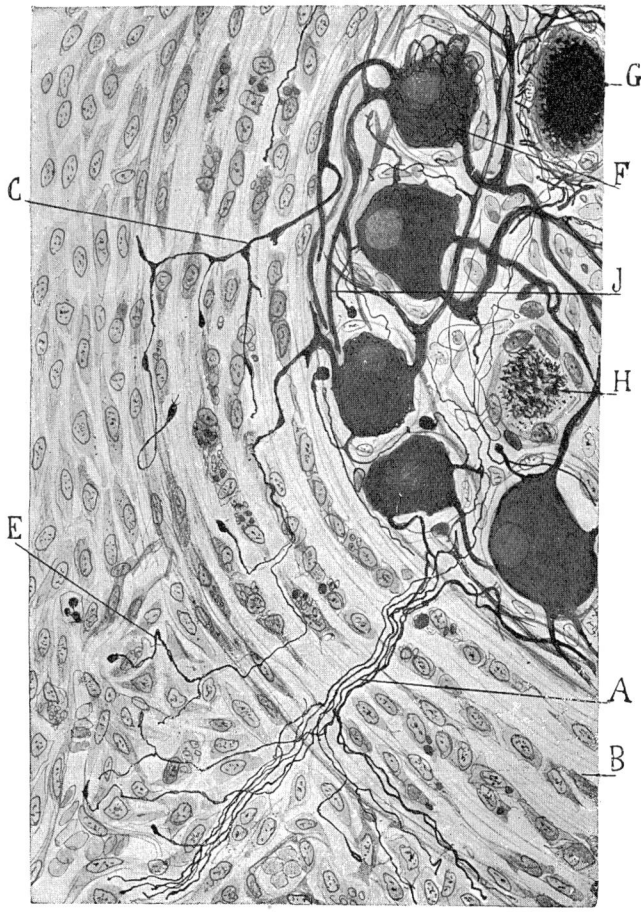

FIG. 169.—Graft of a ganglion of a dog a few days old, killed five days after the operation. *A*, small nerve which crosses the ganglionic capsule ; *B*, capsule infiltrated by embryonic connective cells ; *C*, a perforating fibre which is ramified at the level of the connective interstices of the capsule ; *E*, new fibre which is wandering through the connective tissue of the host ; *F*, cell which has sent branches into the capsule ; *G*, dead neurone, surrounded by a nest ; *H*, other dead neurone.

sprouts which, in their push of growth, pierce through the connective capsule of the nerve centre, creating what are indeed artificial or aberrant nerves (Fig. 169, *A*).

Such somatic appendices are not in any way distinguished from those which issue from the axon. One is thus unable to maintain in this case the distinction introduced by Nageotte between *tropho-paraphytes* and *neurophytes*. All the expansions that are formed merit the title of *neurophytes*, since they all end in clubs or pointed cones of growth, are equally fine and long, ramify in the same way, have a tendency to unite in small bundles and, finally, become surrounded with embryonic cells of Schwann.

A good example of this is shown in Fig. 169, *C*, *F*. One can see how some very long somatic appendices, or their branches, test the weak points of the capsule, trace zig-zags between the latter's concentric fibrous mantles, often dividing within it, and how, finally, their last projections overcome the obstacle and break right into the periganglionic embryonic connective tissue, that is, into the cicatricial tissue formed at the expense of the host animal (*C*). The passage of the capsule is sometimes very laborious, and one often finds arrested branches with strings of varicosities indicating detention (Fig. 166, *b*, *c*). As can be seen in Fig. 166, *d*, autotomy is not infrequent. If instead of one or two branches, many of them have crossed the obstacle, a more or less closely set nerve bundle is formed (Fig. 169, *A*), whose conductors are entirely like true axons in their thinness, smoothness of outline, maintenance of diameter, formation of cones, and even small rings. Later, on the sixth, seventh, and eighth days, they become even more like real axons. At that time nerve bundles are formed right in the periganglionic connective tissue, that is, in the tissues of the host, which bundles are surrounded by adventitial cells and loose axons accompanied by fusiform cells ; these elements entirely remind one of the components of the sheath of Schwann. *The host is thus neurotised, there being established between the intrusive nervous elements and the connective vascular tissue of the former a symbiosis which is more or less lasting.* There is no doubt that, as also occurs in nerve transplantations, the young fibroblasts that wander through the periganglionic tissues or are accumulated round the invading axons are the progeny, at least in part, of those which were brought by the grafted organ. They mix and live perfectly well with the congenerous mesodermal elements of the host animal (Fig. 160).

What is the fate of these strange improvised nerves. It would be very interesting to ascertain whether, with time, they are able to form myelin sheaths, and to persist in the scar, constituting, in union with their neurones of origin, a kind of aberrant nerve centre adapted to the region. Unfortunately, in spite of many experiments of transplantation, we have been unable to discern these nerves beyond the ninth day. We may have been unfortunate. At any rate, when the animal was killed after this interval, the ganglia constantly

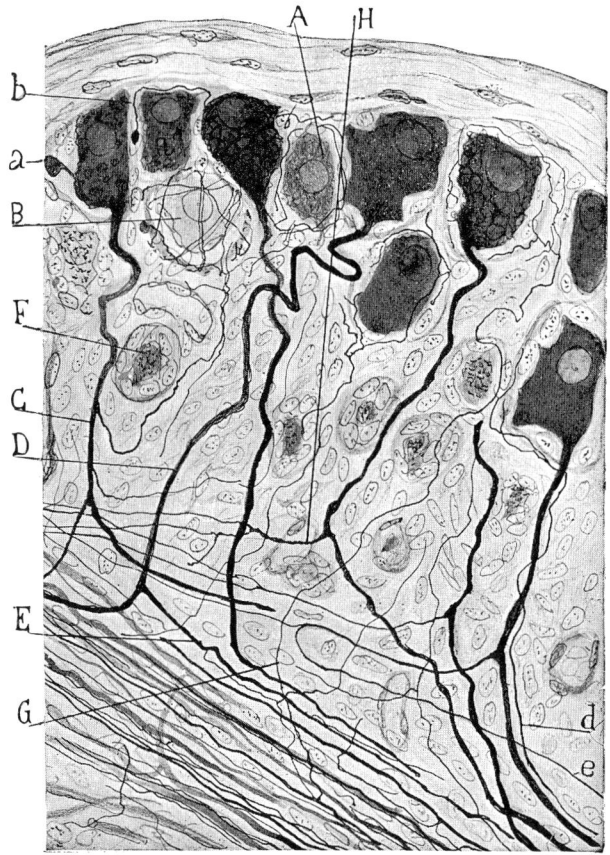

FIG. 170.—Transplanted ganglion of a young cat, killed nine days after the operation. *A*, mantle of surviving ganglionic cells; *B*, cell with spool of Dogiel; *C*, axon from which issues a collateral with spools; *D*, nearly normal axon, whose external bifurcation has given rise to a collateral; *E*, another analogous collateral; *F*, residual nodule; *G*, collateral arriving from the white matter; *a*, *b*, appendices terminating in clubs; *e*, retrograde bifurcation of an axon.

appeared resorbed and converted into a vast mass of cicatricial tissue, in which even the remnants of the ganglionic capsule were beginning to disappear. Since Marinesco, in experiments of auto-transplantation, has seen the survival of the gangliform plexus twenty-two days after the operation, we do not think it impossible that new attempts at grafting, in somewhat different conditions may furnish the proof of the production of more or less persistent artificial nerve tubes from somatic sprouts.

It is very possible that, in the grafts of which we are speaking, the cause of the growth of the nerve sprouts of somatic origin to the point of crossing the natural obstacle represented by the connective capsule, and invading the tissue of the host, is no other than the trophic action exercised by the embryonic connective cells of this fibrous mantle and of the immediate periganglionic scar. As can be seen in Fig. 169, *B*, the connective cells of the capsule do not remain indifferent; they become turgid; they partially retract their expansions, and they actively proliferate ; their immediate progeny forms interlaminar series or strata. Some of the elements produced in this way become amoeboid and, escaping from the fibrous tissue, invade the tissues of the host. The methods that impregnate fats (Sudan III, Osmic acid) show within such elements numerous lipoidal granulations, which are an indication of their phagocytic activity. Under such conditions there is formed around the ganglion, and even within its sheath, some cicatricial connective tissue which, like the intermediate scar of cut nerves, is propitious to the progression and nutrition of the recently-formed fibres. It is clear that, in these processes of expansional growth, the oxygen of the surrounding plasma and the nutritive renovation also collaborate very directly. There is a reason for the fact that the majority of the paraphytes proceed towards the plasmas of the host from the ganglionar periphery, that is, along the shortest path. We may note, in passing, that the newly-formed blood-vessels—the ganglionic *capillary sinuses*—of the connective tissue never attract the sprouts.

Phenomena occurring on the border of the transplanted ganglion.— As Nageotte and Marinesco and Minea experimented very largely with relatively large ganglia in which, as we noted above, the entire white substance, including the roots, becomes necrosed, they were unable to see the curious regenerative phenomena that occur on both sides of the roots which are interrupted when the ganglion is cut out. Fortunately, the survival of small ganglia extends to almost the whole of their texture, the horizon of observation being thus widened. When the vitality of the axon and its internal and external branches is maintained, one easily recognizes, days after the lesion, the well-known phenomena of traumatic degeneration and regeneration of the central stump, characteristic of ordinary nerve wounds. As a consequence of this *the tissues of the host are neurotised much more richly and constantly than across the capsule*, which does not always lend itself to being crossed by the fibres (Fig. 160, F, G).

We need not here give in detail the easily understood stages of aberrant nervous reunion. We will only note that nearly all the sprouts are collaterals that issue, at some distance from the wound, from the cut axons, and that, as occurs in sectioned nerves, many of these branches, which are intratubal, ravel out to form small bundles of very fine fibres. Nor are there lacking extratubal sprouts which are divided along their course and which may arise, ordinarily, from non-myelinated axons. The sprouts originating in the white matter—the *peripheral branch* of the ganglion—lead to the scar which is formed at the expense of the tissues of the host. Here newly-formed fibres debouch and ramify, and are quickly converted into wandering nerves. Nevertheless the majority of these sprouts, on nearing the embryonic connective tissue of the host, which forms the scar, divide into two branches: one is fine and goes out into the newly-formed connective tissue; the other is thicker, is a real continuation of the fibre, and, after tracing an arc and becoming retrograde, resolutely turns back to the ganglion (Fig. 160, E). In the internal branches of the ganglion—the radicular portion situated between the ganglion and the spinal cord—these retrograde prolongations appeared to us infrequent. This may be due to the small number of living conductors that are sufficiently long to assault the scar.

As we have noted above, and as the studies of Nageotte and Marinesco prove, the living portion of the axon which is far from the wound also emits direct and retrograde collaterals. These are especially numerous in the bifurcating branches. One may note in passing, in Fig. 170, the perfect conservation of the division, and one may also see how, after a short path, one of the branches, sometimes both, emit sprouts at an acute angle which divide and subdivide repeatedly, a few branches turning back to the cortical substance (E). Several of them, as we show in Fig. 170, C, emanate from the extracapsular portion of the axon. Sometimes the internal bifurcation becomes divided into two equal branches: one represents the primitive, the other the newly formed branch. The latter may again be broken up into new branchlets. One sees, not infrequently, the branches that are newly formed in the white matter turn back to the grey matter, being in close contiguity to an axon (d). Finally the internal bifurcation, recognizable by its thinness, occasionally gives rise to a conductor thicker than itself which travels in an opposite direction, that is, towards the peripheral nerve (Fig. 170, e).

Modern studies have convinced us that the survival of the bifurcations of the sensory axon in small grafts is not a constant phenomenon. In general, one may say that the majority, or perhaps, all of the thick axons belonging to peripheral branches of voluminous neurones, degenerate from forty-eight hours after the graft onwards. Their sheaths of Schwann evolve progressively, and there appear within them, from the fifth or sixth day on, small bundles of sprouts. This degeneration extends to almost the entire white matter, which, in the grafts, is the region of poorest nourishment. The fine and small tubes resist to a much greater extent, remaining alive to within a short but variable distance of the wound. Consequently the small bundles of fibres present in the voluminous degenerated tubes of the white matter must be considered as collateral or terminal fibres of the axonic trunk or of the crotch of one of its divisory branches. The frequent absence of bifurcation in these axons of large diameter seems to result from the fact that, once their divisory segment has disappeared, the branches which are formed direct their course preferably towards the periphery, which constitutes the path of least resistance. One may remember that the peripheral branch of the sensory axon is wider than the central branch, and its sheath of Schwann, therefore, offers a wider path to the newly-formed fibres.

Experiments of cultivation of ganglia " in vitro."—The interesting experiments of Nageotte, Marinesco and Minea relating to the transplantation of ganglia have demonstrated the great resistance of the sensory neurone to changes of temperature, and its adaptability to regions that are relatively poor in oxygen and dissolved nutritive materials. This ready adaptation led us to suspect that the transplanted sensory neurones, during the first two or three days after their dislocation, extract from themselves or from the intraganglionic environment, reserve substances, at the expense of which they create the newly-formed expansions.

In order to prove this theory [1] we have tried some experiments of cultivation *in vitro*. The method used was to take pieces of spinal cord with uncovered ganglia, but still partially protected by the vertebral column, and to moisten them with indifferent salt

[1] Cajal: " Algunos experimentos de conservación y autolisis del tejido nervioso," *Communicación á la Sociedad española de Biología, Trab. del Lab. de Investigaciones biol.*, tomo 8, Dec. 1910.

solution or with Locke's or Ringer's solution ; they were then quickly placed in test-tubes within which had been previously inserted a wad of sterile glass wool, intended to support the piece and to keep it easily exposed to the air. The tube was closed with sterile cotton, and kept at a temperature of 37° C. in the oven for twenty-four or more hours. After twenty-four hours, if there is no infection, the phenomena of survival have begun and in certain cells have already developed in a marked degree. The best preparations are made from cats recently born or three to four days old. In dogs eight or fifteen days old the phenomena are less accentuated and are often entirely lacking. When survival does not occur, autolysis takes place, and the cells and nerve fibres become notably altered. Putrefaction often impedes the process. This, however, is recognized easily by the bad odour of the tube.

In cats a few days old there are two neuronal categories in the sensory ganglia. Certain cells are large or medium-sized and appear intensely stained by reduced silver nitrate ; others, ordinarily smaller, are not stainable, that is, they have a reticulum that is indifferent to the colloidal silver or attracts it very feebly. It is only in the large and black neurones, which are provided with a well-marked neurofibrillar net, that one can see phenomena of sprouting. These phenomena, beginning after twenty-four hours, reach their maximum, as we have found in subsequent observations, between the second and the third day.

They are of three classes : cellular lobulations, formation of clubs of somatic origin, and formation of clubs of axonic origin.

Lobulations.—These appear principally in the superficial neurones, and they consist in the emission of wide appendices, which are fungiform, polyp-shaped, hemispherical, quadrilateral, etc., and whose volume approximates in some cases to that of the rest of the nucleated protoplasm. We show in Figs. 171, *A* and *B*, and 172, *E*, *G*, the principal forms that are seen in our preparations. The lobule or protuberance has the same structure as the soma ; sometimes the neurofibrillar meshes come out with special clearness. The axon not infrequently emerges from the newly-formed appendix, but more usually from the pedicle intermediate between the lobule and the soma (Fig. 172, *C*, *D*). As for the nucleus, it encloses vacuolizations, takes on a lobuliform aspect, and shows argentophilous spheres in course of fusion which are hardly perceptible.

In short, the excrescences of the protoplasm entirely remind one of the lobulations described some time ago by Pugnat in the ganglia of Chelonians, which were confirmed and well drawn by Levi, and which were also observed in transplanted ganglia by Nageotte and Marinesco.

They are similar to the excrescences mentioned so often in connection with wounded and transplanted ganglia. The clubs that

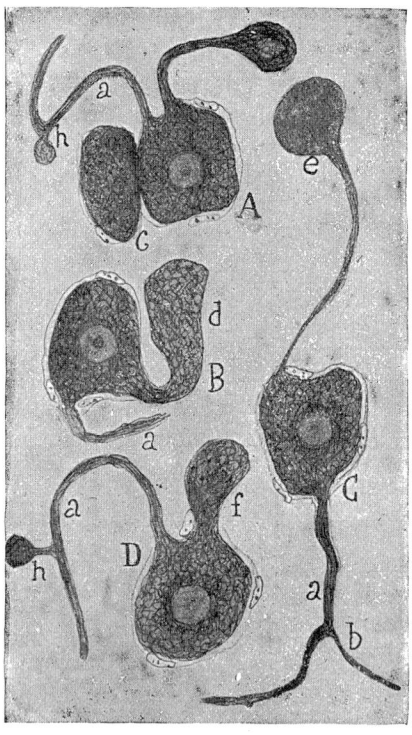

FIG. 171.—Ganglionic cells of a cat, kept for two days in cerebrospinal fluid. a, axon; the lobules d, f, and the expansions ending in balls, e, h, etc., are neoformations due to the culture medium.

appear in the ganglia kept in an oven differ from the ordinary clubs in three respects: they are usually much more voluminous, they have a thicker pedicle, and they never show a capsular sheath. One guesses that they are improvised formations, a kind of cellular lobule whose pedicle has become progressively narrower and longer, and whose terminal thickening, excessively robust, has broken through the capsule before there was time to elaborate a protecting structure. Another special point in such masses is that they show a perfect reticular texture, entirely analogous to the neurofibrillar armour of the soma, instead of the homogeneous, or almost homogeneous, aspect characteristic of the terminal balls that have been described by the authors up to now.

In Figs. 171 and 172 we show some examples, taken from three or four sections of a ganglion in which the appendices in question

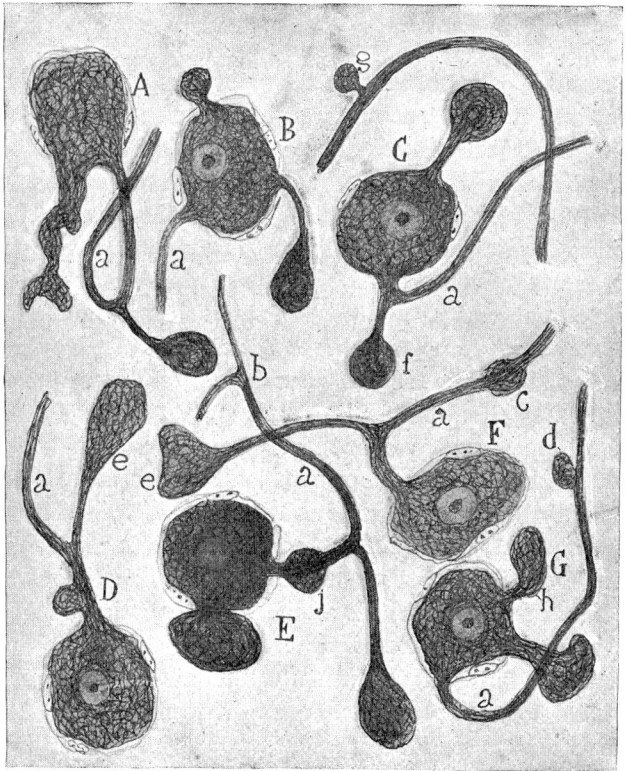

FIG. 172.—Ganglionic cells of a cat a few days old. *a*, axon; *b*, normal bifurcation; *e*, pyriform expansions originating in the axon; *c*, *d*, *g*, phases in the formation of axonic appendices; *j*, spheroidal appendix generated near the cell; *A*, cell with a branched expansion; *B*, *C*, cells with somatic appendices ending in balls; *E*, cell provided with a large lobule; *G*, cell with two lobules.

were abundant. The most common case is where there are medium-sized clubs, with a short and thick pedicle (Fig. 172, *B*, *C*); at other times the club is enormous, and has an ovoidal or spheroidal shape (Figs. 171, *A*, and 172, *E*); finally, the club is sometimes smaller and hangs from a long pedicle which tends to become thin in the portion next to the cell (Fig. 172, *C*).

Appendices of axonic origin.—In sections of ganglia kept in the oven we see all the phases of the budding and growth of axonic prolongations, whose morphological attributes entirely coincide with those of somatic expansions. The emission of the new branch begins by a tuberose enlargement, usually monolateral, at the level of which the neurofibrillar net appears relatively lax and rich in neuroplasm (Fig. 172, *c*, *d*), and later the enlargement grows out, hanging from a relatively short pedicle ; finally the pedicle lengthens out (Figs. 171, *h*, and 172, *g*) and the terminal lobule travels between the surrounding cells, becoming more or less separated from the axon of origin, until it encounters an obstacle (Fig. 172, *e*). Any segment of the axon can give rise to these appendices. But one region is preferred : the extracapsular portion next to the cell. In some cells (Fig. 172, *f* and *D*), these expansions arise nearly at the point where the axon leaves the soma so near the capsule that they often appear like protoplasmic lobules. Frequently the branch which bears the terminal lobule is so thick that it equals or is even greater than the ulterior diameter of the axon. One would say that one was dealing with a normal bifurcation, one of whose branches had become retracted, ending in a ball (Fig. 172, *E*, *F*). But this is simply an appearance, promptly dissipated when one observes the subsequent course of the axon, in which one can always detect the well-known division into internal and external branches (Fig. 172, *b*). Exceptionally one sees axons with two lobules or branches ending in a club. One finds even more complicated dispositions, like that shown in Fig. 172, *E*, where the axon, before emitting a thick branch ending in a sphere, produces a thick lobule.

In the nerve fibres of the white ganglionic substance and nerve roots we have not observed phenomena of ramification. In general they take the stain perfectly, and they appear normal ; in some, however, there are varicosities.

The preceding observations thus show that in certain favourable conditions—such as particular species of animals, developing ganglia, asepsy, aeration, immersion in physiological plasma or in the natural medium of the tissues, etc.—the ganglionic neurones separated from the body of the animal are able to survive *in vitro*, in the oven, twenty-four hours or longer, while neuroformative phenomena take place.

The survival is proved by the very sprouting, which in this case does not consist solely in the production of purely plasmatic appendices, formed through the action of elastic forces, such as variations in the surface tensions or the osmotic pressure, but in the organization, through assimilation, of all the components of the protoplasm and especially of the neurofibrillar skeleton.

A short time after the publication of our investigations there appeared the interesting attempts at cultivation of ganglia on blood and other media by Legendre and Minot.[1] In a first communication these investigators were unable to demonstrate neuronal survival *in vitro*. They observed some important alterations, such as the vacuolization of the nervous protoplasm, the creation of superficial pits, into which neuroglia cells insert themselves, the tendency to homogeneity of the protoplasmic chromatin and, when the culture is prolonged twenty-four hours, total achromatosis. These alterations, observed in cultivations in lymph and blood, which coincide with those noted by us in ganglia preserved in an indifferent salt solution, appear to us to be autolytic in character.

In a second series of experiments, however, these authors were more fortunate.[2] Ganglia of rabbits, which had been preserved one or several days in defibrinated blood and which were then stained by the method of reduced silver nitrate, gave abundant signs of survival. As in transplanted ganglia, only the marginal neurones survived the ablation.

An indication of this survival is afforded by the pictures obtained by ordinary methods. Thus, after three or four days, the Nissl stain shows the persistence in the marginal cells of the chromatic grumes, which have become smaller and more or less pale, unlike the central ganglionic region where this substance has disappeared. The satellite neuroglia cells are abundant and are intensely neuronophagous. With the method of silver nitrate some of these tangential cells, in adult rabbits, show fine sprouts generated from the glomerulus; these sprouts travel beneath the capsule, forming

---

[1] R. Legendre et H. Minot : " Essais de conservation hors de l'organisme des cellules nerveuses des ganglions spinaux," *Compt. rend. Soc. Biol.*, 7, 14, et 21 mai 1909, t. 68.

See also: "Formation de nouveaux prolongements par certaines cellules nerveuses des ganglions spinaux conservés hors de l'organisme," *Anat. Anzeiger*, Bd. 38, Nos. 20-21, 1911.

[2] R. Legendre et H. Minot : " Influence de la température sur la conservation des cellules nerveuses des ganglions spinaux hors de l'organisme," *Compt. rend. Soc. Biol.*, 24 déc. 1910, t. 69 (published in Feb. 1911).

pericellular nests. In ganglia of adult dogs, after twenty-four hours in the oven, there were observed also : (*a*) appendices arising from the glomerulus as well as from the soma, and terminating in buds and rings ; (*b*) residual nodules with nervous arborizations ; (*c*) phenomena of cellular lobulations and of the creation of large balls already observed by ourselves, etc.

Thus the investigations of Minot and Legendre complete our own and show that the sensory neurones are able to survive for several days in defibrinated serum, in the oven, and that they are able to form, to a greater or less extent, the atypical structures that were described by Nageotte and Marinesco in transplanted ganglia.

Lastly, Marinesco and Minea [1] in an excellent memoir confirmed the facts that had been made known by us, and by Legendre and Minot ; they used the method of culture in blood plasma, a method which has given splendid results in the growth of various tissues, when used by Harrison, Burrows, Carrel, Oppel, Hada, Lewis, etc. Marinesco and Minea also discovered surviving neurones in the periphery of the ganglion, and discerned in them, from the second day on, lobulations, short and long appendices which were amply ramified, and, finally, nervous nests. The most interesting fact observed by them, however, consists in the growth of nerve sprouts from the ganglion to the surrounding plasma, across which they grow and ramify freely, like the amphibian neuroblasts cultivated by Harrison. Among the emerged axons some are relatively thick, and grow isolated ; the majority, however, are very fine and grow by supporting themselves on fusiform cells and embryonic connective tissue cells, thus showing a marked stereotropism. The fusiform connective cells, which are disseminated throughout the plasma, emanate from the ganglionic capsule, and arrange themselves in bundles and divergent trabeculae.

We may say in conclusion that the investigations of Marinesco and Minea show that, under favourable circumstances, the sensory nerve cells not only are able to grow within the ganglion, as we and Legendre and Minot had observed, but can emerge from it, growing indefinitely in an appropriate medium. This growth, which is difficult if the fibres have no purchase, becomes easy and rapid when the sprout is able to lean on mesodermal support. Moreover, we

[1] Marinesco et Minea : " Essai de culture des ganglions spinaux de mammifères *in vitro*. Contribution à l'étude de la neurogénèse," *Anat. Anzeiger*, Nos. 7 and 8, Bd. 42, 1912.

had already proved, in grafting experiments, the ability of sensory neurones to project nerve fibres outside the ganglion. We have spoken of these artificial nerves above.[1]

Hypotheses to explain the production of cellular appendices.—In the actual state of knowledge, we are unable to explain the physico-chemical mechanism of the growth of sensory neurones, or that of protoplasmic assimilation and growth, of which this sprouting is but a particular case. We may, however, set forth the attempts at explanation put forward by Nageotte, Marinesco, and other authors.

Conjecture of Nageotte.—Nageotte holds that the principal cause of the formation of neuronal expansions is the rupture of the osmotic equilibrium between the plasmatic surrounding of the neurones and the cellular protoplasm. Inspired by the ideas of Traube and Leduc concerning osmotic vegetations, and the studies of Giard on the influence of carbonic acid in augmenting the cellular osmotic pressure and growth, he submitted the ganglia, before grafting them, to a light desiccation or to the action, during an hour and a half, of a hypertonic solution of chloride of sodium. In ganglia thus treated, seven days after the transplantation, the sprouts are exceptionally long and complex. In the case of grafts in which there has been no previous modifying action, the condition that promotes intraprotoplasmic hypertonicity and therefore the creation of expansion is perhaps the accumulation of carbonic acid or products of catabolism retained in consequence of the sudden rupture of the blood vessels from the rest of the organism.

Conjecture of Marinesco.—Marinesco objected to the theory of Nageotte certain facts which are incompatible with it. Such is the fact that intraganglionic injections of distilled water and of a hypertonic solution of sodium chloride do not bring about any of the characteristic vegetations in grafted ganglia. Marinesco affirms that the disturbance of equilibrium in the osmotic pressure, without being a factor to be neglected, is an accessory physical condition to the neurocladic process. He believes that modifications in the surface tension of the protoplasm and an attraction exerted by certain chemotactic substances of the surroundings are more decisive influences in this neoformative phenomenon.

He says : " The suppression of the vascular and nervous connections of the cells in transplanted ganglia results in the formation of modifications in the chemical structure of the cell ; phenomena of autolysis probably occur which bring about an increase in the number of molecules, thus attracting a certain quantity of water.

[1] See additional note on p. 480.

"Even more important changes, however, supervene in the surface tension, which, as shown by Berthold's researches concerning the mechanics of protoplasm, modify the form of the cell. It will be remembered that Berthold has proved that protoplasm is comparable to a drop of liquid, and that its movements and morphology constitute the expression of the modifications of its surface tension, that is, of the energy of cohesion, owing to which, in a drop free from contact, the various parts attract each other. If the tension is equal on all the points of the surface, the drop takes on a spherical shape. If, however, for any cause, this tension diminishes at some point, there is produced in that region, in consequence of the pressure exercised on the other sides, a liquid eminence which elongates until there is established a new state of equilibrium. Thus the spherical shape of an amoeba, like that of any other round cell, is the expression of the equality in surface tension over the entire surface ; the production of expansions on various points on it indicates a diminution of tension at the level of each of them. But the question arises what are the causes of these changes in surface tension. In accordance with the experiments of Verworn, we must admit that this may result from the affinity of certain parts of the protoplasm for oxygen, which has the property of lowering the surface tension at certain points and of bringing about, therefore, the formation of pseudopods. Owing to the unilateral action of oxygen, this principle must lead to a positive chemotaxis, like that shown by Stahl in naked protoplasmic masses. One must, then, believe with Verworn that the introduction of atoms of oxygen into the molecules of the biogen diminishes the cohesion between the latter's various molecules. In other words, the penetration of oxygen diminishes the molecular attraction, and therefore the surface tension ; on the contrary, the destruction of the molecules of biogen brings about an increase in the cohesion. When we apply these data to our problem we may say that once the oxygen reaches the superficial cells of the ganglion, the surface tension diminishes at some point on the protoplasmic cortex, and the neuroplasm makes an irruption at that place, through which a part of the neurofibrillar reticulum subsequently advances. As new molecules of neurobiones place themselves in contact with the surrounding oxygen, a more or less lengthy prolongation would be formed, according to the circumstances. We may add that since the process of decomposition is very slight as compared with that of assimilation, the appendix, instead of withdrawing as occurs with amoeboid pseudopods, becomes permanent."

The attempts of Nageotte and Marinesco to reduce to physical phenomena the initial moment of the production of expansions in grafted ganglia—and through an extension of this, in all nervous neoformations—are very plausible ; the problem, however, is unfortunately too complex to be attacked with hopes of a definite solution. Besides physical influences, the initiative of the living units constituting the neuronal protoplasm, that is, acts of assimilative synthesis whose mechanism is as yet unknown, doubtless enter into the process of the emission of expansions. The formation of a protoplasmic sprout, far from being a mere effect of the peripheral accumulation of a dissolved colloid, a *sol*, whose form and movements no longer obey physical laws, represents more probably the result of the transformation of proteins which pass incessantly from the *sol* to the *gel* state, and of an intricate morphological organization, by virtue of which the semi-solid materials remain definitely incorporated in the reticulum, the neuroplasm, and the membrane. As Levi notes, this process of expansional creation is entirely comparable to the production and growth of the nervous expansions in the embryo. On the other hand, one cannot justly, in order to explain the origin of the cellular appendices, liken the extremely simple structure of an amoeba, whose very soft consistency easily yields to the physical and chemical conditions of the medium (such as hypo and hypertonicity, electrical and thermal energy, and the action of the oxygen and carbonic acid), to the neurones, cells that have a high consistency and fixity, a great structural complexity, and an armour of neurofibrils, which necessarily must oppose a serious resistance to the physical violence of the surroundings.

Besides, at no time in the formation of sprouts are the neurones exclusively composed, like the pseudopods, of a liquid centre surrounded by a tenuous cuticula. From the beginning one sees in them a reticulated skeleton of neurofibrils or, at least, a fibril ending in a ring. Everything leads one to believe that the neoformative initiative is of a chemical nature, residing in the neurobiones of the reticulum, on which must therefore act the physico-chemical stimuli of the surroundings.

It is also important to note that the creation of expansions often occurs as the mere effect of a commotion propagated from a long distance, as in the case of the appendices produced in the ganglia through the stretching of the roots, or those caused at a distance from the wound in the central stump of cut nerves, without there being any justification for invoking an initial variation in the surface tension of the protoplasm or of the osmotic tonus of the surroundings. It appears as though the stimulus that awakens the divisory action of the neurobiones is nothing else than a mechanical vibration transmitted to the reticulum by the surrounding liquids. Thus one might imagine that the neurofibrillar region where the commotion has its greatest repercussion is the point where the neurobional division is begun. We believe, however, that besides the mechanical vibrations, instantaneous compressions, etc., chemical stimuli must figure among the causal conditions. In favour of their influence, we have the fact, referred to above, that the paraphytes of transplanted or cultivated ganglia are developed, as a rule, on the side of the neurone that is tangential to the ganglionic capsule, and are drawn along so strongly in this direction, that they finally perforate the membrane in question, as though a strong trophic stimulus reached the cell along that path, such as oxygen, enzymes that stimulate nutrition, etc.

The attempt to explain the cellular morphology by purely physical conditions of the environment has had enthusiastic upholders. Apart from the well-known studies of Vries and Verworn, the experiments of Koltzoff,[1] concerning the influence of osmotic pressure on the form of crustacean spermatozooids, are very suggestive and interesting.

This investigator submitted the spermatozooids of *Inarchus scorpio* and other decapod crustacea to the action of hypo and hypertonic solutions of sodium chloride, and observed great variations in the form of the soma and appendices of these cells. We shall not give these experiments in detail here. It suffices to say that hypotonic solutions bring about the retraction, and sometimes the disappearance of the expansions; the hypertonic solutions, while they augment the turgescence of the pre-existent protoplasmic appendices, *never create new appendices*.

One should note the doctrine of Koltzoff concerning the qualities that must be present in the protoplasm if the physical conditions of the environment—hypo and hypertonicity, etc.—are to alter its form in a marked degree, for it concurs perfectly with what we know of the fixity of neuronal expansions. Basing himself on the old experiments of Plateau regarding the shape taken by drops adhering to solid filaments, such as rings, straight fibres, spiral threads, etc., he distinguishes the elements into cells that are provided with a skeleton and cells in which there is none. As regards the second type, physical conditions, especially variations in surface tension and osmotic processes, bring about decisive changes; in the first type, on the contrary, the modifications are attenuated or become impossible, because of the resistance that this internal skeleton offers to deformations; the cellular sap becomes firmly adherent to this internal skeleton.[2] In

[1] Koltzoff : " Studien über die Gestalt der Zelle," etc. *Archiv. f. mikros. Anat.*, Bd. 67, 1906.

[2] Cajal : " Tipos celulares de los ganglios sensitivos," etc. *Trab. del. Lab de Investig. biol.*, t. 4, p. 27, 1905. See also : " Mecanismo de la regeneración de los nervios," *Trab. del Lab. de Investig. biol.*, t. 4, p. 201, 1905-06.

short, the fixed and stable form of highly differentiated elements is a function of the protoplasmic skeleton.

Since the neurone is the prototype of cells with a semi-solid and persistent skeleton, and since its very special morphology depends on the extension and ramification of this skeleton, it is natural to suppose that any modification in the form or number of the appendices results, as we stated above, from the growth or diminution of this skeleton itself, which is a living organ integrated by neurobiones susceptible of assimilation, division, and growth.

It thus appears that the dynamic agents capable of awakening the neoformative property of the neurobione and the chemical agents that give them materials for assimilation, are the essential condition of any neoformation. We do not, however, pretend to deny the possible intervention of osmotic disequilibrations or of changes in surface tension.

Hypothesis of the disequilibration of the neuro-neuroglial symbiosis.— On various occasions we have pointed out the fact that the neurone, far from living independently, becomes dynamically and trophically associated with certain cells of a special nature, among which we include the *protoplasmic neuroglia* of the centres, the *satellite cells* of the ganglia (*amphicytes* of v. Lenhossék) and the *cell of Schwann* of the nerves.[1] The two categories of elements are mutually serviceable, and there is established between them something like a symbiosis comparable to the well-known symbioses of fungi and algae to form lichens, or of the hydra and its chloroplasts.

In a normal state, that is, when the reciprocal actions are in equilibrium, the satellite cells are few. They abstain from proliferating and they respect the neuronal morphology. This quiescence is perhaps due to the paralyzing action of some principle which is liberated, under normal conditions, by the young and robust neurones. When these become fatigued, however, or when they weaken or die, the antimitosogenic check is moderated or suspended, and the satellite cells therefore multiply and press upon the periphery of the neuronal soma, forming in it pits and even holes, handles, fenestrations, etc. Moreover, the growing pressure of the satellite cell, or of the daughter cells proliferated from it, also brings about, through a mechanical or chemical stimulus,

---

[1] Marinesco has also proved that, while living, nervous protoplasm lacks Brownian movement, and must therefore be considered as a very viscous medium, a *gel*, and not a *sol*.

See Marinesco : " Sur la structure colloïdale des cellules nerveuses et ses variations à l'état normal et pathologique," *Congrès intern. de Neurol. et de Psychiatrie*, Gand, 20-26 août 1913.

more or less important neoformative processes. Thus are perhaps formed, for example, the pits and appendices of the frayed cells and the sprouts of the soma and glomerulus of the weakened elements, whether this weakening be by toxins, vascular perturbations, or various traumatic processes. Once the neurone is destroyed the division of the satellite cell continues, and there are formed those pericellular accumulations of cells which were described by Van Gehuchten and Babés in the ganglia in hydrophobia, and by Nageotte and other authors in tabetic and otherwise sick ganglia—the *residual nodules*.

This hypothesis was devised long ago to clear up the origin of the sprouts of the axon of the central stump and the atypical appendices of the sensory neurones of old individuals, etc. It is clear that it can be applied also, without great violence, to the growths occurring in wounded or transplanted ganglia. In this last case one might conceive that the nutritive perturbations provoked in the neurones by grafting have suspended the liberation of paralyzing substances. As a consequence the satellite cells proliferate, stimulate the neurofibrils trophically or mechanically, and these in turn, are compelled to multiply and to form new expansions.

Opinions of Bielschowsky and of K. Schaffer.—These scientists have admitted our conjecture of the *neuro-neuroglial symbiosis*, though with important modifications and with special reference to the production of expansions in certain pathological states, such as sclerosis, tabes, etc.

Bielschowsky [1] believes that the formation of expansions is in intimate relation with the state of the capsular or satellite cells, which, owing to the action of pathological stimuli, provoke the birth of new fibres. But this production of atypical appendices is possible only in neurones that are weakened or gravely diseased. Degeneration and regeneration are correlative processes. Without the first the second cannot exist. In presence of the chemotactic actions of the satellite cells the neuronal protoplasm loses its cohesion and is reduced to the more or less ephemeral formation of paraphytes. Once the cell is destroyed, the satellite cells take its place.

According to K. Schaffer,[2] there is in the normal state a certain equilibrium of reciprocal influences (reciprocal chemotaxis) between the sensory and the satellite cells. When the neurone is diseased this equilibrium is disturbed, and the satellite cells, with no controlling

---

[1] Bielschowsky : " Ueber den Bau der Spinalganglien unter normalen und pathologischen Verhältnissen," *Jour. f. Psychol. u. Neurol.*, Bd. 11, 1908.

[2] K. Schaffer : " Ueber Fibrillenbilder tabischen Spinalganglienzellen," *Zeitschrift für die gesamte Neurol. u. Psychiatrie*, Bd. 11, H. 4, 1910.

check, multiply, destroying through autolysis the companion cell. The capsular cells are without any phagocytic action, but they act as dissolvents on the nervous protoplasm. Finally, K. Schaffer compares the satellite cell to the *protoplasmic neuroglia cell* of Alzheimer, which it resembles in respect of its faculty of proliferating in the sick nervous tissue, and of its cytolytic properties.

We shall not make a critique of our theory nor of its derivatives, the theories of Bielschowsky and K. Schaffer. They all have the defect of explaining satisfactorily only certain special cases of creation of expansions in sick and weak neurones. There are cases, such as the production of appendices in a normal state or through mere neuronal commotion, without any apparent perturbation of the soma or of the capsule, to which this conception is difficult to apply. Even as regards transplantations, it has not been proved as yet that the proliferation or any other type of alteration of the satellite cells always precedes the creation of the appendices. The formation of these seems to be, at times, a direct effect of the physical or chemical stimuli on the neurofibrillar skeleton.[1] The question is therefore far from having reached a fully satisfactory solution. We shall return to it later.

There are authors for whom the problem before us, so to speak, does not exist. The dispositions above referred to are according to them simply normal and constant, and they reach, according to the animal species, a proportion that is always more or less equal. As is natural for these scientists, the dispositions in question, such as paraphytes and nests, have not only a trophic character, as Levi states, but also a specific nervous activity. Besides Dogiel, we must cite, among the authors who hold this view, Huber and Guild [2] and Ranson [3] who have examined, respectively, the ganglia of young and foetal rabbits, and those of adult dogs. Ranson states, in order to prove the

[1] Our observations on grafted and wounded ganglia to determine whether the proliferation of satellite cells precedes the formation of sprouts have not given precise results. Sometimes nerve cells with sprouts appear surrounded by great numbers of satellite cells, to house which they provide pits of impression. But there are also neurones furnished with appendices where it is not possible to recognize with clearness an increased number of capsular cells. It is true that the staining methods following precipitation with silver, such as haematoxylin and the basic aniline dyes, leave much to be desired as regards the demonstration of the satellite cells.

[2] C. Huber and S. R. Guild : " Observations on the histogenesis of protoplasmic processes, etc., of the neurones of peripheral sensory ganglia," *Anat. Record*, vol. 7, No. 8, 1913.

[3] Ranson : " The structure of the spinal ganglion and of the spinal nerves," *Journ. Comp. Neurol.*, vol. 22, 1912.

constancy and normality of such forms, that section of the sciatic brings about no qualitative or quantitative variation in the neuronal appendices of the corresponding ganglion.

We feel certain that Ranson would decidedly modify his opinion had he practised direct ganglionic lesions, or cut the nerve near the ganglion, or, finally made experiments of extirpation of roots. Besides, on such a hypothesis, how can we explain the prodigious abundance of sprouts and lobulated dispositions in tabes and in the cases of grafting and cultivation of the ganglia ?

It also appears that the above-mentioned American scientists forget that in well impregnated silver preparations negative are as valid as positive results. Thus when the atypical dispositions are lacking, as occurs in the majority of the ganglia of dogs, cats, rabbits, etc., it is not prudent to attribute this absence to an imperfect impregnation, any more than it would be to present as common and constant, dispositions that had been laboriously collected by examining hundreds of sections of ganglia. We understand full well that this error, in which we all participate somewhat, is due to the comparison of the neurofibrillar methods with the inconstant methods of Golgi and Ehrlich. An experience of many years with the neurofibrillar methods entitles us to affirm that, in a good impregnation, every formula always stains, with greater or less intensity, the fibres that have an affinity for colloidal silver, and that when there is absolutely no staining we may confidently assume that these do not exist.[1]

GRAFTS OF SYMPATHETIC GANGLIA

Summary of the typical and atypical normal structure of sympathetic neurones.—It is important to remember that the sympathetic ganglia of mammals—the intervertebral chain, semilunar ganglia, etc.—are composed of multipolar cells of great size, 50 to 60 μ. Each neurone shows : a *soma* made up of a fine *neurofibrillar net*, which has less affinity for colloidal silver than the similar net in spinal ganglia ; a *spongioplasm* through which are scattered small *chromatic grains* of Nissl ; a *nucleus*, or sometimes two of them, formed as in the sensory neurones ; and, finally, certain *pigment granules*, which are brown or yellow, which stain a dark grey with colloidal silver, and which are especially accumulated on one side of the protoplasm. Around the soma appears a delicate fibrillar membranous *capsule*, which is bordered internally with an endothelium, beneath which

[1] See additional note on p. 480.

stand out a few satellite cells. These subcapsular cells are especially abundant under the cover of certain sympathetic neurones of man (Fig. 173).

Like the neurones of the nerve centres, the sympathetic neurones possess two kinds of expansions : the *dendrites*, which are successively divided, and which end freely in the thickness of the ganglion, and the *axon* or *neurite*, a relatively thick expansion, which maintains its individuality, without any ramifications, up to its emergence

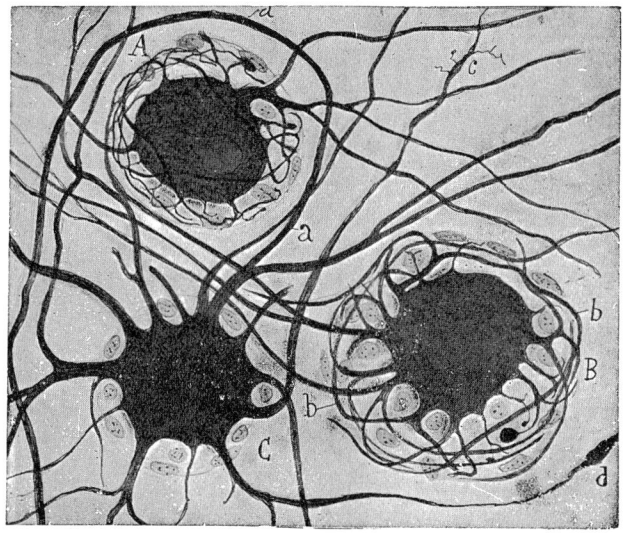

FIG. 173.—Sympathetic cells of the superior cervical ganglion of adult man. Reduced silver nitrate. *A*, type with short dendrites arranged in a crown ; *B*, type whose subcapsular dendrites are arranged in a nest ; *C*, common stellate type.

from the ganglionic centre, and which is nothing else than the *non-medullated fibre* or *fibre of Remak*. As it comes out of the soma it receives a very fine covering, which is a continuation of the capsule, and at intervals it shows elongated nuclei surrounded by a small quantity of protoplasm. A transversal section of the fibre thus shows, from without inwards : first, the afore-mentioned thin covering ; then a clear space which is partly filled by the perinuclear protoplasmic mass ; and, finally, the axon, which is entirely like the axon of medullated tubes. In preparations made with silver nitrate, only the axonic neurofibrillar bundle stands out clearly, as we show in Figs. 173, *a*, and 175, *A*.

464 DEGENERATION AND REGENERATION OF THE NERVE CENTRES

The dendrites proceeding from various cells, contiguous or far from each other, combine to form complicated bundles or plexuses, among which ramify and terminate numerous nerve fibres that have come from the spinal cord with the *rami communicantes*—the *motor fibres* of the first order of Kölliker. These afferent fibres are easily recognized in preparations made with osmic acid or Weigert's stain,

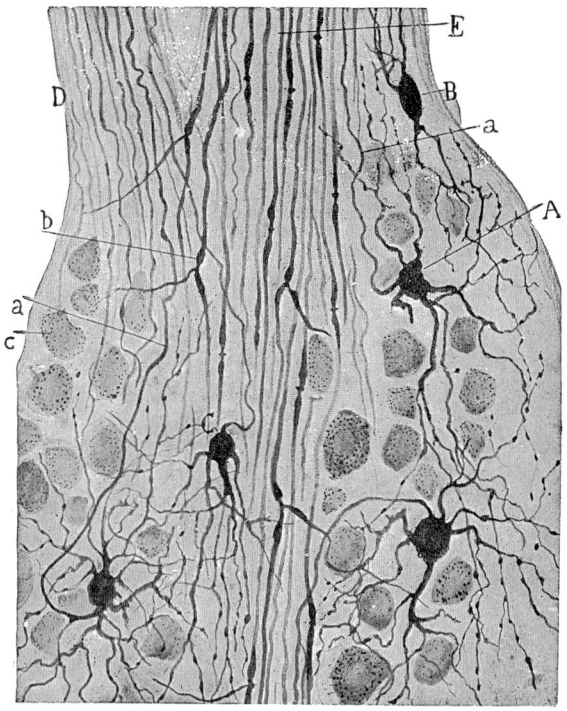

FIG. 174.—Cells of superior cervical ganglion of a cat. Methylene blue stain. A, B, C, sympathetic nerve cells; a, axons, b, bifurcations of afferent motor fibres (motor fibres of the first order); D, communicating cordons.

since they have a myelin sheath and nodes of Ranvier, and in neurofibrillar preparations, because of the black or deep grey tone that they ordinarily take, very different from the coffee-coloured shade characteristic of non-medullated fibres (Figs. 174, b, and 175, b).

Such is, in general, the structure of the sympathetic ganglia of superior vertebrates such as dogs, horses, cats, etc. We show this normal structure in Fig. 178, where we reproduce the interstitial cells and plexuses of the superior cervical ganglion of the horse.

One will notice that, apart from slight variations as regards the length of the expansions and the form and size of the soma, all the neurones are star-shaped and have long dendritic appendices. A similar picture is seen in Fig. 174, A and C, where we show a few ganglion cells of the cat, stained by the method of Ehrlich—methylene blue.

The same condition is not present in man. There is no doubt that here also the multipolar stellate cell predominates. But our investigations [1] carried out with reduced silver nitrate have shown us that, besides this predominant type, the sympathetic centres of

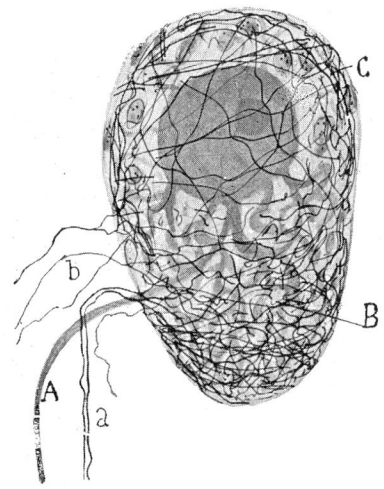

FIG. 175.—Cell in the shape of a comet. A, axon ; B, glomerulus ; a, afferent nerve fibres ; C, subcapsular nerve plexus.

man, and especially the *superior cervical ganglion*, which is a kind of brain of the sympathetic system, show three variants.

(*a*) *Cell in the shape of a crown and provided almost exclusively with short intracapsular dendrites.*—The capsule is very wide and separated from the circumference of the protoplasm, and the intermediate space, which is full of plasma and of satellite cells, is overrun by a multitude of appendices which are short, ramified, divergent, like the cogs of a wheel, and which terminate beneath the capsular membrane. Some are thin, others thick, some are short, others long ; these last sometimes turn back beneath the capsule

[1] Cajal : " Las celulas del gran simpático del hombre adulto," *Trab. del Lab. de Investig. biol.*, fasc. 1 and 2, t. 4, 1905.

and give rise to complicated spools around the cell from which they arise. Some appendices may end in clubs or balls, like those of sensory ganglia. The axon crosses the capsule and behaves in the usual manner (Figs. 173, *A*, and 177, *A*).

(*b*) *Comet-shaped cell.*—This is like the preceding type with subcapsular dendrites, but differs from it in that the capsule has a bag-shaped prolongation, from the end of which the axon may emerge, and sometimes also a long dendrite. The pericellular space is furrowed with fine, radiated appendices, while in the bag or comet-like

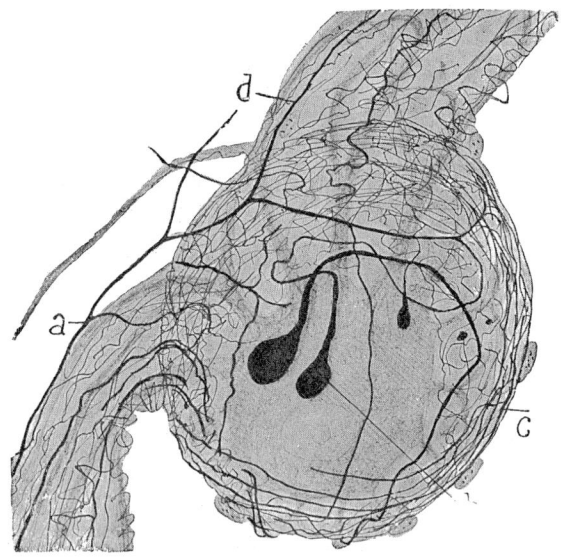

FIG. 176.—Pericellular nerve plexuses of a sympathetic neurone of man. *a*, afferent fibres ; *b*, terminal clubs ; *c*, pericellular plexus ; *d*, branch about to meander among the dendrites.

tail there is a concourse of other thicker protoplasmic appendices, which are longer, ramify repeatedly, and arrange themselves in a complicated plexus. We have designated this closely-pressed subcapsular plexus, made up of thick dendrites, the *sympathetic glomerulus* (Fig. 175, *B*). It is not unusual to find, especially in old individuals, monstrous dendritic branches with enormous local thickenings and even true terminal balls, as though these fibres were the seat of acts of growth and neoformation.

(*c*) *Stellate cell provided with long and short appendices.*—This is similar to the predominant multipolar type, but differs from it in

NORMAL STRUCTURE OF SYMPATHETIC NEURONES   467

that, besides the long dendritic expansions, it has others that are short, fine, and divergent, and end freely beneath the capsule. The axon behaves as in the other sympathetic types (Fig. 173, B). These as well as the preceding types of cells have within their cytoplasm, though not always, pigment granules that are stained by silver nitrate a dark grey.

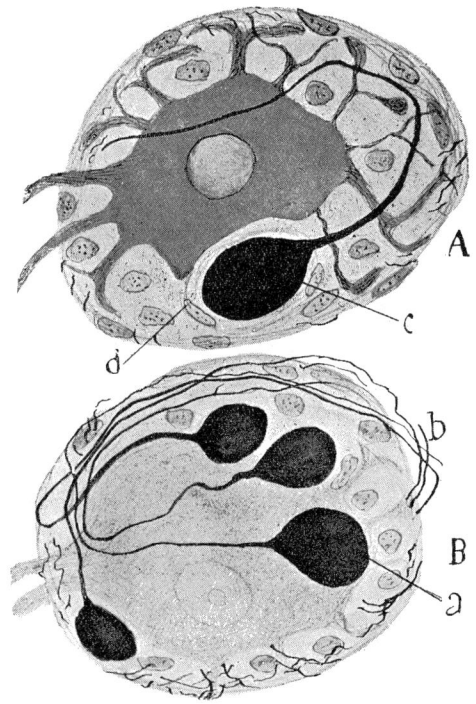

FIG. 177.—Sympathetic cells provided with colossal perisomatic nervous balls. a, nervous ball; b, nervous spool; d, capsule around the ball. Old man.

(d) *Argentophobic cells.*—These elements, ordinarily less common than the preceding types, are characterized by the fact that they contain large quantities of pigment and have expansions that are not stained by silver nitrate. These unstained cells are found in man as well as in the animals, and although they appear multipolar, their true morphology is in reality unknown to us, in consequence of their defective impregnation.

(e) *Atrophic cells.*—These are pale and argentophobic cells, contracted and diminished in size, usually surrounded by a thick mantle of satellite elements, stuffed with pigment that is strongly stained by silver, and apparently without expansions. They probably constitute the last phase of a process of slow and progressive neuronal atrophy. As the animal becomes older (man, horse, ox) the number

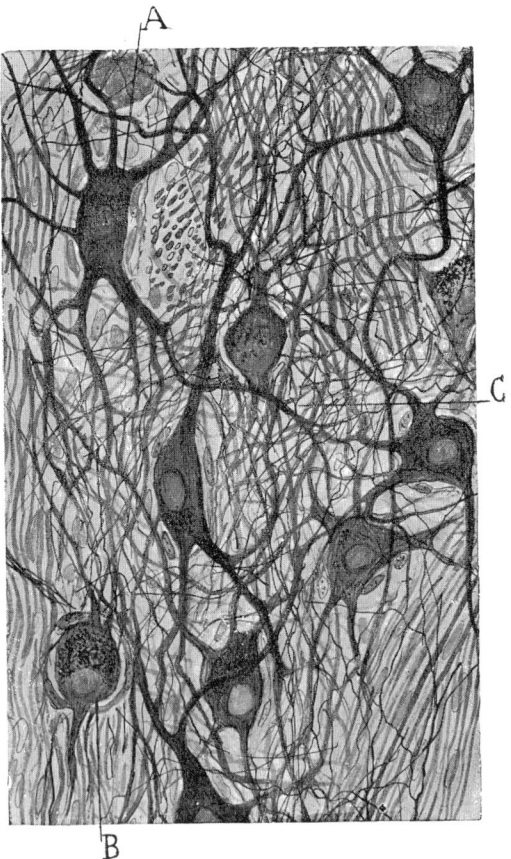

FIG. 178.—Sympathetic cells of a normal horse; superior cervical ganglion. Note the absence of nests and atypical neurones.

of this type of cells increases. In adults they are completely absent or are found only exceptionally.

(*f*) *Pericellular and peridendritic nests.*—All the comet-shaped nervous elements, many of those which are provided with a crown (subcapsular dendrites), and some of the typical stellate cells, show compact nerve plexuses which trace, beneath the capsule or within the capsule itself, complicated turns entirely similar to those which were pointed out previously in sensory ganglia. These afferent fibres penetrate into the subcapsular space, accompanying the dendrites, upon which they often describe spirals and intricate loops. When they come in contact with the short dendrites and satellite cells they dispose themselves in diffuse and complicated plexuses.

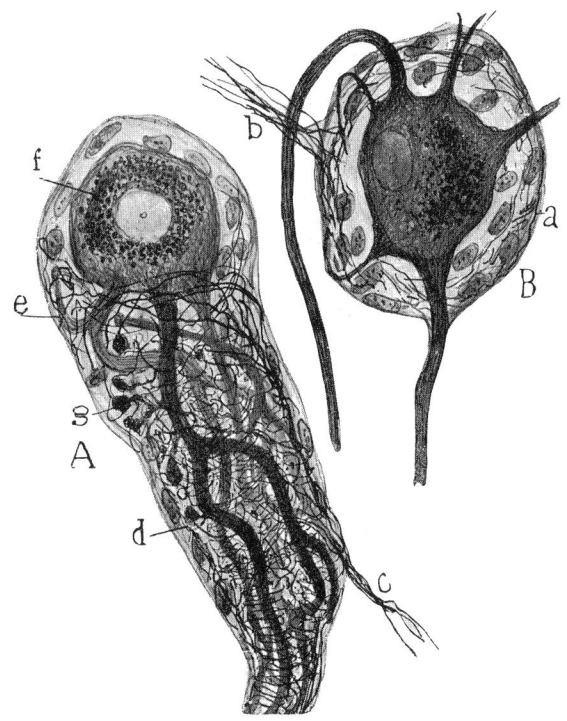

FIG. 179.—Atypical cells of an old horse. *A*. comet-like type with nests: *B*, stellate type with pericellular nest; *c*, afferent fibres; *d*, capsule; *g*, bulbs and terminal clubs of certain fine dendritic appendices.

In Figs. 175 and 176 we show two variations of these curious pericellular plexuses, whose complication is apt to be so great as to defy any attempt at precise analysis. Sometimes the terminal portion of the fibres constituting these nests (Fig. 176, *b*), becomes dilated into a bud or club of greater or less volume. In Fig. 177, *a*, *c*, which reproduces two ganglionic cells of an old man, there appear enormous clubs, one of them capsulated (*c*), which are entirely like those seen in the central stump of regenerating nerves. The filaments of all these plexuses originate, as we think we have demonstrated, from medullated axons that have ramified in the thickness of the ganglion and have come from the spinal cord—fibres of the first order. In Fig. 179 we show some plexuses and subcapsular nests of the horse.

The above sympathetic types, especially the crown type, where there are radiated subcapsular expansions, and the pericellular nests, have been confirmed by all those neurologists who have investigated the sympathetic system of man, in modern times, by the neurofibrillar methods. We may cite Marinesco,[1] who has studied the ganglia of the vertebral chain and the cephalic centres of the human sympathetic system ; Müller,[2] who has made various studies based on the method of Bielschowsky, of the ganglia of the general chain, the cardiac, cephalic (ciliary, otic, sphenopalatine, submaxillary, etc.), and intestinal ganglia ; G. Sala,[3] who has investigated with success the *ciliary ganglion* of man and of the dog, finding not only the neurones with short expansions and the nerve nests, but also complicated fenestrated systems in the dog ; J. Biondi,[4] who has made a good analysis of the cranial sympathetic ganglia, especially the *submaxillary ganglion* of man ; and, finally, N. Achúcarro,[5] who has successfully explored the relative proportions

---

[1] Marinesco : " Quelques recherches sur la morphologie normale et pathologique des cellules des ganglions spinaux et sympathiques de l'homme," *Le Névraxe*, vol. 8, fasc. 1, 1906.

[2] Müller : " Studien über die Anatomie und Histologie der sympathischen Grenzstrangen," *Verhandl. des Kongreses für innere Medizin*, 26th Congress, Wiesbaden, 1909.
  Idem : " Die Darminnervation," *Deutsch. Arch. f. klinische Medizin*, Bd. 105, 1911.
  Idem : " Die Betheiligung des sympathischen Nervensystems und den Kopfinnervation," *Deutsch. Arch. f. Klinische Medizin*, Bd. 99, Leipzig, 1910.
  Idem : " Beiträge zur Anat. Histol. u. Physiol. des Nervus vagus," etc. *Deutsch. Arch. f. klinische Medizin*, Bd. 101, 1910.

[3] G. Sala : " Sulla fina struttura del ganglio ciliare," *R. Instituto lombardo di scienze e lettere*, vol. 21, fasc. 4, Milano, 1910.

[4] Biondi : " Sulla fina anatomia dei gangli annessi al simpatico craniano nel uomo," *Labor. di Anat. normale della Reale Università di Roma*, vol. 16, fasc. 3 and 4, 1912.

[5] N. Achúcarro : " El ganglio cervical superior del gran simpático en diversos procesos patológicos del hombre," *Boletín de la Sociedad Española de Biología*, Nov. 1913.

of the various neuronal types, nests, etc., in the sympathetic system of epileptic, alcoholic, insane, and paralytic individuals.

In animals the types that are crown-shaped, comet-like, or glomerular, are extremely rare, as are also the nests and spirals. It is sufficient to state that in numerous preparations of the sympathetic vertebral chain of the normal cat, rabbit, and dog we have not been able to see a single example of these dispositions. It is only in the horse that we have seen the comet-shaped type, with the subcapsular glomerular plexus, and various types of nerve nests. These were found so rarely, however, that the great majority of the sections of the superior cervical ganglion showed only the typical stellate or multipolar type. Nevertheless, other authors seem to have been more fortunate. Thus Michailow,[1] in a series of interesting investigations, made by the method of Ehrlich-Dogiel, saw in the ganglia of the heart and bladder of the horse neuronal types with short and thick expansions (the *rosettenformige* of this author), which appear to be homologous to the type with a subcapsular crown in man. Michailow also saw cells with long or short dendrites terminating in voluminous clubs or free balls. Pitzorno,[2] on the other hand, saw in the sympathetic ganglia of chelonians true comet-like forms with spiroidal plexuses and characteristic pericellular nests. This same author [3] observed sympathetic neurones of the glomerular type in selaceans. V. Lenhossék,[4] who has studied the *ciliary ganglion* of birds, did not recognize the crown type, but he observed cells provided with ensiform dispositions and nerve nests which seemed in this case true terminations of the common oculomotor nerve. Finally Arcaute,[5] who has investigated the great sympathetic system

---

[1] Michailow: "Zur Frage über den feineren Bau des intracardialen Nervensystems der Säugethiere," *Inter. Monatschr. f. Anat. u. Physiol.*, Bd. 25, 1908.

See also: *Arch. f. mikros. Anat.*, etc. Bd. 72, 1908. *Anat. Anzeiger*, Bd. 33, 1908.

[2] M. Pitzorno: "Su alcune particolarità delle cellule del cordone simpatico dei Cheloni," *Monit. Zool. ital.* anno 21, No. 9, 1910.

[3] *Monit. Zool. ital.* anno 21, No. 3, 1910.

[4] v. Lenhossék: "Das Ganglion ciliare der Vögel," *Arch. f. mikros. Anat.*, Bd. 76, 1911.

[5] Arcaute: "Tipos morfológicos del gran simpático de los mamíferos de gran talla" (buey, caballo, asno, etc.), *Boletín de la Sociedad Española de Biología*, November, 1913.

of large-sized mammals, found the nests and short expansions only very exceptionally.[1]

Possible significance of the atypical cells and dispositions.—The absence of the above-mentioned dispositions in the sympathetic system of the majority of mammals, their exceptional presence in certain large mammals, such as the horse, and the extraordinary variability in their abundance in man, constitute a difficult problem. Nageotte has already put forward the view that the nerve nests described by us in the great sympathetic system of man represent, like the spools of Dogiel in sensory ganglia, pathological dispositions brought about by the formation and aberrant growth of incongruent nerve sprouts. The dispositions like gear-wheels, which are neurones with short subcapsular expansions, are also perhaps abnormal, as well as the cells that throw out subcapsular glomeruli, the pictures of which remind one of the frayed cells peculiar to human sensory ganglia in *tabes* and other pathological states.

We are thus confronted by the same doubts that arose as a result of finding in the sensory ganglia forms and dispositions of a sporadic and conditional character, whose frequency is governed by circumstances that are not clearly determined. The question is doubtless embarrassing. In order to reach a definite conclusion it would be necessary to explore the sympathetic ganglia of man in the various phases of their development, to analyse the lesions of this system in the various nervous diseases and, above all, to study the sympathetic chain in large mammals. We have carried out this comparative investigation, though incompletely, in certain animals and in man of various ages ; Achúcarro has likewise studied the ganglia of paralytics, epileptics, lunatics, etc., while Arcaute has studied large mammals.

While incomplete data do not warrant absolute conclusions, we may be allowed to express here our opinion. Like Nageotte we think it certain that the nests and subcapsular nerve plexuses—the bundles and spirals of afferent fibres—have a pathological or regenerative character. This assertion is supported by the following facts :

[1] There has appeared a paper by C. Riquier concerning the otic ganglion in the ox and man ("Sulla fina struttura del ganglio otico," *Riv. di Patol. ner. e. mentale*, vol. 18, fasc. 10, Oct. 1913). Riquier found in the ox, both foetal and adult, some cells with short subcapsular expansions, sometimes terminated in balls, as well as true comet-like types. He also found in the otic ganglion of an eight months old little girl cells with subcapsular dendrites, some of them monstrous and terminated in clubs. Riquier does not state the proportion of these forms to the stellate type. Neither does he describe nests.

(a) The frequent presence in human ganglia of thick hypertrophied fibres, with enlargements due to detention, and, especially, of rings, balls, and voluminous terminal clubs.

(b) The incongruence of position of these nests, which often come in contact, not with the soma or dendrites, but with the capsular

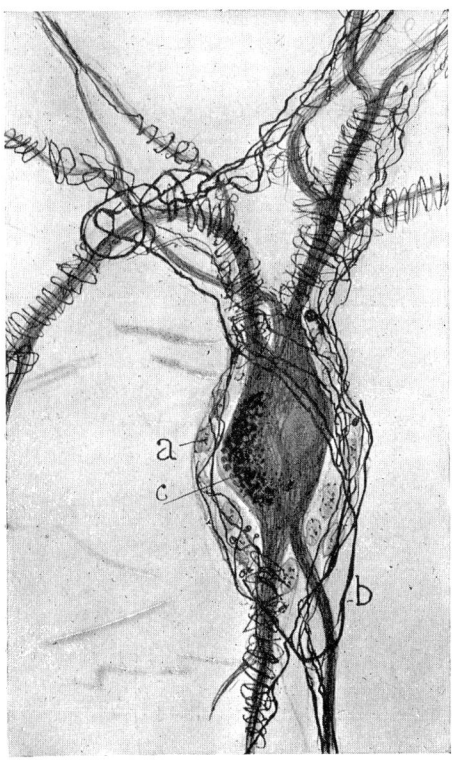

FIG. 180.—Cells of the superior cervical ganglion of a horse which died as a result of diphtheric toxin. *a*, capsule; *b*, afferent nerve fibres which form extra and intracapsular nests; *c*, pigment.

elements. Sometimes these spools describe circles above the capsule or at some distance from the expansions.

(c) The perfect analogy of these nests with those produced experimentally in the sensory ganglia of animals.

(d) Occasional presence of complicated nests and of clubs in the voluminous sympathetic ganglia of the horse and other mammals. In this animal (Figs. 179 and 180), the bundles and spirals assume three principal shapes: perisomatic bundles, peridendritic spirals, and intra and periglomerular plexuses (connective cells).

(e) The complete absence of the nests and plexuses in question (at least in neurofibrillar preparations) in laboratory animals, such as the cat, rabbit, dog, guinea-pig, etc.

(f) The very remarkable abundance of nests in the sympathetic system of aged alcoholics, persons suffering from general paralysis, etc., as found by Achúcarro.

We also hold that all those cells with short subcapsular appendices, as well as the comet-like types and the cells with an internal dendritic glomerulus, which are constantly associated with the presence of plexuses and spools of afferent fibres, are *accidental*, although not absolutely atypical. One may remember the concept of what is physiologically abnormal, which was set forth above. We believe that a ganglion may be normal while containing, nevertheless, neurones that are accidentally deviated from their ordinary form. In such a case their atypical state represents a new mode of trophic and functional equilibrium, which is temporary or definitive, and which is provoked by conditions to which only particular elements are sensitive.

The accidental, and in many cases, pathological character of such formations, seems to be proved by the following observations:

(a) The total absence or very exceptional presence of these cellular types in healthy laboratory animals, such as dogs, cats, rabbits, guinea-pigs, mice, etc.

(b) The usual absence of such elements in the sympathetic system of large mammals, except old or sick horses, where we have exceptionally seen the comet-like type (Fig. 179 A). In this animal we have not up to now observed the crown-shaped type.

(c) The not infrequent presence of terminal clubs and balls in the short dendrites.

(d) The notable similarity of the subcapsular appendices of the crown-shaped neurones of man with the short expansions of the frayed sensory elements, elements whose pathological significance is beyond doubt.

(e) The formation of more or less complicated subcapsular nests at the expense of short dendrites, reproducing a condition that is frequent in transplanted and wounded ganglia.

(f) The considerable reduction in the number of such atypical forms in children and adults who have died through accident, and their relative abundance in the aged.

(g) The artificial production, in grafted sympathetic ganglia, of crown-shaped cellular types, as we shall see below.

(h) While Müller, in the cranial and visceral ganglia of man, and Michailow in the cardiac and vesical ganglia of the horse, have observed abundant crown-shaped neurones, that is, cells with short subcapsular expansions, a comparison of their observations with those of other scientists, and also certain unequivocal signs of regeneration shown in the illustrations given by these two authors, allow one to state that the presence of such types varies according to the cases; and to suppose that often, and perhaps always, Müller and Michailow observed pathological ganglia. The enormous terminal balls and excrescences frequently depicted by Michailow in the short dendrites and even in some long dendrites of the horse are very significant in this direction. Analogous dispositions appear in the drawings of Müller, G. Sala, and Biondi, of human cranial ganglia.

(i) The notable differences observed by Achúcarro in the proportion of the comet-like types, the crown-shaped cells, and the atrophic cells full of pigment, according to the sick individuals examined.

As to the reasons why some cells of the sympathetic ganglia of healthy and sick men assume the curious atypical dispositions noted above, we can state nothing precise. To invoke the fatigue, through over-use, of certain neurones, or the selective action of digestive toxins, or the perturbatory influence of alcohol and other stimulants, of which man makes such great abuse, without adducing exact experimental data or systematic anatomico-pathological investigations, is to point out what may prove a profitable path for thought and investigation, but is not to deliver a fundamental attack on this arduous problem.

The knot of the difficulty lies in the existence, normally, although in small proportion, of some of the atypical dispositions, not only in adult men, but also in children.

Among the purely theoretical hypotheses, which are, therefore, premature and more or less applicable to the case, we may mention the hypothesis of *functional neurono-neuroglial symbiosis*, which we have exposed above. Owing to fatigue, to some selective influence of digestive toxins, to imperfect vascularization, to old age, etc., the paralyzing action that the neurone exercises on the proliferation of satellite elements becomes weakened and the latter therefore divide and return to the phase of secretory activity. The catalytic agents thus produced in excess would awaken the assimilative activity of the neuronal protoplasm, and the creation of appendices would be promoted. These appendices usually originate in the most active portion of the cell, that is, in its cortical region [1] and in the regions where the

---

[1] Achúcarro has shown that in some pathological ganglia, where one sees that the appendices arise from a thin tangential mantle which is in the phase of neurofibrillar hypertrophy, one can clearly distinguish the existence of a

smallest amounts of pigment and nutritive refuse are present. The remainder of these catalytic agents would pass out of the capsule, and would stimulate the nutritive acts of the nerve fibres of the interstitial plexus—the terminal fibres coming from the spinal cord. These fibres, their morphological equilibrium being disturbed, grow in the direction of the capsules and form plexuses, whose richness and concentration are closely bound up with the number of congregated satellite elements. Stereotropism also intervenes decisively in the turns and wanderings of the sprouts.

When a morphological phenomenon occurs in various animal species it rarely is of value. Thus this production of appendices and of afferent nervous ramifications represents a compensatory process which is essentially hypertrophic in nature. As a consequence of this, the exchanges with the surroundings would become more pronounced and the contacts and reciprocal reactions between the sympathetic neurones and the afferent fibres would be greatly amplified and perfected. The neuronal protoplasm, transformed into a centre of intense life, would augment its functional output, which would compensate, not only the previous decadence, but perhaps also the loss or death of those nerve cells which were worn out by overwork or other more or less pathological conditions. This would explain, in particular, the notable increment of crown-shaped cells, of glomerular cells, of nests, etc., in old age, progressive paralysis, insanity, epilepsy, etc., as noted by Achúcarro.

But we repeat that we should have no illusions concerning the extent of the preceding explanation, which has the fault of being complicated and too ingenious. While it is plausible when used to clear up the possible mechanism of the atypical forms in the old and the sick, it is applied with difficulty to those seen in normal children and adults.

certain contrast, from the point of view of the vital and regenerative capacity, between the neuronal protoplasmic cortex, on the one hand, and its perinuclear region and especially the territory occupied by the pigment, on the other. In transplanted ganglia it is also easy to observe that the neurofibrils of the sprouts always emanate from the cortical region of the somatic skeleton, and preferably from the regions where there are no pigment granules. There are thus indications that the central and intermediate regions of the protoplasm, full of the pigment inclusions and other products of catabolism, represent something like an old protoplasm, in contrast with the cortical zone and the axon, where a young protoplasm is present which is able to produce, according to circumstances, adaptive and compensatory neoformations. It is clear that, in this peculiar activity of the frontier region of the soma, one must regard the greater ease of nutritive exchanges as an important factor.

Experiments of grafting of sympathetic ganglia.—Various authors, especially Marinesco, have tried to transplant sympathetic ganglia. Marinesco has several times grafted with success the superior cervical ganglion of the cat under the skin of an adult animal of the same species.

In a first series of experiments made in collaboration with Minea,[1] these authors note the relatively good conservation of the sympathetic cells, whose neurofibrils remain unharmed for several days while those of the contiguous plexiform ganglion, grafted contemporaneously, are entirely destroyed. It was only some subsequent experiments of autotransplantations in the liver that allowed Marinesco[2] to see certain interesting changes in the protoplasmic reticulum, such as : degeneration of the neurofibrillar net, the appearance of numerous unstainable granulations in the protoplasm, the atrophy of the nucleus, the diminution in the number of expansions. In some less degenerated cells he observed a neurofibrillar skeleton, sometimes arranged in flexuous bundles, which are deeply stained, and separated by wide meshes ; at other times in hypertrophic cordons, which are undulated and very acid in relation to the colloidal silver. Finally, there are neurones in which the marginal protoplasmic zone has no affinity for silver ; bundles of robust neurofibrils stand out around the nucleus. The expansions display a simplified texture, showing at times a single central fibril, and terminating frequently in reticulated clubs. Marinesco does not describe newly-formed sprouts or appendices.

Since the experiments of Marinesco, Cardenal and ourselves have made some attempts at grafting sympathetic ganglia, with not very brilliant results.[3] In general, if the ganglion comes from a young animal, the cells retain their condition well until eight or ten days after the operation. As in the spinal ganglia, the central neurones become necrobiosed ; on the other hand, two or three rows of the

[1] Marinesco et Minea : " Changements morphologiques des cellules nerveuses survivant à la transplantation des ganglions nerveux," *Compt. Rend. Acad. Sci. Paris*, 25 fev. 1907.

[2] Marinesco : " Plasticité et amiboïdisme des cellules des ganglions sensitifs," *Revue neurol.*, No. 21, Nov. 1907.

[3] The investigations of Cardenal, made in our laboratory some years ago, were not published. The description that appears in the text is based on preparations by him and others made by ourselves from ganglia of young rabbits and cats grafted in animals of the same age.

marginal cells maintain their normal stainability and structure, and fine and pale neurofibrils are visible. The method of Nissl shows in the protoplasm delicate chromatic granules.

It is difficult to establish whether among the expansions seen some are newly formed. Their variable number for each neurone,

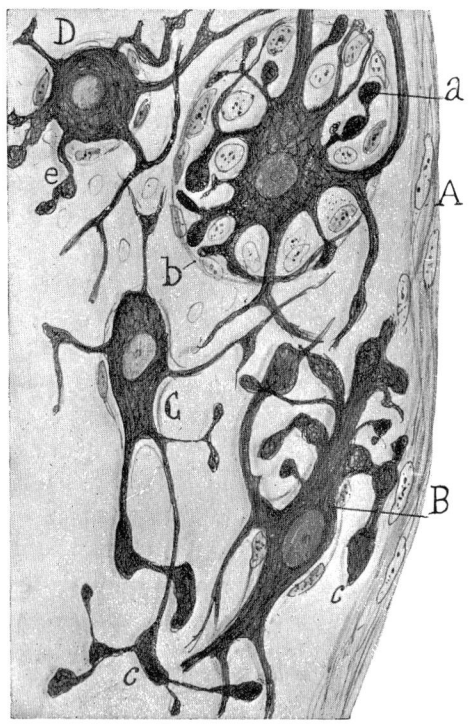

FIG. 181.—Cells from a sympathetic ganglion grafted in a young cat, which was killed seven days after the operation. A, capsule of the ganglion; a, subcapsular excrescences and newly-formed appendices ending in clubs; b, pericellular capsule; B, C, D, cells whose appendices show tuberosities and terminal thickenings; some of these appendices appear to have been recently formed.

and their notable paleness when stained by colloidal silver, make it difficult to determine which are the new sprouts, and whether, in the normal appendices, there are neoformative phenomena. Here, then, the criterion of survival cannot be based on an increase in the number of appendices, but on the presence of projections which, because of their unusual thickness, exceptional shortness, and strange mode of termination, stand out perfectly from the normal prolongations.

In accordance with this method of interpretation we have been able to recognize, in sympathetic ganglia of a young cat transplanted to an animal of the same species and age (*homochronotransplantation*), besides the indubitable survival of the cells, some phenomena of sprouting and certain structural changes that are somewhat different from those indicated by Marinesco. The principal dispositions found by us are as follows :

1. Cells of almost normal appearance, from one of whose sides issue one or more thick expansions, which are varicose, short, and which end in large intracapsular clubs (Fig. 181, *B*).

2. Cells that have, besides their normal extracapsular appendices, a multitude of thick and fine expansions, sparsely divided and ending

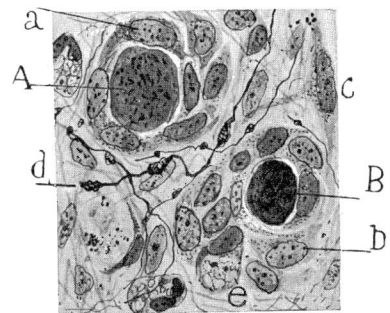

FIG. 182.—Residual nodules in course of formation in transplanted sympathetic ganglia. *A*, *B*, calcified remnants of the neurone ; *a*, proliferated satellite cells ; *e*, granular cell ; *d*, fibres that are being vacuolized. Seven day old graft.

beneath the capsule in olive-shaped eminences, clubs, or veritable balls (Fig. 181, *a*). The presence of this type in mammals, where it is never found normally, has a real theoretical importance. Thanks to this discovery, it is permissible to interpret the elements of this category, which were described by ourselves in man and confirmed by Marinesco and other authors, as atypical or accidental forms, that is, as resulting from phenomena of protoplasmic reaction, which occur even in healthy individuals. We may recall, moreover, that these forms are common in old men, or in adults suffering from various diseases.

3. Cells from whose circumference issues a thick extracapsular expansion, which appears normal, and which ends in a tuft of monstrous hypertrophic branches, which are themselves crowned by thick excrescences of variable size and appearance (Fig. 181, *C*).

4. Neurones that are elongated, as though they were in process of division, or furrowed by the clefts between lobulations.

5. Finally, in the deep portion of the ganglion one finds true residual nodules which are entirely comparable to those described by Nageotte and Marinesco in transplanted sensory ganglia. In sympathetic grafts, on the seventh and eighth day, one can discern all the transitions in the process (Fig. 182), from the phase of dead soma with calcareous deposits, surrounded by a crown of hypertrophic satellite cells, up to the phase of genuine residual nodule, that is, that state in which, the neuronal remnants having disappeared, the space corresponding thereto becomes filled with subcapsular elements, or amphicytes. Around such nodules there are no nerve bundles. Neither have we verified any evident phenomena of neuronophagy. The neuronal protoplasm seems to be progressively destroyed by the cytolyzing action of the amphicytes. It is possible that in the large cells of big mammals this takes place in a different way.

To sum up : the sympathetic cells survive grafting, like the sensory cells of spinal ganglia. Like them also they are capable of producing, though less abundantly, sprouts, balls, and other structures and phenomena that reveal an attempt on the part of the neuronal protoplasm to accommodate itself to the abnormal environment and to turn it to the best account. Perhaps it is the satellite cells that take the initiative in this compensatory reaction ; their number is much increased in the cells in which subcapsular expansions are formed.

ADDITIONAL NOTE TO CHAPTER III.

During the printing of this book in its Spanish edition there appeared another important work by Marinesco and Minea [1] on the subject of culture of ganglia. Their observations show that these sensory cells, preserved outside the organism, besides producing a large number of dendrites and expansions ending in balls, also bring about the formation in the cellular body of handles and complicated fenestrated systems like those which we pointed out in our first treatise on normal spinal ganglia of man and mammals.

[1] Marinesco et Minea : " Nouvelles recherches sur la culture *in vitro* des ganglions spinaux des mammifères," *Anat. Anzeiger*, Bd. 46, 1914.

In a work which appeared after our investigations on the transplantation of ganglia, Ranson [1] affirms that the expansions brought about by grafting, in the sensory cells, are transitory forms, and that after a few days the multipolar elements become apolar. This return to the normal shape occurs, according to him, after fifteen days.

Such observations, made on the rat, are not convincing, because after seventeen days the majority of, if not all, the neurones become necrobiosed, and it is impossible to stain them by the neurofibrillar methods. We may note also that Ranson is ignorant of all my numerous treatises on ganglionic cells as well as of my larger recapitulatory books. He not only is ignorant of my extensive work, *Histologie du système nerveux*, but also of my basic communication on sensory ganglia which appeared in Merkel's *Review*,[2] and which has been the starting point of all later investigations on this point.

[1] Ranson : " Transplantation of the spinal ganglion with observations on the significance of the complex types of spinal ganglion cells," *Jour. Comp. Neurol.*, vol. 24, 1914.

[2] Cajal : " Die Struktur der sensiblen Ganglien des Menschen und der Thieren," *Ergebn. Anat. u. Entwickelungsgeschichte v. Merkel u. Bonnet*, Bd. 16, 1906.

On ganglionic transplantation see Cajal : " Algunas observaciones favorables á la hipótesis neurotrópica," *Trab. del Lab. de Investig. biol.*, t. 8, 1910 (13 figs.).

SECOND PART

DEGENERATION AND REGENERATION OF THE SPINAL CORD AND NERVE ROOTS

At all times neurologists have been interested in the problem of degeneration and regeneration of the nerve centres. If we confine ourselves to the spinal cord, which forms the subject of this chapter, there have been numerous scientists who, desirous of exploring the mechanism of the degenerative reactions and of the possible reparatory acts of the central nerve paths, have studied the histological alterations of the spinal cord, either of men suffering from traumatic myelitis, sclerosis, secondary degenerations, commotions, etc., or else of animals that had been traumatized or submitted experimentally to poisonings, local anaemias and infections, etc. It would be a long list that included all the authors who have distinguished themselves by some original contribution in this difficult field. We may recall the following, whose investigations are closely related to ours, and who have worked almost exclusively on traumatized animals. Among the older authors it is important to remember Dentan (1873), Eichhorst and Naunyn (1874), Schiefferdecker (1876), Kahler (1884), Homen (1885), Lowenthal (1885), Ziegler (1888) Coën (1888), Barbacci (1891), Kerestszeghy and Hanns (1892), Stroebe (1894), etc.; and among the more modern Minor,[1] Nageotte,[2] Lugaro,[3]

---

[1] L. Minor: "Traumatische Erkrankungen des Rückenmarkes, etc.," *Handbuch der pathol. Anat. des Nervensystems v. Flatau-Jacobsohn, u. Minor*, Bd. 2, Berlin, 1904.

[2] Nageotte: *Compt. Rend. Soc. Biol.*, 20 mai, 1905, and 3 mars, 28 avril, 12 mai, 1906.

[3] Lugaro: "Sulla presunta rigenerazione autogena delle radici posteriori," *Riv. di pat. ner. e ment.*, vol. 11, fasc. 8, 1906.
See also: Same review, vol. 11, fasc. 7 and 8.

Cajal,[1] Marinesco,[2] G. Sala and Cortese,[3] O. Rossi,[4] Dustin,[5] Forster,[6] and Jakob.[7]

We shall speak of the discoveries and conceptions of the above-mentioned neurologists in connection with our exposition of the facts.

During the last few years this theme has been much studied. Investigators, possessing in the neurofibrillar methods a means of showing clearly the behaviour of the axon and its progressive growth, have attempted to examine once more, experimentally, the old dogma of the irregenerability of the central paths. They have not hoped to refute this conception, which is based on a fatal and inexorable fact, but to ascertain in virtue of what perturbatory conditions this process of axonic restoration, which is so active and rapid in peripheral nerves, breaks down lamentably in nerve centres, or produces minute and incongruous results.

In order to give an ordered account of the effects of traumatism in the spinal cord, we shall divide this question into three chapters. In the first we shall speak of degeneration and regeneration in the white matter ; in the second we shall describe acts of regression and progression that occur in the grey matter ; and in the third we shall analyze the changes occurring in the spinal roots when they, or their region of origin in the spinal cord, are cut.

---

[1] Cajal : " Notas preventivas sobre la degeneración y regeneración de las vías nerviosas centrales," *Trab. del Lab. de Investig. biol.*, t. 4, 1906-7.

See also : Same review, t. 8, 1910.

" Algunos hechos favorables à la hipótesis neurotrópica," *Ibidem*, t. 8, fasc. 1 and 2, 1910.

[2] Marinesco : " Recherches sur la régénérescence de la moelle," *Nouvelle Iconographie de la Salpêtrière*, No. 5, 1906.

[3] G. Sala and Cortese : *Sui fatti che si svolgono nel midollo spinali in seguito allo strappo delle radici*, Pavia, 1909.

[4] O. Rossi : " Processi rigenerativi e degenerativi consequente a ferite assetiche del sistema nervoso centrale," etc. *Riv. di patol. ner. e mentale*, anno 13, fasc. 11, 1908.

Idem : " Nuovi ricerche," etc. *Riv. di patol. ner. e mentale*, vol. 15, fasc. 4, 1910.

[5] Dustin : " Le rôle des tropismes et de l'odogenèse dans la régénération du système nerveux," *Arch. de biol.*, t. 25, 1910.

[6] L. Forster: "La degeneración traumática de la médula espinal de las aves," *Trab. del Lab. de Investig. biol.*, t. 9, 1911.

[7] A. Jakob : " Ueber die feinere Histologie der sekundären Faserdegeneration in der weissen Substanz des Rückenmarks," etc., *Histol. u. Histopathol. Arbeiten u. die Grosshirnrinde, etc. von Nissl u. Alzheimer*, Bd. 5, Heft 1, 1912.

I

DEGENERATION AND REGENERATION OF THE WHITE MATTER

Technical indications.—Summary of the normal structure of the white matter.—Traumatic degeneration.—Initial phenomena.—Appearance of the granular cells and destruction of the myelin and axon.—Secondary degeneration.—Precocious acts of regeneration.—Late examination of the lesions.—Break-down of regeneration.—Formation of the scar.—Creation, under special conditions, of very long fibres which abandon the spinal cord.

Technical indications.—When one partially interrupts the continuity of the bundles of the spinal cord, with a cutting instrument, in a young animal, such as a dog, cat, or rabbit, from eight to thirty days old, one immediately provokes a haemorrhage and a traumatic phlogosis, which includes, besides the spinal axis, the meninges and the vertebral periosteum. This inflammation is always aseptic and is reduced to the smallest expression when, as is our practice, instead of operating on the spinal cord after it has been exposed through ablation of the vertebral rings, punctures or cuts are made in it through the surrounding tissues which have been previously washed with bichloride of mercury. With a little practice, and by using regions of the cord, such as the lumbar and sacral, in which, in young animals, the vertebral column remains largely cartilaginous, one can interrupt as one wishes and with certainty the spinal cord as well as the roots. Besides, since the latter are almost parallel to the spinal axis and arranged in a bundle, the *cauda equina*, a simple transversal section made with a fine scalpel interrupts simultaneously various anterior and posterior roots. The posterior roots are usually cut between the ganglion and the spinal cord. The only bandage that one need use is a small bundle of cotton saturated in collodion, which is placed on the wound after the latter has been washed in bichloride of mercury and wiped dry.

The animal is killed two, six, twenty or more hours after the operation. Among the neurofibrillar methods we use preferably *formula G*; this includes fixation in pyridine (Section 1, p. 30), and has the advantage of lending to the fibres that are regenerated or in course of transformation a deeper colour than to normal conductors.

Structure of the normal white matter.—When one examines microscopically a cross-section of the spinal cord stained with carmine or haematoxylin one observes two parts of different appearance. One is peripheral and is constituted by longitudinal and parallel tubes ; it is called *white matter*. The other is central, made up of

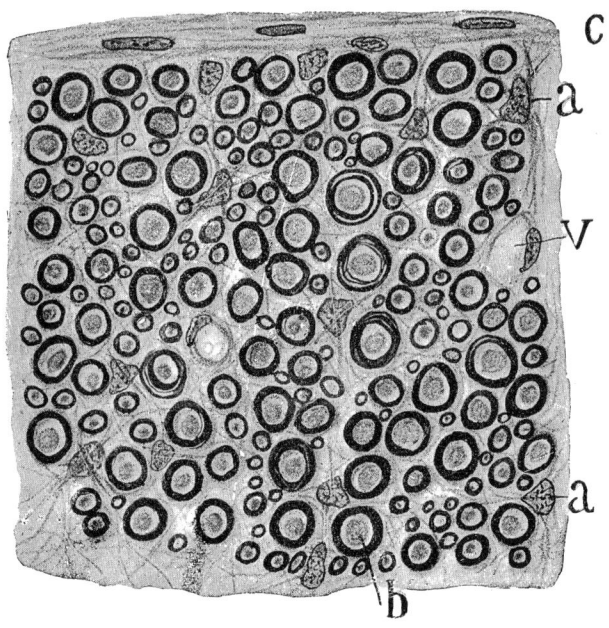

FIG. 183.—Transversal section of the white matter of the spinal cord of the ox; osmic acid stain. *a*, neuroglia cell ; *b*, axon ; *c*, capillary.

cells, and is called *grey matter*. The white matter is composed of two structural factors : the nerve tubes and the neuroglia cells.

The *nerve tubes* are the prolongation of the axons that originate in the neurones of the spinal grey matter, except those of them which are exogenous, that is, which arise from remote centres, such as the *pyramidal bundles* from the cerebral cortex, sensory conductors originating in the ganglia, etc. A good many of these fibres are medullated, but they have no sheath and cell of Schwann. On the other hand they have nodes of Ranvier, and the most robust have true incisures of Schmidt-Lantermann. The strangulation of the axon, which can be seen in a preparation made with methylene blue, is surrounded by a cementing disc, often elongated in the form of a muff, which joins the two contiguous ends of the medullary sheath. The collaterals that originate from the axon issue, as we show in Fig. 185, *a*, from its strangulated portion.

But the white matter also encloses, as we have shown by the use of neurofibrillar methods, a great number of fine fibres arranged in bundles, the majority of which lack a medullary sheath. Fig. 184, *a*, showing the white matter of a rabbit, testifies to the number of these delicate conductors.

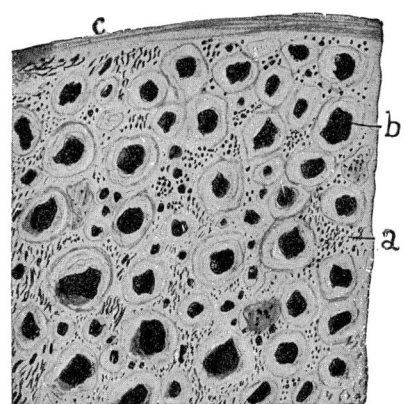

FIG. 184.—Piece of the lateral bundle of the spinal cord of the rabbit; reduced silver nitrate. *b*, thick axon; *a*, fine non-medullated fibres which are not seen in preparations made with osmic acid.

Between the nerve tubes are neuroglia cells, that is, stellate cells whose body has crests which accommodate themselves to the surrounding elements, and from which issue very long filaments which circulate among the conductors and constitute a thick interstitial plexus. These cells belong to the type of *neuroglia cells with long radiations*. Many of these appendices crowd around capillaries and even terminate, in the form of clubs, on the endothelial surface.

Finally, the white matter is crossed in a radial sense by a great number of nervous collaterals which arise from the strangulated portions of the tubes and penetrate into the grey matter. Many of the fine longitudinal fibres also represent collaterals or delicate bifurcations, which arise at the region where the axons coming from the grey matter turn back to become longitudinal in the white matter. We may add that the small veins and arteries that cross the bundles have with them an adventitious tunic provided with collagen bundles and connective cells. These latter are the only elements of mesodermal origin present within the nerve centres.

We add no further details in order not to lengthen the description unduly. The figures herewith will complete our description and remind the reader of details that we have omitted.

THE WHITE MATTER

Degeneration of the nerve tubes.—The alteration of the axons, following on traumatisms, is very precocious in both stumps of the white matter. One must distinguish here two kinds of degeneration, *Wallerian* or *secondary*, which occurs relatively late and is produced in all the fibres that are separated from their trophic centre; and *traumatic degeneration*, which is extremely rapid, and was first described by Schiefferdecker; this extends to a variable, but always small distance, from the lips of the wound, in the distal as well as in the proximal stumps. Since the white matter of the cord contains ascendant and descendant fibres, Wallerian degeneration is seen only partially in both stumps, although it usually predominates in the central one. On the other hand, traumatic degeneration attacks indistinctly all the interrupted fibres, equally in the central and peripheral stumps.

Traumatic degeneration.—This has the same or almost the same character in the central as in the peripheral stump, extending for a variable distance from the wound. Ordinarily it extends over 1 or 2 millimetres, but this varies, of course, with the size of the animal, the amount of contusion of the wound, haemorrhages, etc.

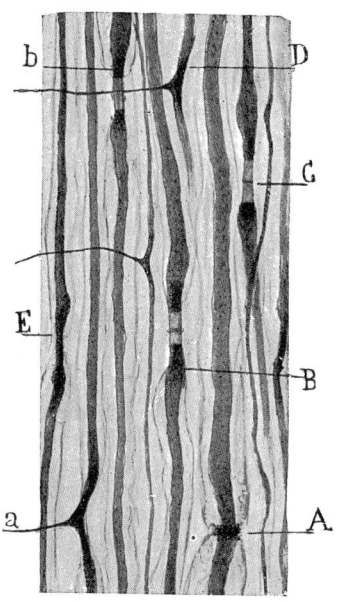

FIG. 185.—Nerve tubes of the white matter of the spinal cord of a cat one month old; methylene blue. *A*, node and cementing disc; *B*, muffs of Nageotte; *C*, *E*, nodes of thin tubes; *a*, collateral issuing from a node.

The examination of the altered portion of the axon allows one to recognize two regions, which are not always sharply delimited: the *necrotic segment* and the *degenerated segment*. Between the two segments lies the terminal stump or mass.

Necrotic portion.—A more or less extensive piece of the axon contiguous to the wound is destroyed by the traumatic violence, being reduced to a granular *tractus* which, three hours after the operation, disappears almost entirely through resorption. In order to see it the preparation must be examined from the first to the second hour after the operation. As can be seen in Fig. 186, *a*, *c*, this dead portion is formed of a series of granules which, starting from the end of the living axon, lose themselves among the fibres adjacent to the wound. Rapid necrobiosis is the more extensive, the more robust the fibre. Thus in non-medullated tubes or those with a thin covering of myelin, the living tip, at least during the hours following the operation, ends near the wound itself. The necrotic portion is thus reduced to an almost imperceptible minimum.

The morphological and structural aspect of this portion that is suddenly necrosed shows many variations. In some thick tubes this segment takes on the form of a wide and granular *tractus*, which is more or less spiroidal. We are here dealing with a precocious necrosis (Fig. 186, *D*), which is comparable to that described in the central stump of nerves, and which can advance cellulipetally twenty or more hundredths of a millimetre in an hour. After six hours we have seen it extend to half a millimetre in some exceptionally thick conductors. Finally, in medullated fibres of small calibre, this necrobiosis remains limited during the first two days to a few hundredths of a millimetre from the wound.

In the traumatised spinal cord one also often sees the *preserved fibres* of which we spoke when we were dealing with the necrosis of wounded nerves. We show a few of them in Fig. 186, *d*. They are characterized by their indifference to autolysis, the deep colour that they take with reduced silver nitrate, and the more or less arciform or glomerular aspect of their free end adjacent to the wound.[1] Towards their deep portion they pale progressively, ending in a point. Further on begins the necrotic segment which is pale or softened, that is, susceptible of rapid autolysis. We shall speak at greater length of the preserved fibres when we study spinal contusions.

Degenerated segment.—This was well studied by the older authors who used osmic acid (Marchi's method) and Weigert's method. It is characterized by two joint phenomena : (1) varicose swelling of the medullary sheath, which finally becomes resorbed into ellipsoids and fatty droplets, and (2) bead-like appearance of the axon, whose argentophilous material leaves certain points where the fibre becomes thin, concentrating in others where fusiform or ovoid thickenings of variable size are formed. We are here speaking, of

[1] Cajal : " Fibras conservadas y fibras degeneradas," etc. *Trab. del Lab. de Investig. biol.*, t. 9, 1911.

course, of those nerve tubes which have retained their continuity with the trophic centre. In the peripheral stumps this degenerative process becomes mixed up with a degeneration called secondary degeneration, of which it represents, in a way, a more rapid initial phase.

Retraction bud.—It is important to study the behaviour of both ends of this degenerated portion of the interrupted axon. The

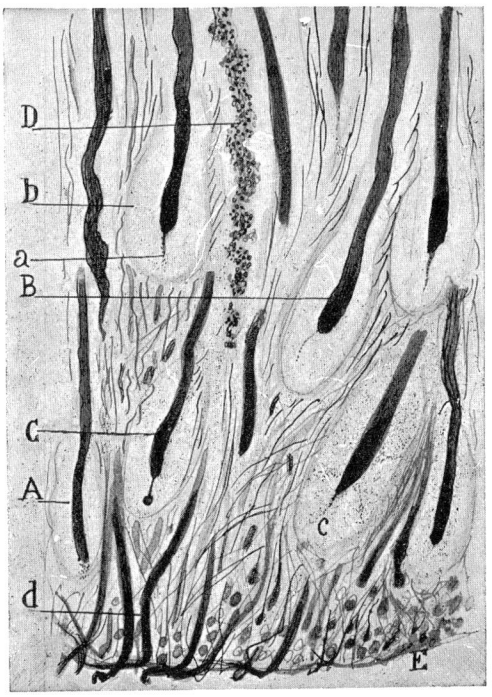

FIG. 186.—Central stump of a wound of the spinal cord of a cat, killed one hour after the operation. *A, B*, thick medullated fibres ending like the tip of a sound; *C*, axon ending in the same way, but provided with a terminal appendix and small ball; *D*, disintegrated axons; *E*, wound; *a*, remnants of the necrosed portion; *b*, plasmatic chamber; *d*, preserved axons.

distal portion, that is, that portion which is next to the necrotic segment, undergoes many transformations through protoplasmic retraction and accumulation. Taking account of this property of progressive withdrawal and separation from the necrotic segment, we have called this intumescence *retraction bud*. This terminal mass or thickening was already seen, more or less clearly, by Homen, Schiefferdecker, Stroebe, and Minor. It has been seen more recently by Nageotte in the white and grey matter of the spinal cord of tabetics, and by ourselves, Marinesco, Sala and Cortese, O. Rossi, Dustin, and L. Forster in the wounded spinal cord of animals. We think it indubitable that such buds are homologous with the terminal buds of the sterile tubes of cut nerves.

These terminal thickenings are large and ovoid in robust axons, but are small and spheroidal in fine axons. The most delicate

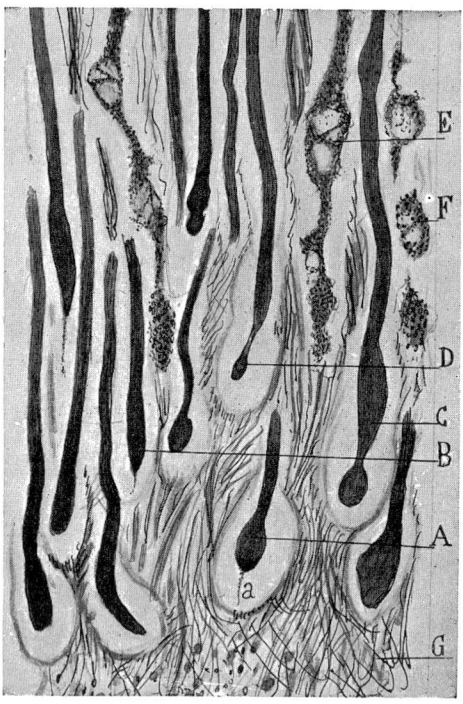

FIG. 187.—Piece of the proximal stump of a wound of the spinal cord of a cat which was killed an hour and a half after the operation. The terminal clubs are beginning to form.

among them belong to the finest non-medullated axons and collaterals, and enclose a neurofibrillar ring which takes the stain very deeply (Figs. 187 and 188). Usually these delicate clubs and rings are found near the wound, owing to the extreme shortness of the necrosed segment. In general *the size of the bud and its distance from the wound are greater in proportion as the fibre is more robust.* This involves the idea that *the extent of the traumatic degeneration perhaps is in direct relation to the diameter of the axon.*

THE WHITE MATTER 491

In preparations made with osmic acid one can see that the ball of retraction, as well as the preceding axonic thickenings, is ensheathed in thick medullary accumulations, a circumstance that was observed by the older authors and upon which Jakob has insisted in more recent times. There is thus a close correlation between the

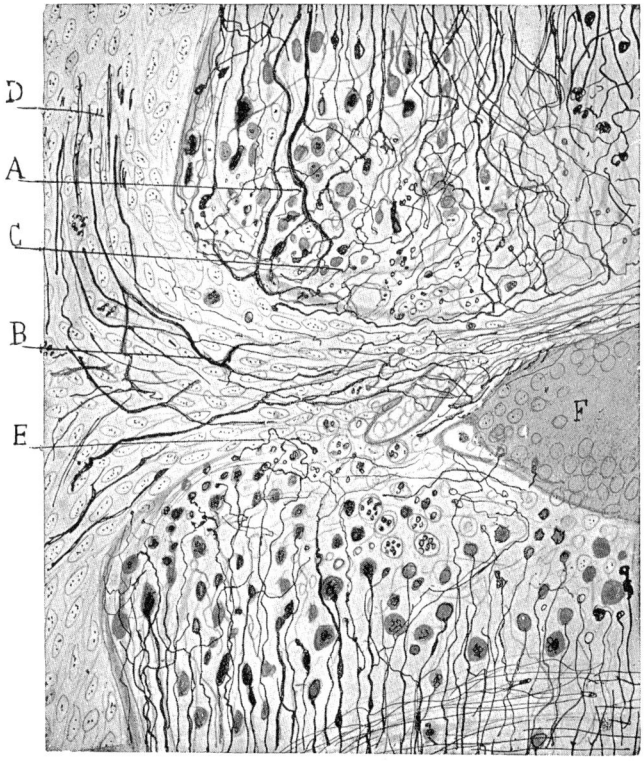

FIG. 188.—Lips of a complete wound of the spinal cord of a dog which was killed six days after the operation. *A*, *C*, fibres from the bundles, which have ramified in the necrotic portion of the white matter; *B*, newly-formed fibres coming from a regenerated anterior root; *D*, remnants of this anterior root; *E*, cyst in formation. One may note next to the wound a multitude of fine fibres ending in rings or small balls, while the thick fibres end in voluminous rings or clubs.

myelin thickenings and those of the axon. The space which is occupied by the myelin and its remnants is seen in neurofibrillar preparations as a transparent chamber (Fig. 187, *A*), which has an even contour. Between the terminal ball and the borders of the clear space one can see certain divergent granular trabeculae, which are perhaps homologous with the neurokeratin of Ewald and Kühne

492 DEGENERATION AND REGENERATION OF THE NERVE CENTRES

(Fig. 186, c). In preparations made with osmic acid, however, one can see that the whole of the space surrounding the terminal club is not full of myelin. This is arranged only in a thin peripheral mantle, and a large space remains between it and the club which is full of plasma devoid of lipoid substances (Fig. 189, I). This hollow space, within which one can see the remnants of the axon, corresponds to the *digestive chamber* of the central stump of peripheral nerves. In such preparations one can often see the terminal club or ball, vacuolated in appearance, or reduced to granular detritus (Fig. 189, C, h). The evolution and progressive withdrawal of the retraction mass may be studied in Figs. 186 and 187.

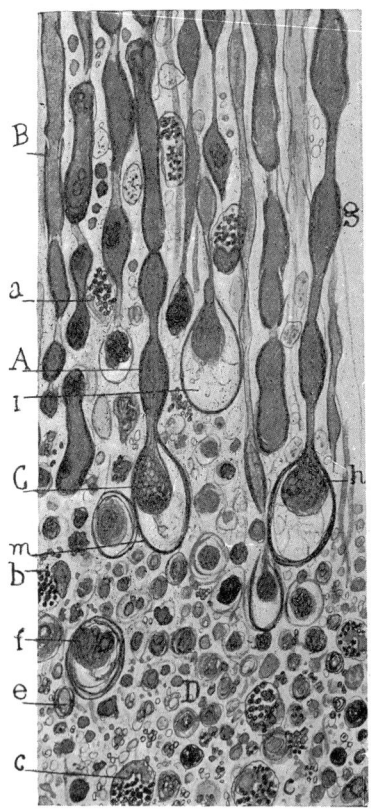

FIG. 189.—Edges of the wound in the spinal cord of a rabbit which was killed three days after the operation; osmic acid. A, beaded appearance of the myelin in the degenerated portion; B, tube only slightly altered, in which one can see the incisures of Lantermann; C, h, terminal buds of the axon; I, plasmatic chamber which surrounds the terminal bud; m, mantle of myelin which limits the chamber; D, fatty and protein detritus of the edges of the wound; e, f, lipoid balls; c, granular cells.

One hour after the lesion the axon of thick tubes shows, not far from the wound, a point which is slightly thickened in the shape of the end of a sound, and surrounded by an ellipsoid digestive chamber. In some axons the terminal stump is prolonged in a fine pale appendix which is still united to the necrotic segment (Fig. 186, B, a, c).

An hour and a half after the lesion one can see the same phenomena, but more accentuated. In the robust nerve tubes there are numerous terminations shaped like the end of a sound, or slightly swollen, with or without a terminal spine. But one can also see, as we are shown in Fig. 187, A, D, terminal clubs and buds that are already formed and entirely comparable to those of peripheral nerves.

In the following hours, up to one day, the terminal club is completely formed, often taking on the shape of a bud or sphere (Fig. 188) which subsequently persists. Apart from this type, various other dispositions may be seen, such as that in the shape of an exclamation mark (Fig. 196, *B*), that is, of a club with a small sphere pendent to it, and also that of a terminal glomerulus (Fig. 196, *C*), whose coils seem finally to combine into a more or less homogeneous mass. The ends not infrequently consist of series of two or more spheres soldered together and of a different size, as Forster has shown in the case of

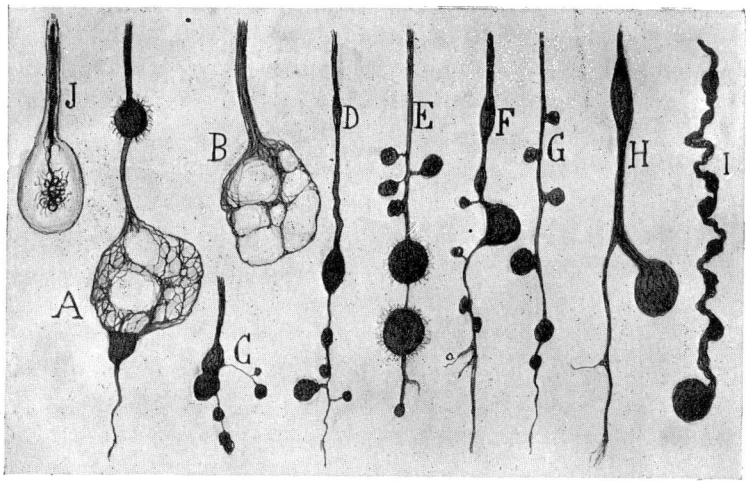

FIG. 190.—Various forms of alteration and regression of the retraction balls of the tubes of the white matter.

birds. In some instances the terminal portion of the axon, besides showing a succession of thickenings, has collateral excrescences which remind one of branches bearing fruit (Fig. 190, *D*, *E*, *G*). Finally, after four or more days, the voluminous balls are often the seat of destructive processes, autolytic in nature, combined with acts of resistance and neoformation on the part of the neurobiones.

We may cite, among other phenomena, the central vacuolization of the sphere, associated with the creation of cortical membraniform neurofibrillar nets (Fig. 190, *A*, *B*), and, especially, the well-known phenomenon of superficial hyalinization, with the persistence of central neurofibrils which may hypertrophy and become arranged in complicated nets (Fig. 190, *J*).

(a) *Autotomy and retraction of the fine and non-medullated conductors.*—The fine fibres generally terminate in clubs or small balls which are slightly granular and form very rapidly. In many of them, as a result of an act of autotomy, the terminal balls become detached, and are piled up near the wound. (Fig 196, *D*). A new club or ball is then formed at the end of the axon. In this way the fibre becomes successively shorter, although always to a less extent than the thick tubes.

(b) *Autotomy of the terminal buds and of the varicosities of thick tubes.*—In thick fibres autotomy is likewise frequent and brings about, to a greater extent than in non-medullated axons, the shortening of the conductor. This shortening takes place, not only through a successive elimination of the last thickening or ball of retraction, but also through a continuous thinning and consequent rupture of the bridges intermediate between the preterminal varicosities. The free balls may retain a remnant of vitality, but this is promptly dissipated through a progressive hyalinization of the neurofibrillar cortex. The centre of the ball, which often attracts colloidal silver very intensely, sometimes shows neurofibrillar nets, meandering fibrils, and other dispositions, which denote the relative survival of the axial group of neurobiones.

Observation of the degenerated segment at its transition to the normal segment.—If, instead of exploring the portion next to the wound, we observe the region of transition between the part of the axon that is degenerated traumatically and its normal portion, we see the same processes of beading and fragmentation, but less accentuated and with a slower evolution. This zone, 1 to 2 millimetres from the wound, where after six or eight days the destructive process is still maintained, is the seat of morphological dispositions that show the remarkable resistance of the neurobiones to destruction. We may note a fact that is seen with difficulty in the regions near to the wound—that the large varicosities often develop on both sides of the node (Fig. 191, *D*). We may also observe that, next to the smooth fusiform varicosities, there exist others which are gibbous and complicated by secondary thickenings (Fig. 191, *c*). One sees, not infrequently, in the intercalary bridge next to the varicosity, a certain hyaline zone and a dark neurofibrillar axis, which is flexuous or spiroidal (Fig. 191, *a*, *b*), and from which fine projections sometimes arise. Another frequent disposition is that in which the isolation of the balls is effected by the successive thinning and paling of the intermediate bridges. This progressive decrease in diameter occurs unequally, and of the two threads on which each bead of the axon hangs, one is finer than the other, so fine at times, in fact, as to be almost invisible (Fig. 191, E, g). Thus rupture which, near the wound, occurs quickly, appears, at a distance from it, to be the consequence of a process of slow lengthening or of retraction through centralization of the neurobiones and neuroplasm. Around each sphere or fusiform eminence there is never lacking, as noted above, the circular chamber for the myelin (Fig. 191, d), which has its interruptions precisely at the level of the axonic thinnings. In Fig. 198 we show the aspect of the myelin in the degenerated portion three days after the lesion.

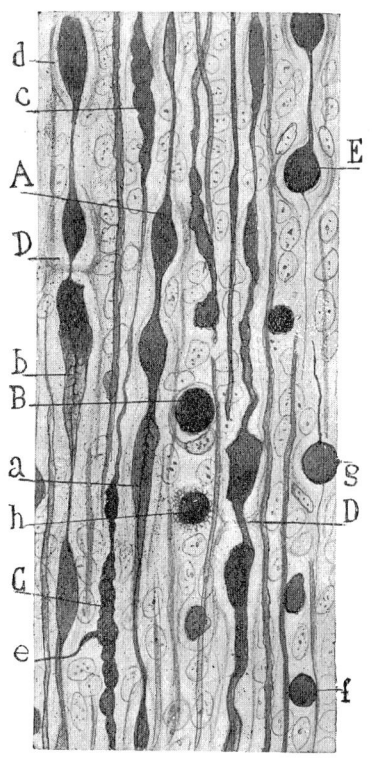

FIG. 191.—Degenerated segment of the centra stump, some distance from the wound. A, fusiform thickenings of the median axons; B, free capsulated ball originating from a robust fibre which has been destroyed; D, axonic thickenings near the nodes; E, double balls with very fine intermediate bridges; a, b, central neurofibrillar threads which are growing within thickenings; f, g, h, free balls; e, collateral which issues from a knotty thickening.

Finally, we may mention as occasional dispositions: glomeruli, in lieu of a varicosity, formed by closely pressed axonic coils, susceptible of being ulteriorly transformed into thick varicosities; thickenings, whether terminal or along the course of the fibre, provided with short appendices; and finally, the presence, between the last eminence and the healthy portion of the axon, of a long segment which is uniformly thickened and greedy of colloidal silver. Such modalities are inconstant and constitute precocious phenomena, which occur during the first few days and disappear when the varicose state becomes consolidated.

All these processes of axonic metamorphosis denote the survival of the neurofibrils and their reactions or movements of defence, represented principally by their dislocation at the level of the segments that are devoid of myelin, and their concentration in the regions where the myelin ovoids are accumulated. It appears difficult to exclude the multiplication of the neurobiones in the hypertrophic state of certain fibres, in the elaboration of colossal clubs, and in the other acts of neurofibrillar transformation of which we have spoken.

Metamorphosis of the myelin.—In the portion of the tubes that has degenerated through traumatism we find repeated the process of formation of ellipsoids and the successive fragmentation of the myelin that we have already pointed out in connection with the degeneration of nerves. Here also the process begins by the swelling of the nodes of Ranvier and the incisures of Schmidt-Lantermann; but here, since there are no cells of Schwann, the task of filling up the intercalary spaces between the myelin masses and of preparing the latter's transformation and resorption devolves, as we have stated, on the neuroglia cells.

Granular cells.—Since we are dealing with a phlegmasia occurring in an essentially vascular organ, we may be sure that the edges of the wound will appear permeated with extravasated plasma, during the two days following the lesion, and that the white and grey matter will be full of migrating white blood-cells. In the wound itself, besides the erythrocytes and the coagulated exudates, one finds abundant white cells, especially large cells with a lobulated nucleus.

The leucocytes introduced into the white matter very soon begin their phagocytic action. After twenty-four hours many of them contain large and small drops of fat, which can be seen by the use of osmic acid (Fig. 189, *c*). Later the protoplasm of these leucocytes grows and becomes vacuolized, and within them are found not only lipoid drops, but also pieces of axon, autotomized balls, and other proteid remnants. These leucocytes are nothing else than the *granular cells* of the authors. On the third and following days after the operation the white matter also contains, as many authors have recognized, neuroglia cells which, like the blood phagocytes, are full of lipoid remnants. Both cellular types thus co-operate in the process of absorption of the remnants of the necrosed nerve tube.

The *granular cells* or *bodies* have been well studied by the older anatomico-pathologists. Since their discovery by Gluge in 1841, they have received various names. Thus Nissl, Boedecker, and Juliusberger call them *Gitterzellen* (cells in the shape of a grate), Merzbacher [1] described them under the generic name of *Abräumzellen*; Jakob [2] differentiates various types of granular cells of different physiological function (*myeloclasts, myelophages*, etc.).

As to their origin, there is an almost general belief in two types. Certain of the cells arise from the mesoderm, and represent leucocytes or connective elements; others, of ectodermal origin, are nothing else than neuroglia cells, mobilized and transformed into amoeboid phagocytes. This is the opinion, among other modern authors, of Merzbacher, Marchand,[3] Held,[4] and Achúcarro.[5] There are nevertheless some authors who believe in a single origin. Thus Stroebe attributes to the cells an exclusively mesodermal origin, and he distinguishes two classes; polynucleated leucocytes which invade the sick region from the first day, and certain cells with an oval nucleus, which come from the endothelium or the perivascular connective tissue. Minor also believes in two classes of phagocytes; one class composed of mesodermal and connective cells, the other of leucocytes. Finally, Cerletti,[6] Marinesco and Da Fano, who hold similar views, deny to the *glia-cell* any phagocytic power.

For our part, without denying that the connective cells which accompany the adventitious mantle of the spinal blood-vessels may possibly collaborate in the above processes of engulfing of the myelin remnants, we believe that the principal role is played, during the first days of spinal phlogosis, by the leucocytes, and on the following days by the leucocytes and the neuroglia elements as well. All the granular cells of the exudate and the immense majority of those which appear on the edges of the wound (*necrotic* segment) are, we believe, leucocytes.

The connective cells of the scar participate also, not by attacking directly the nerve tubes, but by picking up the *detritus* which is taken out of the spinal cord by the exudates.

---

[1] Merzbacher: "Untersuchungen ueber die Morphologie und Biologie der Abräumzellen," etc., *Histol. u. Histopatholog. Arbeiten*, Bd. 3, 1909.

[2] *Loc. cit.*

[3] Marchand: "Untersuchungen ueber die Herkunft der Körnchenzellen des Zentralnervensystems," *Beitr. zur pathol. Anat.*, etc., Bd. 45, 1909.

[4] Held: "Ueber die Neuroglia marginalis der menschlichen Grosshirnrinde," *Monatschr. f. Psychiatr. u. Neurol.*, 1909.

[5] Achúcarro: "Cellules allongées et Stäbchenzellen, cellules névrogliques et cellules granulo-adipeuses à la corne d'Ammon." *Trab. del Lab. de Investig. biol.*, t. 7, 1909.

[6] Cerletti: "Sopra alcuni rapporti tra la cellule a bastoncello," etc., *Rivista Sperimentale di Frenatria*, 1905.

498 DEGENERATION AND REGENERATION OF THE NERVE CENTRES

Examination of the degenerated segment in preparations stained by the ordinary methods.—Investigation of longitudinal sections of the white matter, stained by the methods of Nissl, Heidenhain, Unna's polychrome blue, etc., yields pictures that recall fairly closely those shown by the central stump of interrupted nerves. Between the nerve tubes appear cellular columns composed of neuroglia cells, in mitotic division. We give various examples of this in Fig. 192, *a, d*. On the myelin ellipsoids and within them certain cells stand out (*A*) which, by their thickness, quadrangular figure, predilection for the strangulated regions of the myelin sheath, and by the form and structure of their nucleus (which is provided with a thick nucleolus), etc., are very similar to proliferating cells of Schwann of traumatized nerves. A careful examination with a 1·30 apochromatic objective of Zeiss allows one to distinguish the two. Around the nuclei one can see some protoplasm, which is somewhat stained by methylene blue, and which extends in radiated and independent expansions like the neuroglial appendices. If one carefully focuses the plane occupied by the cells in question, one sees that many of them lie outside the ovoids, which they surround with their protoplasmic arms (Fig. 192,*c,h*). Others, however, perhaps the majority, are lodged in the intervals or median junctures between two fatty ellipsoids, assuming quadrangular shapes through mechanical accommodation (Fig. 192, *A, B*), and also sending to the contiguous myelin expansions which enfold it. One frequently finds that this space is occupied by two or more cells

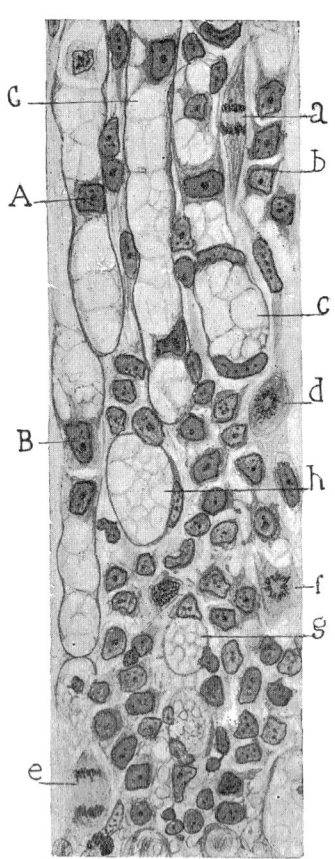

FIG. 192.—Edges of the wound of the white matter of a rabbit which was killed three days after the lesion was made. *A* and *B*, neuroglia cells insinuated between the myelin ellipsoids; *C*, a long ellipsoid, which is surrounded by an amoeboid neuroglia cell; *a, d, e*, neuroglia cells in mitosis; *b*, neuroglia cells arranged in a series; *h* and *c*, ellipsoids surrounded by elements of the same type; *g*, granular cell.

in series (Fig. 192, *B*). Finally, the nucleus is large, oval or slightly triangular, and contains, besides a thick nucleolus, a pale and loose chromatic network which is especially accumulated beneath the membrane.

As we show in Fig. 192, *a*, some perimyelinic elements are in mitotic division. Early anaphase (Fig. 192, *a*, *e*) shows, by its direction, that the plane of division may be perpendicular to the axis of the tubes. Later, from the third day on, these perimyelinic cells become full of lipoid particles or enclose relatively large drops, becoming converted, as we noted above, into true *granular bodies*.

All these observations show that the engulfing and digestive function of the cells of Schwann of the nerves is here taken over by the elements of the *Glia*. This incidentally supports the doctrine, which we have already exposed, of the functional identification of the cells of Schwann with the satellite cells of the sensory neurones and the neuroglial elements of the centres. The form and position —the quadrangular form and the position between the myelin segments, which are so similar to those of cells of Schwann in degenerating tubes—simply result from the fact that, as the membrane of the tube is lacking, the multiplied neuroglia cells, which are in an amoeboid phase, occupy the longitudinal spaces produced by the retraction and fragmentation of the medullary sheath and pieces of the axon.

Traumatic degeneration of the peripheral stump.—The preceding observations relate especially to the central stump of interrupted medullated tubes. The traumatic degeneration of the peripheral stump of axons separated from their trophic centre follows the same plan, with very slight differences. Each tube has a necrotic and a degenerated segment. The terminal ball of retraction of the large tubes appears to be already well formed a few hours after the wound, as do also the rings and delicate grumes of the thin fibres. One can likewise see that the club or bud of the large conductors lies at some distance from the wound, while that of the fine tubes is at its borders. The myelin also shows, at first, moniliform thickenings and a terminal accumulation with a plasmatic chamber. Finally, the neuroglia cells proliferate and enclose the lipoid segments and drops.

At any rate, the characteristics of the traumatic degeneration of the peripheral stump are not as well known as those of the central stump. What hinders one from analyzing the differences that the two stumps may show in this respect is the difficulty of distinguishing in the white matter a conductor united to its cell of origin from another that is separated from it. It is clear that if degeneration occurs nearly in the same way in all the conductors of the distal portion of the interrupted spinal cord (in whose white matter there exist many descending fibres, which are representatives of a peripheral stump), there are grounds for inferring that there is an essential identity of the phenomenon in both categories of fibres. This is precisely what has been observed.

There is fortunately a category of conductors that are undoubtedly peripheral, where one can make these observations with full confidence. We refer to the collaterals that arise from the posterior fasciculus and are distributed in the anterior horn and intermediate substance. Such fibres, sensory by nature, are sometimes cut. More often, however, in the experiments of spinal traumatism, they degenerate through destruction of the white matter from which they proceed. In such fibres there is rapidly formed in the axon a *necrotic* and a *degenerative* segment. The necrotic segment is resorbed from the first to the second day. The segment that is degenerated through traumatism, represented at first by a few varicosities and a terminal bud, is seen after three to six days, owing to the autotomy of the beaded segment, as a more or less retracted terminal ball within the grey matter. As we show in Fig. 193, *b*, *f*, this club sometimes appears more or less doubled. Its size is in relation with the diameter of the collateral. The rest of the conductor, that is the segment situated between the ball and the terminal arborization, is maintained apparently unchanged five, six, and eight days after the lesion, up to the time when it becomes the seat of a secondary degeneration. This secondary degeneration, contrary to the view with regard to myelin held by Van Gehuchten and Molhant, is retarded in the collaterals and fine fibres much more than in the large medullated tubes. As to the myelin of collaterals, it also takes on, from the third to the sixth day after the lesion, the appearance of a terminal globe, which is or is not preceded by a moniliform thickening.

It is clear that what we have said concerning the collaterals cannot be unreservedly generalized to the thick tubes of the fasciculi. In these traumatic degeneration is more extensive. Thus, in the posterior fasciculus we have seen that the varicose state and the consequent autotomy sometimes extend for nearly a millimetre in the ascending branch of the sensory roots. The extension of the degenerative reaction is greater in proportion as the conductor is larger.

Sometimes, nevertheless, of two conductors of the same calibre, one shows a longer degenerated segment than the other. The great

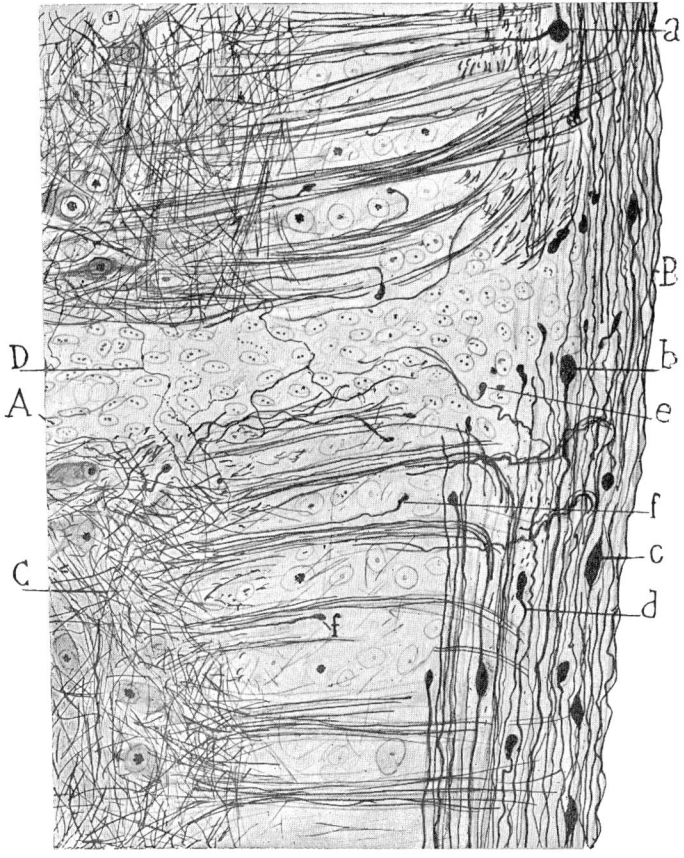

FIG. 193.—Partial section of the spina lcord of a young dog which was killed six days after the operation; region of the posterior fasciculus and substance of Rolando. *A*, scar; *B*, posterior fasciculus; *C*, nerve plexus of the posterior horn; *D*, perforating nerve fibre; *a*, ball from which issues a collateral; *b*, retraction balls of the white matter; *c*, beads of degenerated fibres; *f*, terminal ball of sensory collaterals.

differences visible in this respect in the fibres of the spinal cord may be explained by imagining that the energy and extension of the degenerative reaction bear a proportion, under the same circumstances, not only to the diameter of the axon, but also to the proximity of the lesion to the cell of origin, or, in other words, to the quantity of protoplasm segregated from its trophic centre. According to this concept, a sensory collateral of the posterior fasciculus would degenerate much less than the radicular trunk. We shall speak further of this conjecture below.

Late observations of traumatic degeneration.—One or one and a half months after the operation the degenerated portions of the axon next to the wound have disappeared. The appearance is so normal that a superficial examination would lead us to believe that nothing grave has occurred in the white matter. One sees no varicosities nor terminal clubs. The phagocytes or granular cells have much diminished. Nevertheless a careful examination with a good apochromatic objective allows us to recognize profound changes. One sees that the axons are separated, loose, and are less numerous the nearer we approach the lesion. The files of the conductors that have disappeared have been filled by compact columns of neuroglia cells, among which one can see, here and there, by using procedures which stain fats such as Sudan III and osmic acid, lipoidal vestiges, contained in granular cells. The balls have disappeared almost entirely. If one examines carefully a series of sections, however, one sees a few free balls which are being resorbed, that is, which have a hyaline cortex and a granular centre of a more or less dark colour. Remnants of balls will be found mostly next to the scar and in the scar itself (Fig. 194, c). Some of these are enclosed within granular cells. Finally, one sees exceptionally a few thick fibres terminating in a retraction club not far from the wound (Fig. 194, b).

But the most important change, to which we have already alluded, is the total transformation, near the wound, of the axons into arciform fibres which penetrate into the grey matter (B, C). It is impossible to see in these regions, in the course of axons coming from the spinal horns or the posterior root, the well-known bifurcation into an ascending and a descending branch. All these conductors, as they encounter the fasciculi, are simply deflected so as to become longitudinal and ascendant if one is dealing with the proximal spinal segment, descendant if one is dealing with the distal segment.

How can one explain so important a metamorphosis ? Very simply. By virtue of the eliminatory traumatic degeneration the whole axonic segment directed towards necrosed or gravely impaired regions of the grey or white matter has become resorbed.

Three principal cases occur, of which we give schemata in Fig. 195.

The traumatism has rendered useless the descending branch of posterior roots. This branch is radically destroyed, so that after a

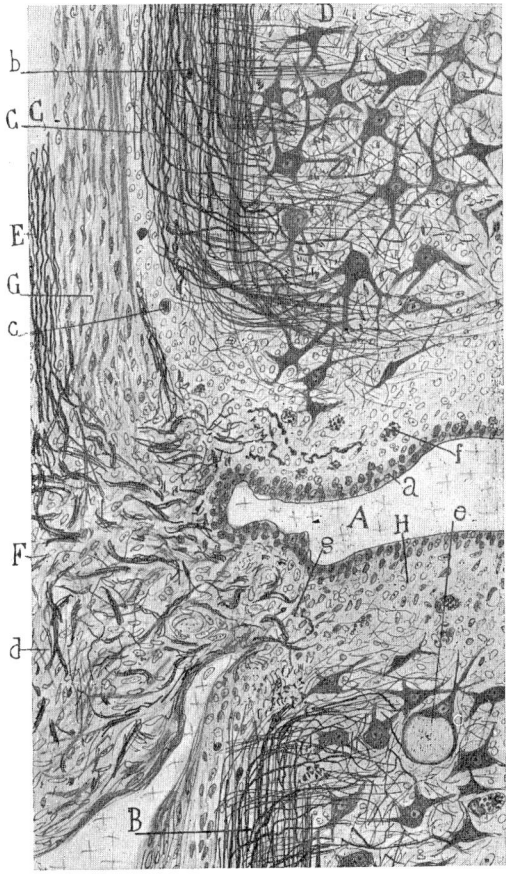

FIG. 194.—Complete section of the spinal cord of a rabbit which was killed a month and a half after the operation. *A*, cyst invested with ependyma; *B*, *C*, arciform fibres in the two stumps of the white matter of the wound (anterior fasciculus); *D*, cells of the grey matter; *E*, piece of an anterior root; *F*, connective scar which is invaded by sprouts issuing from this root; *c*, free balls; *f*, granular bodies.

month and a half it is impossible to see any sign of bifurcation, not only in the roots adjacent to the lesion, but also in some situated at a certain distance (Fig. 195, *A*).

In a second case the lesion has rendered useless the terminal portion of a longitudinal fibre of the fasciculi. As a consequence, we see the disappearance of so much of the axon as is situated beyond the last collateral that has retained its terminal connections (Fig. 195, *C*). This collateral, accordingly re-enforced through a compensatory hypertrophy, now represents the terminal branch.

In a third case a funicular axon, which is bifurcated in the white matter into an ascending and a descending branch, has its descending prolongation mutilated and thus rendered useless. *Ipso*

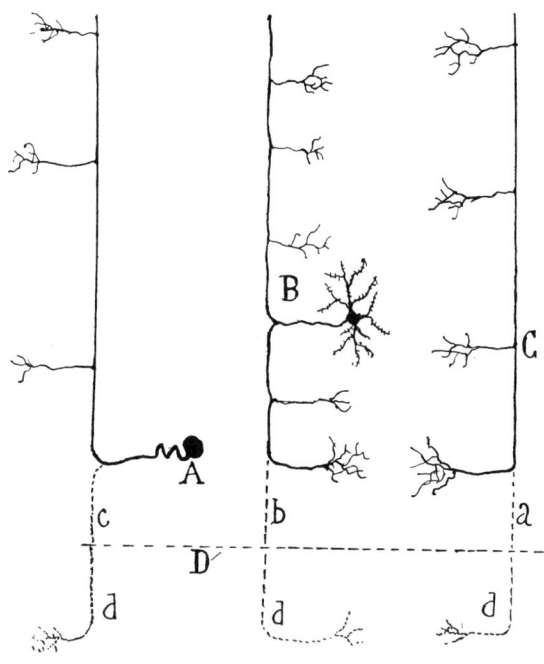

FIG. 195.—Schematic drawing designed to show the resorbed portion of the mutilated conductors of the white matter. *A*, fibre of the posterior or sensory fasciculus; *B*, fibre in continuity with the axon of a funicular neurone; *C*, fibre in continuity with the axon of a neurone situated in superior centres (pyramidal tract of the cerebrum, etc.); *D*, plane of the wound; *a*, *b*, and *c*, segments which have disappeared.

facto, as a result of traumatic degeneration, the ascending branch alone subsists, that is, the branch retaining dynamic relations with the grey matter (Fig. 195, *B*).

This interesting process of simplification, followed by a compensatory hypertrophy, shows us that traumatic degeneration represents a curious mechanism of reaction of an exquisitely economical and utilitarian character. Thanks to it, nature gets rid, so to speak, of useless mouths of protoplasmic segments that serve no useful purpose.

THE WHITE MATTER 505

This eliminating process enters into play very early. Already during the third, fourth, and fifth days after the operation the traumatic degeneration of the useless axonic branches directed towards the wound is very much advanced. In Figs. 193 and 196 we show the phases of the destruction of the terminal portion of the funicular axons beyond the origin of the collaterals. One may note how this stump becomes thinner concurrently with the hypertrophic thicken-

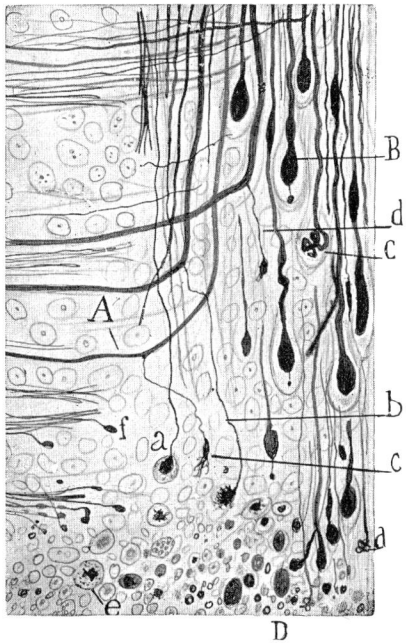

FIG. 196.—Piece of the central stump of the spinal wound of a young cat, three days after the operation. *A*, thickened collaterals which will be transformed into terminal fibres; *a, b, c*, longitudinal portion of axons destined to disappear; *B*, club with an appendix; *C*, final glomerulus; *D*, edges of the wound with axonic and lipoid detritus; *e*, free balls which are becoming hyaline.

ing of the last collateral. The retraction ball shows a variety of degenerative aspects, such as gibbosities, internal vacuolizations, hyalinization, transformation into a granular grume, etc.

Finally the pedicle, which is very fine, becomes pale and vanishes, while the terminal granular grume becomes invisible. After six days perfect arches are already to be seen, as appears in Fig. 193. In other cases, where the axons are thick, the destructive process requires six to eight days.

Sometimes, nevertheless, one finds not far from the scar, within the central stump of the white matter, some robust longitudinal axons, terminating in voluminous clubs, a month and even three months after the lesion (Fig. 194, *b*). Some of them are not infrequently preceded by flexuous hypertrophic segments, showing a knotty or tuberose contour, like those described by Dustin under the name of *nodose fibres*. Conductors showing this recalcitrance to atrophy, which are probably homologous to the thick sterile axons of the central stump of the nerves, appear to be especially abundant in adult animals, perhaps because of the slowness with which regressive phenomena take place in these. They persisted in an adult rabbit four months after the lesion, and Dustin observed them in the dog even three years after the spinal interruption.

Without discussing at present the nature of these tenacious fibres, it is important to know that the white matter of the cord contains, besides axons that are docile to eliminatory degeneration, other *conductors* or *central ends that are refractory to, or extremely tardy in, the fulfilment of the law of utilitarian atrophy.*

In fine, the maintenance of the connections, and therefore the continued functioning, of a collateral, constitute a hindrance to traumatic degeneration. We see here once more confirmed the law, which is so obvious in the degeneration of the nerves, of atrophy through disuse. There is the difference, however, that in the nerves this process of destruction of disconnected conductors takes months and perhaps years to complete, while in the nerve centres it is a matter of a few days.

Metamorphosis of the free balls that result from axonic fragmentation.—We have seen how the autotomy of the traumatically degenerated portions of the axons brings about the formation of free balls, in the centre of which the colony of neurobiones, which is beset by the hyaline degeneration, retains a remnant of vitality. But, we repeat, after one to two months the majority of the spheres disappear.

The fine balls are destroyed through phagocytosis and autolysis. The large balls offer much greater resistance to autolysis, they are not phagocytized, and they undergo important metamorphoses. As was found by the older authors, especially Homen,[1] Kerestszeghy

[1] Homen: "Experimenteller Beiträg zur Pathol. u. pathol. Anat. des Rückenmarks," etc., *Fortschrift. der Medizin*, 1889.

and Hanns,[1] and Stroebe,[2] and as was confirmed by Achúcarro and Catola,[3] ourselves, etc., these free balls take on a stratified texture, they change their chemical affinities, and they become more or less avid of iodine and certain aniline compounds. From them finally emanate the *amilaceous bodies*, which were pointed out some time ago in the degenerative foci of the centres. Some of them become surrounded in course of time with nucleated capsules, as was seen by Stroebe.

Wallerian or secondary degeneration.—Apart from the peripheral stump of interrupted fibres, this form of degeneration begins where traumatic degeneration ends, appearing simultaneously, as was shown by Knick, along the entire extent of the conductor that is separated from its trophic centre.

It is not our plan to study secondary degeneration. Readers who wish to know in detail the histology of this important process, on which are based important methods of investigation of the central paths, like that of Marchi, should consult the excellent monographs of Schiefferdecker, Bouchard, Kähler, Barth, Phylipeaux and Vulpian, W. Müller, Westphal, Hofrichter, Lowenthal, Thooth, Barbacci, Stroebe, Ziegler, Kerestszeghy and Hanns, Marinesco, van Gehuchten, and Jakob. The recent and very extensive study of this last author [4] contains, with a complete bibliography, the details of structure of the metamorphosis of the axon, myelin, and neuroglia, in the light of the most modern methods of staining. We may speak of this matter later from the point of view of alterations of the axon.

We shall confine ourselves now to referring briefly to some observations on the fibres of the fasciculi in the traumatized spinal cord, especially on the posterior fasciculus. The alterations of the axons

---

[1] Kerestszeghy und Hanns: "Ueber Degenerations- und Regenerations-Vorgänge am Rückenmarke des Hundes nach Durchschneidung," *Ziegler's Beiträge*, Bd. 12, 1892.

[2] H. Stroebe: "Experimentelle Untersuchungen über die degenerativen und reparatorischen Vorgänge bei der Heilung von Verletzungen des Rückenmarks," etc., *Ziegler's Archiv.*, Bd. 50, 1894.

[3] Catola und Achúcarro: "Zur Entstehung der Amyboidkörperchen im Zentralnervensystem," *Virchow's Archiv.*, 1906.

[4] Jakob: "Ueber die feinere Histologie der sekundaren Faserdegeneration," etc., *Histol. u. Histopath. Arbeiten über die Grosshirnrinde*, etc., *v. Nissl u. Alzheimer*, Bd. 5, H. 1, 1912.

are relatively tardy, as many authors have already observed. Nevertheless, according to our own observations, one recognizes great differences as regards the time at which the metamorphoses begin, and one may distinguish in this respect three orders of conductors: the *large*, the *medium-sized*, and the *fine*, which are non-medullated in part.

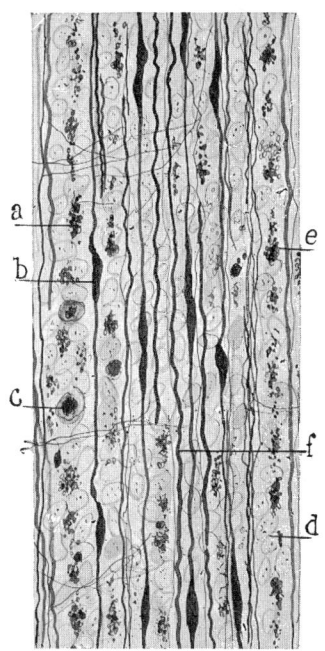

FIG. 197.—Piece of the lateral fasciculus of a young rabbit which was killed ten days after section of the spinal cord; this picture is taken two centimetres above the wound. *a*, *e*, remnants of the large axons which were destroyed early; *b*, thickenings of the medium-sized axons; *f*, unharmed axons; *d*, series of neuroglia cells occupying the place of the robust fibres that have disappeared.

The *most robust tubes*, with exceptions, degenerate very early (Fig. 197, *a*, *e*). It is not after seventy-three hours, in a few axons, as Jakob maintains, but after thirty hours that one sees in them the varicose state followed by extreme constriction of the intermediate bridges to the point of rupture. From the fourth to the eighth days nearly all the constricted segments have disappeared, and large balls remain (*c*), or granular grumes which are more or less stained by colloidal silver. After fourteen and twenty days there still persist some balls and conglomerates of dark grains, which disappear from the twenty-fifth or thirtieth day on. The remnants of the axon are destroyed, partly through phagocytosis of the proliferated neuroglia cells, partly through a slow liquefaction and granular disintegration. In place of the disintegrated tubes one finds columns of proliferated neuroglia cells, some of them with myelinic remnants—the *myeloclasts* and myelophages of Jakob.

As we show in Fig. 197, *d*, the regions that were occupied by those fibres which were destroyed earliest are marked by a series of granular remnants lying in the midst of masses of neuroglia.

The *medium-sized medullated* fibres are preserved better. After the first week (Fig. 197, *b*) they are in the beaded phase, but there is as yet no creation of balls nor ruptures. The interruptions begin from the fourteenth to eighteenth day on, after the intercalary bridges have undergone constriction and shown extreme paleness.

Finally, the *fine fibres* are preserved perfectly during eight or ten days (Fig. 197), showing no other modification than a granular appearance and a certain special paleness, by which they can be distinguished from normal fibres. Later, but at a much more advanced date than the other conductors, they take on a varicose aspect, being finally destroyed through liquefaction and phagocytosis.

Regeneration of the fibres of the white matter.—Pathologists consider it an unimpeachable dogma that there is no regeneration of the central paths, and therefore that there is no restoration of the normal physiology of the interrupted conductors in the spinal cord. A vast series of anatomico-pathological experiments in animals, and an enormous number of clinical cases that have been methodically followed by autopsy, serve as a foundation for this doctrine, which is universally accepted to-day. Nevertheless, some neurologists, setting on one side the incontestable disturbing fact that functional damage is irreparable, have made known histological observations of the partial regeneration of neurones and nerve fibres. Thus Masius, Vanlair, Müller, etc., noted some time ago in lower vertebrates such as reptiles and amphibians what appeared to be positive evidence of sprouting of the axons. Similar phenomena were described in the spinal cord of mammals by Bikeles, Finckler, Stroebe, Miyache, etc., who used the old methods of histological staining. The neurofibrillar methods have placed the problem on a precise basis, and brought the solution much nearer, thanks to the fact that they bring out with exquisite contrast and clearness the real end of the axons and any transformations that may occur. By means of them it has been demonstrated, beyond doubt, that there is a production of new fibres and clubs of growth in the spinal cord of tabetics (Nageotte and Marinesco) and of cones and ramified axons in the scar of spinal wounds of man and animals (Cajal, Marinesco, Lugaro, Bielschowsky, O. Rossi, G. Sala and Cortese, Dustin, Perrero, L. Forster, etc.). These investigations, while they have brought out unquestionable signs of repair, which are comparable in principle with those of the central stump of the nerves, have also confirmed the old concept of the essential impossibility of regeneration, showing that, after a more or less considerable period of progress, the restoration is paralyzed, giving place to a process of atrophy and definitive break-down of the nerve sprouts.

Without insisting on some historical phases of the question, we shall briefly set out here some of the progressive phenomena that have been observed in the white matter of the cord of animals after operation.

We may distinguish two phases in the process : the phenomena of creation and the acts of atrophy.

Phenomena of progression.—The generative acts occur only in a small number of fibres which are usually of moderate and small diameter. The immense majority of the conductors of the white matter, and especially those of large calibre, undergo degeneration and atrophy exclusively. The phases of destruction described in the preceding paragraphs refer especially to these. We may add that the sprouting of which we speak is more general and vigorous in young animals such as cats and dogs a few days old than in adult animals, and that it has some relation with the intensity of the lesions. Thus, in small spinal wounds with an exiguous neuroglial scar the neoformation is insignificant, even in young animals ; while in complete interruptions with a wide gap, into which penetrate first the exudates and later the connective tissue of the scar, the reparatory movement attains a great intensity. These latter are, of course, the cases chosen for the analysis of regeneration.

Initial phase, or formation of the cone of growth.—Let us place ourselves under the best conditions, and suppose that in a dog four to eight days old a complete interruption of the cord and its meninges has been effected, and that the animal was killed twenty-four or forty-eight hours after the operation. An examination of the edges of the wound shows already at that time, in the white matter, a great number of axons that end in more or less retracted balls, and a few terminal glomeruli (Fig. 198, *e, d*). All these axons are probably incapable of regeneration, and confine themselves to displaying the degenerative phases that were noted above. It is certain axons, few in number, ordinarily fine or of a medium calibre, free from buds, that initiate regeneration (Fig. 198, *a, b, c*). At first such conductors are characterized by their avidity for colloidal silver, by a considerable increase in diameter, and by the fact that they are clearly striated. Sometimes the neurofibrils are not only seen very plainly, but initiate the phase of ravelling of the nerves. This hypertrophic and striated portion is prolonged distally several hundredths of a millimetre, sometimes more than a tenth of a millimetre, gently merging into the normal segment. During this phase the end of the axon, which has the shape of a thin brush, progressively assumes a lanceolate aspect, developing a small cone of growth (Fig. 198, *a*). In this way the phase of divisory turgidity is prepared.

Appearance of the ramification.—During the first two days the axon becomes thicker, its neurofibrils become more numerous, but no ramifications are formed, nor does it perhaps grow in a longitudinal direction. It is only between the third and fourth days that

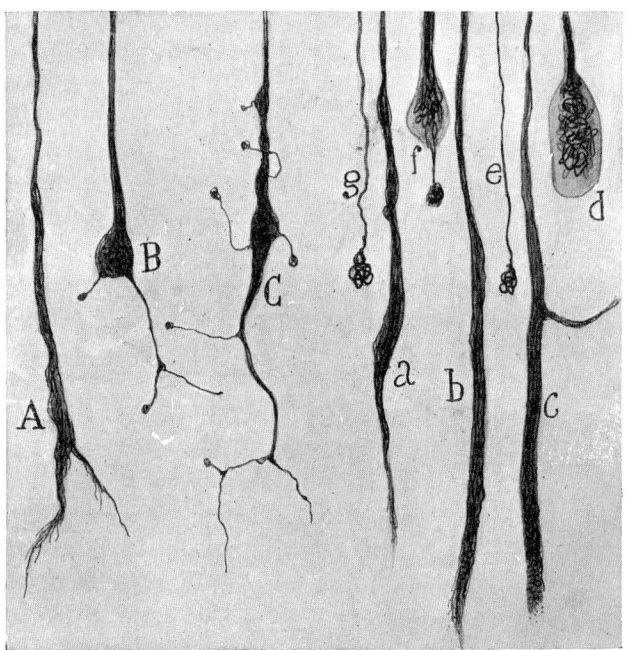

FIG. 198.—Phases of creation and ramification of the cone of growth in the fibres of the white matter. The fibres on the right of the figure are from the spinal cord of a cat which was killed twenty-four hours after the operation; those on the left (*A, B, C*) are from a cat which was killed four days after the operation.

one sees endeavours on the part of the cone of growth to bifurcate, this cone being now thicker and better shaped. (Fig. 198, *A*). One even sees the production of thin branches, which issue either from the vertex of the terminal thickening (Fig. 198, *C*) or from its sides, or else from the pre-terminal regions. As the sprouts grow the mass of the cone unfolds and disappears, passing to the projections, which have, at times, terminal rings or grumes.

It is only after six days that one observes rich and extensive ramifications, which invade the borders of the wound. The form, extent, and orientation of the arborization, as well as the thickness, number, and length of its branches vary remarkably for the various fibres of the same section. The principal types may be studied in Figs. 198, B, C, and 188, A, but especially in Fig. 199, where the branches are drawn on a large scale.

The most frequent disposition appears to us to be that of certain hypertrophic axons, which are clearly striated longitudinally ; at the edges of the necrotic region, or somewhat above it, these divide into two thick branches, set almost at right angles to one another and directed, at some distance apart, towards the scar. Each thick initial projection is apt to bifurcate in its turn and to give rise to an extensive descending ramification. At the level of the bifurcations one can see a certain chiasma or loose neurofibrillar latticework (Fig. 199, D, E). Often from each divisory branch there arise retrograde branches, sometimes of enormous length (Fig. 199, A, B). Ultimately, the finest terminal branchlets usually end in a pale point which is difficult to see, or in a ring, bud, or neurofibrillar grume of irregular configuration (Fig. 199, b). When collaterals arise from the main fibre itself, the sprouting occurs also at the level of a triangular dilatation.

Alongside of this type, which is probably the most abundant, one sees thick axons that are moderately ramified and have relatively short projections (Fig. 199, B, F). They perhaps are early phases of the preceding type. We are dealing here with thick fibres, more or less ravelled out, whose terminal cone breaks up into two or more irregular conic projections, while branchlets issue from the trunk (Fig. 199, A, F). The thickening from which the projections arise sometimes initiates perfectly those ramified cones of growth which we have described in embryos, and which have been well displayed by Harrison in his tissue cultures of nervous tissue. Sometimes the branches which arise either from the cone or from its preterminal portion, instead of being thin and long, are unusually short and thick, showing a loose, easily perceptible neurofibrillar net.

Another type, which is less common, is where the axon, ending in a large ball, emits above this a thick collateral which becomes progressively thicker and more ramified and is converted into a true continuation of the conductor-roots. This variant, already reproduced by Stroebe, (Fig. 199, G), reminds one of regeneration of the collateral type in interrupted nerves. It is very possible that, as occurs there, the terminal ball suffers atrophy of its pedicle, and finally becomes separated from the branch.

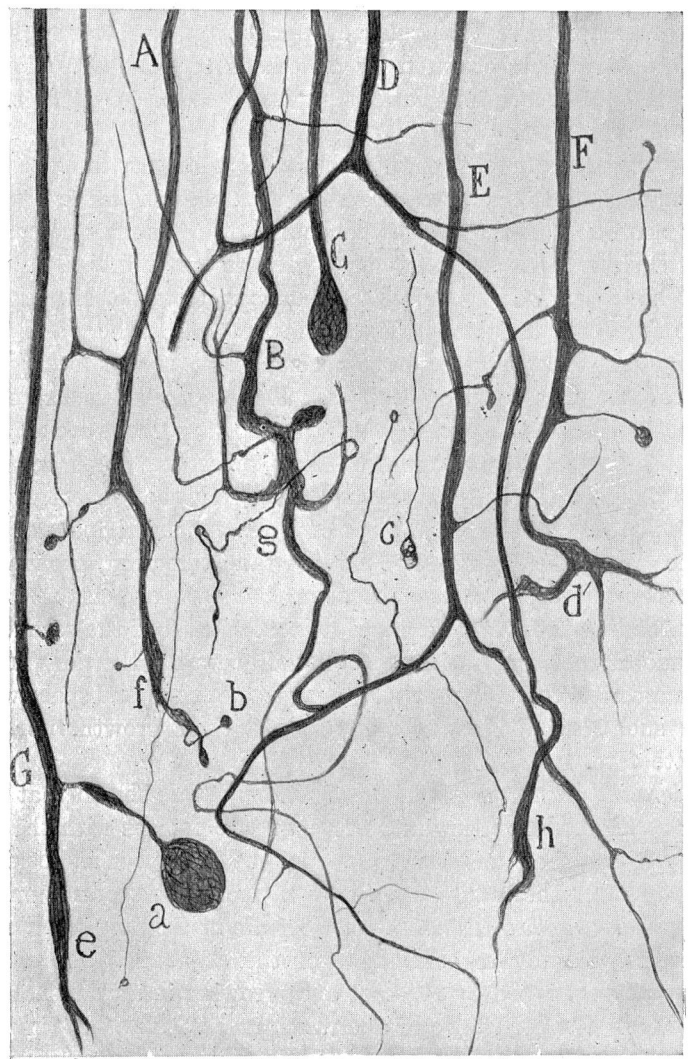

FIG. 199.—Various types of arborizations in the white matter of the spinal cord of a young cat which was killed six days after the operation. *A, F. G*, arborizations of small extent; *D, E*, axons that have ramified copiously and whose final projections approach the edges of the wound; *e, h*, cones of growth of thick branches; *a*, ball of detention; *c*, sterile axon ending in a retraction bud.

Still less frequent than the above are certain types of arborization which were pointed out by Sala and which we might name bulbous, because they remind one of the erect bulbs of the rootlets of certain plants. At times we have axons provided with successive thickenings, from which issue appendices ending in small balls or rings; at other times we have triangular or pyriform protuberances which emit fine branchlets crowned by delicate rings or buds. Finally, there exist many other variations, which one can see in Figs. 188, 198, and 190, *G, H*.

The ultimate branches of the arborizations in question, especially of those of the first type, grow from the third day on in the direction of the necrotic zone, where the concourse of fibres may be so great from the sixth to the ninth day as to give rise to an intricate plexus, which has been well described by Marinesco and Rossi. In this plexus numerous terminal balls and rings stand out here and there, showing that many sprouts have become paralyzed in their growth or have been detained by obstacles. These sprouts penetrate very rarely into the wound itself. When they do so, perhaps accidentally, they succumb, becoming converted into preserved fibres or undergoing autolysis. Neither do they usually invade the connective scar.

Finally, a considerable number of fibres which originate at some distance from the lesion, take a retrograde direction, growing between the tubes of the cordons along the path of least resistance and extending in favourable cases up to the level of the second and third motor root, or turning off obliquely towards the grey matter. It is impossible to state precisely the limits of time and space within which such deviated conductors suspend their growth, nor their ultimate fate.

Migrating branches.—Our investigations [1] have shown that when the zone of formative turgidity of an axon coincides with the level of emergence of an anterior root, and the latter, as an accidental consequence of the traumatism, is in a phase of degeneration (formation of the *bands of Büngner*, etc.), certain bifurcating or collateral branches, belonging to conductors of the adjacent white matter, are strongly attracted by the root and, growing in an unusual way, emerge from the cord to form aberrant nerves. At other times the sprouts or the entire axon cross the *pia mater* and circulate freely through the perispinal cicatricial connective tissue. We shall speak further of these interesting facts, whose theoretical value is very great, in another chapter.

[1] Cajal: " Algunos hechos favorables à la hipótesis neurotrópica," *Trab. del. Lab de Investig. biol.*, t. 8, fascs. 1 and 2, 1910.

The state of divisory turgidity and the creation of new fibres occur in all the fasciculi. Perhaps the posterior fasciculus which, as is well known, is largely in relation with the sensory roots, has more than any other the capacity to ramify and to create long sprouts. On the other hand, the collateral branches of the white and grey matter, as well as the original portions of the neuronal

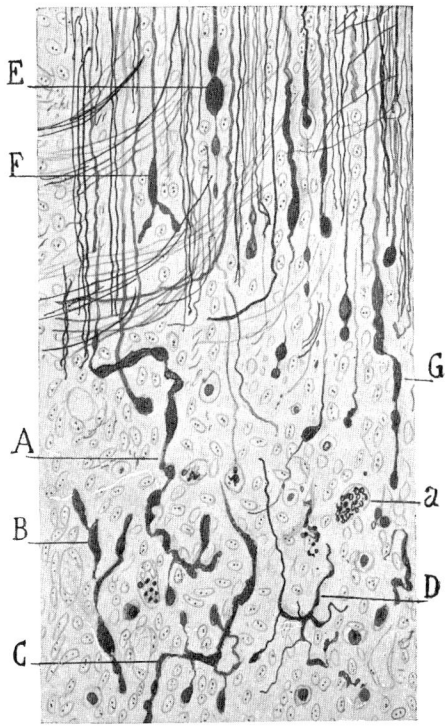

FIG. 200.—Neuroglial scar with an arborization which is in course of resorption. *A*, varicose arborization; *B, C, D*, pieces of the ramification which have become detached from the axon; *E, G*, retraction balls with remnants of the preterminal varicose state; *a*, granular body.

axon (course of the axon of the funicular nerve cells across the grey matter) form no portion, or at most a very small and scarcely perceptible part, of the newly-formed plexus at the edges of the wounds.

Progressive phenomena and atrophy of the regenerated fibres.—The neoformative action decreases or is arrested from the tenth to the fourteenth day. During the following days the newly-formed branches undergo a process of successive atrophy and resorption which entirely destroys the work of restoration of the white matter.

How this destruction is effected has not, as yet, been thoroughly elucidated. Our observations, however, furnish certain details which may help us somewhat to understand the process. As early as the twelfth day, and sometimes before, there is initiated in some branchlets or in the generating axon a certain state of tuberose hypertrophy, in which the fibres become retracted and transformed into a series of balls. Other branches become flexuose, as it were, knotty, and take the silver nitrate stain with great intensity. After thirty days all normal ramifications have disappeared from the edges of the wound and adjacent regions. In their place one sees accumulations of dead balls, and especially certain tuberose and winding pieces of mutilated arborizations which have severed their connection with their fibre of origin.

In Fig. 200 we show some of these atrophic and monstrous arborizations, in which series of balls and complicated paths are seen in abundance. Finally, after a month and a half or two months, all traces of the arborizations have disappeared. The edges of the wound, containing only a few free balls or remnants of balls, enclose a neuroglial scar and a few granular cells which are still swollen with lipoidal remnants. Thus, the regeneration of the white matter, so laboriously organized, ends in a complete break-down. We shall speak below of the hypotheses that have been put forward to account for this lamentable issue.

II

DEGENERATIVE ALTERATIONS OF THE GREY MATTER

Summary of the structure of the spinal neurones.—Necrotic and degenerative phenomena occurring in them—granular state, chromatolysis, neurofibrillar hypertrophy, hirudiform state, etc.—Perturbations of the endocellular Golgi apparatus.—Regenerative phenomena—regeneration of the dendrites and of the fibres of the grey substance.—Neuroglial and conjunctive scars.

Degenerative alterations of the grey matter.—The neurones adjacent to the wound become altered as a consequence of two perturbatory conditions : the physical action of the traumatism, such as pressure, commotion, lacerations, etc., and the pernicious influence of the inflammatory exudate. Naturally the changes brought about in the neurones are proportional to the extent of the wounds and the violence of the traumatism. Small and partial interruptions of the grey and white matter, made with a fine scalpel, have very little effect on the vitality of the neighbouring neurones, which, some days after the operation, appear almost entirely normal even up to the edge of the wound itself. In such cases, once cicatrization has set in, the grey matter appears interrupted by a thin scar of neuroglial tissue, as we show in Fig. 206. When, however, the cord is completely cut and the edges of the wound are inundated by blood and exudates, the neighbouring nervous elements undergo important modifications.

These modifications have been well studied, especially by Stroebe, Minor, Marinesco, Sala, Rossi, etc. Our investigations confirm nearly all the lesions that have been described, besides adding some others, thanks to the method of reduced silver nitrate. Before setting out these observations we may give a brief summary of the normal structure of the spinal neurones.

Normal cells of the grey matter.—Besides the neuroglial elements and a complicated plexus of nerve fibres, formed principally of the arborizations of the collaterals from the white matter, the grey

518 DEGENERATION AND REGENERATION OF THE NERVE CENTRES

matter encloses numerous multipolar neurones with long axons. These neurones may be grouped into two principal categories: *motor cells,* gigantic in size, whose dendrites, long and ramified, are distributed through the anterior horn, so that their robust axons cross the antero-lateral fasciculus to form the anterior or motor roots ; and *funicular cells,* present in both horns of the cord, medium-

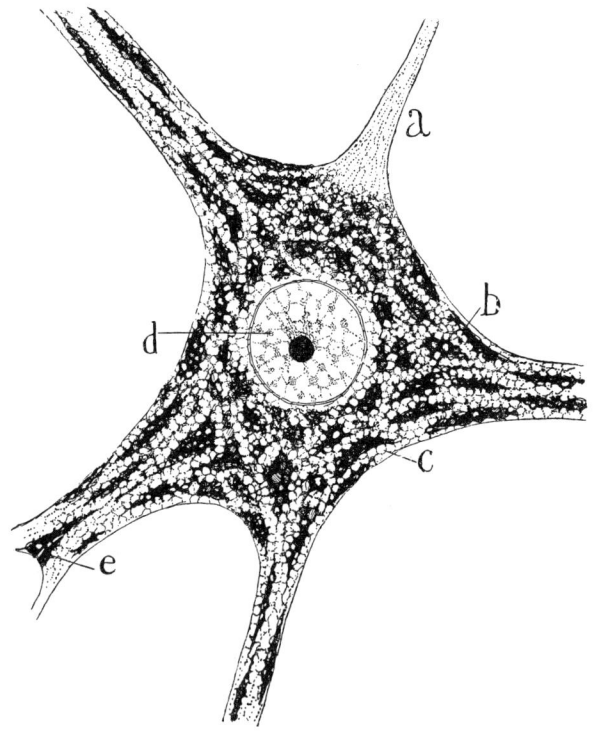

FIG. 201.—Motor cell of the spinal cord of a rabbit ; Thionin stain. *a*, axon ; *b*, chromatic grume ; *c*, spongioplasm ; *d*, nucleus ; *e*, bifurcation mass.

sized and even small, provided with dendrites which spread throughout the grey matter, and with an axon which is no finer than usual, and is directed towards the white matter, where it constitutes, sometimes through a simple flexion, sometimes through a bifurcation, a longitudinal conductor. Both the motor and the *funicular* cells possess a soma which is rich in protoplasm and in which, by employing various methods, one can see: a nucleus, carrying a thick nucleolus which is stained very deeply by colloidal silver, the *neurofibrillar reticulum*, fasciculated, condensed into a bundle at the level of the axon and expansions; the *reticular apparatus of Golgi*, composed of numerous trabeculae and widened areas (Fig. 204, *A*); and, finally, the *Nissl grumes*, which can be stained with the basic aniline dyes. As we show in Fig. 201, *b*, these grumes, which are elongated and fusiform at the level where the dendrites arise and in the protoplasmic cortex, become shorter and smaller in the central regions of the soma and neighbourhood of the nucleus. We may add

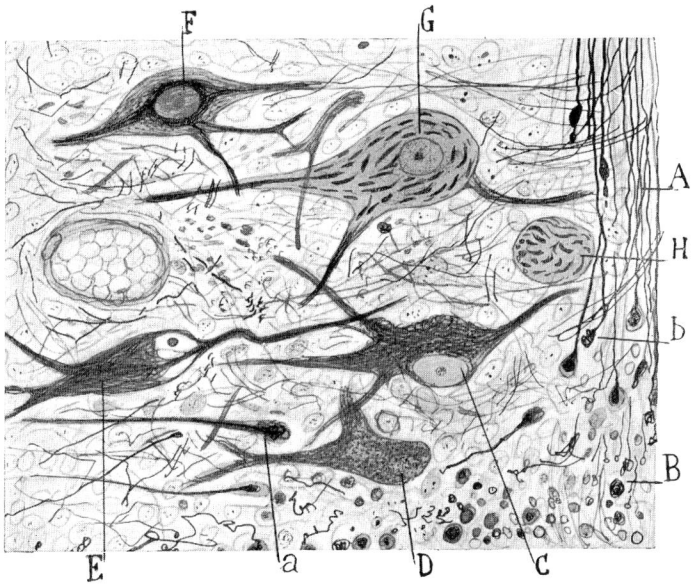

FIG. 202.—Nerve cells in the grey matter of the spinal cord of a young cat which was killed twenty-four hours after the operation. *A*, white matter; *B*, edges of the wound; *C*, neurone with granular neurofibrils; *D*, necrotic cell; *E*, pisciform type of neurone; *F*, hirudiform type; *G*, neurone with fusiform neurofibrils; *a*, interrupted collateral.

that, around the cell one can see by the method of silver nitrate the ends of the sensory collateral fibres, in the shape of a cone or a reticulated cup, intimately applied to the cellular membrane. After this brief summary, we may expose the principal alterations brought about by the traumatism.

(*a*) *Granular state of the cells.*—From the twelfth hour after the operation, and sometimes earlier, the border elements which have felt directly the physical action of the cutting instrument become necrobiosed, appearing either pale or deeply stained and in any case, showing a discontinuous reticulum which is granular and in a phase of disintegration (Fig. 202, C, D). In such cells the nuclei and the grumes of Nissl stain badly. One can often see in the protoplasm the rupture of expansions, the projection of the nucleus, etc. Everything leads one to believe that these neurones died quickly and that the disorders in the reticulum are autolytic in nature.

(b) *Type with neurofibrillar hypertrophy.*—In regions that are less close to the lesion one can discern, though only between twenty and forty-eight hours after the lesion, certain cells whose reticulum

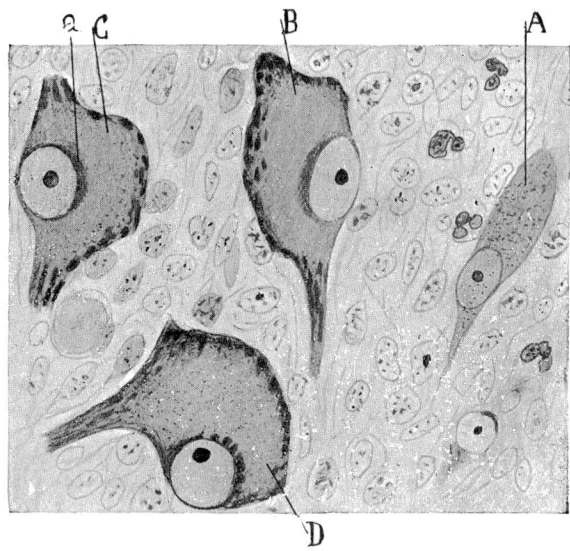

FIG. 203.—Motor cells in chromatolysis taken from the regions next to the spinal wound; cat killed three days after the lesion. A, granular cell with dissolution of the Nissl bodies; B, C, D, various types of cells in chromatolysis; a, perinuclear chromatic mass.

appears ramified and spattered with fusiform thickenings entirely comparable to those which have been described by ourselves, Garcia, and others in animals suffering from hydrophobia (Fig. 202, G, H). Such a lesion is a characteristic sign, as we shall show below, of contusions and commotions of the grey matter. Its production in this case shows that the cutting instrument caused a vigorous shaking in the regions next to the wound. In such cells the nucleus is often, but not always, central in position.

(c) *Hirudiform type of cells.*—In the same region where cells with hypertrophic neurofibrils are found one can also see neurones whose fibrillar skeleton is preserved only around the nucleus. From this perinuclear net fine tracts emerge, which penetrate into the dendrites, where the beginnings of a cortical hyalinization may also be observed (Fig. 202, *F*). All the gradations between this disposition and the normal are met with.

The last two lesions, which are compatible with the maintenance of the neuronal vitality, can be considered as primary reactions of cells which are perhaps destined to an ulterior destruction. They are no longer found, even thirty or forty-eight hours after the traumatism. The following well-known perturbations are prolonged

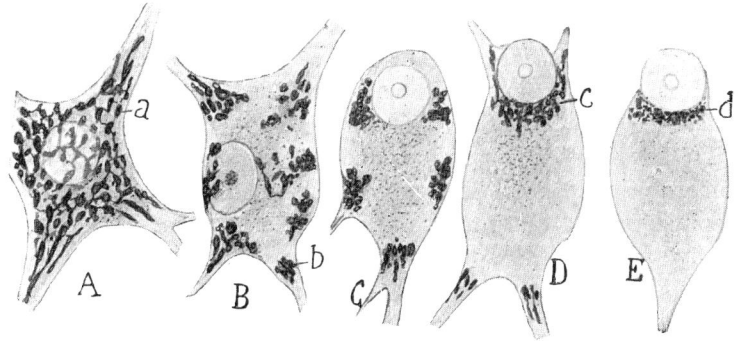

FIG. 204.—Various destructive phases of the reticular apparatus of Golgi of the motor neurones next to a spinal wound; young cat killed three days after the operation. *A*, normal reticulum; *B* and *C*, phase where the reticulum is broken up and marginal; *D* and *E*, remnants of the reticulum preserved beneath the nucleus.

during a much longer period, and they can be seen from the third or fourth day after the operation onwards.

(*d*) *Cells with chromatolytic alterations.*—These have been well described, especially by Minor. They appear at a certain distance, often as much as one millimetre or more from the wound. As we show in Figs. 203, *D*, and 205, *D*, we are dealing here with neurones in which all the characteristic signs of Nissl's chromatolysis are present. The protoplasm appears swollen and almost spherical through absorption of liquid. The chromatic grumes, dissolved or much reduced in the central protoplasmic regions, subsist beneath the membrane and at the issue of the expansions. Finally, the nucleus, tangential in position, and very prominent, seems about to tear through the membrane. This organ is frequently dislocated in an axial direction and placed at the origin of an anterior or posterior dendrite. This dislocation, occurring preferably in the fusiform elements of medium and small size, lends to the soma a strange appearance, which, because of its general resemblance to a fish, we have named *pisciform metamorphosis* (Figs. 202, *E*, and 205, *D*). Finally, between this organ and the somatic centre a more or less homogeneous chromatolytic zone is apt to appear (Fig. 203, *a*). Such is the aspect of chromatolysis in the preparations stained with the basic aniline dyes. In those stained with reduced silver nitrate one naturally does not see the basophilic grumes. But one observes the neurofibrils which, at the level of the central protoplasmic region, lose the characteristic fasciculated disposition and take on the form of a diffuse net, with very narrow and barely perceptible meshes. Often the neurofibrils are invisible as a consequence of the lack of avidity of the soma for colloidal silver. The soma then has a finely granular aspect, except in the periphery and expansions, where the characteristic fibrillation is maintained (Fig. 205, *C, D*).

The transformations of the endocellular apparatus of Golgi in the chromatolytic elements are curious. Impregnation of the edges of the spinal wound of a young dog, killed three days after the operation, by the method of urano-formol reveals, among other lesions, the following :

At first the reticulum is broken up and distributed into isolated groups, which remind one of those depicted by Marcora [1] in the cells of origin of the hypoglossus nerve after extirpation (Fig. 204, *B*). Later the central portion of the reticulum is destroyed, and thin marginal conglomerates are produced beneath the membrane, at the point of issue of the dendrites, and around the nucleus, whose dislocation has begun or is very much advanced (Fig. 204, *C*). When this nuclear eccentricity reaches its maximum the tangential lobules or colonies of the net become pulverized, and there remains only a characteristic subnuclear plaque, formed by the junction of small grumes or clubs (*D* and *E*). Finally the juxta-nuclear plaque becomes pulverized and destroyed, and the protoplasm, much swollen, merely shows fine granules here and there, presumably remnants of the reticular apparatus, imitating the state of resolution and disintegration which has been well described by J. R. Fañanás [2] in the giant

[1] Marcora : *Bolettino della Soc. med. chir. di Pavia*, No. 2, 1908.

[2] J. R. Fañanás : " Alteraciones del aparato reticular de Golgi en las células gigantes y otros elementos del tubérculo," *Trab. del Lab. de Invest. biol.*, t. 11, 1913.

cells of the tubercle, and by F. Tello [1] in aseptic granulomas brought about through the injection of *kieselgur*.

(*e*) *Cells that have gone back to the phase of neuroblasts.*—We must interpret in this way the modification undergone by certain fusiform funicular elements, of medium or small size, which take on the shape of a pear, similar to that of the neuroblasts, and which have preserved, among the expansions, only the axon, which is directed, as usual, towards the contiguous white matter. This return to the primitive type has been seen by us only in the spinal cord of dogs and cats recently born or a few days old. Ordinarily such elements show the nucleus dislocated towards the wide part of the soma and have a neurofibrillar reticulum which is weakly stained by colloidal silver. They are nearly always situated near the wound.

(*f*) *Cells with ansiform dispositions.*—These were noted by Sala and Cortese [2] and by O. Rossi.[3] They are very much like those described above in spinal ganglia. From the edges of the soma, and preferably near the nucleus, there arise threads or cordons in the shape of bundles, or again complex reticulations which form an eminence on the cellular contour (Fig. 205, *D*). Usually, although not always, this alteration is associated with the chromatolytic state, that is, it occurs in cells which, since they have a tangential and prominent nucleus, are considered to be undergoing chromatolysis.

(*g*) *Vacuolated cells.*—These have been well described by various authors. They are generally found during the fifth, sixth, and following days after the operation. Few in number, and often solitary, they abide near the lesion. They are easily recognized by their spheroidal form, the peripheral position of the nucleus and, especially, by the presence of a large vacuole full of plasma. The dendrites and the axon, dislocated through dilatation of the soma, maintain their characteristic striation (Fig. 207, *e*). When the vacuoles are small and numerous the neuronal configuration changes but little, and there may even be no nuclear dislocation.

---

[1] F. Tello : *Bol. Socied. españ. de Biol.*, Febr. 1913, and *Trab. del Lab. de Investig. biol.*, t. 11, 1913.

[2] G. Sala e Cortese : *Sui fatti che si svolgono nel midollo spinale in seguito allo strappo delle radici*, Pavia, 1909.

[3] O. Rossi : *Loc. cit.* and " Sopra alcune apparenze morfologiche che si riscontrano nelle cellule nervose del midollo," etc., *Riv. di. pat. nerv. e mentale*, . 14, fasc. 8, 1909.

Regeneration of the grey matter.—We have spoken of the active though frustrated regenerative phenomena that occur in the white matter. One may now ask: since traumatic stimuli are very efficacious in producing neurocladism in the neurones of the ganglia, are they not also capable of producing new dendrites, that is, true

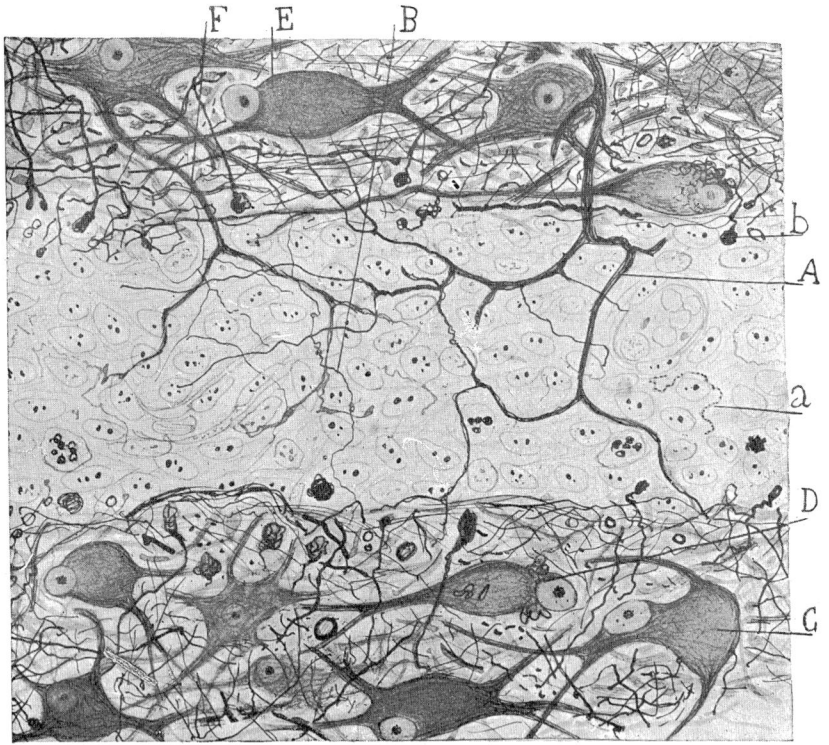

FIG. 205.—Wound of the grey matter of the spinal cord of a young dog which became cicatrized after nine days by means of a neuroglial lamina. *A*, newly-formed protoplasmic expansion ; *B*, perforating nerve fibre ; *D*, neurone with bulging nucleus and hypertrophic neurofibrillar bundles ; *C*, neurone in which the nucleus has migrated towards a dendrite.

paraphytes, in the cells of the wounded spinal cord ? Some authors, especially O. Rossi, reply in the affirmative, since they think they have recognized in some neurones the neoformation of true short, ramified dendrites, which are intensely stained by colloidal silver.

For our part, we must confess that in the case of spinal wounds that were not complicated by contusions or tearings we have not been able to recognize with certainty, in the nerve cells next to the wound, new dendritic appendices. Neither have we been able, at early periods, to see the sprouting of nervous collaterals in that path which all functional funicular expansions follow across the

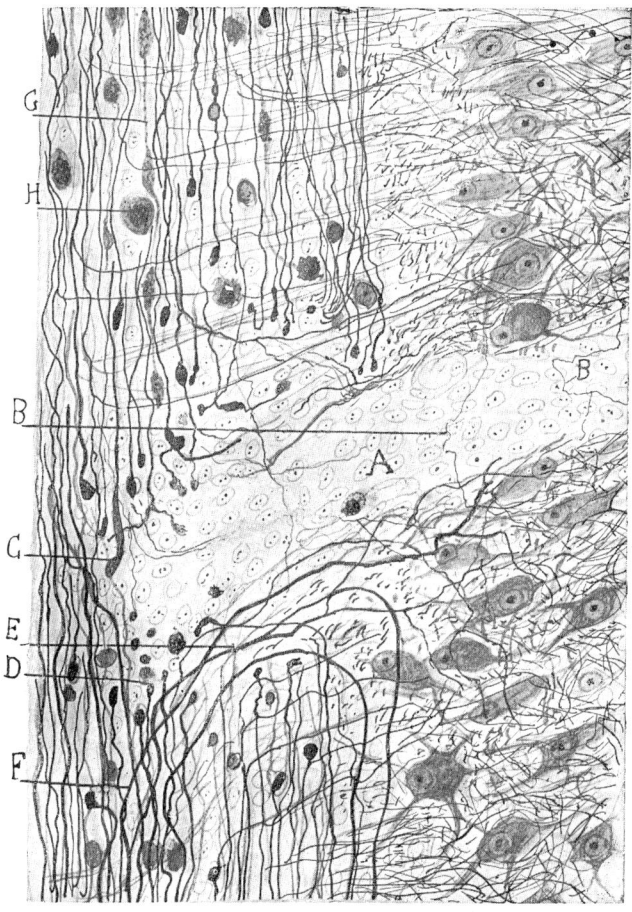

FIG. 206.—Partial section of the spinal cord of a young dog which was killed six days after the lesion. *A*, neuroglial scar; *B*, perforating fibres; *C*, *D*, balls at the end of the tubes of the interrupted white matter; *G*, beaded fibres; *F*, collaterals of motor roots.

grey matter. We do not deny, however, the possibility of these neoformations. In fact we [1] have ourselves seen them in two cases.

[1] Cajal: "Sobre algunos fenómenos de regeneración parcial de la substancia gris," *Trab. del Lab. de Invest. biol.*, t. 8, 1910.

In the case of small wounds in which a scar had been quickly formed by means of neuroglial tissue, we once saw at a late stage, in neurones next to the interruption of the cord which were little affected by the traumatism, certain thick appendices which might very well have been new formations. And in precocious phases we have seen also dendritic sproutings and even new dendrites ; but this was only after contusions, triturations, and rough shakings of the grey matter.

We shall give details of the second case below, when we study the effects of trituration and commotion of the spinal cord. We give here some instructive figures of the first case (Fig. 205, A). One may note how the scar, fifteen days after the lesion, is crossed through and through by certain robust dendrites, ramified like a stag's horns, which strongly attract colloidal silver, as though they were but recently differentiated, and lose themselves in the opposite lip of the wound.

Analogous communicating bridges, which, however, are not ramified, are formed also at times in the small neuroglial scars of the grey matter by means of nervous collaterals (Figs. 205 and 206, B). In this case the fibres were very thin, they took a flexuose course across the scar, they were moderately ramified, and they finally established communications between peripheral nerve plexuses. Such perforating fibrils might result from late sprouting of collateral arborizations of the grey matter. Nevertheless we do not affirm this interpretation with full certainty. There is a cause of error, of which we were not aware at the time when we made known this fact, in the possible persistence in the wounds, and tardily in the scars, of fine *preserved fibres*, which are more or less resistant to autolysis.

Without insisting for the moment on the problem of the regeneration of the grey matter, concerning which we shall have something to say in another place, it seems probable that in some rare circumstances, and in a precarious and pitiful manner, the dendrites are capable of sprouting, and perhaps of restoring, when the neuroglial scars are very short, the interrupted connections between the mutilated neurone and certain systems of collaterals which have ramified in neighbouring regions. In any case, this restoration for short distances is always very incomplete in comparison with the loss involved in the definitive interruption of long nervous paths which have disappeared through degeneration.

Late examination of the grey matter.—One and a half to three months after the lesion the edges of the wound show only normal neurones. The granular nerve cells, as well as those with an altered reticulum, have entirely disappeared, while those in which chromatolysis had occurred seem to have recovered their normal state. Among them one sees a very rich nerve plexus, organized in great part by terminal axons. A few balls undergoing hyalinization, and a few granular bodies containing lipoidal grumes, remind one of the disorders of the first few days.

Formation of the scar.—The authors who have studied the genesis of the cicatricial tissue of spinal wounds, agree, *mutatis mutandis* that, when the lesion is not very extensive the reunion of the edges of the nervous substance is effected by means of neuroglial tissue. If the interruption is total and very wide, involving important bloodvessels, ependyma, meninges, etc., two scars are formed. One of these is *internal* and covers directly the interrupted stumps of the nerve centre; it is composed of neuroglia. The other, *external*, is in the form of a sheath around the wound, into which it often penetrates in the form of a wedge. This latter scar is in continuity with the meninges, especially the *pia mater*; it is from their connective cells that it originates. The cells of the first scar are ectodermal in origin; those which produce the second belong to the mesoderm. The two scars are always separated by more or less well marked lines of demarcation. We may add that in all wide wounds which involve the ependyma there is produced in time, within the neuroglial scar and in continuity with its cavity, a more or less anfractuous cyst, at whose walls the mesodermal formation always stops.

Our studies confirm entirely this classic conception of the neuropathology of the spinal cord. In Fig. 207 we show the disposition of the scar of a complete spinal wound, in a rabbit killed a month and a half after the operation. One may note the characteristic ependymal cyst (A), invested with a row of epithelial cells which, as seen in the left side of the figure, border upon the over-abundant connective scar. It will be observed that the neuroglial scar, which is characterized by its small ovoid nuclei and delicate and almost invisible fibrillar tissue (H), limits itself to investing the spinal stumps, being in continuity with the scar of the old necrotic regions, in which there are now no nervous formations. The connective scar, on the other hand, recognizable through its fusiform cells and its collagenous bundles, appears clearly fused with the meninges (G).

It is difficult to trace a precise demarcation between the two scars. Nevertheless, apart from the structural details that we have noted, there is a characteristic that distinguishes them with sufficient contrast, although without sharply defined frontiers. The meso-

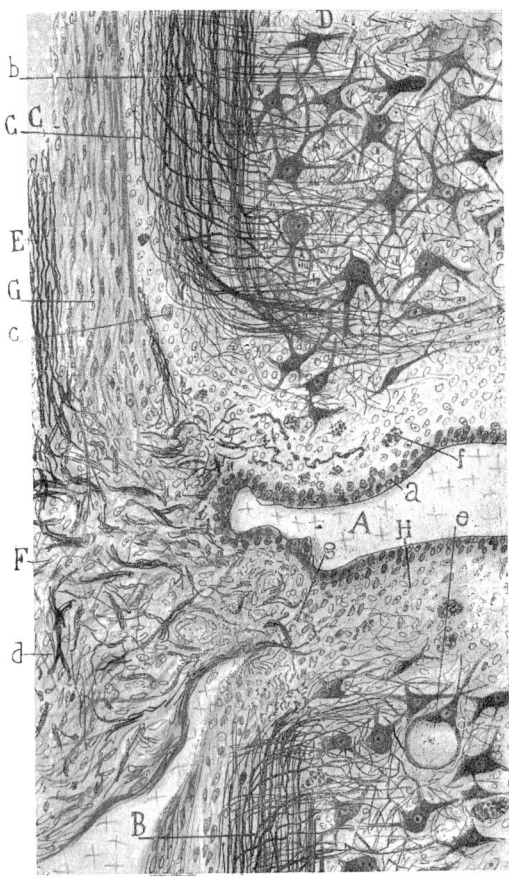

FIG. 207.—Complete section of the cord of a rabbit, one and a half months after the operation. A, cyst invested by ependyma; B, C, arciform fibres in both stumps of the white matter of the wound (anterior tract); D, cells of the grey matter; E, piece of an anterior root; F, connective scar invaded by sprouts arising from this anterior root; c, free balls; f, granular bodies.

dermal scar almost always contains nerve bundles that proceed from the sprouting of the roots (E) (in Fig. 207, the continuity of this cicatricial neurone with an anterior root is evident); while the neuroglia contains no large fibres, and encloses only a few mutilated axons, which are granular and monstrous, and remnants of balls.

Interesting details with regard to the capacity of the aforementioned connective scar, as well as of radicular sprouts, to penetrate into the wound, can be seen also in Fig. 208, *B*. One may note how, coincidentally with the invasion of mesodermal cells, various fibres

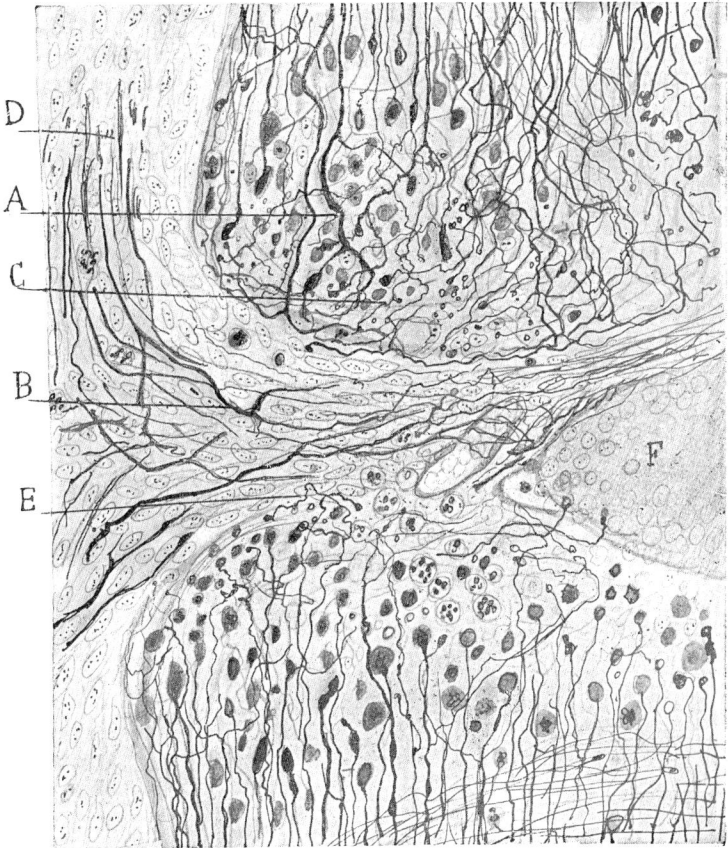

FIG. 208.—Edges of a total spinal wound of a young dog which was killed six days after the operation. *A*, *C*, tract fibres ramified in the necrotic portion of the white matter; *B*, newly-formed fibres arriving from a regenerated anterior root; *D*, remnants of this anterior root; *E*, cyst in process of formation. Note next to the wound the multitude of fine fibres which end in rings or little balls, while the large ones end in buds or voluminous clubs.

of the contiguous white matter are in the phase of excitatory division (*A*) and display a tendency to migrate from the spinal region.

We shall not dwell upon the structure of the scar, a matter which has been well elucidated by the descriptions of the neuropathologists. We shall limit ourselves to calling attention to a fact that has some interest in connection with the doctrine of regeneration of the central paths. There exists a certain parallelism between the regenerative reaction of the white matter and the presence and proximity of the cicatricial mesodermal formations. Very small punctures and fine wounds which are partial, in the grey and white matter, and which are rapidly cicatrized by means of neuroglial tissue (Fig. 206, *A*) hardly ever bring about sprouting of axons ; even the traumatic degenerative process is precarious and of slight extent. On the contrary, complete interruptions of the cord, with an irruption of exudates and an abundant proliferation of the mesodermal cells of the *dura* and the *pia mater*, followed by an application and even a partial penetration of the connective scar into the lips of the white matter (Fig. 208, *B*), are apt to bring about, not only the appearance of numerous nerve sprouts, but even their active migration from the region of the cord into the connective scar, and in certain cases even into the nerve roots. It thus seems natural to conjecture that the regenerative process of the white matter, which is so remarkably faint and sluggish under ordinary conditions, *can be powerfully stimulated by means of active or trophic substances liberated by the mesodermic scar and diffused in the spinal wounds and their edges.*

III

DEGENERATION AND REGENERATION OF THE SPINAL ROOTS

Degeneration and regeneration of the anterior roots.—Their invasion by endogenous and exogenous sprouts.—Degeneration and regeneration of the posterior roots.—Invasion of the connective scar by funicular sprouts.—Partial restoration of the posterior fasciculus.

It is not our intention to speak here of the effects of the section or extirpation of the anterior and posterior roots. Excellent descriptions of the traumatic degeneration and regeneration of spinal roots interrupted at a greater or less distance from the spinal cord have been given, not only by the older authors (Stroebe, Bethe, etc.), but also by Lugaro, Marinesco, O. Rossi, Sala and Cortese, and Dustin. We also have said something of these processes, which do not differ essentially from those occurring in cut peripheral nerves, in Chapter XIV of Section I of this work.

In order to avoid repetitions, we shall deal in this treatise exclusively with the degeneration and regeneration of the intraspinal segment of the roots, which are usually brought about by myelitis or grave alterations of the spinal cord.

Degeneration and intraspinal sprouting of the anterior roots through the influence of the traumatic inflammation of the neighbouring white matter.—The proximity of the inflammatory process often finds a repercussion in the intraspinal paths of the motor roots. It is peculiar that this repercussion is seen, not only in roots that are near, but also in others that are at a considerable distance from the lesion.

When the root is contiguous to the wound nearly all the axons succumb in a few hours, undergoing autolysis. After two days many necrotic segments have already been absorbed. Sometimes relics of axonic grumes persist, among which a few independent spheres stand out. If the roots are at a distance from the wound the degeneration is partial, becoming progressively limited to a smaller number of conductors. Among the degenerated tubes in the central stump, one distinguishes two kinds : axons that have lost their extramedullar portion and terminate in spheres or large buds lying not far from the surface of the organ (Fig. 209, *E*) ; and axons that remain normal, but show a thick and fusiform thickening under the basal membrane. It appears as though the formative turgidity that has developed in the intraspinal segment of the neuroplasm and neurofibrils has found a grave obstacle to its cellulifugal diffusion in the narrow opening of the basal membrane (Fig. 209). In certain cases, nevertheless, this thickening is smaller and is found outside the basal membrane.

Regenerative phenomena.—From the fourth day after the lesion onwards, evident signs of sprouting already appear in the central stump of degenerated and interrupted axons. As occurs in the white matter, a lanceolate end is found, from which projections develop. Ulteriorly these projections, which are short and terminate in a point, are transformed into branches of varied length.

In Fig. 209 we show diverse types of ramification in the spinal cord of a dog a few days old. The sprouts that are shown are in two stages : those which have been able to cross the basal membrane and to penetrate into the roots, and those which still remain within the white matter.

The radicular fibres of the first category, besides bifurcating or ramifying in a complicated way within the root, send out in the neighbourhood of the basal membrane a few collaterals, which are often recurrent and penetrate into the grey matter. To this type of branches belong, in particular, certain robust descending or ascending fibres, which are ramified and prolonged (Fig. 209, *A*), sometimes up to the lips of the scar.

The radicular fibres of the second category are more numerous than the above, and at first sight are distinguished from normal fibres by their greater thickness and avidity for colloidal silver. These conductors travel along the first portion of their path in union with the normal spinal root fibres. Arrived at the superficial region of the anterior bundle, they are resolved into an intracordonal terminal arborization, in which there is an abundance of branches following a retrograde or tangential course. It is curious to note that the majority of such branches take a chance direction, availing themselves of the interstices which they find in their path. Not a few of them encounter the basal membrane and become retrograde after having emitted a few branches (Fig. 209, *E*).

In general, the obstacle formed by the basal membrane, when it is not rapidly crossed, brings about axonic ramifications and agglomerations, as we show in Fig. 209, *F*. Finally, some branches which are more fortunate succeed in perforating the basal membrane and invading the corresponding anterior root, where they occasionally

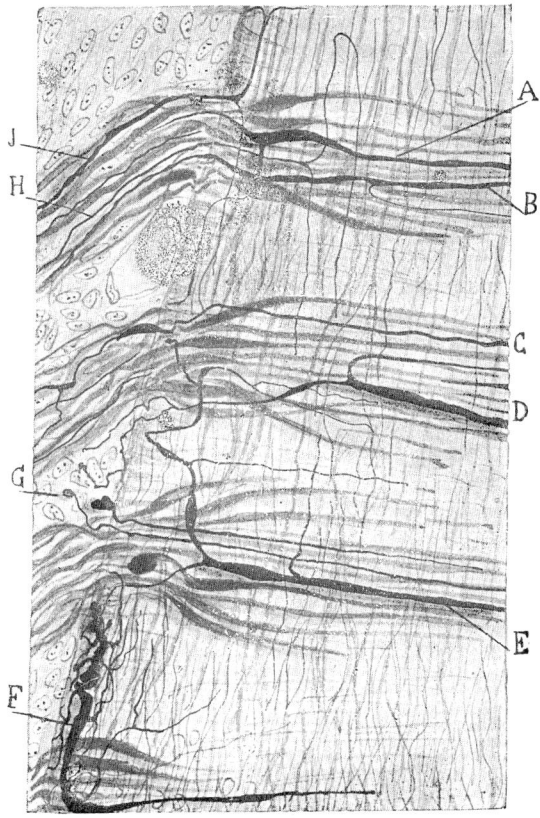

FIG. 209.—Phenomena of regeneration in anterior roots close to spinal wounds; dog, a few days old. *A, B, C, D, E,* regenerating fibres; *F,* fibre agglomerated under the *pia mater*; *G,* fibres lost in the connective tissue; *H,* fibres arriving from the exterior.

ramify (*C*). It sometimes occurs that it is not the continuation of the axon, but one or two of its collaterals that effect their escape from the anterior bundle, falling right into the root, or again wandering in the perispinal connective tissue (*G*). In these preparations moreover, one does not see those interesting spools and agglomerations of collaterals and terminal branches which G. Sala and Cortese have observed in the intraspinal course of extirpated motor roots.

From the present observations one may especially deduce two things. First the fact that, without any traumatism of the roots, and at a distance from a small and aseptic lesion of the spinal cord, certain motor axons degenerate nearly to the point of origin and prepare themselves for the restoration of the lost portion. And second, the singular lack of orientation of the axon and its branches while they grow within the cord and have not crossed the basal membrane.

One may add to the above two kinds of regenerative fibres those axons which are entire but stimulated, and from whose intraspinal course there arise recurrent collaterals. In Fig. 210 we show some conductors of this kind. One may note that only a few branches issue from the intraspinal portion of the roots (a), usually not far from the basal membrane. Once formed, several of these collaterals travel forwards among the motor axons, to lose themselves in the anterior bundle, while others turn in a longitudinal direction, abandoning the radicular current to proceed towards the wound.

Retrograde collaterals of the extraspinal path of the roots.—On various occasions we have alluded to the singular fact that a large number of the sprouts formed in the central stump of nerves that are cut at a great distance from the spinal cord become retrograde. They travel beneath the sheaths of Schwann or through the nervous interstices. Once they have reached the cord, instead of stopping their growth, they resolutely invade the white matter, within which they bifurcate repeatedly.[1]

A similar phenomenon occurs when, instead of sectioning the nerves or cutting and compressing the anterior roots, one allows these to degenerate through the diffusion of the neighbouring traumatic myelitis. Such is the case shown in Fig. 211, where the exudates of the immediate inflammatory centre, or perhaps also some slight compression of the root caused by the scalpel, has occasioned in many axons the formation of retrograde collaterals. One may note how, once the branches have reached the cord, they grow actively along the path of least resistance, dividing repeatedly. Although there is a great variety of orientations, two great currents predominate, doubtless a result of mechanical accommodation to

---

[1] Cajal: " Algunas observaciones favorables á la hipótesis neurotrópica," *Trab. del Lab. de Invest. biol.*, t. 8, 1910.
See also: *Trab. del Lab. de Invest. biol.*, t. 11, 1913.

the region traversed, or else through stereotropism : the *radial current*, which follows the path of the roots to lose itself, either near the grey matter or in different regions of the spinal cortex (Fig. 211, *H, I*) ; and the *longitudinal current*, formed by those branches which, when they encounter an obstacle, fold back so as to enter the contiguous anterior bundle and associate themselves with the longitudinal conductors (Fig. 211, *C, F, G*). There are some bifurcated sprouts in which each branch chooses a different path, one growing

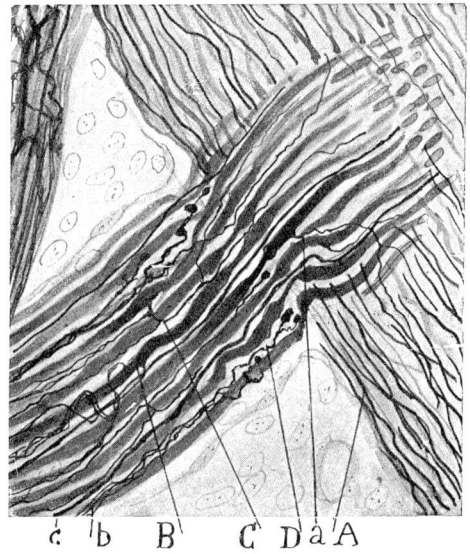

FIG. 210.—Details of a radicular bundle which is in full production of direct and retrograde branches ; young cat, killed four days after ligation of the anterior roots. *A*, antero-lateral bundle of the cord ; *B, C*, axons of the anterior root in full divisory activity ; *D*, branches detained at the edge of the cord ; *a*, small branch arising within the antero-lateral bundle ; *c*, fine fibre penetrating into the cord.

longitudinally, the other radially. Neither is it rare to find newly-formed fibres which are divided into an ascending and a descending branch, incorporated in the tubes of the anterior bundle. When the collaterals emanate from the axon in regions close to the basal membrane they are apt to arise, in accordance with the law enunciated in another chapter, from the frontier thickenings of the first node of the radicular tube (Fig. 211, *E*). Finally, since the basal membrane forms a narrowed point in the path of the root, and therefore an obstacle before which the wandering exogenous fibres waver, one not infrequently observes clubs and buds detained outside it (Fig. 210, *D*).

536 DEGENERATION AND REGENERATION OF THE NERVE CENTRES

Invasion of the anterior roots by newly-formed bundle fibres.—We have stated above that, among the new conductors of the roots next to the spinal wound, some are also met with that are of a centrifugal

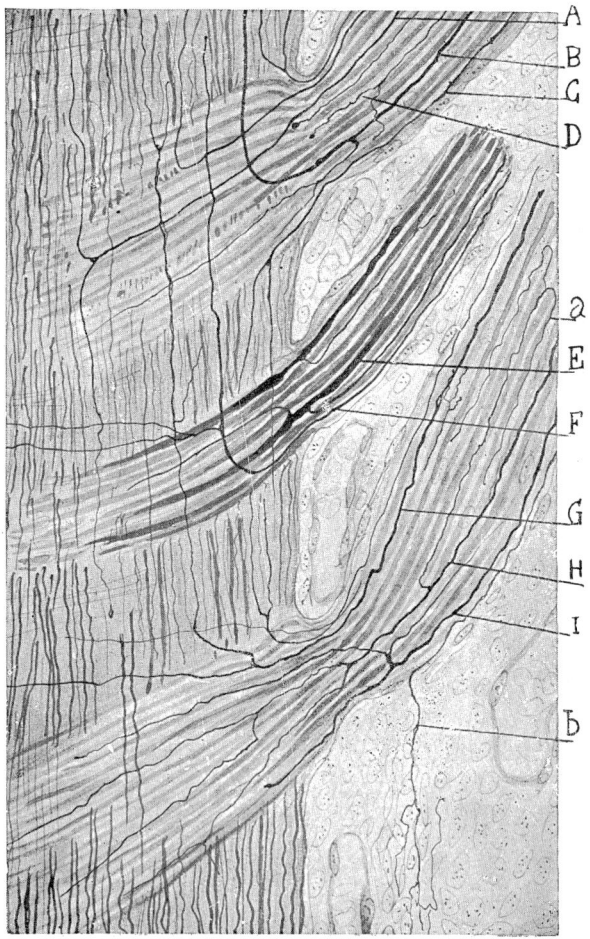

FIG. 211.—Invasion of the spinal cord by motor collaterals which are retrograde and originate from the extraspinal path of the anterior roots; cat a few days old, killed four days after section of the spinal cord. *A, B, C, D,* recurrent motor branches which invade the spinal cord; *E,* almost normal axon from which issue two collaterals; *F,* branch which becomes longitudinal; *H, I,* invading branches which are divided repeatedly; *a,* arciform branchlets; *b,* nerve branch which crosses the membrane of the root and becomes distributed in the perispinal connective tissue. (This semi-schematic figure depicts the fibres found in three successive sections.)

character and originate from the fibres of the anterior bundle. Such strange migrating sprouts are the more abundant the nearer the root is to the wound, provided always that the degenerated roots have been largely replaced by *bands of Büngner*. This phenomenon, which begins from the fourth to the fifth day, culminates during the seventh and eighth. The principal forms may be seen in Fig. 212.

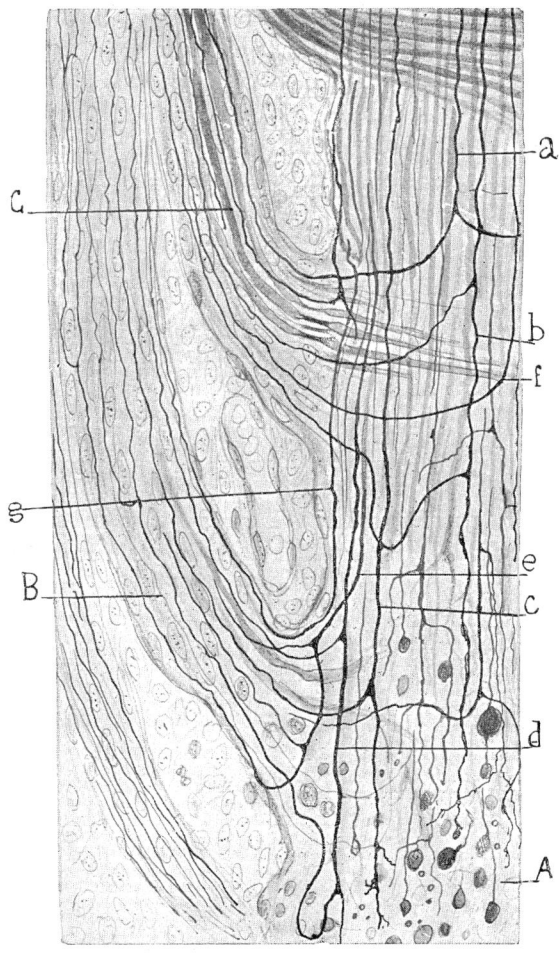

FIG. 212.—Longitudinal section of the antero-lateral bundle of a cat a few days old, in which the spinal cord was sectioned in the lumbar region. *A*, edge of the wound of the antero-lateral bundle; *B, C*, degenerated anterior roots which are invaded by newly-formed fascicular branches; *a, b*, funicular fibres which send out branches to the motor roots; *e*, axon which sends out three branches to a root; *g*, migrant non-ramified axon; *d*, axon which gives out a retrograde branch, etc. (In this figure are combined the fibres of three successive sections.)

The most common case is that shown in Fig. 212, *c*. A robust funicular fibre, which is in the state of divisory excitation, arrives in front of the motor root and then bifurcates; one branch, frequently thinner, continues its original course up to the point where it reaches the edges of the spinal wound or its neighbourhood, where it ramifies ; the other, directed outwards, traces a curve whose concavity faces towards the cells of origin, and unhesitatingly enters into the anterior root, within which it follows a lengthy course.

Another common case, although less frequent than the last, is that shown in Fig. 212, b, d. Instead of a bifurcation the funicular axon sends two robust branches to the root, generally with a considerable interval between them ; while the continuation of the stem pursues its downward course towards the wound, often ending at a short distance in a terminal cone or ball. Finally, at times, the last migrating collateral adopts a retrograde direction (d).

Another interesting example is that of the fibres from the bundles that migrate integrally through the motor root (Fig. 212, g, f), where they sometimes bifurcate or ramify in a complicated way (e). Cases of this kind are also shown in Fig. 213, D.

If one follows these migrating branches along the root, one sees that they are interstitial, that they bifurcate from time to time, and that they end in cones, fine grumes, or rings. Their growth in the new region must be very rapid, since five days after the operation they have already advanced nearly a millimetre in the root.

It would be very interesting and significant, from a theoretical standpoint, to determine the fate of these strange deviated conductors. It is to be supposed that once the first week is passed and when the spinal neoformations have begun to wilt or break down, they atrophy and disappear. It would also be of great doctrinal value to determine whether such axons, introduced into the motor root, become covered with embryonic cells of Schwann (cells of the endoneurium), behaving, even though for only a short time, like motor conductors. Our investigations are not sufficient to give a categorical answer to these questions. The field is still open for fresh research.

Degenerated motor roots which are assailed by wandering sensory sprouts.—We have already spoken of this interesting phenomenon at p. 318 of Section I of this work, when we were assembling the facts that support the theory of neurotropism. Here we shall limit ourselves to reproducing Fig. 130 (213). Further, in this case, the wandering sprouts assail the motor root through its proximal stump, which is degenerated and disintegrated as a consequence of the propagation of the traumatic myelitis. When, however, one multiplies the operations of section of the cord and anterior roots, one not infrequently sees wandering sensory sprouts that also innervate the roots through their distal stump (in cases of section or contusion somewhat removed from the cord), and therefore travel centripetally.

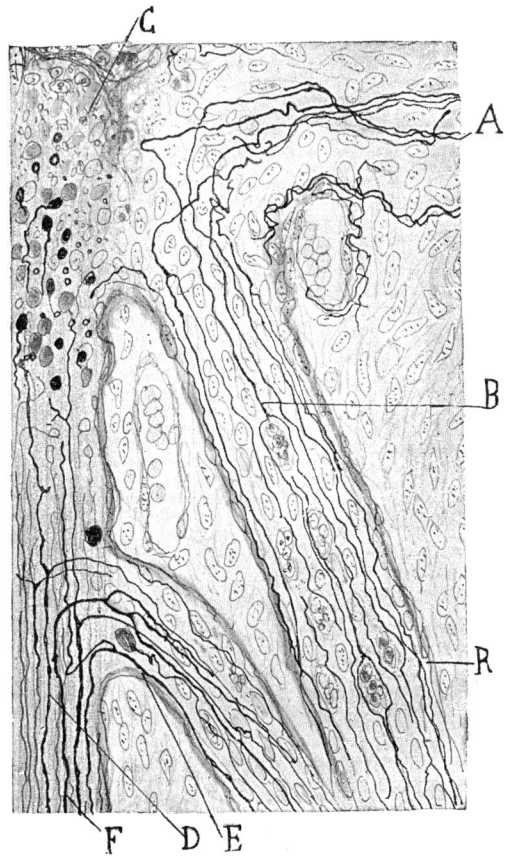

FIG. 213.—Longitudinal section of the anterior roots of a cat whose spinal cord was wounded. *A*, sensory fibres of the scar which are invading a degenerated anterior root; *B*, invading fibres which are ramifying at the level of a fatty accumulation; *C*, necrosed portion of the anterior bundle in the vicinity of the wound; *D, E*, bundle fibres penetrating in a radicular motor fascicle.

Moreover, among the retrograde fibres described in the preceding pages, and especially at pp. 322 and 323 of Section I, motor and sensory conductors are shown indifferently.

An important conclusion follows from the preceding observations: that the degenerating radicular tubes—formation of ellipsoids, proliferation of cells of Schwann, etc.—elaborate some non-specific trophic principle which is rapidly diffused, on one side towards the cord, and on the other towards the scar. This principle would act as an exciting and attracting agent to the wandering sprouts, no matter what the physiological category or derivation of the latter. In favourable cases such a catalytic agent might awaken the divisory amoeboidism of the axons in the white matter and bring about in them extraordinary phenomena of growth and orientation. The catalytic agents given out by the roots would exert a much more energetic trophic influence than those elaborated by the scar.

Degeneration and regeneration of the posterior roots.—Stroebe, among the older, and Lugaro [1] among the more modern histologists, have produced striking proof of the regenerative capacity of the posterior root—the portion between the ganglion and the cord. Lugaro has devoted a conscientious and penetrating study to this question, in connection with the pretended autogenous regeneration and the problem of neurotropism. Later, we ourselves, Marinesco, Sala, O. Rossi, Dustin, etc., have confirmed the most essential points in Lugaro's descriptions. Concerning this point we need only remember at present that a nerve root cut near the cord and in continuity with the ganglion, which is its trophic centre, behaves in degeneration and regeneration exactly like the central stump of a peripheral nerve. And when, as often occurs with the sensory roots, one likewise interrupts the spinal cord partially or totally, a good many of the sprouts that are formed invade the connective scar surrounding the spinal lesion, approaching very close to the neuroglial scar, where the newly-formed fibres of the white matter also at times collect.

The richness in sensory sprouts of the mesodermal scar juxtaposed to the spinal cord has more than once led to the supposition that the fibres of the bundles emerge freely from the region of the bundle to invade the connective formations of meningeal origin. This may occur, as we shall point out below, but only under very special conditions which are difficult to reproduce.

In the present treatise we shall set out certain data concerning these two points : degeneration and regeneration of the sensory

---

[1] Lugaro : " Sul Neurotropismo e sul Trapianti dei Nervi," *Riv. di Pat. nerv. e ment.*, vol. 11, fasc. 7, 1906.

See also : " Rigenerazione delle radici posteriori," *Ibid.*, vol. 11, 1906.

" Sulle presunte rigenerazione autogena delle radici posteriori," *Ibid.*, vol. 11, fasc. 8, 1906.

root through disorganization or serious inflammation of the spinal cord; and partial regeneration of the posterior bundle, following its traumatic degeneration and the sprouting of the roots.

Degeneration and regeneration of the posterior roots through destruction of the spinal cord, or grave disorganization of the grey and white matter.—The suppression of the spinal cord, in order to study the behaviour of the sensory roots, is accomplished by the method of d'Abundo,[1] that is, by separating, in recently-born animals, a more or less lengthy piece of this centre and respecting as much as possible the subdural path of the roots. But it is far simpler and more efficacious to cause, by contusions and lacerations, an extensive traumatic myelitis, which is likely to cause necrobiosis of a large part of the posterior bundle, as well as of the grey matter.

We may cite a few cases of this type, carefully analyzed by ourselves and published in a special work[2] in which we criticized the doctrines of d'Abundo and Dustin concerning the predestination of the form of the axonic divisions.

In one of these we were dealing with a cat ten days old, whose spinal cord was almost completely sectioned in the lumbar region, with aseptic precautions. The animal was killed five days after the operation. The wound was converted into an enormous longitudinal cyst of somewhat crooked form. On the ventral side this hollow was surrounded by a fairly thick mantle of the antero-lateral bundle, which thinned out progressively on the lateral sides. Behind, the cavity opened full into the subdural space. Various sensory root fascicles which had been attacked by the inflammation, and perhaps also by the cutting instrument, were interrupted and in full traumatic degeneration—moniliform state, retraction balls, formation of empty sheaths of the bands of Büngner, myelin ovoids, etc. As was natural in a peripheral stump, the new fibres found in it came from the central stump, having crossed the scar.

In Fig. 214, C, D, we show the path of these newly-formed fibres.

[1] D'Abundo: "Di nuovo sul potere rigenerativo del prolongamento midolare dei gangli intervertebrali nei primi tempi della vita extrauterina," *Riv. ital. di Neuropat. Psichiatria e Elettroter.*, vol. 2, fasc. 7, 1909.

Ibid.: "Dottrina metamerica e rigenerazione consecutiva allo strappo contemporaneo di molteplici gangli intervertebrali," etc. *Riv. ital. di Neuropat.*, etc. vol. 1, fasc. 8, 1909.

Ibid.: *Arch. italiennes de Biol.*, vol. 50, fasc. 2, 1909.

[2] Cajal: "Observaciones sobre la regeneración de la porción intramedular de las raíces sensitivas," *Trab. del. Lab de Investig. biol.*, t. 8, fasc. 4, 1910.

One may note that they come from a nerve bundle of the scar, across which they travel alongside of a spinal cyst. When one followed this small bundle in a series of sections one saw that it arose from the central stump—that portion of the root which was united to the ganglion—of a degenerated posterior root.

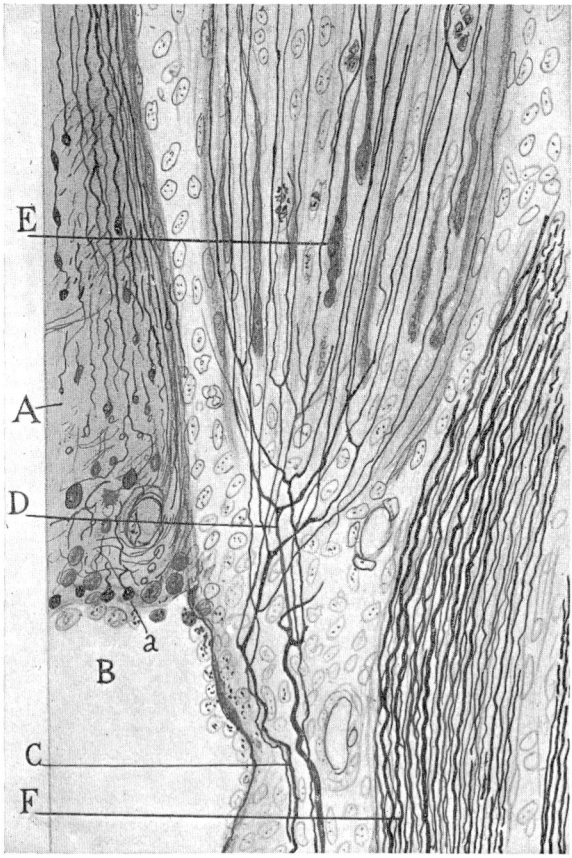

FIG. 214.—Synchronous section of the spinal cord and of a posterior root in a young cat which was killed five days after the operation. *A*, posterior bundle of the cord; *B*, cyst formed in the wound; *C*, nerve fibres of the scar which have penetrated into a central stump of a cut posterior root; *D*, branches produced at the edges of the root; *F*, normal sensory root.

It is interesting to note that these sprouts, solicited at once by numerous degenerating sensory tubes (of the peripheral stump united to the cord), break up successively into many branchlets, all of them ascendant and penetrating into the old sheaths of Schwann (Fig. 214, *D*).

THE SPINAL ROOTS 543

It is important to find out how such invading fibres terminate on coming near to the cord. As we show in Fig. 215, *C*, *D*, the majority of these conductors, when they approach the posterior bundle, lose their orientation, rapidly turn back, and form long

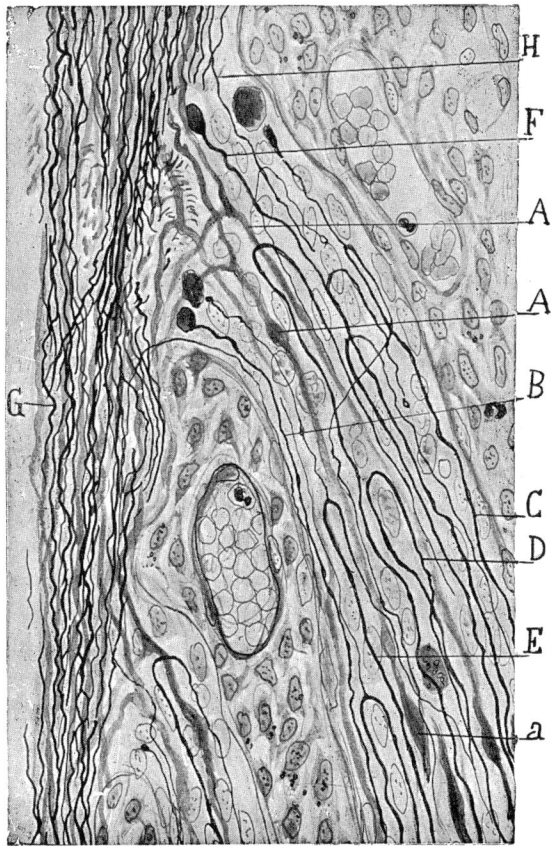

FIG. 215.—Portion united to the cord of a posterior root which has been sectioned within the ganglion; cat a few days old, killed five days after the operation. *A*, old fibres of the posterior root; *B*, *F*, new branches terminating, next to the posterior bundle, in a bud of growth; *C*, *D*, retrograde branches; *E*, retrograde fibre which emits a fine collateral directed towards the cord : *H*, fibril which penetrates into the cord.

retrograde branches. From the arch thus formed there issues at times a fine collateral, which terminates near the cord in a fine spherule or free bud.

A few conductors reach the posterior bundle, where they appear to be detained, showing a large terminal club of disproportionate size (Fig. 215, B, F). Finally, an occasional fine fibril crosses the spinal frontier, going right into the posterior bundle, in whose fibrillar complexus it loses itself in an unknown way (H).

In the preceding case, the interruption of the sensory roots is effected at a certain distance from the cord. But in the same animal in which the preceding observations were made, roots could also be seen that were not cut, but were disorganized by the traumatic inflammation in the very place where they entered the degenerated posterior bundle. In such roots the stump that is in continuity with the cord has completely disappeared. There remains the central stump which is very close, cut at the level of the cord and in a phase of divisory excitation. (See Fig. 216.)

The ends of these stimulated fibres are very varied in their appearance. They appear as though floating on the embryonic tissue above the pia (Fig. 216, B, C). Some are of an unusual thickness, are capriciously curved, and terminate in a kind of truncated cone which gives to the whole the appearance of a leech. Others, also voluminous and, as it were, ravelled out, are in full divisory excitation, showing short, divergent ramifications which have no tendency to grow towards the cord (Fig. 216, F). Finally, a great number of root fibres, after having sent some weak collateral towards the cord, give rise to robust retrograde branches which appear to flee from the inflamed zone towards the ganglion. The abundance of arciform fibres is as great as in the preceding case. There are some axons that give rise to two or more recurrent branches (E). Such branches may even ramify on their retrograde path, travelling for long distances. The majority lie between the tubes of Schwann, right in the intrafascicular connective tissue.

In the examples that we have cited the regeneration of the posterior bundle breaks down. This may result from the fact that the cord is gravely disorganized. One may suppose that the sensory sprouts which have come in by way of the root lack the natural *terrain* in which they find the normal stimulants of their nutrition and orientation. When, however, as we show in Fig. 217, E, the superior bundle persists in large part, the newly-formed fibres have also to cross great obstacles. The break-down, in this case, is almost as complete. One may note how the majority of growing axons are detained outside the basal membrane, forming large buds of various forms. Sometimes one sees enormous agglomerations of arrested balls which are crowded on the basal membrane, either because they cannot pass through its substance or because of inflammatory disorganization of the pre-established paths. An occasional fibre succeeds in laboriously penetrating the basal membrane and the mass of the posterior bundle; it is nearly always an appendix that has branched from the arrested bud.

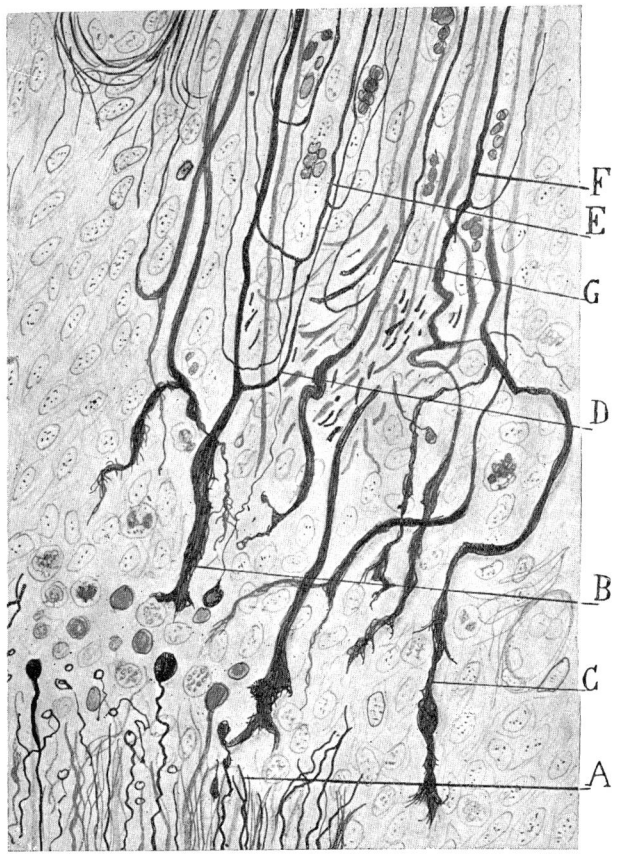

FIG. 216.—Juxtaspinal portion of a sensory root which is intact, but whose entrance into the posterior bundle was intercepted by destruction of the white matter. *A*, remnants of the posterior bundle; *B*, large roots ending in hirudiform stumps; *B*, *C*, other ramified axons; *E*, *F*, axons which give out retrograde fibres.

All these attempts at innervation of the posterior bundle are precarious; they give one the impression that the sensory axons possess a potential, but not an actual, regenerative capacity. We do not know whether such attempts would eventually meet with better success. At any rate, the short time between the operation

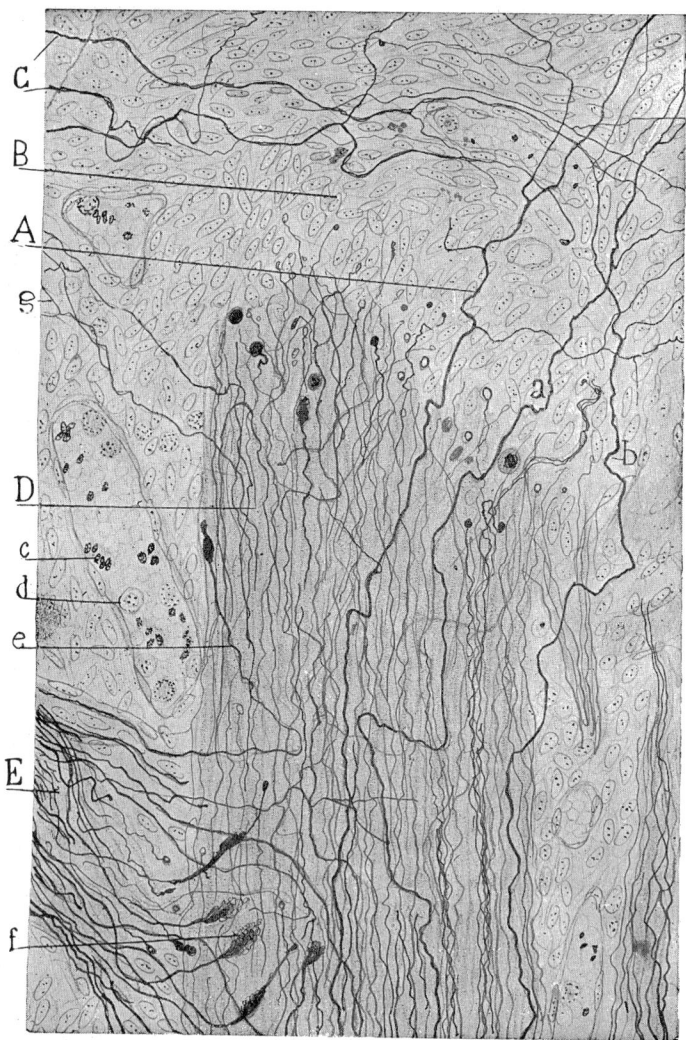

FIG. 217.—Longitudinal and tangential section of the posterior bundle of a dog a few days old. *A*, fibres of the posterior bundle in divisory excitation ; *B*, wound of the posterior cordon, filled up by the scar ; *C*, nerve fibres coming from a sensory radicular branch which are penetrating into the scar ; *D*, posterior bundle ; *E*, regenerated posterior root ; *a, b*, other large fibres, also ramified in the scar ; *c*, elements in a blood-vessel ; *f*, terminal clubs of regenerated root fibres ; *g*, fine fibres of the posterior bundle that have migrated.

and the autopsy (five days) prevented us from finding out whether the sensory axon is able, notwithstanding the obstacles, to reestablish the final bifurcation and to elaborate, as d'Abundo claims

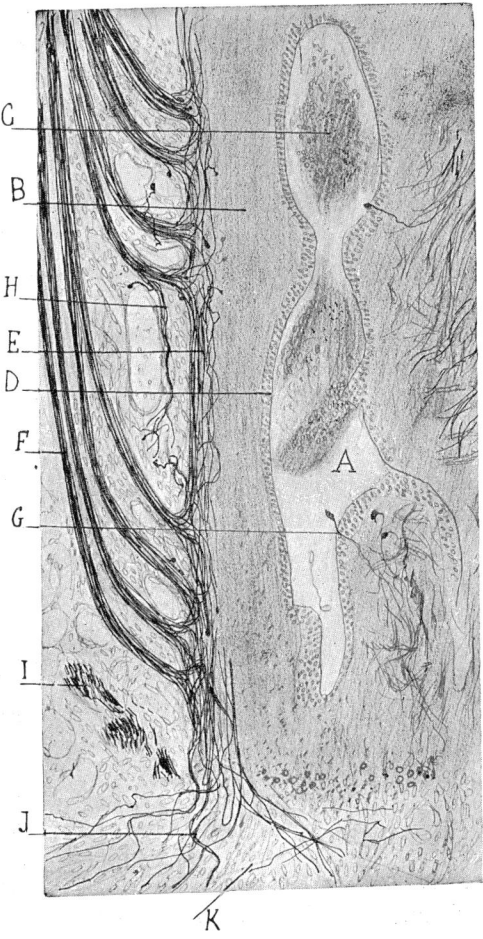

FIG. 218.—Longitudinal section of the posterior bundle; terminal portion of the cord of a ten-day old dog, killed six days after the operation. *A*, spinal cyst; *B*, degenerated posterior bundle; *D*, pericystic epithelium; *E*, regenerated portion of the posterior bundle; *F*, posterior roots; *I*, posterior root cut across; *J*, fibres of the posterior bundle ramified in the scar; *H*, bundle of deviated root fibres; *G*, clubs that have fallen into the spinal cyst; *K*, wound of the cord.

for the regenerated roots in the empty vertebral tube of the cord, a rough appearance of a posterior bundle.

The following observation appears to us decisive, as regards the essential capacity of the root fibres to penetrate into the cord and to restore the posterior bundle partially and in a somewhat incongruent manner. We shall describe it in some detail, as it certainly deserves.

Two causes of confusion ordinarily prevent one from ascertaining, in good preparations, whether the sprouts that have reached the edges of the cord have really penetrated into the posterior bundle and transformed themselves into its constituent fibres : (1) The relative persistence, days after the operation, in the roots, of many conductors as yet undegenerated (peripheral stumps) ; and (2) the formidable mass of axons of the posterior bundle among which the recently penetrated fibre may or does penetrate. It is thus necessary to operate in such a way that the posterior bundle is destroyed, but without harming more than the terminal portion of the roots. One must also be careful to preserve the basal membrane and the general morphology of the cord, so that the physical conditions of the region through which the nerve sprouts have to travel are not too much altered. In order to do this we have performed on dogs several spinal punctures—two or three in an interval of half a centimetre—by means of a fine scalpel. The result of this was that, six to eight days after the operation, the white and grey matter showed grave regressive processes, manifested through the almost complete unstainability of their nerve fibres, a partial disappearance of the neurones, and the formation of cysts full of exudates and leucocytes (Fig. 218, *A*, *B*, *C*).

The examination of cords from such animals, killed at successive periods after the operation—three, four, five, and six days—showed that the propagation of the phlogosis is capable of producing degeneration of the intraspinal portion of the roots (ascending and descending branches) and of a portion of its extra-central path, without the lesion appearing to have impaired the ganglia and the greater portion of the internal neuronal prolongation.

In the case shown in Fig. 218, coming from an animal that was killed six days after the traumatism, two of the punctures had completely interrupted the spinal axis. The intercalary space, which was about half a millimetre long, showed, as can be seen in Fig. 218, *A*, a large irregular longitudinal cyst, invested with an ependymal neoformation. The greater part of the posterior bundle appeared pale, because of the unstainability and perhaps the degeneration of its conductors ; towards the anterior bundle there were remnants of fibres which were regenerating, with ramifications and buds of growth. Some of them, in their impulsive movement, had fallen right in the cyst (Fig. 218 G). Finally, on the side of the roots one recognizes in the posterior bundle a thin fibrillar cortex, which is stained black, is bespattered with clubs, and stands out wonderfully well on the pale yellow background of the white matter (E). Into this cortex there penetrated, intermingled, the sprouts of various

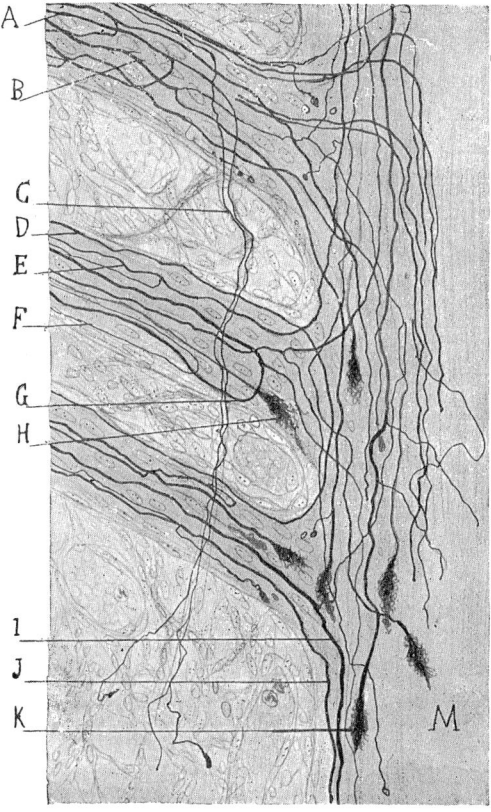

FIG. 219.—Piece of the posterior bundle and regenerated roots of a dog a few days old, whose terminal cord was lesioned in several places. A, sensory roots; C, deviated sensory fibres; D, penetrating fibre which abandons the cord; H, terminal club; E, fibre which puts out recurrent branches; G, arciform fibre which supplies a collateral to the cord; J, ascending fibre; K, intraspinal clubs from penetrating root fibres; M, spinal cord.

neighbouring sensory roots. We reproduce some details of this radicular neoformation in Figs. 219 and 220.

One notices at once that not all the regenerating root axons have reached the edge of the cord. Some of them, after having crossed the neurilemma, deviate and wander through the connective tissue, as we show in Figs. 219, *C*, and 220, *C*. Some of these deviated axons end in clubs which are variously placed in the arachnoid spaces, while others grow actively, giving rise to branches which travel blindly across the perispinal connective tissue. Nor is it rare to see various axons or branches of axons abandoning the root simultaneously and forming a nerve bundle which wanders along diverse paths in the subdural connective tissue (Fig. 218, *H*). Finally, some fibres abandon the root next to the cord, wandering in an aimless way round it and above the basal membrane (Fig. 220, *S*).

The fibres that are afferent to the cord may be grouped into three categories : those which are retrograde, those which are detained at the edge of the cord, and those which penetrate.

A. *Retrograde fibres.*—In preparations of the inflamed terminal cone of young dogs they are less numerous than in the central stump of cut roots, but they are never lacking. One meets with a variety of cases. Sometimes the axon becomes entirely retrograde, tracing an arc whose concavity is external ; more often a thick branch turns back, which may be considered as the continuation of the trunk (Fig. 219, *G*), while from the arc there arises a fine branch which is directed towards the cord. Sometimes, on the contrary, the recurrent fibre is the collateral of the trunk.

The arches of retrograde fibres are commonly situated near the cord ; nevertheless one finds them also at a certain distance, as we show in Fig. 220, *D*. Lastly, the retrograde fibre not infrequently emerges beneath the *pia mater*, right in the posterior bundle or on its edges.

B. *Detained fibres.*—These are constant, as we show in Fig. 219, *H*. They are recognized by the fact that they have a prolonged club which is more or less angular and provided with short expansions, paler than its centre (Fig. 220, *O*). Sometimes the club emits a fine appendix which penetrates into the cord (Fig. 220, *N*). Finally, the presence of clubs that are folded back, from whose base a penetrating branch issues (Fig. 220, *H*), shows that, when the obstacle cannot be crossed, the protoplasm of the club emits a compensatory appendix, capable of correcting the effects of detention.

C. *Penetrating branches.*—These behave in several ways. The most common varieties are the following :

(*a*) The majority of these conductors, once they have reached the external basal membrane of the cord, proceed, without any bifurcation, almost always in an ascending, less often in a descending, direction. The former represents the path most resembling that of the radicular trunk, owing to the general inclination upwards of the lumbo-sacral roots; it is thus the path of least resistance. Some

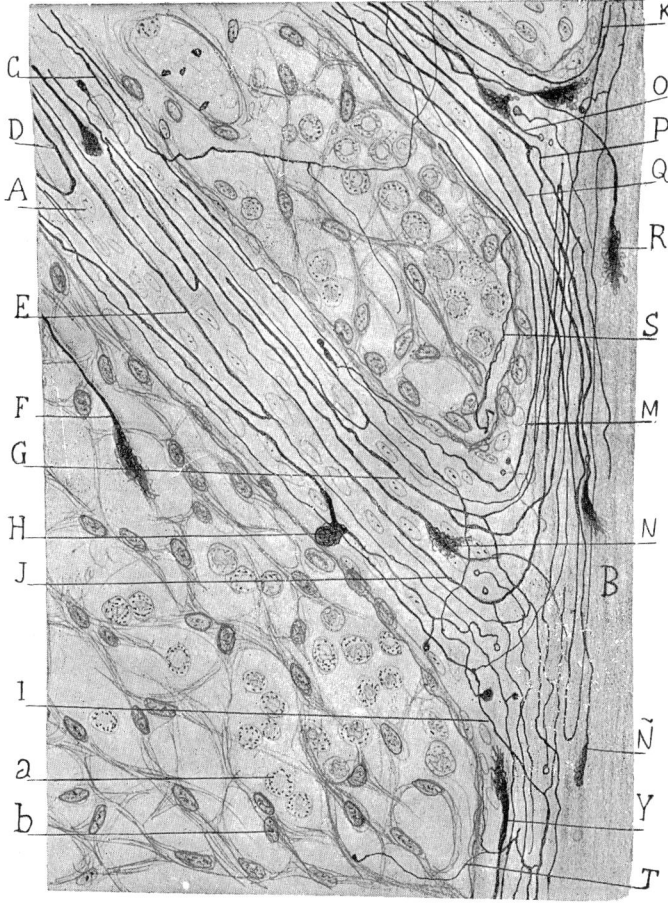

FIG. 220.—Same preparation as in the preceding figure. *A*, regenerated sensory root; *B*, spinal cord; *C*, deviated fibre; *D, E,* arciform fibres; *F*, deviated club; *G*, root fibre which ramifies in a complicated way on its entrance into the cord; *H, N, O*, clubs from which arise penetrating branches; *J*, bifurcated root fibre; *Q*, club with a short branch; *P*, root fibre divided into two ascending branches; *Ñ*, intraspinal clubs; *T*, fibre which emerges from the cord.

fibres, nevertheless, before becoming ascendant, travel horizontally and even downwards, tracing an arc whose concavity is superior (Fig. 219). In Fig. 220 we show a peculiar fibre which, after a long ascendant path, becomes suddenly descendant. In their extensive itinerary along the posterior bundle the root fibres occasionally send out collaterals, which often terminate at a short distance in the form of rings or small buds. Finally, the trunk, after a variable course, ends in a club or prolonged thickening, of diverse shapes, often covered with crests and villosities (Figs. 219, K, and 220, Ñ).

(b) A small number of root fibres, perhaps less than 6 per cent., bifurcate into an ascending and descending branch when they reach the posterior bundle (Fig. 220, J). Ordinarily the descending fibre is finer than the ascending, although there are exceptions. In a certain case (Fig. 220, I) the ascending fibre, of the same thickness as the descending one, has emitted two collaterals. We may also mention that, occasionally, the initial collateral becomes recurrent and goes back to the root.

(c) One also sometimes observes root fibres that are divided into two ascending or two descending branches (Fig. 220, P). Sometimes the root fibre breaks up into three or more longitudinal fibres, varying in their direction (Fig. 220, G).

(d) A singular fact, which shows that there is no neurotropical influence of the spinal tissue on the new root fibres, is that sensory fibres, arriving through a root, escape from the posterior bundle to become centrifugal, taking advantage of other roots, neighbouring or distant (Figs. 219, D, and 220, M). It is also curious to note, though this is a very rare feature, that an occasional sensory fibre, travelling along the bundles, sends out a collateral to lose itself right in the connective tissue, which it reaches after having crossed the basal membrane of the cord (Fig. 220, T).

In fine, the preceding observations prove that newly-formed root fibres which penetrate into the cord *proceed along the path of least resistance, blindly impelled by the incessant growth of the terminal point*. The details of the itinerary of the fibres within the posterior bundle do not suggest the idea of the presence within the cord of orienting and attracting substances, but neither do they imply, as Lugaro believed, the repulsive action of negative neurotropic stimuli.

As opposed to the views of d'Abundo and Dustin, the preceding facts show that the bifurcation of the sensory axons within the posterior bundle is not *a necessary result of internal tendencies of the nervous protoplasm*. This bifurcation is often lacking, and when it exists it can be simply explained, as in any growing peripheral axon, by the capacity that the newly-formed conductor possesses of breaking up into two or more branches in presence of a mechanical obstacle.

Ultimate fate of the regenerated root fibres.—Not having observed the injured animals beyond the sixth day after the operation, we do not know the ultimate fate of the newly-formed intraspinal root fibres. It is possible that, as occurs with interrupted axon bundles, these fibres degenerate and die, as the establishment of connections with the neurones of the bundles supposes the pre-existence of free paths as well as of orienting neurotropic substances. At any rate, within the six days following the operation the penetrating branches have developed to a great length, and show as yet no signs of degeneration. One often sees in the region of the posterior bundle clubs whose fibres may be followed longitudinally along the space covered by four root fascicles.

Capacity of the regenerated fibres of the posterior bundle to invade the embryonic connective tissue.—In a special work [1] and in various passages of this treatise we have called attention to the property possessed by young sensory and motor root fibres of growing and ramifying preferably in the embryonic connective tissue, as though they found in it some substance that stimulated their metabolism and growth. In the light of that fact one may ask whether the regenerated root fibres that have made their way into the posterior bundle have retained their appetite for young connective tissue. Has their passage through the spinal tissue modified their receptivity in respect of neurotropic stimuli ?

This theme has been the object, on our part, of numerous observations, with very significant results. Here are the most interesting :

(a) *Capacity for innervation shown by the regenerated intraspinal sensory fibres.*—Nothing is easier than to prove this curious property when, as occurred in the case shown in Fig. 218, *J*, the sensory fibres which have penetrated into the posterior bundle reach the cicatricial tissue of a spinal wound. When this scar lies near a regenerated root, one sees clearly that the sensory intraspinal fibres, ascendant or descendant, enter the embryonic connective tissue, thicken in its interior, ramifying repeatedly, and behaving generally like sensory branches that have developed from the end or along the path of a cut posterior root. Among the branches that are destined for the scar, some travel towards the interior, as shown in Fig. 218, others towards the exterior (*J*), reaching by divergent paths connective regions far removed from the spinal cord. Along its path each sensory axon emits numerous ramifications which appear

[1] *Loc. cit.* : *Trab. del Lab. de Invest. biol.*, t. 8, fascs. 1 and 2.

to be attracted by the colonies of embryonic connective tissue cells. We may add that some of the oldest intra-cicatricial branches appear at times bordered by elongated nuclei and fusiform cells, rudiments of the future lemnoblasts or cells of Schwann.

(b) *Capacity for innervation shown by the sensory fibres of the posterior cordon.*—The property of bundle fibres to ramify and invade the connective tissue of spinal scars was more or less clearly observed, according to the methods used, by various authors, such as Stroebe,[1] Cajal,[2] Marinesco,[3] Henneberg, O. Rossi, etc.[4] We believe, however, that we were the first [5] to demonstrate clearly and finally this phenomenon of cicatricial ramification and innervation, thanks to a method that reveals in an exquisite way the young non-medullated fibres and their divisions in the connective tissue and necrotic zone of the edges of the wound.

This migratory property of the bundle fibres had been noted by the above-mentioned authors and by ourselves, but always as exceptions and on a small scale. Our investigations, however, regarding the invasion of the posterior roots by extraneous fibres, and those concerning the regenerative capacity of the posterior bundle, show that this regenerative and migratory power may attain, in certain cases and under somewhat undetermined conditions, an extraordinary development, producing extraspinal arborizations of great abundance and extent. Figs. 217 and 221 show two typical examples of the regenerative capacity of the thick sensory fibres of the posterior bundle when these, abandoning the surrounding neuroglia, find their support right in the embryonic connective tissue.

Fig. 217 represents a sectioned spinal cord, together with several posterior roots. At the level of the wound one finds, as is well known, many bundle fibres that are moderately ramified, and many more

[1] Stroebe : *Loc. cit.*

[2] Cajal : " Notas preventivas sobre la regeneración y degeneración de las vias nerviosas centrales," *Trab. del Lab. de Invest. biol.*, t. 4, 1905-06-

[3] Marinesco : " Recherches sur la régénérescence de la moelle," *Nouvelle Iconographie de la Salpêtrière*, No. 5, 1906.

[4] O. Rossi : " Processi rigenerativi e degenerativi consequenti a ferite assetiche del sistema nervoso centrale," etc. *Riv. di patol. ner. e mentale*, year 13, fasc. 11, 1908.

Idem : " Nuove ricerche sui fenomeni di rigenerazione che si svolgono nel midollo spinale," *Riv. di patol. ner. e mentale*, vol. 15, fasc. 4, 1910.

[5] Cajal : " Regeneración intramedular de las raíces sensitivas," etc. *Trab. del Lab. de Invest. biol.*, t. 8, 1910.

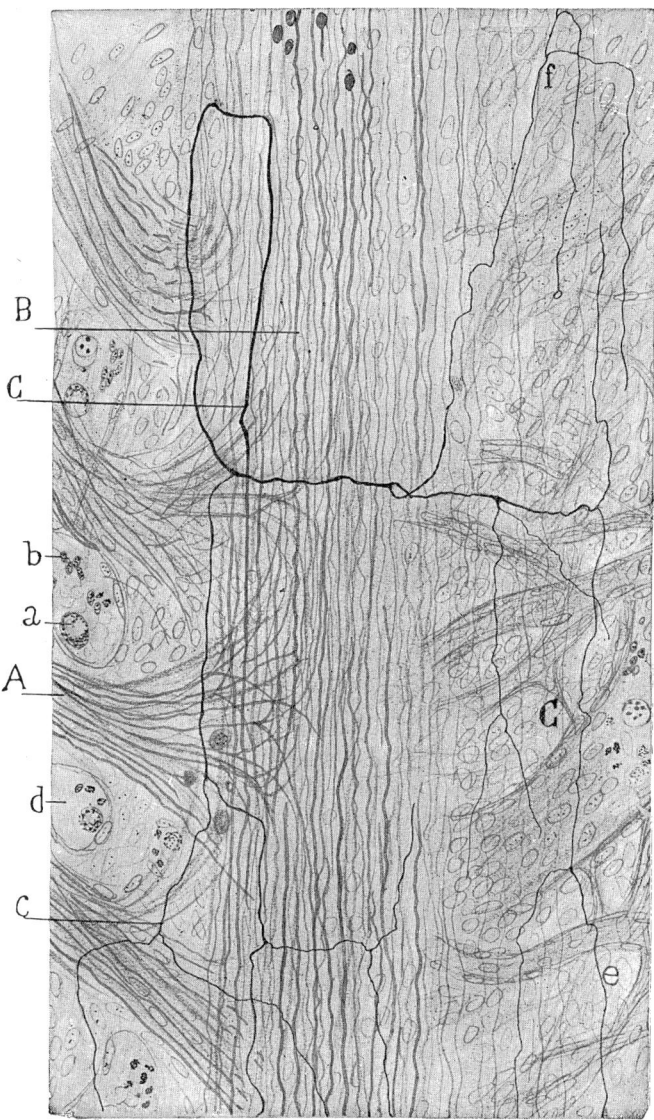

FIG. 221.—Tangential and longitudinal section of the posterior bundle near a spinal wound in a young dog. *A*, almost normal root fibres; *B*, posterior bundle; *C*, thick nerve fibre which, emerging from the posterior bundle, gives rise to an enormous terminal arborization; *c, e, f,* branches of this arborization *a*, leucocytes; *b*, elements in a blood-vessel.

conductors that end simply in retraction balls (Fig. 217, D). The majority of these fibres do not cross the spinal necrotic region. But next to these axons of short growth, tangential sections parallel to the posterior bundle show three or more vigorous bundle axons in full divisory excitation, and which have grown remarkably (Fig. 217, A). These robust fibres, in continuity with descendant branches of healthy roots, become progressively thicker before reaching the necrotic zone of the spinal wound, cross at various points the basal membrane, and, after reaching the connective tissue of the *pia mater*, invade the scar, forming finally an extensive arborization of ascendant and descendant extraspinal branches. The majority of these branches travel towards the scar, where they subdivide repeatedly, augmenting the number of the sensory axons distributed about it. Often the retrograde or ascendant branches travel on the *pia mater* for long distances. In Fig. 217 we show only a part of the extensive terminal arborization.

Fig. 221 shows an even more remarkable case of arborization of a sensory bundle fibre. In a region that is fairly distant from a spinal wound and where the sensory roots, seen along their length, are normal and very little stimulated, a certain robust conductor (C) suddenly abandons the cord, making an angle (not very apparent in the figure owing to the direction of the loop) ; it then places itself on the *pia mater*, gaining in thickness and stainability and travelling towards the wound. It becomes retrograde, after describing an arc, and it finally resolves itself into a very extensive supra-pial arborization, in which the fine ascending and descending branches predominate. The last branchlets were so long that the entire arborization covered a perispinal area extending between six radicular fascicles. In Fig. 221, C, we show barely two-thirds of this ramification. During their long itinerary the nerve branches lack any nuclear escort and show no preference for the scar. It is true, however, that the *pia mater* was infiltrated with connective cells and a few migratory leucocytes.

This case thus constitutes a notable example of neurocladism through traumatic stimulation or, what seems more probable, through the influence of substances given out by the cicatricial connective tissue.

From all the preceding observations we may deduce the following conclusions :

1. The intraspinal portion of the posterior roots, that is, the

posterior bundle, regenerates with difficulty, as Lugaro already believed. This, however, is due, not to a negative neurotropism, but to the absence, within the cord, of trophic materials, and to the presence of mechanical obstacles at the entrance. For this reason the majority of the sensory axons that regenerate are detained or become retrograde at the edges of the posterior bundle.

2. Notwithstanding what we have just said, in young and recently born animals, and under specially favourable conditions (such as the preservation of the neurilemma, inflammation of the roots without their section, etc.), a considerable portion of the regenerated root fibres penetrate into the cord, travelling through the region of the posterior bundle in an ascendant or a descendant direction. We do not know whether this restoration of the posterior bundle is subsequently consolidated or whether, as appears more probable, it is frustrated and suspended.

3. In the penetration and intraspinal course of the sensory root fibres attracting or repelling substances appear to exercise no influence. The clubs of growth proceed along the path of least resistance and the divisions occur when insuperable obstacles are encountered.

4. Contrary to the doctrine upheld by d'Abundo and Dustin, the root fibres that have arrived at the posterior bundle do not necessarily divide, by virtue of internal tendencies, into an ascending and a descending branch. It is inadmissible, on the other hand, to compare the intrarachidial neuroma shown by d'Abundo to be a consequence of the extirpation of the cord, to a regeneration of the posterior bundle, as observed by ourselves, since in the examples given by us the restoration took place without the help of the cells of Schwann and beneath the perispinal basal membrane, and not freely as in d'Abundo's experiments.

IV

PHENOMENA OF NECROSIS, DEGENERATION, AND REGENERATION BROUGHT ABOUT BY SPINAL CONTUSION AND LACERATION

Necrotic and degenerative forms of the nerve fibres.—Necrotic and degenerative disorders of the neurones.—Regenerative acts of the axons and dendrites.—Historical notes concerning regeneration of the spinal cord.

In order to distinguish that which, in the degenerative processes of axons and neurones, is merely an effect of the interruption and consequent phlogosis, from the disorders that may be imputed to commotion and contusion, physical acts inseparable from any traumatism, we have systematically subjected the spinal cord to various treatments, such as compression, laceration, and trituration.

For this purpose we chose young animals, such as cats, dogs, and rabbits from fifteen days to two months old. We exposed the lumbar cord and we introduced, either in an ascending or in a descending direction, a channelled sound, in order to crush the nerve substance and to split it into longitudinal pieces. With a view to combining this triturating effect with an experiment of transplantation, in other mammals, most often cats, we introduced into the vertebral tube and spinal matter a sensory ganglion with its root, taken from an animal of the same age and species. The animals were killed two, three, five, and six days after the operation. The pieces, fixed in 60 per cent. pyridine, then underwent neurofibrillar silver impregnation.

Necrotic phenomena of the white matter.—The violence of the traumatism causes, at first, laceration in the bundles, the formation of small fascicles and loose fibres, and a few days later of vast cysts, in which float, with the detritus of neurones and neuroglia cells, leucocytes full of lipoids, etc., a multitude of dead axons of the type that we have called *preserved*. We may say something of these, since their abundance is one of the characteristics of the lacerations and contusions of the nerve centres.

These *preserved axons* appear either free and floating, or else arranged in large masses.

Free axons.—Torn axons, which have been pulled out by the cutting instrument and which are often assembled in tangled bundles and skeins, are characterized by their black colour and clean contour, almost homogeneous aspect, and by the fact that they are devoid of buds and thickenings. They are found in great numbers in the exudates of spinal wounds where there has been crushing and laceration from the fourth or sixth hour up to many days later. Subsequently the ends become pale and granular, and the entire fibre undergoes a process of progressive autolysis. Phagocytosis does not seem to be involved in their disappearance. The cephalo-rachidial liquid does not accelerate the autolysis of preserved fibres ; on the contrary it appears to retard their destruction. Once the exudate is resorbed, one occasionally finds preserved fibres floating unchanged, eight and ten days after the operation, in the cysts which are formed at the expense of the softened spinal region.

Preserved fibrillar masses which are united to the living portion of the white matter.—Whenever one produces a trituration and laceration of the white matter, the wound in the latter appears crowned with locks or wads of preserved fibres, intimately connected with the living portion. This is shown in Fig. 222, G, which represents the cord of a cat which was killed two days after the operation.

The longitudinal sections show two very distinct regions : the *living* portion, formed by axons that still react, the majority of which end in buds, balls, or rings (Fig. 222, A), and the *dead* or *preserved* portion, composed of a multitude of axons and neuroglia cells arranged in an irregular bunch. In Fig. 222 we show these two regions of the contused white matter. One may observe, at the level of the wound, the flexuose aspect of the dead axons (Fig. 222, D), their termination in a hook or glomerulus, while towards the healthy region they become progressively pale, ending in points of corrosion (B). This segregation of the dead portion is very rapid, as we have observed it even in animals killed six hours after the operation.

The marginal bundles of preserved fibres are found as well in the proximal as in the distal edge of the interrupted white matter of the cord. Occasionally, and when the scalpel has not wounded, but only contused transversally, a bundle of the white substance, the preserved fibres of the compressed point are not interrupted, but are arranged in a loose swab connecting two living and metamorphic regions which are full of clubs. In this case each preserved axon thus possesses two opposite points of corrosion.

Regeneration of the living portion of the white matter.—This occurs exactly as in ordinary spinal wounds. Besides the buds and balls of retraction one finds, three to six days after the lesion, true cones of growth and more or less extensive arborizations. We therefore need not repeat what is already known.

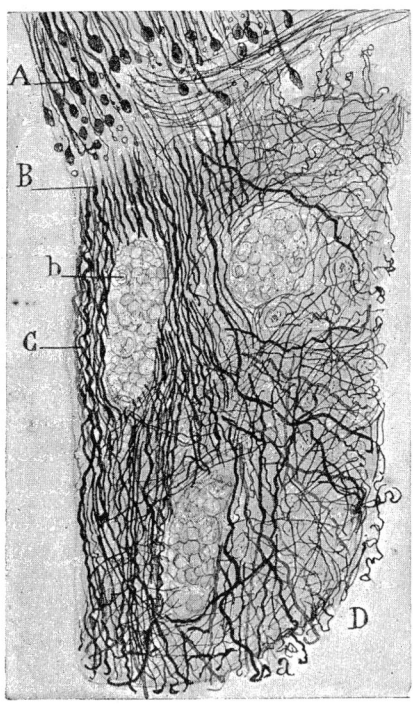

FIG. 222.—Longitudinal section of the proximal edge of a spinal wound, complicated by extirpation; cat one month old, killed two days after the operation. *A*, white matter reacting and showing clubs; *B*, points of corrosion of the preserved fibres; *C, D*, edges of the preserved block; *a*, glomeruli of preserved axons; *b*, blood-vessels.

Necrotic and degenerative phenomena of the grey matter.— Observation of the exudate of the cyst and of the torn edges of the irregular wound allows one to note a great number of alterations, brought about by the death and autolysis of the elements. It is difficult to distinguish, at times, the autolytic lesions shown by the dead neurones from those of cells in course of degeneration but still capable of reacting. Leaving aside, for the present, the deeper analysis of this problem, we shall enumerate the most important perturbations found in the nerve cells.

If one examines, three or four days after the operation, the central stump of a spinal cord which has been triturated by the penetration of a channelled sound, one sees that the grey matter is torn in pieces and that the relatively sound portion of the edges is split up into lobules or longitudinal fringes, whose intervals are filled with the inflammatory exudate, with haemorrhagic remnants and floating islets of grey and white matter. The spinal wound thus takes on a great irregularity. One nevertheless finds in it with some

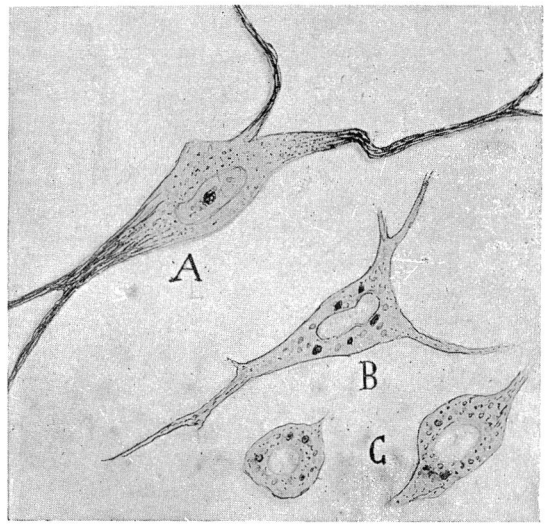

FIG. 223.—Cells wandering in the exudate of a wound caused by laceration, in the spinal cord of a cat killed six hours after the operation. *A*, floating neurone with fasciculated dendrites; *B*, *C*, granular neurones of the necrotic zone.

degree of constancy certain regions, starting from the interruption, which have the shape of concentric bundles as follows : (*a*) *zone of isolated nervous tissue*; (*b*) *necrotic zone*; (*c*) *living metamorphic zone*.

(*a*) *Zone of the isolated nervous tissue.*—This involves an extensive region of the cord which is furrowed with plasmatic gulfs, loose or floating bundles of white matter, and isolated portions of grey matter, separated by the traumatism from the spinal tissue.

One notes immediately that, both in the floating islets of grey matter and in those which are only partly separated from the spinal trunk, the fibres of the interstitial plexus are perfectly preserved. They appear flexuose, smooth in their contours, turned back on themselves, intensely stained, and with an aspect recalling elastic fibres.

The cells of the isolated pieces vary much in their aspect, according to the damage they have suffered. If the sequestrated piece is small and its neurones have been brutally compressed and lacerated, the protoplasm loses its staining reactions, taking on a granular appearance. Its nucleus, almost unstained, appears full of irregular granulations. Its dendrites are hardly recognizable. If the sequestrated piece is large, and if the trauma has broken it off without grave internal disorders, the neurones are preserved better, showing an almost normal reticulum and nucleolus. Sometimes the soma appears pale, while the dendrites attract intensely the colloidal silver. It may be added that this tenacity of the dendrites to preserve their neurofibrils when the soma is in granular degeneration has been observed by Marinesco in various pathological states.

The isolated piece may be so small that it encloses only one or a few floating neurones. In such a case, as we show in Fig. 223, *A*, the large neurones show a pale, more or less altered soma, and dendrites that are clearly fasciculated and well stained. Some elements of medium or small size appear extremely altered, showing a lacerated contour which is cotton-like in appearance and bristling with floating neurofibrils. We shall deal with this type of cell below.

(*b*) *Necrotic zone.*—Leaving the isolated tissues and lacerations of the spinal contour, and penetrating into the edges of the firm portion, that is, of the spinal region that has preserved its vascular and dynamic connections, there is a zone of varied extent, characterised by the unstainability of its neurones and by the relative preservation of its nerve fibres. In this gravely degenerated region the nerve cells appear pale, showing a nucleus full of remnants of nucleolar argentophilous portions and a cytoplasm in which two classes of granulations are found : *fine* or *colourless*, and *thick* or *stained*, greyish yellow or slightly red. In some cells the dendrites still show neurofibrillar remnants. Sometimes the dendrites are invisible or else assume a pale hyaline granular appearance.

In the transitional region between the necrotic and the metamorphic zones one often sees neurones in whose cytoplasm colonies or blocks of neurofibrillar substance persist. Such cells, which we shall call *cells with neurobional remnants or residua*, are usually lacking after the fourth or fifth day from the operation; but they are relatively frequent in the spinal cord of animals killed from the second to the fourth day after the traumatism. In Fig. 224, *A, B, c, d,* we show some elements of this type, taken from the cord of a cat which was killed two days after the operation. It will be seen that near the nucleus lies a lobulated, irregular mass, intensely stained, which is composed of neurofibrils folded back on themselves and of uncertain outline. It appears as though the trabeculae of the net were coalescent, having fused or joined into an irregular block. In some cells (Fig. 224, *A*) the stained neurobional block

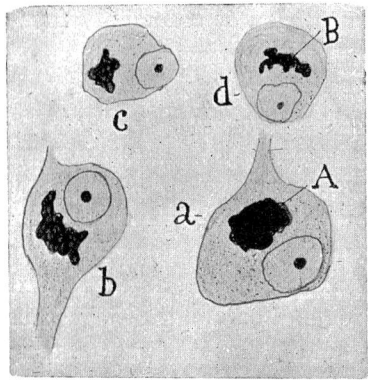

FIG. 224.—Cells of the necrotic region of a wound caused by trituration of the spinal cord of a cat which was killed two days after the operation. *A, B,* remnants of the neurofibrillar skeleton concentrated into a mass.

is fairly extensive; in others the colony is small and shows fine peripheral lobulations (*B*). Finally, in some cells all the neurofibrillar residuum is reduced to a small black grume, irregular in shape, without any appearance of internal filaments (Fig. 226, *D, E*).

The transitions between these elements and normal ones, on the one hand, and between the granular and unstainable cells, on the other, show that they represent phases of a destructive process of the neurofibrillar reticulum, which, under the influence of external violence, becomes hyaline and is progressively destroyed, beginning with the protoplasmic periphery.

We have noted that these neurones with a residual reticulum are temporary structures. Indeed, from the fourth day after the operation, they have largely disappeared, and the few subsisting cells show only very small grumes stainable with colloidal silver. After six days they are completely lacking.

(c) *Metamorphic zone.*—One finds, deeper than the necrotic region, and united to it by transitions, neurones whose protoplasm is more or less intensely stained by colloidal silver and which appear to have retained their vitality. This is shown by various transformations of the reticulum, as well as by morphological changes of the somas and of the position of the nucleus, which are never seen in cells that are suddenly necrosed or preserved. The alterations that may be detected in this zone vary. The zone may be of considerable dimensions, extending to more than half a millimetre, while the necrotic zone does not usually exceed a few hundredths of a millimetre. Among the types most commonly found we may mention the following :

(a) *Cells with marginal vacuoles and ansiform neurofibrillar dispositions* (Fig. 225, A, B, C).—Here we are dealing with neurones that are more or less swollen through the absorption of liquids, and are provided with well stained dendrites and with a soma that is pale in its central, but intensely stained in its cortical, region. The latter appears broken up into a multitude of neurofibrillar bundles which are divergent, anastomosed, and arranged in an arc. These neurofibrillar arcs remind one entirely of those pointed out by G. Sala and Cortese [1] and O. Rossi [2] in the neurones of the cut spinal cord, which were confirmed by ourselves.[3] At first sight the system of peripheral anastomotic loops seems to extend freely around the cellular body. A careful analysis, however, allows one to see that these bundles and loops lie beneath the neuronal membrane and between wide and clear communicating vacuoles. It is possible, however, that in some cases the rupture of the membrane, through excessive pressure of the internal fluid, liberates some of the loops. There are certain cells, like that shown in Fig. 225, A, where this phenomenon seems to have occurred, at least on one side of the protoplasm.

[1] G. Sala e Cortese : *Sui fatti che si svolgono nel midollo spinale in seguito allo strappo delle radici*, Pavia, 1909.

[2] O. Rossi : "Sopra alcune apparenze morfologiche che si riscontrano nelle cellule nervose del midollo," etc., *Riv. di pat. ner. e mentale*, vol. 14, fasc. 8, 1909.

[3] Cajal : " Algunos hechos de regeneración parcial de la substancia gris," *Trab. del Lab. de Invest. biol.*, t. 8, 1910.

The number, form, and dimensions of the cortical vacuoles and of the ansiform intercalary bundles vary much in the different neurones examined. Naturally those neurones which are richest in loops and intervacuolar nets are the motor neurones, as can be seen in Fig. 225, *B, D*. The median bundle neurones show vacuoles that are less numerous and ample (Fig. 225, *C*). In some elements the vacuoles are enormous and threaten to break up (Fig. 225, *A*).

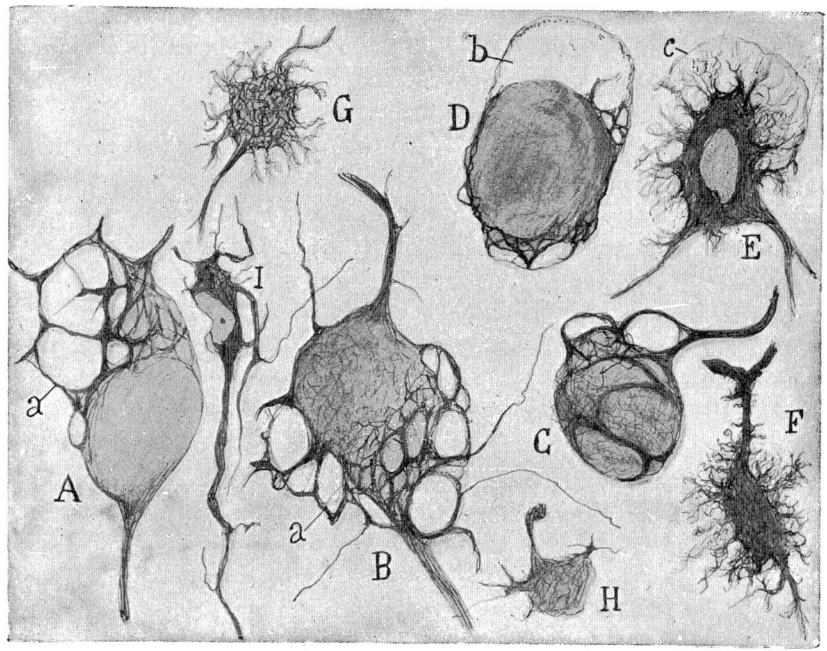

FIG. 225.—Cells taken from the metamorphic region of a spina wound which had been caused by trituration in a cat twenty days old ; the cat was killed five days after the operation. *A, B, C, D*, neurones with loops and marginal vacuoles ; *G, F, E*, cotton-like neurones ; *H, I*, deformed cells with dendrites torn out ; *a*, marginal cordons of the reticulum ; *b*, vacuole beneath the membrane.

Finally, instead of various spaces separated by loops, one sometimes observes a single marginal vacuole of very large dimensions. Almost always, no matter what the size of the vacuole, it lies peripherally, separated from the membrane by a few tangential neurofibrils (Fig. 225, *b*).

(*b*) *Hirudiform type of cell*.—In Fig. 226, *C*, we show a small hirudiform cell which is fairly typical (funicular neurone), and which is comparable to the cells found in ordinary spinal wounds.

In some hirudiform cells the dendrites stain well, while the soma remains colourless and in a granular state. One occasionally sees, in these cells, a group of neurofibrils, which has come from an expansion, ending near the nucleus in thickened rings and loops. Such a disposition, which might be interpreted as a destructive phase of the hirudiform type, is rather exceptional.

(c) *Cell with a hypertrophic reticulum.*—Near the necrotic zone one sees, here and there, large neurones from bundles, whose neurofibrils are considerably thickened and separated by clear spaces which are poor in filaments (Fig. 226, *B*). The thick fibrils are condensed around the nucleus, giving rise to a closely-pressed plexus. The dendrites appear almost normal. This type of cell, which had already been seen by Rossi and ourselves in spinal wounds, is not as frequent here as in the traumatised and compressed cerebrum. As to the cell with a fusiform reticulum, we have not as yet found it in the spinal cords that have been compressed and lacerated.

(d) *Spheroidal neurone with a marginal nucleus.*—This variety of cell, which appears to correspond to the chromatolytic or tigrolytic alteration of such authors as Marinesco, van Gehuchten, Minor, Jakob, etc., is remarkably abundant. It is so abundant, in fact, that it often occurs from the second day after the operation in all the motor and bundle cells, large and medium-sized, in the metamorphic region. It appears in the metamorphic zone as early as forty-eight hours after the traumatism.

As may be seen in Fig. 226, *A*, these cells are rounded and larger than the normal. Its dendrites stain well, showing the neurofibrils very clearly. It is not so with the principal mass of the soma, where the reticulum, extremely intricate and compact, hardly allows one to see its constituent fibrils. The nucleus is marginal, being notably bulky under the membrane. Very often this again becomes dislocated along a thick dendrite, as is shown in Fig. 226, *a*. One may note in this same figure that, between the nucleus and the neuronal covering, a thin mantle of neurofibrils is interposed. Sometimes this intercalary piece of the reticulum bristles with small loops. We have not been able to see nuclei that have been expelled through the tearing of the membrane, as described in other lesions by Marinesco, van Gehuchten, etc. The nucleolus is ordinarily invisible. Nevertheless, in some cases it attracts strongly the colloidal silver, showing then its characteristic spherules.

All the authors who have studied the effects of traumatic violence in man and animals mention *hematomyelia*. In our preparations it is always present. Here we are dealing with punctiform haemorrhages localized around the capillaries of the grey as well as of the white matter. The extravasated blood forms globular, ovoid, elliptical, or wounded accumulations, which displace the nerve fibres eccentrically, and lend to the grey matter, as a result of small enlargements, a characteristic spongy aspect. Such punctiform

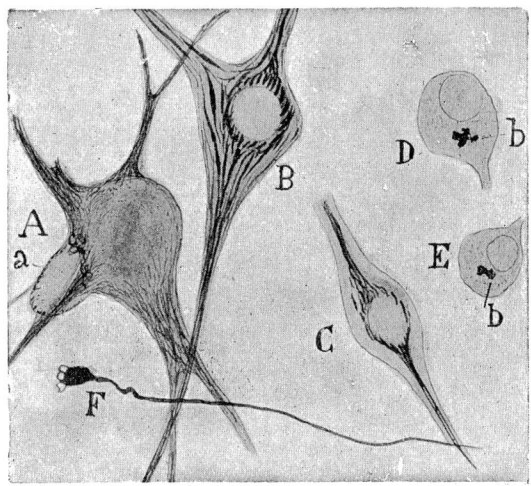

FIG. 226.—Cells taken from the metamorphic region of a contused wound in the cord of a cat twenty days old, which was killed four days after the operation. *A*, large neurone with a marginal nucleus ; *B*, *C*, hirudiform types ; *D*, *E*, cells close to the necrotic zone with a residual neurofibrillar reticulum ; *F*, peripheral end of an axon, terminating in a club crowned with loops.

haemorrhagic foci extend above the wound for nearly half a millimetre, up to regions in which the neurones and nerve fibres appear normal. Those neurones which are enclosed in each haemorrhagic centre and which are thus bathed in the extravasated blood (Fig. 227, *B*), generally show the chromatolytic state two to six days after the operation. It is interesting to observe how intensely these cells are stained ; their dendrites and axon, deep grey or black, can be followed for long distances.

In many of them, although they are bathed in blood, there persist the grumes of Nissl, as Minor notes.

The lesions of hematomyelia, due to lacerations or contusions of the cord in man and in animals, were pointed out some time ago by

Westphal, Pitres and Sabracés, Bailey, Lépine, Lange, Goldscheider and Flatau, Oppenheim, etc., and lastly by Minor (1904) and Jakob (1913).

We may add that the interstitial haemorrhagic centres also enclose plexuses of nerve fibres, as well as bundles of dendrites which are compressed by the masses of erythrocytes. Finally, here and there, pale neurones (Fig. 227, D), of small size stand out in the coagulum.

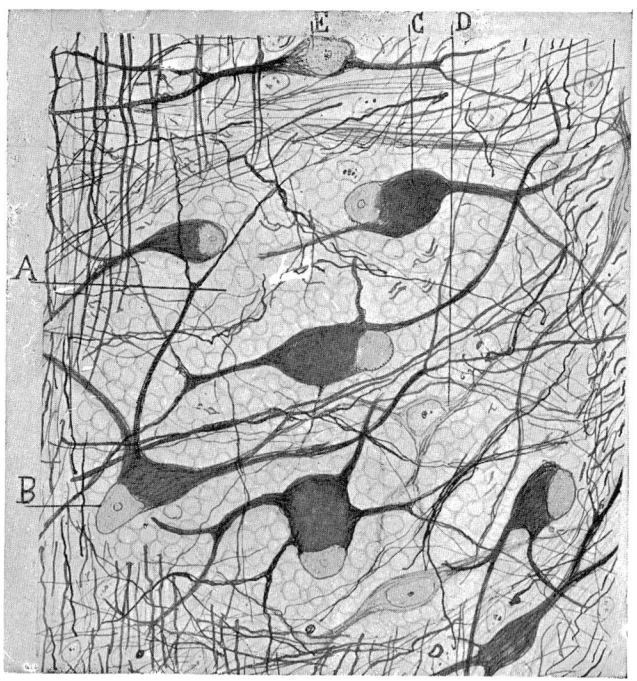

FIG. 227.—Cells lying in an interstitial haemorrhagic centre of the grey matter of the cord of a cat twenty days old, killed four days after the operation. A, deposit of blood ; B, C, cells with a marginal nucleus ; E, fusiform cells of the margins of the blood mass.

(e) *Cotton-like cells.*—We give this name to certain elements, probably dead, which are found in the metamorphic zone, near the necrosed region, and are characterized by the fact that their soma is torn peripherally, is without a membrane, and bristles with an infinite number of delicate neurofibrillar appendices. In Fig. 225, F, G, we show some of the most frequent cotton-like types. Nearly all of them belong to medium-sized and small funicular cells. One may note the absence or unstainability of the nucleus, the irregular shape of the soma, and above all the multitude of pale locks that spring from the border of the protoplasm and appear to ravel out, diverge, and end at liberty. The most delicate of these floating fibrils are yellow, and doubtless represent loose neurofibrils.

The lack of a membrane denotes its destruction during some anterior degenerative process. In cell E of Fig. 225 we seem to have this phase preliminary to the cotton-like state, since the nucleus still subsists, and the membrane also in part. One may note that the

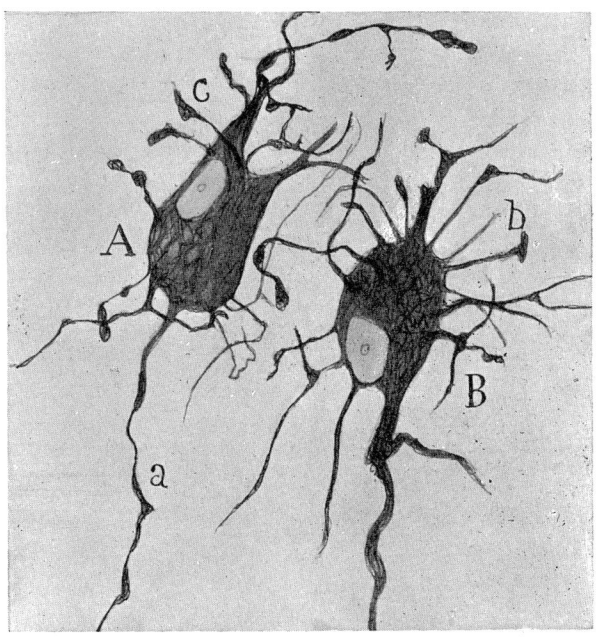

FIG. 228.—Two thick funicular neurones in the phase of emission of new dendrites; young cat, killed six days after trituration of the lumbar spinal cord. *a*, axon; *b*, newly-formed dendrites; *c*, terminal bulbs.

locks, which are free in certain somatic regions, are in others inserted in the covering (*c*). It is to be presumed that, during the preliminary phase, an active vacuolization was first produced in the protoplasmic periphery. Later, the increasing tension of the accumulated liquid tore the membrane, and the neurofibrillar loops and locks which were intercalated between the vacuoles remained free. The nucleus might also have been expelled with the membrane. It is not infrequently seen, some time before its migration, lodged in a superficial vacuole.

The cells with which we are dealing are also found, as we have already pointed out, in the exudates that separate the torn pieces of the grey matter, around the floating sequestered pieces, and in all the regions where the nervous tissue has undergone some great

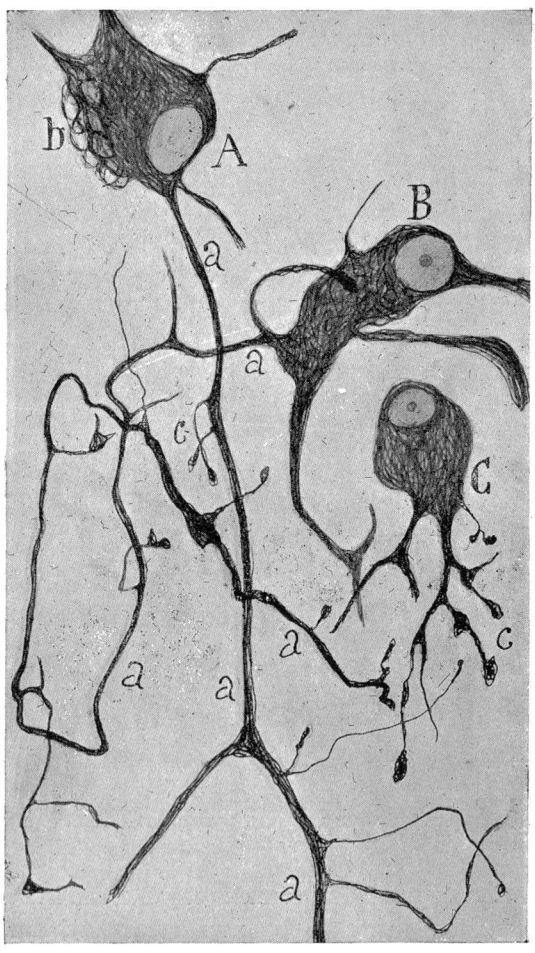

FIG. 229.—Large funicular cells from the base of the posterior horn, provided with axons along whose course arise sprouts. *A*, large neurone, whose bifurcated axon emits various branches ending in buds ; *B*, cell whose axon has a very sinuous and convoluted path, with reticulated thickenings and bulbous branches ; *C*, neurone whose neucleus is tangential and whose dendrites are varicose and apparently newly-formed ; *a*, axon ; *b*, ansiform dispositions.

violence. We consider the cotton-like neurone as a dead cell. But the mechanism of the formation of its locks shows that, in an anterior phase, it retained some remnants of vitality, and was the seat of degenerative processes.

In fine, laceration and crushing of the cord produce, among other disorders, grave structural modifications of the neurofibrillar reticulum. These transformations are not specific, since they may likewise be the result of other pathogenic conditions.

Of all the lesions that we have mentioned, those which are more particularly due to compression are: the *hirudiform state*, the formation of *residual neurofibrillar masses*, and *superficial vacuolization*. *Chromatolysis*, the *hypertrophic* and *fusiform* state of the reticulum appear as well in a great number of morbid conditions of the grey matter.

Regenerative phenomena in neurones stimulated by contusion.— From time to time one finds in grey matter that has been strongly shaken by the traumatic violence, but is little degenerated, motor or funicular neurones showing evident signs of neoformation. This occurred in the cord of a young cat, killed six days after an attempt to graft a nerve within the cord, which had caused grave contusions and lacerations. A short distance from the necrotic zone the neurones appeared deeply stained, furnished with expansions, thick or fine, but clearly striated, and displaying signs of a fresh neoformation. One could see sprouting in the dendrites as well as in the axon.

The new dendrites are preferably produced in large-sized funicular cells situated in the anterior horn. As may be seen in Fig. 228, *b, c*, besides the thick and long somatic appendices, which very probably were pre-existent, these cells emit certain radiated, filiform expansions, which have a strong affinity for colloidal silver and end in grumes or reticulated thickenings, of variable configuration and size (*b*). The aspect of the entire newly-formed radiation reminds one to some extent of certain cells of the " frayed " type in the sensory ganglia.

Bielschowsky and Gallus [1] have also described somewhat similar neoformations in the human brain affected with *tuberose sclerosis*. Pick and Bielschowsky [2] also showed in the nerve cells of a cerebral *ganglio-neuroma* similar dendritic sprouts.[3]

[1] Bielschowsky und Gallus : " Über tuberöse Sclerose," *Journal f. Psychol. u. Neurol.*, Bd. 20, 1913.

[2] L. Pick und M. Bielschowsky : " Ueber das System der Neurone u. Beobachtungen an einem Ganglioneurome des Gehirns," *Zeits. f. d. ges. Neur. u. Psych.* Bd. 6, 1911.

[3] Rodríguez Lafora, when examining in our laboratory Ammon's horn in senile dogs, saw in the body of the giant cells of this organ numerous dendritic vegetations, arranged like the barbs of a feather and submerged in a hyaline mass. *Trab. del Lab. de Investig. biol.*, t. 11, fasc. 4, 1914.

Axonic sprouts.—We attribute this character to certain fine, short, nodose collaterals that spring from triangular swellings, although they are less evident than the dendritic neoformations. They end in buds, reticulated grumes, or lanceolate eminences (Fig. 229). The thickened axons, in a state of divisory turgidity, reproduced in Fig. 229, belong to neurones of the base of the posterior horn. Such axons, besides the remarkable abundance of their collateral projections, were characterized by their clearly striated aspect, almost ravelled in certain regions, and finally by the fact that they showed, at the level where the branches issued, perfectly marked neurofibrillar nets.

Might not these branches represent pre-existent collaterals, which had been more or less altered by the traumatic commotion? While admitting the fallibility of the morphological criterion in distinguishing the new from the old in a nervous arborization, there are two reasons which lead us to consider nearly all these projections as recent sprouts. These are their considerable number—in normal preparations of young cats there is no axon with such a number of collaterals; and their free termination, at a short distance, in buds of growth—in the normal state a neurofibrillar method has never shown clearly a free termination in the interstitial plexus of the grey matter.

Therefore, even though this be exceptional, we must admit that in certain conditions *the axons as well as the dendrites and the soma of spinal neurones that have been shaken by traumatic violence are able to emit ramified sprouts.* We can say nothing concerning their fate.

Historical notes concerning regeneration of the spinal cord.—The subject of the regeneration of the nerve centres has for a long time attracted the attention of histologists and physiologists. After the experimental attempts of Brown-Séquard, Vanlair, Masius, Müller, etc., designed to show the regenerative capacity of amphibians, reptiles and birds, we come among the observers of the end of the nineteenth and beginning of the twentieth centuries to Bikeles,[1] Finckler,[2] Eischort[3]

---

[1] Bikeles: " Zur Frage der Regeneration," *Neurol. Centralb.*, 1904.

[2] Finckler: " Zur Frage der Regeneration des Rückenmarks," *Neurol. Centralbl.*, 1901.

[3] Eischort u. Naunyn: " Ueber die Regeneration und Veranderungen am Rückenmark, nach stellenweise totalen Zerstörung derselben," *Arch. f. exper. Pathol. u. Pharmak.*, Bd. 2.

and Naunyn, Stroebe, Minor,[1] Parhon and Goldstein,[2] Henneberg,[3] and Bethe;[4] these have given us somewhat precise observations concerning the formation of new fibres in the roots and spinal cord of mammals that had undergone various traumatic actions.

If we make an inventory of the positive facts of regeneration collected by these observers, allowing for the errors due to the insufficiency of their technique, we get the impression that none of them was able to discern clearly the sprouting of a fibre of the white substance. On the other hand, nearly all of them were able to observe, months after the lesion, and in preparations where the medullary sheath was exclusively stained, new fibres disseminated throughout the mesodermal scar. For some of them, such regenerated fibres proceed from the white matter of the cord; others, more numerous, believe that they originate in the spinal roots that have been interrupted by the traumatism.

The observations of Stroebe[5] merit particular notice. He used an axonic stain which, while imperfect, allowed him to see with relative clearness the presence of nerve sprouts in the scar, and the production of bulbs or voluminous thickenings at the ends of some axons of large diameter. He observed besides that the branch newly formed in the roots results sometimes from the growth of the interrupted axon, while at others it arises as a collateral, above a more or less degenerated bulb or thickening of the axon. The fibres end according to him in the form of the tip of a sound, showing that by Stroebe's method the terminal bud or cone could not be seen.

---

[1] Minor: "Traumatische Erkrankungen des Rückenmarkes," etc., *Handbuch des Pathol. Anat. des Nervensystems, v. Flatau, Jacobsohn u. Minor*, Bd. 2, Berlin, 1904.

[2] Parhon et Goldstein: "Recherches sur l'influence exercée par la section transversale de la moelle sur les lésions secondaires des cellules motrices sousjacentes," etc. *Rev. de Neurol.*, 1905.

[3] Henneberg: "Nervenfasernregeneration bei totalen Querläsion des Rückenmarkes," *Charité Annalen*, Bd. 31, 1907.

[4] Bethe: *Allgem. Anat. u. Physiol. des Nervensystems*, Leipzig, 1903.

Idem: "Neue Versuche über die Regeneration der Nervenfasern," *Arch. die gesamt. Physiol.*, Bd. 116, 1907.

[5] H. Stroebe: "Experimentelle Untersuchungen ueber die degenerativen und reparatorischen Vorgänge bei der Heilung von Verletzungen des Rückenmarks," etc. *Ziegler's Arch.*, Bd. 50, 1894.

Idem: "Die allgemeine Histologie der degenerativen und regenerativen Prozesse im zentralen und peripheren Nervensysteme nach den neuersten Forschungen," *Centralbl. f. allg. und pathol. Anat.*, Bd. 6, 1905.

Stroebe, however, was not so fortunate in his analysis of the regenerative phenomena of the white matter of the cord. His descriptions show that aniline blue does not stain the non-medullated axons well and thus does not elucidate the first phases of the process of ramification of the old conductors. As a matter of fact, he claims to have been able to see right in the white matter and some distance from the wound, as early as the second week after the lesion, certain fine non-medullated fibres, more or less sinuous, arranged in plexuses prolonged up to the scar, where they ended freely like the tip of a probe. But he was unable to establish the continuity of these new fibres with the healthy pre-existent tubes, far from the wound. Neither does he appear to be better informed concerning the determination of the origin of certain plexuses of nerve fibres, seen in the scar forty-five days after the operation and which, according to all the evidence, should be fine pre-existent axons. Against the theory that they might be newly formed militates the fact that, forty-five days after the operation, the immense majority of really regenerated fibres in the white matter have disappeared through atrophy and resorption, without reaching, therefore, the phase in which they become medullated. Stroebe believed, however, that they were medullated already in the second week.

The question of regeneration and degeneration of the spinal cord could make no serious progress without methods which would present clearly, in their initial period, the sprouts of the old conductors, as well as the branches which were free from myelin. We began this work in 1906, when we applied to spinal lesions of young cats and rabbits the method of reduced silver nitrate, which had been used some time before by Perroncito in the analysis of regeneration of the nerves. As a matter of fact, Nageotte,[1] some little time before, had used the same technique for his study of the lesions of the roots and spinal cord of tabetics, in whose white matter he discovered bundles of fine sprouts and pre-existent axons ending in terminal buds or clubs homologous with the terminal masses observed by ourselves and Perroncito in the central stump of interrupted nerves.

[1] Nageotte : " Régénération collatérale des fibres nerveuses terminées par massues de croissance à l'état nor.," etc., *Nouvelle Iconographie de la Salpêtrière*, No. 3, mar-juin, 1906.

Idem : " Un cas de tabes amyotrophique étudié par la méthode à l'alcool ammoniaque de Ramón y Cajal," etc., *Société de Biol.*, 20 mar, 1905.

Idem : " Note sur le régénération amyélinique des racines postérieures dans le tabes et sur les massues d'accroissement qui terminent les fibres néoformées," *Soc. de Biol.*, 3 mars, 1906.

Idem : *Soc. de Biol.*, 28 avril, 1906.

The recognition in spinal wounds, as a general and constant disposition, of these terminal buds, in the medullated as well as in the non-medullated axons of the white matter, in old interrupted conductors as well as in recently-formed sprouts, was one of the first results of our researches at that time.[1] Moreover, our investigations revealed the existence, in the wounds of the white matter, of axons that were undergoing neurofibrillar hypertrophy, with non-medullated ramifications penetrating into the edges of the wound and ending in points or terminal grumes. We showed that the regenerative phenomena stop some weeks after the operation, the sprouts disappearing even from the neuroglial scar. We finally demonstrated that in the central stumps of many interrupted axons the degeneration and resorption end at the level of the last collateral, which is thus transformed into a terminal branch.

Later research [2] allowed us to supplement the first communication with other observations, already referred to in the text. We may note now: the sprouting of the dendrites of the spinal cord; the excitatory action of the mesodermal scar on the white matter; the partial reconstruction of the posterior bundles following on the destruction of the proximal stump of the sensory roots; the migration of the bundle fibres across the degenerated motor roots which liberate the trophic or attractive substances; the capacity of the recurrent axons, sensory or motor, to innervate the anterior root and to penetrate into the spinal cord; and, to sum up, the demonstration that the irregenerability of the cord is not an immanent and fatal property of the neuronal architecture, but the result of the absence in the neuroglial scar of a trophic and orienting environment similar to that produced in the peripheral stump of the nerves by the proliferated cells of Schwann.

Naturally, these new investigations, besides amplifying the first results, corrected some opinions of too narrow a character that we had put forward in our first paper. Such was, for example, our primitive conception of the terminal bud. At first, under the influence of the morphological analogy between the spinal axonic bud and that

[1] Cajal: "Notas preventivas sobre la regeneración y degeneración de las vías nerviosas centrales," *Trab. del Lab. de Invest. biol.*, t. 4, 1906.

[2] Cajal: "Algunas observaciones favorables á la hipótesis neurotrópica," *Trab. del Lab. Investig. biol.*, t. 8, 1910.

Idem: "Regeneración intramedular de las raíces sensitivas," *Trab. del Lab. de Invest. biol.*, t. 8, 1910.

Idem: "Algunos hechos de regeneración parcial de la substancia gris," *Trab. del Lab. de Invest. biol.*, t. 8, 1910.

of interrupted nerves, we believed that this intumescence was a true cone of growth, capable of lengthening and ramifying in order to give rise to new conductors. Later, we perceived that while there are clubs and rings at the ends of true nerve sprouts, they are found specially abundantly at the ends of sterile axons and degenerating conductors. To-day, we believe that the pre-existent axons which may give rise, during early phases, to cones of growth, do not always go through the phase of terminal buds or bulbs. And when the fibre that carries a bud goes into divisory turgidity, the sprouts arise, with exceptions, not from the bud itself, but above this and at a variable distance from the axonic stump.

One of the first authors to take advantage of the new method was Lugaro,[1] who, in a series of works which were essentially polemical, (it was the epoch of auto-regeneration), definitely refuted the catenary theory, especially the interpretations of Bethe as regards auto-regeneration of the posterior bundle and proximal stump of the sensory roots after ablation of the ganglia. He moreover confirmed, in his experiments of section of the roots, the formation of buds and sprouts, their ramifications and plexuses invading the scar, and especially the principle of the topical indifference of the fibres that wander in the mesoderm, and which frequently penetrate into the peripheral stump of the anterior root or into the proximal stump of the posterior root. Finally, Lugaro also observed, as noted above, many facts favourable to the theory of neurotropism.

We owe to Marinesco and Minea [2] a good analysis of the degeneration and regeneration of the fibres of the white matter ; of their eventual penetration into the connective scar, where these authors admit the possible migration of apotrophic cells separated from the nerves ; of the sprouting of the posterior roots after their section or extirpation ; of their capacity to innervate the mesodermal scar, and especially of the degenerative phases of the free balls and voluminous terminal

---

[1] Lugaro : "Sulla presunta rigenerazione autogena delle radici posteriori," *Riv. di patol. nerv. e mentale*, vol. 11, agosto 1906.

Idem : "Rigenerazione delle radici posteriori," *Riv. di patol. nerv. e mentale*, vol. 11, 1906.

Idem : "Sul neurotropismo e sui trapianti dei nervi," *Riv. di patol. nerv. e mentale*, vol. 11, fasc. 7, 1906.

[2] Marinesco et Minea : "Recherches sur la régénérescence de la moelle," *Nouvelle Iconographie de la Salpêtrière*, 19ᵉ an., No. 5, 1906.

Idem: "Note sur la régénérescence de la moelle chez l'homme," *Compt. rend. de la Soc. de Biol.*, 22 juin, 1906.

See also—Marinesco : *La cellule nerveuse*, 1909.

buds. These authors state that spinal regeneration (sprouting of the white matter), occurs towards the seventh day after the section; that the penetration into the scar of the newly-formed branches and small bundles takes place after about sixteen days; and that such branches, which are sometimes a continuation of the axonic trunk, while at other times they form collateral projections, persist in the scar a long time, even ninety days later.

Rossi,[1] for his part, after confirming the phenomena of regeneration as described by ourselves and Marinesco, calls our attention to the fact that the sprouting of the white matter is a rapid process, ordinarily occurring during the first week, while degeneration and resorption of the sprouts that have penetrated into the scar then follow. This strange regression of the new fibres is very much advanced fifty days after the operation, and it is especially due to the destruction, through lack of vascularization, of the neuroglial scar and to the production of the spinal cyst. Since the sprouts lack sustenance or appropriate nutritive environment, they finally become resorbed.

Rossi analyses carefully the reactions of the grey matter. He notes that the neurones near the wound show various alterations such as: *vacuolizations, superficial fenestrated* state, with formation of tangential loops and nets, *neurofibrillar hypertrophy*, and, in some cases, *vegetation* or sprouting of the dendrites, which emit short and fine expansions. As regards the mechanism of regeneration, Rossi, like Dustin, concedes a great importance to the trophic action of the connective or sustaining tissue.

In a later study [2] he endeavoured to supply a lacuna in his observations—the ulterior fate of the destructive focus of neuroglia. He examined the cord of an animal that was killed two hundred and fifty days after the operation, and saw that the neuroglia had proliferated, filling nearly the entire cyst, subministering the sprouts to the point that an appropriate nutritive environment had disappeared. As a consequence of this restoration of the neuroglial support the fibres grow, show buds, and ramify afresh. It remains to be determined, however, whether this tardy rejuvenescence is more efficacious than

---

[1] O. Rossi: "Processi rigenerativi e degenerativi consequenti a ferite asettiche del sistema nervoso centrale (midollo spinale e nervo ottico)", *Riv. di pat. nerv. e mentale*, vol. 11, 1908.

Idem: "Nuove ricerce sui fenomeni di rigenerazione che si svolgono nel midollo spinale," *Riv. di pat. nerv. e mentale*, vol. 15, 1910.

Idem: "Sulla rigenerazione del sistema nervoso," *Riv. di pat. nerv. e ment.*, vol. 16, fasc. 4, 1911.

[2] O. Rossi: *Loc. cit.* and *Anat. Anzeiger*, Bd. 39, March 26, 1909.

that which occurs at an early stage. Finally, he also adds a curious study on regeneration of the cord in hibernating animals.

Pariani [1] desired to investigate to what extent the suspension of the arrival of the cortical and sensory stimuli disturbs the regeneration of the nerves and roots. Like Parhon and Goldstein, he cut, in the dog, the roots and spinal cord—the latter above and some distance from the interruption of the roots. He had observed that in such circumstances regeneration of the central stump of the motor roots is very feeble and is notably retarded, appearing only after twenty-three days, owing to the interruption of the sensory and cortical discharges. Even the chromatolytic phenomenon of the motor neurones is arrested, while a restoration of the Nissl bodies takes place.

Sala and Cortese [2] studied the subject of regeneration of extirpated motor roots. They observed phenomena of intraspinal sprouting of the motor axons, their growth and penetration into the anterior roots, and their terminal dispositions consisting, not only of rings and clubs, but also of complicated helicoidal structures, already referred to in the text. They add interesting details concerning the perturbations occurring in the neuronal soma—formation of cortical loops, neurofibrillar hypertrophy, peripheral position of the nucleus, etc.

D'Abundo [3] made several interesting reports on the regeneration of the posterior bundle after destruction of the roots. He cut out in recently-born cats large segments of the cord, leaving the *dura mater* in place. Months later he saw, in preparations made with osmic acid or by Weigert's method, that the meningeal hollow space, placed in front of the interrupted posterior roots, was filled by a kind of newly-formed posterior bundle, in which one could even discern the well-known bifurcation into an ascending and a descending branch. In a special work we believe that we have proved that this supposed regenerated bundle must be a simple cylindrical neuroma, formed by

---

[1] Pariani: "Ricerce sulla rigenerazione dei nervi," *Riv. di pat. nerv. e ment.*, vol. 15, 1910.

[2] Sala und Cortese: "Ueber die im Rückenmark nach Ausreissung der Wurzeln eintretenden Erscheinungen," *Folia neurobiologica*, Bd. 4, 1910. (Congreso della Società italiana di Neurologia in Genova, 22-23 October, 1909).

[3] D'Abundo: "Di nuovo sul potere rigenerativo del prolongamento midolare dei gangli intervertebrali nei primi tempi della vita extrauterina," *Riv. ital. di Neuropat., Pschiatria e Elettroter.*, vol. 2, fasc. 7, 1909.

Idem: "Dottrina metamerica e rigenerazione consecutiva allo strappo contemporaneo di molteplici gangli intervertebrali," etc. *Riv. ital. di Neuropat.*, etc., vol. 1, fasc. 8, 1909.

Idem: *Arch. italiennes de Biol.*, vol. 50, fasc. 2, 1909.

sprouts of the posterior root, which take on a myelin sheath, cells of Schwann, and all the structural characters of cicatricial neuromas. As to the supposed constant bifurcation of the root fibre, on which d'Abundo and Dustin base the conception of the predetermination of the form of the axon, it is an illusion, which can be explained by the fact that the neuroma is drawn out longitudinally and the newly-formed axons are consequently distributed in two opposite directions. The methods used by d'Abundo do not allow one to observe with certainty divisions of the nerve tubes. At any rate, these curious experiments show us the great regenerative power acquired by the posterior roots when they move in an environment free from obstacles, and also the persistence of the neoformation, even though there are no connections between the sprouts and the central organs.[1]

Dustin,[2] in his experiments of section and grafting of the cord, has confirmed nearly all the above-described phenomena of regeneration of the roots and white matter. This author recognizes the terminal clubs in the bundle fibres, as well as the production of branches which penetrate into the scar, often accompanying capillaries. His most interesting investigation, however, is his analysis of the late phenomena of spinal regeneration and degeneration. He saw in a dog killed as late as three years after the operation acts of recent neoformation— new collaterals— and he observed degenerative lesions in the central stumps of pre-existent axons, showing that the resorption of the useless portion of the conductor does not always occur rapidly (varicose and nodose state, vacuolated axons, terminal globes). Finally he notes that, no matter what the lapse of time, the nerve sprouts do not cross the scar, and cannot, therefore, restore the paths that have been destroyed, perhaps owing to absence of *odogenesis*.

Lastly, in order to be complete, we must mention Perrero[3] who, in a case of fracture of the vertebral column, with consequent myelitis, saw, twenty-nine days after the lesion, newly-formed fine fibres ending

---

[1] D'Abundo subsequently adduced new observations in support of his thesis that regeneration of the intraspinal portion of the sensory roots depends in a preponderating degree on the creative potentiality, according to a preestablished plan, of the ganglion cell. The influence of the environment, and especially of neurotropism, is of secondary importance in the process.

See: "Ulteriori osservazioni sulla rigenerazione del tratto midollare dei gangli intervertebrali," *Riv. di Neuropat.*, etc., vol. 4, 1911.

[2] Dustin: "Le rôle des tropismes et de l'odogénèse dans la régénération du système nerveux," *Arch. de Biol.*, t. 25, 1910.

[3] Perrero: "Contributo allo studio della rigenerazione delle fibre nervose del sistema nervoso centrale," *Rivista di pat. ner. e ment.*, vol. 14, 1909.

in rings or buds near the focus ; Guido Sala,[1] who also saw evident neoformations in the white matter, in a patient suffering from transversal section of the cord ; Miyake Koichi,[2] who observed in rabbits, whose cord had been sectioned, swelling of the axons and acts of restoration in the white matter ; Bielschowsky,[3] who studied foci of softening of the cord in a Cercopithecus and in various pathological states in man, noting the existence of rings, clubs, and bifurcations in new fibres, many of which had a tendency to encircle the capillaries ; Marinesco,[4] who saw, both in a patient suffering from Pott's disease and in a syphilitic, foci of spinal softening, with invasion by nerve sprouts, as well as rosettes of clubs (*senile plaques* of Fischer) and helicoidal dispositions ; Laura Forster,[5] who demonstrated in our laboratory the precocity of traumatic regeneration of the axons of the white matter in chicks and pigeons, pointing out curious phases of transformation of varicose balls and axons, and recognizing, in the roots, acts of regeneration a few hours after the operation ; Donaggio and Fragnito [6] who, with Donaggio's method, saw interesting lesions in the motor neurones of the extirpated sciatic nerve, etc.

ADDITIONAL NOTE TO CHAPTER IV

In the larvae of amphibians, and even in adult amphibians, regeneration of the spinal cord is more complete than in mammals, as was shown by the old researches of Müller (Triton), Colucci, Barfurth,

---

[1] Guido Sala : " A proposito di un caso di sezione trasversa completa del midollo spinale," *Boll. della Soc. Medico-chirurgica di Pavia*, 10 Giugno, 1910.

[2] Miyake Koichi: "Zur Frage über Regeneration der Nervenfasern zum zentralen Nervensysteme," *Arbeiten aus dem Neurol. Institut. an der Wiener Universität*, Bd. 14, 1907.

[3] Bielschowsky : " Ueber Regenerationerscheinungen an zentralen Nervenfasern," *Jour. f. Psychol. u. Neurol.*, Bd. 14, H. 3-4, 1909.

Idem : " Über Verhalten der Achsencylinder in den Geschwülsten des Nervensystems," etc. *Jour. f. Psychol. u. Neurol.*, Bd. 12, 1906.

Idem : " Zur Histologie der Kompressionsveränderungen des Rückenmarkes bei Wirbelgeschwülsten," *Jour. f. Psychol. u. Neurol.*, Bd. 17, 1910.

[4] Marinesco : " Nouvelles contributions à l'étude de la régénérescence des fibres du système nerveux central," *Jour. f. Psychol. u. Neurol.*, Bd. 17, 1910.

[5] L. Forster : " La degeneración traumática de la médula espinal de las aves," *Trab. del Lab. de Investig. biol.*, t. 9, 1911.

[6] Donaggio e Fragnito : " Lesione del reticulo fibrillare endocellulare nelle cellule midollari per lo strappo dello sciatico e delle relativi radici spinali," *Riv. sperim. di Freniatria*, vol. 31.

Caporaso, Harrison (grafting in amphibian larvae), Hooker (frog larvae). This last author [1] records the union in the scar of the two stumps by means of axons of growth, associated to connective cells and to fibres arising from the ependyma. After eighteen days cicatrization is almost perfect. He affirms that in the re-establishment of the spinal integrity the axons intervene, but not the neurones, which are incapable of division.

These investigations, however, were made by methods which are not capable of clearly revealing the axons and their balls of growth. Hence the difficulty of interpreting histologically the effects of regeneration.

It was Lorente de Nó [2] who successfully applied the neurofibrillar methods to this problem, and definitely solved many doubtful points with regard to spinal regeneration in amphibians.

He cut the spinal cord in larvae 20-35 mm. long, making an incomplete section always at the level of entrance of the eighth and ninth pairs. He made histological examinations from the fifth to the twentieth day after the operation.

We shall not here give details of this careful work, which is enriched by numerous figures. Suffice it to say that, according to Lorente, the axons of the lesioned white matter become crowned with clubs, and many of them cross the peripheral portion of the wound and re-establish the spinal continuity. Before this repair the ependyma appears dilated and full of liquid ; but, little by little, this kind of cyst becomes resorbed and the grey matter of the two stumps—distal and proximal—comes into contact. The neurones do not divide, but they accommodate themselves in form and position to the new state of things.

When the spinal section involves some *posterior root* (cut within the ganglion) the mutilated axons, preceded by a club, penetrate into the white matter, but without bifurcating ; as a rule some proceed above and others below, this being due to the profound modification that has occurred in the cord at the injured point owing to the scar. If the section is effected beyond the ganglion, the sprouts grow within the pre-existing tubes. The same occurs when the anterior roots are cut.

---

[1] D. Hooker : " Studies on regeneration in the spinal cord," *Jour. Comp. Neurol.*, vol. 25, 1915.

See also : *Jour. Comp. Neurol.*, vol. 27, 1917 : and *Anat. Record.*, vol. 24, 1922.

Of great interest also are the studies by Duesberg : " Sur la régénération des ganglions et de leurs connexions médullaires dans la queue des Urodèles," *Compt. rend. Soc. Biol.*, t. 90, 1924.

[2] Lorente de Nó : " La regeneración de la médula espinal en las larvas de batracio," *Trab. del Lab. de Investig. biol.*, t. 19, 1921.

It is curious to observe, as we have already stated in another place, that the newly-formed sensory fibres of the cord travel freely within the latter and even across the intraventricular liquid, without the necessity of any guides or supports; this, while not being an absolute proof, is a point in favour of the theory of neurotropism. In fine, we may say that in amphibian larvae regeneration is much more active than in mammals, and to a great extent efficacious and congruent.

Raposo [1] also, in a very interesting study on regeneration of the spinal cord and ganglia in the tail of Urodeles, shows the great regenerative power of the spinal axis of amphibians. The character of the present work does not allow us to give details concerning Raposo's observations and inferences, which are especially related to the problem of neurogenesis. We may observe, however, that this investigator affirms, though with reserves, that all the newly-formed neurones of the mutilated cord, as well as the ganglionic cells and the cells of Schwann, are descended from the ependymal elements which proliferate at the central stump. In accord with Hooker, he also observes mitotic divisions, especially in the developing ganglia. The classic theory of His concerning the two races of *neuroblasts* and *spongioblasts* appears, at least in lower vertebrates, hardly reconcilable with these facts.

[1] L. S. Raposo: "La régénération de la moelle épinière et des ganglions rachidiens chez les amphibiens adultes," *Trav. du Lab. de Rech. Biol.*, t. 13, 1925.

V

TRAUMATIC DEGENERATION AND REGENERATION IN THE OPTIC NERVE AND RETINA

As is well known, the *optic nerve* is a central path, organized anatomically like the white matter of the cord or cerebrum. The sheaths and cells of Schwann are thus wanting in its medullated tubes. Instead of the endoneurium of ordinary nerves, one sees in its interstices true neuroglia cells—*glia* of large radiations. With such an organization, it is to be presumed that the optic nerve and retina will react to traumatic violence, not like peripheral nerves, but like the spinal cord, that is, by small and frustrated regenerative acts, because of the absence of cells of Schwann, which emit powerful neurotropic agents. This expectation has been fully confirmed by the concordant investigations of F. Tello,[1] O. Rossi,[2] and Leoz and Arcaute.[3] These authors have cut the optic nerve at various distances from the retina in the rabbit, cat, dog, etc., and studied in it on successive days, by the method of reduced silver nitrate, the degenerative and regenerative reactions in both nerve stumps. Our own observations on the variously traumatized optic nerve and retina of the rabbit fully confirmed the facts and inferences of these authors. We shall first set forth the reactions that occur in the two stumps of the cut optic nerve, and subsequently those in the retina.

[1] F. Tello : " La régénération des voies optiques," *Trab. del Lab. de Invest. biol.*, t. 5, 1907.

Idem : " La influencia del neurotropismo en la regeneración de los centros nerviosos," *Trab. del Lab. de Invest. biol.*, t. 9, 1911.

[2] O. Rossi : " Processi rigenerativi e digenerativi consequenti a ferite asettiche del sistema nervoso centrale " (Midollo spinale e nervo ottico), *Riv. di patol. ner. e ment.*, vol. 13, fasc. 11, 1908.

Idem : "Sulla rigenerazione del nervo ottico," *Riv. di patol. ner. e ment.*, vol. 14, fasc. 4, 1909.

[3] Leoz Ortin y L. R. Arcaute : " Procesos regenerativos del nervio óptico y retina, con ocasión de ingertos nerviosos," *Trab. del Lab. de Invest. biol.*, t. 11, fasc. 4, 1914.

DEGENERATIVE AND REGENERATIVE PHENOMENA OF THE OPTIC NERVE, AFTER ITS SECTION

The degeneration is to be distinguished into traumatic and secondary degeneration.

Traumatic degeneration.—Twenty-four hours after the wound of the optic nerve its two segments show, over a more or less extensive region, all the signs of *traumatic degeneration* of which we have spoken in connection with our study of the white matter of the cord, namely, formation near the wound of a necrotic zone, where the axons are reduced to detritus ; the establishment of a metamorphic axonic region, where the neurofibrils appear thickened and deeply stained with the colloidal silver ; and, finally, the creation, between the necrotic and the metamorphic regions, of a varicose segment, more or less long, which ends in a club or retraction bud. As occurs in the cord, this varicose segment becomes successively shorter on the following days, coming to a stop at various levels, according to the calibre of the fibre and the nerve segment under investigation. At any rate, the phenomena of traumatic degeneration are essentially the same in both stumps, as Tello noted and reproduced perfectly. Thus, in both portions of the optic nerve one sees clubs, rings, bead-like arrangements, disruption of the myelin, proliferation of neuroglia cells, phagocytosis of lipoids and of axonic remnants by leucocytes and glia cells, etc., etc.

Secondary degeneration.—This occurs only in the proximal stump, that is, in that portion of the optic nerve which is connected with the brain. It was studied, some time ago, by Gudden, Ganser, Singer and Münzer, Monakow, Bechterew, Kölliker, etc. We have ourselves investigated it [1] by Marchi's method in the rabbit and the guinea-pig. We subsequently made an analysis of it, by the method of reduced silver nitrate.[2]

Our investigations showed that the axon, separated from its trophic centre, is destroyed very late. Thus, three or four days after the interruption, one can scarcely distinguish the sectioned from the normal optic nerve. The former merely shows some irregularity in the contour of the axons and some local thickenings

---

[1] Cajal : " Estructura del kiasma óptico y teoría general de los entre-cruzamientos de las vías nerviosas," *Rev. trim. microgr.*, t. 3, 1898.

[2] Cajal : " Notas preventivas sobre la degeneración y regeneración de las vías nerviosas centrales," *Trab. del Lab. de Invest. biol.*, t. 4, 1905-1906.

in these, with a tendency to neurofibrillar granulation. After seven or eight days the lesions become accentuated, the fineness of the neurofibrillar impregnation disappears, and the neurofibrils take on a truly granular appearance (*granular degeneration* of Bethe) while the axon becomes varicose or bead-like. Fusiform thickenings alternating with pale bridges begin to be produced in the large tubes.

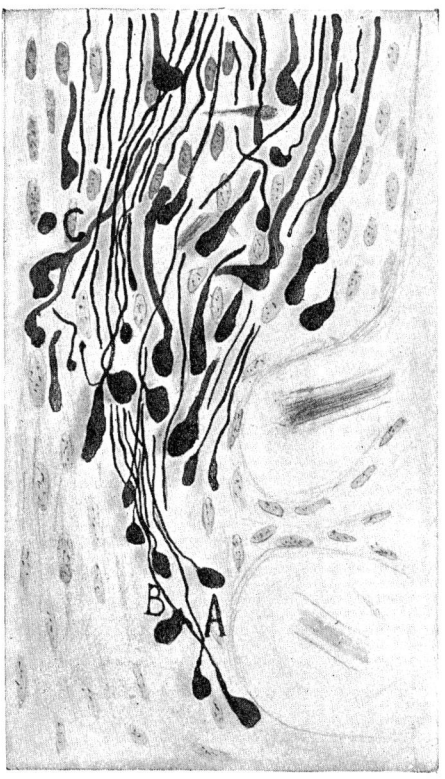

FIG. 230.—Piece of the cerebral stump of the optic nerve three days after the section. *A*, group of fibres penetrating into the scar and ending in clubs. (After Tello.)

Later the varicose phase manifests itself in the fine conductors, among which some appear to be unaltered. Then, from the fifteenth day on, the pale intercalary bridges between the thickenings begin to break asunder. Subsequently the majority of the tubes are marked by a succession of globular or fusiform masses, more or less deeply stained by colloidal silver, which become successively smaller through slow dissolution. Phagocytosis does not appear to enter into this process. As in traumatic degeneration, after a month or a month and a half one still sees axonic balls in process of autolysis, with a stainable centre and a hyaline cortex.

During this time the myelin, broken up into ellipsoids, has been successively phagocytized by neuroglial elements and by migratory leucocytes. The medullary remnants are absorbed, and series of proliferated neuroglial elements are now found in the region previously occupied by the tubes, where a few granular cells stand out, and some axonic spherules that have resisted destruction.

Regenerative phenomena.—These occur in the peripheral and the central stumps, although naturally with more intensity in the latter than in the former.

In the *peripheral stump* (proximal or connected with the brain) there occur (Fig. 230, *B*), as Tello showed, frustrated regenerative acts comparable to those described by Perroncito and ourselves in the distal segment of cut nerves. Once the necrotic zone has disappeared through resorption, thirteen or more days after the operation, the metamorphic portion of the axons grows across the neuroglial scar, and small bundles are formed which are crowned with buds and rings. Some fibres debouch and ramify in the mesodermal scar. But, as Tello observed, after forty days these sprouts have completely disappeared, owing, no doubt, to a degenerative process with consequent resorption.

At any rate, this observed fact shows that even the peripheral stumps of interrupted central paths, when they are near embryonic connective tissue, are capable of developing metamorphic phenomena, of growing and ramifying, even though only ephemerally.

As may be expected, the regeneration of the central, or retinal, stump shows greater strength and activity (Fig. 231). This sprouting would be more energetic still if, as Tello observes, the section of the optic nerve near the retina did not irremediably disturb, through the lesion of the central artery, the normal nutrition of the neurones or trophic centres. To avoid this grave disadvantage, O. Rossi cut the optic nerve near the chiasma and he obtained, as it appears, regenerative acts in the central stump of a more vigorous character than those described by Tello. At any rate, and notwithstanding the bad nutrition which is inherent in the interruption of the circulation of the retina, one always observes a greater or less quantity of conductors which, three, four, or more days after the operation, are in active regeneration. The superficial axons, bathed in the surrounding plasma and little disturbed by the arterial lesion of which we have spoken, take the initiative, rapidly crossing the necrotic zone to finally invade the scar. On the other hand, the axons that are deeply placed, whose necrotic zone, owing to the above-mentioned circulatory deficiency, is often extended to the retina itself, have to travel a longer distance along the axis of the nerve. They

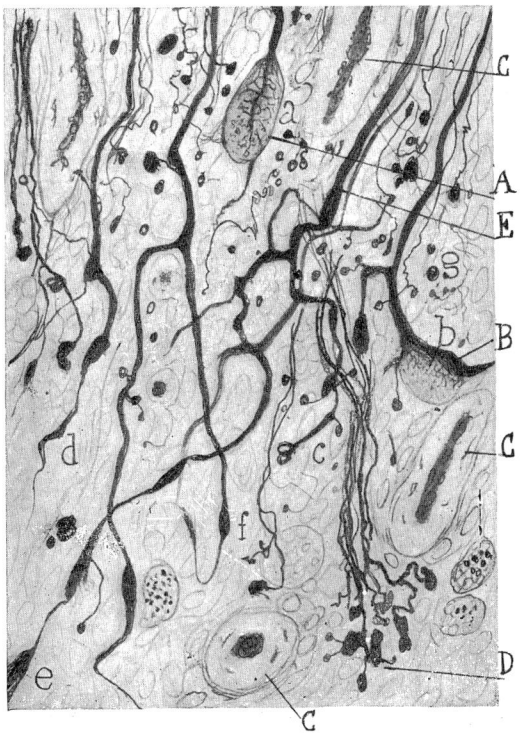

FIG. 231.—Retinal stump of the optic nerve of a rabbit, which was killed seven days after the operation. *A, B*, terminal balls undergoing hyaline degeneration; *C*, blood-vessels obstructed by anaemia and consequent proliferation of the adventitial layer; *D*, bundle of fibres ending in balls and penetrating into the scar; *E*, richly ramified fibre; *d*, cone of growth; *e*, terminal thickening in the form of a brush.

are therefore delayed, and one often sees their cones of growth, eight or ten days after the lesion, still far from the scar. They are all preceded by cones, truncheons, or rings. Arborizations are also common, in groups of short and thick branchlets, each one of which ends in a bud, small ball, or ring. Tello, who discovered this disposition, compared it to the raceme of certain fruits; Rossi has also reproduced it well. Finally, as we show in Fig. 231, one often sees the dispositions that terminate in a cone, a fine, ravelled, and pointed grume, or in reticulated balls or clubs from which spring appendices ending in rings, etc. (Fig. 231, *A, B*). The frequent presence of voluminous balls and buds in the nerve and in the edges of the scar, together with the hyalinosis, partial or total, of such masses, shows that the progress of the sprouts is very difficult, and that it suffers at times continual detentions and delays, atrophy occurring before they are able to get past the first third of the scar. This is due, in part, to the bad vascular irrigation, since the majority of the blood-vessels are obliterated and provided with a sclerosed adventitial membrane (Fig. 231, *C*). We may add that in the scar, as well as in the optic nerve itself, there are many free rings and balls, showing the frequent changes of course and the formation of exploratory or compensating fibres (Fig. 231, *d, e*). Neither is it rare to see conductors that turn back on encountering the scar, near which they accumulate, forming complicated plexuses, as though the edge of the nerve presented an obstacle that the cones find it very difficult to cross. When an axon or axonic bundle has found a practicable opening, numerous sprouts escape by it, as occurred in the preparation shown in Fig. 232. There the nerve stump had only two accessible openings.

Break-down of regeneration and possibility of stimulating neurocladism through nerve grafts.—As we stated above, the sprouts from the retinal stumps of the optic nerve, on arriving at the scar, undergo in the latter a certain neurocladic stimulation, but are unable to cross it entirely and to reach the central stump. Nervous reunion thus breaks down, very likely because the cerebral stump of the optic nerve, besides being very far from, and not always in a line with, the retinal stump—since the movements of the eye dislocate the axis of the latter and are a cause of the exceptional extension and irregularity of the scar—does not give out in its region substances to stimulate axonic growth. Thus, after twenty and thirty days, many sprouts disappear through degeneration and resorption, and those which remain show arrested balls in course of being hyalinized. Other signs of these destructive phenomena are the free, semi-destroyed balls disseminated in the scar. Nor does late examination of the cerebral stump give hopes that, with time, the situation improves. Rossi,[1] to clear up this point, made an intra-

[1] O. Rossi: "Sulla rigenerazione del nervo ottico," *Riv. di patol. ner. e ment.*, vol. 14, 1909.

cranial section of both nerves in the rabbit. He killed the animals seven months later, and he still saw, persisting in the retinal stump, newly-formed fibres and terminal ramifications and buds, and even spiroidal dispositions. But he was unable to find any sprouts in the scar, and therefore, any fibres that had reached the cerebral optic stump.

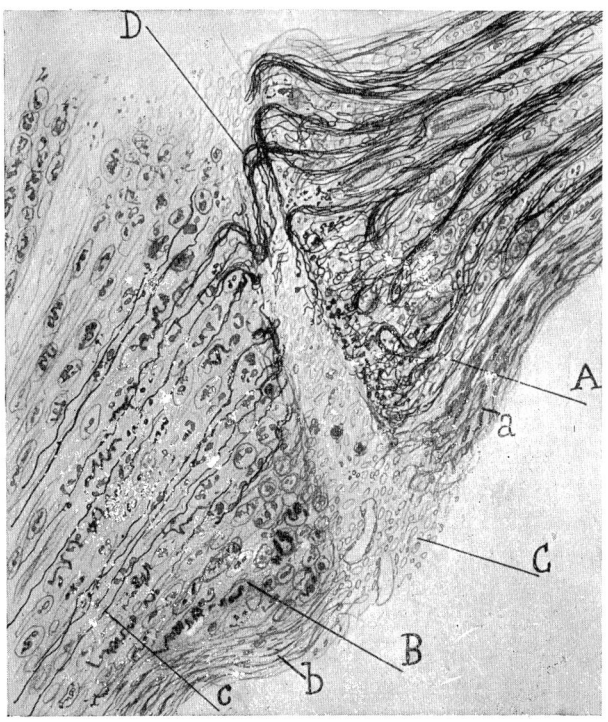

FIG. 232.—Graft of a sciatic nerve on the retinal stump of the optic nerve of the rabbit; experiment and preparation by Leoz and Arcaute. *A*, optic nerve with numerous sprouts; *B*, end of the transplanted sciatic nerve; *C*, intercalary scar; *D*, sprouts which cross the scar; *a*, fibrous sheath of the optic nerve; *b*, "neurilemma" of the sciatic nerve; *c* new fibres penetrating into the graft. (After Leoz and Arcaute.)

Tello, noting this poor regeneration of the optic conductors, undertook experiments of grafting nerves in the wounds of the optic nerve of the rabbit, with a view to investigating if, as occurs with the bundle fibres of the spinal cord (Cajal), the visual sprouts also, wandering through the scar, can be nourished and oriented by the cells of Schwann that are forming bands of Büngner in the grafted nerves. Tello, in collaboration with Leoz, operated for this purpose on ten rabbits. They cut the optic nerve, and then intercalated and fixed, by means of a suture, a piece of sciatic nerve of the same animal, the nerve having or lacking bands of Büngner, according to the cases. The animals were killed fourteen days later. One then saw that the graft had become enormously dislocated, owing, as noted above, to the movements of the eye. Thus, the retinal stump of the optic nerve, far from coinciding with the stump or edge of the graft, often corresponded to its neurilemma, which forms, as we already noted in another chapter, an almost impermeable obstacle to neurotropic substances. In some cases one saw, nevertheless, a marked tendency of the sprouts to orient themselves towards the graft, even though they did not penetrate into it. One could frequently see the latter being innervated by little newly-formed bundles originating from small muscular nerves.

This relative break-down of the animation and orientation of the sprouts of the visual fibres, notwithstanding the nerve grafts, has also been observed by Leoz and Arcaute in their experiments of section of the optic nerve combined with grafts in the wound of pieces of sciatic nerve and sympathetic and sensory ganglia. Although these authors operated with the strictest aseptic precautions (union by first intention between the transplanted nerve and the retinal optic stump), they were unable to avoid, in nearly all the cases, the dislocation of the graft and the entrance into the scar of external disturbing factors, such as adipose and muscular tissue, suture threads, etc. Nevertheless, in one case in which, by chance, the graft remained very close to the edge of the optic nerve stump, by means of an embryonic bridge of small extent, one could clearly see some bundles of sprouts which had grown considerably and which, after a few turns, crossed the scar and insinuated themselves into the graft, within which they travelled for long distances. Such sprouts ramified in the new region, pushed aside the ellipsoids of myelin, and grew intra- as well as extratubally (Fig. 232, D, c). Finally, in this example, some bundles which had become detached from the sciatic nerve and were wandering through the scar, received contingents of muscular nerves, as occurred in the experiments of nerve grafting carried out by Tello and ourselves.[1]

Thus the observations of Tello, Leoz and Arcaute, and our own give the impression that if the eye could be fixed and if one could

[1] Cajal: " El neurotropismo y la transplantación de los nervios," *Trab. del. Lab. de Invest. biol.* t. 11, fasc. 11, 1913.

thus avoid deviation of the transplanted nerve, the sprouts of the retinal stump, stimulated by the cells of Schwann, would notably augment their force of growth and would virtually be capable of innervating long nerve grafts. This is a new indication of what we have repeatedly stated, namely, that the irregularity of the central

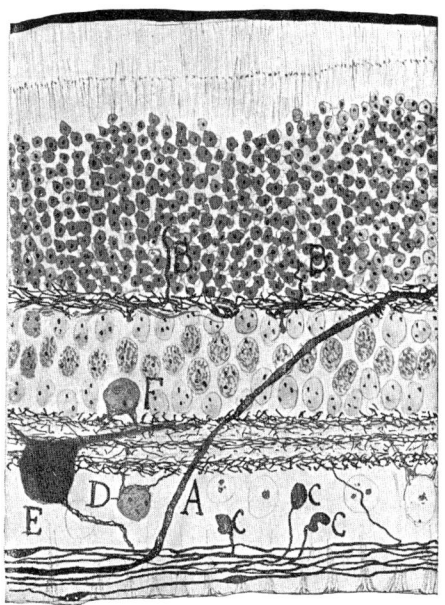

FIG. 233.—Retina of a rabbit forty days after section of the optic nerve. *A*, robust sprout which crosses the deep zones obliquely, becoming horizontal in the external plexiform layer; *D*, *E*, ganglionic cells; *c*, small sprouts ending in clubs in the zone of the ganglionic cells. (After Tello.)

paths is not a fatal result of the immanent organization of the axonic protoplasm, but an accidental condition, due to the conditions of the neuroglial environment, in which, since the embryonic period, all excitatory activity of neuronal trophism and neurocladism has definitely ceased.

DEGENERATIVE AND REGENERATIVE PHENOMENA OCCURRING IN THE RETINA

When the optic nerve is cut near the eye the consequent traumatic inflammation and degeneration sometimes propagate themselves in a retrograde direction up to the retinal papilla or even further; the metamorphic or living portion of the axons goes back to the visual membrane and to variable distances from the emergence of the nerve.

As a consequence of this fact, Tello has observed curious and interesting phenomena of intra-retinal regeneration, and of dislocation and deviation of the sprouts. The new fibres originate in the fibrillar retinal layer, and their terminal buds can be seen ten, fourteen, and more days after the operation, disseminated not only in the above-mentioned zone, but also in those superposed, where

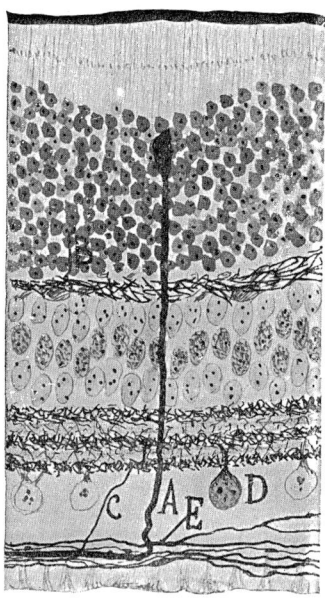

FIG. 234.—Section of the retina forty days after section of the optic nerve. *A*, large newly-formed fibre which crosses nearly the entire retina. (After Tello.)

they ramify profusely. One portion of the branches naturally follows the direction of the optic fibres, and emerges through the papilla, not without showing deviations and retrograde and capricious courses—some sprouts accidentally invade the opposite side of the retina ; other fibres, less numerous, and ordinarily robust, form a right angle before reaching the papilla (Fig. 233, *A*) and, resolutely crossing the ganglionic and plexiform layers, travel horizontally, that is, along the plane of these strata, for long distances. There are some which, divided or not divided on their way, change their direction, turning parallel within the external plexiform layer. Finally, there are some which, crossing all the retinal strata perpendicularly or obliquely, do not cease to grow until they meet the impediment of the pigment zone, where they take the shape of a detention club or bud (Fig. 234). There are numerous ramifications of the perforating fibres at the level of the obstacles, as can be seen in Fig. 235, *n*, where the sprouts encounter the pigment layer. As we show in Fig. 234, *c*, some of these perforating fibres are really collaterals of pre-existent optic fibres.

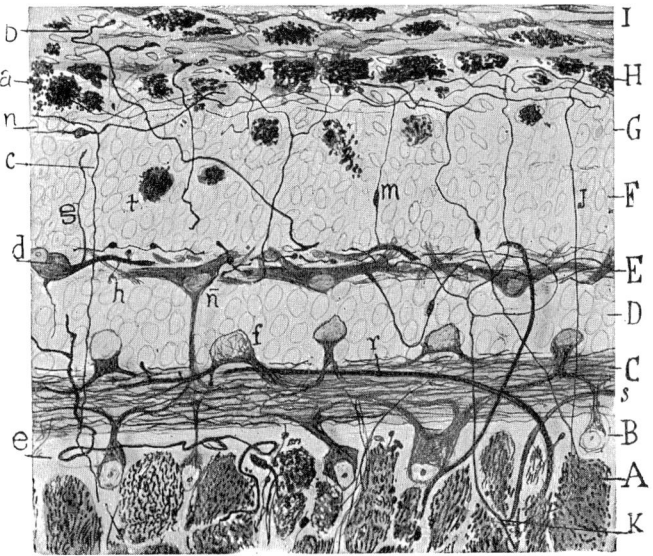

FIG. 235.—Phenomena of neoformation and dispersion of the optic fibres after traumatic inflammation of the sclerotic and choroid coats. *A*, layer of optic fibres that is full of sprouts; *B*, ganglion cells; *C*, internal plexiform layer; *D*, internal granular layer; *E*, external plexiform layer and horizontal cells; *F*, external granular layer; *G*, layer of rods and cones, disorganized and invaded by pigment cells; *e, k, j, s*, dispersed nerve sprouts; *b*, axon whose branches penetrate into the sclerotic coat; *d*, horizontal cell provided with an ascending sprout; *m*, another similar branch. (After Leoz and Arcaute.)

The investigations of Leoz and Arcaute fully confirm the above-mentioned discoveries of Tello and add some interesting details. As we show in Fig. 235, *b*, taken from the work of these authors, certain perforating axons, in their blind impulse across the retina, traverse even the pigment layer, and penetrate resolutely into the sclerotic coat, where they ramify, attempting to leave the eye, and taking advantage of the channels or interlaminar caverns. Leoz and Arcaute have also seen, as results of the inflammation, degenerative and destructive phenomena in the horizontal cells, rods and cones, and pigment cells, and they have observed in the external plexiform layer indubitable dendritic vegetations comparable to those pointed out by Rossi and ourselves in the neurones of the spinal cord. Some of these branches represent collaterals issuing at a right angle, which travel in an ascendant direction and end in buds within or in the neighbourhood of the pigment layer (Fig. 235, *g, m*). One also sees descendant dendritic vegetations, formed in the shape of angular loops (Fig. 235), which are reincorporated anew into the external plexiform layer. The vegetations of the amacrine cells are less frequent and important (Fig. 235, *f*). Finally, in the regions where the formation of sprouts has reached a great intensity, all the layers of the retina appear invaded by ramified fibres arranged in

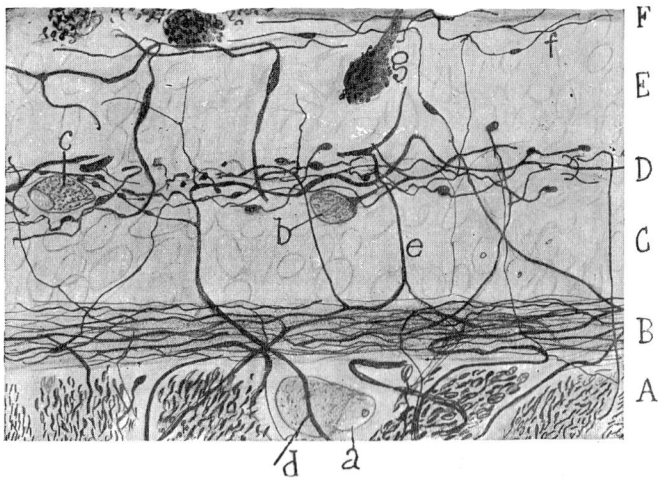

FIG. 236.—Regions of the retina from which nearly all the neurones had disappeared, being replaced by layers of optic sprouts. *A*, layer of optic fibres ; *B*, internal plexiform layer ; *C*, internal granular layer ; *D*, external plexiform layer ; *E*, external granular layer ; *b, c*, horizontal degenerated cells ; *e, d*, optic fibres which are dispersed and ramified ; *f*, horizontal plexus at the level of the pigment layer. (After Leoz and Arcaute).

complex plexuses, whose branches, more or less varicose, become associated with the normal dendrites that occupy those layers. There are some regions, like that shown in Fig. 236, where the plexiform layers are almost entirely replaced by regenerated fibres, the neurones having been destroyed, with the exception of a few degenerated cells, which are spheroidal, granular, and provided with a tangential nucleus (*a, c*).

The most interesting part of the investigation of Leoz and Arcaute is their determination of the efficient conditions of these processes of neoformation and dispersion of intra-retinal sprouts. Ordinarily it is not sufficient, in order to bring them about, to cut the optic nerve in immediate proximity to the eye. One must cause an inflammation of the sclerotic coat, by a contusion or wound, or by leaving on it a foreign body, such as a ligature thread, etc., and one must bring about the propagation of the phlogistic process to the retina. In the neurocladic excitations of the optic sprouts, and in their decisive orientation towards the sclerotic coat, the creation within the sclera and choroid, by multiplication of their cells, of embryonic connective tissue would, in the opinion of these scientists, exercise a great influence. This connective tissue apparently has trophic and attractive properties for the newly-formed fibres.

The formation of the above-mentioned perforating conductors, their neurocladic force, and their impressive penetration of the retinal layers, are facts of great theoretic interest. Among other important inferences, they make it clear that : (1) notwithstanding the assertions of Held and Dustin, the new axons do not need pre-established paths in order to grow and travel over long distances within or without the nerve centres ; (2) mechanical stimuli, or perhaps the consequent inflammation, may, in certain cases, increase considerably the energy of growth of the cut central axons (retinal stump), even in the absence of cells of Schwann, and provoke complicated phenomena of ramification ; (3) it is very probable that, in the growth or escape of the newly-formed axons in a perpendicular direction towards the retinal layers, there co-operates a trophic action of the numerous newly-formed connective elements of the choroid coat ; one must not exclude, however, the action of the laws of least resistance and of stereotropic growth.

ADDITIONAL NOTE TO CHAPTER V

After the impression of the Spanish edition of this book some histo-pathological studies have been published on the alterations of the optic paths and retina after section of the optic nerve. Those of Muñoz-Urra [1] and of Cattaneo [2] are well worthy of mention.

Muñoz-Urra has carried out his investigations on the hen, in which at times he causes retinal wounds and at others he cuts the optic nerve. The alterations observed in the retina of birds coincide essentially with those seen by Tello and by Leoz and Arcaute ; that is, he saw : a notable growth (and invasion of the retinal layers) by many interrupted axons of the layer of optic fibres ; buds of growth and detention of these

[1] Muñoz-Urra: *Archivos de Oftalmologia*, 1923.

[2] Cattaneo : " I fenomeni degenerativi e regenerativi nelle vie visive in seguito a lesioni del nervo ottico," *Rivista di patol. ner. e mentale*, Firenze, Marzo-Aprile 1923.

axons in various zones and even in that of the pigment cells ; alterations of the reticulum of the various retinal neuronal types, etc.

Cattaneo has studied more especially the aborted regenerative phenomena of the two stumps of the cut optic nerve; he saw there axon-balls, some with a central neurofibrillar axis and a hyaline cortex ; aberrant tuberose ramifications ; helicoidal dispositions that remind one of those seen in the central stump of ordinary nerves, etc. In the retina he saw alterations of the soma of the ganglionic cells, among which certain forms of neurofibrillar thickening and concentration are of special interest ; these remind one of the *hirudiform* types of cerebral neurones described by ourselves and confirmed by Miscolczy. One also finds bundles and neurofibrillar glomeruli isolated within the hyaline protoplasm of the axons. Finally, examining the *optic lobe* in the chick, and the external *geniculate* body of mammals by the method of reduced silver nitrate, he saw degenerated fibres ending in a ring and small clubs. These lesions appear to be localized in birds in a single lobe (that on the other side of the cut nerve) and in the rabbit in both primary optic centres.

Thus, in harmony with all the research carried out by neurofibrillar methods, Cattaneo has been unable to see a true efficacious regeneration, but only abortive attempts at regeneration and degenerative processes of fibres and cells.

In Urodeles, if one is to believe Weissfeiler,[1] the regeneration of the retinal stump of the optic nerve is more active and extensive. Although the results obtained are very variable, the extirpation of the chiasma and of part of the optic nerves gives rise to a new chiasma, from which many new optic tracts originate (examination 80 to 250 days after the operation). In general these tracts are arrested in their growth under the cerebrum ; but in a few cases he has seen the penetration of fibres into it. Weissfeiler does not state which methods of axonic coloration he used nor whether the sprouts which are joined to the cerebrum encroach upon the optic lobe, the normal place of connection of the visual paths. At any rate, these experiments are interesting and merit to be confirmed by more precise methods.[2]

---

[1] Weissfeiler : " Régénération du nerf optique et du chiasma chez le Triton," *Compt. rend. Soc. Biol.*, t. 92, p. 1412, 23 mai, 1925.

[2] Concerning the entrance of optic nerves, experimentally induced, into the nerve centres of amphibian embryos, see: May, R. M., and Detwiler, S. R., " The relation of transplanted eyes to developing nerve centres," *Jour. Exp. Zool.*, pp. 83-103, vol. 43, 1925, and May, R. M., " Modifications des centres nerveux dues à la transplantation de l'œil et de l'organe olfactif chez les embryons d'anoures," *Arch. de Biol.*, p. 335-395, t. 37, 1927.

THIRD PART

I

DEGENERATIVE PHENOMENA CONSEQUENT ON CEREBELLAR TRAUMATISMS

Technical notes.—Degenerative processes in the white matter.—Degeneration of the central stump.—Degeneration of the peripheral stump.—Elimination of the axonic segment beyond the collaterals, and transformation of the cells of Purkinje into elements with a short axon.—Details of this transformation in the pathological human cerebellum.—Absence of regenerative phenomena.

THE cerebellum is an especially appropriate organ for the analysis of expansional alterations of the traumatized neurones. The admirable regularity of the architecture of the grey matter, and the typical and constant orientation of the cells and axons in relation to the axons of the cerebellar laminae, allow one to recognize with certainty, on interruption of the fibres, which are the conductors connected with the trophic centre and which are those separated from it, and therefore destined to secondary degeneration. This case of interruption justifies the predilection with which we have studied, for many years, the traumatisms of the cerebellum and the curious metamorphoses of its neurones. Among other theoretical results, we think it of value to have demonstrated for the first time the capacity of all neurones to remain alive, after extirpation of their axon, on condition that the mutilation has been effected beyond the region of emergence of the recurrent collaterals and that the nervous impulse received by the dendrites can consequently be deflected towards the congenerous nerve cells. In virtue of this strange accommodation to circumstances, the Purkinje cells, which are neurones with a long axon, become transformed into cells with a short axon.

Technical notes.—The reactional phenomena of the grey matter of the cerebellum can be studied in adult laboratory animals. After a few trials, however, with adult rabbits, cats, dogs, and pigeons, we have found it preferable to use cats and dogs from fifteen days to a month old. At that age cerebellar wounds are wonderfully supported, and the technique may be reduced to a simple puncture across the skin, by means of a scalpel recently flamed in a camphor flame, so that the carbon black may later show up the lesion of the cranium and cerebellum. The wound ought to be very oblique, so as to involve several cerebellar laminae.

Besides this operatory simplicity, young cerebella possess two inestimable advantages. One is the great resistance of the Purkinje cell to the effects of traumatism, against which its neurobiones boldly react, forming before their death singular and tenacious constructions, which are of some value from the point of view of the general biology of protoplasm. The second advantage is that, since the development of the grey matter is not complete, only the Purkinje cells, with their axons and nervous collaterals, are intensely stained by the neurofibrillar methods, the injured fibres standing out beautifully on the background, diaphanous and scarcely coloured, of the molecular or granular layers, like the black lines of a drawing. Naturally, as development proceeds, the molecular and granular zones have more of their elements impregnated, and it is therefore more difficult to follow the conductors effectively.

As the cerebellar reactions are very rapid, the animals are killed from the twelfth or sixteenth hour onwards after the lesion. The most instructive preparations are obtained two or three days after the operation. After fifteen and twenty days the majority of the degenerated balls and axons have disappeared. The best formula of impregnation is that with pyridine of 50 to 60 per cent. (fixation in pyridine for twenty-four hours, washing for six, alcohol for twelve hours, silver nitrate three to four days, etc.). As complementary procedures we also use the method of Nissl, Ehrlich's and Mallory's haematoxylin, Unna's polychrome blue, osmic acid, and the method with gold to stain the neuroglia.

The most interesting lesions are seen in wounds that involve the white granular and axon layers of the cerebellar laminae. In these regions the neurones are more or less altered, as a result of the traumatic commotion and the influence of the inflammatory exudate, and show peculiar phenomena of reaction and metamorphosis. One must distinguish two types of alterations : those which occur in the axons, especially in those of Purkinje, and those which are localized in the neurones. All these reactions are degenerative in character, although some of them are compensatory or are designed to make the best of the circumstances, eliminating the useless portion of the mutilated conductors.

DEGENERATIVE PHENOMENA OF THE AXONS OF THE GREY AND WHITE MATTER

1. Central stump.—Whenever the wound involves the white matter, or the deepest portion of the grey matter, one sees in the edge corresponding to the central stump the three zones that we have so often noted: the *necrotic*, the *traumatic degenerative*, and the *metamorphic*. Since the central axons are incapable of regeneration, this last segment shows exclusively, as we shall note below, *reactions of accommodation* or of anatomico-functional adaptability to the circumstances.

Necrotic zone.—If one makes an examination after two or three days, it is impossible to discover remnants of the axons which were necrosed by the traumatic crushing; all the axons end in the retraction bud or ball. If the observation takes place, however, from the sixteenth to the twenty-fourth hour, one can then discern below the living portion of the central stump certain granular masses, remnants of the pieces of axon that were suddenly necrosed by the traumatic agent. As we show in Fig. 237, *a*, *B*, this necrotic segment appears pale, conic in form, tapering progressively, and in course of resorption. In many fibres this granular portion has already entirely disappeared, or has become reduced to a thin cap surrounding the terminal bud that is being formed. As in the spinal cord, it is the thickened axons that have the longest necrotic segment.

Preserved fibres are never absent in cerebellar wounds. They are found at the edges in the form of free fibres, curled up, and often united in considerable blocks and masses, intimately mixed with the living portions of the white matter. Where interstitial haemorrhage occurs, all the fibres and cells involved in the coagulum succumb, showing the staining reactions, the autolytic indifference, and other signs of preserved axons.

Finally, the edges of the wound, from twenty-four hours after the lesion onwards, appear spattered with free axonic balls and full of leucocytes and granular cells, a great many of which float in the exudate.

Degenerated zone.—This corresponds to the traumatic degeneration of the white matter of the spinal cord, and it shows essentially the same features (Fig. 237).

From the twelfth to the twenty-fourth hour, or even before, the living portion of the axon can be well distinguished from the necrosed portion, for it becomes notably thicker and shows in sections an exceptional avidity for colloidal silver. This thickening, which is somewhat accentuated towards the axonic stump, there takes the shape of the *tip of a sound*, forming, twenty to thirty-six hours after the wound, a *retraction club* or *ball*. There are various dispositions premonitory of the creation of a retraction club. Some of them are seen in Fig. 237. One may notice, among other configurations, clubs prolonged into spindles or very fine long appendices (C); balls from which hang delicate and very long filaments crowned by a granular and ovoid grume (F); terminal buds from which arise fine and short filaments ending in small (E) or relatively large balls, etc. The preceding dispositions perhaps represent phases of contraction and retrograde movement of the neurobiones, which seem to flee from the wound. Owing to this sudden retrogression neurobional groups may remain behind which isolate themselves from the rest and constitute free balls and rings (*nervous autotomy*). As a consequence of this phenomenon of retraction the terminal stump of the axon, besides becoming thicker, withdraws progressively from the wound.

As a rule, the terminal ball appears well formed from the second to the third day, but there are exceptions. Starting from the ball and proceeding in a cellulipetal direction, one finds those varicosities alternating with strangulations which are characteristic of traumatic degeneration. They are present in the cerebellum for many days, at least from the third to the sixth or seventh. As we show in Figs. 238 and 239, the varicose disposition here is shorter than in the white matter of the cord, consisting of one, two, or three fusiform thickenings. It is clear that the extent of this degenerated portion depends on the proximity to the wound or the necrosis of the cells of Purkinje. If the wound is far off, right in the white matter, the varicose segment is relatively long and provided with two or more thickenings besides the terminal bud. But when it involves the granular layer there is only a terminal club, preceded by some axonic thinning. The varicosities may extend in a retrograde direction beyond the collaterals and may even affect the collaterals themselves, as we shall see below.

What is the fate of this varicose segment, that is, of the portion of the axon that is degenerated traumatically? If one studies the central stump during the period between the third and tenth days after the lesion one perceives that, in the majority of interrupted fibres, the principal part of this varicose portion progressively

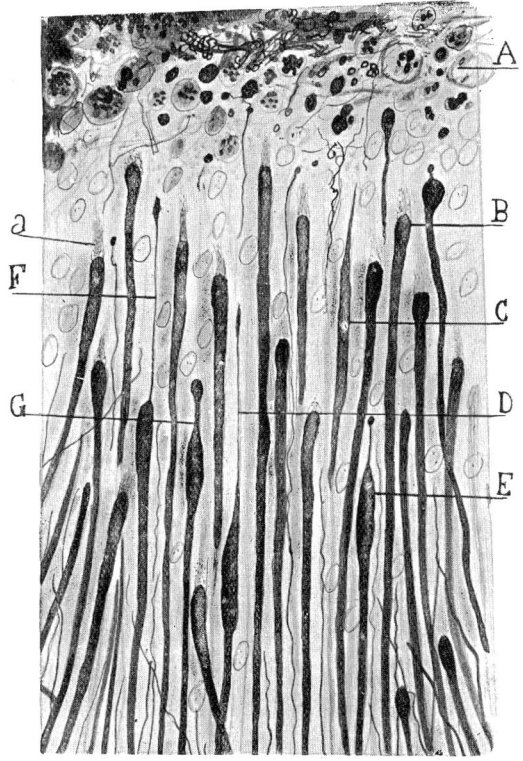

FIG. 237.—Section of the white matter of a cerebellar convolution of a cat, twenty-five days old, twenty-four hours after the operation; the wound A is at the point of convergence of the axons of Purkinje of a lamina. B, axon ending like the tip of a sound; C, axon ending like the point of a lance; D, F, pyriform terminal eminences from which long thin fibrils emanate; E, G, axons ending in a fine ball preceded by a fusiform thickening; a, pale substance of the necrosed axon, directed towards the wound.
Nearly all the fibres are the central stump of axons of Purkinje.

disappears. The pre-collateral varicosities of the axon are an exception to this.

As happens in the spinal cord, *this resorption is arrested at the level of the last collateral*. Apart from exceptional cases, this destructive process comes to an end fifteen days after the traumatism, sometimes much before, and there remains of the old fibre only the segment situated above the recurrent collaterals. Naturally, when the lesion occurs in the white matter, at a great distance from the cells of Purkinje, the traumatic degeneration does not extend, at least at first, to the axonic segment within the granular layer. In such cases it probably develops in a retrograde direction up to the point of emergence of some collateral of the white matter. (It is known that the axons of Purkinje emit collaterals and bifurcations in the axis of the cerebellar laminae, at a great distance from the cell of origin.)

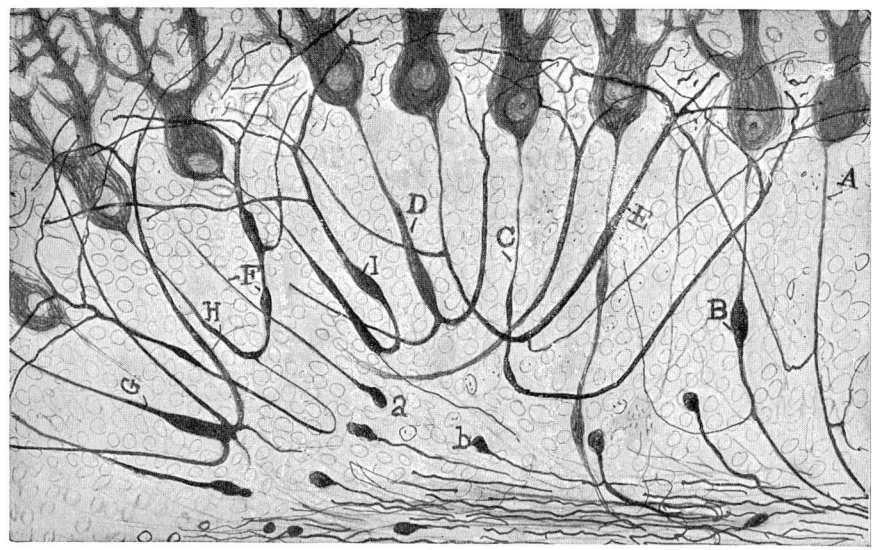

FIG. 238.—Principal types of axons of Purkinje in the cerebellum of a cat twenty days old, two days after the traumatism; this zone is near the wound and the axons belong to two successive sections of the same region. *A*, normal axon *B*, axon with a varicosity; *C*, *D*, *E*, *G*, axons of the arciform type; *F* terminal club.

The phases of this curious disappearance of the extra-collateral axonic portion can be seen in Figs. 239 and 241. As we show in Fig. 283, *C*, *E*, after two days one already sees axons of Purkinje whose course extends only up to the last collateral. In others the terminal axonic portion is short, thinned, and crowned with an ellipsoid bud (Figs. 239, *a*, *F*, and 241, *b*). In short, all the transitions between total resorption and the phase of a fine and free appendix can be clearly observed. Exceptionally, when the wound occurs right in the white matter, this extra-collateral portion subsists for fifteen or more days. One is led to believe that, if the examination were made months later, the disappearance of this axonic segment would be confirmed. Finally, when the axon lacks a collateral, as occurs in *H*, Fig. 242, the varicose degeneration may come up to the Purkinje cell. It seems to us probable that in this case the ulterior resorption reaches the soma and that the cell itself is gravely impaired.

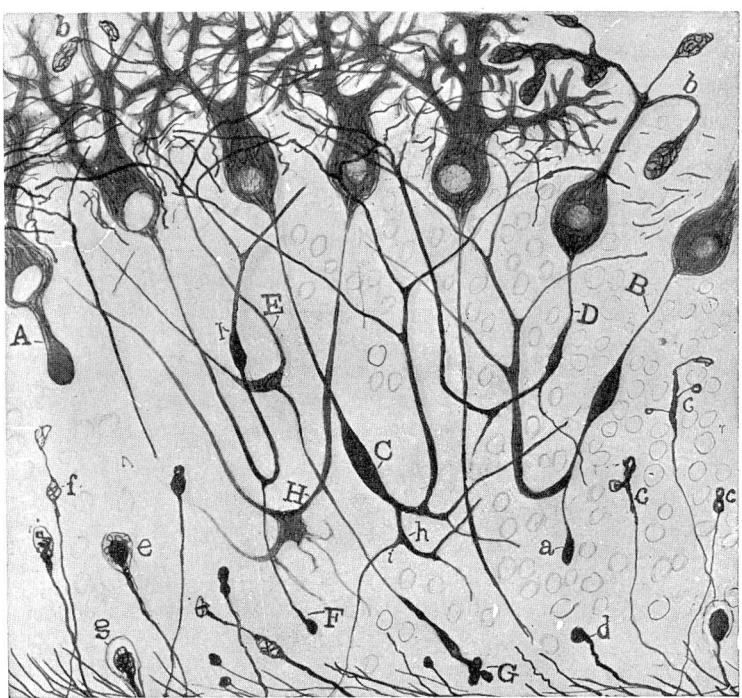

FIG. 239.—Disposition of the Purkinje axons in the cerebellum of a cat, twenty days old, which was killed fifty-two hours after the operation. *A*, short club; *B*, *I*, hypertrophic collaterals from which hangs the axon, terminating in a club; *C*, *H*, arciform thickenings from which many branches issue; (*h*) *F*, terminal ball of a Purkinje axon; *a*, *G*, other balls of the same type; *b*, contracted dendrites (rosaliform type); *c*, altered moss-like fibrils; *d*, *e*, *g*, various type of clubs connected with fibres of the white matter; *f*, reticulated varicosities of fine fibres.

In the above examples we have supposed that the section occurs beyond the collaterals, right in the white matter or near it. What happens in the central stump when the lesion takes place near the Purkinje cells, that is, in the very region of the collaterals or else above them ? When this occurs (Figs. 240 and 242, *a*), the central stump undergoes traumatic degeneration along its entire short path, forming a club which retracts progressively until it hangs near the soma. This typical *retraction club* may subsist for a long time without showing signs of regeneration or destruction, as we showed in our first experiments of traumatic lesion of the cerebellum. At other times, however, and as early as the first day, the terminal bud runs up to the cell, appearing as a short, hardly swollen appendix (Fig. 241, *G, H*). We think it probable that on the following days this exiguous appendix is entirely resorbed, and that the Purkinje neurone remains completely unprovided with a functional expansion. It is very possible that many of the cells without axon, which have been observed from the third to the fifth day after the lesion, have lost their axon in this way. Nevertheless these neurones remain

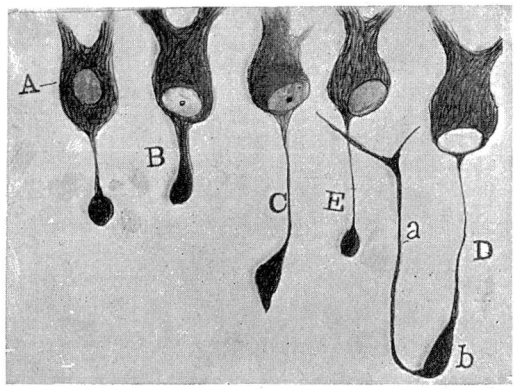

FIG. 240.—Cells of Purkinje of the cerebellum of a cat, twenty days old, three days after the operation. *A, B, C, E*, cells with a club devoid of collateral; *D*, cell whose club is prolonged as a collateral.

alive for some time, as we shall note below, although, in the end, they may finally degenerate and die.

These phenomena and others of which we shall speak at the proper time, show that *indefinite conservation of the neurones, after mutilation of the axon, is certain only when the initial region of the latter and some of its recurrent collaterals have been respected by the traumatism.*

Metamorphic portion, or portion of compensatory reaction, of the injured axon.—When the interruption of the axon occurs in the inferior plane of the granular layer, or in the vicinity of the white matter, one sees that the axonic segment, as well as the collaterals situated above the region suffering from traumatic degeneration, is the seat of an interesting hypertrophic process. The diameter of these portions augments considerably, and may attain twice and three times its normal thickness. Its stainability with colloidal silver becomes more pronounced and, finally, the neurofibrils undergo a certain swelling and coalescence which renders them hard to see. This hypertrophy is propagated, in a retrograde direction, through the axonic trunk up to near the initial strangulation, and on the side of the collaterals up to the secondary branches, inclusive, of the molecular layer. Once the peripheral portion of the axon has disappeared, it seems as though all its mass has become concentrated in the living portion of the functional expansion and of its emissions.

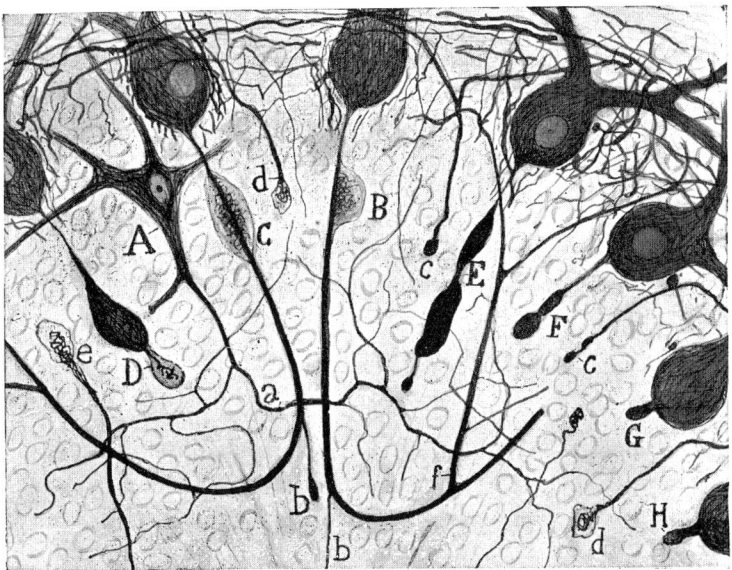

FIG. 241.—Section of a cerebellar lamina; cat, twenty-five days old, one day after the section. *A*, cell with a short axon; *D, E, F*, varieties of double clubs; *G, H*, axon reduced to a digitiform appendix; *b*, continuation of the Purkinje axon, ending in a club; *c, d*, recurrent collaterals of the Purkinje axons with a retraction ball in their peripheral stump.

It is curious to note the frequent presence of solitary thickenings, which are fusiform, and sometimes very voluminous, and are thus true varicosities, at certain points along the hypertrophic course of the axon and collaterals. Such thickenings lie preferably near the nodes, and thus represent processes of growth of the axonic swelling next to the ring. As we show in Figs. 242, *E*, and 239, *B*, this localization explains the almost constant appearance of a fusiform enlargement in the centre of the axonic path (pre-collateral portion) as well as of another of a singularly robust character (Fig. 239, *C*), placed a little above the origin of the hypertrophic collaterals.

Finally, along the course of the collaterals themselves, one sometimes sees thickenings which correspond also to the vicinity of nodes of Ranvier (Fig. 239, *I*). We may note that the preceding varicosities are distinguished from those found in the segment undergoing traumatic degeneration in that they persist almost indefinitely, are situated in specific regions, and are not subject to processes of vacuolization or hyalinization. Evidence of their power of resisting destruction is furnished by H. Rossi, Nageotte, and Marinesco, who observed them in human cerebella affected with various chronic diseases.

The axon of Purkinje has such a tendency to form varicosities next to nodes that the former are found at times in uninterrupted axons that are simply stimulated by the vicinity of an inflammatory process, as D. García and ourselves [1] pointed out some time ago. They occur even in normal animals. Finally, we may note that the varicosities of the hypertrophic portion of the axon and collaterals frequently show, as can be seen in Fig. 241, *B*, *C*, processes of cortical hyalinosis, with ravelling and a cotton-like disposition of the axial neurofibrils.

A result of the disappearance of the extra-collateral portion of the axon and of the compensatory hypertrophy of the collaterals and initial portion of the axon is the transformation of the cell of Purkinje into a neurone with a short axon. Apart from its faithful conservation of the type of a normal Purkinje cell, one recognizes this form at first sight by the singular avidity of the axon for colloidal silver and, above all, by the sudden continuation of the axon in one or more retrograde arciform branches, which repeatedly divide and are very robust, much more so than the congenerous normal collaterals.

There is great variety in the number, dimension, and position of the curved prolongations of the functional expansion, according to the number of collaterals previously existing, and the retrograde extent of the traumatic degeneration and consequent resorption. As can be seen in Fig. 242, *B*, *F*, the most common case is where an axon is simply prolonged in a curve by a very robust retrograde collateral, which appears to be its continuation. But there are also cases of axons from which two arcs spring in different planes with corresponding collaterals. An example of three arcs is very rare. These collaterals divide already in the granular zone, and ascend to

[1] R. Cajal y D. García : " Las lesiones del retículo de las células nerviosas en la rabia," *Trab. del Lab. de Invest. biol.*, t. 3, 1904.

the molecular layer, where they take a direction parallel to the axis of the laminae, becoming connected, as we showed some time ago, with the trunk and large bundles of the Purkinje cells.

True regenerative phenomena are never seen in the metamorphic portion of the axon and collaterals of the Purkinje cell. Neither does one see them in the other cerebellar axons. Regeneration is here an intraprotoplasmic function, occurring in the neurobiones and other

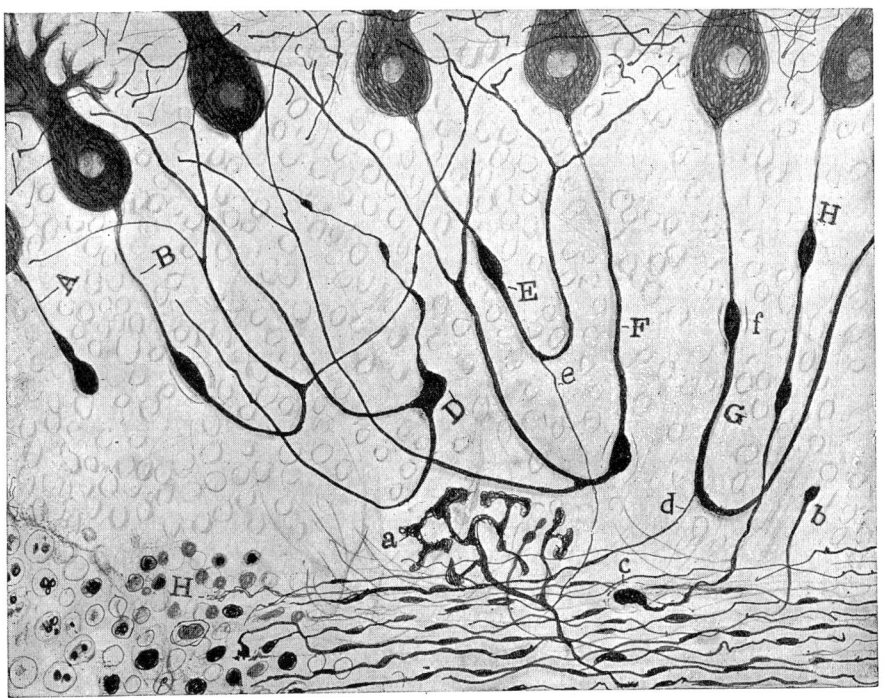

FIG. 242.—Section of the granular layer of the cerebellum of a cat, one month old, which was killed ten days after the operation. *A*, axon with a short club; *B*, *D*, *F*, various types of arciform axons; *E*, *G*, hypertrophic arcs from which issues the thinned peripheral portion of the axon; *H*, normal axon with two varicosities; *H*, free balls near the wound; *a*, abnormal arborization of a fibre arriving from the white matter; *f*, varicosity surrounded by a fusiform vacuole.

axonic constructive factors. Exceptionally one sometimes observes (Fig. 239, *H*) indications of new branches, rudimentary in character, and as it were aborted, issuing from the thickening of origin of an arciform fibre. The branches shown in Fig. 239, *h*, also appear to be newly formed, although it would be possible to explain their presence by the fact that two robust collaterals, abruptly divided, may arise from the same point on an axon. Thus the hope originally entertained by us, and subsequently shared by H. Rossi, that the *retraction ball* is transformed into a *cone of growth*, turns out an impossibility, or at any rate an extremely rare occurrence.

2. **Degeneration of the peripheral stump.**—As occurs in the spinal cord, the axons which are separated from their trophic centre likewise show, twenty-four to forty-eight hours after the lesion, three segments : the *necrosed* or granular segment, that which is *degenerated through traumatism*, and the segment of *secondary degeneration*.

The necrosed segment is rapidly resorbed. That suffering from traumatic degeneration becomes varicose and, at a variable distance from the wound, ends in a retraction ball which is frequently preceded by fusiform thickenings and strangulations. Finally, the portion that undergoes secondary degeneration extends up to the trunk of the axon and is the only one to show the characteristic signs of Wallerian degeneration—granular appearance, formation of pale fusiform masses, rupture of the intercalary bridges, etc.—eight or ten days after the lesion.

The free balls resulting from autotomy of the portion that is degenerated traumatically are preserved for many days near the wound, showing the well-known superficial hyalinosis. In preparations made with osmic acid one sees that each varicosity, as well as the terminal club, is surrounded by a myelin sheath.

When the interruption of the fibres occurs in the grey matter, the peripheral stump appears to offer a remarkable resistance to degeneration. Three or more days after the operation one still sees its axons, which are fairly well stained, as we show in Fig. 238, *b*, crowned with large more or less retracted balls, some of them showing signs of vacuolization and hyalinosis (Fig. 239, *e*).

The most instructive wounds, however, are those which affect the zone itself of the cells of Purkinje (Fig. 243). When the lesions are relatively deep, one may have some doubts concerning the condition of the peripheral stump of an interrupted axon ; for, as is well known, the climbing and the moss-like axons have been interrupted along with the axons of Purkinje. When, however, as we show in Fig. 243, *D*, the wound has clipped the axons of Purkinje next to the cell, there is no difficulty in identification ; the thickness of the fibres, their absolutely radial orientation, their relative parallelism, and, especially, the persistence of their collaterals, would allow us easily to distinguish such axons from the other fibres. In these axons we shall see, in a very superficial plane, thick masses or terminal balls in course of degeneration. If the examination is carried out in good time—after twenty-four hours—we shall still perceive within the clubs, apart from the cortical hyalinization (*B*), peculiar formations of neurofibrillar nets, loops, and glomeruli. Among other shapes, one often discerns two glomeruli of thick neurofibrils united by a thin filament (Fig. 243, *C*, *E*).

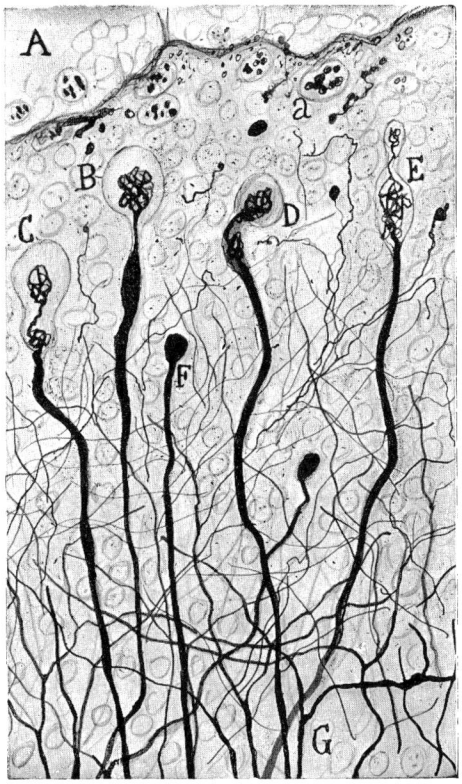

FIG. 243.—Section of the granular layer of the cerebellum of a cat, twenty-five days old, one day after the operation; the Purkinje cells have disappeared owing to a haemorrhagic centre. *A*, coagulum; *B*, *C*, *D*, peripheral stump of Purkinje axons each terminated by a ball containing a neurofibrillar glomerulus; *G*, moss-like fibres, little altered; *E*, glomerular ball provided with a small terminal lobule.

The varicosities of the axonic remnant may subsist for several days; after a week one still finds peripheral stumps that are hardly altered.

We see another curious example of this resistance in recurrent collaterals that are clipped at some distance from the Purkinje cell. As we show in Fig. 241, *c*, *d*, these branches, which end in a club in the granular zone, resist autolysis and show secondary degeneration for many days. We may note that the same occurred with the sensory collaterals of the spinal cord.

Arciform transformation of the Purkinje axons in man.—The transformations of the Purkinje axon that are provoked experimentally in traumatized animals have been observed in man by various pathologists, such as H. Rossi, Nageotte, and Marinesco.

Before speaking of these observations, however, we must say something of a preceding study. The application to the pathology of the cerebellum of neurofibrillar methods was begun by us in 1907.[1] We saw the production, in axonic stumps, after wounds in the rabbit, cat, and dog, of voluminous balls, as well as of strings of varicosities. The most interesting fact brought out by our researches, however, was the discovery in the interrupted Purkinje axons, of the *retraction club or bud*, situated very often near the neuronal soma, even though the section may have been made in the white matter, far from the cell.

Subsequently H. Rossi[2] published a case of human cerebellar sclerosis in which curious alterations appeared. The Purkinje cells were less numerous than usual, and, next to cells that could be considered normal, there were others which were characterized by the interruption of the axon within the granular layer. In some cases the terminal stump of the axon, mutilated through degeneration, showed a free club or ball, without appendices, and entirely comparable to those seen by ourselves in the cerebellum of traumatized animals. But in other elements this terminal club emitted a thick recurrent branch which, after tracing an arc and sometimes bifurcating, extended up to the molecular layer, where it was lost. Such appendices, in the opinion of H. Rossi, might be the result of the regeneration of normal recurrent collaterals. In this way the retraction club would become converted into a bud or growth.

The Purkinje cell, whose axon appears injured and provided with a retraction ball or club, would thus be unable to regenerate anything more than the initial collaterals which, from the functional point of view, would be very important dispositions. It is curious to observe, as we had already noted, that the Purkinje cells with a terminal bud are found at times very far from the cerebellar lesion, and among cells that are completely normal.

[1] Cajal: "Note sur la dégénérescence traumatique des fibres nerveuses du cervelet et du cerveau," *Trav. du Lab. de Recherches biol.*, t. 5, 1907.

[2] H. Rossi: "Per la rigenerazione dei neuroni," *Trab. del Lab. de Invest. biol.*, t. 6, 1908.

In a later paper H. Rossi, in collaboration with G. Garbini,[1] confirmed these formations in various nervous diseases, furnishing certain details on the normal and pathological histology of the cerebellum—among others the twin Purkinje cells with a joint basketwork.

In a very interesting note presented to the Société de Biologie, Nageotte and Kindberg [2] also recognized, in two cases of cerebellar atrophy and in various patients suffering from motor disturbances, tumefactions along the course of the Purkinje axons, and hypertrophy of the collaterals. In some cells the ultra-collateral portion of the axon had disappeared, the Purkinje cell being finally transformed into an element with a short axon. As the recurrent collaterals become connected with the immediate Purkinje cells, the impulses reaching the soma and dendrites would thus form something of a vicious circle. At any rate, the functional connection of these peripherally dissociated cells suffices to explain, according to Nageotte and Kindberg, the good conservation of the protoplasmic soma and arborization. The axonic nodosities were also observed by Straussler in cerebellar atrophy, and by Bravetta, who saw them in paralytic dementia. This latter author [3] has been able to impregnate the axonic tumefactions, as well as the arciform dispositions and retraction balls, both by our method and by that of Golgi.

Marinesco and Minea,[4] examining in man degenerations brought about by cerebellar tumours, have confirmed the lesions described by H. Rossi and Nageotte, with some variations that have a certain interest as contributing to the better interpretation of terminal balls. Marinesco and Minea have observed, besides the clubs that had no appendices and were evidently terminal in character, axons of Purkinje from whose clubs arose one or two recurrent expansions, which divided along their course and terminated in the plexiform layer. The most

---

[1] H. Rossi e G. Garbini: "Intorno a speciali connessioni tra alcuni neuroni cerebellari," *Annal. della Facoltà di Medicina di Perugia*, serie 4, vol. 1, fasc. 1, 1912.

[2] Nageotte et L. Kindberg: "Lésions fines du cervelet. I. Nodosités des prolongements protoplasmiques des cellules de Purkinje, etc. II. Tuméfaction fusiforme des cylindre-axes de Purkinje," *Séances de la Soc. de Biol.*, 25 nov. et 5 déc. 1908.

[3] E. Bravetta: "Sopra alcune alterazioni degli elementi nervosi nella demenza paralitica," *Boll. della Società Medico-Chirurgica di Pavia*, Seduta 2 Julio 1909.

[4] Marinesco et Minea: "Nouvelles contributions à l'étude de la régénerescence des fibres du système nerveux central," *Jour. f. Psychol. u. Neurol.*, Bd. 17, 1910.

significant discovery, however, was that of axons continuous with the white matter, showing on their way through the granular layer a large dilatation from which issue hypertrophic recurrent collaterals. The ball or thickening is sometimes found, not in the course of the parent axon, but in that of the hypertrophic collateral. It thus seems certain that the presence of varicosities in the axon and collaterals of Purkinje does not necessarily imply a destruction of its peripheral portion.

Finally, we may also cite Ottorino Rossi,[1] who has demonstrated, in pellagra, degenerative phenomena in various nerve organs, and true retraction balls in the axons of Purkinje.

We have also observed axonic metamorphoses similar to those pointed out by H. Rossi, Nageotte, Kindberg, and Marinesco, in the cerebellum of old people and of relatively young persons who died through accidents.[2] As we show in Fig. 244, where we have assembled the dispositions most frequently found in various sections, the axons of Purkinje show three types of dispositions:

(*a*) More or less complete hypertrophy of the axons with thickenings along their path, but without apparent collaterals.

(*b*) Axonic hypertrophy with a thick recurrent collateral which ends in the molecular layer. The ulterior course of the axon is reduced to a fine collateral, which loses itself in the white matter (Fig. 244, *E, H*).

(*c*) Arciform axon provided with a robust terminal ball; a thick recurrent collateral emerges from this and ramifies in the molecular layer (*F*). The varicosity lies at a variable distance from the cell, and at times the collateral first descends for a certain distance, and then ascends. Sometimes this hypertrophic collateral also shows some voluminous varicosity. Finally, it is not unusual for the axon to show two contiguous balls (Fig. 244, *D*).

(*d*) Axon ending in a ball before the region of emergence of the collateral. In this case the recurrent branch is naturally lacking, and the axon ends at various distances from the cell in a sphere of variable size (Fig. 244, *A, B*). As Rossi and Marinesco and Minea have shown, the descending brush of the pericellular basket accompanies the axon up to near the terminal ball, making it difficult to perceive the initial portion of the latter, which in adult man is very thin and pale.

[1] Ottorino Rossi: " Klinischer und anatomo-pathologischer Beitrag zur Kenntniss der sogen. Pellagratyphus," *Jour. f. Psychol. u. Neurol.*, Bd. 20, H. 1-2, 1913.

[2] Cajal: " Los fenómenos precoces de la degeneración neuronal en el cerebelo," *Trab. del Lab. de Investig. biol.*, t. 9, 1911.

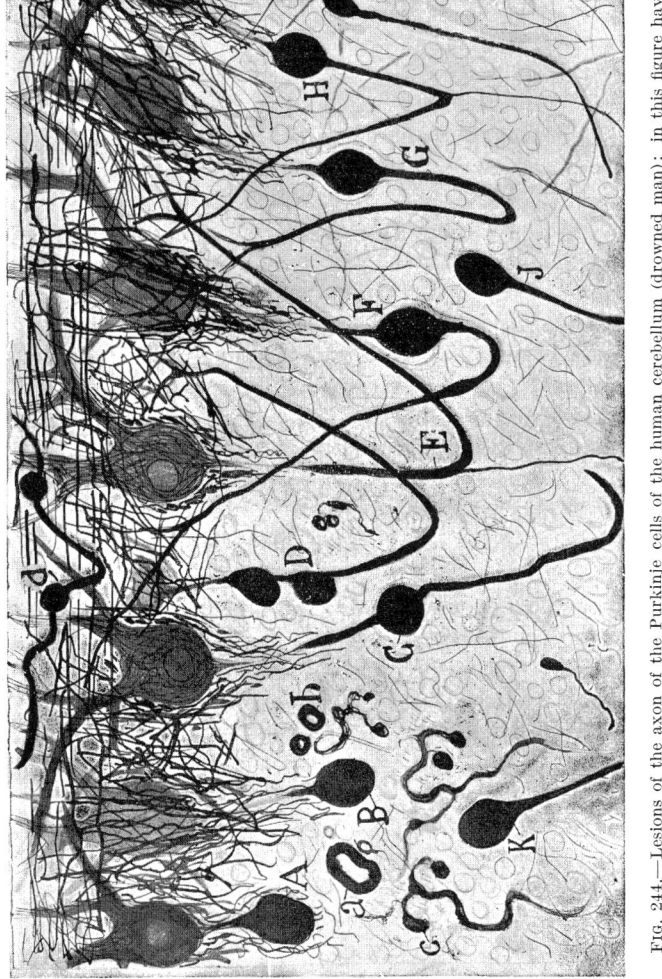

FIG. 244.—Lesions of the axon of the Purkinje cells of the human cerebellum (drowned man); in this figure have been drawn the principal lesions found in a single section. A, B, terminal balls situated near the cell; D, arciform axon with a double ball; C, G, arciform axon whose ball lies at some distance from the arc; E, H, arc formed by the recurrent collateral, in which the axon appears to be a collateral of the collateral; J, K, fibres ending in a club.

(e) Hypertrophy of the bunches of moss-like fibres, whose terminal thickenings appear very dark and voluminous, and constitute terminal balls. Sometimes these thickenings break loose from their pedicle and, becoming independent, give rise to enormous rings (Fig. 244, a, b, c), which stain very deeply with colloidal silver.

(f) Hypertrophy of some fibres of the plexiform layer (Fig. 244, d). These fibres, which are very voluminous and ramified, show thick balls along their course or at their extremity.

(g) Disappearance of numerous Purkinje cells, at the level of which, as the authors have recognized, the terminal baskets still subsist.

(h) Finally, terminal clubs and balls that are centripetal, or in other words that end right in the granular layer, and that belong to fibres coming from the white matter (Fig. 244, J, K).

The examination of these dispositions of the human cerebellum, which have been in great part very accurately described by H. Rossi, Nageotte, and Marinesco and Minea, suggests an interesting problem. Are the above-mentioned recurrent collaterals the result of regenerative phenomena having their seat in the retraction ball, as H. Rossi believed, or are we dealing with pre-existing collaterals which are hypertrophied and have resisted the degenerative process, the latter ceasing precisely at their point of origin ?

Can the fact that the club sometimes has collaterals and sometimes not, result from the greater or less extent of the traumatic degeneration, which ends sometimes above, sometimes below the point of origin of these branches ?

The answer to these questions appeared in an experimental study of which the preceding description is but a summary.[1] Our observations showed, without any possible doubt, that the arciform dispositions shown by H. Rossi, Nageotte, Bravetta, and Marinesco and Minea in the human cerebellum are not neoformations of the retraction club, but the persistence of hypertrophied collaterals, after elimination of the peripheral axon, which has been seriously affected or perhaps destroyed by toxic substances (alcoholism, etc.).

It can be seen from the preceding descriptions and from the neuronal metamorphoses which we are about to discuss that all the modifications occurring after traumatisms are degenerative in character. If there is a new creation, it is always intimate, that is, intracellular. The neurobiones multiply, arrange themselves in new groups, but lack sufficient energy to cross the line of the interruption of the axon and to give rise to new sprouts. The *retraction ball*, which at first we

[1] Cajal : " Los fenómenos precoces de la degeneración neuronal en el cerebelo," *Trab. del Lab. de Invest. biol.*, t. 9, 1911.

believed might with time become transformed into a cone of growth, represents an act of sedentary reaction, without any power of vanquishing the surrounding obstacles, or energy to form new paths. Something appears to be lacking, such as food or a stimulant of the activity of the club, capable of rousing it from its apathy and quiescence. The neurobiones doubtless become more numerous under the influence of the traumatic stimuli, and this explains the notable

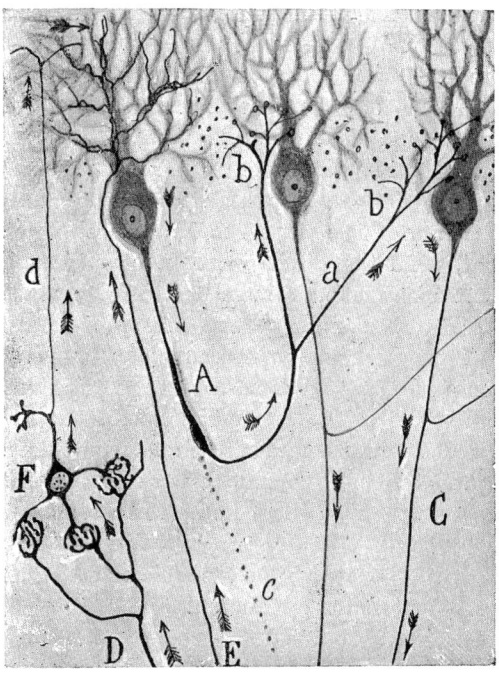

FIG. 245.—Schematic drawing designed to show the path of the currents in the Purkinje cells that are deprived of the peripheral portion of the axon. *A*, arciform Purkinje cell; *D* moss-like fibres; *E*, climbing fibre; *F*, granule; *C*, normal Purkinje axons; *c*, position previously occupied by the axon that has disappeared.

hypertrophies of axons and collaterals, as well as the appearance of buds and strings of balls; but that *something* which in peripheral nerves disturbs the equilibrium of the nervous protoplasm and traces a path by which the neurobiones emerge in the shape of fibres, that *ignotum quid* which at once nourishes and directs the assimilation and growth of the stump of the axon, is absent in the cerebellum, which appears to us as an essentially immutable organ, incapable of any process of reconstruction. Finally, we must not forget that we are dealing with a centre of reflex phenomena, where all must be perfect, ended, definite;

unlike the cerebrum, where, as we shall note below, the plasticity of axons and neurones is much greater, although it never reaches the regenerative power of the nerves.

Conjecture as to the physiological significance of the Purkinje cells provided with arciform axons.—Since arciform fibres are found with relative frequency in the cerebellum of the aged who have no apparent nervous diseases, it seems very probable that, as occurs in the ganglia, fatigue or other pathological causes, such as toxins and poisons of intestinal origin, alcohol, etc., bring about after a long time the irreparable destruction of some Purkinje fibres. The cells with a short axon thus produced would be unable to reconstitute the lost functional expansion. But, nevertheless, they would not prove completely useless, as Nageotte and Kindberg believe, with their conjecture of the vicious circle. The impulses arising in elements which are dissociated peripherally would fall back upon cells with a normal axon, thus increasing the energy of the efferent currents. In this way there would be established, even though imperfectly, something like a dynamic compensation, which up to a certain point is comparable with cardiac, glandular, and muscular compensations, provoked by permanent deficiencies of congenerous organs. It is very possible that such functional compensations are formed through the same mechanism in the brain and spinal cord. As we shall point out in later chapters, the traumatized cerebral cortex also contains pyramidal cells with a short axon, produced in the same way, and entirely similar to those described above in the cerebellar laminae. In the schematic Fig. 245, we show the dynamic effect of the disappearance of the axon of a Purkinje cell, in harmony with the probable plan of the normal path of nervous impulses across the cerebellum.

II

CONTINUATION OF THE DEGENERATIVE AND METAMORPHIC PROCESSES CONSEQUENT ON CEREBELLAR TRAUMATISMS

Degenerative phenomena occurring in the neurones and their dendrites—aneuritic cells and rosaliform, hirudiform, etc., dispositions of the neurofibrillar reticulum. —Swelling of the soma and dendrites.—Destruction of the reticulum.—Creation of aberrant expansions.—Alterations of the basket cells, moss-like fibres, and other elements in the cerebellum.

THE immediate reactions of the Purkinje cells are of many varieties, and their importance, form, and character depend very largely on the proximity of the soma to the wound. In general, from twenty-four hours after the operation, the edges of the wound appear necrosed and present a granular aspect. If anything remains alive of its fibres and cells, colloidal silver is incapable of revealing it. Indeed the stainable portion of the cerebellar tissue, whose cells show active or reactional structural modifications, is always, or almost always, situated at some distance from the traumatism. The necrosed region often involves half the thickness of a cerebellar lamina, or even more. After the first series of stainable cells there follow, with a certain order, in the direction of the healthy regions, various types of neuronal metamorphoses, which we may distinguish under four heads.

(1) *Anaxonic cells, that is, cells without axons.* (2) *Cells with short axonic masses.* (3) *Cells with a clubbed axon and with hypertrophic recurrent collaterals.* (4) *Cells whose axon is in continuity, in the form of an arc, with hypertrophic recurrent collaterals.* Having already spoken of the last three cellular types, in connection with the alterations of the axon, it now remains for us to study the first type, that is, the Purkinje cells deprived of axons—in consequence of a retrograde necrosis—which are remarkable for the surprising metamorphoses that occur in the neurofibrillar skeleton.

Aneuritic cell, that is, without a neurite or axon.—Nothing is more usual than to find near the wound Purkinje cells that are perfectly stainable but in which one cannot detect the least trace of an axon. This absence of a functional expansion, compatible with the temporary maintenance of cellular life, occurs, not only in cells in the vicinity of a wound or of exudates and haemorrhagic foci, which necessarily cause a necrosis of this fibre near the soma, but also in Purkinje cells situated far from the traumatism, although at no great distance from the pale or necrobiotic region.

These Purkinje cells, lying in an inflamed region or near it, behave in different ways, according to the route by which the exudates invade them, and other as yet unknown circumstances. Leaving aside, for the present, the productive mechanism, a problem very difficult to elucidate, and confining ourselves to objective facts, we may say that the anaxonic Purkinje cell is seen under the following forms : (*a*) *a cell with soma and dendrites hardly altered* ; (*b*) *a mallet-shaped cell or cell of a rosaliform type* ; (*c*) *a hirudiform cell* ; (*d*) *a glomerular cell* ; (*e*) *a cell with dendritic neoformations* ; (*f*) *a necrotic or granular cell*.

(*a*) *Scarcely altered Purkinje cell.*—Notwithstanding the vicinity of the lesion, the cellular soma is sometimes little modified, showing after twenty-four or forty-eight hours a well-stained dendritic arborization, which seems normal in its texture. The nucleus is frequently situated at the inferior pole of the cells, but at other times occupies a central position. A necrosed region is seen under the soma, without the least indication of a functional expansion. In such elements neither the incipient nests, nor the terminal balls of the recurrent collaterals, attract the colloidal silver.

(*b*) *Rosaliform disposition.*—In this cellular type the form of the soma is little altered, but the neurofibrillar network takes on a greater density and stainability than usual, and the nucleus is situated at the inferior pole, with its chief axis transversal, and leaning heavily on the membrane. On the other hand the trunk, and especially the secondary dendritic branches, assume a curious and elegant shape. Instead of showing thick, pale trunks and robust secondary branches emerging from triangular chiasmas or thickenings, and dividing up into digitiform branchlets, pale in colour and ending in a point, as occurs in normal Purkinje cells, the cells, in the form of a rose-bush, have thin dark trunks, without chiasmatic thickenings, which break up into a great number of very fine branches ; these take the stain intensely and end in a kind of club or bulb, which is remarkably swollen and deeply stained (Fig. 246, *a*). These terminal bulbs lend to the protoplasmic branchings the aspect of a pot of flowers. A careful analysis of these terminal buds reveals in them very clearly a network of wide meshes entirely comparable to that shown by the terminal thickenings of the arborization of motor plates, a network lying within a hyaline material which corresponds to the old necrosed protoplasm.

If one compares, as may be done in Fig. 246, these peculiar dendritic arborizations with normal examples, one recognizes not only the existence of an intradendritic retraction of the neurofibrillar

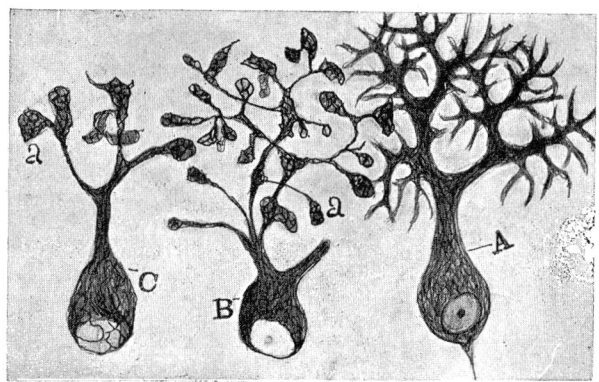

FIG. 246.—Purkinje cells of a cat, twenty days old, killed two days after a traumatic lesion. *A*, normal cell; *B, C*, cells whose dendrites are retracted and end in reticulated clubs; *a*, terminal bulbs.

network, but also its reconstruction on new bases. In some cells this metamorphosis is associated with a notable diminution of the number of terminal dendrites, which, by way of compensation, end in bulbs, triangular, ovoid, or voluminously lobulated (Fig. 246, *C*, and Fig. 239, *b*). The old dendrites, now devoid of neurofibrils, persist for various periods under the form of granular tracts.

The above observations with regard to the rosaliform type relate to animals killed two or three days after the operation. It was of interest to determine how this lesion behaved on the following days. For this purpose we killed some cats one week and ten days after the traumatism (Fig. 247). This afforded confirmation of the persistence of the above-mentioned disposition of the dendrites in those cerebellar laminae whose molecular layer, little altered, touches the necrotic zone or adjoins the blood clot or exudate of the wound. One may note that not all the cells of a same region, nor all the dendrites of a same cell, show the rosaliform disposition. Usually it is the higher expansions, that is, those nearest to the traumatism, which are metamorphosed. The details of the metamorphosis show some variation. The contrast between the thickness of the dendrite and the terminal bulb is less great. Finally, in some tangential dendrites near to the lesion we find, from time to time, an enormous

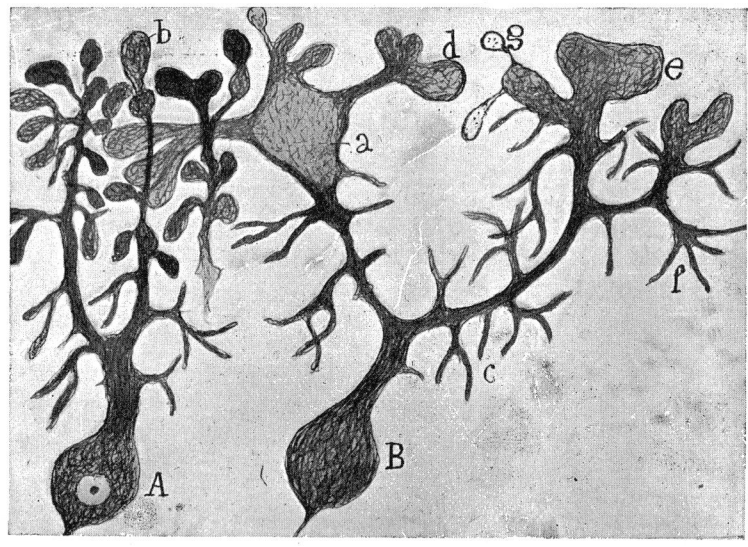

FIG. 247.—Purkinje cells of a cat, one month old, killed ten days after the traumatism. On the uninjured molecular layer was an unresorbed coagulum, situated near the wound. *A*, cell with numerous terminal balls situated high up; *B*, cell with enormous grumes and triangular dilatations; *a*, triangular dilatation at the level of a dendritic chiasma; *b, d*, terminal bulbs; *e*, considerable terminal dilatation; *g*, fine diverticula full of cytoplasm; *c*, normal dendrites.

hypertrophy with colossal swellings, of which Fig. 247, *B*, gives an idea. At the level of these monstrous dilatations the neurofibrillar network becomes pale (*a, d, g*), and in the largest of them one notices a central hyaline vacuole and a peripheral cortex, more or less stained by the colloidal silver, a remnant of the neurofibrillar framework. This curious alteration shows that the exaggeration of the rosaliform disposition may lead to the partial necrosis of the dendrites.

We have stated that, ordinarily, the axon is lacking in neurones undergoing the rosaliform reaction. Nevertheless, in cats killed seven and ten days after the traumatism one finds, now and then, cells of this type, in which the axon is still present (Fig. 247, *B*), especially among those partially affected by the lesion. The rosaliform disposition is therefore not special to anaxonic neurones, but it seems to be a local reaction of the dendrites in presence of stimuli diffused through the molecular layer and usually arriving through its surface.

Various authors have spoken of a local dendritic dilatation that recalls to some extent the facts noted above. Limiting ourselves to the observations made by neurofibrillar methods, we may say that K. Schäffer found cystic formations in the dendrites of pyramidal cells

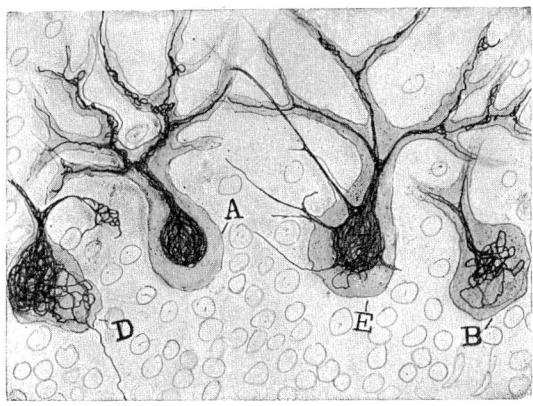

FIG. 248.—Purkinje cells of the cerebellum of a cat, fifteen days old, thirty-six hours after the operation; these elements were situated not far from the necrotic region. *A, E,* cells of the hirudiform type; *B, D,* glomerular cells.

in *amaurotic idiocy*. This same author [1] described pale terminal tumefactions in the dendrites of Purkinje cells in *Tay-Sachs' disease*. Similar tumefactions have been seen by Sach and Strauss,[2] and Schob [3] in family amaurotic idiocy. Nageotte and Kindberg [4] also describe, in a case of *ordinary idiocy*, Purkinje cells whose dendrites show hollow nodosities containing numerous argentophilous granules, especially at the level of

[1] K. Schäffer: "Zur normalen und pathologischen Fibrillenbau der Kleinhirnrinde," *Hirnpathol. Beiträge aus dem hirnhistol. Institut der Universität Budapest*, 2 Heft, 1913.

[2] Sach and J. Strauss: "The cell changes in amaurotic family idiocy," *Jour. of experim. Med.*, vol. 12, 1910.

[3] Schob: "Zur pathol. Anat. der juvenilen Form der amaurotischen Idiotie," *Zeitsch. f. die Gesamt. Neurol. u. Psych.*, Bd. 10, 1912.

[4] Nageotte et Kindberg: *Loc. cit.*

their bifurcations. From the walls of these dendritic tumefactions or from their immediate surroundings there arise numerous fine branches, which Nageotte believed to be newly formed. Finally, Straussler,[1] in *cerebellar atrophy*, and Ruiz de Arcaute,[2] in *hereditary syphilis*, also note the existence of similar intraprotoplasmic cavities, full of products of disintegration that are more or less stainable by colloidal silver.

(c) *Hirudiform type*.—This metamorphosis, described by ourselves in the cerebrum and spinal cord, also occurs in the Purkinje cells of the traumatized cerebellum thirty-six hours after the operation and onwards. As can be seen in Fig. 248, the alteration consists in a concentration of the neurofibrillar network around the nucleus and

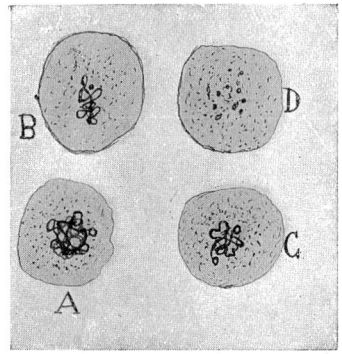

FIG. 249.—Cells in which the reticulum, in course of destruction, is reduced to a few loops situated near the nucleus which is half destroyed (*A*, *B*, *C*). *D*, cell in which only argentophilous granules remain, apparently remnants of the reticulum that has disappeared.

in the axis of the dendritic trunks (*A*). At the level of the cortical regions of the soma and dendrites one sees only a pale protoplasm of a slightly granular character. In general, the persistent neurofibrillar network reveals a certain tendency to the coalescence and fusion of its elements, and because of this one cannot always discern the individual threads of the network. In other cases the neurofibrils stand out better, and even appear to have undergone a process of hypertrophy and of reconstruction.

[1] Straussler: " Ueber einenartige Veränderungen der Ganglienzellen und ihrer Forsätze im Zentralensystem eines Falles von kongenitaler Atrophie," *Neurol. Centralbl.*, 1906.

[2] Ruiz de Arcaute: " Sobre algunas alteraciones de las células de Purkinje del cerebelo en un caso de sífilis hereditaria," *Boletín de la Sociedad Española de Biología*, sesión del 16 de Febrero de 1912.

An examination of the various phases of this process shows that we are apparently dealing with a neurobionic necrobiosis, which extends from the somatic and dendritic cortex towards the central portions, where the living units of the protoplasm resist for a longer or a shorter time, reacting against the stimuli by new reconstruction of the neurofibrillar skeleton. The *hirudiform alteration* probably leads to the total destruction of the Purkinje cell. As early as two days after the operation one sees cells in which the neurofibrillar colony displays signs of approaching destruction. As we show in Fig. 248, *B*, the neurofibrils successively abandon the dendrites,

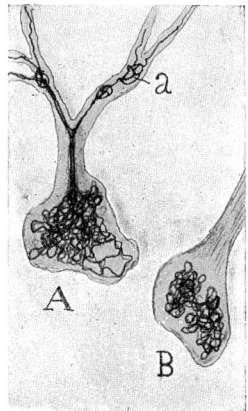 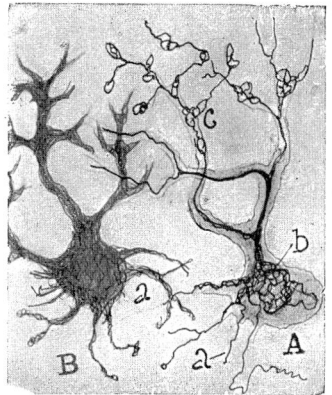

FIG. 250.—Purkinje cells with a glomerular reticulum (cat killed two days after the operation). *a*, intradendritic glomeruli.

FIG. 251.—Cells provided with descending dendrites (cat fifteen days old, killed thirty-six hours after the operation). *b*, glomerular reticulum; *c*, intradendritic nets.

confining themselves exclusively to the perinuclear region, where they form loose reticulations and capricious ansiform dispositions. Later on the network becomes even simpler, forming a structure which reminds one very much of the spireme thread in mitosis (Fig. 250, *A*, *B*); finally, when the process is almost ended, a very small neurofibrillar colony stands out in the soma, and soon disappears (Fig. 249, *C*, *D*), breaking up into scattered granules.

The *hirudiform alteration* seems to be a transitory process. Six days after the operation cells of this type are very rare, and after ten days the examination of more than thirty sections of a cat's cerebellum revealed only one example (Fig. 252, *A*). In it the perinuclear net was very thin, and its meshes were loose and irregular.

(d) *Glomerular metamorphosis.*—In certain cells, which are usually less involved in the inflammation than the cells of the *hirudiform* type, the reticulum takes a deep black stain and its neurofibrils, which are considerably hypertrophied and relatively isolated one from the other, form a kind of glomerulus or spool of sinuous threads. At the proper time, as occurs also in the *hirudiform* type, one sees under the membrane a more or less thick zone of neuroplasm which is pale and lacks filaments, crossed by a few loops and knots of neurofibrils (Figs. 250 and 251, and Fig. 248, B and D).

The most common dispositions of the glomerulus are shown in Figs. 248 and 250, where one sees that the neurofibrillar skeleton often forms small secondary lobules or glomeruli or isolated peripheral loops. One also frequently sees that the somatic glomerulus is continuous with a system of intradendritic axial neurofibrils similar to those of the hirudiform type. Finally, one finds within the dendrites, at times, thickenings of the reticulum formed by loose nets of few meshes (Fig. 251, c, and 250, a). One finds many transitions between the glomerular, hirudiform, and rosaliform types, which often render classification difficult, as may be seen by comparing Figs. 248, 250, and 251.

The structural peculiarities of the *hirudiform, glomerular,* and *rosaliform* types are interesting in several ways. They show that destruction of the neurofibrils, at least their unstainability or hyalinization, constantly begins at the cortical layer of the protoplasm and is propagated towards the centre, where the reticulum resists for a certain time. It appears as though the cortical portion of the reticulum, in presence of some noxious substance arriving from the inflammatory zone, undergoes necrobiosis, the central portion reacting with compensatory or reconstructive sprouts. Above all, however, these alterations show how erroneous is the doctrine of those neurologists for whom the neurofibrils are a fixed and stable element, incapable of other variations than those which result from their mechanical approximation or separation, consequent on the action of endosmotic currents or of nutritive disturbances.

(e) *Vacuolated Purkinje cells.*—Vacuolations have been seen by numerous authors in pathological nerve cells and even in normal cells (Athias, Mencl, etc.). Such alterations are very frequent after traumatisms, being especially abundant in the neurones adjacent to the region where substance has been lost. In Fig. 252 we show some varieties of vacuolated Purkinje cells. In *A* the process begins, and a spheroidal hollow space is formed of no great size; in *B* the vacuole notably distends the soma, pushing aside the nucleus and the neurofibrillar network. Finally, in the cell *E* there remain only the membrane, more or less wrinkled, and granular remnants of the reticulum spread like a dark limbo within this covering. The vacuolation thus ends in the total destruction of the cytoplasm and nucleus.

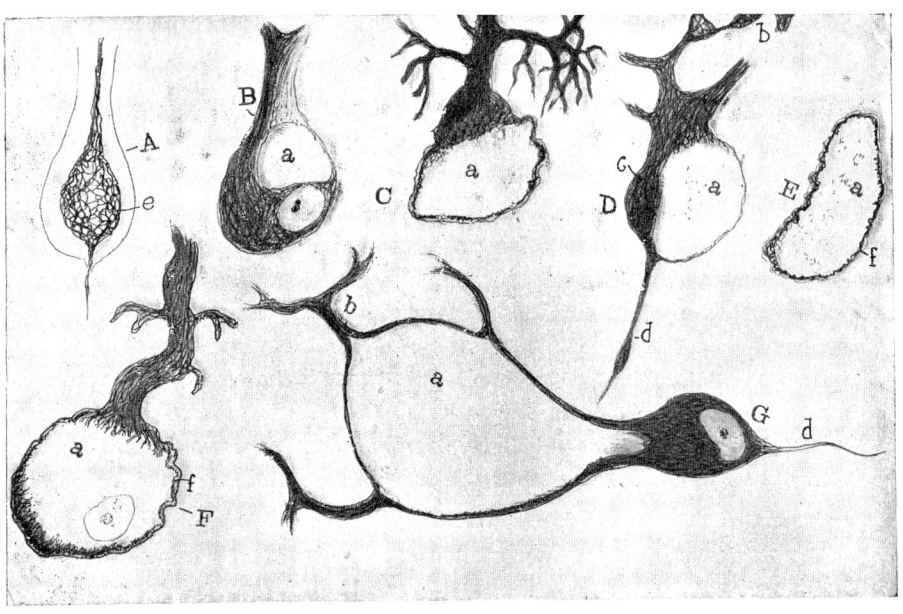

FIG. 252.—Vacuolated Purkinje cells from the cerebellum of a cat, twenty-five days old, ten days after the operation. *A*, hirudiform cell; *G*, colossal vacuole situated in the dendritic trunk; *C*, *D*, *F*, large vacuoles; *E*, cell transformed into a bladder; *f*, remnants of the reticulum; *d*, axon.

The vacuoles may also be situated in the principal trunk and dendrites. In Fig. 252, *G*, we show a cell in which the trunk has been enormously hollowed out owing to a great amount of liquid, part of which appears to open up and to try to penetrate within the secondary branches. Under the irresistible pressure of these liquid masses the neurofibrillar net atrophies rapidly, becoming deliquescent.

In the majority of cases the axon is unstainable; at other times it is impregnated by the colloidal silver, appearing thick and showing fusiform thickenings.

Such a vacuolar alteration implies the presence, around the soma and dendrites, of a solid and elastic membrane, which is capable of offering a long resistance to great pressures.

Purkinje cell with newly-formed dendrites.—In the glomerular type one not infrequently sees neurofibrils which, abandoning the inferior and lateral part of the soma, lose themselves in the granular layer. In Fig. 251, *A*, we reproduce a cell of this type, which represents, in respect of the disposition of the dendrites, a transition between the rosaliform and the hirudiform cells. The descending dendrites also appear in cells in which there is no axon, whose soma and dendrites show little or no alteration (Fig. 251, *B*).

Necrosed Purkinje cells.—The traumatism rapidly brings about a necrosis of the Purkinje cells that are close to the wound. Twelve hours after the operation there are often lacking, on the edges of the lesion, series of six, eight, and more cells of this type. And the curious thing is that one cannot see even their remnants. Active autolysis and resorption seem to have consumed even the remains of the protoplasm. Sometimes the cell-bodies cannot be seen, while a few pieces of the dendritic arborization take the stain, showing a granular reticulum. At the point of transition from the necrosed zone to the metamorphic, stainable zone, one finds a few pale Purkinje cells, which are very granular and in course of disruption and autolysis. Among the protoplasmic granulations, some are large and are impregnated by the colloidal silver. Nests of such elements survive, more or less, the necrobiosis of the soma (Fig. 254, *B*, *D*).

Alterations of other constituent factors of the cerebellum.—We have hitherto spoken almost exclusively of the perturbations occurring in the Purkinje cells and their nervous and dendritic expansions. Such a preference is justified by the fact that it is these elements which are mainly impregnated by the colloidal silver in young and recently-born animals. The same preparations, however, also show, although less pronounced, some changes in the pericellular baskets, in the moss-like fibres and axons of the white matter, etc.

Baskets of the Purkinje cells.—While these are perfectly formed in animals from twenty to thirty days old, they are constantly altered in the vicinity of wounds, although they never react so actively and energetically as the axons of the Purkinje cells.

The lesions most commonly found are as follows :

(*a*) Baskets whose descending appendices have terminal balls. We have found this disposition only precociously in young animals whose baskets seem to be well formed. As can be seen in Fig. 253, *A*, the Purkinje cells have been resorbed, and the descending branches of the baskets, notably thickened and intensely stained, end in a terminal ball or in a series of clubs. Such varicosities may also be seen in the course of the descending branches. When the lesion of the nests is very severe, these branches assume a granular aspect and undergo necrobiosis. The transversal fibres or axons from which the baskets proceed nearly always appear fairly normal ; at most they show some irregularities in their thickness and a granular aspect. Nevertheless, in the cerebellum of a cat twenty days old, which was killed twenty-four hours after the lesion, we have found them here and there showing varicosities and ending in clubs right in the molecular layer.

(b) *Loose and contracted baskets.*—The baskets resist pathological influences much more than do the Purkinje cells. Some time ago D. García and ourselves [1] observed that in dogs and rabbits suffering from hydrophobia the descending branches which form the nest survive the atrophy and destruction of the Purkinje cell, undergoing modifications of position and resisting perfectly the effects of the infection. Similar lesions are found in the pip of dogs. In man Nageotte and Kindberg, Marinesco and Minea, have also seen persistent baskets in regions where the Purkinje cells were wanting or had undergone grave alterations.

The baskets in young traumatized animals appear nearly normal, even at the level of regions where the cells have disappeared. The only appreciable modifications consist in the proximity of the descending branches which tend to invade the region formerly occupied by the absent neurone, and a certain disposition to constitute flakes or flexuous descending brushes. In cats and dogs from fifteen to twenty days old these brushes rarely have a varicose aspect (Fig. 254, *D*).

Fibres with balls in the molecular layer.—On different occasions, and especially in preparations of the cerebellum of dogs which were suffering from distemper (*Hundertaupe*), we have seen transversal fibres in the molecular zone.

One also finds them in sections of the traumatised cerebellum, not far from the wound. But it is commoner to find clubs at the end of certain radial fibres that come from the granular layer and probably represent recurrent collaterals in a degenerative phase.

[1] Cajal y D. García : " Las lesiones del retículo de las células nerviosas en la rabia," *Trab. del Lab. de Invest. biol.*, t. 3, 1904.

In old and alcoholic men one not infrequently observes hypertrophic fibres terminated by balls in the molecular layer (Fig. 244, d).

Moss-like bunches.—In sections of the cerebellum of cats from fifteen to twenty days old the bunches of moss-like fibres stain badly, perhaps because they are not completely formed. On the other hand, in cats, dogs, and rabbits that are more than a month old they stain better, showing here and there hypertrophic branches and bunches, the extremities of which assume the appearance of buds and even of rings, supported by a fine pedicle (Fig. 239, c).

This exaggeration of the terminal bulbs of the rosaceous fibres and the formation of robust free rings is notably accentuated in the

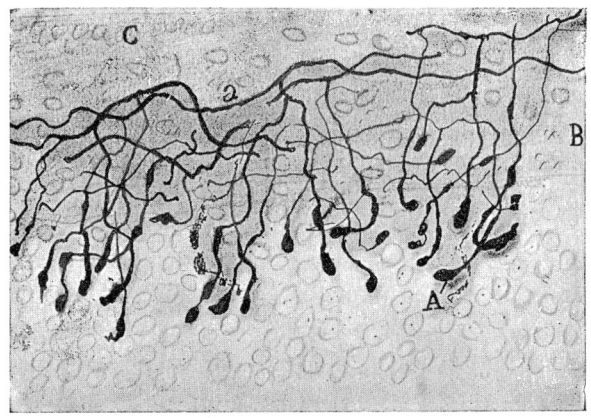

FIG. 253.—Baskets of the Purkinje cells of a rabbit, two months old, thirty hours after the operation. *A* terminal clubs; *B*, molecular layer; *a*, transversal fibres of this zone.

human cerebellum. As we show in Fig. 244, b, the terminal branches of the rosaceous fibres, in their hypertrophic movement, finally detach themselves and constitute independent neurobional colonies, which at times take on colossal dimensions (a).

Persistence of the climbing fibres.—In the same way that the baskets survive the soma of the Purkinje cells, the terminal arborization of climbing fibres subsists when it is impossible to discern the slightest remnants of the dendritic ramifications of these elements. This persistence occurs near the wound and can be especially well seen twenty-four hours, and at most three days, after the operation. The ramification of the moss-like fibre stands out vigorously on the pale plexiform zone, showing all its secondary and tertiary ramifications intact. As we have found no climbing fibres subsisting after three days where the molecular layer is devoid of even the slightest sign of cells, it appears that, at the end of a few days, hyalinization and resorption occur in them also.

The fact of the survival of baskets and climbing fibres, when the Purkinje cells have disappeared through hyalinization and resorption, constitutes a serious argument against the opinion of those authors who, like Bielschowsky, Wolff, and others, still believe that there are communications between these arborizations and the neurofibrils of the cytoplasm of the cells that they surround.

Hypertrophic axons of the Golgi cells of the granular layer.—Apart from the axons of the baskets, the axons of the cerebellar short-axon

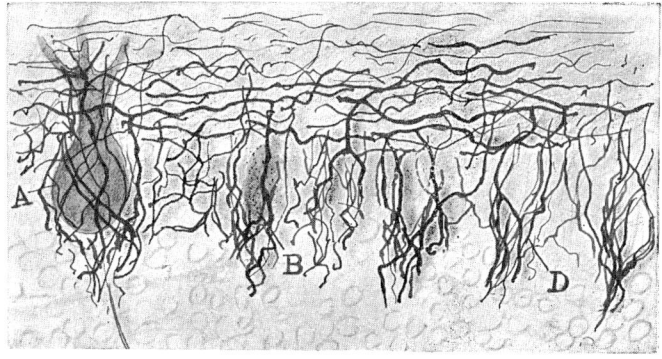

FIG. 254.—Cat, twenty-five days old, twenty-four hours after the operation. *A*, almost normal Purkinje cell; *B*, Purkinje cell undergoing atrophy and granular in appearance; *D*, baskets surrounding the empty space previously occupied by Purkinje cells that are now destroyed.

cells do not attract the colloidal silver. Nevertheless, exceptionally and thanks to the hypertrophy brought about by the traumatic stimulus, we have occasionally found, within the granular layer, Golgi cells whose hypertrophic axon could easily be followed in its secondary and tertiary ramifications. The last branchlets, however, were imperceptible (Fig. 241, *a*).

This peculiar property of colloidal silver to render visible in a pathological state axons that are scarcely discernible under ordinary conditions is also confirmed in certain pericellular plexuses that we have pointed out [1] as being normal dispositions in the granular layer (Fig. 255, *B*). By reason of the hypertrophy of its plexuses, they appear in the vicinity of the traumatism with unusual clearness,

[1] Cajal: " Sobre ciertos plexos pericelulares de la capa de los granos del cerebelo," *Trab. del Lab. de Invest. biol.*, t. 10, 1912.

confirming the fact that recurrent collaterals of the Purkinje cells are instrumental in forming such nests. It is very possible that some of those plexuses or fascias, coming from the baskets, which H. Rossi describes as joining certain pairs of Purkinje cells, correspond to such nests, whose surrounded neurones are sometimes

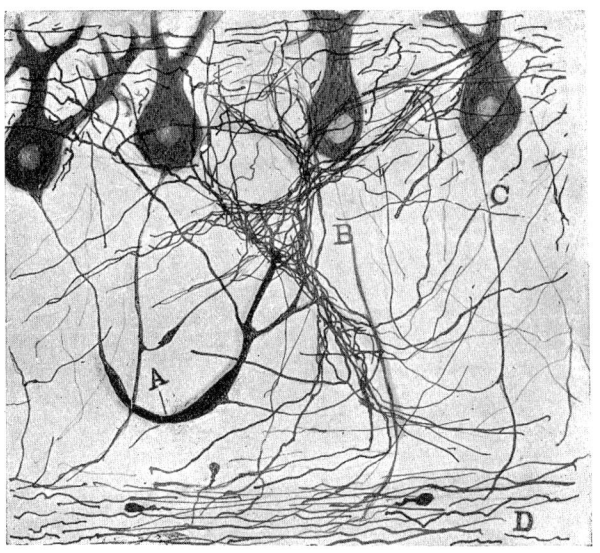

FIG. 255.—Piece of the cerebellum from a cat, twenty-five days old, three days after the operation. *A*, hypertrophic collateral, whose branches end in a nest; *B*, nest around a special triangular cell of the granular layer; *C*, normal Purkinje axon.

found at the same level as the above-mentioned cells. We may also recall that in the normal state uniting bundles between neighbouring baskets are met with sporadically, as we and Illera [1] noted some time ago, and as K. Schäffer [2] has confirmed in man.

[1] Cajal et R. Illera: "Quelques nouveaux détails sur la structure de l'écorce cérébelleuse," *Trav. du Lab. de Recher. biol.*, t. 5, 1907.

[2] K. Schäffer: *Hirnpathol. Beiträge*, etc., 2 Heft, 1913.

FOURTH PART

I

TRAUMATIC DEGENERATIVE PROCESSES OF THE CEREBRAL CORTEX

Necrotic phenomena consequent on wounds.—Preserved nerve fibres.—Preserved dendrites.—Preserved neurones.—Corrosion and autolysis of the axons and dendrites.—Degenerative metamorphoses of the peripheral stump.—Autotomy of the terminal spheres and their metamorphic phenomena.—Formation of neurofibrillar plexuses and buckles.

WHEN one wounds the cerebral cortex of a young mammal, such as a cat, dog, rabbit, etc., under the conditions indicated in our study of lesions of the spinal cord and cerebellum, the degenerative and reactional processes are repeated which were observed in the other nerve centres, but with variations of intensity and form which endue them with a special character. The axons of the central stump, although incapable of effective regeneration, testify, by their neurofibrillar transformations, to a surprising activity, far superior to that shown by the cerebellar neurones. The separation between the living and the necrosed portions is established with extraordinary rapidity and the processes of adaptive elimination begin immediately. The most characteristic fact, however, is the exquisite susceptibility of the cerebral fibres and cells to the mechanical effects of the traumatism. The least commotion, stretching or compression, especially when they are accompanied by diffusions of blood beyond the edges of the wound, bring about the almost instantaneous death of the nervous protoplasm and the peculiar phenomenon of *preservation*, that is, necrosis associated with the most perfect morphological integrity. The unusual development that this phenomenon may attain in cerebral wounds, and its transcendent importance and utility for the purpose of a correct appreciation of particular acts of supposed regeneration, as set out by certain authors, in lesions of the human cerebrum, make it necessary for us to describe the *preserved* fibres and cells in some detail.

Preservatory necrosis.—We may distinguish three variations of this curious process, corresponding to the three cellular segments in which it occurs : (*a*) *preservation of the axons* ; (*b*) *preservation of the dendrites* ; (*c*) *preservation of the neuronal bodies.*

(*a*) *Preserved axons of the white and grey matter.*—These are seen in great numbers in any cerebral wound, from the first hours after the operation; but their number increases enormously and involves large portions of grey and white matter when, owing to the hazards of the operation, the scalpel causes slight compressions, lacerations, or dislocations of the grey matter.

In Fig. 256, *C*, we reproduce a typical example of preserved axons. We are here dealing with the cerebrum of a cat, killed twenty-one hours after the lesion. In the central stump, which was somewhat compressed, and therefore necrosed, there clearly appear two regions : a marginal region, or region of indifferent axons, and a deep region, where the axons show reaction. Irregular series of terminal balls act as a somewhat ill-defined frontier between these two territories.

The marginal territory corresponds to the zone which was most strongly contused by the scalpel (Fig. 256, *C*) and which was most thoroughly permeated by the inflammatory exudate. In this region all the fibres without exception are *preserved*, that is, they retain their normal or almost normal calibre, they show no thickenings, and they stain very deeply with colloidal silver. Their path presents a disposition which at first sight differentiates them from living fibres. Their course is flexuous, frequently spiroidal, describing great curves to and fro, which give them a peculiar resemblance to elastic fibres. Their calibre, which is perfectly uniform, is variable, corresponding both to that of large medullated axons and to that of medium and fine non-medullated axons. Finally, and this is the most characteristic thing about preserved axons, of its two stumps, that which is cut or submerged in the exudate is without terminal ball, showing a point in the shape of a hook, which is semi-circular or, more commonly, doubled and bundled up in the form of a glomerulus (*D*); while the opposite or proximal stump, after a course of greater or less length, when it reaches the region of the terminal buds (the frontier of the degenerative reaction), tapers off, becomes progressively paler, and finally disappears completely.

As a rule the zone of the preserved fibres encloses no stainable neurone. Most of the cells that were energetically contused not only succumbed, owing to the traumatic violence, but also underwent lacerations and disruptions of the reticulum, rupture of the membrane, projection of the nucleus, and other very grave disorders, incompatible with the maintenance of the stainability of the cytoplasmic and nuclear factors.

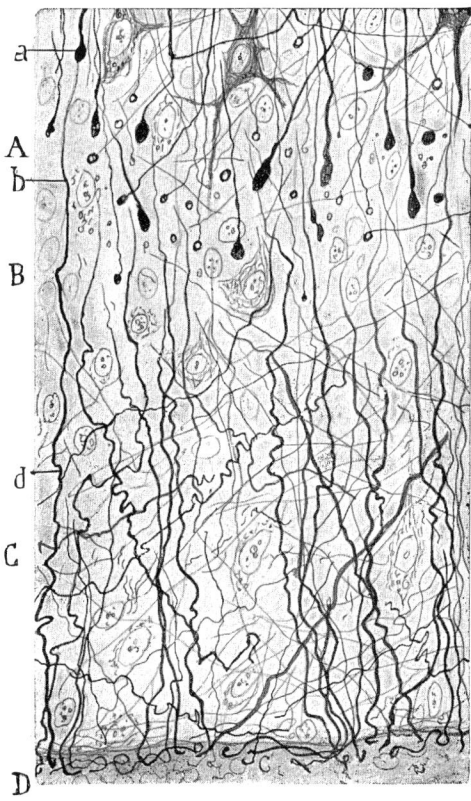

FIG. 256.—Proximal edge of a transversal wound of the cerebrum of a cat, one month old, which was killed twenty-one hours after the operation. *A*, living or reacting zone; *B*, zone of corrosion; *C*, zone of preserved fibres; *D*, exudate from the wound; *a*, reaction club; *b*, point of corrosion of a preserved fibre, which is still united to a healthy axon; *c*, floating points of preserved fibres.

Above the zone of the preserved fibres one finds the living region of the grey matter, the frontier which separates that which is degenerated from that which is merely preserved. This frontier can be seen as early as four hours after the lesion and perhaps before (we have no experiments to indicate what occurs earlier) and shows, as is well known, the terminal clubs and hypertrophic stumps of surviving axons.

In this intermediate region one sees that the preserved axon becomes gradually thinner and paler, until it ends in a *point of corrosion*.

A scrupulous examination of the point of union between the necrosed and the living tubes in wounds from three to five hours old allows one to detect the moment of segregation, that is, the phase in which the living segment detaches itself from the preserved segment. In Fig. 256, *a, b*, we show this phenomenon. We have there

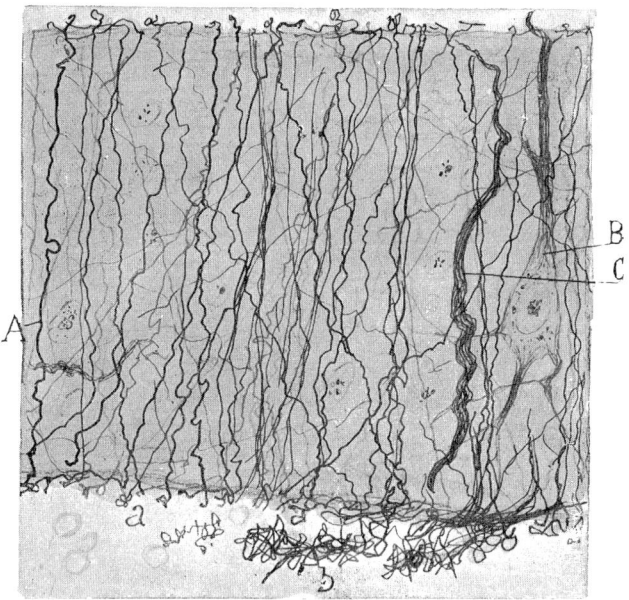

FIG. 257.—Transversal floating block of grey matter; cat, fifteen days old, killed two days after the operation. *A*, preserved axons; *B*, neurone whose soma is beginning to fade away; *C*, loose dendrite, serpentine in character, and ending in two points of corrosion; *a*, terminal glomeruli of the preserved axons.

a fine preserved fibre, whose distal stump is extended towards the exudate. On its deep side this axon tapers and fades away so as to form a fine point of corrosion ; before it breaks off, however, one can see it united, by means of a very slender bridge, to the terminal club of the living segment lying in the metamorphic zone. A few moments later the separation would have been complete and the club would have appeared as a retraction bud.

The small pieces of grey or white matter torn by the scalpel from the circumvolutions, which remained floating in the inflammatory coagulum or exudate, enclose fibres which are typically preserved

THE CEREBRAL CORTEX 635

and which show all the signs already noted when we discussed the contused edges of spinal wounds.

As can be seen in Fig. 257, *A*, which reproduces a thin transversal block, torn from the deep portion of the grey matter and fixed two days after the operation, the axons appear normal, completely crossing the block and coming out on both surfaces. These stumps, often arranged in the shape of hooks, or glomeruli, float in the exudate, appearing very dark, and having a spiroidal course and a perfectly clean outline. Naturally, the contrast that we noted above between the distal and the proximal stumps of the preserved axons is here lacking. This is inevitable, since in the present example both ends were from the first in similar conditions, that is, they were separated from the cell of origin and bathed in the same way in the exudate, which permeated and preserved them, strengthening their affinity for colloidal silver.

After two or three days, some fibres become pale and granular. The stumps become paler and more pointed. But the majority of the axons still subsist, with few variations, four, five, and six days after the lesion. Some of them, the thickest, become somewhat thicker, but do not form terminal balls or clubs. Among them all, the darkest and most persistent are always those which float isolated in the plasma or remain included in the exudate. Finally, complete hyalinosis of the sequestered pieces takes place only two or three weeks later.

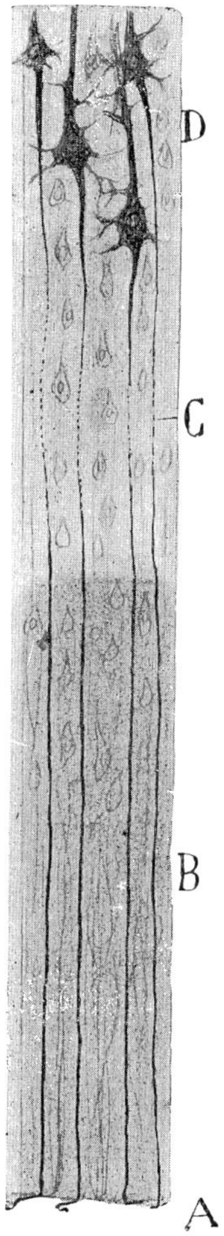

Another curious form of conservation of the axon is that observed in grey matter permeated owing to an interstitial haemorrhage. The sudden compression due to the haemorrhage, and perhaps also the absence of oxygen, cause the rapid death of the axons, while the neurones of origin remain alive for a longer or shorter time.

FIG. 258.—Schematic drawing showing the appearance of the grey matter of a large preserved block whose deep portion was infiltrated with blood. Dog, twenty days old, killed seven days after the operation. *D*, dead portion which appears normal; *B*, region preserved through infiltration by blood; *c*, intermediate region with signs of autolysis.

This phenomenon is shown schematically in Fig. 258. Here we have an extensive oblique section which had isolated almost an entire cerebral circumvolution and whose deep region (dark in Fig. 258) was infiltrated with blood. The axons were intensely impregnated, arranged in radiating bundles or in plexuses of small fascicles; in their midst, separating or rather dissecting them, one discerns a granular yellowish material containing remnants of erythrocytes and sprinkled with leucocytes. This substance is extravasated blood which has been modified by the action of the tissues. Here and there, right in the interstitial haemorrhage, there stand out admirably numerous free neuroglia cells and not a few neurones, which for the most part are fusiform and triangular, and belong to the zone of polymorphic cells. They are full of a granular material, which is stained a greyish yellow by the colloidal silver. All the axons, thick and thin, myelinated or non-myelinated, which are present in the interstitial coagulum, are free from signs of degeneration and are perfectly preserved, taking the stain with unusual intensity. If one follows them towards the cells of origin one sees them fading and thinning out at certain points which probably correspond to the nodes of the myelin, and extending in a proximal direction up to beyond the infiltrated or haemorrhagic zone. Once they have reached the edge of the nervous tissue which is free from the haemorrhagic infiltration, these fibres become pale and granular. That is to say, where the coagulum ends the preservation of the axons tends to be less effective, and something like a point of corrosion is formed (Fig. 258, C).

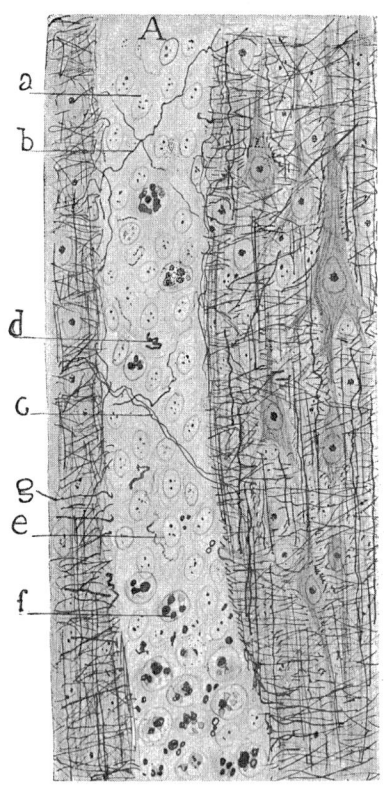

FIG. 259.—Cerebral wound of a young cat, with a thin neuroglial scar. A, scar; b, c, passing fibres; d, folded piece of axon; e, other piece which is granular and semi-resorbed; f, granular cells.

This and other cases of maintenance of the morphology of the axon in consequence of haemorrhage show that, as we said in connection with the preserved fibres of the nerves and spinal cord, *in the phenomenon of preservation a great part is played by some antiautolytic principle which proceeds from the sanguineous exudate and is fixed in the protoplasm of the axon.* It is perhaps due to this material that the axons in question have a special affinity for colloidal silver.

Finally, preserved fibres are found, though in smaller numbers, in all perpendicular or oblique wounds of the grey matter, even when the nervous contusion has been very small, on condition that the inflammatory exudate has infiltrated the edges of the lesion. This is what occurred in the cases shown in Figs. 259 and 260. The fine fibres that cross the exudate at *c* (Fig. 259), are necrosed non-medullated axons, which the scalpel had pulled towards the wound, where they remained unharmed during eight days. In Fig. 260, taken from a cat on which the operation was performed twelve days before the autopsy, the clipped fibres show

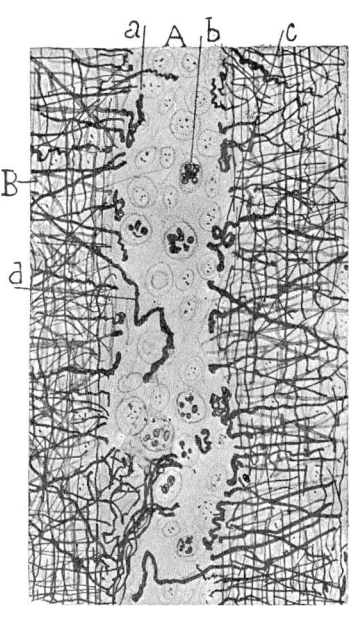

FIG. 260.—Scar in the wound of the white matter of a young cat's cerebrum. *A*, scar; *B*, white matter; *c, d,* fibres ending in a glomerulus, but without balls.

swollen and flexuose ends floating in the remnants of the exudate and incipient cicatricial tissue.

One can well understand how many errors may occur, when the observer, without being put on his guard, finds himself confronted with preparations in which he cannot see a single club nor any sign of a degenerative or regenerative process. Deceived by appearances, he might imagine, as happened to us at first, either that the peripheral stumps of the interrupted axons remain alive, thus falling into an absolute degenerative apathy, from which perhaps they may be able to emerge later; or else, on the contrary, that, after very rapid degeneration and absorption, they were immediately replaced by sprouts issuing from the central stump. To-day, taught by experience, we know with certainty that, not only the perforating fibres, but also all the apparently normal plexuses and neurones visible on the edges of certain wounds (see Figs. 259 and 260) represent necrosed and preserved parts. One may note especially (Fig. 259) the total absence of retraction clubs and of varicosities

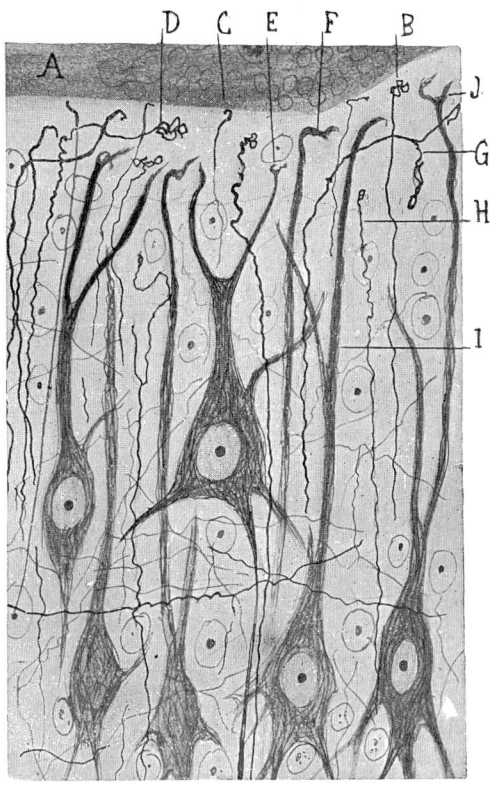

FIG. 261.—Pyramidal cells of the cerebral cortex of a cat, two months old, in which a horizontal cut was made. *A*, wound with remnants of the exudate; *B, C, D*, hooks and glomeruli which form the ends, in the wound, of the axons ascending towards the molecular layer; *E, F, J*, traumatized ends of the dendritic trunks.

along the fibres in the grey matter that is shown, although many interrupted collaterals—both transversal and oblique fibres—are included, and although seven or eight days have passed since the operation. The terminal glomerular swellings floating in the exudate, as shown in Fig. 260, are very significant.

(*b*) *Preserved dendrites.*—On several occasions we have tried to ascertain whether section of the dendrites belonging to the cerebral pyramidal cells is followed by the degenerative phenomena characteristic of axons. For this purpose the cerebral cortex affords us particularly easy technical conditions. Owing to the enormous length, the parallelism, and the exquisite radial orientation of the trunk of the pyramidal cells, nothing is easier than to divide their dendrites transversally, by tangential sections, causing the formation

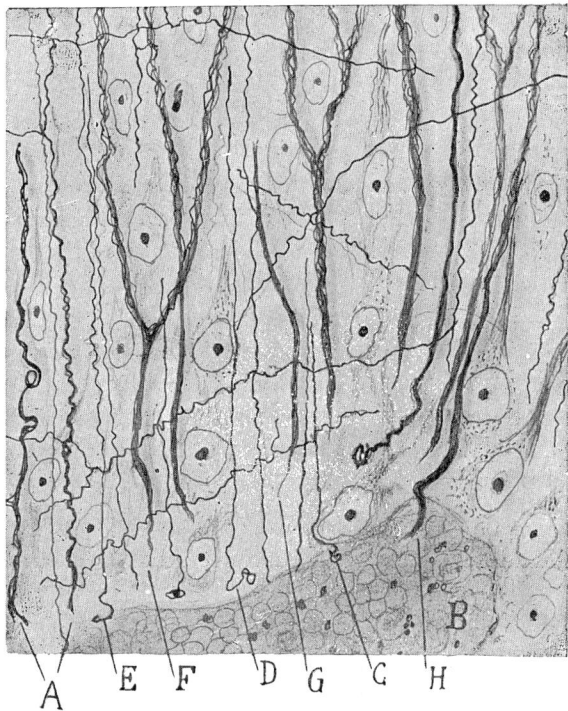

FIG. 262.—Superficial part of the cortex of the same wound as in Fig. 261 (cat two months old). *A, E, C, D*, terminal glomeruli of nerve fibres at the edges of the wound; *G, F, H*, deep corroded stumps of dendritic trunks; *B*, wound with haemorrhagic remnants.

of a central stump, that is, of a portion united to the neurone of origin, and of a peripheral stump which is cut off from its trophic centre.

The result of these experiments, made repeatedly by ourselves, is that *neither the central nor the peripheral stump of the cut dendrites is able to form buds, balls, or other phenomena of neurofibrillar reaction peculiar to traumatized axons.*

In Fig. 261 we show the appearance of the central dendritic

stump of several mutilated pyramidal cells. Here we were dealing with a cat, two months old, in which a wound was made which passed immediately above the layer of the large pyramidal cells, in the motor region. The animal was killed sixteen days after the operation. The hollow space of the wound was occupied by clear exudate, with remnants of erythrocytes and a few granular cells.

One may note that the trunks of the pyramidal cells and ascending protoplasmic branches connected with the trophic centre appear almost normal, as also the pyramidal cells on which they depend. One only remarks that as they reach the wound the dendrites become somewhat denser and darker, and end in various ways. Most of them fold back in a transversal direction and end in a brush-like point which is to some extent ravelled out and paler (Fig. 261, *F*). Others, after bending, show at their ends two pale terminal branches or brushes which are very short (Fig. 261, *J*) and of unequal length. In no case do they present a spiroidal course and a terminal spool as often occurs in the cut ends of nerve fibres (Fig. 261, *B*, *D*). Finally, many trunks and branches end in a point of corrosion.

In the peripheral stump (Fig. 262, *G*) the dendrites appear more or less altered and as though used up at their proximal ends. The majority of them terminate, at a certain distance from the lesion, in a pale point which at times is somewhat flexuose (point of corrosion). One may note that, near the wound, the neurofibrillar bundle of each trunk appears compact and deeply stained by silver nitrate; but as one recedes from the lesion the neurofibrils of the bundle become paler and looser, taking a sinuous form and thus enlarging the diameter of the radial trunk, which may be followed more or less well up to the first or plexiform layer. There thus takes place, in the proximal stump of all dendrites that are separated from their trophic centre, a process of atrophy or corrosion even more concentrated than that suffered by the stump which is joined to the cell of origin.

The absence of retraction clubs, varicosities, and sprouts, the passive conservation of the neurofibrils, their indifference in presence of the exudates and, finally, the appearance of a *point of corrosion* characteristic of preserved fibres, lead one to think that both the peripheral and the central stumps of the interrupted dendrites constitute a particular case of death followed by *preservation*. It is probable that the traumatic commotion caused the immediate necrosis, not only of the dendrites, but also of the neurones themselves, and that the exudate which rapidly penetrated and, as it were, embalmed them, transformed them into inert fibres, indifferent to autolysis. And as this phenomenon of neuronal death and preservation often occurs, even in cerebral wounds that are little contused, we must admit that, so far as the maintenance of cellular life is concerned, *the lesion of the large dendrites and especially of the radial trunk is much more serious than that of the axon.*[1] This seriousness may be a contingent phenomenon, due to the proximity of the lesion to the cellular soma.

(c) *Preservation of the neurones.*—The morphological preservation *in toto* of the nerve cells may be well studied in sequestered portions of the cerebrum by means of reiterated punctures or successive cuts in the cortex of young animals.

The most instructive portions are the voluminous and superficial ones, which have been completely separated from the subjacent cerebral mass, so that its deep vascular connections have disappeared. One of the most expressive examples seen by ourselves is that reproduced in Fig. 263. In this the sequestered portions were two, placed concentrically. One was superficial (A) and included the molecular layer, and the other deep (B), completely isolated, and corresponded to the zones of large and medium-sized pyramidal cells. The animal, a cat one month old, was killed six days after the operation.

That which first strikes one's attention in this cerebral islet, is

---

[1] Up to now, all efforts to recognize phenomena of active reaction in cells whose radial trunk has been extirpated (mitral cells of the olfactory bulb, pyramidal cells, etc.) have proved fruitless. According to the operation, the mutilated neurones either become rapidly necrosed, or remain for some time in the preserved state.

Rapid cellular death appears to be a consequence of propagation to the soma of the brutal mechanical commotion caused by the traumatism. To suppose, for example, that this destruction is due to the suppression of the principal afferent path of the stimuli is a hypothesis that can hardly be reconciled with the speed of the process. We believe, however, that the last word has not been said on this question. We think it possible, and even probable, that if the mutilation of the dendrites took place very far from the soma, and if one avoided as much as possible contusion of the wound, the neurone would preserve its vitality, and would do so the more in proportion as the part of the trunk in continuity with the soma was still able to receive nervous impulses. Moreover, do we not know that the neurones of spinal ganglia remain alive, although they lose, through section of the nerves, a large portion of their peripheral expansion or cellulipetal prolongation?

the excellent preservation of some of the neurones, as well as of their dendrites (Fig. 263, *B*). Their neurofibrils appear strongly stained and apparently completely normal. Nevertheless, a few neurones that were next to the interruption appeared granular, and their expansions hardly attracted the colloidal silver (Fig. 263, *g*). It is curious to note that in the cells that are best preserved the nucleolus has suffered no change, appearing composed of a conglomeration of

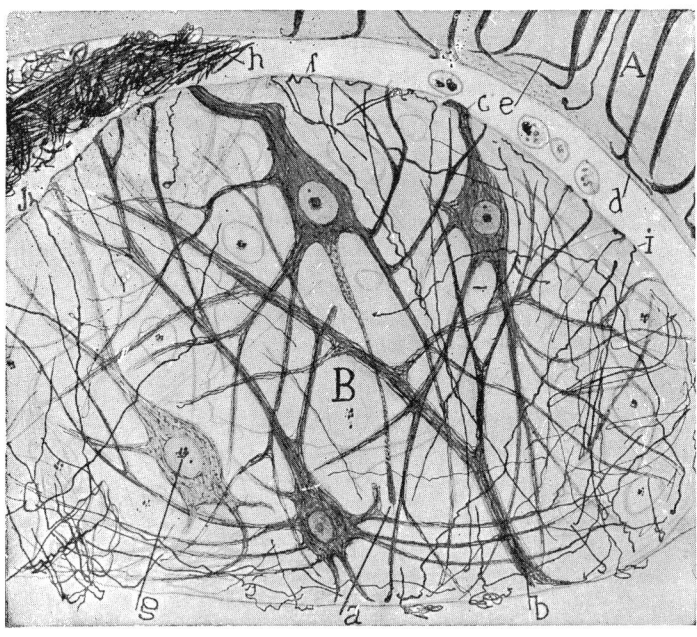

FIG. 263.—Cerebral sequestra of a cat, one month old, which was killed six days after the operation. *A*, superficial portion in which the deep stumps of the dendritic trunks are being corroded ; *B*, deep portion with an isolated cellular colony ; *a*, degenerated axon ; *b, c*, isolated trunks ; *d*, bifurcated dendritic stump ; *h*, block of dislocated nerve fibres ; *g*, disintegrated nucleolus.

deeply-stained spherules. Even the accessory granule is easily seen. At the same time, in the granular and pale neurones, the spherules of the nucleolus appear as though broken up and smaller than usual. The non-medullated nerve fibres are well preserved, taking various directions and frequently presenting a spiroidal appearance.

The behaviour of the axon of the elements present in the sequestered portion especially deserves attention. Where one could with certainty recognize the axon as such (Fig. 263, *a*), it appeared granular, as also did its cone of emergence ; after a pale and tapering course, it became somewhat thicker, showed a greater affinity for colloidal silver, and ended, not in a club of growth or of retraction, but in a blunt point, slightly thickened and comparable to the tip of a sound (Fig. 263, *a*). Sometimes, from this dark stump a short thread emerges, very fine and pale, a remnant of the vanished segment of the axon, which appears to undergo a process of corrosion.

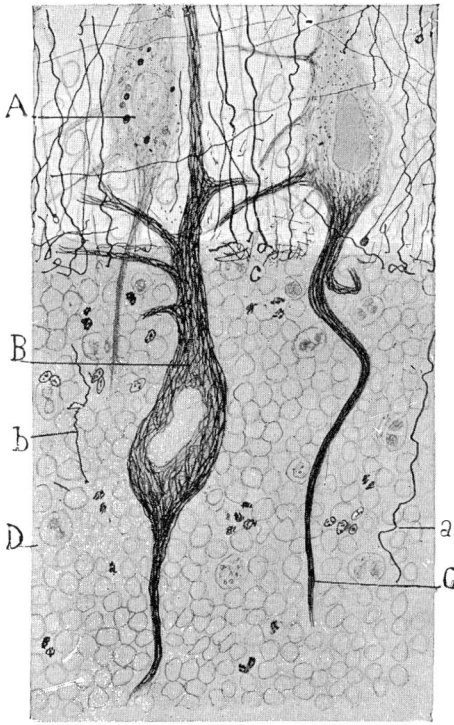

FIG. 264.—Two neurones preserved as a result of being mechanically drawn within a haemorrhage; cerebral wound of a cat, thirty days old, which was killed six hours after the operation. *A*, necrosed and granular neurone; *B*, preserved pyramidal cell.

That this axonic resorption or digestion is a real phenomenon is easily proved by the fact that the end of the axon appears almost constantly retracted a few millimetres from the edge of the wound.

The dendrites show the same phenomena as already described above, that is to say, all of them, in both the central and the peripheral stumps, end near the wound in a point of corrosion.

One may deduce from what has been said that the neurones, as well as the nerve fibres, die rapidly in sequestered fragments, owing to the traumatic commotion and the lack of oxygen, and that the cellular cadavers, with their expansions, remain several days in a state of morphological preservation and of resistance to autolysis.

The same thing occurs in the cerebral pyramidal cells that are pulled towards the exudate by the violence of the traumatism. We give an example of this in Fig. 264. It occurs also in the neurones that are asphyxiated as a consequence of diffuse and extensive haemorrhages of the cerebral cortex.

In Fig. 258, *D*, we reproduce schematically a case where certain neurones were surrounded at some distance by an interstitial coagulum, and where the neurofibrils remained indifferent several days. It is only in a few cells that the autolytic fragmentation of the axon and dendrites has begun.

DEGENERATIVE PHENOMENA OF THE PERIPHERAL STUMP

With some variations, the projection axons from cerebral pyramidal cells, when they are separated from their trophic centre, either within the grey cortex or in the white matter, reproduce the reactional and destructive metamorphoses that we have so often described. It is therefore superfluous to describe them afresh. We shall confine ourselves to a few new details concerning the medullated axon of large and medium-sized pyramidal cells in traumatisms of the cerebral cortex of young animals. As a general thesis, one may affirm that the peripheral segment of an axon interrupted near the pyramidal cell reacts more intensely than that of an axon clipped at a great distance from it, for example right in the white matter. These differences are sufficiently marked to justify a special study of the degenerative processes occurring in the two classes of peripheral stumps.

1. Degeneration of the peripheral stump when the section occurs in the white matter.—Apart from the portion that degenerates secondarily, the distal stump of the pyramidal axon includes two successive regions : the *necrotic* portion, and that undergoing *traumatic degeneration*.

Necrotic segment of the peripheral stump.—This represents, as we have repeatedly stated, that portion of the axon which is instantaneously disorganized by the mechanical violence and is resorbed very quickly in the absence of the preservative action of the autolytic substances. This process of liquefaction is so precocious that two hours after the traumatism the necrosed segment has very largely disappeared, the living or degenerated portion of the stump ending near the wound in the shape of the tip of a sound. A series of grains, which becomes successively thinner, shows at times the remnants of the necrotic segment in course of autolysis.

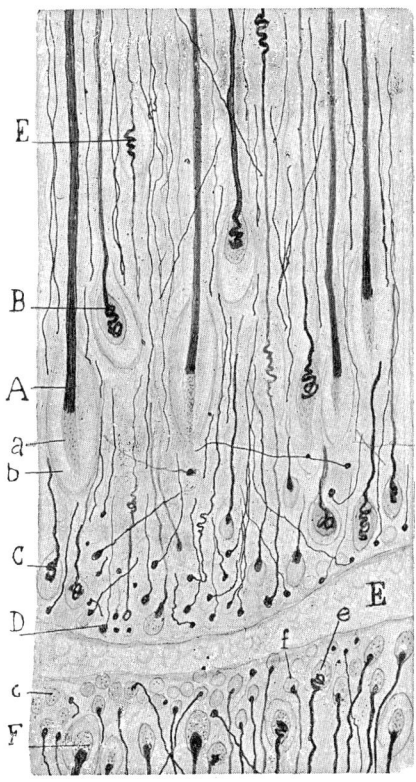

FIG. 265.—Cerebral wound of a cat, two months old, which was killed four hours after the operation. *A*, termination of the thick axons; *B*, stumps ending in glomeruli; *C*, *D*, ends of fine fibres; *E*, wound; *F*, peripheral stump; *E*, spirals along the course of the fibre.

We may add that the edges of the wound enclose semi-disintegrated axonic grumes and a great quantity of free balls and rings; in sections stained by osmic acid one may see that the largest balls possess a sheath of myelin. Needless to repeat, the preserved fibres, whether few or many, are never lacking.

Segment affected by traumatic degeneration.—From five to eight hours after the operation, the initial retraction balls or rings are formed, and one can see in many of them the well-known concentric layers : the *hyaline*, or peripheral, and the *central*, whose neurofibrils, perfectly stained, are arranged in complicated nets and loops. As a rule this neurofibrillar focus, in continuity with the axon, withdraws progressively towards the pedicle, where it remains a certain time.

The neurofibrillar focus of the terminal club does not always end in a homogeneous grume ; sometimes it appears replaced by a glomerulus surrounded by hyaline substance. It would seem as though, once the club is formed, the axon grew within it, trying to innervate it secondarily (Fig. 265,*e*). This peculiar folding of the axon appears, as we shall note below, much more developed in the central stump.

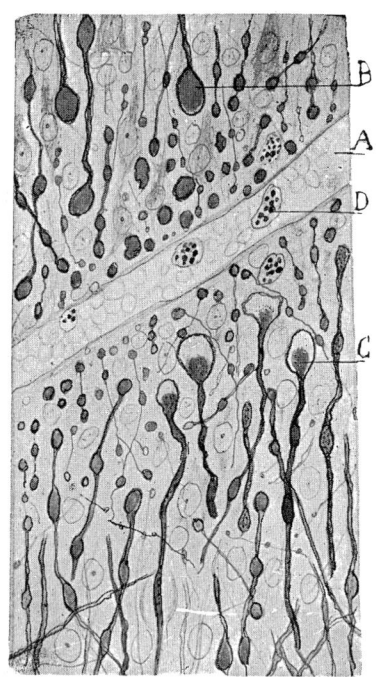

FIG. 266.—Cerebral wound of a dog, twenty days old, which was killed six hours after the operation. *A*, wound ; *B*, terminal balls of the central stump ; *C*, balls of the peripheral stump ; *D*, granular cells. Osmic acid stain.

After six or eight hours one already finds varicosities along the fibres near the terminal ball. In some of these tumefactions one can also discern the characteristic glomeruli or flexuosities, surrounded by a more or less thick hyaline mass.

One also not infrequently finds varicosities in the course of the fibres, having an unstained cortex and a neurofibrillar axis, from which issue very fine threads and numerous fine and flexuose filaments. Sections stained with osmic acid are of particular interest for the study of the terminal ball and the varicosities (Fig. 266, *C*). As in the spinal cord, these sections show that the balls as well as the varicosities are surrounded by a myelin sheath, and that between this and the axonic dilatation there exists the plasmatic chamber of which we have so often spoken. In these same preparations one observes, moreover, the great precocity of appearance of the granular bodies or cells (Fig. 266) ; six hours after the lesion they are already full of black granules, in the exudate as well as in the edges of the wound (*D*).

The convolutions of the axon within the varicosities and terminal balls are still present seven and eight hours after the operation, as we show in Fig. 267. In some of them one notes a tendency for the coils to fuse (*E*) so as to constitute compact fusiform thickenings. After the first day all, or nearly all, the terminal glomeruli and convolutions along the fibres have disappeared. This also occurs in the central stump. One may thus state as a very probable conclusion that *in the majority of medium-sized and fine axons the terminal axonic grumes and the axonic varicosities result respectively from the fusion of the terminal glomeruli and of the spirals along the course of the fibres.* Since the spirals disappeared with a certain regular periodicity, with some exceptions, we think it probable that they occur at the level of the nodes of Ranvier (Fig. 267, *A*).

As we shall note when we deal with the central stump, the varicosities of the most robust axons are produced by another mechanism—retraction of the axonic protoplasm into a mass.

After two or three days the degenerative lesions become accentuated, and the series of varicosities begin to resolve themselves into free spheres which are digested successively, as already described in respect of the nerves and spinal cord, within ample plasmatic chambers.

In Fig. 268 we show the principal types of alterations that can be seen in the white matter of dogs killed two days after the operation.

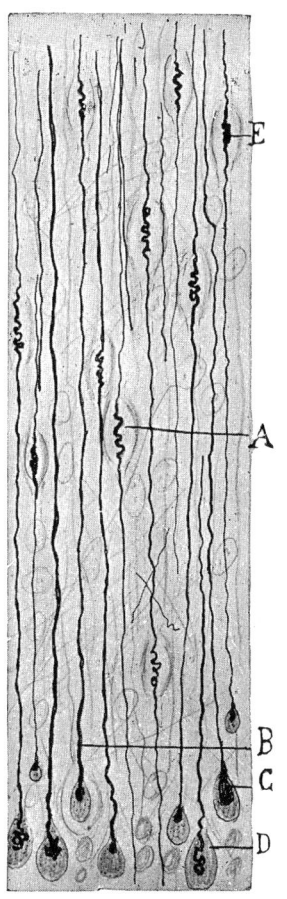

FIG. 267.—Peripheral stump of a cerebral wound in a cat, one month old, which was killed seven and a half hours after the operation. *A*, spirals along the course of fibres, situated in a plasmatic space; *B*, axonic stump provided with a terminal bud; *D*, axons ending in a glomerulus; *E*, spirals whose turns coalesce so as to produce a varicosity.

One may note that there are axons which are attacked rapidly, over long distances (*C*, *E*), by granular disintegration. Another characteristic that can also be observed in this figure is that the large medullated tubes are more altered than the fine tubes. Indeed, many of the former terminate in an enormous ball, more or less retracted in a distal direction, besides showing thick

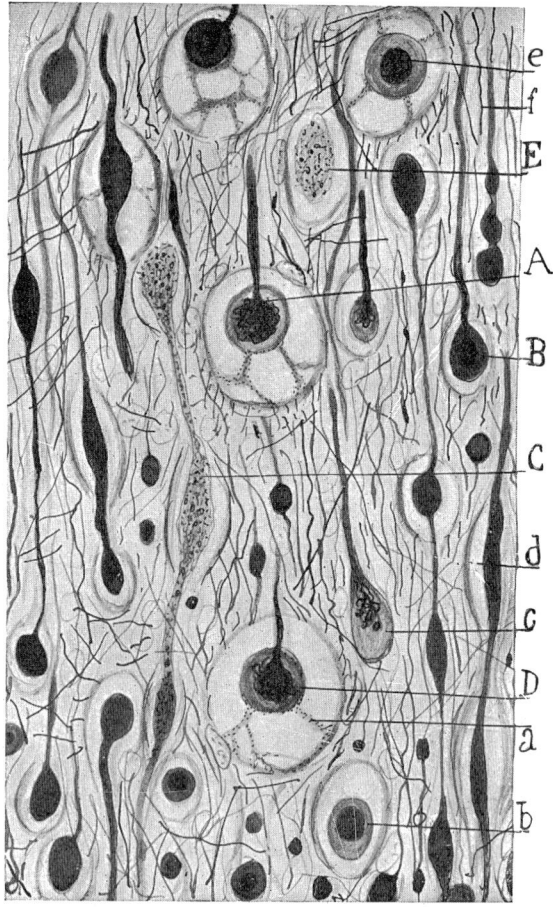

FIG. 268.—Section of the white matter of a dog, two months old, which was killed two days after the operation; the portion reproduced corresponds to the distal edge of the wound. *A, D*, gigantic terminal balls surrounded by a digestive chamber; *B*, terminal ball of an axon of medium-sized calibre; *C*, varicose fibre degenerated precociously; *E*, ball necrosed precociously; *a*, granular lines which traverse the digestive chamber of the ball; *b, e*, free balls which are being digested; *f*, non-medullated fibre.

varicosities along their path and a few fusiform tumefactions. In other conductors, which as a rule are less voluminous, after the terminal sphere and two or three varicosities, the normal segment begins almost without transition. The widest digestive chambers (*D*) lie round terminal balls; but they are also present round free balls (*b*) and varicosities along the course of the fibres. As we have stated in another place, these chambers contain, besides the ball, which is more or less hyaline cortically, a certain clear liquid (in the fresh state), granular trabeculae formed by some coagulated protein (*a*), and, finally, a tangential layer of myelin which is visible only in preparations made with osmic acid or by Weigert's method.

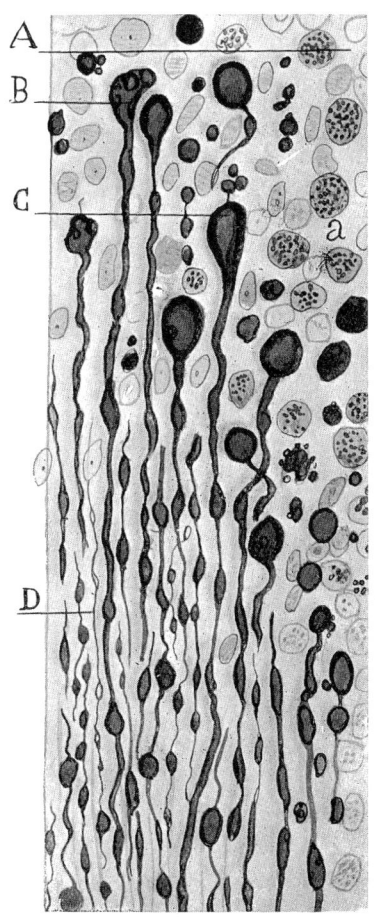

FIG. 269.—Peripheral stump of a wound four days old, in a cat two weeks old; osmic acid stain. *A*, region near the wound; *B* and *C*, terminal clubs of myelin; *D*, fine medullated fibre; *a*, granular cell.

The terminal balls and varicosities along the fibres persist for a considerable time, being found in preparations made four or five days after the operation. In Fig. 269 we show such structures impregnated with osmic acid; they are from a cat, fifteen days old, which was killed four days after the operation. We shall not repeat what we have described so often, but confine ourselves to pointing out that the fine fibres (*D*) have the medullary sheath less altered than the large fibres, which end near the wound in very voluminous myelinic balls or masses (Fig. 269, *B, C*). One may also note the presence of series of myelin droplets at the level occupied by disintegrated fibres.

Segment undergoing secondary degeneration.—Among the nerve tubes reproduced in Figs. 267 and 268, there are some which doubtless are centripetal and therefore in continuity with uninjured cortical neurones of other cerebral lobules or of the optic thalamus (ascending sensory fibres). But since all are undergoing traumatic degeneration, it is impossible to differentiate physiological or topographical categories of conductors. Such a distinction would be possible only if one examined the fibres 1 to 2 millimetres from the wound; for example, at the level of the corpus striatum. But to distinguish such contrasts it would be indispensable to explore the median and intermediate parts of the brain fifteen to twenty days after the operation, since after five or six days the secondary or Wallerian degeneration has not yet begun, at least not with well-marked characteristics. If this degeneration is advanced, and one examines regions of the peripheral stump situated very far from the lesion, one sees that only a small number of the fibres emerging from the wound are bead-like and therefore are distal ends of interrupted projection fibres. The great majority of the peripheral stumps formed by section of the white matter are in continuity with the association fibres and cannot be counted among the degenerated fibres of the corpus striatum or internal capsule.

2. **Degenerative phenomena of the peripheral stump of axons cut right in the grey matter, that is, near the cell of origin.**—As in the previous case, the conductor rapidly differentiates into a *necrotic segment* and a segment that is *degenerated traumatically*; but, as we have already noted, its neurobiones react with unusual vigour and undergo, especially at the level of the terminal ball, curious metamorphoses. Since such structural mutations constitute a decisive argument for the relative autonomy of the ultramicroscopic units of the reticulum, we shall describe them here in some detail. The phenomena observed between the twenty-fourth and the forty-eighth hours are as follows.

Leaving aside the *necrotic segment*, since it shows nothing of special interest, except the rapidity with which it is absorbed, we shall examine the retraction ball. In Fig. 270 we show some phases of the retraction itself, relating to the peripheral stump of giant axons (*pyramidal cells of Betz*, from the motor region of a dog one month old). One is at once struck by the fact that, near the wound, autotomized balls attached to fine tubes are very frequent. The large terminal balls, in continuity with robust axons, lie at some distance, as though they shunned the inflammatory exudate. In each of these robust axons which are crowned with a gigantic retraction ball one can recognize three parts or segments: the *sphere* itself, a *thin segment* or appendix which is directed towards the wound, and a *hypertrophic segment*, or distal portion.

(*a*) The *ball* or *club* may be terminal, and so it is in many fibres shown in Fig. 270 (*b*, *c*), usually very close to the lesion. More

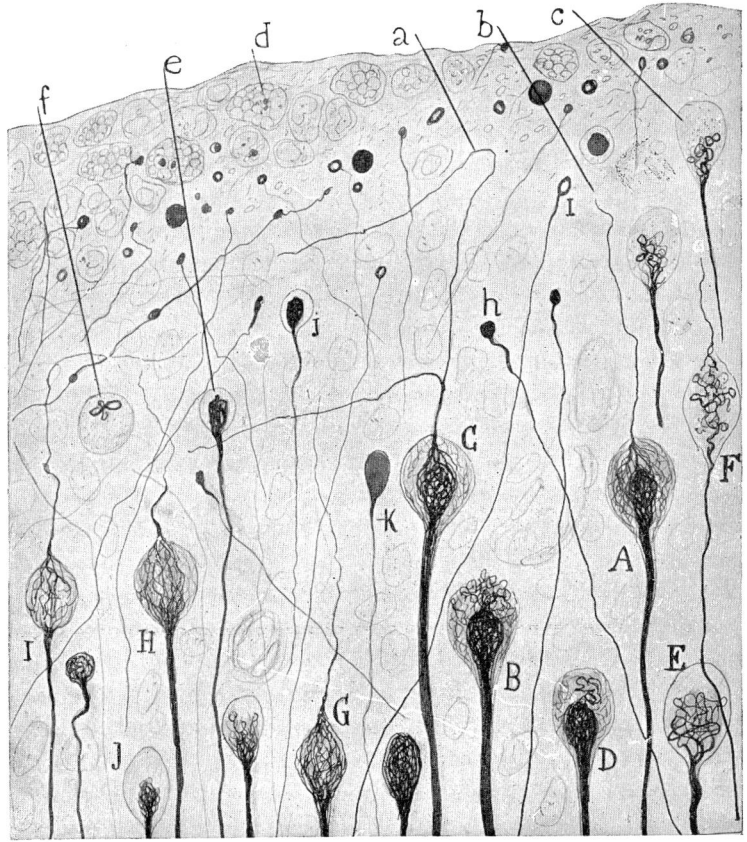

Fig. 270.—Distal edge of a cerebral wound of a dog, one month old, which was killed forty-two hours after the operation. *A, C, G, H, I*, retraction balls with a tenuous filament directed towards the wound; *B, D, E*, terminal balls which are provided with a dense central focus and a peripheral neurofibrillar glomerulus; *F*, ball provided with a neurofibrillar axis, from which issue branchlets ending in rings; *c*, hyaline sphere with nets and rings at its distal pole; *e*, sphere of a non-medullated fibre; *d*, granular cells; *f*, free ball with neurofibrillar remnants arranged like handles. (*Note*: The edges of the wound were contused.)

usually, however, this excrescence is intercalated, as we have stated, between a terminal axonic segment and another hypertrophic segment. In general the axons of large diameter show robust spheres, while the medium-sized and small ones have expansions which are proportionate to their thickness (Fig. 270, *C*).

The majority of the large balls or clubs show a reticulum divided into two concentric zones : a dark central zone which is compact and made up of a dense neurofibrillar framework ; and a cortical region, rich in neuroplasm and made up of a loose neurofibrillar skeleton, whose trabeculae are relatively robust and at times flexuose. One may note that some fibrils of the cortical network are arranged in loops, whose convexity stands out on the periphery of the club (Fig. 270, B). One frequently sees that from the dense central net there arise two small converging neurofibrillar bundles, one of them wide and continuous with the distal segment, the other fine and connected with the proximal segment (Fig. 270, A, C, F).

The fine central segment is lacking in many medium-sized fibres and in all the small ones (e, j) ; it is present, however, although not constantly, in the most robust spheres when they have not yet become hyalinized (A, C, I, H).

Ordinarily this segment, which resembles a fine appendix arising from the centre of the sphere, advances towards the wound, in the edges of which it terminates in a pale point, without showing any thickening along its path. At other times, from the course of this segment a collateral issues at right angles (Fig. 270, C), which is somewhat thicker than the ascendant filament. At any rate, these appendices are much finer than the distal segment of the axon.

How should these fine proximal appendices of the large spheres be interpreted ? At first sight one might explain their presence by imagining that these spheres, like the terminal balls of the peripheral stump of the nerves, are capable of forming agonal neoformations, which tend vainly to re-establish their neuronal connection. But when we remember : that the central axons are almost absolutely incapable of giving rise to free branches directed towards the wound ; the presence at the end of these fibrils, of points of corrosion instead of fine buds and rings ; their direction, which almost always is that of the vanished axonic trunk, etc. ; we incline to the view that these proximal fibres represent the remnant of the axon between the ball and the wound, and that the neurobiones of this piece of the axon, in harmony with the theory of retraction, withdraw progressively towards the focus of attraction or terminal clubs. This interpretation, besides explaining the proportionality between the terminal sphere and the diameter of the axon, also enables one to understand why the spheres that are most retracted and distant from the wound are of considerable size.

(b) The segment of the axon that precedes in a distal sense the terminal sphere is frequently hypertrophic. At the same time, this disposition, which we show in Fig. 270, A, B, C, may be lacking. When this hypertrophy exists the diameter of the axon progressively diminishes until it reaches a completely normal region. On

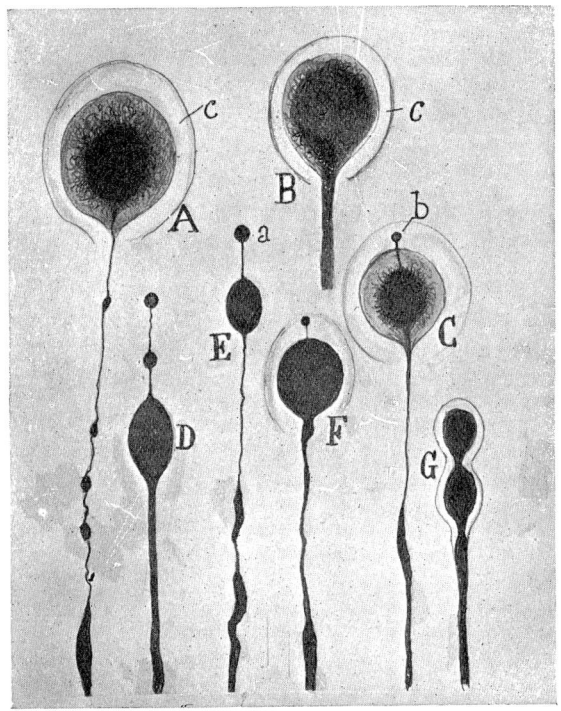

FIG. 271.—Some terminal balls from the distal stump of a cerebral wound of a dog, fifteen days old, killed three days after the operation. A, B, gigantic balls with a clear space around them (c) and a loose marginal zone; C, D, F, large terminal balls from which issues an appendix with a terminal sphere (a); G, twin balls. The wound was complicated by contusion.

the other hand, the fusiform and varicose states are rare in sections from wounds twenty-four hours old.

Examination of the peripheral stump two or three days after the operation.—The phenomena that we have just described vary somewhat after the second day from the operation. The ball becomes more and more hyaline, and there appears a clear limbo, absolutely devoid of neurofibrils, while the fine segment or proximal appendix becomes shortened and retracted. The hypertrophic region also becomes transformed, the axon assuming a fusiform or varicose disposition, according to the cases. At times a long fine neck joins the ball to the first fusiform eminence or to a hypertrophic segment that is exceptionally persistent (Fig. 271, *C*, *E*). Finally, round the ball one sees a digestive chamber, with its plasma and myelinic cortex.

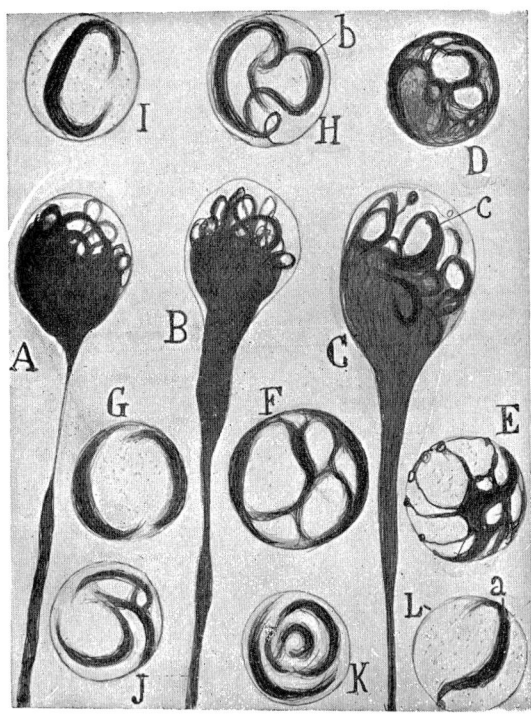

FIG. 272.—Dispositions found in many free balls and terminal spheres of the distal edge of a cerebral wound of a dog, fifteen days old, which was killed three days after the operation; the wound was contused and triturated owing to attempts at grafting a ganglion. *A, B, C*, terminal balls in whose hyalinized cortex metamorphic phenomena are taking place (formation of neurofibrillar loops, buckles, etc.); *D, E, F, H, I, J, K, L*, hyaline free balls with buckles or locks of neurofibrils arranged in various ways.

The autotomy of the terminal ball is very curious. In some cases, beneath the sphere, and by virtue of a retraction towards it, the hypertrophic portion of the axon becomes thin, varicose, and finally breaks (Fig. 271, *A*). *In this way large independent spheres are produced, whose neurobiones may be preserved for several days, giving rise to extremely varied reticulated structures* (Fig. 272).

On the other hand, the fine segment which is prolonged up to the wound becomes progressively thinner and disappears. It appears as though its entire mass has been attracted by the terminal ball. During its contraction one may frequently observe in this appendix local neurobional accumulations which have the shape of fine spherules (Fig. 271, *a*, *b*).

The colossal free balls produced through absorption of both pedicles show at times, besides the well-known cortical hyalinization, curious metamorphoses, which we depict in Fig. 272.

This metamorphosis, which reminds one very much of the phenomenon described by Alzheimer in senile dementia, confirmed by various authors (Perusini, Achúcarro, Sinchowicz, Lafora, etc.), consists in the production of certain neurofibrillar loops, which are vividly stained by colloidal silver, and which stand out against the hyaline or colourless background, more or less granular, of the sphere. As we show in Fig. 272, *A*, this degeneration into loops occurs as well in terminal as in free balls. Very probably it begins in the former, usually at the level of the distal or free pole of the axon, and continues and becomes exaggerated after nervous autotomy. There are hyaline balls that are crossed only by a tangential neurofibrillar bundle, which is arranged in the form of a *C*, with pale and ravelled points (Fig. 272, *I*, *L*); other balls contain two or three marginal bundles in the form of locks or loops (*G*, *H*, *J*); in some of them the bundles sometimes occupy concentric layers and have a spiroidal configuration (*K*). These locks assume the form of a net with large intercalary hyaline masses (*F*), that is, masses of protoplasm that is stainable and not yet entirely hyalinized (*D*). Exceptionally, one sees plexuses of locks from which arise relatively fine branches, which terminate peripherally in rings (Fig. 272, *E*). In the neurofibrillar plexuses one not infrequently finds free neurofibrils, ramified and terminated by rings (Fig. 272, *C*).

The balls with neurofibrillar loops represent agonistic neurofibrillar reactions, destined shortly to cease. Progressively the small central bundles disappear, and there is a corresponding increase of the hyaline matter; the neurofibrils become pale and more or less granular, and, finally, the entire sphere is seen to be composed of a pale substance of granular appearance. The *phenomenon of Alzheimer* represents, as is well known, a process of necrosis of the neurones. But as the neurofibrillar locks appear within the soma, which is still connected dynamically with other neurones, the necrobiosis perhaps develops more slowly.

II

STUDY OF TRAUMATIC DEGENERATION IN THE CEREBRAL CORTEX (*Continued*)

Degenerative phenomena of the central stump in wounds of the white matter.—Degenerative phenomena of this stump when the interruption is in the grey matter.—Compensatory eliminations.—Transformation of the cerebral pyramidal cells into cells with short axons.—Degenerative phenomena in the nerve collaterals and in some intrinsic fibres of the cerebral cortex.

In an analysis of the morphological and structural perturbations occurring in the central stump of the nerve fibres originating in the grey matter, one should consider two important subjects : (1) degenerative lesions of the neurones ; (2) degenerative lesions of the axons.

As in our exposition of the cerebellar lesions, we shall deal at first with the metamorphoses of the central stump of the axon of pyramidal cells, reserving for a separate chapter the analysis of the degenerative reactions of the pyramidal neurones themselves.

TRAUMATIC DEGENERATION OF THE CENTRAL STUMP

The cerebral axons, from the point of view of neuronal survival and secondary production of compensatory hypertrophies, behave in different ways, according as the interruption occurs in the white matter, in the region of the collaterals, or again between these and the pyramidal cells. One must therefore examine separately the effects of these three kinds of section.

Metamorphosis of the central stump when the interruption occurs in the white matter or the deep region of the grey matter.—We may immediately distinguish the reactions of the fine tubes and non-medullated fibres from those of the thick conductors.

Non-medullated fibres and thin tubes.—As we stated with regard to the white matter of the spinal cord, so also the central stump of the finest conductors of the cerebrum possesses a very short *necrotic segment* which is quickly resorbed, and a *degenerated segment* which is so short that one can usually see only a *terminal* or *retraction ball*. This ball appears almost entirely formed four to six hours after the lesion. The finest fibres end in rings, as G. Sala demonstrated.

The early phases of the formation of the balls appear in Fig. 265, where we have reproduced preferably fine medullated axons and tenuous non-medullated fibres, in a cat two months old. One may note how, four hours after the operation, many fibres of fine and medium calibre have a terminal ball composed of a colourless hyaline mass and central glomerulus (*C*). As we described in connection with the peripheral stump, one sees here also that the neurofibrillar bulk of the terminal club is at first arranged in convolutions and spirals, later to melt into a compact grume. Finally, certain fine tubes show in addition glomeruli along their course (*E*), situated precisely in the regions where the varicosities will subsequently appear.

In the most delicate terminal fibrils the final sphere displays, during the second to the third hour after the operation, a detail that perhaps explains the mechanism by which terminal rings are produced. This consists in the appearance of a certain colourless vacuole which gradually throws back the argentophilous substance towards the membrane, while the neurobiones concentrate along the equator of the ball so as to form a hoop in continuity with the axon.

The retraction balls and rings of the fine conductors are preserved several days near the wound, losing hardly any ground in a cellulipetal direction. Finally, the autotomies of terminal rings and tumefactions sprinkle the edges of the wound with pale balls within which foci of living neurofibrils subsist for a time.

In Fig. 273 we show, greatly enlarged, the appearance of the terminal portion of the fine fibres, three days after the lesion. In addition to the lesions that we described when we were studying the degenerative metamorphoses of the spinal cord and cerebellum, one must note here large rings at the end and along the course of the fibre, somewhat reticulated internally (*a*); double rings or double loops (*c*); autotomized rings of large size. There are, besides, within the wound, and right in the exudate, floating masses, in which one may observe complicated glomeruli and arcs (*F*, *D*), and many granular cells containing preserved axons intricately coiled.

Traumatic degeneration of the thick tubes.—As the phenomena that occur in the central stump coincide in their general lines with those already described in the peripheral stump, we shall note here only certain points peculiar to the former, or which, without being original, show some special feature. As in the peripheral stump, one sees here also a pale *necrotic segment*, which breaks down rapidly (Fig. 265, *a*), and a *living segment*, which is the seat of the actual traumatic degeneration.

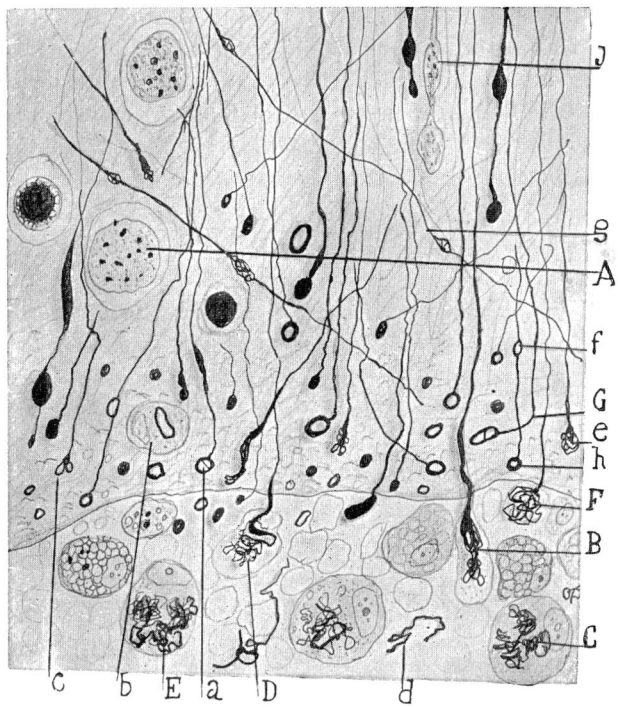

FIG. 273.—Central stump of the wound of a dog, two months old, which was killed three days after the operation; in this figure we show only the edge of the wound that contains the thin fibres and balls. *A*, granular spheres belonging to axons that have been destroyed precociously; *B, D*, hyaline masses floating in the wound and furnished with a neurofibrillar glomerulus showing ansiform dispositions; *C, E*, phagocytes that have engulfed fine non-medullated axons; *d*, free piece of an axon, well preserved in the exudate; *a, G*, terminal rings with oblique trabeculae; *F*, fine fibril terminated by a ball within the exudate; *b*, phagocyte which contains a ring; *f*, rings along the course of fine fibres; *c*, fibre ending in a double ring; *g*, collaterals with reticulated varicosities.

We shall examine, chronologically, the changes occurring in the living segment.

From the first hour after the traumatism the axonic reaction begins with the well-known thickening in the form of the tip of a sound, preceded by a slight hypertrophy (Fig. 274, *A*). After six hours the terminal thickening is accentuated and an interesting detail appears, which is peculiar to the central stump, and which we reproduce in Fig. 275, *a*. It consists in the progressive hyalinization of that part of the hypertrophic segment which is situated immediately above the terminal bud (*a*); only a fine central neurofibrillar bundle subsists, which often follows in a spiral or flexuose course. Such an axial thread debouches at its lower end in the stainable axis of the club, while in a proximal direction it thickens progressively until it merges into the normal axon (Fig. 275, *b*). We may mention that this axial thread sometimes begins to form within three or four hours; but its full development takes place after

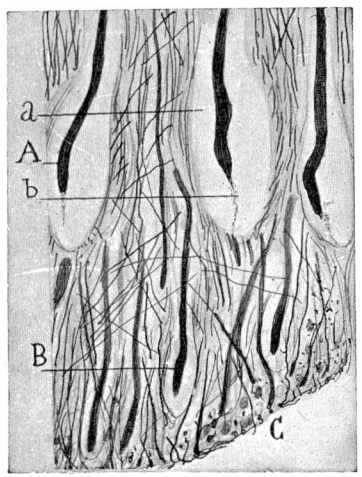

FIG. 274.—Piece of the central stump of a cerebral wound of a cat, killed one hour after the operation. *A*, thick axon ending in the form of the tip of a sound; *B*, thinner axon; *a*, plasmatic chamber; *b*, granular appendix emerging from the axon.

six to eight hours. Occasionally (Fig. 276, *A*), innumerable tenuous branchlets issue from the axial filament, flexuose in character, and extended through the hyaline matter. They are entirely like those described in the peripheral stump of nerves.

We think it probable that this cortical hyalinization, situated above the club, spreads to the axis, and that in this way a piece of the hypertrophic portion, as well as of the original terminal ball, is destroyed. Later, and nearer the cell, a new bud would be formed, and in this way the hypertrophic process would be propagated cellulipetally.

But the most interesting phenomena occur eighteen to thirty-six hours after the operation. The axonic destruction has progressed, the vaginal or cortical necroses of which we spoke above have become eliminated, the argentophilous substance has retired in a cellulipetal direction, and the living axon is now affected over a long portion of its course. One can now see clearly in it the four segments called : *terminal bud or ball, varicose segment, hypertrophic segment, and normal segment.*

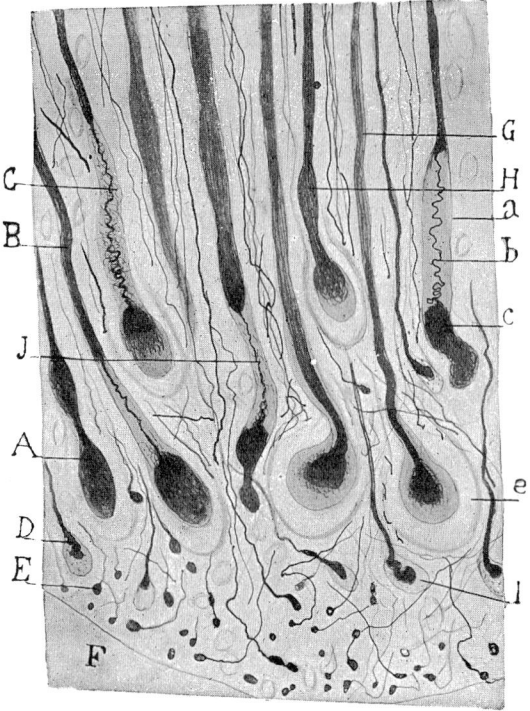

FIG. 275.—Central stump of a cerebral wound in a dog, twenty days old, which was killed six hours after the operation. *A*, stumps in the form of balls ; *B, C*, balls preceded by a pale neck through which runs a spiroidal neurofibrillar axis ; *E*, ends of fine fibres ; *F*, wound ; *I*, medium-sized fibre ending in a glomerulus ; *e*, plasmatic cavity.

In Fig. 277, and in a schematic way in Fig. 278, we show the morphology and situation of these segments.

(*a*) *Terminal or retraction ball.*—This has a volume proportional to the axon and, twenty-four hours after the operation onward, has the shape of a ball, bud, or pear. Around it one sees a wide plasmatic space, outside which the nervous tissue appears as though compressed. From the terminal ball often hang fine threads extending towards the wound. Sometimes they are short and end within the plasmatic chamber in a fine sphere; at other times they are longer (Fig. 277, g), and lose themselves in the nerve tissue. Every transition is found between the short and the long terminal appendices. We think it probable that such appendices, arising from the retraction ball, are phases in the centripetal withdrawal of

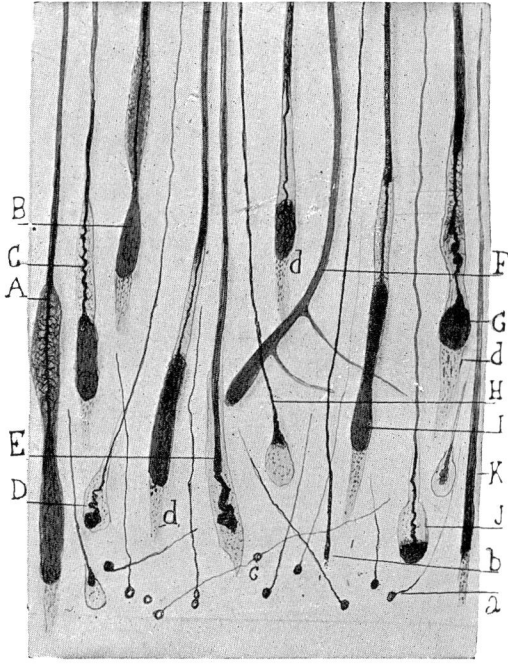

FIG. 276.—Central stump of a cerebral wound of a cat, one month old, which was killed sixteen and a half hours after the operation. *A, B, C*, large fibres terminating like the tip of a sound and whose preterminal portion shows a pale reticulum and a dark neurofibrillar axis; *D, E*, thin axons ending in a glomerulus; *F*, axon ending like the tip of a sound; *a*, small terminal balls of very fine axons; *d*, necrotic appendix hanging from the terminal club.

the neurobiones. As occurs in the peripheral stump when the section is made right in the grey matter, the terminal ball would, according to this view, result from a growing congregation of the living ultramicroscopic units that have escaped from the portion of the axon next to the wound, other than those which have succumbed to the mechanical commotion or undergone autotomy (the free balls).

(*b*) *Varicose segment.*—This extends further towards the neurone the larger the diameter of the axon, and has the characteristics that we have described so often. Examination of Figs. 277 and 278, *E*, will render unnecessary the repetition of well-known morphological facts.

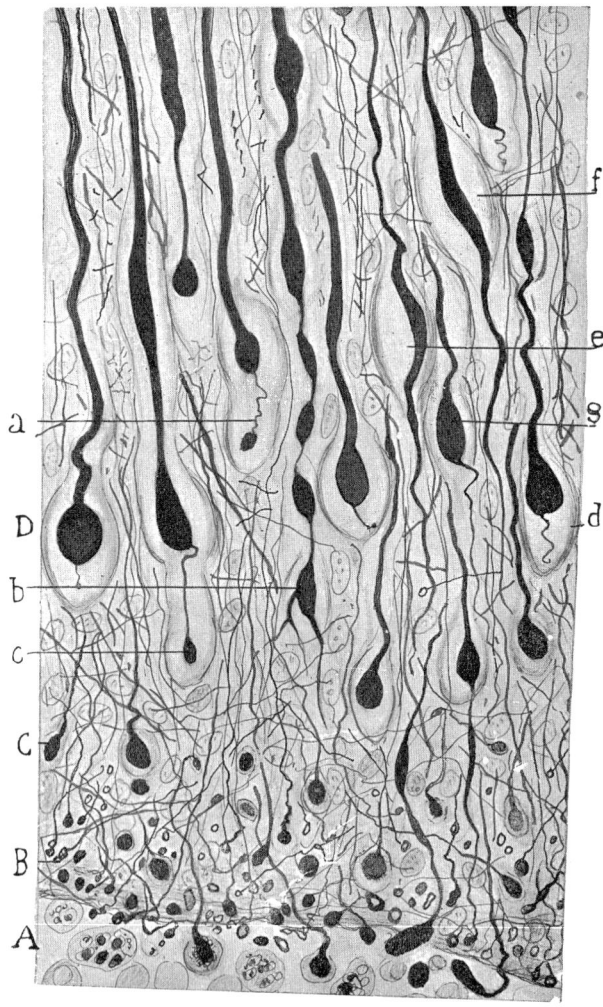

FIG. 277.—Central stump of a cerebral wound of a dog, two months old, which was killed one day after the operation. Section of the white matter: *A*, wound with granular cells and masses floating in the exudate; *B*, region of the small clubs and rings; *C*, region of the medium-sized clubs; *D*, region of the clubs of the axons of giant pyramidal cells; *a, c*, fine ball hanging from a large club; *b*, varicosity with expansions; *d*, clear space which surrounds the balls; *e, f*, similar spaces round the varicosities; *g*, club from which a long fine appendix starts, which is lost in the edges of the wound.

(*c*) *Hypertrophic segment.*—This is a primordial phase chronologically, almost always contemporaneous with the formation of the

THE CEREBRAL CORTEX 663

first retraction club, since it appears as early as sixteen to twenty-four hours after the traumatism. From the first to the second day it makes headway in a centripetal direction, giving place to the phase of varicosities. Once these are formed, the hypertrophic state forms the alteration that is nearest to the unimpaired segment of the axon, and therefore furthest from the retraction ball. There are, however, some exceptions (Fig. 278, B).

We call *hypertrophic state* a certain longitudinal swelling of the axon, extending over a variable length (which is usually greater for thick than for medium-sized axons), and characterized by an increase in the stainability of the neurofibrils and a certain re-arrangement of their neurobionic architecture (Fig. 278, B). Indeed, one can see by careful observation of this thickened region that instead of being compact and fasciculated, as usual, it has a finely reticular, as it were sponge-like, disposition. The neuroplasm has increased, dilating the meshes of the reticulum; at the same time, however, the neurobiones appear more numerous, forming a certain dense mass, which is frequently looser towards the cortex. Sometimes one clearly discerns a central axis of narrow meshes with a deeply stained skeleton, and a cortex with a loose and pale reticulation. The picture reminds one of the boa furs with which women adorn themselves. Finally, at times the hypertrophy is unaccompanied by any well-marked structural change. The *hypertrophic state* has been seen by G. Sala, who also noted its propagation up to the initial collaterals and the clearly striated appearance of the axonic protoplasm.

(d) *Unimpaired or normal segment of the axon.*— No matter how violent the traumatism, if it occurs in the white matter beneath the grey matter, one always observes a considerable piece of axon which,

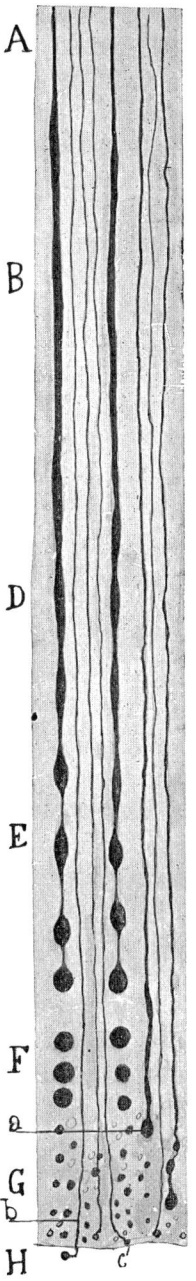

FIG. 278.—Schematic drawing showing the various segments which form the degenerated portion of a robust medullated axon; three days after the section. *A*, normal region; *B*, hypertrophic region; *D*, fusiform region; *E*, varicose region; *F*, free balls; *G*, region of the medium-sized and fine terminal balls; *a*, medium-sized terminal ball; *b*, *c*, fine balls.

neither by its stainability, thickness, nor structure, seems to have suffered any alteration. The myelin sheath also remains normal, as may be seen in preparations made with osmic acid. The collaterals are also unchanged (Fig. 278, *A*).

Naturally, the piece of normal axon varies with its distance from the wound. It is large if the wound involves the white matter, far from the grey cortex; it is small if the lesion occurs in the deep zone of the cortical substance. By a gentle transition one passes, in the direction of the wound, to the hypertrophic segment, which indicates a movement of neurobional neoformation in the axon.

The segments described, arranged in a radial direction, also succeed each other in time. The process begins by the appearance of the terminal bud; then follows immediately the hypertrophic state. The varicosities are formed at the expense of the latter. Finally, while these changes occur successively within a single segment, they are also propagated in a cellulipetal direction to a distance that varies for each fibre. No doubt the varicose state presents at times a character of relative stability; nevertheless, in the regions next to the wound, it often constitutes the antecedent of axonic autotomy. The process of protoplasmic concentration becomes successively exaggerated, the varicosities become converted into large spheres, and the uniting threads become pale, granular, and end by breaking. In this way large balls are produced, which are completely isolated and surrounded by a spacious vacuole. Often the series of balls are arranged along a straight line, showing the position previously occupied by the axon from which they were formed. Some spheres form couples, and the uniting thread subsists for a certain time. Finally, the majority of the balls undergo a process of regression, which we shall not describe, as it is identical with that referred to in the corresponding description of the spinal cord.

The phase of balls in series is maintained, more or less completely, in the large cerebral axons from the third to the sixth or seventh day. On the tenth day remnants of the largest axons alone subsist.

Late retraction ball.—The preceding phenomena often lead, as we have stated, to the destruction of the varicose portion of the axon. As a consequence of this necrobiosis the remaining central segment, which is normal or but little altered, forms a more or less lasting terminal thickening; this has the shape of a club or bud of variable dimension, which we shall call *late retraction ball*, in order to distinguish it from the initial traumatic club. It is very possible that this ball, which remains fifteen and twenty days after the operation, also finally disappears.

One may suppose also that, as occurs in the cerebellum, this terminal retrograde degeneration is propagated in a centripetal direction up to the last bifurcation or collateral of the axon arising in the white matter.

Axons that are destroyed precociously.—Alongside of axons in course of metamorphosis, but stainable and furnished with balls or varicosities, one always finds, from the first day after the lesion, and more abundantly on the following days, robust axons—apparently projection fibres—which are completely destroyed and in process of disintegration (Fig. 273, *A*). These conductors, which are so exquisitely vulnerable, appear for the most part broken up into free and voluminous balls, surrounded by a large cavity. In presence of the colloidal silver, these spheres either do not stain, or present a greyish, coarsely granular appearance.

Metamorphosis of the axon when the lesion occurs right in the grey matter, below the collaterals.—Where the cut is oblique to the cerebral cortex, and traverses the zone of polymorphic cells, the majority of axons are interrupted beneath the region of the collaterals or at the level of origin of some of the deeper branches. Under such conditions these expansions undergo, more or less, the changes that we have so often described, forming finally a *retraction club*, preceded by a more or less extensive *hypertrophic segment*. When the animal is very young, one sees after twenty-four hours that the hypertrophic region (Fig. 279) is of great length, often extending up to the last uninjured collaterals, and affecting them in turn. These become exceptionally thick and deeply stained by colloidal silver (*a*). The varicose state is not displayed, or is reduced to the smallest possible manifestation (Fig. 279).

Of more interest are the phenomena occurring in somewhat older animals, such as cats and dogs from twenty-five to thirty days old, where the sections pass, as in the previous case, beneath the two or three initial collaterals. The most important fact observed is that, in consequence of the retraction of the terminal ball, of its detention at the level of, or near the emergence of the collaterals, and of the latter's consequent hypertrophy, the pyramidal cells, which are, as is well known, *cells with a long axon, are transformed into cells with short axons*, absolutely like the arciform type described in the Purkinje cells of the cerebellum. In Fig. 280 we show this interesting disposition, which has great theoretical importance. The cells which are shown are medium-sized and large pyramidal cells. The dispositions of the arciform pyramidal cells most commonly found,

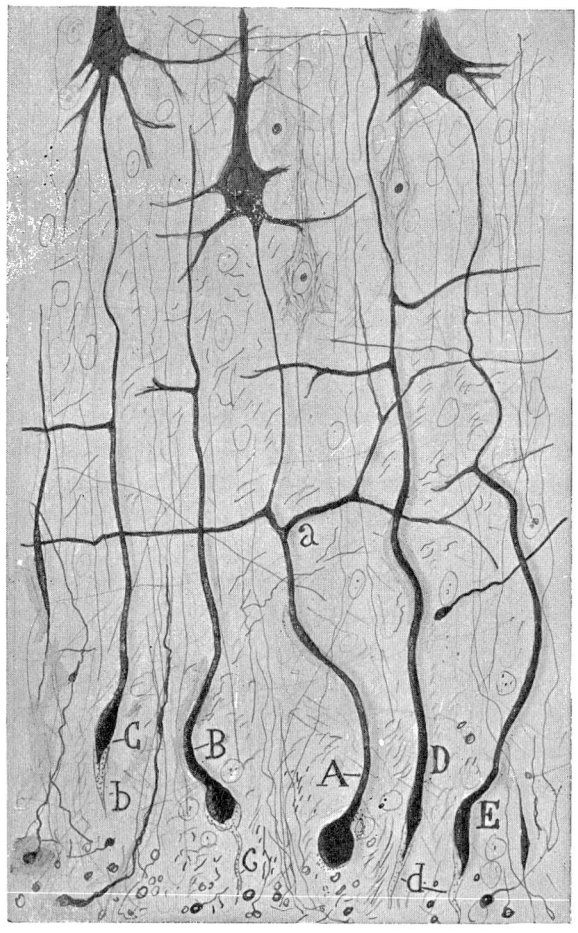

FIG. 279.—Section of the motor cortex of a cat, four days old, killed one day after the operation. *a*, hypertrophic collaterals; *A*, retraction clubs.

according to our investigations [1] of the cortex of young cats, are as follows :

(*a*) Pyramidal cell furnished with a hypertrophic axon in con-

[1] S. R. Cajal: " Los fenómenos precoces de la degeneración traumatica de los cilindros-ejes del cerebro," *Trab. del Lab. de Invest. biol.*, t. 9, 1913.

tinuity with the first collateral. Between the axon and the latter there are no clubs or thickenings, nor any vestige of the peripheral course of the axon. From the collateral issue recurrent horizontal

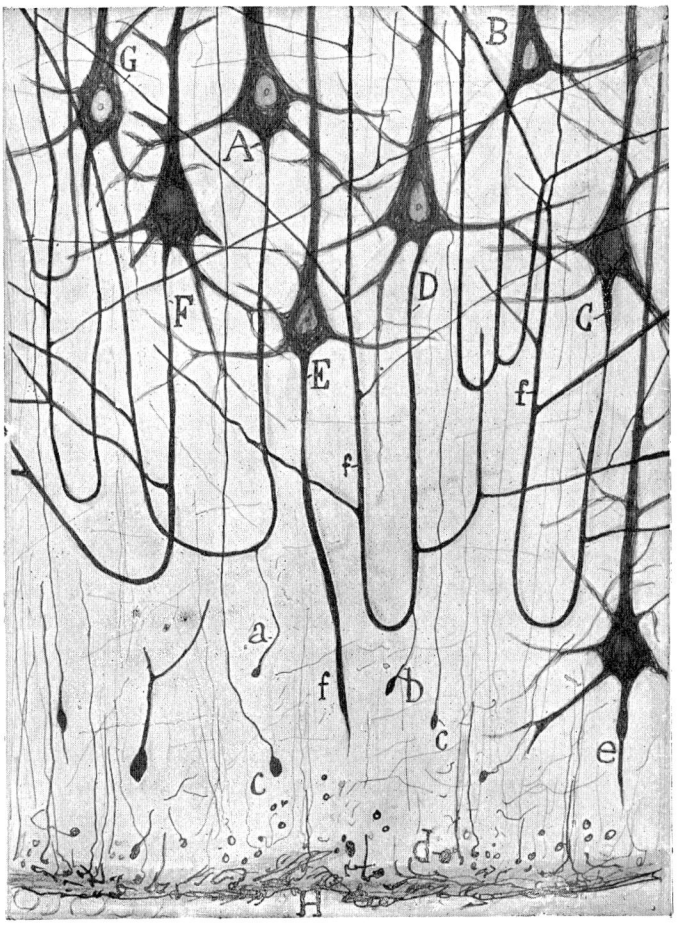

FIG. 280.—Section of the motor cortex of a cat, twenty-five days old, which was killed twenty-four hours after the operation. A, D, medium-sized pyramidal cells with hypertrophic arciform collaterals and a fine atrophic axonic stump (a, b); C, F, G, arciform pyramidal cells whose peripheral portion of the axon has disappeared; B, pyramidal cell whose axon resolves itself into two recurrent arches; H, wound; c, axons terminating in a club whose cells of origin are probably situated in the zone of small pyramidal cells; e, axon cut above the collaterals and ending in a point of corrosion.

or oblique branches, which are notably thick, deeply stained, and which may be traced for long distances. This type of neurone is a perfect reproduction of a cell with a short axon, except that the terminal arborization is composed of hypertrophic branches which involve an enormous part of the cortex (Fig. 280, *A*, *C*, *F*).

(*b*) Cells of a similar type, but from whose axon two or more arciform branches emanate, which start at slightly different levels or on different planes (Fig. 280, *B*, *D*). The thick recurrent fibres that are thus produced emit very long horizontal or oblique branches.

(*c*) Pyramidal cells of a similar type, but having, at the level where the axon merges into the arc or collateral branch, a fine descending fibre, which ends in a small club or bud, not very far from the wound (Fig. 280, *A*, *D*, *a*, *b*).

The existence of transitions between this type, which is still provided with a peripheral axonic member, and those previously described, where this prolongation of the axon is lacking, gives the key to the mechanism of the transformation that is effected in the pyramidal cells. The cutting instrument interrupted the axon below the first collaterals. These were not harmed, but, on the contrary, underwent a considerable hypertrophy, as did also the portion of axon situated between them and the soma. But the portion of the axon next to the lesion behaves in two different ways. Sometimes, gravely affected by the traumatic action, it is rapidly destroyed by necrobiotic hyalinization, which stops, as we have also seen in the cerebellum, at the point of origin of the last collateral. At other times it is preserved in part, but immediately undergoes a traumatic degeneration, becoming gradually thinner and being resorbed until it totally disappears.

The compensatory collateral hypertrophy is a phenomenon difficult to explain. We can only form an idea of it by comparing it to the effects of an arterial ligature. In the same way as, when an artery is obstructed, the collaterals situated above the obstruction, and in part the trunk itself, undergo an adaptive hypertrophy and an increase of calibre, so also the segment of the axon between the cell and the last efficient collateral grows in thickness and is the seat of an active neurobional multiplication. It seems as though, super-stimulated by the excess of current, it undergoes a compensatory hypertrophy, in order to adapt itself to the overwork occasioned by the deflection to these projections of all the nerve currents that were previously carried by the axon.

As in the *arciform Purkinje cells*, this accommodation may also serve a utilitarian purpose, constitute a passable *modus vivendi*, having regard to the gravity of the lesions. Certainly the projection fibre is not repaired; but the nervous impulse that reaches the mutilated neurone is not absolutely lost, since it is now diverted, through the enlarged channel of the collaterals, towards other congenerous neurones, and may increase the energy of the motor reaction. However, in order definitely to accept this idea, it would

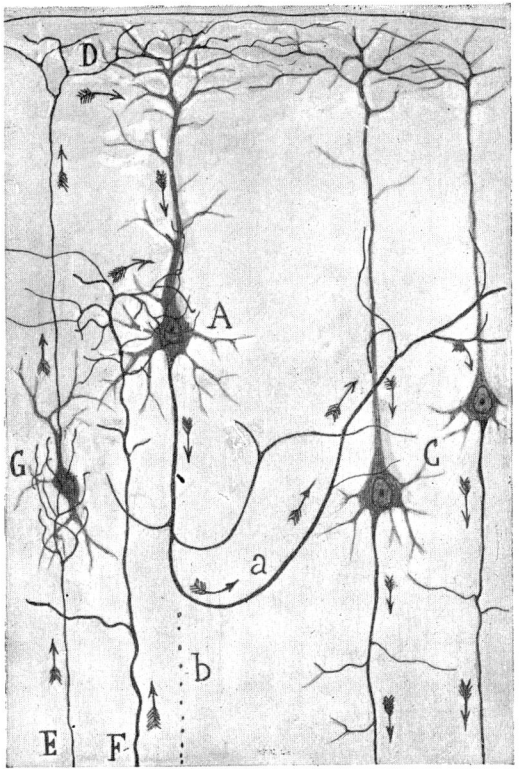

FIG. 281.—Schematic drawing showing the possible track of the currents across the arciform pyramidal cells. *A*, arciform pyramidal cell; *C*, normal pyramidal cells; *D*, plexiform layer; *E, F*, afferent fibres; *G*, cell with an ascending axon, called Martinotti's cell; *a*, hypertrophic collateral; *b*, part of the axon that has disappeared.

be necessary to prove that the arciform pyramidal cells subsist indefinitely without becoming atrophied, and maintain their original connections. In Fig. 281 we show schematically the flow of currents in a mutilated pyramidal cell furnished with hypertrophic recurrent collaterals. One may note that the sensory stimuli brought by *F*, having reached the soma and trunk of the arciform pyramid, are then propagated to the uninjured neurones (*C*), from which they descend towards the spinal cord in the *pyramidal bundles*. Stimuli arriving from association fibres take the same path (*E*); we believe them, hypothetically, transmitted to the terminal tuft of the pyramidal cells through the medium of the cells of Martinotti (*G*).

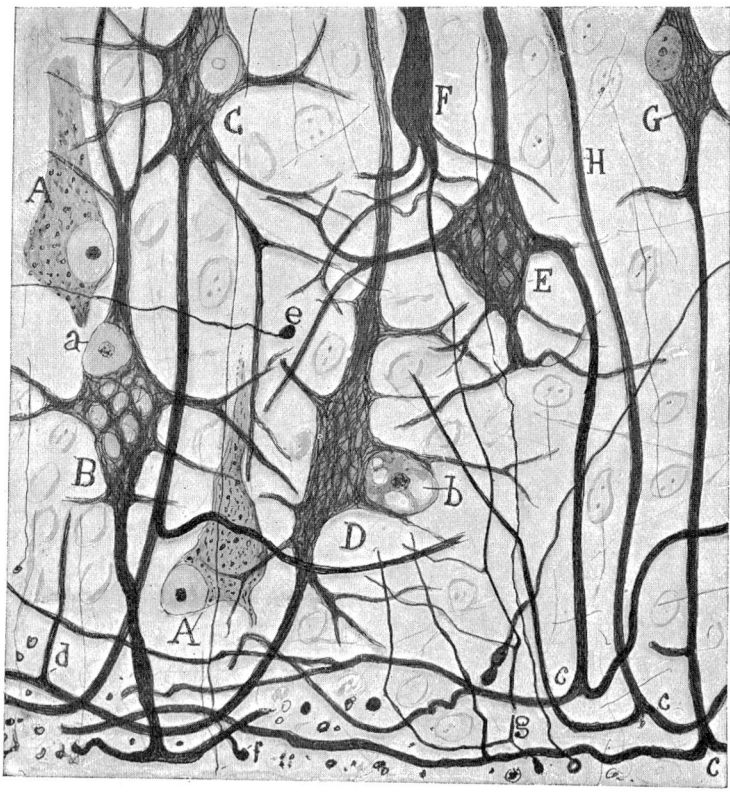

FIG. 282.—Section of the cerebral cortex of a dog, two days old (motor region); the animal was killed twenty-four hours after the operation. *A*, gigantic necrosed pyramidal cell; *B*, pyramidal cell whose axon appears to be bifurcated in the wound; *C*, *D*, pyramidal cells whose axons form an arc, and are prolonged by horizontal or recurrent collaterals; *E*, *G*, *H*, cells whose axon is prolonged by two hypertrophied ramified collaterals; *F*, small cell whose axon ends in a ball below the point of origin of a hypertrophied arciform collateral; *a*, marginal nucleus; *b*, nucleus with vacuoles bulging between two appendices; *c*, bifurcation of the axon; *d*, secondary branches of nerve collaterals.

The arciform cells appear to subsist for some time, maintaining the hypertrophy of their collaterals and showing a soma and dendrites which seem normal. The stem of the axon also retains its course and connections with the molecular layer. We do not know the fate reserved for the pyramidal cells with short axons. Perhaps they persist indefinitely, like the arciform Purkinje cells. On this point our observations cannot provide a definite solution, since they do not extend beyond twenty-five days after the operation.

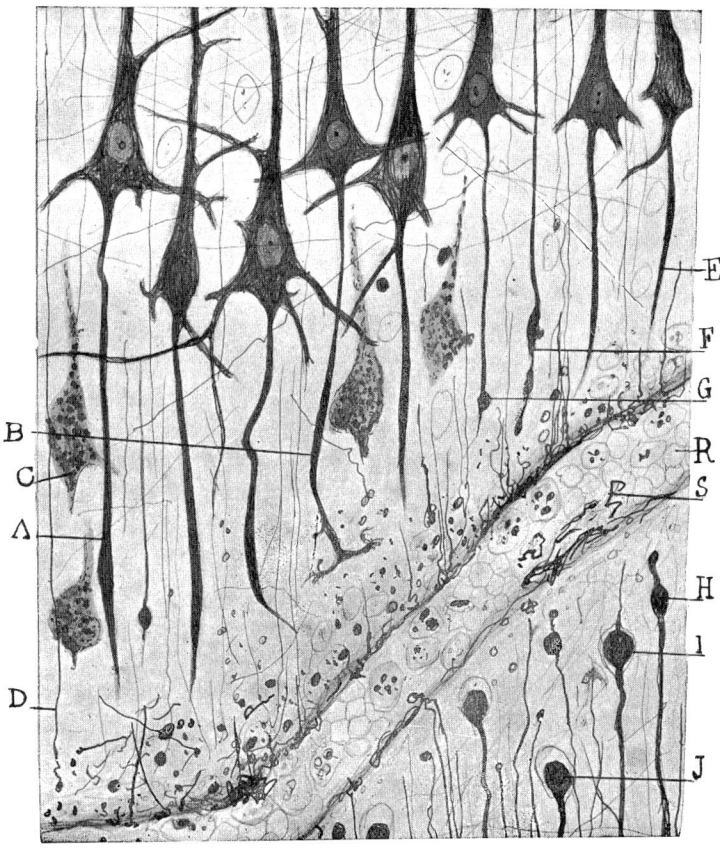

FIG. 283.—Section of the cerebral cortex of a cat, twenty-five days old, which was killed twenty-four hours after the operation ; the oblique wound passed beneath the median pyramidal cells, involving the region of their collaterals. *A*, *E*, axons ending in spindles ; *B*, axon bifurcated at its end ; *c*, dead and granular cell ; *D*, fine axon ending in a ball next to the wound ; *F*, axon provided with granular terminal varicosities ; *G*, axon from whose terminal club a pale point emerges ; *H*, *I*, *J*, peripheral ends of cut axons, with large balls.

The pyramidal cells defend the integrity of the uninjured collaterals with singular tenacity. It is surprising to observe the immunity of these branches to the growing traumatic degeneration. This is very apparent in the giant pyramidal cells of recently-born mammals, when the traumatism involves the region of the collaterals and when it has violently affected the neurones. One may see in Fig. 282 how, despite the proximity to the wound, the initial necrotic destruction of the axon remains circumscribed to the small portion of it situated between the collaterals and the wound. The elimination of this segment is so complete from the first day that one may look in vain below the collaterals for the least sign of a functional expansion. It is only in those axons whose pyramidal cells lie very high (Fig. 282, *g*) that one may detect a fine axonic stump undergoing traumatic degeneration and furnished with a retraction ball. One may also note in the figure the enormous hypertrophy of these branches, as well as of their secondary projections, their transversal path, a path that is more or less parallel to the edges of the wound, and, finally, the retrograde thickening of the axon which often extends up to the pyramidal cell.

Thus, as we noted also in respect of the cerebellum, the point of origin of the collaterals often constitutes an insuperable obstacle to the propagation of traumatic degeneration. After the interruption of the axon in their vicinity the collaterals react by the hypertrophic state, and exceptionally display a few varicosities. These distant tumefactions may well, as shown by lesions of the Purkinje cells of the cerebellum, be perfectly compatible with the preservation of the neuronal vitality.

Phenomena occurring in the axon when the section is effected above the initial collaterals.—As a general rule, whenever the traumatism involves the initial portion of the axon, there is a notable absence of the terminal balls, of the hypertrophic segment, and, in general, of all phenomena indicative of the survival of the neurobiones.

In proof of this we reproduce the giant pyramidal cells of a cat twenty days old (Fig. 283). The reader will observe the swollen axonic stump, of an almost uniform diameter, the initial node being almost entirely absent. He will also note how the majority of these stumps end near the wound in a pale, sharp point, which is preceded by a slight fusiform thickening. Exceptionally (*G*, *F*), this point is preceded by a varicosity or ends in a bifurcation (*B*). One undoubtedly is dealing here with the point of *corrosion* characteristic of the preserved dendrites and axons. We believe to-day, contrary to our early opinion, that all these cells, whose pointed axon, without terminal bud or retractions, ends near the wound under the influence of traumatisms which have destroyed the region of the collaterals and involved the precollateral region, are really cells that have suddenly been killed and *preserved*. In corroboration of this assertion one may consider the perfect normality of the soma (Fig. 283), in which the nucleus has not become tangential nor have the neurofibrils changed in appearance, in spite of the proximity to the wound and the violence of the traumatism. As we shall see presently, the survival of neurones under such severe conditions is always manifested by some reactional modification of the axon or soma.

It is to be presumed that such neurones, which have suddenly died, subsequently undergo autolytic processes and finally disappear.

Central stump of the medullated and non-medullated fibres of the grey matter. Collaterals and axons of the Martinotti cells.—When the section of the cerebral cortex, instead of being horizontal or oblique, is in a direction perpendicular to the circumvolutions, one sees fewer pyramidal cell axons. The greater part of those involved by the lesion are found to have been destroyed *ab initio* as a result of the traumatic contusion, without producing terminal clubs (examination after twenty-four hours). On the other hand, many medullated and non-medullated fibres, both oblique and horizontal, of the grey matter, are interrupted in these perpendicular wounds; among which are included : the collaterals of the pyramidal axons, the tangential axons continuous with the Martinotti cells of ascendant axons, and finally, the terminal branches of centrifugal fibres.

From twenty-four to forty-eight hours after the lesion, the central stump of all these fibres constantly shows a retraction club which is situated at a variable distance from the wound, generally at a much shorter distance than the terminal balls of the large pyramidal axons are usually placed. This terminal thickening is small, as we show in Fig. 284, *f*, when it belongs to collaterals of pyramidal axons, and it is finer in proportion as the nerve branch from which it depends is more tenuous.

Among the autochthonous fibres of the grey matter whose interruption always gives rise to terminal clubs and balls one must cite, above all, the medullated and non-medullated axons of the molecular layer. As we show in Fig. 284, *a*, *d*, the dimension of the terminal club of such axons is in relation with the diameter of the fibre, and one can also see that this terminal bud retracts and withdraws further from the wound the more voluminous the conductor that carries it. In the segment before the terminal club, a few tangential fibres show signs of hypertrophy and even fusiform and varicose thickenings (*c*). One also sees, not infrequently, double clubs in the shape of a gourd (Fig. 284, *J*) and enlargements showing phenomena of cortical hyalinization. In Fig. 284, *a, d*, we reproduce some of these metamorphic clubs, in which one can discern a certain central neurofibrillar net, filled with divergent loops, which seem to invade the cortical hyaline region. As in the case of the axons of small pyramidal cells, one can also see that the delicate tangential fibres end in rings.

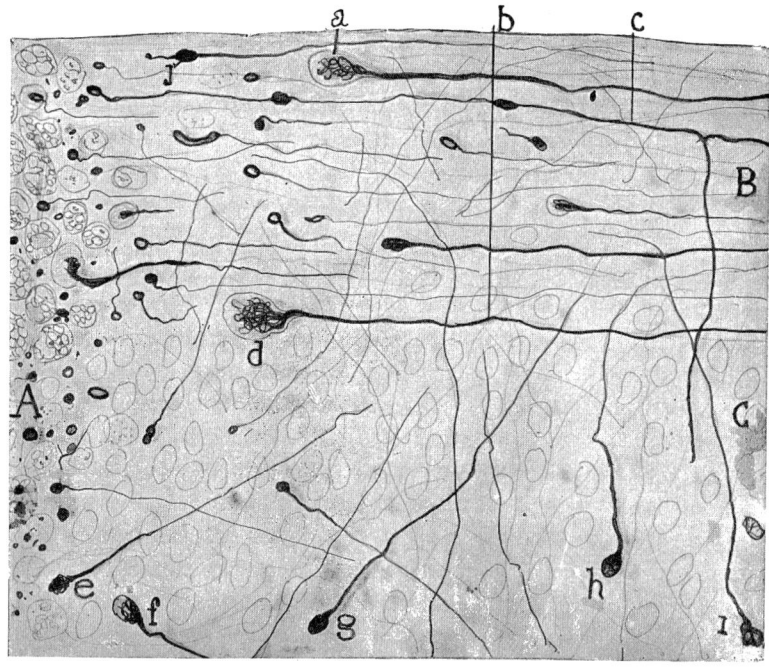

FIG. 284.—Perpendicular section of a cerebral circumvolution of a dog, two months old, which was killed one day after the operation. *A*, edge of the wound; *B*, molecular layer; *C*, layer of the small pyramidal cells; *a, d*, central stump of interrupted tangential fibres; *c*, varicose Martinotti fibre ending in a ring; *h, i*, peripheral stump of degenerated Martinotti fibres with retracted club.

It is difficult at times to distinguish, when one is dealing with fine fibres cut in the grey matter, whether the terminal club that we are considering belongs to a central or a peripheral stump. This is because, as we have often remarked, the peripheral stump of all interrupted fibres also forms, at a very early stage, a retraction club. Nevertheless, certain tangential branches, which were followed up to their continuation with ascendant Martinotti fibres (Fig. 284, *c*) had unquestionably the character of central stumps. One also may be sure of this as regards many collaterals of pyramidal cells (*f*). Other fibres, for example those designated in Fig. 284 by the letters *g, h, i,* seem to us to be peripheral stumps of Martinotti fibres, which have degenerated along their ascendant path.

To the same category of peripheral stumps doubtless belong a considerable number of conductors of the molecular layer that end in fine clubs or rings.

To sum up : the central stump of the collaterals of pyramidal cells or secondary branches of ascending arborizations (cells of Martinotti), behaves essentially in the same way as the axons of the pyramidal cells, except that the terminal club retracts very little and that the varicose and hypertrophic segments are reduced to their smallest expression, or are completely absent. We believe that we are not far from the truth when we say that, *under equal conditions, the importance of the traumatic degeneration and the extent of retrograde propagation* of the latter

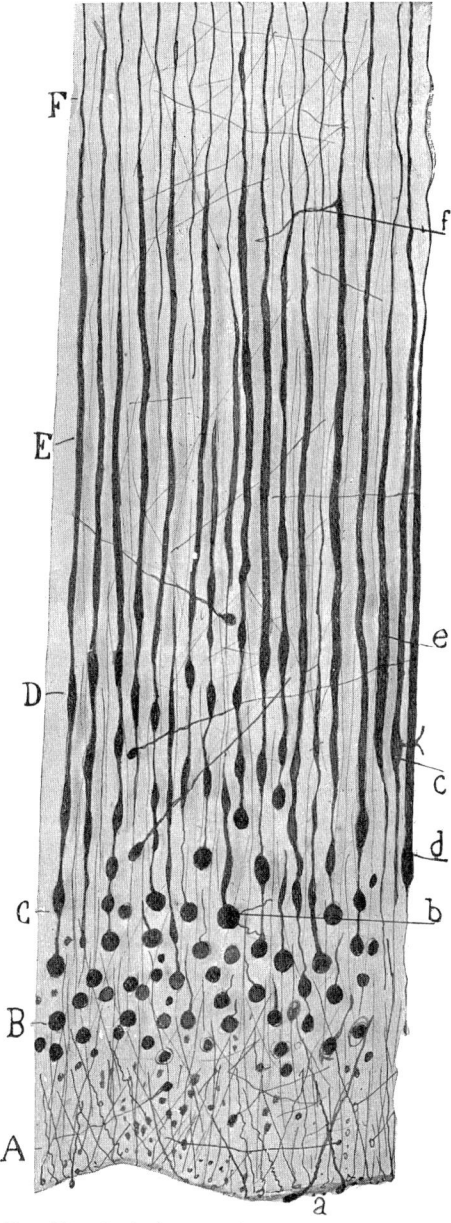

FIG. 285.—Cerebral wound in the white matter of a recently-born dog, killed one day after the operation. *A*, edge of the wound with the region of the fine fibres and clubs ; *B*, region of free balls of large size ; *C*, region of the large varicosities ; *D*, region with fusiform degeneration ; *E*, hypertrophic region; *F*, normal region of the axons ; *a*, balls fallen in the exudate ; *b*, terminal club with appendix ; *c, d*, terminal clubs from which hangs a long delicate appendix ending in a point or grume ; *e*, hypertrophic axon without a club, from which starts a long terminal fibre.

are proportional to the thickness of the medullated fibre. In the non-medullated fibres these phenomena are less extensive than in fine medullated fibres.

Degenerative phases of the peripheral stump in animals just born, or a few days old.—In order to see whether the degenerative phases of the traumatized axon that we have described occur likewise in animals recently born, or a few days old, or are subject to important variations, we have undertaken a series of experiments of cerebral lesion in recently-born cats and dogs, and in similar animals from four to fifteen days old. The animals were killed, in some cases, twenty-four hours after the operation, in others forty-eight and fifty-six hours.

In Fig. 285 we show the appearance of the white matter and contiguous portion of the grey matter in the centre of a circumvolution of a dog, four days old, which was killed after twenty-four hours. The wound here involved the white matter of the motor region at a short distance from the grey matter. One may note the thinness of the axons as compared with adult axons (*F*), and the great extent of the metamorphic segment of large and medium-sized pyramidal cells, which appear almost exclusively impregnated in the section. One may also remark, next to the wound, a zone where fine non-medullated fibres appear almost in a pure state, ending in small balls, rings, or hooks (Fig. 285, *A*).

In many of the large axons, whose terminal stump has retracted a considerable distance from the lesion, one sees, from the periphery to the centre, the *varicose, fusiform,* and *hypertrophic* phases (*D*). Nervous autotomy, or the formation of series of *free balls,* has hardly begun (*B*), and, naturally, the state of late retraction balls is lacking, as it will develop only later.

Of special interest, in this figure, is the enormous extension and unusual robustness of the hypertrophic segment of the axon, which is prolonged in many cases beyond the last collateral (*E*). This great length of the hypertrophic portion is intelligible if we remember that we are here at the beginning of the degenerative process, and that a considerable portion of the thickened axon will, in the following days, become fusiform and varicose. The texture of the hypertrophic axon can be clearly discerned, and there often appears in it a dense neurofibrillar axis and a somewhat paler and looser marginal reticulation.

Thus, although our experiments are not as yet sufficient to furnish definite conclusions, we may affirm that in young animals the degenerative phenomena in medullated tubes develop with great speed and pass through essentially the same phases as adult conductors.

ADDITIONAL NOTE TO CHAPTER II.

Among the studies which have appeared during the last few years on traumatic degeneration of the cerebrum, special mention should be made of that of Miscolczy.[1]

His observations were made on sixteen dogs whose cerebrum was cut obliquely so as to section transversally the axon of the pyramidal cells. Observations were made from fifteen minutes after the operation up to thirty hours and, some, fifteen days after the surgical intervention.

His descriptions confirm our *preserved fibres* of the edges of the wound; the *retraction balls*, with various degenerative phenomena of their protoplasm; the spiroidal dispositions of certain axons; the colossal masses along the course of cut neurites, in their central stump; axons with a neurofibrillar axis and a necrosed cortex, etc. In some degenerative axonic masses he discovered, in addition, neurofibrillar arrangements that recall Alzheimer's lesion in senile dementia, and finally, he observed, in many more or less contused neurones, granular somas that were absolutely mortified; others provided with hypertrophied and spindle-shaped neurofibrils; large vacuoles situated either in the cellular body or in the radial sprout; hypertrophy of the recurrent collaterals, when the axon had been sectioned near their point of emergence; our type of pyramid with a perinuclear reticulum similar to that of many neurones of Hirudo; and many undescribed lesions which we have not the space to enumerate here. He believes, with reason, that the *retraction ball* is a degenerative phenomenon. In a schematic figure he draws a scale of the structural morphological perturbations of the pyramidal cells according to the height at which the axon is cut.

He has not seen any mitoses of neurones, agreeing in this with Borst and ourselves, but differing from the opinion of Saltykow and others, who have admitted them. There thus does not exist in the cerebrum of mammals a real process of effective regeneration.

[1] Miscolczy: "Ueber die Frühveränderungen der Pyramidenzellen nach experimentellen Rindeverletzungen," *Travaux du Lab. de Recherches Biol.*, t. 23, 1925.

III

ALTERATIONS OF THE NERVE CELLS IN CEREBRAL TRAUMATISMS

Neuronal metamorphoses occurring after wounds that entail little or no contusion. —Disorders occasioned by contusions and commotions that are accompanied by traumatisms.—Granular degeneration, chromatolysis, hirudiform state, fusiform hypertrophy and alteration of the neurofibrils, and neurofibrillar pycnosis.

WHEN cerebral wounds occur, the pyramidal cells near the lesion, whether they are mutilated or not by the traumatic agent, undergo, owing to pressures and disturbances, various degenerative changes, which frequently end in the annihilation and resorption of the protoplasm. Since they are essentially the same as those described in connection with the spinal cord and cerebellum, we shall here speak of them only briefly. One must distinguish, to begin with, between the changes occurring in wounds when the contusion has been moderate (simple sections or punctures of the cerebrum) and those occurring after grave lacerations, contusions, and crushings.

Lesions seen in simple wounds.—No matter how thin and sharp the scalpel that penetrates into the grey matter, the wound always shows, from twelve to twenty-four hours after the lesion, a zone of ruins, granular and pale in appearance, in which one sees a great number of free axonic balls and rings, myelin drops, granular cells, leucocytes, and finally, neurones and neuroglia cells that are dead or in process of disorganization and autolysis. Among the neurones, the most frequent anatomico-pathological types are as follows:

1. *Granular neurones.*—Already twenty-four hours after the operation, and even before, there appear on the edges of the wound, and sometimes at a certain distance from it (Fig. 283, *C*), nerve cells that repel the colloidal silver and are granular in appearance. Among their granulations, some are large, grey or black, while others are fine, numerous, and colourless. The nucleus, which frequently has an almost normal nucleolus, may be situated at the side or end of a neurone (Fig. 287, *A*). Finally, the dendrites, granular and pale,

cannot be traced, and appear as though disintegrated. It seems probable that at least the neurones furnished with a marginal nucleus of an ovoid or spheroidal shape (Fig. 287, *A*) have survived the traumatic action for some hours, and have subsequently fallen into granular degeneration. As to those which have a central nucleus and normal appearance one may suppose that they fell victims to the violence of the cutting instrument.

2. *Hirudiform cells.*—These are similar to the hirudiform cells described in the spinal cord and cerebellum. They are rare, and may even be entirely lacking when the wounds are thin and there has been a minimum of traumatic commotion. In Fig. 286 we show two cells of this type, belonging to a cat, fifteen days old, which was killed three days after the operation. They were situated near the lesion, to which they sent their axon; the latter, because it appeared to be doubled back, could not be followed to its end. One may note that, at the level of the dendrites, the neurofibrillar axes show, from place to place, certain nodosities composed of loose meshes (*a*). Within the soma the net usually surrounds the nucleus; but the neurofibrils are not infrequently seen to be concentrated exclusively outside it, in a lateral region of the protoplasm (Fig. 286, *B*). The nucleus may be eccentric, or at times tangential (*B*). Finally, on the following days (third to seventh), the cortical hyaline zone advances and the neurone succumbs. The hirudiform state has been recently confirmed by Bianchi in cerebral wounds studied by Donaggio's method.[1]

3. *Cells with fusiform neurofibrillar bundles.*—These entirely reproduce the alteration described by ourselves and D. García in hydrophobia, which consists in the production, through dislocation and congregation of the neurobiones, of large bundles which are more or less fusiform and deeply stained by colloidal silver. This lesion is seen only during the first two days after the operation, and passes rapidly into the granular state.

As is well known, the *fusiform state* of the neurofibrils is found in many pathological states. Marinesco has observed it even in cases of cerebral softening through haemorrhage. Bianchi also saw it in cerebral wounds two months after the operation.

[1] Bianchi: "Alterazione istologiche della corteccia cerebrale in sequito a focolai distruttivi e a lesioni sperimentali," *Annali di Neurologia*, fasc. II. 1912. This author does not seem to know our studies of neuronal changes consequent on traumatisms, which appeared in 1911.

4. *Vacuolated neurones.*—Among the large pyramidal cells that have lost their axon at the level of, or somewhat beyond, the collaterals, and therefore undergo a slight traumatic commotion, one frequently perceives somas containing many vacuoles full of a transparent fluid, and in which the neurofibrils are arranged in anastomotic bundles or fascias. In such neurones the nucleus is tangential,

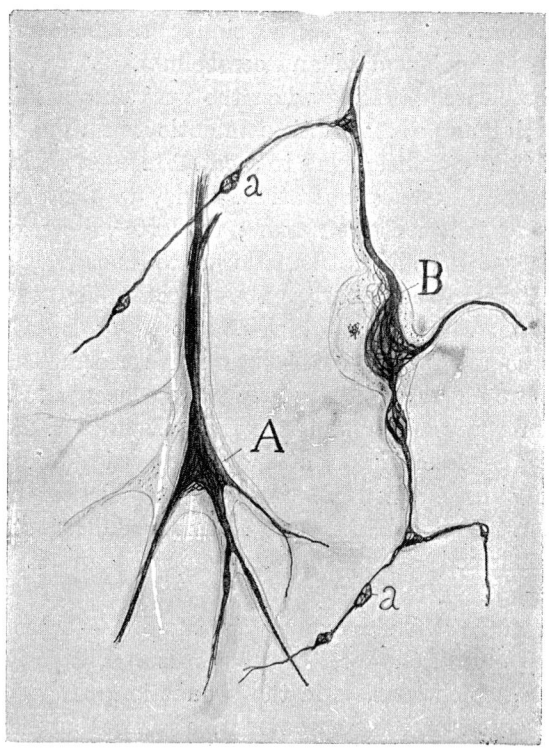

FIG. 286.—Section of the cerebral motor cortex of a cat, fifteen days old, three days after the lesion; proximal edge of the wound. *A*, median pyramidal cell with necrotic cortex and neurofibrillar axis; *B*, hirudiform type of cell with a short axon; *a*, nodosities, at the level of which large nets are to be seen.

bulging out on the edge of the cell, as in the cells that are undergoing chromatolysis (Fig. 287, *B*). At other times vacuolization is less marked; the neurofibrils are almost normal, while the nucleus, which is dislocated laterally, bulges out among the dendrites, as though striving to escape. In all these neurones the nucleolus appears more or less disintegrated and its spheres stain with difficulty. The vacuolated alteration has been described by numerous authors in the most diverse pathological states.

ALTERATIONS OF NERVE CELLS IN CEREBRAL TRAUMATISMS 681

5. *Pycnotic neurones.*—These cells are deeply stained by colloidal silver; their neurofibrils, very close to each other, hardly leave any intermediate spaces. One can easily recognize these cells, not only by their dark colour, but also because they have a soma which is

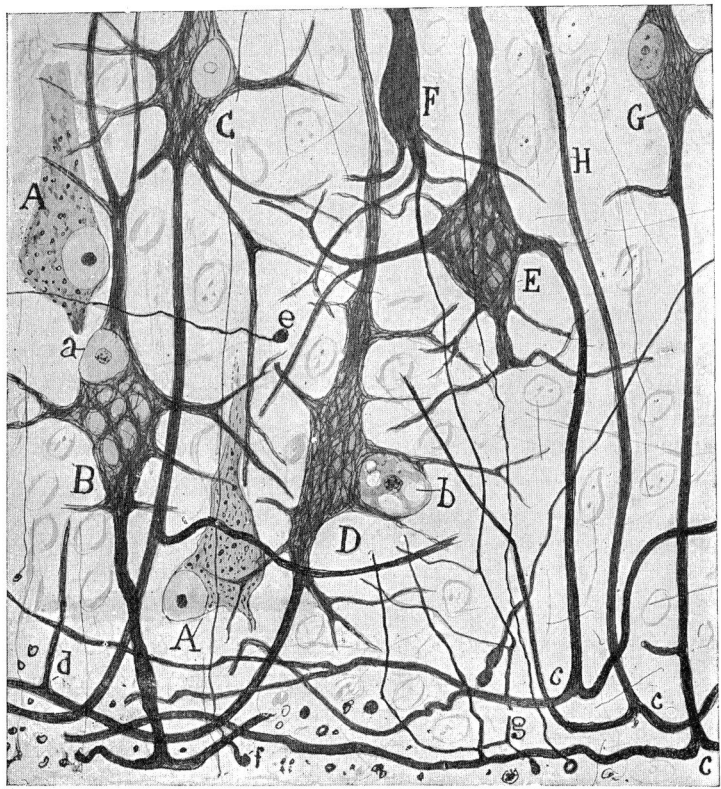

FIG. 287.—Section of the cerebral cortex of a dog, two days old, in the motor region; the animal was killed twenty-four hours after the lesion. A, gigantic necrosed pyramidal cell; B, pyramidal cell whose axon is bifurcated in the wound; C, D, pyramidal cells whose axons form an arc, being prolonged by horizontal or recurrent collaterals; E, G, H, cells whose axon is prolonged by two hypertrophied ramified collaterals; F, small cell whose axon ends in a ball beneath the point of origin of a hypertrophic arciform collateral; a, marginal nucleus; b, nucleus bulging between two appendices and vacuolated; c, bifurcation of the axon; d, secondary branches of nervous collaterals.

peculiarly elongated and a certain unusual thinness of the radial trunk and basilar dendrites. There usually springs from these an almost normal axon, furnished with collaterals which are little altered. As an exception, the cell of this type shown in Fig. 287, F, lay at a certain distance from the wound and showed an arciform axon.

6. *Cells in chromatolysis.*—These are mentioned by all the authors who have occupied themselves with nervous traumatisms. They are constantly present at some distance from the wounds. In order to see them one must, of course, use Nissl's method.

7. *Transformations of the reticular apparatus of Golgi.*—When one examines by appropriate methods, such as our process of impregnation with previous fixation in uranium nitrate-formol, the edges of a cerebral wound of a young cat or dog, killed two to four days after the operation, one sees various phases of disintegration of the Golgi apparatus, related to the amount of commotion or contusion undergone by the neuronal soma. These metamorphoses, which are very accentuated when the wound is accompanied by some contusion (such as angular pressure of the scalpel) are very restricted, being limited to a very narrow band, in simple sections.

The elements situated on the very edges of the wound—the necrotic zone—are not stained by colloidal silver. They probably correspond to the granular cells in course of disintegration and autolysis.

Somewhat beyond, that is, in the zone where neurofibrillar methods reveal cells with neurofibrils and a tangential or vacuolized nucleus, the reticulum of Golgi is fragmented, granular, sometimes reduced to a very fine dust, which is disseminated through nearly the entire soma (Fig. 288, *A*).

If one penetrates further into the living regions, this reticulum is broken, not into granules, but into relatively long cordons and even into groups of loops and meshes which remind one of the fragmentations described by Marcora and ourselves in the medulla and cord respectively (*B*). Not infrequently the nucleus, dislocated towards the periphery, leaves on one side the entire mass of the Golgi apparatus.

There finally follow regions where the apparatus appears without appreciable alteration (*A*). They coincide with the cells in which neurofibrillar methods reveal a normal neuronal structure.

All these alterations are found in a relatively narrow strip situated radially next to the radial edges of the wound. It sometimes happens, in the superior edge of the wound, that, instead of the stages of fragmentation that we have noted, the only manifestations are a notable paling and thinning of the reticulum (*C*). This rarefaction gradually disappears as one advances towards the normal regions.

Thus, in the dead cells the Golgi apparatus disappears rapidly through autolysis; in those which are degenerating it sometimes breaks down and becomes pulverized, while at other times it gradually thins down and is resorbed. We do not know exactly to what degree of neurofibrillar metamorphosis or chromatolysis these alterations correspond. At any rate, the lesions described show that the Golgi apparatus contains a granular material which may become

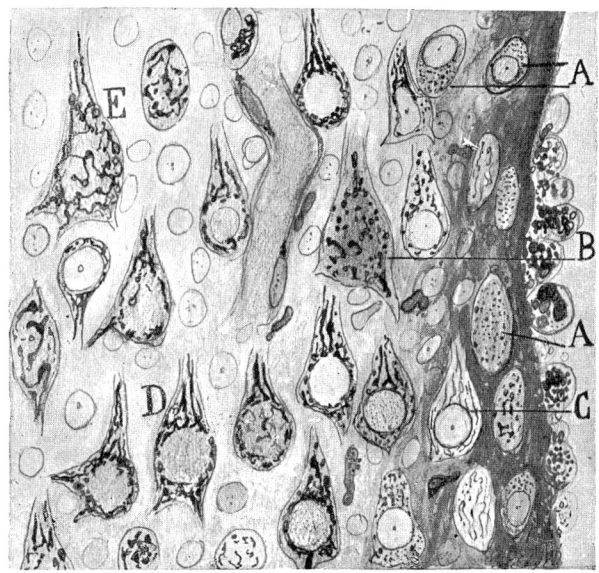

FIG. 288.—Edge of a cerebral wound of a cat, twenty days old, which was killed three days after the operation. *A*, cells with Golgi apparatus fragmented into fine grains; *C*, cell with atrophy, through thinning, of the cordons; *B*, pyramidal cell whose Golgi apparatus is segmented into cordons and large grumes; *D*, *E*, normal or nearly normal cells. Formol-uranium process.

disorganized and resorbed when the soma succumbs or undergoes grave trophic disorders.

Neuronal disorders produced by strong commotions and instantaneous crushing of the grey matter.—In connection with the study of the degeneration and regeneration of nerve centres in man, several authors have examined, by neurofibrillar methods, certain effects of slow and continued pressure on the white and grey matter. It was nearly always a question of lesions caused by compression, due either to the growth of tumours (gliomas), or to chronic inflammations (gliomas, syphilomas, tubercles, *Pott's disease*), or else to the presence of foreign bodies. From the investigations of this type undertaken by Bielschowsky,[1] Herxheimer und Gierlich,[2] R. Pfeifer,[3] Miyake,[4] Marinesco,[5] Bianchi,[6] etc., one reaches the conclusion that a compression in the spinal cord, cerebellum, or cerebrum of man, due to tumours, chronic inflammations, or Pott's disease, brings about the necrosis of the nervous tissue and causes the formation around the necrobiotic masses of terminal clubs and buds, ramified fibres, perivascular nerve plexuses, etc.

The experiments of commotion without traumatism, undertaken on animals by Schmaus, Luzenberger, Kirschgasser, Bikeles, Paracandolo, Scagliosi, Gudden, Jakob,[7] etc., show that blows and light contusions without wounds are capable of bringing about nutritive disorders in the cells (vacuolations, chromatolysis, etc.), as well as degeneration of the medullary sheath.

We shall not here analyze the effects of simple commotions without wounds or of slow and progressive experimental compression. We shall merely mention the lesions occurring in the neurones when instantaneous compression and commotion are combined in the same operation. This occurs, for example, when, having introduced a scalpel in the cerebrum, one imparts to it angular movements in order to crush and violently shake, in a tangential direction, the cortical grey matter. The lesions thus produced evolve very rapidly, and the animal should be autopsied from six to twenty-four hours after the operation. After a few days nearly all the neurones

[1] Bielschowsky: "Ueber das Verhalten des Achsencylinders in Geschwülsten des Nervensystems," etc., *Jour. f. Psych. u. Neurol.*, vol. 7, 1906.

[2] Herxheimer u. Gierlich: *Studien über die Neurofibrillen im Zentralnervensystem*, etc., Wiesbaden, 1907.

[3] R. Pfeifer: "Ueber die traumatische Degeneration und Regeneration des Gehirns erwachsener Menschen," *Jour. f. Psych. u. Neurol.*, Bd. 12, 1908.

[4] Miyake: "Zur Frage der Regeneration der Nervenfasern in zentralen Nervensystem," *Arbeiten aus dem neurol. Institut an der Wiener Universität*, Bd. 12, 1908.

[5] Marinesco: "Sur la neurotisation des foyers de ramollissement et d'hémorrhagie cérébrale," *Rev. neurol.*, déc. 1910.

Idem: "Nouvelles contributions à l'étude de la régénérescence des fibres du système nerveux central," *Jour. f. Psych. u. Neurol.*, Bd. 17, 1910.

[6] Bianchi: *loc. cit.*

[7] Jakob: "Experimentelle Untersuchungen über die traumatischen Schädigungen des Zentralnervensystems," etc., *Histol. u. Histopath. Arbeiten über d. Grosshirnrinde*, von F. Nissl und A. Alzheimer, Bd. 5, 1913.

affected by the instantaneous contusion or compression have fallen into necrobiosis, and are unstainable.

Six hours after the operation conditions are as follows : On the edges of the cerebral wound, which are, therefore, the seat of maximum compression, no neurones are stained ; the somas and dendrites reject the colloidal silver, and it is only the nuclei that stand out in the midst of a pale, grey, granular substance, traversed by spaces full of liquid. On the other hand, there still subsist some nerve plexuses which attract the silver strongly, showing that the resistance of the fine non-medullated fibres to traumatic violence is much greater than that of the neurones. From this region, where the alterations are extreme, up to regions where the neurones are absolutely normal there are transitions which take the form of degrees of simplification and metamorphosis of the reticulum. Not all the lesions, however, undergo a morphological cycle. Some of them appear to be more or less permanent states, although our investigations on this point are far from being exhaustive. At any rate, the most common changes, beginning with the regions of the slightest alterations, are as follows :

(a) *Contracted and pycnotic pyramidal cells.*—These are exceptional in wounds that are free from commotion, but numerous when the compression has been violent ; they are always situated at a certain distance from the lesion. Their characters coincide with those already referred to when we were dealing with neuronal effects in simple wounds. We may note again the transversal contraction of the soma, the intense colourability of the reticulum, and, finally, the thinning of the dendrites, which appear to be formed by a thick neurofibrillar bundle. Owing to this excessive colourability of the reticulum, the nucleus is hardly seen ; the hollow spaces which correspond to the grumes of Nissl are very narrow, and the neurofibrils, very close to each other, can with difficulty be detected. As we show in Figs. 289, *H*, and 290, *B*, the dendrites are compact from their origin, and the secondary and tertiary branches are so thin that they appear to be constituted by a single neurofibril. The axon forms a very dark and thick bundle. The pycnotic state may be partial and occur only in the dendrites and axon. Fine dark expansions, in which no neurofibrils can be distinguished, are then seen issuing from a soma that has a loose and normal, or almost normal, reticulum.

(b) *Hypertrophic neurofibrillar state.*—This is more frequent than the previous type, and much more characteristic of cerebral compression. It is a pyramidal cell whose reticulum, in full metamorphosis, reminds one very much of the initial phases of the fusiform alteration in hydrophobia. It is characterized by the local thickening, with intense stainability, of some neurofibrils, most of them longitudinal (Fig. 289, J), accompanied by the thinning and paling

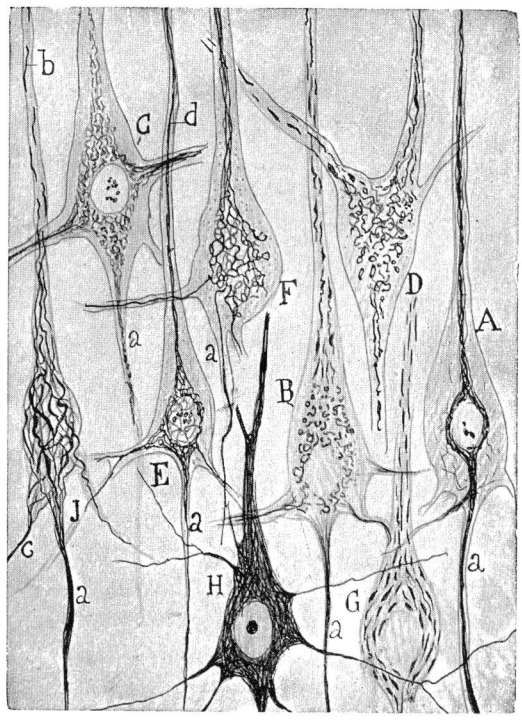

FIG. 289.—Edges of a contused cerebral wound in a cat, twenty days old, which was killed twenty-one hours after the lesion. A, E, F, hirudiform neurones; B, C, D, phases of granular formation of the hirudiform type; G, type with neurofibrillar spindles; J, type with hypertrophic neurofibrils; a, axon; b, neurofibrillar spindles.

of others, which hardly attract the colloidal silver. In addition, the interfibrillar spaces are dilated, the secondary neurofibrils are resorbed or hyalinized, and there is formed, in this way, a net of spacious longitudinal meshes, whose trabeculae stand out vigorously, converging in the axon and dendrites. Some of the neurofibrils follow a serpentine course. The dendrites, as in the preceding type, are thin, dark, and compact, except where they originate; there their neurofibrils are clearly separated and much reduced in number.

The hypertrophic state occurs very precociously. As we show in Fig. 290, C, it is found as early as six hours after the operation, and perhaps earlier, and it lasts for at least a day after the lesion

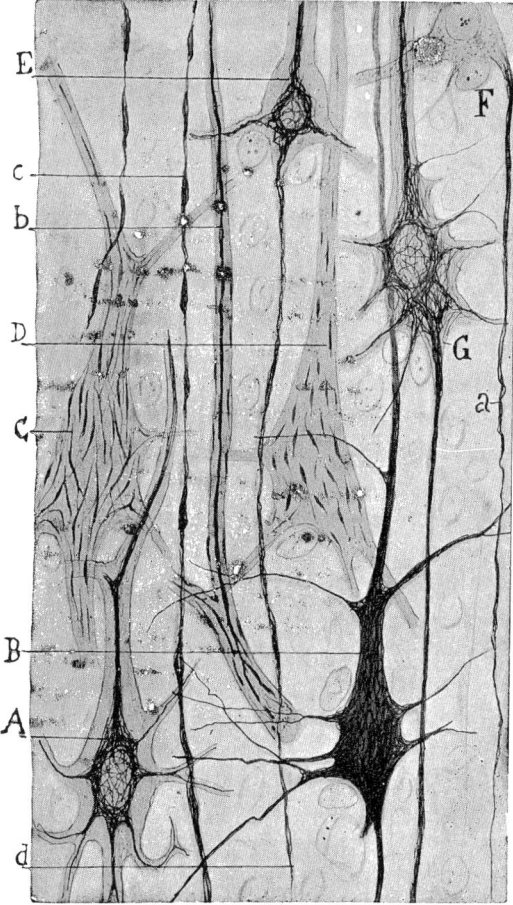

FIG. 290.—Piece of grey matter situated near a contused cerebral wound in a dog twenty-five days old, six hours after the operation. A, E, hirudiform types; B, hyperchromatic neurone; C, D, neurones with neurofibrillar spindles; F, hyalinized neurone with altered axon; a, axon; b, neurofibrillar axis of a dendritic trunk; d, atrophied point of an axon; c, altered dendrite.

(Fig. 289, J). After two days this cellular type becomes rare, and then disappears.

(c) *Fusiform state of the neurofibrils.*—This is even more frequently met with than the preceding type, especially if one examines brains of cats or dogs killed ten to twenty-four hours after the compression. It reproduces the disposition described above (Figs. 289, *G*, and 290, *D*), appearing constantly in contused brains.

The fusiform state is retained for a short time. After two days nearly all the cells that exhibit that state fail entirely to stain. Before losing their stainability and falling into necrobiosis the spindles shorten and become pale, attracting less and less the colloidal silver. At the same time the pale intercalary spaces become larger. Finally, the spindles nearest to the nucleus fade away and the neurone becomes granular.

Two interesting peculiarities distinguish the fusiform state of cerebral neurones due to traumatism or compression from that brought about by cold or infections. As we show in Fig. 290, *D*, the spindles are very thin and small—in pyramidal cells in hydrophobia they are apt to be larger—and, above all, these thickenings do not lie exclusively in the soma, but extend throughout the radial trunk and the principal somatic dendrites (Fig. 289, *G*). In the trunk the argentophilous material often shows up as a continuous central axis almost devoid of thickenings (Fig. 289, *d*), while the marginal zone displays longitudinal spindles (Fig. 289, *b*). As a rule there is only a line or series of such tangential thickenings. In some cells, where the fusiform somatic state is little advanced, the radial trunk has no neurofibrillar axis, and appears sprinkled with spindles. The fusiform state may start at the dendrites and subsequently extend to the soma, or on the contrary, may begin in the soma and spread into the protoplasmic expansions. One frequently notices that while certain dendrites have spindles, others are almost normal. The fusiform state is thus a local reaction of the reticulum, which may spread to almost the whole of the soma and dendrites, but which is also capable of subsisting for some time without any tendency to diffusion in particular neuronal regions. This peculiarity has already been noted by us some time ago in the axons of the peripheral stump of cut nerves.

The axon of the cerebral pyramidal cells never shows the fusiform alteration, and this is a curious point which distinguishes well the dendrites from the axon.

(*d*) *Hirudiform state.*—This has been described by us on various occasions,[1] and also above in connection with the effect of simple

[1] Cajal: "Los fenómenos precoces de la degeneración neuronal en el cerebelo." "Los fenómenos precoces de la degeneración traumática de los cilindros-ejes del cerebro," etc. *Trab. del Lab. de Invest. biol.*, t. 9, fascs. 1, 2, and 3, 1911.

cerebral wounds. This pathological type is especially abundant in the contusions and lacerations of the grey matter. There are reasons for thinking that its abundance is in direct proportion to the violence and diffusion of the mechancial waves. Preparations from cats and dogs that have been killed six, twelve, and twenty-one hours after the operation indicate, moreover, that this metamorphosis is very precocious, appearing preferably in neurones that are near to the necrotic regions, and leading, by gradual transitions, to another state, which we shall call *granular metamorphosis of the reticulum*.

The forms assumed by the hirudiform alteration in the cerebral neurones are very varied. In all the types the stainable reticulum is concentrated around the nucleus, but there is much variation in the extension and thickness of the preserved skeleton, as also in the disposition of the neurofibrillar net. A somewhat uncommon variation is that shown in Fig. 289, *A* (cat twenty days old), where this skeleton is reduced to two bundles of fibres which, after surrounding the nucleus and ramifying so as to produce a net, connect respectively with the axis of the radial trunk and the axon, along which they extend for a long distance.

Apart from some of the dendrites, the basilar and lateral expansions of the soma appear devoid of stainable filaments. In less advanced phases of this metamorphosis one may discern, within the protoplasmic cortex of the soma, a few pale and loose neurofibrils.

Very close to this disposition is that shown in Fig. 290, *A*, *E*, found in the cortex of a dog six hours after the traumatism. The neurofibrillar cortex concentrated round the nucleus is thicker, and the trunk as well as the fine dendrites has a neurofibrillar axis constituted by a bundle of fine fibres.

Another hirudiform type, shown in the cell of Fig. 289, *F*, is somewhat more common, especially in the cortex of cats, twenty-one hours after the operation. The perinuclear net is very thin, being formed of relatively thick trabeculae, clearly anastomosed, which enclose rounded or polygonal meshes, some large, some narrow, the latter usually congregated in little groups. A neurofibrillar bundle penetrates into the axis of the trunk, while in the axon as well as in the basilar dendrites may be seen fine compact cordons, which are formed at times of a single neurofibril. The number of fibres entering into each expansion, as also their thickness, vary greatly, according to the case under examination.

The nucleolus of the hirudiform type is almost always altered.

As a rule, its argentophilous spherules are unequal and disintegrated, reminding one of the dispositions pointed out by us in hydrophobia, and well observed and described by Achúcarro [1] in this infection and in other morbid conditions.

(e) *State of discontinuous or granular reticulum.*—This lesion consists in a coarse or fine fragmentation of the somatic reticulum, whose pieces, concentrated principally in the perinuclear region, mark the position occupied in an earlier phase by the principal filaments of the hirudiform state. As may be seen in Fig. 289, B, C, D, this fragmentation, which is seen in all its phases, sometimes exhibits the form of large pieces like bacilli, commas, or rings; at other times it is composed of finer pieces, which are ovoid or spheroidal, and arranged in a series, like seeds. The granules still delineate the old meshes of the reticulum. As we show in Fig. 289, the disintegration of the reticulum proceeds unequally in each cell. Usually it appears less advanced in the axon than in the dendrites, and less in the latter than in the soma. One commonly sees (Fig. 289, B) in the basilar dendrites and the axon a manifestly fasciculated appearance, when the net of the soma has been reduced to fine grains. One may also frequently observe in the dendrites fusiform neurofibrillar fragments which remind one somewhat of the *fusiform* state described above. In the more advanced phases of the process the entire reticulum is pulverized into more or less pale, grey granules, which are concentrated in the central regions of the reticulum. It is very possible that the granular alteration of the reticulum coincides with the necrosis of the hirudiform cell.

One must not confuse this granular fragmentation of the reticulum with the pulverization or *granular degeneration* that various authors, particularly Marinesco and Dustin, have described in neurones subjected to the effects of anaemia and other nutritive disturbances. In the lesion that we are now studying we have, not a direct disintegration of all the reticulum into very fine granules, but a fragmentation of the perinuclear skeleton characteristic of the hirudiform state, with pieces that are relatively large.

Precocious alterations of compressed cerebral axons.—In general one may affirm that compression rapidly alters the soma and dendrites, but not the axon, which resists, without obvious modification, relatively large commotions and pressures. One therefore often sees

[1] Achúcarro: " Zur Kenntniss der path. Histologie des Zentralnervensystems bei Tollwut," *Nissl-Alzheimer Arbeiten*, Bd. 3, H. 1, 1909.

in sections of the cerebra of cats, twenty-one hours after the operation, large neurones with their reticulum in granular disintegration, while the axon remains more or less normal in the first part of its course. In Fig. 290, *F*, we show some cells of this type, in which the neurofibrils of the axon seem to end within the soma in series of granulations. The axon extends a long way in a cellulifugal direction, apparently retaining its normal aspect. Nevertheless, when one follows it sufficiently far, one notices that, once it has reached the region of the collaterals, it undergoes a certain abnormal thinning, as though certain superficial neurofibrils had been resorbed (Fig. 290, *a*).

A common alteration of the axons that extend from the hirudiform type of cell in its various modalities is a rarefaction of the reticulum, associated with the presence of fine thickenings in the course of the remaining filaments. These thickenings, which have a certain parallel character, and are fairly prolonged, give a peculiar double effect to the axon (Fig. 290, *a, d*). The doubled or trebled parts, that is, the regions constituted by two or three thickened and intensely stained neurofibrils, alternate irregularly with segments that are little stained and almost invisible. If one follows the axon sufficiently far, one reaches regions where it becomes so pale and thin as to be almost invisible (Fig. 290, *d*).

Alteration of the dendrites.—The dendrites that are subjected to instantaneous compressions also atrophy and disappear, after displaying phenomena of simplification and metamorphosis. We have spoken of radial trunks sprinkled with elongated spindles which are characteristic of the hirudiform types and of those in the fusiform state. We must speak of other alterations occasioned by the compression or its results. One of them is the *moniliform state*, with breaking down of the neurofibrils. We reproduce various cases of it in Fig. 290, *c*. Sometimes the neurofibrils of the trunk subsist, but they are unequally impregnated, and dark and pale zones alternate irregularly. In other trunks the dark segments are seen in a simplified form, so that, instead of one bundle of fibres there are two or three, more or less thickened, which penetrate into the pale segment, where they become thin and hyaline or invisible. There are also dendrites that are absolutely disintegrated, in other words devoid of apparent neurofibrils. These have been replaced by a substance that stains grey and is finely granular and is arranged in bead-like varicosities, within which a vacuole is at times discernible.

In fine, one may deduce from the above that the lesions brought about in the grey matter by instantaneous movement and compression, associated with traumatisms, are the same, *mutatis mutandis*, in all the nerve centres. There is thus confirmed once more the concept of the uniformity of reaction of the reticulum and of the grumes of Nissl. These reactions (hirudiform state, fusiform state, chromatolysis, etc.), are not specific in any way, nor are they associated necessarily with particular affections, nor bound up with particular chemical or physical stimuli. The neurone responds to the most varied stimuli by uniform reactions, which succeed each other in a regular order, from the slight thickening of the neurofibrils up to the granular destruction of the reticulum and liquefaction of the chromatophilic material.

As regards the components of the reticulum, these alterations also corroborate the concept frequently maintained in the course of this work, namely, that in presence of destructive causes the neurobiones defend their life, retreating and succumbing from the periphery to the centre, or, in other words, from the cortical to the perinuclear region; the same occurs in axons and autotomised balls. Before dying, however, they nearly always form, as ephemeral adaptations, new neurofibrillar constructions such as nets, loops, rings, spindles, etc. The last point of resistance is in the vicinity of the nucleus, as though the neurobiones found in it some nutritive material capable of sustaining for a certain time their threatened lives.

IV

PHENOMENA OF ABORTED REGENERATION IN THE CEREBRAL CORTEX

Regenerative inefficiency of the central paths.—Internal and external productions of the central stump of the axon.—" Cephalopodic " structures and neurofibrillar spools.—Radial or " testudinoid " formations of the varicosities.—Aspect of these neoformations in the cerebrum of recently-born individuals.—Incongruence and break-down of these neoformations.

ON various occasions, basing ourselves on precise observations by ourselves and others, we have recorded the radical incapacity of central axons, medullated or non-medullated, young or old, to restore interrupted paths of the white and grey matter. In the spinal cord, however, under propitious circumstances, one sees from time to time cones of growth connected with axons of the white matter and capable of ramifying and growing across the scar. But in the cerebellum and cerebrum this vigorous, though ineffective, attempt to innervate the cicatricial connective tissue is always lacking.

Nor is there anything to hope from the beneficial effects of time. In the nerves the restoration is a revolutionary work, begun with the utmost rapidity and activity, and apparently stimulated by obstacles. In the centres, on the contrary, the apathy or precarious productive attempts of the first few days are succeeded by the most absolute inactivity. After one, two, or more months the neuroglial or connective scar has united the edges of the wound, but no sprout crosses the scar, connecting the two sides. Those perforating fibres first pointed out by us, and whose regenerative character appeared probable, have been shown, by a scrupulous analysis, to be *preserved fibres*. One must recognize that the axons of the cerebrum and cerebellum are far less plastic than those of the cord, and more refractory to the action of the neurocladic stimuli of the connective tissue.

We do not hold the view, however, that the interrupted cerebral axons have absolutely no neurocladic activity. Various authors have seen partial and incongruent acts of regeneration of axons in the cerebrum of man after haemorrhages, softening, and tumours, and, as we shall point out below, the axons of young animals are also capable, in the presence of traumatisms, of attempting the production of sprouts. It is true that such reactions are ephemeral, aborted, and purposeless; but, although ineffective, they merit careful study. No matter what their significance, these productions have a positive biological interest. Besides fortifying the doctrine of neurobional autonomy, they definitely refute the fatalist concept of the essential irregenerability of central paths.

The progressive mutations of the pyramidal axons may be grouped into two categories : *intra-axonic* and *extra-axonic neoformations*.

Extra-axonic neoformations.—Leaving aside here the production of clubs and the hypertrophic phenomena of the axon and collaterals, of which we have spoken above, one may affirm that the only positive act of production of sprouts consists in the radial or testudinoid neoformations pointed out by us [1] in the cerebrum of cats and dogs. We are speaking here only of spontaneous productions, thus excluding the extraordinary arborizations and growths obtained by Tello in his admirable experiments of intracerebral grafts of nerves. We shall deal with these later.

Radial or testudinoid neoformations.—These are very precocious productions, appearing from the twentieth hour and reaching their climax between the second and the third days after the operation. They are found in the central stump of the medullated axons of large pyramidal cells, in the region of the *traumatic degeneration* (varicose segment), and at a certain distance from the wound. They consist in divergent branches which are repeatedly divided, and which spring from the axonic spindles and varicosities, in the second and third phases, somewhat like terminal balls. The aspect of such varicosities, with their radiations, reminds one of a spider, or rather of a turtle with extended legs. It is for this reason that we have named them *testudinoid structures*. The branches are the longer and more numerous in proportion as the medullated axon is larger.

[1] Cajal : " Algunos hechos de regeneración parcial de la substancia gris de los centros nerviosos," *Trab. del Lab. de Invest. biol.*, t. 8, 1910.

Idem : " Note sur la dégénérescence traumatique des fibres nerveuses du cerveau et du cervelet," *Trav. du Lab. de Rech. biol.*, t. 5, 1907.

These newly-formed appendices are collateral and terminal or, in other words, they spring sometimes, and more frequently, from varicosities along the course of the fibres, and sometimes from terminal varicosities or clubs. The latter seem to represent spheres of late retraction, since below them and towards the wound one always finds series of more or less independent balls.

In Fig. 291, *E*, *F*, we show various types of these interesting formations. One may note the divergent direction of their appendices, their division into secondary branches, and the extreme paleness of their last branchlets, which seem to end in a point. In certain cases the stumps that are very visible (Fig. 291, *a*) assume the appearance of terminal buds or grumes. As a rule the voluminous varicosities have thick and abundant appendices, as one can see in Fig. 291, *F*, where the testudinoid structure reminds one of the soma of a pyramidal cell. On the other hand, the small varicosities, which usually lie on medium-sized fibres, are poor in branches (Fig. 291, *J*, *R*, and 292, *c*, *d*).

There also are differences between the testudinoid dispositions of adult animals and of those recently born or a few days old. While in the robust medullated axons of the cerebrum of dogs three months old these divergent appendices are thick and abundant, in the thin axons of young cerebra they are short and few, and are often entirely absent. Sometimes, two days after a cerebral traumatism in cats, rabbits, and dogs less than one week old, one can discern no testudinoid structures, even though the various degenerative phases of the axons can be recognized. The presence of a medullary sheath and an axon of large diameter appear to be necessary conditions to the production of numerous testudinoid figures rich in divergent appendices. In Fig. 294, *G*, we show a ball, situated on the course of a fibre, which has ramified appendices; in *i* we reproduce a terminal club which emits a prolongation ending in a bulb (Fig. 294).

Finally, in a few days the neoformative dispositions just described disappear. After the first week they are already very rare, and after fifteen days they are completely absent. All the varicosities, where they could be seen, have become transformed into free spheres, and many of them have completely disappeared.

Newly-formed branches springing from non-thickened regions of the axon.—When examining the central stump of the axon of pyramidal cells in connection with the study of wounds from thirty-six to fifty-six hours old, we have seen, here and there, a few short branches issuing at a right angle, and ending in small clubs or varicosities. In Fig. 292, *f*, for example, we show two branches issuing from the thin portion of an axon, near a terminal ball. Similar branches appear in Fig. 291, *b*, in a portion of the axon which is situated between varicosities. These appendices ended in sharp points. We cannot at present determine whether such branches are true neofor-

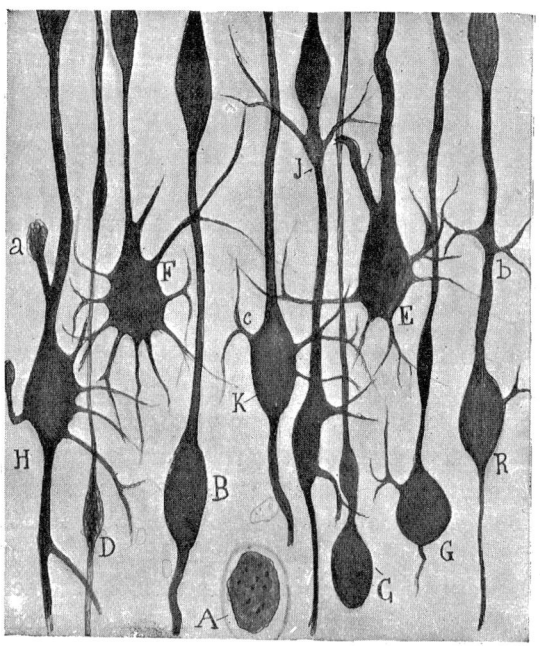

FIG. 291.—In this figure have been assembled various types of testudinoid structures as seen in a cerebral section of a dog, two months old, fifty-six hours after the operation ; region of the varicosities of the giant axons. *A*, granular ball of axons that have been precociously destroyed ; *B*, large varicose fibre ; *D*, thin varicose fibre ; *E*, *F*, *G*, terminal testudinoid structures ; *H*, *J*, *K*, *R*, collateral testudinoid structures ; *a*, appendix ending in a reticulated ball ; *c*. appendices ending in a pale point.

mations or whether they are remnants of pre-existent collaterals in process of atrophy, although we incline towards the first opinion.

Intra-axonic neoformations.—These consist of ramified sproutings of the neurofibrils within the necrosed portions of the axon. The central stump of the axon, in its degenerative segment, often undergoes, owing to the traumatic commotion, cortical necroses confined to a varicosity or tumefied region more or less distant from the wound. Such vegetations, which are very tangled and end in balls of various dimensions, arise from a neurofibrillar axis which

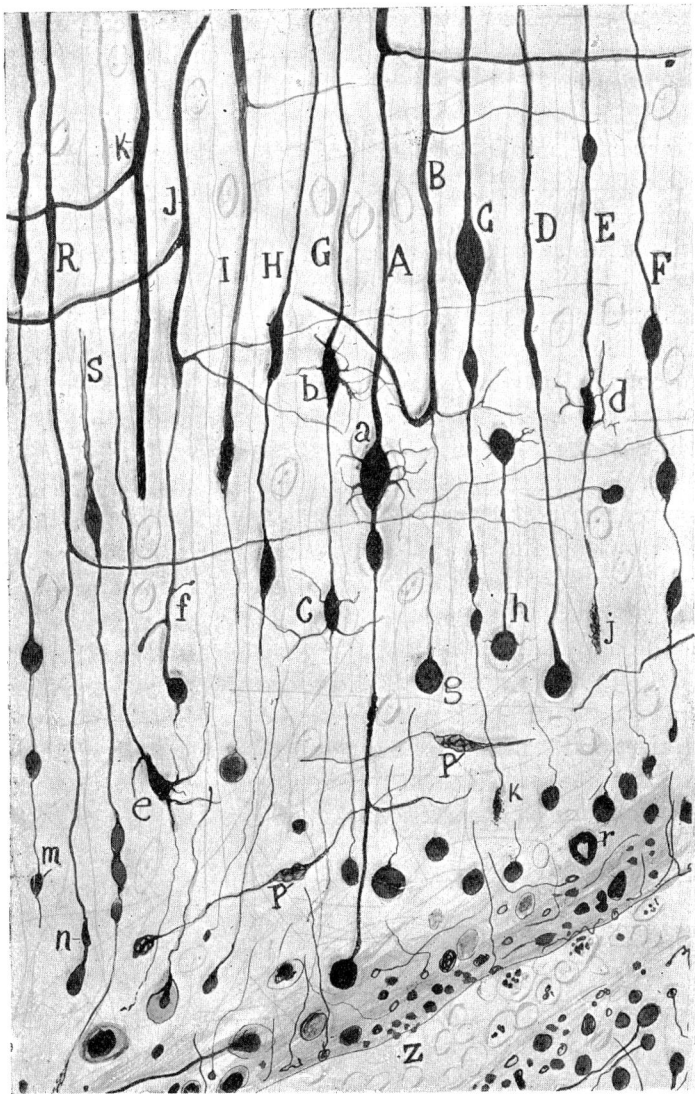

FIG. 292.—Cerebral wound of a dog, from fifteen to twenty days old, fifty-six hours after the operation.—A, B, C, D, E, F, various morphological types of degeneration of the large axons; G, axon with two testudinoid structures (b, c); H, I, fibres whose club emits delicate fibres ending in a grume or small ball near the wound; J, K, R, axons with hypertrophic collaterals; Z, oblique wound of the deep portion of the grey matter; h, coupled free balls; j, terminal grume of an axon; p, free collaterals with reticulated varicosities; r, gigantic independent ring. (Semi schematic figure.)

subsists in the semi-necrosed varicosity. The peculiar and interesting figures which result often roughly resemble a calamary. For this reason, and for the sake of brevity, we shall call them *cephalopodic structures*.

The *cephalopodic structures* are *collateral* and *terminal*.

The most common type of terminal cephalopodic structure is that shown in Fig. 293, *A, B, C*. We are dealing with an axon in the varicose state. One of the varicosities has become detached from the series of balls, but is still united to the central stump of the axon. Above the terminal varicosity the phenomenon of local necrosis previously mentioned has occurred. The cortical neurofibrillar zone has disappeared, and there remains a fine axis stainable by the colloidal silver, while the neuroplasm and remnants of the destroyed framework form a voluminous mass of a spheroidal or semi-ellipsoidal shape; it is perfectly transparent, its outline is difficult to discern, and within it, as though in a good culture medium, the neurofibrils now grow. The varicosity, which is more or less hollowed out on the side of the neuroplasmic mass, receives the terminal stump of the axonic axis, and sometimes gives rise to ramified appendices.

All these appendices springing from the terminal club, and the other more numerous ones that issue at a right angle from the axis of the axon, divide and subdivide successively in the region of the neuroplasm, and remnants of the necrosed axon wind and turn and end in spheroidal thickenings. The branches, relatively thick, end in thick, finely reticulated or granular bulbs; the most delicate may end in rings. They are all, however, confined within the borders of the neuro-plasmic dilatation. Sometimes the pedicle which supports the large terminal grumes is so tenuous or so pale as to be hardly visible, and the thickenings seem to be free balls.

A careful analysis of the pedicles, as also of the axis of the cephalopodic structures, clearly reveals a neurofibrillar texture. This axon is composed of a bundle, more or less ravelled out, of fibres that stain well, and each branch is composed of one or more neurofibrils. In the bifurcations of the appendices we can clearly see the division of the neurofibrils and, less distinctly, the reticular arrangement of their terminal bulbs. Finally, having regard to the direction of many branches, it appears as though the colossal ball attached to them were the centre of nutritive energy that has been used up in the creation of the cephalopodic structure.

In certain cephalopodic structures the large varicosity that precedes them may be wanting or may be reduced to a very small

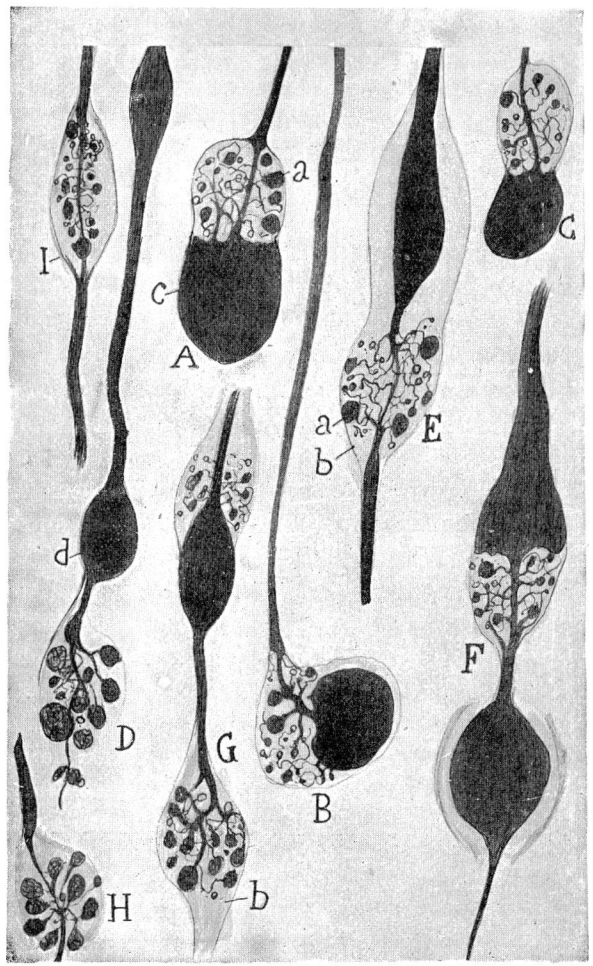

FIG. 293.—In this figure have been assembled various cephalopodic structures found in two successive sections of a cerebral wound of a dog, two months old, which was killed fifty-six hours after the operation. Region of the varicose axons— *A, B, C,* terminal cephalopodic structures along the fibres; *D, H,* structures in which the hyaline portion of the axon tends to disappear, the nerve sprouts remaining free; *a,* grumes in which the intra-axonic appendices terminate; *b,* hyaline portion of the axon in which the sprouts grow; *d,* thick varicosity from which the newly-formed appendices emanate.

volume, a disposition that is sometimes associated with an almost complete invisibility of the contour of the hyalinized axonic region. The resulting aspect, which recalls somewhat the terminal arrangements of the moss-like fibres of the cerebellum, is that of a radial and multiple arborization springing from the free central stump of a voluminous axon (Fig. 293, *D*, *H*). One would think that one was dealing with a vegetation of independent nerve sprouts. As appears from Fig. 293, *D*, it is difficult not to believe that, after the destruction of the segment of the axon, within which some of these divergent branches were nourished, these have recovered their independence, growing more or less in the interaxonic spaces.

Collateral cephalopodic structures are perhaps more frequent than terminal ones and are formed on the same lines. As may be seen in Figs. 293 and 294, the neoformative process occurs indifferently at the central or peripheral ends of a voluminous varicosity. In some cases (Fig. 293, *F*) the thickening furnishes appendices to the terminal spool, and the former appears more or less hollowed out to receive it; in others (Fig. 293, *E*) the varicosity lies somewhat separated, and all the intra-axonic branches arise from the neurofibrillar axis of the cephalopodic structure. Finally, there are fibres whose cephalopodic structure lies at a great distance from the varicosities, this being rather exceptional (Fig. 293, *G*, *I*). In some thick axons there are two and even three cephalopodic structures.

Is the disposition that we are studying something transitory, or is it the point of departure of ulterior neoformative processes ? At first sight, and considering certain characteristics, such as crowding of spheres, radiating pedicles, etc., one might believe that these cephalopodic structures are the primordial phases of the curious lesion described in man by Fischer under the name of *senile plates*, and confirmed by Perusini, Achúcarro, etc., who stained them by ordinary methods; they were subsequently impregnated with colloidal silver in the cerebrum of old men by Simchowicz, Marinesco, etc.

To establish between these two phenomena a connecting link one need merely suppose that, once the neuroplasm and the terminal ball are resorbed, the appendices of the cephalopodic structure become free, grow in all directions, trace complicated turns, and finally give rise to a kind of colony of terminal balls. But in order to be certain of the identity of the senile plates of Fischer (*colonies of clubs of* Marinesco) and the structure described by us, it would be necessary to follow its metamorphoses from the third day after the lesion on, and to show its transformation into a wide colony of divergent terminal balls. Unfortunately, the investigations undertaken up to now in animals that were over two months old or adult, and whose traumatisms were investigated fifteen to twenty days after the operation, have never shown us anything similar to the *senile plates* of Fischer, or the *colonies of clubs* of Marinesco. Besides, the buds and fibres of the *senile plates* of man are such complicated and altered dispositions, perhaps owing to a process of resorption and atrophy, that it is nearly always very difficult to follow the path of the pedicle and to see where it is implanted.

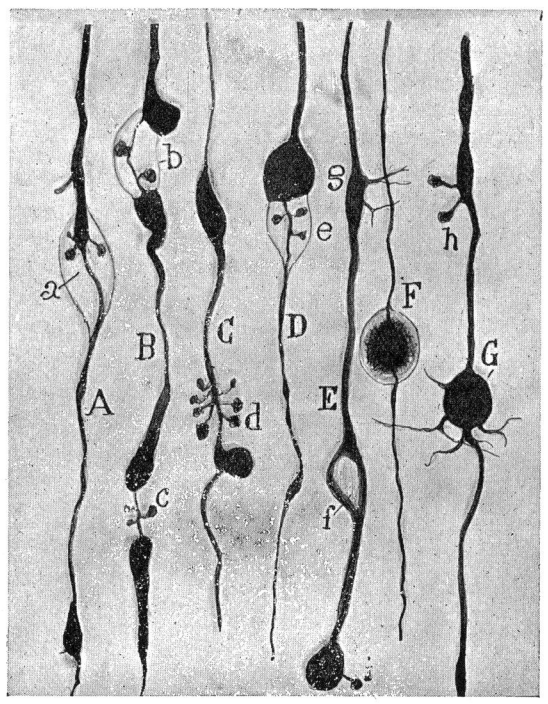

FIG. 294.—Cephalopodic and testudinoid structures found in various sections of a cerebral wound of a dog, twenty-four days old, killed three days after the operation. *A, B, D,* axons with cephalopodic structures along their course ; *C,* axon whose cephalopodic structure appears free (*d*) ; *E, G,* axons with testudinoid structures ; *a, b,* hyaline portion of the axon ; *c, d,* sprouts which appear free through resorption of the hyaline portion ; *f,* vacuole in a varicosity ; *h,* sprouts of a small thickening ; *i,* terminal ball with an appendix ending in a spherule.

We have seen the testudinoid and cephalopodic structures only in cats and dogs. In adult rabbits wounds of the white matter have given us, and that rarely, only indications of the cephalopodic disposition. As a rule, the thicker the axons the more abundant and complicated are these dispositions. One may well believe that in man, whose white matter contains robust axons, a study of fibres recently injured (thirty-six to forty-eight hours before) would yield an abundant harvest of testudinoid and cephalopodic structures.

Recently-born animals, as well as animals a few days old, display very few cephalopodic structures. As we show in Fig. 294, *a, b, e*, the branches that innervate the hyalinized portion of the axon are few in number; they are very short, without curves, and end in a granular

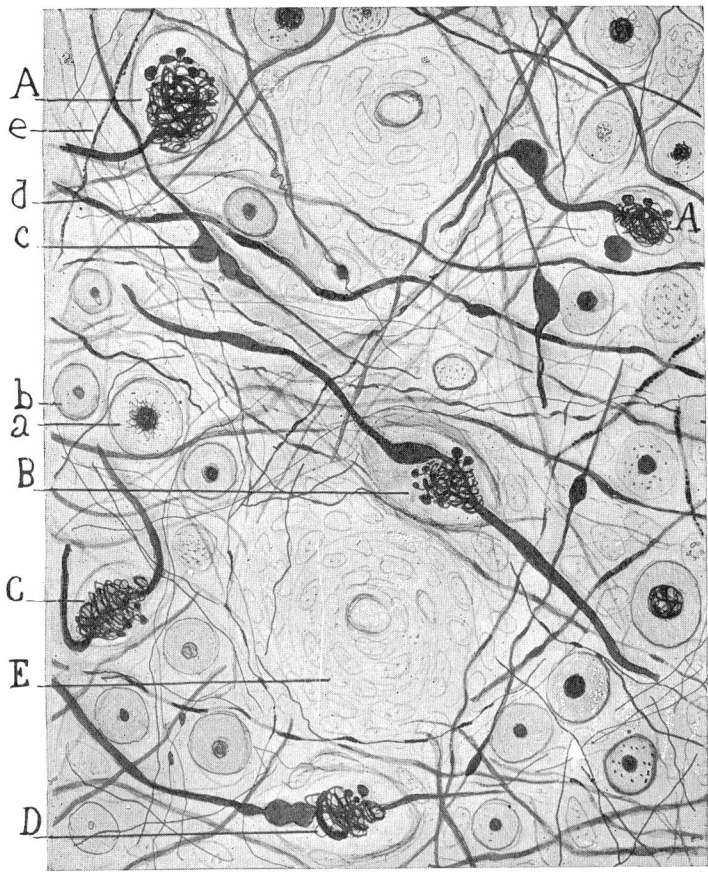

Fig. 295.—Central portion, very largely degenerated, of a wound of the white matter in a dog, twenty-five to thirty days old, killed one week after the operation. *A*, terminal spools; *B, C, D*, spools along the fibres; *E*, embryonic nodules situated around blood-vessels; *a*, free balls whose central portion still stains with colloidal silver; *b*, other ball whose centre appears granular; *c*, varicosities along the fibres; *d, e*, degenerated axons.

or reticulated grume or bulb (*a, b, e*). The majority of these arborizations are collateral in character.

Finally, in some cephalopodic structures of this type, the hyaline substance that supports them is invisible, and the terminal bulbs appear to lie freely among the axons (Fig. 294, *c, d*), an appearance that has already been pointed out in the congenerous dispositions of dogs two months old.

We lack sufficient observations to enable us to say how long the ramifications of the cephalopodic structures last. We believe, however, that in some cases these structures are preserved one or more weeks, undergoing some interesting modifications. The case shown in Fig. 295 is instructive in this respect. Here we were dealing with a dog, thirty days old, killed seven days after the operation.

The metamorphic region of the white matter in which such structures were present was very extensive and full of fragmented axons. One could see in it numerous free balls in a phase of hyalinization, that is, with a neurofibrillar focus that was more or less reduced and in course of neurolysis (Fig. 295, a, b). Here and there one observed embryonic islets that were free from fibres and composed of concentric layers around small blood-vessels (E). Among the subsisting axonic bundles not a few conductors might be seen with stainable segments, which were more or less varicose, and pale, somewhat granular, intercalary portions (d, e). These were probably fine axons in process of degeneration as a consequence of having lost their connections with the trophic centre.

Finally, along the course of the more robust axons, probably continuous with the giant pyramidal cells, appear the spiroidal structures of which we have spoken (Fig. 295, A, B, C). Within a large transparent space a kind of spool stands out, formed by various branchlets which describe loops and circles around the axon, and end in fine or medium-sized balls in the periphery. The plexus formed by such spiroidal branches is so complicated that it is impossible to follow the individual path of each fibre. The axon shows, sometimes near the spool, sometimes far from it, a varicosity of no great size (B), which is simple or double (D). One can see no remnants of the necrosed axonic portion within which the helicoidal branchlets were formed. They have perhaps disappeared through autolysis within the vacuole or fusiform space which is the frame of the degenerative figure. Finally, even though some of the spools seem to be terminal (A), the majority are collateral.

We feel sure that these spools represent late phases of the cephalopodic structures. One can easily understand the relation between the two structures by supposing that, from the third day on, the mortified piece of the axon has been resorbed, and the nerve sprouts, having regained their liberty, make remarkable growth, circling round the axon or some large appendix of the terminal spool.

V

ATROPHIC PHENOMENA CONSEQUENT ON CEREBRAL WOUNDS

Aspect of the traumatised grey cortex in late periods, that is, some weeks and months after the lesion.—Relative immunity of the neurones in radial wounds.— Late atrophies and necroses in transversal wounds.—Calcified pyramids and residual nodules.

THE majority of the phenomena that we have described in the preceding chapters are early neuronal reactions, manifested during the two or three days following the traumatism, and possibly prolonged up to the end of the first week. We shall now investigate the behaviour of the grey and white matter two or more weeks after the operation. In order to do this we must distinguish the *radial wounds* (simple puncture or sections) in which there was hardly any destruction of axons, from *transversal and oblique wounds*, as a consequence of which extensive nerve regions were entirely separated from the inferior centres and even from other cerebral spheres.

Late effects of radial wounds.—When the scalpel penetrates parallel to the axis of the pyramidal cells, simple lineal interruptions are formed, followed by the degeneration of a few series of neurones (two or three). Similarly the number of axons and collaterals rendered useless is very small. In young animals these moderate losses of substance, when they are not complicated by haemorrhages, are rapidly filled up by a very thin scar, at the level of which, as shown in Fig. 259, *G*, a few preserved fibres may subsist for a certain time. This soldering of the edges appears to be complete five to seven days after the lesion. When the scar is formed and one studies sections stained with silver, the marginal neurones are found to be deeply stained, displaying a normal nucleus and soma and a continuous axon, without any signs of varicosities or other alterations. The interstitial plexus of collaterals and centrifugal fibres of the grey matter also appears normal and very full.

Finally, twenty-five and thirty days after the operation, the thin lineal scar can with difficulty be recognized in certain regions, owing to the gradual approximation of the opposite nerve plexuses. But the lack of parallelism between the plexuses and series of neurones on the two sides of the wound helps one to distinguish it, as also does the persistence at the level of the interruption of a few granular cells which are still full of lipoidal remnants or of ruins of axonic balls.

A scrupulous examination of the axons next to the region where substance has been lost shows, as was to be expected, the disappearance of some nerve collaterals directed towards the wound. All the others, however, are perfectly preserved. This examination is instructive only in young animals such as cats and dogs operated on a few days after their birth and studied thirty or more days later. Here, besides the advantage of structural simplicity, one can see clearly by neurofibrillar methods the origin and ramifications of the nerve collaterals.

The fact that the frontier neurones of the wound are preserved perfectly is also confirmed in preparations made with formoluranium. As we show in Fig. 307, *B*, eighteen days after the operation the endocellular net of Golgi appears normal or almost normal even in the pyramidal cells situated full in the cicatricial band. It is only here and there that one sees neighbouring pyramidal cells with a pale or finely fragmented reticulum. In view of these facts we think it probable that those neurones which, two or three days after the operation displayed a granular or fragmented reticulum, have been able to restore it. Exceptionally, some frontier pyramidal cells may be detected which possess a hypertrophied and strongly stained Golgi apparatus, a peculiarity that is more frequent at the edges of transversal sections.

It is useless to add that, at this time—two or more weeks after the operation—young animals now show no clubs or balls at the edges of the wound. The immense majority of these formations, which were already very scarce after seven days, disappear from the tenth or twelfth day after the operation. Nor does one see any varicose or degenerating axons in the corpus striatum, medulla, and spinal cord.

Late aspect of the grey matter in transversal wounds.—Any traumatism of this type causes the necrosis of a large number of pyramidal cells, interrupts numerous axons whose direction is radial, severs a large part of the centripetal conductors coming from the inferior centres, and, finally, sections numerous radial blood-vessels of regular calibre, bringing about more or less important haemorrhages and a consequent asphyxia of large regions of the grey matter. We shall not stop here to analyze, as has so often been done, the effects of haemorrhages in contiguous regions. It will suffice to note once more that the extravasated blood is apt to swell the wound considerably, forming great spaces which are subsequently converted into serous cysts; these forcibly compress the frontier neurones, whose degeneration occurs at once, and impede and delay considerably the organization of the scar.

Leaving now the cicatricial process and turning our attention to the late effects of these grave interruptions in the superposed cortical sector, it is important to note the great variety of neuronal mutations observed, which are doubtless related to the quality of the nutritive disorders, and the extent and depth of the axonic mutilations. In order to fix our ideas, we may cite two typical examples.

(a) Let us imagine a long and extensive wound which involves transversally or obliquely the region of the large pyramidal cells, and is complicated by haemorrhage. Once the degenerative phenomena, whose details we shall not give here, have occurred, the arc of cortical substance that is situated above the lesion undergoes belatedly a more or less rapid atrophy, which finally leads to the disappearance of almost all the pyramidal neurones (Fig. 296, *A*). After fourteen and seventeen days it is already impossible to impregnate any of them by neurofibrillar methods. Neither does the Nissl method allow one to recognize the chromatic grumes, nor the method of formol-uranium the Golgi reticulum. Nevertheless, basic aniline dyes bring out a large number of large nuclei, which correspond to neurones of normal or small size (cells with short axons ?) and other medium-sized and small nuclei, which doubtless belong to neuroglia cells. The radial axons have disappeared without leaving in the grey matter any ball, club, or remnant of a degenerated conductor. On the other hand one may see a diffuse plexus of fine, not very abundant fibres which, by reason of their direction and size, may be identified with collateral nerve branches travelling in a tangential direction from other adjacent cortical regions (*a*) and, especially, with oblique or horizontal projections of centripetal tubes (perhaps sensory). In the plexiform layer it is only exceptionally that a few fine tangential fibres are preserved, and in that of the small pyramidal cells a few fine ascending axons of Martinotti. The survival of these nerve plexuses is analogous to the preservation of basket and climbing fibres of the cerebellum, simultaneously with the disappearance or grave degeneration of the neurones, with which they have contact relations.

After two or more months these arciform areas become thinner and smaller, and the neighbouring normal regions draw gradually

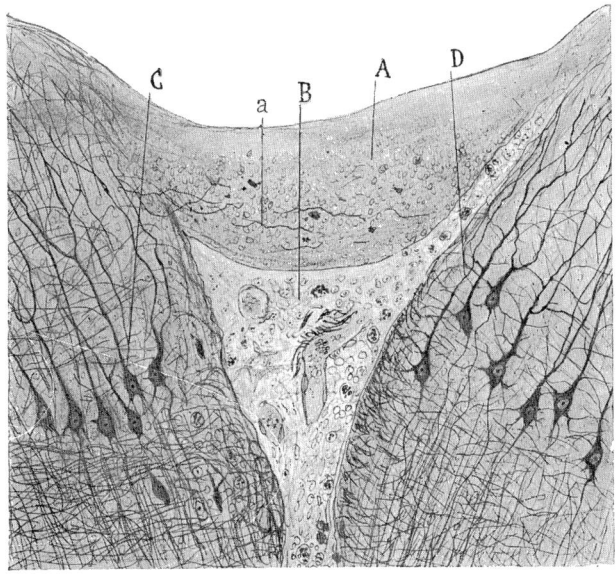

FIG. 296.—Transversal wound of the cerebrum of a young cat, killed fourteen days after the operation. *A*, superficial portion of the grey matter, which is atrophied and sunk in relation to the general plane of the neighbouring circumvolutions; *B*, wound in process of cicatrization; *C, D*, neighbouring cortical portions which have retained their nerve cells; *a*, persistence of a few exogenous fibres in the atrophied cortex.

closer together in a transversal direction. In the dissociated regions there stand out fewer and fewer fine fibres. At this period it is very easy to recognize the frontier which separates the atrophied territory from that which is normal and well nourished. In contrast to the paleness and fibrillar poverty of the former, the latter shows, besides robust and brilliantly stained neurones, an intricate nerve plexus in which the axons of the medium-sized and large pyramidal cells stand out, arranged in bundles. If one follows the collateral dendrites of the apical trunk or of the soma towards the atrophic region, one sees them diminish in thickness and end in a point. Thus a part of the course of the dendrites that originate in healthy regions and extend to the morbid one disappears through atrophy, perhaps brought about through poor nutrition. The axonic collaterals, directed towards the dissociated region, undergo the same fate. We may add that the wound tends to become narrower in a transversal direction, and that it often forms an acute inferior angle, by the increasing convergence of the axonic bundles of the normal regions. To this there are exceptions, due, above all, to the persistence of the traumatic cyst.

(b) The example just cited is an extreme case of cerebral atrophy. Usually the destructive process does not advance so far. The transversal wound, although it involves a large contingent of radial axons, is deep enough for numerous association and callous conductors to escape mutilation. This same depth of the traumatism contributes to preserve the superposed cortex from the grave effects of vascular interruption, since the superficial and intermediate circulation of the superposed grey sector is maintained through the anastomoses of the radial blood-vessels and a good preservation of the *pia mater*. Such was the case shown in Fig. 297, where the scalpel, having passed through the centre of a circumvolution, brought about the formation of a spheroidal cyst (C) which involved, on various planes, the radial fibres of two neighbouring cortical sectors. In Figs. 297 and 298 we show a few details of the structure of these sectors. In order to distinguish them we shall name them sector A, which was little affected by the vascular disorders, and sector B, which suffered more from asphyxia and poor nutrition.

One may note in the neighbouring healthy regions the series of large and medium-sized pyramidal cells, well impregnated, with their radial nerve fibres, and the neuronal and fibrillar poverty of the ill-nourished cortical areas (E). The sector A is particularly poor in stainable plexuses and cells; in it all the large pyramidal cells and the majority of the medium-sized cells have disappeared. There still subsist a few small and medium cells and an interstitial plexus composed principally of collaterals and centripetal fibres. In some sections one finds a few small or medium solitary pyramidal cells whose axon, stainable for a long distance, ends far from the wound in a retraction ball. Sometimes this terminal bud, and also the axon, are very pale and finely granular, as though an obviously destructive process had begun in them.

Of special interest is sector B, which is more distant from the wound; owing to this fact the zone of the polymorph cells has escaped almost intact. One may note in Fig. 298, B, that, after twenty days, notwithstanding the relative immunity of this region, all the giant neurones, as well as their axons, have disappeared. On the other hand there subsist, apparently little altered, a certain number of medium-sized and small pyramidal cells, whose functional prolongation, followed up to the white matter or its vicinity, curves

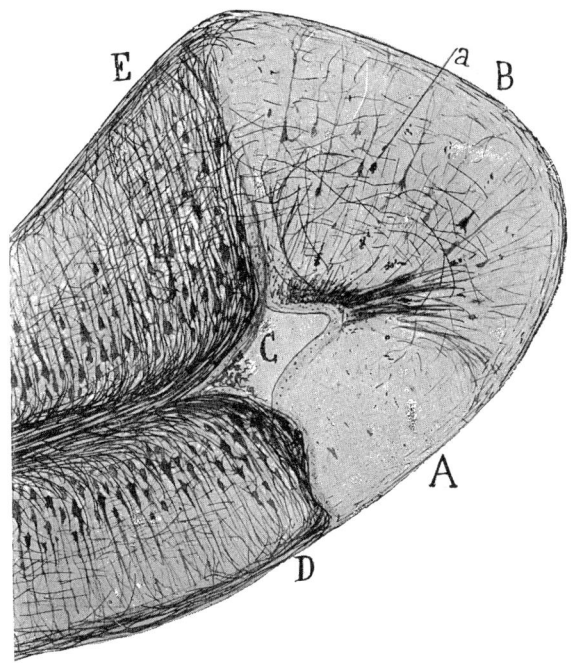

FIG. 297.—Transversal wound of a circumvolution of a young cat, killed seventeen days after the operation; schematic figure. A, much atrophied region; B, segment from which the large neurones have disappeared; D, E, normal cortex; C, cyst of the wound; a, necrosed pyramidal cells.

round so as to connect, at times, with an association or callous fibre. Some pyramidal cells of medium size have hypertrophic recurrent nerve collaterals. Others, less voluminous, have a fine axon of great length, which describes an arc owing to suppression of its ultra-collateral course. There are also some axons terminating in a small pale retraction bud (g). One sees important changes in the soma of these cells. In some it appears normal; in others the nucleus is dislocated in the direction of the trunk, fixing itself in its

710 DEGENERATION AND REGENERATION OF THE NERVE CENTRES

root. Sometimes the neuronal body is divided in two regions : one is superior, vacuolated, with a neurofibrillar axis from which spring fine divergent fibrils ; the other is basal, compact, formed of a dense net (Fig. 299, *E*). The interstitial nerve plexuses are preserved

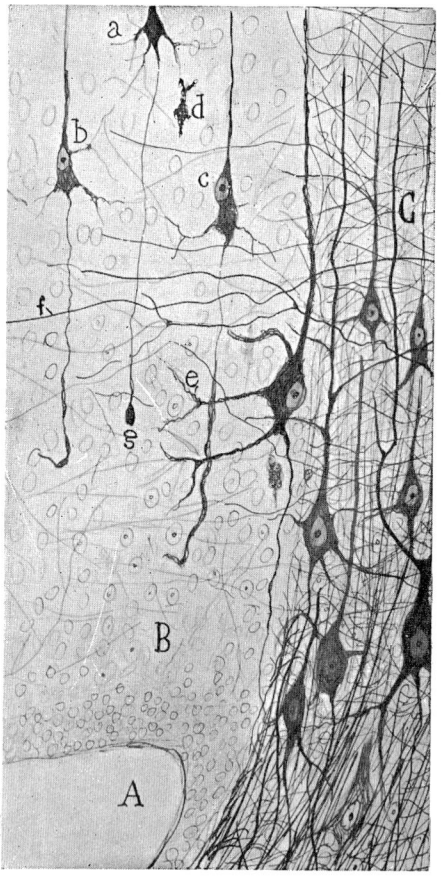

FIG. 298.—Details of the transition region between territories *B* and *E* of the preceding schematic figure. *A*, wound ; *B*, zone without stained neurones ; *a*, medium-sized pyramidal cell whose axon ends in a retraction ball ; *b*, other cell with an arciform axon ; *e*, other cell with an axon that is ravelled and hypertrophied in its inferior region ; *f*, subsisting centripetal fibrils ; *C*, healthy region of the cortex ; *c*, ravelled and atrophic dendrites which penetrate into the poorly-nourished sector.

fairly well, although impoverished as compared with the normal regions (Fig. 298, *B*).

Thus, in the relatively unharmed regions, *the giant or Betz cells that are in continuity with interrupted projection fibres alone disappear* ;

the association neurones, whose axon has undergone no mutilations or has suffered them at a great distance from the soma, are very largely preserved.

We do not assert, however, that all cerebral neurones whose axon is mutilated in the grey matter must necessarily disappear. We have noted several examples that prove the contrary. In the

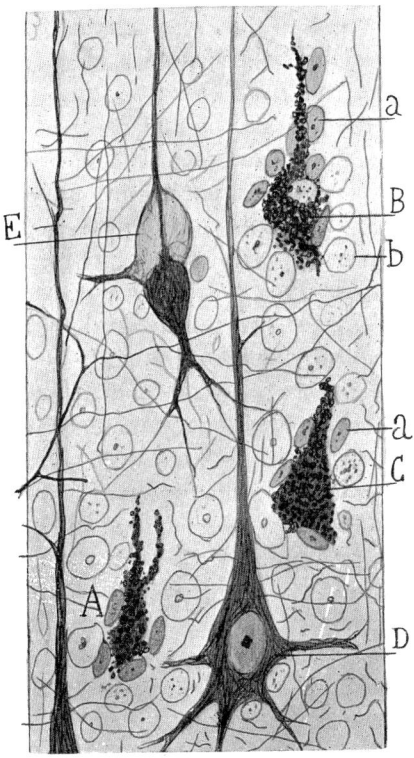

FIG. 299.—Details of a few cells of sector B from Fig. 297. *A, B, C*, necrosed pyramidal cells, reduced to disintegrated granules; *a*, proliferated satellite cells; *D*, normal neurone; *E*, neurone vacuolated in its apical portion.

case before us the neuronal atrophy that followed seems to us to be a mere consequence of the circulatory and trophic disorders. We must not forget that the above-mentioned pyramidal cells were situated in sectors A and B, very near the wound. They must, therefore, have suffered, much more than the small and medium pyramidal cells, the ravages of vascular asphyxia and haemorrhage, besides the perturbatory effect of the mechanical commotion. Perhaps among the pyramidal cells that have disappeared there were some that survived a few days and even attempted an arciform compensation. But the deficiency of nourishment rendered such reactions useless.

We are of opinion—but this is a conjecture which must be tested by experiment—that the definitive preservation of an arciform pyramidal cell requires, besides the integrity of its afferent nerve paths, favourable conditions of irrigation and oxygenation. Otherwise, after the elimination of the extra-collateral portion of the axon, atrophy and destruction of the neuronal soma will follow.

Calcified pyramidal cells and residual nodules.—There are doubtless various types of autolytic necrosis and destruction of the neurones affected by traumatism or circulatory disorders. We have already spoken of sudden death accompanied by *preservation,* immediate destruction or disorganization through *granular disintegration,* and slow death following on progressive lesions of the reticulum (hirudiform and fusiform states, etc.). To these types we must add another, which is late in appearance, occurs in cerebral pyramidal cells situated at a great distance from the wound, among perfectly normal cells, and manifests itself by the presence of calcareous deposits, easily discernible by the black colour they assume, owing to the formation with silver of silver phosphate reducible by pyrogallic acid.

In Fig. 299, *A, B, C*, we show details of this mortification, followed by calcification. Neuronal death must have occurred at an early period, since this process of calcareous infiltration, which reaches its climax from the twentieth to the twenty-fifth day, can be seen after fourteen days. Of the neuronal soma and its expansions there remains only a finely granular material which is semi-liquefied, partly resorbed, and so transparent as to be frequently invisible. The calcareous grains are deposited on it, especially at the level of the soma and root of the radial trunk (Fig. 299). These earthy precipitates appear very stable, as we have seen them also in cerebral neurones and neurones of the corpus striatum two months and a half after the production of many deep wounds.

In the presence of so grave a process the peripyramidal satellite cells become active, corroding and digesting the remnants of the soma. As we show in Fig. 299, *a*, such elements are numerous and possess a protoplasm which is parallel to the elongated somatic contour. Instead of being one or two, as in the normal state, the satellite cells multiply, numbering five, six, or more, and forming an aggregation that in all respects recalls the residual nodule described by Nageotte in transplanted ganglia. These elements, by reason of their size, protoplasmic paleness, and exiguity of the nucleus, may be identified with the *adendritic satellite cells*, which we have recently discriminated round the pyramidal cells, in a careful study of neuroglia.[1] Some more voluminous nuclei, which are occasionally found in the perineuronic conglomerates, might, however, correspond to the satellite neuroglia cells (Fig. 299). Various authors, and especially Marinesco,[2] have described, in destructive lesions of the human cerebral cortex, accumulations of satellite cells situated round remnants or in the region previously occupied by the neurone. (See works on *neuronophagy* in the cerebrum.)

[1] Cajal: " Contribución al conocimiento de la neuroglia del cerebro humano," *Trab. del Lab. de Invest. biol.*, t. 11, 1912.

[2] Marinesco: *La cellule nerveuse*, t. 2, 1909.

VI

CORTICAL INFLAMMATION CONSEQUENT ON TRAUMATISMS

Invasion of the grey substance by migratory elements—granular cells, rod-like cells, plasma cells, etc.—Behaviour of the neuroglia in presence of the inflammation. —Formation of the scar.—Neuroglial and mesodermal scars.—Organization of exudates and haemorrhagic foci.—Gigantic granular cells.

Inflammation of the grey matter after traumatisms.—As this subject is well known, we shall refer to what was said in connection with wounds of the nerves and spinal cord, and merely describe here briefly, on general lines, the progress of the inflammatory process. A few hours after the lesion, when a more or less considerable haemorrhage has occurred, the cerebral blood-vessels in immediate proximity to the wound, and especially those of the *pia mater*, are the seat of a great congestion. An abundant plasmatic exudate, coming from the capillaries of the grey matter and from the meningeal blood-vessels, accumulates at the place where the wound occurred, mixes with the blood coagulum, and sometimes dilating the wound, forms considerable cysts or enlargements. Together with the plasmatic exudate, a large number of migratory cells from various sources, make their way into the pial tissue, into the cavity of the wound, and into the thickness of the grey matter; these cells increase progressively from the sixth to the forty-eighth hour after the operation, and even longer. They comprise: the *poly- and mononucleated leucocytes, granular cells, rod-like cells, fibroblasts,* and finally, in late periods, *cyanophil cells* (plasma cells). The majority, if not the whole, of these invading cells break up and digest the dead neurones and fibres, and clean the wound of products of disintegration and autolysis, so that later a systematic organization of the scar is possible. The more extensive and contused the wound, the larger is the affluence of phagocytic elements and the longer and more laborious is the process of destruction and absorption of the nervous remnants. Thus, in large transversal wounds in which contusion occurs, three months after the traumatism one still sees, in the exudate or the edges of the cyst resulting from the destruction of the grey matter, a large number of granular cells (*Gitterzellen*). These cells are also abundant when one leaves, as did Borst, Farrar, and Morgenthaler, foreign bodies within the cortex. We shall now enumerate some of the elements which have penetrated into the nervous substance.

Polynucleated leucocytes.—Abundant during the first hours after the operation, they diminish after twenty-four hours. They may be distinguished by the relatively small size of the nucleus, which is divided into lobules, and especially by the intense and almost homogeneous coloration of the latter by basic aniline dyes. In their incursions into the grey matter they usually do not penetrate far, yielding in this respect to the rod-like cells (*Stäbchenzellen* of German authors). Nevertheless, they sometimes go very deep and, as is known, and as Sittig [1] has observed in certain important pathological processes of the human cerebrum, they may form perineuronal accumulations which imitate the satellite cell conglomerates. Their phagocytic power is well known; nevertheless one must recognize that the great majority of the cells that are full of products of disintegration belong to other migratory types.

Granular cells (Gitterzellen).—We have spoken of these already in our study of the spinal cord, considering them as among the earliest phagocytic elements to invade the nervous substance and exudates of the wound. In traumatized cerebra they are very abundant from the twenty-fourth hour, as Farrar and many other authors have observed. They are present in great numbers in the lesioned *pia mater*, within the exudate, and in the edges of the wound, usually avoiding the normal regions. They are also especially abundant, as many neurologists have observed, in the proximity of vascular adventitious tissue (small arteries and veins of the grey matter).

We shall not speak of their structure and morphology, which are well known. We shall merely reproduce in Fig. 300 the principal types of granular cells found in the edges of a cerebral wound of a dog (molecular layer), two days after the operation. One observes among them large vesicular cells with an enormous vacuole and a

---

[1] O. Sittig: "Anhäufung von polynucleaeren Leukocyten um die Ganglienzellen beim epidemischer Cerebrospinal-meningitis," *Zeitsch. f. d. gesamte Neurol. u. Psychatr.*, etc., Bd. 8, 1912.

tangential nucleus (a) ; others that have a central nucleus and a vacuolar crown of divergent trabeculae (b) ; others with a large central cavity and a crown of small areolae (c) ; others with a clear space full of liquid and containing a small spherical nucleus, which perhaps arose through karyorrhexis from the large tangential nucleus

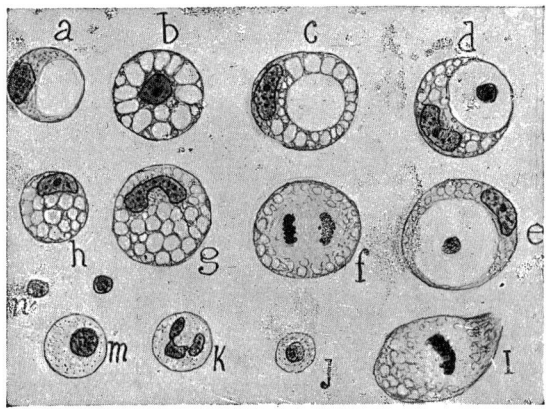

FIG. 300.—Various types of granular cells found in the edges of cerebral wounds in a dog, two days after the lesion (a, b, c, d, e, h, g) ; f, i, granular cells in process of division ; j, k, m, migratory leucocytes ; n, apparently free nuclei.

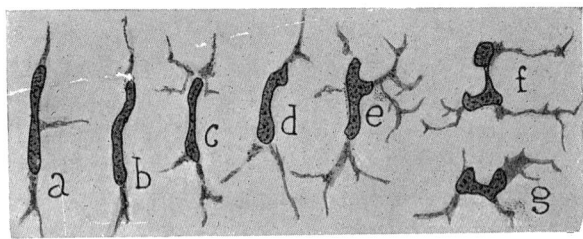

FIG. 301.—Various types of rod-like cells from the edges of a cerebral wound in a dog, two days after the operation. a, b, c, typical forms ; e, f, g, forms that recall leucocytes in an amoeboid phase. (Unna's polychrome blue.)

(d and e). One may also note that the nuclear organ, which is spherical or somewhat irregular in certain cells (f), has a kidney-like, semi-lunar, and even bilobed shape in others (g). Finally, one sees granular cells in course of division (f, i).

Our observations are not conclusive with regard to the origin of the *Gitterzellen*. Their rapid appearance in the exudates, their spheroidal shape, their migratory and amoeboid capacity, incline us to believe that they are a type of leucocyte, perhaps *large mononuclear* or *transitional*. But it is unquestionable that, as many authors admit, the young fibroblasts are also capable of carrying disintegration products, and so of being transformed into granular cells. It is difficult, at times, to distinguish the two types of cells, since when young fibroblasts are full of inclusions they may become spheroidal in shape. At any rate, it seems to us improbable that the granular cells originate in the vascular endothelium, as Farrar

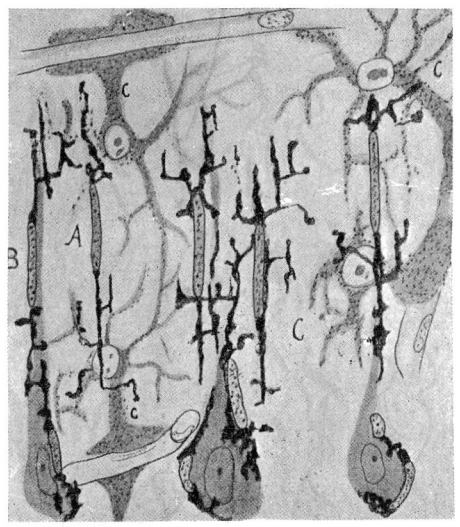

Fig. 302.—Semischematic drawing of the rod-like cells found in the *stratum radiatum* (Ammon's horn) of a rabbit inoculated with Sporothrix; Bielschowsky's method. Mordanted in copper acetate. *A, B,* rod-like cells adapted to pyramidal cells, or free in the tissue, with abundant ramifications.

suggests. We have never seen in our preparations dispositions that would lead one to presume such an origin. The *Gitterzellen,* when next to blood-vessels, always appear as spheroidal and independent.

Rod-like cells (Stäbchenzellen).—These were first described by Nissl [1] in the cerebrum of paralytics and in that of various diseased conditions. They were confirmed by Alzheimer, Cerletti,[2] and

[1] Nissl: "Ueber einige Beziehungen zwischen Nervenzellenkrankungen und gliösen Erscheinungen bei verschiedenen Psychosen," *Arch .f. Psychiatrie*, Bd. 32, 1899.

[2] Cerletti: "Sopra alcuni rapporti tra le cellule a bastoncello e gli elementi nervosi nella paralisia progresiva," *Riv. sperim. di Freniatria*, vol. 31, 1905.

Ulrich,[1] and they have been carefully analysed by Achúcarro,[2] who saw them, not only in progressive paralysis, in hydrophobia, and other nervous diseases of man and animals, but also in the edges of,

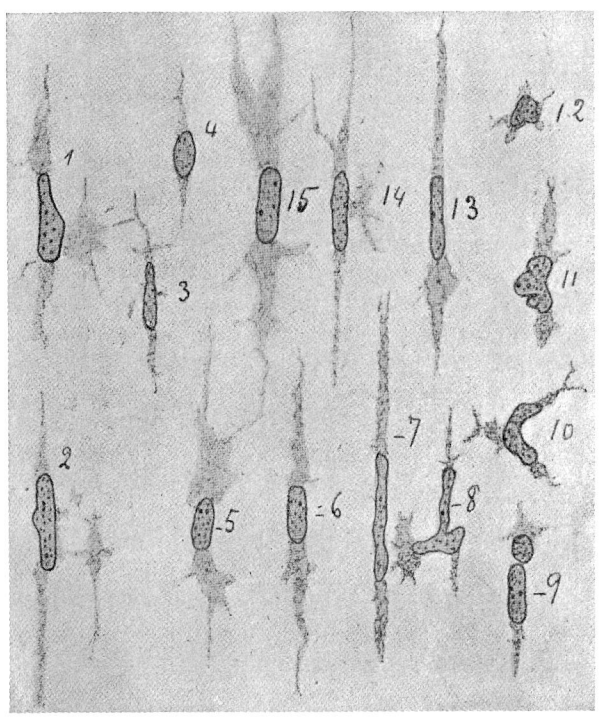

FIG. 303.—Stratum radiatum of a rabbit affected with hydrophobia. Toluidine blue, Im. horn, 1.30, Oc. 12—4, 9, 10, 11, 12, primitive phases of elongation of the interstitial cells; 1, 2, 3, 5, 6, 15, elongated cells; 7, 13, 14, rod-like elements. (After Achúcarro.)

and at some distance from, cerebral wounds (Ammon's horn). They are characterized by the fact that they contain a nucleus which is elongated and often rod-like; by a pale soma, oriented

[1] M. Ulrich: "Beiträge zur Kenntniss der Stäbchenzellen," etc., *Monatschr. f. Psych. u. Neurol.*, 1910.

[2] Achúcarro: "Cellules allongées et Stäbchenzellen," etc., *Trab. del Lab. de Invest. biol.*, t. 7, 1909.

Idem: "Algunos datos relativos a la naturaleza de las células en bastoncito de la corteza cerebral humana, obtenidos con el método de Cajal," *Trab. del Lab. de Invest. biol.*, t. 8, 1910.

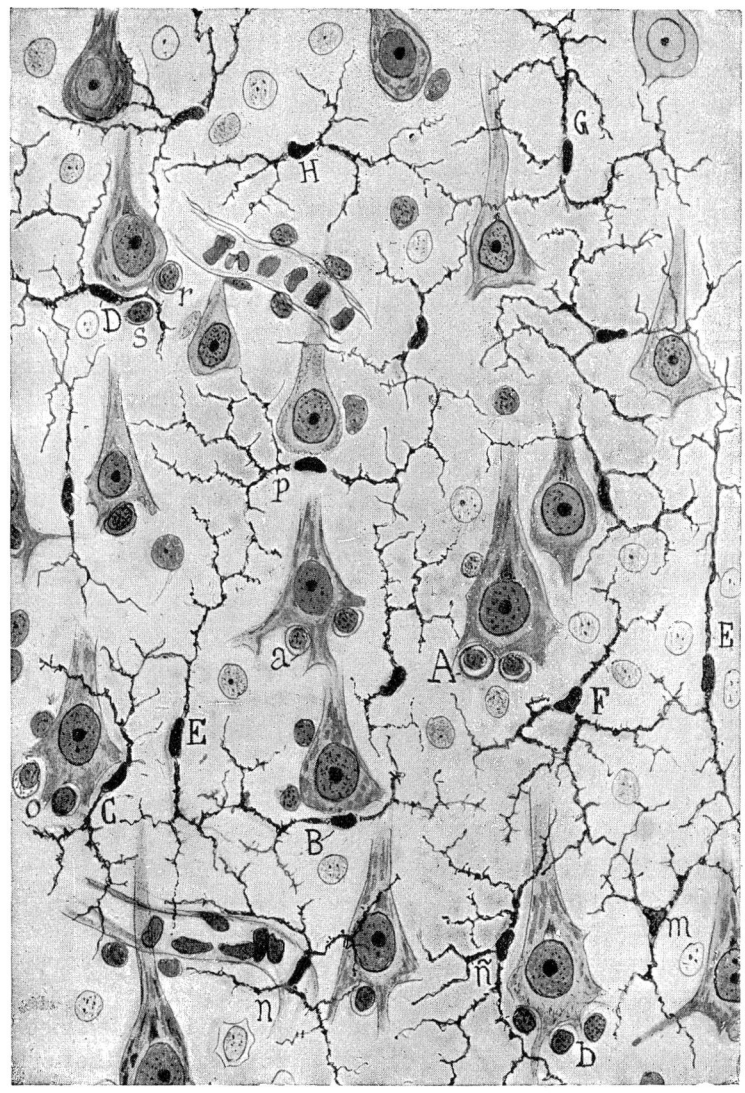

FIG. 303A.—Cerebral microglia. General paralysis.

parallel to the cerebral pyramidal cells, to whose trunk they are often intimately applied ; and, finally, by very pale polar expansions of granular appearance (Fig. 301, *a*, *b*, *c*).

Achúcarro, who has impregnated the *Stäbchenzellen* by a special modification of the method of reduced silver nitrate (fixation in formol, immersion in Weigert's mordant for neuroglia, and reduced silver nitrate), describes them as comprising : a spongy soma whose meshes are tenanted by a considerable quantity of argentophilous granules, fairly similar to the pigment of the neurones (apart from other disintegration products) ; and certain pale polar expansions from which collateral appendices issue at a right angle ; these are relatively short, strongly attract silver nitrate, and end in a round bulb, which is dark and slightly thickened. Fig. 302, *A*, *B*, in which we reproduce a schematic drawing by Achúcarro, gives an idea of the peculiar morphology of these elements.

In our preparations of the cerebrum of cats and dogs killed two to five days after the operation, the rod-like cells are constant and sometimes very numerous. One finds them both in preparations stained with Unna's polychrome blue (Fig. 301) and in those impregnated with colloidal silver (formol-uranium). Their properties concur exactly with those described by Nissl, Alzheimer, Cerletti, and Achúcarro. Figures 301 and 303 make it unnecessary to give a minute description of them. We need only note, in accord with Achúcarro, that these elements contain granules which stain a deep grey with silver (Fig. 307, *d*, *e*).

As the above authors have observed, besides the typical cell with an elongated, rod-like nucleus, one finds morphological and structural transitions with the nucleus of polynucleated leucocytes (Figs. 301, *g*, and 303, 11). These gradations of nuclear configuration, to which correspond transitions in the size and form of the soma, lend great probability to the opinion that the *Stäbchenzellen* are simply large leucocytes with a lobulated nucleus, which have migrated across the interstices of the grey matter and been adapted mechanically, as Achúcarro showed, to the form and direction of the neuronal expansions. This same author has made it clear, moreover, that these elements belong to the great category of *granular cells* in its widest sense (*Abbauzellen* of the German authors), that is, the cells designed to extract disintegration products from necrosed or degenerated parts. Thanks to the exquisite ability of the rod-like cells to insinuate themselves through the narrowest openings, their action has perhaps a wider radius than that of ordinary *Gitterzellen*, since one finds them at a great distance from the wounds, in regions which may be considered, at first sight, as normal. Nor need one be surprised that such elements assume occasionally a stellate appearance, with long ramified appendices, since leucocytes, like young connective tissue cells, are very stereotropic, that is, they adhere along the expansions of other cells, adapting themselves closely to their form and direction. In corroboration of this view one may remember the numerous cells like rods, horse-shoes, stars, etc., with nuclei wrested and drawn out into numerous shapes, seen in leucocytes that have migrated into the inflamed cornea, and, in general, in all dense and fibrous tissues. Alzheimer, Ulrich, and Achúcarro have given very suggestive descriptions and figures of these atypical nuclear forms, which very much remind one of certain leucocytes. E. del Río [1] has also seen typical rod-like cells in many infectious granulomas, and especially in lepromas.

The neurologists are not agreed as to the origin of the *Stäbchenzellen*. Cerletti, repeating Nissl's original opinion, holds them to be of neuroglial, and therefore ectodermal origin, representing a secondary adaptation of the glia to the nervous structures that have disappeared or are being destroyed; but Nissl, Alzheimer, and Achúcarro are in favour of a mesodermal origin. In a study prepared in collaboration with Gayarre,[2] Achúcarro confirms his opinion as to the origin of the *Stäbchenzellen*, noting that they do not attract gold in the specific sublimate-gold process for the staining of neuroglia, and that they cannot therefore be considered as gliomatous elements. Although with reserves, he is inclined to view them as mononuclear leucocytes, which have migrated from the blood-vessels.

As to the corpuscles that Achúcarro calls *interstitial cells*, which are clearly star-like in shape, with divergent expansions, spongy soma full of inclusions, and a relatively large, spheroidal nucleus capable of mitosis, it seems to us, as to him, that they are small glia cells of the grey matter, transformed and phagocytic. At any rate, from the point of view of the origin, the demarcation of the various types of Stäbchenzellen, pointed out by Ulrich and Achúcarro, is a difficult undertaking and likely to lead to confusion. One must remember that *any element*

[1] E. del Río: " Algunos datos concernientes á la anatomía patológica del leproma," *Trab. del Lab. de Invest. biol.*, t. 8, 1910.

[2] Achúcarro y Gayarre: " La corteza cerebral en la demencia paralítica," etc., *Trab. del Lab. de Invest. biol.*, t. 12, fasc. 1, May 1914.

that adapts itself to a given function, adopts, no matter what its origin, the structure and form of the cells organized ex profeso to discharge that function, especially if they both possess the characters of amoeboidism and stereotropism.

Connective cells.—When cerebral wounds are wide and appear to be invaded by the *pia mater*, or rather by the latter's mesodermal formations, one frequently sees, from the second or third day after the operation, connective perivascular cells wandering full in the molecular layer or in that of small pyramidal cells, and often exhibiting evident mitoses. The distinction between such young elements, which have penetrated into the grey matter, and true *granular cells* is at times impossible. The criterion of expansions—lacking in *Gitterzellen*—is of no value, for young fibroblasts are often without them. Neither will the absence of disintegration products be decisive, since between young fibroblasts with a finely granular protoplasm and *Gitterzellen* there are intermediate forms.

Cyanophil cells (Unna's *plasma cells*).—These have been pointed out by several authors, and more recently by Farrar and Bianchi. They occur late—from the eighth day on—in connective scars, and are rarely found in the grey matter. They are usually situated near the blood-vessels. These elements are much more numerous in certain chronic pathological states of human nerve centres, as Alzheimer, Nissl, Vogt, Spielmeyer, Papadia, Cerletti, and Achúcarro have shown—in *progressive general paralysis, syphilitic encephalitis, tuberculous processes, sleeping-sickness, hydrophobia,* etc.

Amoeboid cells of Alzheimer.—Alzheimer pointed out two types of these cells, which were confirmed by Eisath, Rosenthal, Buscaino, Achúcarro, etc. One is that derived through degeneration of the small neuroglial body, and the other that coming from *adendritic cells* (*apolar cells* of many authors). Our preparations of the inflamed cerebral cortex clearly reveal only the latter variety. As we show in Fig. 304, *a, b, c*, which reproduces a piece of the cerebral cortex of a cat, killed three days after the operation, which was stained by formol-uranium, these cells are very abundant in the wounded white matter, and are not rare in the grey. They are small elements, with a spherical and slender nucleus, and they have a protoplasm full of granulations, and drawn out into tuberose, fungiform, divergent appendices which rarely have secondary ramifications. Amoeboid cells of this category are especially abundant near the blood-vessels, the region where the adendritic cells are principally found. They appear to play no part in the formation of the scar. The frequency with which such cells are seen charged with disintegration products entitles us to regard them as a particular type of neurophages, comparable, perhaps, to the various types of *Abbaumzellen* pointed out by Jakob in the white matter of spinal cords undergoing secondary degeneration.

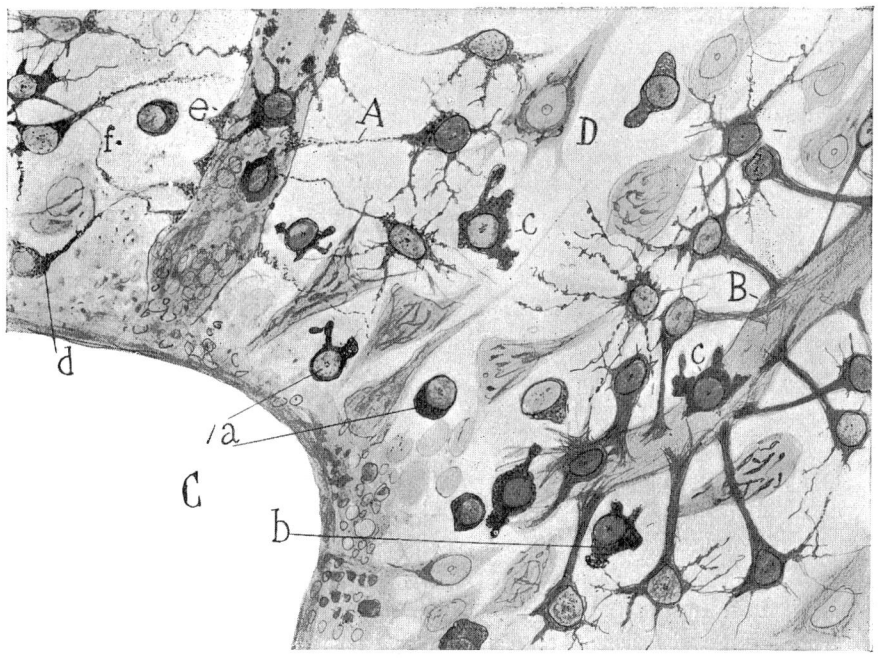

FIG. 304.—Edges of a cerebral transversal wound of a young cat, killed three days after the operation; uranium nitrate method. *a*, adendritic small cells; *b*, *c*, small amoeboid cells; *B*, normal capillary surrounded by neuroglial pedicles; *C*, obstructed capillary whose gliomatous appendices become striated and atrophied; *D*, neurone.

Since in the normal state, and in young animals, the white matter presents, here and there, adendritic elements shaped like a cogwheel, with a few longer tuberose appendices, it is prudent not to exaggerate the pathological significance of this type. The pathological element consists perhaps in their excessive multiplication, in the mobility with which they tend towards degenerating nerve tubes, and, above all, in the fact that they overload themselves with disintegration products.

Alterations of the neuroglia.—Leaving on one side the intervention of the neuroglia stellar cells in the formation of the scar, we shall point out some interesting metamorphoses of the glia, observed near wounds during the first three to five days after a cerebral traumatism. In order to analyze them we have used especially the method of sublimate-gold, introduced by ourselves into neurological technique.[1]

When the scalpel incises the white or grey matter extensively in a transversal direction, the radial vessels situated above the section become thrombosed, at least up to a certain distance from the lesion. As a consequence of this the star-like cells with a firm perivascular footing, which are especially abundant in the white matter and deep layer of the grey matter, modify their shape and chemical composition. The aurophilous substance of the soma and foot implanted in the blood-vessel attracts the gold deposit less vigorously than usual, and the foot becomes progressively paler and thinner, sometimes changing into a series of granulations, and finally, in some cells, breaks off entirely (Fig. 304, *A*). In this way the endothelio-neuroglial symbiosis is interrupted and the glia cell can migrate freely to other regions, perhaps in search of permeable vessels in order to form new symbiotic colonies.

In Fig. 304, *A, B*, we show the notable contrast between the glia cells of a normal blood-vessel, permeable to blood, and those of a thrombosed capillary which is cut at the level of the wound (*A*).

In certain interruptions of the white matter complicated by haemorrhage (where a blood coagulum stops up the sectioned and thrombosed vessels), we have observed, three days after the operation, a curious phenomenon of dislocation of the perivascular glia cells. Their appendices, instead of lying, as usual, in a direction approximately perpendicular to the axis of the vessel, are notably oblique, often almost parallel, at the same time stretching out, so as to attain two, four, and six times their normal length. Some cells are met with that have travelled in this way twenty hundredths of a millimetre. This peculiar migratory movement takes on the character of a flight from the lesioned region, since *the pedicles above referred to orient themselves, without exception, in a direction opposite to the loss of substance.* In Fig. 305, *C. E*, we reproduce this curious migratory process, which, while corroborating once more the amoe-

[1] Cajal: "Sobre un nuevo proceder de impregnación de la neuroglia," etc., *Trab. del Lab. de Invest. biol.*, t. 15, 1913.

boid capacity of the glia cells, shows that these elements are able to change their position when the lack of oxygen or the absence of renewal of the interstitial plasma creates an environment that is seriously harmful to the glia. In the preparation copied in Fig. 305, the lethal condition that brought about the migration was, perhaps, the coagulum, with the consequent suspension of afflux of oxygen (*A*). In regions farther from the lesion, in the direction of the cortex, that is, in regions of normal or almost normal circulation, the glia cells occupy their usual position or are but little displaced.

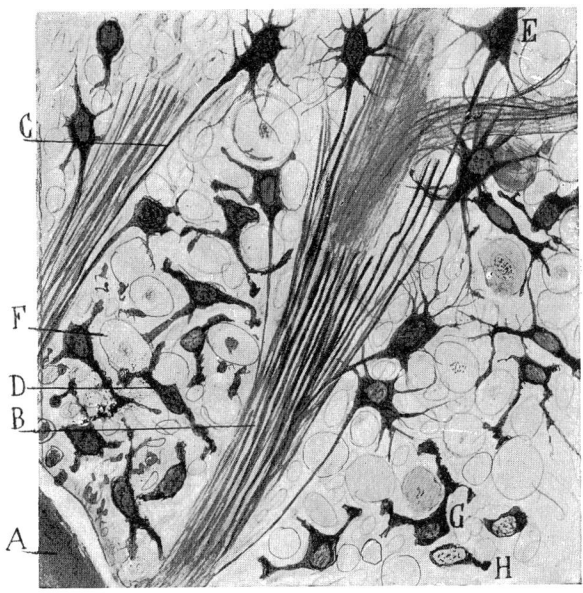

FIG. 305.—Edges of a transversal wound in a young cat, killed three days after the operation. *A*, blood coagulum situated in the wound; *B*, vessel surrounded by neuroglia appendices which are notably elongated and whose cells of origin seem to withdraw from the wound; *C*, one of these appendices; *G*, *H*, emancipated glia cells in course of alteration. Method of sublimate-gold.

If we leave the perivascular neuroglia and examine that of the edges of the wound, we see, among the accumulations of axonic balls and granular cells, numerous free glia cells of strange shapes, accommodated to the irregularity of the interstices, some of them small, others large. We will confine ourselves to observing, in Fig. 306, *a*, *b*, the large number of these free glia cells, poorly provided with expansions, having varicose, angular appendices, which frequently end in granular grumes. Some appendices are prolonged up to the wound itself, where they terminate in granular accumulations. Certain expansions, doubtless to adapt themselves to the balls and colonies of leucocytes and granular cells, describe strange convolutions and show, at the level of their bifurcations or along their path, thickenings which are very rich in aurophilous substance.

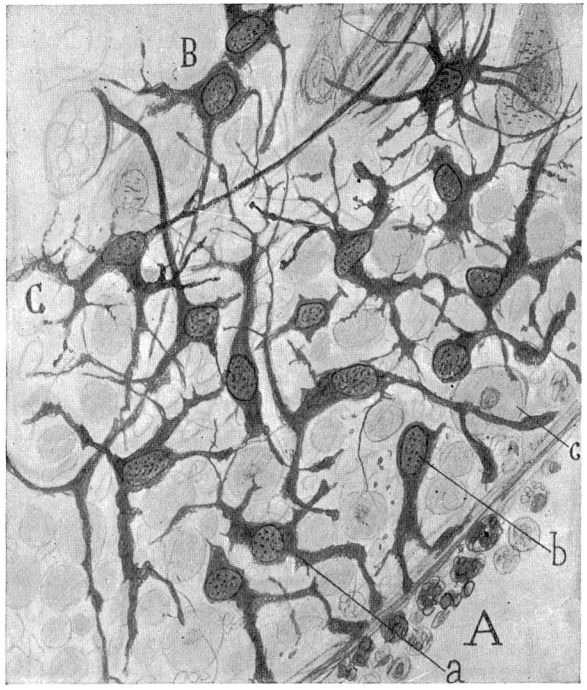

FIG. 306.—Edges of a transversal wound in the cerebrum of a cat, killed four days after the operation. *A*, wound with plasmatic exudate; *B*, pair of glia cells; *C*, neuroglia cells provided with a very long perivascular pedicle; *a*, *b*, detached gliomatous cells situated near the lesion. One sees among them numerous degenerating axonic balls. (Method of sublimate-gold.)

Cavities appear in the protoplasm of some of the glia cells, probably filled with products of disintegration, which the gold does not stain. Finally, pairs of cells, and even binucleated glia cells, are not infrequently seen, although they are not as common as one might presume (Fig. 306, *B*).

It is impossible to say at present whether these free neuroglia cells, unprovided with a vascular pedicle and accumulated near the wound, represent a degenerative or a progressive phase.

CICATRIZATION OF CEREBRAL WOUNDS

The mechanism of cicatrization in the cerebrum is the same as in the spinal cord ; we shall therefore merely summarize briefly the course of the process. There are two types of cortical union : that which is produced through a lineal neuroglial scar after radial wounds without grave contusion or haemorrhage, and that which is produced through extensive mesodermal scars, when there have been extensive transversal wounds, of a complicated character or accompanied by contusion.

Rapid cicatrization of radial wounds.—This type of scar often occurs in young animals, from the third to the fifth day after the operation. It is composed of a thin band of transparent tissue, which is rich in nuclei, poor in leucocytes, sprinkled with a few granular cells, and constituted essentially by neuroglia. Such a rapid union occurs only in those cases in which the scalpel has not interrupted any important vessel, and has injured only a few transversal capillaries of the cortical net, that is, delicate vessels devoid, or nearly so, of adventitial connective cells.

Preparations made by the method of formol-uranium prove that the fine tissue which unites the edges of the wound, and which in ordinary preparations appears as a delicate transparent band besprinkled with nuclei, is composed of neuroglia. In Fig. 307, A, we show the scar of a radial wound in a young cat, killed eighteen days after the operation. Thanks to the silver impregnation, one sees that some elements of the glia dwell right in the scar (C, E), spreading their expansions in a radial direction, while others lie tangentially, emitting transversal appendices which, after crossing the cicatricial septum, ramify on the opposite side. Finally, one sees how glia cells situated at a certain distance, right in the grey matter, contribute with their radiations to interlace and complicate the cicatricial tissue. Here and there a few *granular cells* appear, which are full of lipoidal remnants (D) and, above all, of carbon grains taken from the exudate (it must be remembered that we darken the scalpel in the smoke of burning camphor in order more easily to recognize the position of the cerebral wound).

After thirty days the neuroglia scar is almost definitely organized. Preparations made by means of sublimate and gold supply important data with regard to its formation. As we show in Fig. 308, A, both the edges of the wound and the scar itself contain a large number of newly-formed neuroglia cells, provided with long expansions, among them a very robust foot. One can see that a large number of these perivascular pedicles converge in the endothelium of regenerated vessels situated full in the scar or in the very edges of the wound (*C*). As in the foetus, so in cerebral wounds, where formative processes peculiar to ontogenetic development are repeated, the

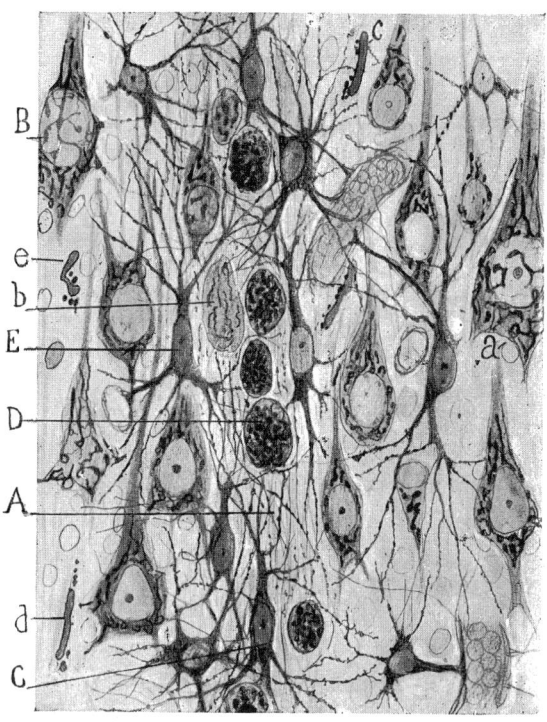

FIG. 307.—Lineal scar of a radial wound in the cortex of a young cat, killed eighteen days after the operation; method of uranium nitrate. *A*, scar; *B*, normal pyramidal cells; *C*, *E*, neuroglia cells of the scar; *D*, granular cell with carbon granules; *c*, *d*, *e*, rod-like cells with inclusions in their protoplasm.

appendices of the glia are attracted by the vessels of the scars to form the well-known glio-endothelial symbiosis, which appears to be a condition *sine qua non* of the physiological activity of the neuroglia. One may observe, moreover, that the greater part of the scar is composed of a plexus of neuroglial appendices, wherein predominate transversal fibres, which often extend from one edge of the wound to the other, and are connected with glia cells lying at the edge of, or entirely immersed in, the grey matter. The glia cells are of the type of those of the white matter. As can be seen in Fig. 308, the Weigert fibrils have already differentiated, standing out at the level of the vascular pedicle, from which they pass to the soma, and penetrate into other appendices. It is thus apparent that the mechanism of production of the fibrils adjusts itself to the ontogenetic standards formulated by Da Fano, Rubaschkin, and ourselves. Finally, here and there, the intercalary spaces of the cicatricial warp show a few granular cells carrying remnants of nerve or particles of carbon (Fig. 308, *a*).

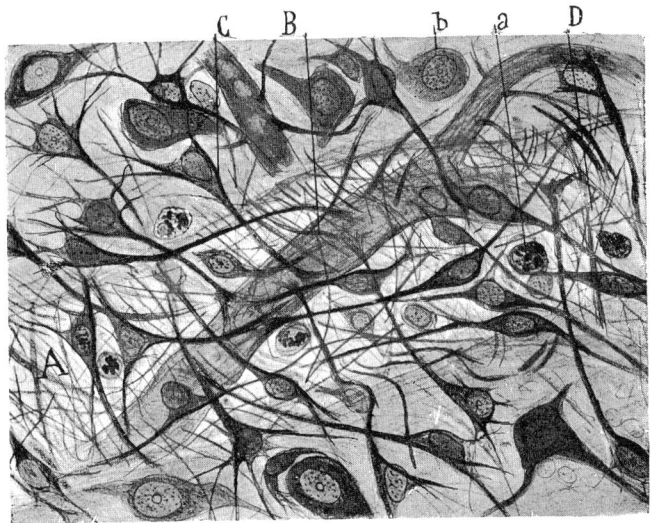

FIG. 308.—Lineal and oblique scar of the cerebral cortex of a cat, which was killed one month after the operation; method of sublimate-gold. *A*, region of the scar; *B*, newly-formed vessel in the scar, to which converge numerous pedicles or feet of neuroglia cells; *C*, newly-formed glia, wherein fibrils have differentiated; *D*, neuroglial plexus; *a*, granular cell; *b*, cerebral pyramidal cell.

When the cortical scar is very thin and radial in direction the gliomatous tissue becomes reduced, months after the lesion, to one or two discontinuous series of fibrous glia cells, which are usually parallel to the direction of the wound. This direction may change if the scar contains a parallel newly-formed capillary.

After forty-five to sixty days the scar, almost entirely free from granular cells, is so elongated as to be hardly perceptible. The fusion of the two edges is thus perfect and effective. Nevertheless, no nerve fibres or dendrites pass across it.

To sum up, we may say that in small cerebral wounds without contusion or haemorrhage, in young animals, the mesodermal tissue of the *pia* does not seem to intervene, and there is a kind of fusion of the edges by a proliferation and migration of the glia cells.

Our observations, made by the new methods of impregnation, once more corroborate the classic law of Weigert (1890), confirmed by Nissl (1894), Alzheimer, and a great number of neurologists, according to which any destruction of nervous tissue is compensated by a neuroglial neoplasm. It has long been known that the gliomatous cells of the scar are due to mitosis of other pre-existent cells ; this was confirmed by Borst, Farrar, Bianchi, Morgenthaler, etc. We have often seen, by Nissl's and other methods, from the second day after the lesion, mitoses in the glia cells of the molecular layer of the cerebrum, when the wound was complicated with contusion. From the architectonic point of view one must recognize that the cicatricial neuroglial tissue is very heteromorphous. Thus we may note that the glia of the grey matter is replaced by glia cells of the white matter, and that the orientation, dimensions, and distribution of the neuroglial appendices do not coincide strictly, as can be seen in Fig. 308, with normal dispositions. The scar, from this point of view, may be conceived as a *reparatory sclerosis* (that is, not *isomorphous*), in the sense given by Storch [1] to this expression, which he used to designate those great mutations of neuroglial organization occurring as a result of grave destructive processes of the cerebral cortex. The term, *anisomorphous sclerosis*, proposed by Bielschowsky,[2] seems to us preferable, since both the typical neuroglial neoformation following on secondary degenerations, and that due to extensive necroses or wounds of the cerebral cortex, assume a reparatory and neoformative character.

We have not found *gigantic neuroglia cells*, that is, the Monstrenzellen of which many German authors speak, in the scar, although some glia cells somewhat larger than the normal were abundant.

Transversal scars complicated by haemorrhage and cysts.—Any extensive cerebral wound, no matter what its direction, but especially if this is transversal or oblique to the cortex, interrupts important vessels, and therefore provokes serious haemorrhage, which is liable to contuse and separate the grey and white matter and to occasion later the formation of cysts or cavities full of plasma, grave obstacles to the cicatricial process. The cicatrization of such losses of sub-

---

[1] Storch : *Virchow's Arch. f. pathol. Anat.*, Bd. 157, 1899.

[2] Bielschowsky : Article I, " Allgemeine Histologie und Histopathologie des Nervensystems " in *Handbuch der Neurologie*, v. Lewandowsky, Bd. I, Berlin, 1910.

stance is due to the *pia mater* with its mesodermal and vascular constituents, as many authors, and more recently Farrar, Achúcarro, Morgenthaler [1] and Bianchi have demonstrated. We shall give no details concerning this process, which is well known to-day. We may merely recall that the fibroblasts of the *pia mater* penetrate, together with newly-formed capillaries (points of growth) and granular

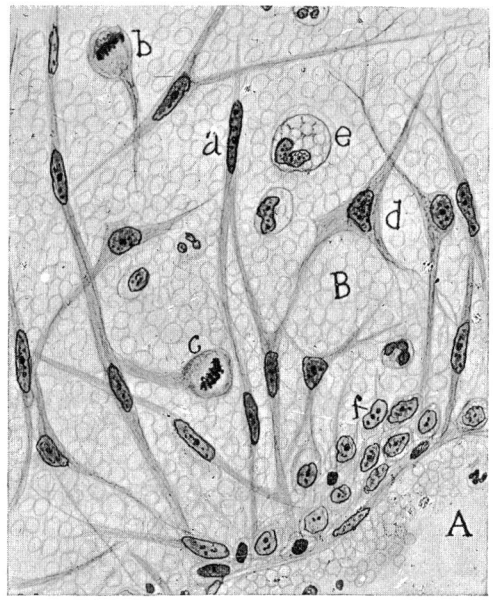

Fig. 309.—Serosanguineous exudate in the entrance of a wound of the cerebra cortex; young dog, killed two days after the operation. *A*, blood-vessel of the *pia mater*: *B*, exudate; *a*, connective cells invading the exudate; *b*, *c*, mitoses in young fibroblasts; *e*, leucocyte transformed into a granular cell.

elements, into the inflammatory exudate and haemorrhagic remnants, and that during their exodus they multiply rapidly. Nothing is easier than to see from the very first day, right in the exudate, series of young fibroblasts, greatly elongated, which traverse this in all directions, although the direction of the wound predominates; they are in all phases of mitosis (Fig. 305, *b*, *c*). Not only the plasmatic exudate, but also the coagula are rapidly penetrated by

[1] Morgenthaler: " Heilungvorgängen in der Grosshirnrinde des normalen und alkolisierten Kaninchens nach Einführung eines Fremdkörpers," *Zeitschr. f. d. gesamte Neurol. u. Psychiatrie*, Bd. 8, 1912.

colonies of wandering fibroblasts. Nevertheless, when the haemorrhage has been very great, the phenomena of liquefaction and phagocytosis of the vascular elements preponderate over the acts of organization and there is produced a cyst of the nervous substance, well known by neuropathologists.

At the same time the edges of the contused and necrosed cerebral substance become softened, and their remnants are taken up by granular cells of various sizes, some of them gigantic. Under such conditions, since a considerable portion of the nerve substance has to be eliminated and the cystic liquid resorbed, the cicatricial process develops very slowly. Thus, sixty-five days after the wound, in a cerebrum of a young cat we have still seen an ample cyst, full of plasma with marginal haemorrhagic remnants, bordered by compact masses of *Gitterzellen* which are full of nervous detritus. Later the connective tissue becomes condensed, leaving, nevertheless, spaces or interstices which in all respects recall the normal organization of the *pia mater*. The granular cells diminish in number; the small connective bundles become differentiated; and, finally, the Ehrlich and cyanophil cells of the plasma make their appearance. If the opening remains dilated the scarred wound tends in time to become organized, as Achúcarro noted, according to the structural type of the anfractuosity, at the bottom of which the *pia mater* forms a fold in which are important vessels.

But outside the mesodermal scar one always finds in the wounds another neuroglial scar of varying thickness. This glial zone always appears perfectly marked off from the mesodermal tissue, as Farrar and Morgenthaler have observed. Needless to say that it results from the multiplication of the neuroglia cells of the white and grey matter. In those cases in which the formation of large cysts has retarded the organization of the mesodermal scar one sees that the seat of the loss of substance is surrounded by a thick neuroglial zone, entirely devoid of regenerated nerve fibres.

If one applies the gold method to the analysis of this neuroglial zone, one sees the majority of its cells lying in a radial direction, and sending to the edges of the mesodermal region a thick appendix, which breaks up into numerous terminal fibrils forming a very complicated perinervous plexus. We find reproduced in this way the well-known disposition of the molecular layer of the cerebrum, where the radial expansions of the glia become resolved into a tangential fibrillar plexus.

Gigantic granular cells.—Months after a lesion followed by serious haemorrhage and considerable contusion of the nervous substance, one often sees in the extensive connective scar a loose collagenous tissue, sprinkled with granular cells, some of them of large size, containing four, six, or more nuclei. Cells of this type are found not infrequently surrounding large accumulations of nerve remnants, and perhaps also remnants of the colouring matter of the blood (haemosiderin ?). Some of these large masses of ruins appear free and are stained red and grey by the reduced silver.

VII

STUDY OF REGENERATIVE PROCESSES OF THE CEREBRUM (*Continued*)

Breakdown of the regeneration of the nerve paths.—Experiments of Tello showing that regeneration fails owing to the absence in the surroundings of substances that stimulate the growth and orientation of the axonic sprouts.—Theories explanatory of the poverty and incongruence of the natural regeneration.—Historical notes concerning regeneration in the cerebrum of man and the higher mammals.

WE have stated in previous chapters that the intra- as well as the extra-axonic neoformations grow for a certain time, sometimes ramify in a complicated way, form terminal buds and wings and, finally, paralyzed by insuperable obstacles, come to a stop not far from the parent axon.

We have also noted that, apart from exceptional cases, these sprouts do not start from true cones of growth, but from varicosities situated far from the wound and included in the portion of the axon that is attacked by the traumatic degeneration. They thus constitute reactions that are in a certain sense pathological and aberrant, since they take place in a diseased segment often destined to be entirely eliminated. One must thus admit that the *testudinoid* and *cephalopodic* structures are absolutely superfluous.

Once the axonic *cul de sac*, or useless portion of the conductor, is eliminated, the secondary retraction bud or ball is formed, which is never converted, at least under normal conditions, into a cone of growth. This retraction ball remains for a certain time, but at last, at times which vary for each mutilated axon, it also disappears, withdrawing and perhaps entering into the formation of the last living collateral, which is markedly hypertrophied. So perfect, months later, is the elimination of the retraction spheres that frequently one finds in the soma or at a distance from it neither free balls, nor terminal tumefactions, nor varicose fibres, nothing, in fact, to show the serious destructive processes that have taken place in the affected territory. Near the lesion one sees only smooth, well-stained axons, presenting all the signs of being normal conductors, that is, uninterrupted by the vulnerating agent. In man affected by various nervous diseases there also occur, though ephemerally, regenerative phenomena comparable to those described by ourselves and G. Sala in young traumatized mammals. Among other valuable observations, establishing this fact, we have : Bielschowsky's discovery of sprouts ramified around syphilitic tumours and gliomas ; the newly-formed fibres observed by R. Pfeiffer near cerebral punctures ; those observed by O. Rossi in the corpus callosum of alcoholics ; those observed by Marinesco in the foci of softening ; and, above all, the colonies of new clubs and fibres (*senile plaques*) discovered by Fischer in the cerebrum in senile dementia, well studied later by Alzheimer, Perusini, Bonfiglio, Achúcarro, Lafora, Marinesco, G. Sala, etc.

Perhaps there is foundation for the doubt expressed by Miyake, Herxheimer, and Gierlich as to the genuine regenerative character of the fine fibres and buds seen around infectious tumours or granulomas. But no reserve seems possible as regards the plaques of Fischer where, as we show in Fig. 310, *A*, *D*, *F*, taken from a study by Dr. Simarro which is as yet unpublished, one may see, besides terminal buds, grumes, and rings, evident divisions of pre-existent axons. It is perhaps because Simarro observed the early phases of formation of *plaques* that one sees very clearly in his preparations the collateral character of many of the nerve branches that penetrate into the plaques, as also the aggregation of terminal clubs and balls, more or less degenerated and monstrous, connected with passing fibres. It appears as if the sprouts had been attracted towards the region of the plaque, under the influence of some special neurotropic substance. Certain colossal clubs, whose reticulum is half disintegrated (*D*), appear to represent centripetal axons brought to an abrupt end.

The dendritic neoformations seen by R. Lafora[1] in the Ammon's horn of senile dogs are likewise incontestable. They appear to have been preceded by the deposit of a certain stimulating substance which is expelled from the expansional protoplasm, and which is destroyed later. Fig. 311, taken from the work of this author, attests this curious neoformation, correlated perhaps to a chemical

[1] G. R. Lafora: "Neoformaciones dendríticas en las neuronas y alteraciones de la neuroglia en el perro senil," *Trab. del Lab. de Investig. biol.*, t. 12, fasc. 1, May 1914.

736 DEGENERATION AND REGENERATION OF THE NERVE CENTRES

or mechanical stimulus. One may note that some of the new dendrites end in bulbs and tumefactions, which remind one of the buds of newly-formed axons.

We may thus infer from what has been said that, in man as in laboratory animals, the regenerative act commences, and may even

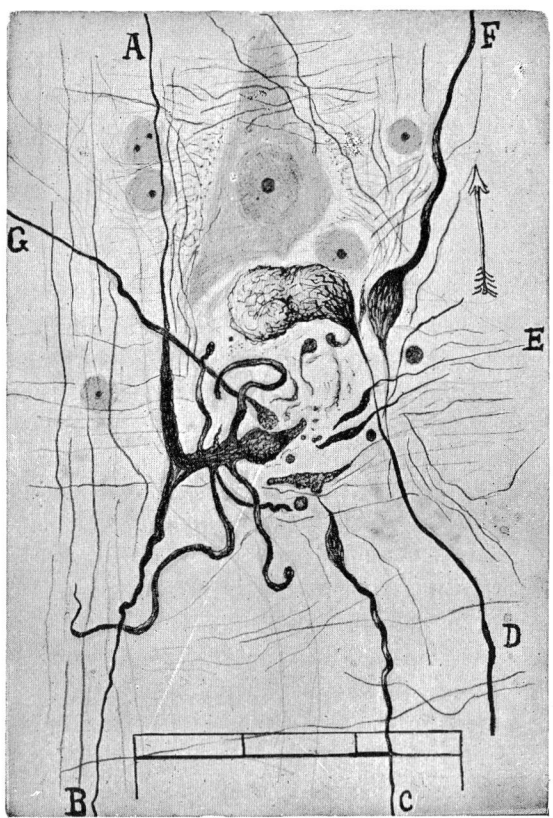

FIG. 310.—Details of a plaque of Fischer in course of formation. *A*, hypertrophied projection axon, next to the plaque, to which it sends a thick collateral ending in a bulb and numerous terminal branches; *D*, *G*, *F*, fibres ending in buds or balls in the region of the plaque. (From a drawing by Simarro.)

attain a certain strength, on condition that the traumatic commotion be sufficient to stir the axons out of their lethargy, or else that toxins or special stimulative principles, as yet undetermined, invade the grey matter. As is known, this tendency to restoration is frustrated by two negative conditions : (1) the lack of substances able to sustain and invigorate the indolent and scanty growth of the sprouts ;

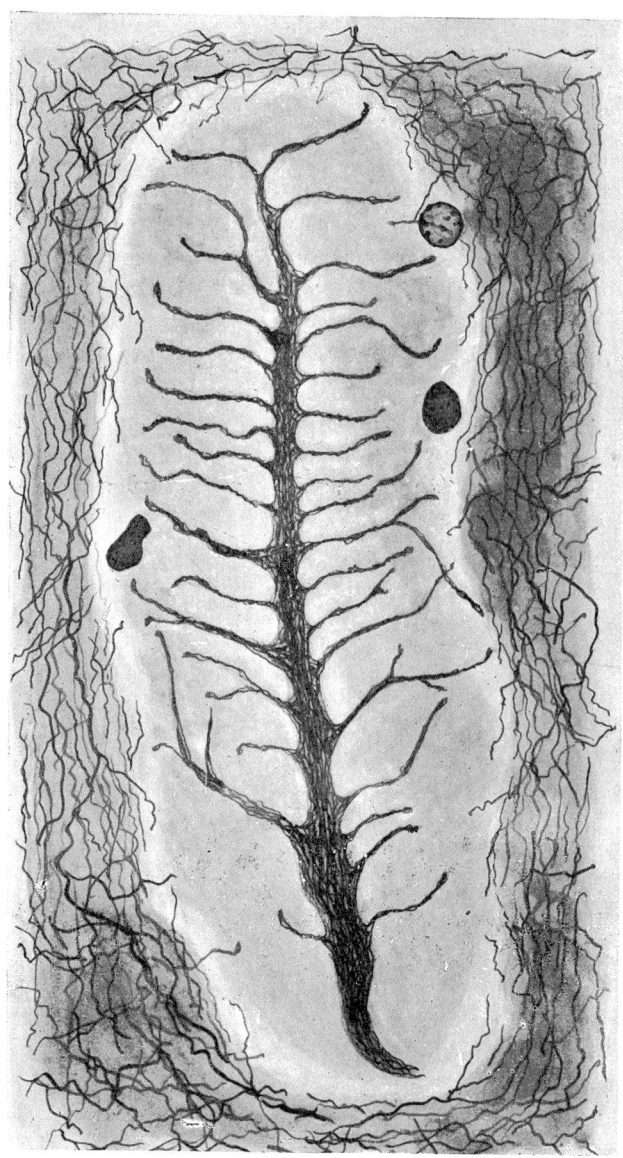

FIG. 311.—Disposition of the dendritic neoformations in the pyramidal cells of Ammon's horn in a senile dog; homogeneous substance which surrounds them, with the few neuroglial nuclei found in it. (Method of Cajal; figure extracted from the work of Dr. R. Lafora.)

(2) the absence in the paths or systems of interrupted nerve fibres of catalytic agents capable of attracting and directing the axonic current to its destination.

From this it may be inferred that, if experimental neurology is some day to supply artificially the deficiencies in question, it must accomplish these two objects : it must give to the sprouts, by means of adequate alimentation, a vigorous capacity for growth ; and place in front of the disoriented nerve cones and in the thickness of the tracts of the white matter and neuronic foci specific orienting substances. This last experimental condition is almost impossible to satisfy. On the other hand the first condition is relatively practicable, as Tello showed in some important experiments undertaken in our laboratory.

Tello placed near these aborted and flagging sprouts powerful chemotactic centres, represented by cells of Schwann in process of division, and found that the axons of the pyramidal cells are capable, under such impulses, of vigorous growth, crossing the mesodermal scar and invading the transplanted nerves ; they behave, in short, like a central nerve stump influenced by the proximity of the peripheral stump in course of transformation. The exceptional interest of these experiments leads us to give some details and figures concerning them.

Experiments of intracerebral nerve grafting carried out by Tello.— Lugaro [1] was the first to attempt to graft the sciatic nerve on the cerebral cortex. He used for this purpose normal nerves of dogs from one to two months old, and he killed the animals after eighteen to twenty-five days. The result was negative ; according to him, the neurotropic substances of the cells of Schwann do not appear to stimulate the neurocladism, or affect the attraction, of the normal axons of the cerebrum. Tello,[2] in his grafts, used adult rabbits and nerves in process of degeneration, that is, peripheral stumps of sciatic nerves cut eight and fourteen days before, and therefore in the phase of the bands of Büngner. But—and this was an essential point—instead of grafting the nerves on healthy cerebra, he made the transplantation on cerebral cortex that had been deeply cut. He made an incision in the nerve centre down to the white matter,

---

[1] Lugaro : " Sur le neurotropisme et sur les transplantations des nerfs," *Riv. di patol. ner. e mental.*, t. 11.

[2] F. Tello : " La influencia del neurotropismo en la regeneración de los centros nerviosos," *Trab. del Lab. de Invest. biol.*, t. 9, 1911.

and in the bottom deposited the piece of nerve. To avoid the possibility of the transplanted nerve containing sprouts that had previously reached it from the central stump of the sciatic—which would have seriously interfered with the interpretation of the phenomena—he took this graft, not near the nerve wound, but at a great distance

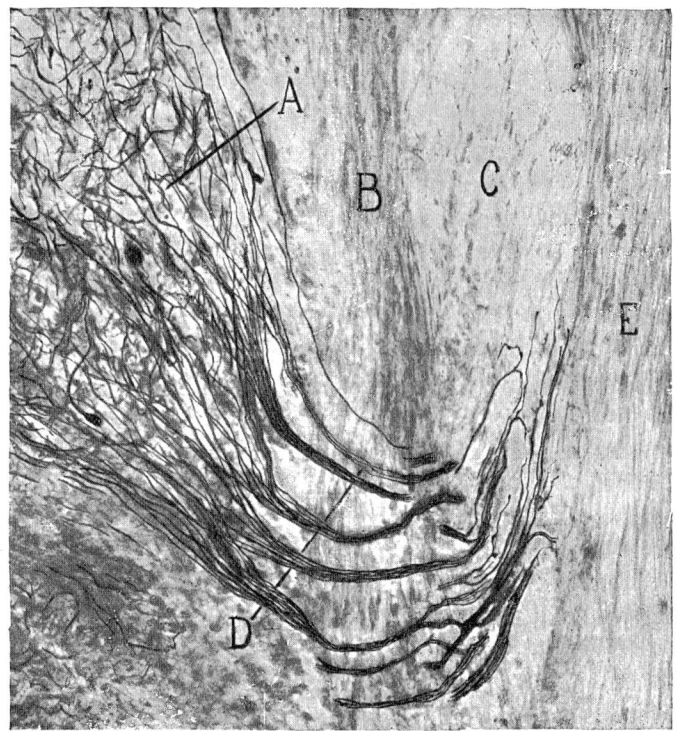

FIG. 312.—Growth of the cerebral fibres towards the nerve graft; retouched microphotograph of a piece of sciatic nerve free from fibres in the cerebral cortex of an adult rabbit, killed fourteen days after the operation. *A*, white matter of the cortex; *B*, limiting membrane formed by the connective tissue; *C*, connective tissue with granular cells at the beginning of the sciatic nerve; *D*, bundles of fibres which cross the limiting membrane and proceed towards the graft; *E*, connective tissue in contact with the neurilemma.

from it. These *empty grafts*, as Tello called them, are especially rich in neurotropic substances, whereas in normal nerves grafted directly, though not entirely absent, these are liberated very tardily. The animals were killed twelve, fourteen, and forty days after the cerebral operation.

In fortunate cases, that is, when the graft remained deep and the cerebral wound cicatrized rapidly, the method of reduced silver nitrate, after fixation in 50 % pyridine, revealed round the transplanted nerve : a thickened and proliferated neurilemma intimately united to the cerebral substance ; the peripheral fibres of the sciatic nerve, alive, free from myelin ellipsoids, and in the phase of the *bands of Büngner* ; the deep fibres retracted, with many lipoidal globes, and apparently necrotic. Between the graft and the cerebral substance, moreover, a connective scar is seen, sprinkled with fusiform cells, in continuity with the *pia mater*, and full of newly-formed capillaries, anastomosed with those pre-existing in the grey matter.

The fibres of the grey matter next to the graft are thickened, divided, and deeply stained. Many of them end in clubs or rings, but they do not seem to increase nor to proceed towards the graft. On the other hand, numerous large medullated tubes of the white matter display unusual activity. Not only are they hypertrophic and in process of neurocladism, but they have branches that are enormously developed, resolutely directed towards the graft, and congregated in compact groups or small bundles. These newly-formed axons reach the capsule or intermediate cicatricial layer continuous with the *pia mater*, perforating it at different points, and approach one of the ends of the graft ; they congregate at the entrance of some superficial sheaths of Schwann, and finally penetrate within them, pushing aside the lipoid remnants, and *behaving in their growth, ramifications, orientation, energetic progress, etc., exactly like the sprouts of the central stump of a cut nerve*. One finds sprouts growing between the bands of Büngner ; others, which did not hit upon the end, skirt the graft longitudinally, sliding along the neurilemma ; others again are held up, either inside or outside the transplanted nerve, forming spheres and buds of various sizes.

Another important fact brought out by the surprising researches of Tello is the following. Among the cerebral sprouts that enter the graft, the majority are young and naked axons ; but among the large and relatively old sprouts that circulate within and outside the transplanted nerve, *there are some provided with satellite cells, that is, with embryonic cells of Schwann*. Notwithstanding their advanced differentiation, the cerebral fibres have not, like the motor fibres of the cord, lost their initial capacity of establishing symbioses with the mesodermal elements present in the peripheral cordons.

The facts quoted above relate to a rabbit killed twelve days after the operation. After fourteen and more days the phenomena of innervation of the graft display still greater activity and power of growth. As we show in Fig. 312, the piece of nerve is assailed by thick bundles of fibres which are in continuity with the axons of the white and grey matter. These newly-formed fibres *converge from*

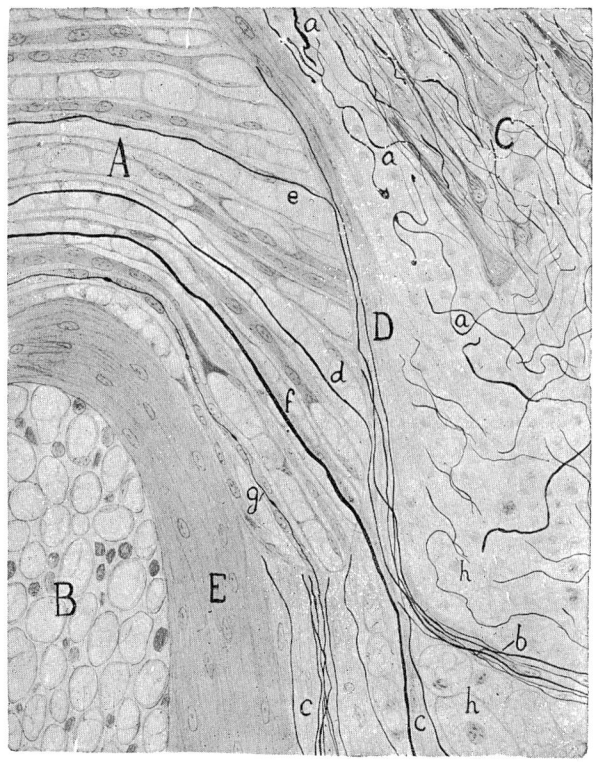

FIG. 313.—Other living graft with perfect preservation of the bands of Büngner in the cerebral cortex of an adult rabbit, killed fourteen days after the operation. *A*, fascicle of the sciatic nerve cut longitudinally; *B*, the same in cross-section; *C*, deep portion of the grey matter; *D* and *E*, limiting membrane; *a*, newly-formed fibres of the grey matter; *b*, fibres of the white matter attracted by the graft; *c*, fibres that have entered lower down and are advancing along the limiting membrane; *d, e, f, g*, fibres advancing along the bands of Büngner; they can be traced on the other side of the limiting membrane.

various points of the cortex, as though they were attracted by an irresistible force. Nearly all these fibrillar bundles pick up along their way, which is sometimes very irregular across the scar, satellite cells, which, at least in this case, do not seem to come from the nerve, but from the mesodermal tissue continuous with the *pia mater*. Some mesodermal elements cross the bundles, follow along the axons and become converted into true cells of Schwann. The sprouts, on their way towards the graft, repeatedly divide, frequently show detention clubs, and trace complicated turns outside of the neurilemma up to the place where they reach the end of the graft. Once there, they become rectilinear and grow very rapidly (Fig. 313, *A*). Nevertheless, it is not unusual to see free bundles and axons that have gone astray and are wandering round the graft, trying in vain to cross the compact cicatricial masses that surround it.

Tello attributes these differences in the fate of the sprouts to the inequality in the structure and permeability of the cicatricial capsule. Its constitution differs somewhat according to the regions. At some points it is composed of collagenous masses poor in fibroblasts; at others the connective mass appears crossed and interrupted by islets and bands formed of stellate or fusiform connective cells. When the bundles of sprouts fall upon these relatively permeable regions, they rapidly reach the graft; if they accidentally fall upon fibrous masses they go astray and trace complicated turns.

What is the fate of these curious cerebral fibres, converted by circumstances into conductors in a peripheral nerve? Tello has attempted to clear up this point, killing the animals on which the graft had been made forty days after the operation. Such a late examination showed the graft diminished in volume, penetrated by the connective tissue of the *pia mater*, and in process of atrophy and resorption. There are regions in which migratory sprouts still subsist, preserved in the old sheaths of Schwann. At any rate, the movement of innervation is tending to decrease. It is probable that, months after the operation, both the transplanted piece of nerve and its newly-formed fibres finally disappear.

The graft, under similar conditions, both of normal nerves and of peripheral segments of sciatic nerve that had been cut and innervated previously to the graft, failed to attract the cerebral axons. In the first case the normal cells of Schwann of the graft must undergo, from the first, all its metamorphic phases, and the precarious nutrition of the graft in a new region doubtless offers serious obstacles to an abundant secretion of neurotropic substances. The sprouts, accordingly, fail altogether or penetrate exceptionally. In the second case, once the secretory power of the bands of Büngner is stopped, so to say, by the previous arrival of abundant sprouts, the trophic substances that may be produced around the graft cease to be liberated, or are liberated only feebly. One can thus easily understand why it is difficult to attract the cerebral axons and rouse them from their apathy.

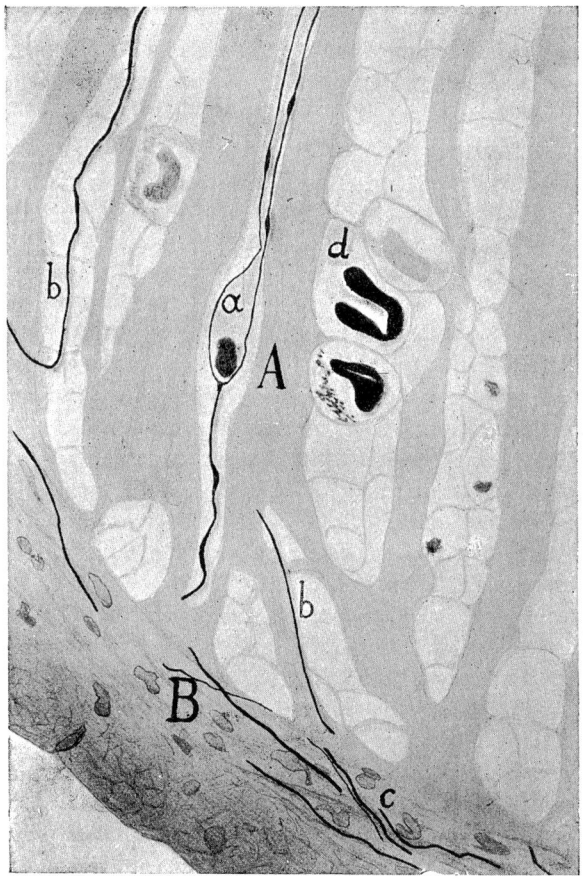

FIG. 314.—Details of the penetration of the sprouts into a graft of sciatic nerve free from fibres; rabbit, killed twelve days after the operation. *A*, sciatic nerve; *B*, remnants of nervous tissue surrounding the ventricular portion; *a*, fibre that has entered an empty sheath and there bifurcates; *b*, undivided fibres within other sheaths; *c*, fibres that follow the edges of the graft, trying to penetrate it; *d*, empty sheaths with remnants of the axons of the sciatic nerve.

Tello has shown, in addition, that the cerebral fibres are also attracted, although less vigorously, by the juice pressed from the bands of Büngner of the peripheral stump of the cut nerve. The following experiment proves this. On the surface of the cerebrum was placed a piece of elder pith, soaked in neurotropic substances.

The animal was killed after eight days, and one saw that the tangential axons of the molecular layer, which are usually so apathetic, had grown notably towards the cells filled with free catalytic agents. As we show in Fig. 315, c, one of the fibres, after crossing an areola, penetrates into the cavity of the next one. It is important to note, however, that in other experiments the results were not so decisive, no doubt because the presence of a small quantity of neurotropic substances, which are rapidly rendered inactive through decomposition or are resorbed, is usually insufficient to maintain the process of growth of a sprout ; the constant secretion of such substances during many days is needed. This is the function of the cells of Schwann of the peripheral stump of cut nerves, and to this is doubtless due their formidable attractive power on the free sprouts in the scar.

Opinions concerning the causes of the breakdown of regeneration of the central tracts.—All the above observations with regard to the phenomena following on spinal, cerebellar, and cerebral traumatisms, lead to the conclusion that, as is well known, the central tracts are incapable of regeneration, for the majority of the regenerative acts described in man and laboratory animals are temporary reactions, aborted restoratory processes, incapable of bringing about a complete and definitive repair of the interrupted paths.

It may also be inferred that this defective capacity for regeneration does not depend on essential, fatal, and unchangeable conditions, but on the absence in the surroundings of catalytic agents able to overcome the osmotic equilibria of the cones of growth, to provoke their vigorous nutrition, and to direct them to the path that they must follow. These views, defended by ourselves, in various treatises, are not held by the majority of neurologists. It is true that many of the authors of explanatory hypotheses did not know of the facts advanced by Tello and ourselves in support of our view. At any rate, it is desirable to record here the opinions in best repute :

Bethe, and with him various auto-regenerationists or polygenists, for whom the cell of Schwann has the property of producing neurofibrils and axonic segments, with independence of the neuronal soma, maintained that the absence of regeneration of the central paths derives logically from the absence of cells of Schwann. Putting aside the assertion, refuted by numerous observations, of the essential inability of the central axon to sprout, there is much truth in this view. Although the cells of Schwann lack the neurogenetic power which Bethe attributed to them, they appear necessary for the nutrition and orientation of the newly-formed peripheral tubes. But this hypothesis, while it contains part of the truth, does not contain it all.

We may recall that the fibres of the nerve centres, especially of the cord, form sprouts, more or less, when they are injured, and they are capable, under special conditions, of leaving the cord and growing

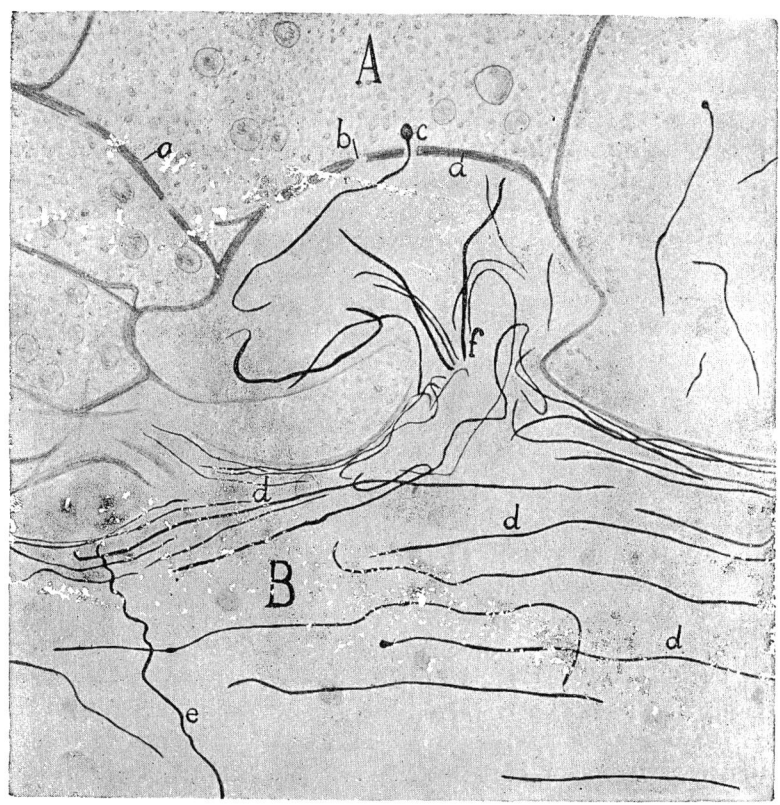

FIG. 315.—Graft of a piece of elder pith steeped in neurotropic substances, in the cerebral cortex of a rabbit which died after two days. *A*, elder pith; *B*, cerebral cortex; *a*, thin walls enclosing the cells of the elder pith; *b*, openings in these walls; *c*, fibre passing from one cell to the other through one of these openings; *d*, tangential fibres; *e*, one of the few persisting vertical fibres; *f*, fibres partly introduced through pressure.

along the roots and right into the embryonic connective tissue. Though on a lesser scale, this sprouting also occurs in the axons of the cerebrum, the optic nerve, and retina. It cannot be denied, therefore, that the central axons have the property of producing new fibres, and what has to be explained is why, once the reconstructive movement is initiated, the nerve sprouts lose their energy and suspend their growth.

Stroebe,[1] who never doubted the restoratory capacity of the central axons, attributed the breakdown of the regeneration to the tendency of these fibres to disperse themselves in a multitude of collaterals within the scar. The energy of growth being thus dissipated, no axon possesses sufficient vigour to overcome the mechanical obstacles and re-establish the interrupted paths. Marinesco,[2] in his first papers on the regeneration of the spinal cord, held a similar opinion.

The fact noted by Stroebe is certain ; but he exaggerates it somewhat. The immense majority of the fibres of the white matter do not ramify at all, and of the axons that divide in the edges of the wound, the greater number have only two, three, or four terminal branchlets, which are not very long, save in exceptional cases which we have pointed out (spinal cord). In the cerebrum and cerebellum, as we have noted, axonic neoformations are extremely rare.

O. Rossi,[3] who has devoted various interesting studies to this subject, has formulated a conjecture that deserves careful attention. In his opinion, the neuronal reaction that causes the regenerative process is in direct ratio to the mass of protoplasm that has been cut off, that is, to the extent of its axonic mutilation. A sensory or motor root severed near the cord displays great regenerative power because a large part of its mass has been taken from it, since the piece of axon cut off is quantitatively superior to its own cellular body ; on the contrary a pyramidal cell of the cerebrum, or a funicular cell of the cord whose axons are cut in the latter centre, lose only a small part of their mass, and therefore the regenerative reaction is absent or insignificant.

Unfortunately, forcible objections to this hypothesis may be put forward, and O. Rossi himself has pointed out some which he has been unable to refute satisfactorily. We may mention certain facts that are contrary to, or not easy to reconcile with, this theory. (a) When, instead of cutting the sciatic nerve near the pelvis, one cuts both its bifurcations in the thighs (in cats, rabbits, etc.), the nervous regeneration

---

[1] H. Stroebe : " Experimentelle Untersuchungen über die Degeneration und reparatorischen Vorgänge bei der Heilung von Verletzungen des Rückenmarks," etc., *Ziegler's Beiträge*, Bd. 15, H. 7, 1894.

[2] Marinesco : " Recherches sur la régénérescence de la moelle," *Nouvelle Iconographie de la Salpêtrière*, No. 5, 1906.

Marinesco et Minea : " Note sur la dégénérescence de la moelle chez l'homme," *Compt. Rend. Soc. Biol.*, t. 40, p. 1027, 1906.

[3] O. Rossi : " Processi rigenerativi e digenerativi consequenti a feriti asettiche del sistema nervoso centrale," *Riv. di pat. ner. e ment.*, anno 13, fasc. 11, 1908.

occurs with the same or greater activity. (b) The section of the posterior roots (internal or spinal portion) in the ganglion itself is not followed by a greater regenerative activity than when the interruption is effected near the cord. The same occurs with a section close to or at a distance from the anterior roots. (c) In the cases of central lesions, in which the axon has evidently been divided near the cell of origin (pyramidal cells of the cerebrum, Purkinje cells, etc.), instead of exaggerated regenerative phenomena, one sees a retraction club formed, which is incapable of emitting sprouts, and the definitive atrophy and destruction of the mutilated cell almost always follows at various intervals. (d) Section of the optic nerve near the papilla necessarily separates a protoplasmic mass superior to that which remains in the retina; nevertheless, regeneration slows down and is quickly frustrated, as has been proved by the experiments of Tello, of O. Rossi himself, and of Ríos and Arcaute.

When one sees the slight regenerative capacity of the motor roots within the cord, of the funicular axons of the latter, of Purkinje axons mutilated near the soma, of the functional expansion of the pyramidal cells of the cerebrum cut right in the grey matter, etc., one is almost tempted to invert O. Rossi's hypothesis, attributing the scanty capacity for regeneration of the central fibres to the notable state of prostration and atony into which all neurones fall when a large quantity of protoplasm is taken from them. This conjecture would harmonize better than that of Rossi with the researches and conclusions, no longer recent, regarding the atrophies provoked in the motor cells by tearing out their axons (atrophy of Gudden) or by their section near their point of emergence (phenomena of chromatolysis, etc.). But such an explanation must not be erected into a general law. As we have noted in various passages of this work, the quantity of protoplasm separated from the cell, especially when the initial collaterals have been cut off with it, may settle the question of the preservation of the neurone and of its functional capacity or aptitude; but this preservation appears, in the majority of cases, to be absolutely independent of the regenerative potentiality of the mutilated central stump. Whether the axon is cut near or far from the initial collaterals one obtains nearly always in the cerebrum and cerebellum, not the emission of new branches directed towards the scar, but traumatic degeneration and the formation of a retraction ball.

Dustin,[1] for his part, propounded another solution of the problem before us. Seduced by the theoretical speculations of Held concerning

[1] Dustin: "Le rôle des tropismes et de l'odogénèse dans la régénération du système nerveux," *Arch. de Biol.*, t. 25, 1910.

pre-established paths in neurogenesis, he attributed the breakdown of regeneration of the central paths, and especially of the spinal cord, to the absence of *odogenesis*, that is, the lack of an embryonic connective tissue similar to that of internervous scars, with spaces or interstices capable of guiding the young fibres. According to Dustin, some influence is also exerted by the presence, in central wounds, of dense and exuberant scars, and by the fact that in the axons of the centres the faculty of growth is more restricted than in peripheral axons.

Dustin is right in claiming as a cause of the regenerative breakdown the absence, in the scars of centres (he especially refers to the spinal cord), of hollow spaces or pre-existent paths. But this deficiency occurs likewise in the connective scar of interrupted nerves and in the thickness of the peripheral stump itself, which is full, as is well known, of lipoid drops and of cellular conglomerates. Nevertheless, the sprouts launch out among all the obstacles from the central stump as far as the remotest terminal structures. When it is a question of the nerves, the prodigious multiplication and growth of the branches provide for and accomplish everything. But when we study the centres we are confronted with a fundamental defect—the absence or initial poverty of the sprouting. Thus the entire problem lies in explaining why there are very few fibres capable of generating *cones of growth*, and why, once these are formed, they are suddenly paralyzed. The hypothesis of Dustin might perhaps partially elucidate the incapacity of the new fibres to reach the terminal organs, but not the niggardly development and rapid breakdown of the nerve sprouts. We may add that the absence of *odogenesis* fails also to explain why in Tello's experiments the sprouts grow exceptionally well, and are capable, owing to the growing tension of their cones, of perforating thick cicatricial masses devoid of paths or interstices that are congruently oriented, in order to reach the graft.

Marinesco,[1] in a paper quoted above, puts forward an explanation that recalls to some extent that of Dustin and to some extent that advanced by us. After confirming the fact that in the central fibres pre-existent sprouts develop a capacity for crossing long distances, he says: " If these newly-formed fibres do not restore the old connections, the cause of this is not intrinsic, but it surely depends on the absence of a conductor adapted to their growth." In other words, the guide, the directing neurotropic action, capable of bringing the nerve sprouts to their points of terminal connection, is wanting.

Some years ago, in connection with experiments on degeneration

---

[1] Marinesco: " Nouvelles contributions à l'étude de la régénérescence des fibres du système nerveux central," *Jour. für Psychol. u. Neurol.*, Bd. 17, 1910.

and regeneration of the spinal cord,[1] we formulated a hypothesis which, while it is founded on postulates different from that of the polygenists, has a certain affinity with the latter.

We said: "To sum up, while these experiments are incomplete, they seem to prove: (1) That the axons of the posterior roots (internal portion) and spinal white matter are capable of regeneration, showing buds of growth and newly-formed arborizations. (2) That the creation of the intraspinal cyst and perhaps also the absence of cells capable of segregating chemotactic substances conducive to the exodus of the new axons, or other as yet undetermined conditions, cause the breakdown of the restorative process, the nerve sprouts becoming atrophied, and only those portions of the conductors which establish interneuronal connections ultimately remaining."

One must recognize that the terms of the problem have changed somewhat, as a consequence of the latest research. Certain supposed conditions of the incapacity for regeneration, such as the presence of cysts and the excessive thickness of connective scars have lost in importance since we know, as indicated above, that white substance in process of sprouting is unable to cross neuroglial scars that are very thin and devoid of cysts. On the other hand, the negative condition of our hypothesis, that is, the absence of catalysers to nutrition, has grown in value since our investigations [2] have shown that in certain circumstances, especially when embryonic mesodermic masses accumulate round the spinal wound or within it, or when there are cells of Schwann in course of division near the sprouts (newly-formed fibres of the bundles, in presence of degenerated anterior roots), the fibres of the white matter at times grow remarkably, giving rise to extensive extracentral arborizations. Finally, Tello's experiments, already referred to, besides confirming the hypothesis of neurotropism, show that the sufficient growth of the central axons depends on the presence of a special food which is produced in effective proportions solely by the cells of Schwann of the nerves.

Thus, the central axons, and in a less measure the dendrites, possess, *ab initio*, the capacity, inherent in the constitution itself of the nervous protoplasm, of increasing their mass intrinsically and extrinsically, that is, of rebuilding their structure and of expanding into new projections. The neurobiones are the principal protagonists of such processes. But in order that the regeneration may attain a certain

---

[1] Cajal: "Notas preventivas sobre la degeneración y regeneración de las vías nervosas centrales," *Trab. del Lab. de Invest. biol.*, t. 4, 1905-06.

[2] Cajal: "Observaciones sobre la regeneración de la porción intramedular de la raíces sensitivas," *Trab. del Lab. de Invest. biol.*, t. 8, 1910.

vigour and utility, the co-operation of mesodermal cells is necessary, either under the form of embryonic connective elements, or under the superior form, particularly adapted to this end, of rejuvenated cells of Schwann. Adult cells of Schwann, ectodermal elements like those of the *glia*, the neurones themselves when they are necrosed or degenerating, the remnants of axons and of the medullary sheath, the exudates with their leucocytes, etc., are impotent to elaborate these stimuli. Perhaps during the ontogenetic process the neuroblasts or neurones had a phase of specific neurotropic secretion; perhaps the ependymal elements also collaborated chemically in the tutorial and orienting process. But the functional specialization of the brain imposed on the neurones two great lacunae; proliferative inability and irreversibility of intraprotoplasmic differentiation. It is for this reason that, once the development was ended, the founts of growth and regeneration of the axons and dendrites dried up irrevocably. In adult centres the nerve paths are something fixed, ended, immutable. Everything may die, nothing may be regenerated.

It is for the science of the future to change, if possible, this harsh decree. Inspired with high ideals, it must work to impede or moderate the gradual decay of the neurones, to overcome the almost invincible rigidity of their connections, and to re-establish normal nerve paths, when disease has severed centres that were intimately associated.

It would be ingenuous to pretend to go farther in the solution of a problem so full of difficulties. We must recognize that, in the matter of neurogenesis and nervous regeneration, we are still in the phase of collection of materials. As a consequence our hypotheses are premature, and they can aspire neither to perfection nor to permanence. They are conceptions to point the way, conjectures thrown out to excite and keep up investigation. It is in this sense that, as regards the regenerative process, we profess and accept the theory of neurotropism. It is the banner under which we are working. We shall follow it so long as it may lead to the discovery of new facts, so long as it may satisfy our tendency to subordinate multiform phenomena to the same principle. We shall abandon it whenever another conception provides a better explanation of the facts of nervous regeneration and degeneration, and ministers more effectively to that desire for unity and system which seems to be an unchangeable consequence of our cerebral organization.

Historical notes concerning the existence of regenerative acts in the cerebral neurones and axons.—In the course of this work we have already alluded several times to the valuable contributions by modern scientists to the resolution of the problem before us. We shall now give more details concerning those researches, and we shall place them in their chronological order.

The present doctrine of the regeneration of the cerebrum is founded on two series of facts : *anatomico-pathological observations* in man ; *experiments on traumatisms* in animals.

We shall not speak here of observations made before the advent of methods for demonstrating neuro *fibrils*, because it is only since the invention of such colloidal silver methods that it has been possible to obtain regular and precise images of axonic sprouts and of phenomena of compensatory hypertrophy.

Anatomico-pathological facts.—It was Bielschowsky [1] who, applying his method to the study of lesions of the white and grey matter caused by tumours, such as gliomas and syphilitic tumours, found in the vicinity of the neoplasms numerous fibres, apparently newly formed, provided with terminal buds, as well as perivascular plexuses and even true spiroidal structures, comparable to those occurring in interrupted peripheral nerves. These regenerating fibres were present, not only around tumours of the spinal cord, but also around neoplasias of the human cerebrum (sphenoidal bulb). Since such axons had no myelin, ramified from time to time, followed atypical paths, and ended in clubs or thickenings, comparable in principle to the *terminal podia* of Held, or the *cones of growth* of Cajal, Bielschowsky was inclined to regard them as resulting from regenerative acts. On the other hand, all the fibres ending in a club, but whose direction and position coincide with those of normal fibres would, in his opinion, be more or less altered pre-existent conductors.

Finally, Bielschowsky also observed fine fibres ending in rings, clubs, or balls affected with superficial hyalinization, neurones with cortical fenestrations, and various other alterations, confirmed later by anatomico-pathological experimentation on animals.

Some time later, using the same analytic method, Herxheimer and Gierlich [2] studied histologically a few cerebral gliomas, and found within the tumour a considerable number of nerve fibres that were more or less altered and terminated in buds. These investigators, while they did not contradict the assertions of Bielschowsky, were inclined to consider the fibres internal as well as external to the neoplasms, not as regenerated conductors, but as pre-existent degenerating axons.

---

[1] Bielschowsky : "Ueber das Verhalten der Achsencylinder in Geschwulsten des Nervensystems," etc., *Journ. f. Psychol. u. Neurol.*, Bd. 14, 1905-06.

Ibid. : *Journ. f. Psychol. u. Neurol.*, Bd. 14, 1905-06.

[2] Herxheimer und Gierlich : *Studien über die Neurofibrillen in Zentralnervensystem*, Wiesbaden, 1907.

R. Pfeifer [1] studied human cerebra that had undergone in life exploratory punctures. He recognized, by Bielschowsky's method, within the scar as well as on its edges, numerous nerve fibres, apparently regenerated and provided with terminal clubs. He also described free balls, ramifications, etc.

The existence of regenerated fibres does not follow clearly from Pfeifer's descriptions, which are very interesting under certain aspects. Those which he regards as regenerated fibres (and which might legitimately be considered such when retraction balls were not well known) are perhaps the central stump of pre-existent axons with a retraction ball. Even the fibres existing within the scar might belong to this type, since the operatory procedure of the puncture tends, better than any other, to push apart and dislocate nerve fibres which are subsequently surrounded and dissociated by the neuroglial tissue.

Miyake [2] has serious doubts as to the regenerative character of the fibres with clubs found around tubercles and gliomas, being inclined to consider them as pre-existent conductors in course of degeneration.

O. Rossi [3] examined the corpus callosum of alcoholics and observed, although rarely, nerve fibres that were ramified, amyelinic, and terminated by very small balls. Some newly-formed fibres seemed to twine round others from the same nerve trunk and had an evident regenerative character.

Marinesco has made several important studies of this problem, using the method of reduced silver nitrate. In one of them [4] he carefully analyzed the foci of softening produced in man by cerebral haemorrhages of long standing, and he found, in the midst of exudates which were being resorbed and which were strewn with macrophages and cellular detritus, bundles and plexuses of axons which were apparently newly formed, since they lacked myelin and ended in buds and balls. The axonic bundles frequently followed the course of the bloodvessels. In recent softenings, sixteen days after the haemorrhage, the regenerative phenomena are little apparent, for the old axons still

[1] R. Pfeifer: "Ueber die traumatische Degeneration und Regeneration des Gehirns erwachsener Menschen," *Jour. f. Psychol. u. Neurol.*, Bd. 12, 1908.

[2] Miyake: "Zur Frage der Regeneration der Nervenfasern in zentralen Nervensystem," *Arbeiten aus dem Neurol. Institut. an der Wiener Universität*, Bd. 12, 1908.

[3] O. Rossi: "Sul istologia patologica di una speciale alterazione descritta da Marchiafava nel corpo calloso degli alcoolisti," *Riv. di pat. nerv. e mentale*, vol. 15, fasc. 6, 1910.

[4] Marinesco: "Sur la neurotisation des foyers de ramollissement et d'hémorragie cérébrale," *Revue neurologique*, No. 24, 30 déc. 1908.

subsist and appear more or less altered, arranged as chains of beads—moniliform—and often very pale and granular. One frequently finds pieces of axons, folded and altered, within macrophages. In the periphery of the focus one comes upon fibres that are swollen and moniliform, and others that are varicose. There are, however, axons that are more or less normal, provided with a round or ovoid club of growth, and these may be taken as expressions of a phenomenon of growth.

In a more recent work in which he attempted to analyze the degenerative effects of spinal compression due to Pott's disease and those brought about in the cerebellum by various tumours, he observed the miliary plaques of Fischer, and recognized the indubitable existence in them of radial sprouts ending in clubs, rings, or buds, and continuous with pre-existent axons.

Fischer himself stated that the miliary plaques commonly found in senile dementia contain plexuses of newly-formed fibres and crowns of more or less degenerated terminal buds and rings. This has been corroborated besides by Simchovicz,[1] who furnished many illustrations and descriptive details. We also owe excellent descriptions of the neoformations occurring in such plaques to Alzheimer,[2] Bonfiglio,[3] Perusini,[4] Achúcarro,[5] Bielschowsky,[6] Marinesco,[7] G. Sala,[8] and Lafora.[9]

[1] Simchowicz: "Histologische Studien über die senile Demence," *Histol. u. histopathol. Arbeiten über die Grosshirnrinde*, etc., von *F. Nissl u. Alzheimer*, Bd. 4, H. 2, 1911.

[2] Alzheimer: "Ueber eine eigenartige Erkrankung der Hirnrinde," 37 *Vers. Südwestdeutsch. Irrenärtze in Tübingen*, 1906, *Zentralbl. f. Nervenheilkunde u. Psych.*, Bd. 18, 1907.

[3] Bonfiglio: "Di speciali reperti in un caso di probabile sifilide cerebrale," *Rivista sperim. di Freniatria*, vol. 34, 1908.

[4] Perusini: "Ueber klinisch. und histopath. eigenartige psychische Erkrankungen des späteren Lebensalters," *Histol. u. histopathol. Arbeiten*, von. Nissl, 1909.

[5] Achúcarro: "Some pathological findings in the neuroglia and in the ganglion cells of the cortex in senile conditions," *Bulletin No. 2, Government Hospital for the Insane*, Washington, 1910.

[6] Bielschowsky: "Zur Kenntniss der Alzheimerschen Krankheit," *Journal f. Psychol. u. Neurol.*, Bd. 18, 1911.

[7] Marinesco: "Etude anatomique et clinique des plaques dites séniles," *L'encéphale*, No. 2, fév. 1912.

[8] G. Sala: "Sopra un caso di demenzia senile," *Società medico-chirurgica di Pavia*, No. 1, 1913.

[9] G. Lafora: "Beitrag zur Kenntniss der Alzheimerschen Krankheit," *Zeitsch. f. die gesam. Neurol. u. Psychatr.*, Bd. 11, 1913.

Catola,[1] who studied the phases of softening and destruction of the cerebrum by Bielschowsky's method, found numerous fibres devoid of balls, serpentine in their course, sometimes ending in hooks and intensely stained by silver.

Catola, with some reserves, is inclined to regard such axons as resulting from a regenerative process. Nevertheless, on studying the descriptions of this author, it seems to us that these were what we have called preserved fibres. To this order of dead pre-existent axons may belong not a few of the sprouts described by Bielschowsky, Herxheimer and Gierlich, Miyake and Marinesco, in softened nerve regions, infiltrated with blood, or where there were haemorrhagic foci.

We may also mention as testifying to the essential regenerative capacity of the human cerebrum the observation by Bielschowsky and Gallus[2] of pyramidal cells provided with numerous fine newly-formed dendrites (*tuberose sclerosis*), a discovery recognized also by Bielschowsky and Pick[3] in the neurones of a cerebral *ganglioneuroma*; also the observations by G. R. Lafora[4] of the appearance of new dendrites in Ammon's horn of senile dogs (*radial trunk* of the large pyramidal cells of the layer subjacent to the *dendata fascia*) as a consequence of the pericellular deposit of foreign stimulating materials. But the discovery of Lafora and that of Bielschowsky and Gallus differ considerably. While the former author observed relatively thick neoformations in the radial trunk, the latter found them in the soma, under the form of very fine threads, divergent, extraordinarily numerous, little ramified, and ending at a short distance.

Positive facts concerning regeneration furnished by experimental pathology.—Among the authors who have studied regeneration of the cerebral nerve fibres in modern times, we may cite Borst[5] who, besides using the methods of Mallory and Nissl, used that of Stroebe for staining large axons. In order to cause neoformative acts in the cerebral cortex of rabbits, Borst introduced into it pieces of sterilized celloidin riddled

---

[1] Catola: "Alcune nuove ricerche sulla struttura delle lacune di desintegrazione cerebrale," *Riv. di patol. nervosa e mentale*, vol. 15, 1910.

[2] Bielschowsky u. Gallus: "Über tuberöse Sclerose," *Journal f. Psychol. u. Neurol.*, Bd. 20, 1913.

[3] L. Pick u. M. Bielschowsky: "Ueber das System der Neurone u. Beobachtungen an einem Ganglioneurome des Gehirns," *Zeits. f. das ges. Neur. u. Psych.*, Bd. 6, 1911.

[4] G. Lafora: Loc. cit. *Trab. del Lab. de Invest. biol.*, tomo 11, fasc. 4, 1914.

[5] Borst: "Neue Experimente zur Fräge nach der Regenerationsfähigkeit des Gehirns," *Beiträge zur pathol. Anat. u. zur allgem. Pathologie von E. Ziegler*, Bd. 36, 1904.

with transversal perforations; examination some weeks later showed not only mitoses in the glia and in the neurones, but also the production of new medullated axons, which, taking advantage of the holes in the foreign body, crossed it more or less completely. It would be advantageous to repeat the interesting experiments of Borst, with the assistance of the neurofibrillar methods, in order to see to what extent the neoformation referred to is well established, and to show whether or not the sprouts in question are merely pre-existent conductors dislocated through hernia of the grey matter before the constant pressure of the foreign body. We may note, moreover, that Farrar,[1] who also operated by leaving in the wounds of the cerebral cortex pieces of elder pith, has never seen a sprout penetrate the openings of the foreign body.

Saltykow [2] made some interesting experiments of re-implantation of pieces of brain in the rabbit. Leaving aside the fact of the relatively good preservation of the neurones of the cut piece during the first week, and of the ulterior degeneration of these neurones and of their axons, it is especially important to note the statement that after twenty-five days from the operation new fibres are found on the edges of the cerebral wound, which are produced concurrently with the neuroglial repair. As such sprouts are found only at the level of the newly-formed glia, Saltykow suspects that the neuroglia cells play some part in the regenerative process of the axons, since in this case it is not possible to invoke the neurotizing influence of the cells of Schwann.

It is unfortunate that the imperfect methods used by Saltykow (those of Nissl, Van Gieson, etc.) are not capable of dissipating our doubts as to the reality of the nerve sprouts, which might very well be *preserved fibres* or living pre-existent neurones that had been dislocated in the scar.

We believe that we were the first to point out the indubitable existence, in the brain of young traumatized animals, of partial and frustrated acts of axonal regeneration, as well as of compensatory hypertrophies occurring in collaterals situated above the interruption of the axon. The extensive descriptions contained in the earlier chapters excuse us from giving details here.

It will be useful, however, to enumerate chronologically and from a purely historical standpoint the most important facts that we have made known.

[1] Farrar: "On the phenomena of repair in the cerebral cortex," etc., *Histol. und histopathol. Arbeiten v. Nissl*, Bd. 2, 1908.

[2] Saltykow: "Versuche über Gehirnreplantation," *Arch. f. Psychatr. u. Nervenkrankheiten*, Bd. 40, H. 11, 1905.

756 DEGENERATION AND REGENERATION OF THE NERVE CENTRES

Our first treatise [1] on this matter disclosed the following :

1. Discovery of the *retraction ball* of the central stump of traumatized axons and the disappearance of the segments of these next to the wound.

2. Hypertrophy and ravelling of the axon above the retraction ball.

3. Compensatory hypertrophy of the initial collaterals of the axon and its branches.

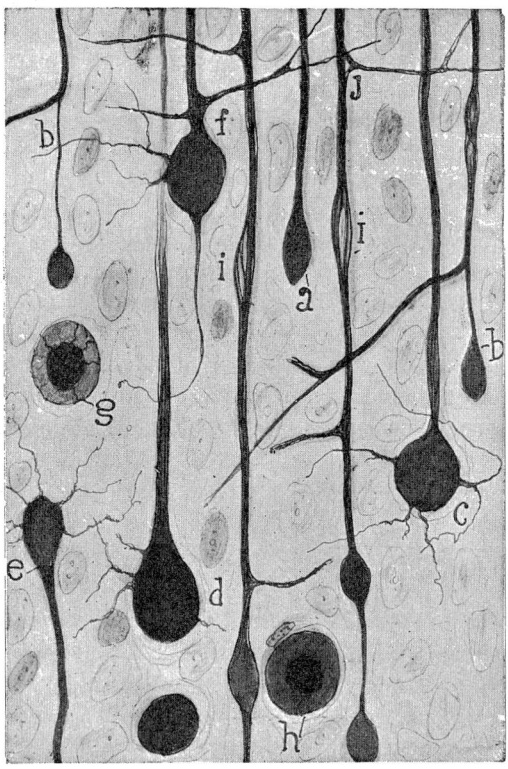

FIG. 316.—Details of the degenerated region of the central stump of the axons of pyramidal cells ; young dog, killed eight days after the operation. *a, b,* retraction buds ; *d, e, f,* retraction balls provided with sprouts ; *b,* axons whose collateral appears hypertrophied a short distance from the retraction ball ; *i,* ravelling out of certain hypertrophied axons ; *g, h,* free spheres (nervous autotomy). Figure taken from our communication of 1907.

4. Successive atrophy of the axonic segment below the last collateral.

5. Eventual appearance of new branches in the retraction balls or varicosities along the fibres.

6. Indication that axonic autotomy (formation of independent spheres) is a sign of traumatic degeneration of the axons ; phenomena

[1] Cajal : " Note sur la dégénérescence traumatique des fibres nerveuses du cervelet et du cerveau," *Trab. del Lab. de Invest. biol.,* t. 5, 1907.

of cortical hyalinization and of agonal neurofibrillar reaction in the free spheres.

Figs. 316 and 317 illustrate the essential facts that we pointed out in that treatise.

In another communication which appeared in 1910 [1] we described the regenerative structures called *cephalopodic* ; we pointed out the reparative incapacity of mutilated dendrites, and we noted the stainability and relatively good preservation of the neurones and free dendritic trunks in isolated pieces of the brain, days after the operation.

The work done in 1911 [2] brought to light, among other data : the incapacity of the axon for any formative reaction when the mutilation occurs above the collaterals ; the preservation of the neurone and production of arciform axons when the interruption occurs beyond the initial collaterals ; and the reactive and metamorphic power of the neurofibrils of the retraction ball of the peripheral stump when the section is effected near the neurones of Betz (*neurofibrillar phenomenon* of Alzheimer, etc).

Later contributions published in the same year completed our investigation of this matter. We may mention : the observation of *preserved fibres and cells*, dead

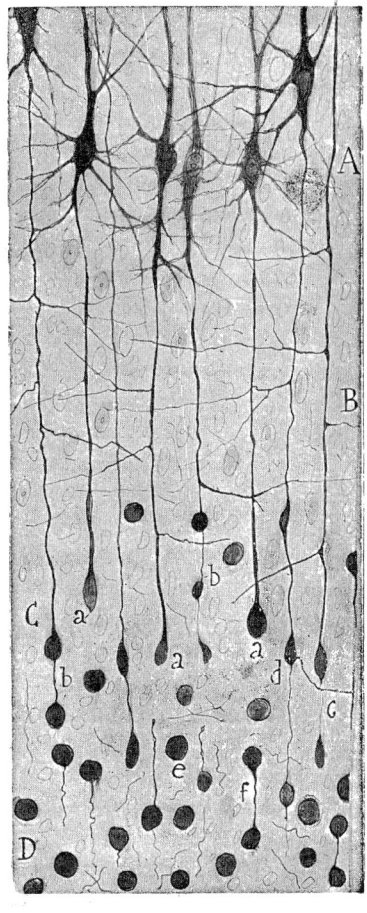

FIG. 317.—Section of the cerebral cortex of a dog, fifteen days old, killed nine days after the operation. *A*, layer of the Betz cells; *B*, healthy portion of the axons; *C*, segment in which traumatic degeneration has occurred; *D*, autotomized balls; *a*, retraction buds. Figure taken from our paper of 1907.

elements, with all the appearance of the most exquisite normality; [3]

[1] Cajal : " Algunos hechos de la regeneración parcial de la substancia gris de los centros nerviosos," *Trab. del Lab. de Invest. biol.*, t. 8, 1910.

[2] *Idem* : " Los fenómenos precoces de la degeneración traumática de los cilindros ejes del cerebro," *Trab. del Lab. de Invest. biol.*, t. 9, fasc. 1, 1911.

[3] *Idem* : " Fibras conservadas y fibras degeneradas," *Trab. del Lab. de Invest. biol.*, t. 9, 1911.

the interesting metamorphic figures of the somatic reticulum,[1] due to cerebral contusions (*hirudiform, fusiform* degeneration, etc., of the neurofibrils); and, finally, certain curious phenomena of reaction that occur in recently cut axons (one to six hours after the operation). These phenomena serve to explain the generative mechanism of balls and varicosities (*glomeruli*, whether terminal or along the fibres, formation of axial neurofibrils in necrosed segments, etc.).

After the appearance of our first note on degeneration and regeneration of the traumatized cerebral cortex of young animals, G. Sala [2] published an interesting work on the same theme, using young cats and the method of reduced silver nitrate.

Sala observed the cerebral wounds of cats killed two and fourteen days after the traumatism, and he confirmed the existence, in the central stump of the axon, of balls, clubs, and divisions, and he noted for the first time the annular ending. He recorded two interesting facts with regard to regeneration itself which it is difficult to reconcile with our descriptions, and concerning the interpretation of which we shall say a few words.

He found first, on the edges of the wound, fourteen days after the lesion, extensive plexuses composed of fine fibres, apparently newly formed, as is to be presumed from the presence of terminal buds and divisions. Some of these bundles invade the scar and run along the blood-vessels.

Without denying absolutely that in such plexuses there may exist a few newly-formed fibres, the comparison of our preparations with Sala's descriptions allows us to suppose that these axons are nothing else than fine fibres previously existing on the edges of the wound after destruction of the large tubes. Guido Sala perhaps made the mistake, as we did at first, of taking *preserved* and dead fibres for living fibres. Those shown by him in Fig. 5, among which there appear no terminal clubs or varicosities, seem to us to belong to this category of dead fibres.

The second fact recorded by Sala concerns the presence in the central axonic stump of pyramidal cells, forty-eight hours after the lesion, of a club-like thickening, intensely stained by silver, and below which there appears a pale, almost colourless segment, directed towards the wound. Sala wonders whether this pale appendix subsequently degenerates, the dark mass preceding it being then converted into a

---

[1] *Idem*: "Alteraciones de la substancia gris provocadas por conmoción y aplastamiento," *Trab. del Lab. de Invest. biol.*, t. 9, fasc. 4, 1911.

[2] G. Sala: "Sui fatti che si svolgono in sequito alle ferite asettiche del cervello," *Nota preventiva*, Pavia, 1908.

true bud of growth. In a later work,[1] published in German, he alludes to the same fact, adding that the club, situated often below a collateral, cannot, in his opinion, be identified with our *retraction ball*, and he conjectures that regenerated appendices perhaps emerge from such a dark tumefaction.

As a matter of fact, the observations of Sala do not demonstrate the regenerability of cerebral axons, and in that sense one may welcome the author's reserves. It seems to us that the clubs described and drawn by him are retraction buds in course of formation, for it is well known that the bud is preceded by a thickening having the shape of the tip of a sound. The pale portion is a piece of necrotic axon in process of elimination, and, finally, the branch which in some of his drawings seems to arise from this club is nothing else than the last pre-existent collateral, more or less hypertrophied.

Bianchi[2] used neurofibrillar methods in traumatizing the brain of rabbits by means of a piston-like mechanism, and he too provoked the formation of clubs and rings on the edges of the necrotic focus; he observed in addition various degenerative processes in the neurones—swelling of the soma, rarefaction of the reticulum, hirudiform state, hyalinosis, etc. He used the methods of Donaggio and of reduced silver nitrate. As regards the regenerative process, he claims to have found around the necrotic region numerous newly-formed fibres, similar to those pointed out by G. Sala. But, months after the lesion, the sprouts undergo involution, disappearing from the scar.

The same criticisms that were directed against the observations of Sala may be applied to those of Bianchi. The supposed nerve sprouts probably are fine pre-existent axons which sometimes persist for many days on the edges of the wound, unlike the thick axons which are rapidly destroyed over long distances and terminate very far from the wound in robust retraction balls. Some of these so-called newly-formed fibres are perhaps really *preserved* fibres.

As to the oft-debated question of the multiplication of neurones, there reigns at present a silence which is equivalent to a denial. For our part we may state that in the course of our prolonged investigations of the effects of traumatisms in mammals we have never seen a case of *indubitable neuronal division*. It is true that in the rabbit and the guinea-pig Borst, Saltykow, and, much earlier, Sanarelli, Mordino, and

[1] G. Sala: "Ueber die Regenerationserscheinungen im zentralen Nervensystem." *Anat. Anz.*, Bd. 34, Nos. 9-11, 1909.

[2] V. Bianchi: "Alterazioni istologische della corteccia cerebrale in sequito a focolai distruttivi ed a lesioni sperimentali," *Anali di Neurologia*, fasc. 11, 1912.

Coën, affirmed the existence of mitotic figures, apparently intraneuronal. Unfortunately, however, none of the methods used by these investigators, such as that of Nissl, are capable of distinguishing absolutely a multiplying neuroglia cell from a small mitotic neurone. It is all the more easy to attribute to the neurones divisory phenomena that are perhaps taking place in the glia, as during the mitotic process the neuroglia cells of the grey matter attain a considerable size and may even show peripherally granules that are more or less basophilic and remind one very much of the Nissl bodies. Everything leads one to think, therefore, that in mammals nervous restoration is a purely expansional act, in which the cellular body never participates. We do not, however, deny the facts, apparently well established, of neuronal division in the lower vertebrates, especially amphibians and reptiles, recorded by Müller, Fraise, Caporaso, Barfurth, Masius, Van Lair, and others ; nor the indubitable existence, in certain pathological cases in the human cerebral cortex, of binucleate pyramidal cells. Of this pathological binucleation, frequently mentioned, Bielschowsky and Gallus [1] have furnished descriptions and figures that are highly convincing.

[1] *Loc. cit.,* p. 754.

INDEX OF SUBJECTS

'Abbaumzellen,' 720, 723
aberrant nerves, 443-6, 447
'Abräumzellen,' 497
acetic acid, glacial, 37
acetone, 37
adendritic cells, 713, 722-3
adipose tissue, 190-1
alcohol, 28-32, 34-7, 39
alveolar tissue, 182
amacrine cells, 594
amaurotic idiocy, 197, 621
amilaceous bodies, 507
ammonia, 33, 38
Ammon's horn, 718, 735, 754
amoeboidism, 170, 171, 176, 179, 180, 181, 329, 364, 722-3
amphicytes, 459
amphibian larvae, 352
amphibians, 580-2
amputated limbs, 327-8
amyelinated fibres, staining of, 35
anaphases, 82, 83
anaxonic Purkinje cells, 618-26
aneuritic Purkinje cells, 618-26
angular cell, 416
anhydrous sodium sulphite, 56
aniline stains, 29, 31, 37, 356, 372
animals used for experiments, 39-40
anlagen, 203
annular apparatus, *see* Schwann cell (cytoplasm)
— system in Wallerian degeneration in peripheral stump of cut nerve, alteration of, 77-9
ansiform cells, 523
apolar cells, 722-3
apotrophic cells, 222, 252. 254, 262, 371, 390
— corpuscles, 21
arciform fibres, 606-7
— pyramidal cells, 665-72
— transformation of Purkinje axons in man, 609-16
argentophobic cells, 467
arrested fibres, 208-17, 310
atrophic cells of sympathetic ganglia, 467-8, 475
Auswahl, 376
autobundles, 439
auto-differentiation, 367
autogenous regeneration, 9, 12, 14, 194-6
autoneurotomy, 256
autotomy, 255, 370, 600, 608
autotransplantations, 432, 445, 477
avalanche phenomena, 154, 162, 292
axon, the (or neurite), 16, 41, 60-2
— alterations in compressed cerebral nerve, 690-1
— amoeboidism, 142-4, 329, 364
— and colloidal silver, 17, 27, 29
— and indifferent neurotropism, 375
— and nerve grafts, 334, 338, 349, 353, 374, 439-42, 740, 742, 744
— and scar, 358

axon and Schwann cells, 366, 392
— and sensory cell, 400
— arrested, 208-17
— assimilation, 302
— cortical mantle, 62
— degeneration of, in cut nerve : peripheral stump, 66-9, 72-7, 80-1, 100-24 ; central stump, 133-40
— — in ligated nerve, 292-3, 302, 304
— — in traumatised cerebral cortex : peripheral stump, 644-55 ; central stump, 656-76
— deutoplasm or neuroplasm, 54, 61, 103, 174
— development in normal neurogenesis, 367
— elective capacity (Auswahl), 376
— growth, 185-7, 302, 363, 365, 370, 373, 386 ; *see also* regeneration, *below*
— in arciform pyramidal cells in cerebral cortex, 665-72
— in degeneration, after cerebellar traumatisms, 597 *sqq.* ; in optic nerve, 584-8 ; of sensory nerve ganglia, 415-16
— in extirpation of nerves, 321-2
— in innervation of peripheral stump of cut nerve, 223-4, 230-44, 246-8, 251, 265-72
— in spinal cord : in nerve tubes of white matter, 486-95, 499, 500, 502-5 ; in white matter, 506-12, 514-16 ; in grey matter, 518, 523, 528, 530
— in spinal roots : anterior, 531-4, 538 ; posterior, 544-5, 547-50, 552-3, 556-7
— in traumatised sensory ganglia, central stump of, 418
— innervation by, retrograde, 305-13
— Martinotti, 707
— Nageotte's double axonic bracelet, 62-3
— necrosis of, in instantaneously crushed nerve, 282-4, 288
— neurocladic stimuli, action of, 358
— neurofibrillar apparatus, 16, 27-34, 101-4, 113-15, 118, 121, 134, 138-9, 147-8, 162, 171, 174
— newly formed, atrophy through disuse, 367-8
— nutrition, 100
— of Golgi cells, 629-30
— of sympathetic neurones, 467
— preserved, in cerebral cortex, 632-8, 642-3 ; in spinal contusion, etc., 558-60, 562 ; *see also* preserved fibres
— Purkinje, *see* Purkinje
— ravelling, 162-3, 190

axon, regeneration, in cut nerve—central stump: preliminary phenomena, 141-4 ; direct and indirect sprouting, 144-50 ; collateral branches, 150-66, 199 ; cones of growth, 176-82
— — in instantaneously crushed nerve, 284
— — in ligated nerve, 291, 300, 304
— — in retina, 593, 595
— — in spinal contusion, etc., 572
— — of cerebral cortex, 694-703, 745 *sqq.*, 750-4
— — of cerebrum, 734-5
— — of spinal cord, 573-6
— — of traumatised sensory nerve ganglia, 408, 418-19
— staining of, 258-9
— *See also* ganglia ; nerve sprouts

balsam, 29, 33, 36, 38, 39
bergamot, oil of, 29
Betz cells. 650, 710
— neurones of, 757
binucleation, 760
blood, influence of, on nerve sprouts, 188, 189, 355, 356
Bombinator, grafting, 352
bracelets, axonic, of Nageotte, 62-3, 78
brain, human, 217
Brownian movement, 459
bud, *see* nerve sprouts (cones of growth)
Büngner, bands of, 84-7, 89, 192-4, 238, 240, 241, 248, 288, 318, 320, 331-3, 335, 340, 346-9, 353, 374, 388-9, 391, 429, 514, 537, 589, 590, 738, 740, 742-3
Bufo vulgaris, grafting, 352

calcified pyramidal cells, 712-13
capillaries, 66, 185
capillary sinuses, ganglionic, 446
carbol-xylene, 37
catenary theory, *see* discontinuity
cauda equina, 442
celloidin, 29, 31, 34, 36, 38, 39
cells of Schwann, *see* Schwann cell
cellular bands, 89
— migrations, primitive, 385
cementing disc, 42, 69, 72, 77, 78, 486
central stump : in cerebellar traumatisms, *see* cerebellar traumatisms
— in extirpation experiments, 320-1
— in multiple nerve hemisection, 317-18
— in spinal cord, traumatic degeneration in nerve tubes of white matter, 487-99
— in transplantation experiments, 316
— in traumatised sensory ganglia, 418

INDEX OF SUBJECTS

central stump: of cut nerve: degeneration, 13, 127-40; modifications after nerve section, 248-9; regeneration, 20, 21, 32, 136, 139, 167-222
— of cut optic nerve, 586-91, 596
— of instantaneously crushed nerve, 285-7
— of ligated nerve, 291-2, 302-4
—of nerve in amputated limbs, 327-8
cephalopodic structures, 698-703, 734, 757
cerebellar atrophy, 622
cerebellar traumatisms: degenerative phenomena, 597-630
— absence of regenerative phenomena, 614-16
— axons of grey and white matter, 599-616; central stump, 599-608; peripheral stump, 609-16
— neuronal metamorphoses, 617-26
— other alterations, 626-30
— technical notes, 597-9
cerebellum, pathology of, neurofibrillar methods in, 610
cerebral cortex: aborted regeneration (axonic neoformations), 693-703
— atrophic phenomena (late) consequent on radial wounds, 704-5; on transversal and oblique wounds, 705-13
— inflammation after traumatisms, 714-33
— traumatic degenerative processes: preservatory necrosis, 632-44; axonic peripheral stump, 644-55, 676; axonic central stump, 656-76; additional note, 677; nerve cells, 678-92
cerebro-spinal ganglia, 397-8; see also ganglia
cerebrum, cicatrization of cerebral wounds, 728-33
— nerve graft on, 332-3
— regenerative processes, 734-60
Chelonia, 428
chemotactism, see neurotropism
chloral hydrate, 30-2, 339, 356
chloroform, 338-9
chromatolysis, 521-3, 527, 682, 747
cicatricial plexus, 168
cicatrization, of cerebral wounds, 727-33
— of nerve grafts, 334
clasmatocytes, 65
cloves, oil of, 29, 36
clubs, terminal, see retraction bud
clubs of growth, 182, 327-8, 333, 349, 370, 371, 509; axonic, 141-2, 145, 148, 171
cocaine, 356
colloidal silver, 28, 29 et passim
collagen bundles, 38, 92
— fibres, 38
comet-shaped cell, of sympathetic ganglia, 466, 471, 474, 475
compensation and regeneration, 15
cones of growth, 172-82, 234, 238-41, 309, 363-6, 374, 386, 388, 392, 510-12, 608, 615, 748, 751
connective tissue, 37-9, 66, 182-92, 358, 372, 553-6, 595
— tissue cells, 182-8, 208, 259, 311, 313, 722; primitive, 387
contact sensibility of retrograde fibres, 207
continuity, theory of (monogenist hypothesis), in regeneration of nerves, 3-7, 389
contracted cells, in severe cerebral commotions, etc., 685
corpuscles, 400; of Erzholz, see Schwann cell (cytoplasm)

corrosion, point of, 634, 640, 672
cortical inflammation, see cerebral cortex
cotton threads and nerve sprouts, 182, 208, 311, 356
cotton-like cells, in spinal contusion, etc., 568-70
cranial ganglia, 402; see also ganglia
— nerves, sensory, ganglia of, 406
crown-shaped cell, of sympathetic ganglia, 465-6, 471, 474-6
crushed nerves, 281-90
cut nerves, passim
— combined with ligatures, nerve sprouts in, 305-13
cyanophil cells, in cortical inflammation, 722, 732
— in embryonic connective tissue, 184
— staining, 37
cytoplasm, of Schwann cell, see Schwann cell
— of sensory ganglia, 399, 401

dead nerves, grafting of, 338-46
deformed cell, in degeneration of sensory nerve ganglia, 416, 420
degeneration: of instantaneously crushed nerves, 281-90; of ligated nerves, 290-304
— see also central stump; distal stump; nerve centres; optic nerve and retina; peripheral stump; sensory ganglia; spinal cord; Wallerian
— and regeneration of nerves: traumatic or inflammatory, historical notes, 1-26; staining methods, 27-39; operatory technique, 39-40
— — of nerve tubes of white matter of spinal cord, 487-507
— — see also regeneration
dendrites: compressed cerebral, alterations in, 691-2
— degenerative phenomena after cerebellar traumatisms, 617-26
— neoformation in cerebrum, 735-7
— — in spinal contusion, etc., 571-2
— of sympathetic neurones, 463-9, 471-2, 474-5
— preserved, in pyramidal cells of cerebral cortex, 638-41, 643
desiccation and nerve grafting, 339
dentoplasm, see axon
digestive chambers, 72, 75, 158, 218, 221, 289, 492, 647-9
discontinuity, theory of (polygenist hypothesis or catenary theory), in regeneration of the nerves, 3, 7-14, 84, 387; refutation of, 14-26
dissociation (ravelling), 162-3, 290, 292
distal stump of cut nerve, functional degeneration of, 13
Dogiel, spools (nests) of, 404, 406, 409, 411
Dominici's fluid, 36, 44, 45
dura, 530

Ehrlich (mast cells), 185, 732
ellipsoids, medullary, see medullary
embryo, 176-82, 216-17
embryonic cells, see fibroblasts
embryonic connective tissue and nerve sprouts, 182-8
endocapsular elements of sensory ganglia, 399-401
endocellular apparatus of Golgi, see Schwann cell (cytoplasm)
endoneurium, 63, 64-5, 97, 98, 132, 160, 282-3, 292, 298, 306, 342, 353, 390

end-organs, arrival of nerve fibres at, 265-80
enzymes, 372-4, 392
eosin, 36, 39
ependyma, 527
epineuron, 393
Erzholz, corpuscles of, see Schwann cell (cytoplasm)
— spherules of, 68, 72
ether-glycerin, 37
extirpation of nerves, experiments in, 320-3
extratubal fibres, 234-5, 245, 249
exudates and nerve sprouts, 188-9

fenestrated cells, in sensory ganglia, 404-5, 411
fibres, see nerve fibres
Fibrillenscheide, 63
fibrillogenous zone of the neuroblast, 376
fibrin, threads of, and nerve sprouts, 182, 208
fibroblasts, 132, 183-5
filaments, longitudinal, in cytoplasm of Schwann's cell, 49, 50-1
fissural rings in cytoplasm of Schwann's cell, 49
formalin, 28, 32-8, 45, 56, 64, 339
formol-uranium, 184
formula G, 484
frayed cell, in sensory ganglia, 405, 409, 411, 415-16, 420
frozen sections, 33, 35
fuchsin, 34, 37
functional degeneration, 7
funicular cells of grey matter of spinal cord, 518
fusiform state of neurofibrils in cerebral cortex, 676, 679, 687-89, 758

galvanotropism, 391, 394-5
ganglia: cerebro-spinal, 397-8
— cranial, 402
— crushed, 407
— excited, 407
— of amputated individuals, 407
— sensory: degeneration, 397 sqq.; cells and tubes of sensory nerve, 414-16; types of cells, 415-16, 420; after extirpation of sensory roots, 419-20
— — regeneration, 397 sqq.; cells and tubes of sensory nerve, 416-19; types of cells, 420-1; after extirpation of sensory roots, 420-5; after crushing, 423-4
— — satellite cells or endocapsular elements, 399-401, 459-61
— — structure and nerve cells, 397-413, 416, 421-5
— — transplanted, types of cells, 427-9; necrobiosis, 432-6; homochronotransplantations, 432, 442-8; cultivation in vitro, 448-62; appendices, 436-53, 455-9; disequilibrium of neuroglial symbiosis, 459-62
— spinal, 397-8, 402, 414
— sympathetic: degeneration and regeneration, 397 sqq.
— — normal structure, 462-76; grafting, 477-80; types of cells, 479-80
— transplanted, 407, 409; see also above, sensory
— wounded, 407
ganglioneuroma cerebral, 754
germinative zone, axonic, 152
Gitterzellen, see granular cells
glia cells, see neuroglia
glioma, 251
glomerular Purkinje cells, 624, 626

INDEX OF SUBJECTS

glomerulus, sympathetic, 466, 471, 476
glycerine, 35
gold solution, 33
Golgi, apparatus of, 47-50, 184, 254, 278, 519, 522, 682-3, 705-6
— cells, 629-30
Golgi-Rezzonico, apparatus of, 50-1, 57-8, 78
grafting (transplantation) of nerves, 192, 316-20, 329-61, 755
— free grafts on to skin and muscles, 351-2
— intracerebral, 738-44
— neurotropic action on nerve sprouts, 353
— of dead nerves, 338-46
— of degenerated nerve exposed to air, 342-6
— of degenerated nerve on healthy nerve, 337-8
— of entire limbs on amphibian larvae, 352
— of nerve immersed in chloroform, 338-9
— of nerve in healthy state, 346-51
— of semi-necrosed crushed nerve, 339-42
— on optic nerve, 590-1
— recent experiments and results, 359-61
— sympathetic ganglia, 477-80; types of cells, 479-80
— *see also* ganglia, sensory (transplanted)
grafts, *see* grafting
granular cells (Abbaumzellen), 497, 720, 722
— cells (Gitterzellen), 496-7, 502, 715-17, 721, 722, 727-9, 732
— degeneration, 585
— neurones, in simple cerebral wounds, 678-9
— reticulum, *see* reticulum
grey matter, *see* cerebellar traumatisms ; spinal cord and nerve roots
gum dammar, 29, 33, 34, 37

haematin, 36
haematoxylin, 34-6, 67, 72, 259
haptotropism, 207, 221
hematomyelia, 567-8
hemisection of nerve : simple, 336-7 ; multiple, 316-18
Henle membrane, 200, 202-4, 221, 266, 271-2, 274
heterochronotransplantation, 432
heteromorphic nervous reunion, 319-20
heterotransplantation of nerves, 330, 334, 352-3, 429-30, 432
hirudiform cells, 415, 416, 520-1, 565-6, 622-4, 679
hirudiform neurofibrillar state, 596, 688-90, 758
Hirudo, neurones of, 677
histodynamic impulse, 366
histomeres, 285, 368
homochronotransplantation, 432, 442-8, 479
homoiotransplantation, 330, 334, 429, 430, 432
homotropism, 183, 221, 369
hyaline change, 668, 672, 674
hyalinosis, 608
hyaloplasm, 102, 104
hydrophobia, 520, 627
hydroquinone, 45, 56
hymenoclastocytes, 385
hypertrophic : neurofibrillar state, 663-4, 676, 685-7
— reticulum, cells with, 566
— segment, 660, 662-3, 665, 672, 676

incisures of Schmidt-Lantermann, *see* Schmidt-Lantermann
inclusions of Schwann's cell, *see* Schwann cell
indigo carmine, 36
infundibula, 67-9, 76-9
Innenscheide, 59, 62, 63, 103, 122
interannular segment of Schwann cell, 44, 78
interrupted nerves, 66 *sqq.*
interstitial cells, 98-9, 721
intratubal fibres, in innervation of peripheral stump of cut nerve, 233-4, 246, 248-9
iodine, 36
iron, 393
iron haematoxylin, 72

Key and Retzius : mantle of, 200 ; sheath of, 132, 241
Kühne : sheaths of, 371 ; spindles of, 74, 273-5, 278, 371

laminar sheath (or perineurium), 64-5
Lantermann, *see* Schmidt-Lantermann
Leitzellen, 259, 263, 376
lemmoblasts, 259, 371, 554
leucocytes, 83, 93-7, 132, 185, 433-5, 496-7, 715, 717, 722
ligated nerves, 212, 290-304 ; nerve sprouts in, 305-13
lipoidal substances of myelin, 54
lobulations, cellular, 449-50
Locke's solution, 123
longitudinal filaments in cytoplasm of Schwann's cell, 49, 50-1
lymphocytes, 97, 185

μ grains of Reich in inclusions of Schwann cell, 51-2
macrophages, 433
macroscopic tertiary fascicle, 306
manganese nitrate, 56
Mann's fluid, 36, 39, 45
Marchi's fluid, 36, 45
Martinotti axons, 707 ; cells, 670, 673, 675 ; fibres, 674-5
mast cells, 185, 733
Mauthner's sheath, 60
medullary sheath, metamorphosis of, in Wallerian degeneration in peripheral stump of cut nerve, 67 *sqq.*
medullary fragmentation, 69-77
medullated fibres of grey matter of cerebral cortex, 673-6
medullated nerve fibre, *see* nerve fibre
membrane of Schwann, *see* Schwann sheath
meninges, 527
metaphase, 82, 83
methylene blue, 24, 29, 36, 39, 80
methylene green, 37
microtome, freezing, 33
mitochondria, 38, 54, 55
mitosis, 99, 721
moniliform state, of axon, 101-2 ; of dendrites, 691
monogenism, *see* continuity
mononucleated or transitional leucocytes, 717, 722
Monstrenzellen, 730
morphine, 356
motor cells, 518
— fibres, 74, 265-72, 322
— nerves, atrophy of, 320
— plates, 371 ; degeneration, 85, 107-8, 267-8 ; regeneration, 268-72
— roots, 322, 538-40, 578, 747
— stump, central, 314

Müller's fluid, 35, 36, 37, 45
muff, germinative, 152-3, 155, 286, 288, 291, 364
muscles, free nerve grafts on to, 351-2
muscular nerve, 265-72
— tissue, 189-90
myelin : action of Schwann cells on, 392
— cells, 53
— composition of, 52-5
— degeneration in central stump of cut nerve, 127-30, 134
— disintegration in peripheral stump of cut nerve near wound (not Wallerian degeneration), 108
— formation of, in new fibres of nerve sprouts of central stump of cut nerve, 200-4
— in degeneration of nerve tubes of white matter of spinal cord, 491-2, 495-6, 498-9, 500
— in degeneration of optic nerve, 586
— in instantaneously crushed nerve, 282, 286
— in ligated nerve, 292-3, 299
— in nerve grafts, 331
— in nervous degeneration *in vitro*, 122-3
— in Wallerian degeneration in peripheral stump of cut nerve, 66-8, 73, 121 ; fragmentation of, 69-79 ; resorption of, 73-5
— nets, 52-4, 59
— sheath, 42, 52-5, 246-9, 327
— staining of, 34-5, 37
myelitis, in spinal cord, 534, 538, 541
myeloclasts, 497, 508
myelophages, 497, 508

necrobiosis, 432-6
necrosed Purkinje cells, 626
necrosis, 487-8, 499-500
necrotic portion of instantaneously crushed nerve, 282-90 ; of ligated nerve, 292-4
nerve bundles, 198-200
nerve cells, 18
nerve centres, degeneration and regeneration of, 397 *sqq.*
nerve fibres (neurofibrils) :
— after cerebellar traumatisms, 627-9
— atrophy through disuse, 367-8
— difficulties of, in crossing membranes, 373-4
— experiments to impede or prevent direct progress of, 323-7
— exploratory fibres (precursors), 380-2
— in cut nerve, 111-21, 123, 128-30, 133-6
— in degeneration : of spinal cord (nerve tubes of white matter), 495-6
— — of cut nerve, 74-7, 99, 128-30, 133-4, 136
— — of optic nerve, 585
— in regeneration : growth of, 363-6, 377 ; mechanical obstacles to, 368-9
— — of cut nerve, 265-80
— — of ligated nerve, 292, 294-304
— — of ligated and cut nerve, 302
— — of retina, 592-4
— — of spinal cord : white matter, 511-12 ; grey matter, 522
— — of spinal roots : anterior, 532-8 ; posterior, 541-57
— in spinal cord, white matter of 485-6, 492

INDEX OF SUBJECTS

nerve fibre: medullated, 41-65, 111-17, 121, 123, 128-30, 133-4, 136
— non-medullated 49, 99, 117-21, 123, 135
— old, absence of iron in, 393
— staining of, 32-4
— see also axon, motor fibres, nerve sprouts, sensory fibres, preserved fibres
nerve grafting, see grafting
nerve roots, 332-3
nerve sprouts:
— aberrant, in homochronotransplantations, 443-6, 447
— in regeneration: attraction of bands of Büngner, 374
— — classification of substances acting on, 372-5
— — dynamic character of trophic influence on, 366-7
— — generic and specific orienting chemical stimuli, 371-2
— — growth, 363 sqq.
— — in experiments in extirpation of nerves, 322
— — neurotropic action on, 329-61
— — obstacles, 191-2, 208, 311, 368-9
— — of anterior spinal roots, 538-40
— — of cut nerve: central stump, 167-222; peripheral stump, 223-64
— — of cut and ligated nerve, growth, etc., 305 sqq.
— — of instantaneously crushed nerve (central stump), 286-7
— — of intracerebral grafts, 740-4
— — of retina, 592-4
— — polarization of, 314-20, 323
— in transplanted sensory ganglia, 439-42
nerve transplantation, see grafting
nerve tubes of white matter of spinal cord, 485-6; degeneration of, 487-509
nervous reunion: heteromorphic, 319-20
— in degeneration caused by pressure, etc., 241-4, 250-1
— of crushed nerves, 285-90
— of ligated nerves, 293-4, 306-13
— of peripheral stump. 323-7, 371
— retrograde, 306-13, 318-19
nervous spools, 217-22
neurilemma, 65, 98, 282, 313
neurite, see axon
neuritic nerve, 252
neurobiones, 61, 101, 108, 121, 284, 368, 600, 607, 615, 749
neurobionic necrobiosis, after cerebellar traumatisms, 623
neurobiotaxis, 390-1, 394
neuroblastic differentiation, 385
neuroblasts, 523, 682
neurocladism, 336, 338, 369, 370, 412, 556, 588
neurofibrillar apparatus of axon, see axon
— autotomy, 370
— nets, 491, 492, 618-20 622-3, 625
neurofibrils, see nerve fibres
neurogenesis (ontogeny), 252-3 375-92. 394
neuroglia cells, 254 262, 497, 502
— in cortical inflammation, 724-33
— in optic nerve, 583
— Nageotte s neurogenetic formula, 251-2
— of white matter of spinal cord, 485, 486, 496, 508
— staining of, 38-9
neuroglial nerve, 252
— sheaths, 257
neuroglial nerve tract, 260

neurokeratin (myelin) nets, 47, 52, 73, 491
neuroma, 251
neurone, 26, 399, 401, 437, 448
neurones: after cerebellar traumatisms, 597 sqq., 617-26
— central, trophic influence on nerve sprouts, 302
— cerebral, 596, 750-4
— in spinal contusion, etc., 562 sqq.
— iron in, 393
— of grey matter of spinal cord, 517-30
— of spinal ganglia, 641
— preserved, in cerebral cortex, 641-4
neuro-neuroglial symbiosis, 459-62, 475-6
neuronophagy, 414, 426, 428, 430, 432-6, 480, 713
neuroparaphytes, 429
neurophytes, 444
neuroplasm, see axon (deutoplasm)
neurospongium, 429, 430
neurotropic action on nerve sprouts, 329-61
— currents, action on cone of growth, 374-5
— stimulus, provokes protoplasmic assimilation, 372
neurotropism, 195-7, 221-2, 318-19, 329, 384, 418, 582, 750
— Harrison on, 380
— negative, 374-5
— reciprocal, 257, 382
— recent work on, 393
— theory of, main difficulties, 373-4
— — summary, 388-92
Nissl bodies, 393, 395, 760
— grumes, 519-20, 567, 685; in neurones of grey matter of spinal cord, 519, 520
nitric acid, 36
nodes of Ranvier, 41, 67-9, 72, 77-9, 104, 246, 248-9, 485, 496, 647;
metamorphoses of, 152-3
nodose fibres, 506
nodules, residual, 414-15, 425, 428-9, 435, 441, 442, 460, 480
non-medullated fibres of grey matter of cerebral cortex, 673-6
— nerve fibres, see nerve fibres
normal organ, 407
— segment, in fibres of central stump of cut axon in cerebral cortex, 663-4
nuclei, staining of 30-2
nucleus: necessary for nutrition of protoplasm, 100
— in Wallerian degeneration in peripheral stump, 68, 72

obstacles, artificial, to growth of nerve sprouts, 191-2, 208, 311, 368-9
odogenesis, 252, 332, 335, 358, 377-8, 579, 748
ontogeny (neurogenesis), 252-3, 263, 376, 385
optic nerve and retina: degeneration and regeneration, 583-96;
optic nerve, 584-91, 595-6; retina, 591-6
organic normal, 407
origanum, oil of, 29, 34
Orth's fluid, 36, 45
orthophytes, 409-10, 412
osmic acid, 16, 34, 67, 72
osmio-bichromate fluid, Marchi's, 36
osmotic pressure, and production of nerve sprouts, 370
oxydases, 253, 393
oxydasophore cells, 393

π grains of Reich (protagonoidal grains) in inclusions of Schwann cell, 51
paraffin, 29, 34; oil of, 37
paraphytes, 409-10, 412, 416
pericellular nests: of sensory ganglia, 421, 425
— of sympathetic ganglia, 468-70 471, 473, 476
peridendritic nests, of sympathetic ganglia, 468-70, 471, 476
perifibrillar substance, 102
perihyalplasmic limiting membrane in axonic fragmentation, 104
perinervous tissues, staining of, 259
perineuron, fibroblasts of, iron in, 393
perineurium, 65, 96, 97, 98, 283
perinodular bundles, 441
perinuclear mass, see Schwann cell (cytoplasm)
peripheral stump: and neurotropic action on nerve sprouts, 353
— causes of nervous reunion of, 371
— experiments to impede or prevent nervous reunion of, 323-7
— in experiments in extirpation of nerves, 320
— in multiple hemisection of nerve, 317-8
— in nerve grafts in a healthy state, 347-51
— in nerve tubes of white matter of spinal cord, 499-507
— innervation of, by central motor stump, 314
— — in cut and ligated nerve, 306-12
— of axon in traumatised sensory nerve ganglia, 418
— of cut nerve, degeneration in, 35, 100-26
— — innervation of, 223-64; arrival of nerve sprouts, 233-4; time required for innervation by sprouts, 224-6; speed of growth, 226-30, 236-44; ramification of fibres and growth of branches, 230-44; rapid nervous reunion, 236-40; modification in fibres, 244-8; recent investigations, 251-64
— — regeneration in, 17-20, 32 (see also innervation, above)
— — resorption of, 366-7
— of cut optic nerve, 586
— of instantaneously crushed nerve: degeneration, 282; regeneration, 287-90
— of ligated nerve, 293-4, 300-2
— rapid growth of axon through, 373
— see also cerebellar traumatisms, cerebral cortex
peritoneum, nerve graft in, 335
peritubular connective tunic, 63-4
peroxydase, 393
Perroncito, apparatus of, 21, 157-60, 163, 205, 218-9, 280, 289, 292
phagocytes, 83, 92-8, 132, 311, 433-4
phagocytosis, 73, 585-6
phlogosis, 548
phosphomolybdic acid, 36, 39, 45
pia mater, 527, 530, 550, 556, 722, 730, 731, 732, 740, 741
picric acid, 36
picric-carmine, 37
picric-indigo, 37
pip, 627
pisciform metamorphosis of neurone in degeneration of grey matter of spinal cord, 522
plaques, senile, 580, 700-1, 735-6, 753

INDEX OF SUBJECTS

plasma cells, *see* cyanophil cells
plasmatic exudates, influence on growth of nerve sprouts, 355-6
plasmatic spaces, in scar in central stump of cut nerve, 185
plasmodesmas, 259-60
plasticity, neuronal, 430
plexiform ganglion, 425
plexuses, pre-terminal, of the embryo, 382-3
polarization of nerve sprouts, 314-20, 323
polychrome blue, 37
polygenist hypothesis, *see* discontinuity
polynucleated leucocytes, in cortical inflammation, 715
potassium bichromate, 35
potassium hydroxide, 37, 45
precursors (exploratory fibres), 380-2
preservation, in cerebral cortex, 631-44; axons, 632-8, 642-3; dendrites, 638-41; neurones *in toto*, 641-4; *see also* preserved fibres
preserved cells, 672-3, 757
preserved fibres, 109-12, 124, 134-5, 293, 488, 514, 526, 558-60, 562, 599, 645, 657, 677, 693, 754, 755, 757-9
prophase, 82
protagonoidal grains (π grains of Reich), *see* Schwann cell (inclusions)
protomeres, 368
protoplasm, mechanics of, 456
— neuronal, 434-5
— nutrition of, 100
protoplasmic annulus, *see* Schwann cell
— marginal net, *see* Schwann cell
— neuroglia, 459
— neuroglia cell, 461
— unfolding, 411
pseudopods, amoeboid, 456, 457
Purkinje axons after cerebellar wounds, 601-3, 605-6, 608; arciform transformation of, in man, 610-16
— cells, after cerebellar wounds, 597-8, 600, 602-4, 606-10, 614, 616-30; baskets of, 626-7
— — in cerebral cortex, 665-72
pus, and nerve sprouts, 311, 354-5, 372
pycnotic neurones in simple cerebral wounds, 681
— pyramidal cells in severe cerebral commotions, etc., 685
pyramidal cells: arciform, 665-72, 712
— calcified, 712-3
— of cut axon in cerebral cortex: in central stump, 673-5; in peripheral stump, 676
pyridine, 484, 598
pyrogallic acid, 28, 31
pyrogallic-formalin mixture, 37
pyridine, 30-3, 56, 64, 258
pyronine, 37

rabies, 428
Ranvier, nodes of, *see* nodes
ravelling, *see* dissociation
regeneration: and compensation, 15
— autogenous, 9, 12, 14
— effect of temperature on, 374
— electrical theories of, 394
— in cerebral neurones, etc., 750-60
— in nerves of amputated limbs, 327-8
— of central nerve tracts, breakdown of, 744-50
— of cerebrum, 734-60

regeneration of cut nerve, 144-66, 276-80
— of instantaneously crushed nerve, 281-90
— of ligated nerve, 290-304
— theory of phenomena of, 362-96; history of explanatory theories, 375-92; additional note, 393-6
— traumatic, central stump, 20-1, 141-66; staining of, 32
— — methods of investigation, 16-25
— — monogenism, 3-7, 389
— — peripheral stump, 17-20; staining of, 32
— — polygenism, 3, 7-14, 84, 387; refutation of, 14-6
— under special conditions, 305-28
— *See also* central stump, peripheral stump
Remak, fibre of, 463
reticulum, 689, 690
retina, *see* optic nerve and retina
retracted cell, in degeneration of sensory nerve ganglia, 416
retraction balls, 677, 756, 757, 759
— bud, 489-94, 499-500, 502, 505, 734
retraction club, 599, 600, 603-4, 608, 610, 614-15, 650-5, 657, 660, 664-5, 673-4, 676
retrograde fibres, 182-92, 204-8
— nervous reunion, 306-13
retrogression of nerve sprouts, 185-7
Retzius, *see* Key
— sheath of, 282
reunion of cut nerves, imperfections of, 276-80
Rezzonico, *see* Golgi-Rezzonico
Ringer's solution, 123
rings in cytoplasm of Schwann cell, 49
rod-like cells (Stäbchenzellen) in cortical inflammation, 715, 717-22
rosaliform Purkinje cell, 618-22, 624
'rosettenformige', type of cell in sympathetic ganglia, 471

safranin, 34
satellite cells, 399-401, 740-1
scar: effect of, on growth of nerve sprouts, 357-8
— formation of, in regeneration of grey matter of spinal cord, 527-30
— region of, in central stump of cut nerve, 167-97
Scarlet R, formula for, 35
Schmidt-Lantermann, incisures of, 6, 45-6, 50, 55-60, 68-72, 76-9, 128-9, 485, 496
— account of, 55-62
Schwann cell: absent from nerve sprouts, in central stump of cut nerve, 168; from nerve tubes of white matter of spinal cord, 485, 496, 498-9
— account of, 41-52
— and nerve grafts, 334
— and neurotropic action on nerve sprouts, 332, 333, 336, 339, 341, 353
— and optic nerve, 583, 589
— and regeneration in retina, 595
— cytoplasm, 44-51, 68-9, 72, 80, 81, 83, 124-6; inclusions of, 51-2, 80
— daughter cells, 95, 97
— formation of, in new fibres of nerve sprouts of central stump of cut nerve, 200-4
— in central stump of nerves of amputated limbs, 327-8
— in degeneration of central stump of cut nerve, 130-3, 134

Schwann cell: in disintegration of cut axon in peripheral stump, 110, 111
— in homochronotransplantations, 444
— in innervation of peripheral stump of cut nerve, 238, 240, 244-9, 251, 254, 257, 262, 263-4
— in instantaneously crushed nerve, 282, 283
— in intracerebral grafts, 738, 740, 742
— in ligated nerve, 292-3
— in nervous degeneration *in vitro*, 123
— in regeneration of motor fibres, 267; of nerves, 6, 10, 12, 16; of posterior spinal roots, 554, 557
— in semi-necrosed crushed nerve, 339
— in transplanted sensory ganglia, 429
— in Wallerian degeneration, 66-7, 73-5, 79-92, 94-7
— interannular segment, 44
— neurotropic action in, 389-92
— neurotropic sources in, 371
— neurotropic weakness or incapacity of sick or dead cells, 374
— not necessary for genesis and growth of axons, 366
— of peripheral stump of cut nerve, 744
— protoplasmic annulus, 46
— protoplasmic marginal net, 46
— regenerative influence of, 744-5, 749-50
— staining methods, 36-7
— syncytium formed by, 36, 46, 83, 89, 90, 92, 130, 252-4, 263; iron in, 393
Schwann sheath or membrane: absent from nerve tubes of white matter of spinal cord, 485
— and nerve grafts, 334
— and neurotropic action on nerve sprouts, 340
— definition, 41
— degeneration of, in central stump of cut nerve, 128
— in axonic regeneration in central stump of cut nerve, 148, 150, 153, 155, 157-8, 160, 162
— in cut and ligated nerve, 306-8, 312-3
— in degeneration of central stump of cut nerve, 128, 136
— in innervation of crushed nerve, 225; of peripheral stump of cut nerve, 237-41, 245, 248, 262
— in intracerebral grafts, 740, 742
— in ligated nerve, 292, 294, 298, 299
— in nervous spools, 218-21
— in nerve grafts in a healthy state, 348-50
— in optic nerve, 583
— in regeneration of central stump of cut nerve, 199-20
— in regeneration of motor fibres, 265-72; of nerve damaged by pressure, etc., 241-2; of posterior spinal roots, 542, 544; of traumatised sensory nerve ganglia, 418, 424-5
— in transplanted sensory ganglia, 440, 441
— in Wallerian degeneration in peripheral stump of cut nerve, 66, 68, 74
— nature of neurotropic substance in, 392
— not interrupted at strangulations, 42

Schwann sheath or membrane: uninterrupted, in instantaneously crushed nerves, 281-2, 288-9
sciatic nerve, grafting on, 333-6
sclerosis, 730
semiligature of nerves, 305-9
senile plates, 580, 700-1, 735-6, 753
sensory : cells, see ganglia
— fibres, penetration into degenerated anterior or motor roots, 319-20
— ganglia, see ganglia
— peripheral stump, innervation by central motor stump, 314
— structures, in cut nerve, regeneration of, 272-6
silk, effect on growth of nerve sprouts, 356
silver nitrate, 17, 20, 27-29, 30, 33, 37, 38, 45, 434
skin, the, and nerve grafts, 335, 351-2
sodium chloride, 122 ; hydroxide, 33, 35, 38 ; hyposulphite, 33 ; sulphite, 33, 45
solitary rings in cytoplasm of Schwann cell, 49
soma, phenomena in homochronotransplantations, 442-8
spermatozoöids, crustacean, influence of osmotic pressure on form of, 458
spheroidal cell, in spinal contusion, etc., 566-8
spinal cord : phenomena of necrosis, etc., after contusion and laceration of, 558-82
— retrograde nervous reunion after section of, 318-9
spinal cord and nerve roots : degeneration and regeneration of : white matter, 484-516 ; grey matter, 517-30 ; spinal roots, 531-57
spinal ganglia, 397-8, 402, 414, 426 ; see also ganglia
spinal roots, extirpated, nervous reunion in, 318-19
spiroidal structures, 703

sponge, effect on growth of nerve sprouts, 356
spongioblasts, 582
spongioplasm of myelin, 53
spools, nervous, in central stump of cut nerve, 217-22
spools or nests of Dogiel, 406, 409, 411
Stäbchenzellen, 715, 717-22
staining, 16, 27-37, 258-9
staphilococcus, 354
stellate cell, 466-7, 471, 486
stereotropism, 155, 186, 207, 221, 252, 254-7, 262, 358, 369, 377, 380, 395, 418, 476
sterile tubes, 163-6, 230, 234, 248
stimulofugal growth, 394
stimulopetal growth, 394
sublimate, saturated corrosive, 36
Sudan III, 35, 72
symbiosis, neuro-neuroglial, 459-62, 475-6, 724, 728
sympathetic ganglia, see ganglia
sympathetic neurones, see ganglia
sympathicord neurones, 437
syncytium of nerve sprouts in scar of interrupted nerve, 250-5, 257, 260, 263 ; see also Schwann cell
syngenesis, 383
syphilis, 38, 622

tabes, 407, 410, 411, 433, 436, 441, 472
tactile adhesion, 186, 207, 221
tactile hairs, 276
tannin solution, 38
Tay-Sachs disease, 621
telophases, 82
temperature, effect of, on regeneration, 374
terminal club, 646-9, 653-5, 657, 659, 660, 665 ; see also retraction club
— masses of nerve sprouts, 174-82
— podia, 751
— rings, 657
testudinoid structures, 694-5, 701, 734
thionin, 29

topographic indifference of nerve sprouts, 308, 310
trabeculae, transverse, see Schwann cell (cytoplasm)
transplantation, see grafting
traumatocytes, 434
trichromic stain, Cajal's, 37
trophic centres, 4
— current, 77
— degeneration, see Wallerian degeneration
trophoparaphytes, 429, 436-9, 444

Urodeles, 582, 596

vacuolization in peripheral stump of axon after cerebellar traumatisms, 608
vacuolated cells, in neurones of grey matter of spinal cord, 523 ; in spinal contusion, etc., 564-5
— neurones in simple cerebral wounds, 680
— Purkinje cells, after cerebellar traumatisms, 624-5
van Gieson's stain, 37
varicose appearance of cut axon, 101-2
— segment, in fibres of central stump of cut axon in cerebral cortex, 660, 661-2
— state, of axon in cerebral cortex, 664, 665, 676
veronal, 30
vis a tergo, 212-13, 220, 227, 229, 363, 373, 376

Wallerian degeneration, 66-99, 101-8, 282, 293, 415, 507-9, 608, 649-50 ; see also Schwann cell
Water, boiling, and nerve grafting, 339
Weigert fibrils, 729
— haematoxylin, 72
— mordant, 38, 39
white matter, in transplantations of sensory nerve ganglia, 446-8, 452 ; see also cerebellar traumatisms, spinal cord and nerve roots

INDEX OF AUTHORS

Abreu, 63
Achúcarro, 38, 470-2, 474-6, 497, 507, 655, 690, 700, 718, 720, 721, 722, 723, 731, 732, 735, 753
Agduhr, 413
Alzheimer, 38-9, 461, 655, 677, 717, 718, 722-3, 730, 735, 753, 757
Anderson, 14, 15
Anglade, 39
Apathy, 4, 61, 415
Arcaute, 249, 471-2, 583, 590, 593-6, 747
Assaky, 330
Athias, 263, 624

Babés, 460
Bailey, 568
Ballance, 4, 10, 11, 13, 81, 84, 93, 94, 96, 97, 99
Barbacci, 482, 507
Bardeen, 382
Barfurth, 580, 760
Barth, 507
Bechterew, 584
Benda, 35
Berblinger, 195
Berthold, 456
Besta, 57, 84, 91, 97
Bethe, 4, 8-14, 16, 19, 21, 22, 25, 26, 59, 61-3, 67, 74, 77, 81, 84, 91, 93, 102-4, 121-2, 127, 130, 180, 192-4, 202-3, 226, 246, 308, 314-16, 320, 324, 332, 335, 358, 362, 379, 531, 573, 576, 585, 744-5
Bianchi, 352, 679, 684, 722, 730, 731, 759
Bielschowsky, 24, 32-3, 38, 45, 159, 195-7, 250, 262, 263, 360, 407, 423, 436, 460, 461, 509, 571, 580, 629, 684, 730, 735, 751, 753, 754, 760
Bikeles, 509, 572, 684
Biondi, 470, 475
Blass, 268
Boedecker, 497
Boeke, 195, 249, 250, 263, 396
Bok, 394
Bolton, 53
Bonfiglio, 735, 753
Bordet, 388
Borst, 192, 677, 715, 730, 754, 755, 759
Bouchard, 507
Boveri, 50, 53, 56, 59, 62
Braun, 10
Braus, 352
Bravetta, 611, 614
Brown-Séquard, 13, 19, 572
Bruch, 4, 5, 148, 246
Büngner, 4, 10, 11, 19, 53, 74, 75, 81, 84-7, 89, 91, 92, 127, 130, 131, 136, 142, 202-4, 224, 245, 246, 248, 290, 292
Burrows, 172, 178, 192, 454
Buscaino, 722

Caporaso, 581, 760
Capparelli, 53, 56, 59
Cardenal, 327-8, 429, 477
Carrel, 454
Castro, F. de, 412, 413, 425
Catanni, 50
Catola, 507, 754
Cattaneo, 595-6
Cerletti, 497, 717-18, 721, 722
Child, 394
Chio, 57
Chittenden, 53
Cipollone, 269
Coën, 482, 760
Colucci, 580
Cornil, 10, 11
Cortese, 23, 320-2, 483, 490, 509, 523, 531, 534, 564, 578
Cox, 13, 16

Daae, H., 404
D'Abundo, 541, 547, 552, 557, 578-9
Da Fano, 179, 407, 497, 729
Darschewitsch, 279
Daszkiewicz, 93
De Arcaute, R., 622
Deineka, 17, 29, 85, 142, 144, 159, 163, 173, 178, 184, 205, 224-6, 249, 374
Delafield, 35
del Río, E., 721
De Nó, L., 196, 197, 263, 413, 581
Dentan, 482
Detwiler, 391
Dickinson, 5
Dickson, 279
Disse, 402
Dogiel, 17, 61, 399, 400, 404, 406-7, 409, 411, 423-4, 461, 472
Dohrn, 25
Doinikow, 33-4, 36-7, 44-7, 51-4, 57, 65, 73, 80, 82-3, 85, 92, 97-8, 142, 159, 163, 166
Dominici, 36, 44, 45
Donaggio, 30-1, 159, 580
Dürk, 53, 54
Durante, 10, 11, 14, 82, 84, 91
Dustin, 17, 18, 23, 159, 163, 166, 180-2, 185, 187, 195, 207-9, 215, 217, 221-2, 224, 238, 249, 252, 290, 312, 326, 332, 335-7, 346, 350, 358, 362-3, 369, 373-4, 377-8, 380, 429-30, 483, 490, 506, 509, 531, 540-2, 557, 577-9, 595, 690, 747-8

Edinger, 196-7, 360
Edmond, 24
Ehrlich, 24, 34-5, 72, 80, 334, 406
Eichhorst, 5, 7, 67, 74, 482
Eisath, 722
Eischort, 572
Engelmann, 53, 127, 136
Erb, 74, 246
Erzholz, 68, 72
Esposito, 407

Ewald, 47, 52-4, 491
Expósito, 436

Fañanás, J. R., 523
Farrar, 715, 717, 722, 730-1, 732, 755
Feiss, 196
Finckler, 509, 572
Fischer, 580, 700-1, 735-6, 753
Flatau, 57, 568
Flemming, 13
Forel, 4, 5, 8, 320
Forssmann, 308-9, 324, 329-31, 333-6, 346, 353, 375, 379, 389
Forster, L., 366, 483, 490, 493, 509, 580
Fragnito, 580
Fraise, 760
Fürst, 57

Gabrichewsky, 388
Gad, 53
Galleotti, 10, 11, 202-3, 269, 272
Gallus, 571, 754, 760
Garbini, G., 611
Garcia, D., 428, 520, 606, 627, 679
Gauser, 584
Gayarre, 721
Gedoelst, 53, 54
Gemelli, 352
Gerlach, 53
Giard, 455
Gierlich, 684, 735, 751, 754
Gluck, 330
Gluge, 496
Goldscheider, 568
Goldstein, 573, 578
Golgi, 15-16, 34, 263
Gudden, 5, 320, 584, 684
Guild, 461
Guyon, Mlle. Dr., 359

Hada, 454
Halliburton, 14, 24, 223, 324, 351-2, 391
Hanns, 482, 507
Harrison, 8, 25, 172, 178, 180, 182, 186, 191-3, 203, 207-8, 221, 252-3, 263, 326, 352, 360, 362-4, 366-7, 369, 377, 379-84, 387-8, 395, 454, 512, 581
Hatai, 53-4
Hedinger, 195
Heidenhain, 25, 36, 61, 77, 217, 278, 285, 302, 326, 366, 368, 382-7, 396
Heizmans, 53
Held, 25, 30-1, 174, 196-7, 203, 212-13, 227, 229, 250, 253, 258, 259-60, 262-4, 326, 362-3, 376-8, 382-4, 386-8, 497, 595, 747
Henneberg, 554, 573
Hensen, 375-6, 383
Hermann, 395
Herzt, 7
Hertl, 93

INDEX OF AUTHORS

Herxheimer, 35, 80, 84, 684, 735, 751, 754
Hesse, 53
Hirudo, 677
His, 4, 8, 25, 258, 362-3, 375-7, 380, 384, 387-8, 582
Hjelt, 246
Hofmann, 268
Hofrichter, 507
Holmgren, 429, 430
Homen, 327-8, 482, 489, 506
Hooker, 581, 582
Howell, 75, 84, 203, 246
Huber, 11, 74, 75, 84, 203, 246, 335, 403, 461
Hunger, 54
Hyelt, 10

Illera, 630
Ingvar, 394
Isuguchi, 196

Jakob, 195, 483, 491, 497, 507-8, 566, 568, 684, 723
Johanson, 56
Johnson, 330
Joseph, 53, 54
Juliusberger, 497

Kähler, 482, 507
Kaplan, 53-4, 56
Kapper, 394
Kappers, A., 253, 390-1, 394
Kennedy, 335, 351
Kerestszeghy, 482, 506-7
Kerr, G., 258, 387, 391
Key, 51, 63, 64, 66, 86
Kimura, 195
Kindberg, 611-12, 616, 621, 627
Kirschgasser, 684
Klippel, 215
Kölster, 223
Knick, 507
Koch, 56
Kölliker, 4, 25, 57, 58, 202-3, 247, 258, 263, 362, 375, 387, 584
Kölster, 7, 9, 14, 127, 142, 198, 202-3
Koltzoff, 458
Korybalt, 93
Kossa, 434
Krassin, 15, 24, 34, 85, 142, 144, 205, 224, 249
Kühne, 52-4, 273, 491
Kühnt, 56
Künme, 47
Küpffer, 25, 362, 375, 387
Kultschitzky, 35

Lafora, 571, 655, 735, 737, 753-4
Landacre, 395
Landowsky, 53
Lange, 568
Langley, 14, 15, 268, 324
Lapinsky, 92
Lantermann, 52-4
Leduc, 455
Leegard, 202
Legendre, 453-4
Lenhossék, see von Lenhossék
Lents, 10
Leoz, 583, 589-90, 593-6
Lépine, 568
Levaditi, 38
Levi, 10, 11, 17, 22, 25, 202-3, 253, 263, 269, 273, 405-6, 410-12, 423, 428, 436, 450, 457, 461
Lewis, M. R. and W. H., 172, 178, 192, 367, 380, 454
Leydig, 53
Loeb, Leo, 186, 207, 221, 358, 369, 377, 380, 395
London, 180
Long, 360
Longet, 4

Lorente de Nó, see de Nó
Lowenthal, 482, 507
Luciani, 10
Lugaro, 14, 15, 22, 29, 142, 195, 215, 222, 224, 226, 249, 258, 263, 278, 280, 314-15, 324, 332-7, 346, 354, 367, 374, 379, 388, 390, 482, 509, 531, 540, 552, 557, 576, 738
Luzenberger, 684

Macallum, 395
Macdonald, 395
Mallory, 37
Marchand, 11, 91, 395, 497
Marchi, 14, 24, 35, 507
Marcora, 522, 682
Marenghi, 50
Marinesco, 11, 15, 17, 18, 20, 21, 23, 29, 61, 75, 85, 97-8, 102, 106, 120, 136, 138, 142-4, 151, 158-9, 163, 166, 168, 171, 173, 178-82, 193-6, 203, 205, 209, 214, 215, 217, 222, 224, 226, 249, 250, 252-4, 262-4, 278-80, 290, 320, 324, 333-5, 339, 346, 353, 359, 360, 362, 367, 371, 374, 379, 381, 388, 390, 393, 399, 405-7, 416, 423-5, 429-30, 432-3, 436-8, 441, 445-8, 450, 454-6, 459, 470, 477, 479, 480, 482-3, 490, 497, 507, 509, 514, 517, 531, 540, 554, 562, 566, 576-7, 580, 606, 610-2, 614, 627, 679, 684, 690, 700-1, 713, 735, 746, 748, 752-4
Martinotti, 670, 673-5, 707
Masius, 509, 572, 760
Massart, 388
Mayer, S., 18, 208
Maximow, 184
May, 276, 391
Medea, 17, 142, 224
Meissner, 372
Mencl, 624
Menten, 395
Merzbacher, 331, 333-4, 353, 497
Metchnikoff, 388
Michailow, 471, 474-5
Michotte, 17, 56
Minea, 17, 22-3, 120, 142, 151, 159, 163, 205, 217, 224, 226, 249, 290, 381, 407, 423-5, 429-30, 446, 448, 454, 477, 480, 576-7, 611, 614, 627
Minor, 482, 489, 497, 521, 566-8, 573
Minot, 453-4
Miscolczy, 196-7, 596, 677
Miyake, 509, 580, 684, 735, 752, 754
Modena, 13, 16, 24, 142, 159
Molhant, 106, 500
Monakow, 5, 584
Monckeberg, 11, 59, 62-3, 67, 77, 93, 102-4, 121-2
Mondino, 50
Mordino, 759
Morgenthaler, 715, 730-1, 732
Mott, 14, 24, 223, 324, 334-5, 351-2, 391
Mourawieff, 84, 91, 97
Müller, J., 4
Müller, W. 470, 474-5, 507, 509, 572, 580, 760
Munöz-Urra, 595-6
Münser, 4, 14, 223, 226, 324, 362, 584

Nageotte, 15, 17, 18, 23, 29, 35, 36, 42, 44-6, 53-8, 60, 62-3, 67, 72, 75-8, 80-1, 85-6, 90-4, 97-8, 102, 104, 106, 121-3, 142, 178, 193-4, 197, 209, 250-7, 260, 262-4, 359-60, 362, 370, 374, 381, 388, 390, 399, 406-12, 415, 416, 423-5, 426-30, 432-3, 435-41, 444, 446-8, 450, 455, 460, 472, 480, 482, 490, 509, 573-4, 606, 610-12, 614, 616, 621-2, 627, 713

Nemiloff, 44-6, 53-4, 59, 62
Neumann, 7, 74, 84, 92, 246
Newmann, 198
Nissl, 497, 521-2, 717-18, 721-2, 730
Nothafft, 5, 67, 75, 130, 144, 202, 223, 330

Olóriz, 399, 400, 424
Oppel, 454
Oppenheim, 568
Ortin, 249

Pacheco, 405, 407, 423, 436
Papadia, 722
Paracandolo, 684
Parhon, 573, 578
Pariani, 578
Penero, 509
Perrero, 579
Perroncito, Aldo, 11, 15, 17, 18, 20-1, 23, 29, 81, 85, 89, 91-2, 97-8, 102, 117-20, 136, 138, 142-5, 150-2, 160, 163, 166, 168, 171. 173-4,178, 181-2, 184, 193, 195, 205, 209, 217, 222, 224, 234, 236, 249, 254, 263, 324, 349, 360, 362, 376-7, 574, 586
Pertik, 53, 56
Perusini, 655, 700, 735, 753
Pesker, 180
Pfeiffer, 388, 684, 735, 752
Phylippeaux, 8-9, 11, 324, 335, 351, 507
Pick, 571, 754
Pitres, 568
Pitzorno, 471
Plateau, 458
Poscharisky, 24, 142, 159, 179, 249
Pugnat, 428, 450
Purpura, 15, 16. 34, 84, 144, 223, 231, 249

Quervain, 361

Ramanow, 195
Ranke, 39
Ranson, 195, 461-2, 481
Ranvier, 5-7, 9, 14, 16, 18, 44, 53, 55-6, 60, 67, 70, 80, 91, 127-8, 130, 136, 138, 141-2, 144, 158-9, 168, 198, 200, 202, 205, 208, 217, 222-4, 234, 238, 245-6, 272, 278, 290, 324, 330-1, 354, 362, 376-80, 383, 387-8, 400
Raposo, 197, 582
Rawitz, 57
Ray, R. M., 395
Rebizzi, 53-4, 56, 58
Reich, 51-2, 56, 75
Remak, 5, 49, 67, 99, 135
Retzius, 8, 17, 25, 61, 63-4, 66, 86, 90, 92, 263, 362, 400
Rios, 747
Riquier, C., 472
Rojas, P., 196
Rosenheim, 51
Rosenthal, 722
Rossi, H., 29, 249, 381, 606, 608, 610-12, 614, 630
Rossi, O., 17, 18, 23, 29, 142, 205, 249, 332, 336, 346, 350, 358, 361-2, 389, 405-7, 419, 423-4, 429-32, 436, 441, 483, 490, 509, 514, 517, 523-4, 531, 540, 554, 564, 566, 577, 583, 586-9, 594, 612, 735, 746-7, 752
Roux, W., 367
Rubaschkin, 729
Ruffini, 63
Ruiz, 249

Sabracés, 568
Sach, 621
Saito, 195

INDEX OF AUTHORS

Sala, G., 18, 22-3, 29, 50, 85, 142, 178, 320-2, 441, 470, 475, 483, 490, 509, 513, 517, 523, 531, 533, 540, 564, 578, 580, 657, 663, 735, 753, 758-9
Saltykow, 677, 755, 759
Sanarelli, 759
Scaffidi, 250, 253, 394
Scagliosi, 684
Schäffer, K., 196-7 405, 407, 423, 433, 436, 441, 460-1, 621, 630
Schiefferdecker, 25, 42, 49, 50, 53, 56, 61, 63, 482, 487, 489, 507
Schiff, 8, 11, 316
Schmaus, 684
Schob, 621
Schültze, O., 10, 11, 34, 148, 382
Scott, 393
Segall, 15, 49, 50
Sittig, 715
Simarro, 735, 736
Simchovicz, 655, 700, 753
Singer, 584
Spencer, Herbert, 368
Spielmeyer, 192-4, 250, 262-3, 360, 722
Spirlas, 402
Stahl, 456
Stefani, 315-16
Stewart, 10, 13, 93-4, 96-7, 99
Storch, 730
Strasser, 391, 394
Strauss, 621

Straussler, 611, 622
Stroebe, 4-7, 9, 24, 53, 67, 74, 80-1, 92, 127, 130, 133, 136, 141-2, 150, 152, 166, 198, 201-3, 217, 223-5, 238, 245-8, 282, 290, 330, 362, 378-9, 387, 482, 489, 497, 507, 509, 512, 517, 531, 540, 554, 573-4, 746

Tello, F., 2, 15, 17, 18, 23, 29, 61, 74, 85, 91, 102, 106-8, 138, 142, 159, 163, 173, 178, 181, 193, 195-7, 205, 249, 252-3, 258, 262, 265-74, 276, 333, 359, 361-2, 372, 383, 388, 390, 395-6, 523, 583-4, 586-7, 589-90, 592-3, 596, 694, 738-44 747-9
Thooth, 507
Tizzoni, 74, 93
Traube, 455
Tsukaguchi, 197

Ulrich, 718, 721
Unger, 195, 360
Unna, 37, 184, 722
Unna-Pappenheim, 37

Valentin, B., 195
van Gehuchten, 11, 13, 17, 25, 75, 106, 215, 226, 263, 460, 500, 507, 566
van Gieson, 37
Vanlair, 5-7, 9, 14, 67, 74, 80, 127, 142, 168, 191, 198, 201, 205-6, 217, 223, 238, 258, 278, 290, 324, 326, 330-1, 354, 360, 362, 378-9, 383, 388, 509, 572, 760
Veratti, 29, 418-19, 424
Verworn, 391, 456, 458
Viale, 250, 253
Villa, 50
Vogt, 722
von Kölliker, 8
von Lenhossék, 4, 8, 17, 25, 172, 176, 203, 258, 263, 259, 362, 364, 371, 382, 384-5, 387-8, 399, 400, 402, 406, 459, 471
Vries, 458
Vulpian, 8-11, 19, 324, 335, 351, 507

Waller, 4-5, 9-10, 13, 16, 26, 148, 362
Walstein, 53
Weber, 53
Wegstrecke, 376
Weigert, 38-9 72, 730
Weigert-Pal, 35
Weissfeiler, 596
Wietting, 10, 11, 81, 84, 91-2, 127, 130, 136, 142, 202-3
Westphal, 507, 568
Wolff, 629

Zalla, 80, 81, 84, 91-2, 97-8
Ziegler, E., 5, 14
Ziegler, P., 67, 80, 130, 142, 223, 482, 507